INTEGRATIVE RHEU
AND INFLAMMATION MASTERY

Third Edition

ALEX VASQUEZ DC ND DO FACN

- Doctor of Osteopathic Medicine, graduate of University of North Texas Health Science Center, Texas College of Osteopathic Medicine (2010)
- Doctor of Naturopathic Medicine, graduate of Bastyr University (1999)
- Doctor of Chiropractic, graduate of University of Western States (1996)
- Fellow of the American College of Nutrition (2013-present)
- Fellow of the Royal Society of Medicine (2013-present)
- Chief Editor, *International Journal of Human Nutrition and Functional Medicine* intjhumnutrfunctmed.org
- Director of Programs, International College/Conference on Human Nutrition and Functional Medicine ICHNFM.org
- Founding Program Director of the world's first accredited university-affiliated graduate-level program in Functional Medicine: Master of Science in Human Nutrition and Functional Medicine
- Former Adjunct Faculty (2009-2013) of Advanced Laboratory Medicine in the Master of Science in Advanced Clinical Practice, National University of Health Sciences
- Former Adjunct Faculty (2004-2005, 2010-2013) and Forum Consultant (2003-2007), The Institute for Functional Medicine
- Former Adjunct Professor of Pharmacology (2011-2012), Doctor of Chiropractic program
- Former Adjunct Professor (2011-2013) of Evidence-Based Nutrition, Immune and Inflammatory Imbalances, Principles of Functional Medicine, Psychology of Wellness
- Former Adjunct Professor of Orthopedics (2000), Radiographic Interpretation (2000), and Rheumatology (2001), Naturopathic Medicine Program, Bastyr University
- Consultant Researcher and Lecturer (2004-present), Biotics Research Corporation
- Private practice of integrative and functional medicine in Seattle, Washington (2000-2001), Houston, Texas (2001-2006), Portland, Oregon (2011-present)
- Author of approximately 100 articles and letters published in *JAMA—Journal of the American Medical Association, BMJ—British Medical Journal, The Lancet.com, JAOA—Journal of the American Osteopathic Association, Annals of Pharmacotherapy, Journal of Clinical Endocrinology and Metabolism, Alternative Therapies in Health and Medicine, Nutritional Perspectives, Journal of Manipulative and Physiological Therapeutics, The Original Internist, Integrative Medicine, Holistic Primary Care, Nutritional Wellness, Evidence-based Complementary and Alternative Medicine,* and *Arthritis & Rheumatism*: Official Journal of the American College of Rheumatology

INFLAMMATIONMASTERY.COM

Title: Vasquez A. *Integrative Rheumatology and Inflammation Mastery, Third Edition*. Barcelona, Spain

Copyright: © 2004-2014 by Alex Vasquez. All rights reserved by the author and enforced to the full extent of legal and financial consequences. No part of this book may be reproduced, stored in a retrieval system, used for the creation of derivative works, or transmitted by any means (electronic, mechanical, photocopying, recording, or otherwise) without written permission from the author.

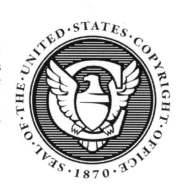

Trademark: ® 2013 by Alex Vasquez. The functional immunology/inflammology protocol discussed in this series of videos/notes/books/audios is recalled by the F.I.N.D.S.E.X. acronym trademarked™ in association with Dr Vasquez's book <u>Functional Immunology and Nutritional Immunomodulation</u> (2012), <u>F.I.N.D. S.E.X. The Easily Remembered Acronym for the Functional Inflammology Protocol</u> (2013). Portland, Oregon; Integrative and Biological Medicine Research and Consulting, LLC. All rights reserved and enforced. For additional information and resources, see InflammationMastery.com, ICHNFM.org, NutritionAndFunctionalMedicine.org, FunctionalInflammology.com

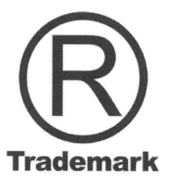

Notices: The intended audiences for this book are health science students and doctorate-level licensed medical clinicians. This book has been written with every intention to make it as accurate as possible, and each section has undergone peer-review by an interdisciplinary group of clinicians. In view of the possibility of human error and as well as ongoing discoveries in the biomedical sciences, neither the author nor any party associated in any way with this text warrants that this text is perfect, accurate, or complete in every way, and all disclaim responsibility for harm or loss associated with the application of the material herein. Information and treatments applicable to a specific *condition* may not be appropriate for or applicable to a specific *patient*; this is especially true for patients with multiple comorbidities and those taking pharmaceutical medications, which are generally associated with multiple adverse effects and drug/nutrient/herb interactions. Given that this book is available on an open market, lay persons who read this material should discuss the information with a licensed medical provider before implementing any treatments and interventions described herein.

Chapter and Introduction	*Pages*

Dedications: I dedicate this book to the following people in appreciation for their works, their direct and indirect support of this work, and for their contributions to the advancement of true healthcare.

- **To the students and practitioners of naturopathic/functional medicine**, those who continue to learn so that they can provide the best possible care to their patients
- **To the researchers** whose works are cited in this text
- **To Dr Alan Gaby and Dr Jeffrey Bland,** my most memorable and influential professors and mentors
  - Of additional note, Dr Bland deserves credit for being the primary developer of the American rendition of "functional medicine", a conceptual framework and clinical model used and discussed in this text. Development and continuous maturation of the functional medicine model has depended upon numerous researchers and clinicians; Dr Jeff Bland was clearly the pioneer for this concept circa 1993 and the nucleus around which many of us have worked (at least initially) in this regard.
- **To Dr Bruce Ames**[1] **and Dr Roger J Williams**[2], for proving biochemical individuality
- **To Dr Chester Wilk**[3,4] **and important others** for documenting and resisting the organized oppression of natural, non-pharmaceutical, non-surgical healthcare[5,6,7]
- **To Jorge Strunz and Ardeshir Farah,** for artistic inspiration

Acknowledgments for Peer and Editorial Review: Most of the sections that comprise the current work have been previously reviewed/published/presented; peer/editorial reviews are acknowledged below. Acknowledgement here does not imply that the reviewer fully agrees with or endorses the material in this text but rather that they were willing to review specific sections of the book for clinical applicability and clarity and to make suggestions to their own level of satisfaction.

- 2013 Edition of *International Journal of Human Nutrition and Functional Medicine*: Annette D'Armatta ND and J William Beakey DOM
- 2012 Edition of *Fibromyalgia in a Nutshell*: Lisa Scholl BA, Annette D'Armatta ND
- 2012 Edition of *Migraine Headaches, Hypothyroidism, and Fibromyalgia*: Holly Furlong DC
- 2011 Edition of *Integrative Chiropractic Management of High Blood Pressure and Chronic Hypertension*: Barry Morgan MD, Holly Furlong DC, Kris Young DC, Erika Mennerick DC, and J William Beakey DOM
- 2011 Edition of *Integrative Medicine and Functional Medicine for Chronic Hypertension*: Erika Mennerick DC, JoAnn Fawcett DC, Ileana Bourland MSOM LAc, James Bogash DC, J William Beakey DOM
- 2010 Edition of *Chiropractic Management of Chronic Hypertension*: Joseph Paun MS DC, David Candelario OMS4 (TCOM c/o 2010), James Bogash DC, Bill Beakey DOM, Robert Richard DO
- 2009 Edition of *Chiropractic and Naturopathic Mastery of Common Clinical Disorders*: Heather Kahn MD, Robert Richard DO, James Leiber DO, David Candelario (UNT-HSC TCOM OMS4)
- 2007 Edition of *Integrative Orthopedics*: Barry Morgan MD, Dennis Harris DC, Richard Brown DC (DACBI candidate), Ron Mariotti ND, Patrick Makarewich MBA, Reena Singh (SCNM ND4), Zachary Watkins DC, Charles Novak MS DC, Marnie Loomis ND, James Bogash DC, Sara Croteau DC, Kris Young DC, Joshua Levitt ND, Jack Powell III MD, Chad Kessler MD, Amy Neuzil ND
- 2006 Edition of *Integrative Rheumatology*: Amy Neuzil ND, Cathryn Harbor MD, Julian Vickers DC, Tamara Sachs MD, Bob Sager BSc MD DABFM (Clinical Instructor in the Department of Family Medicine, University of Kansas), Ron Mariotti ND, Titus Chiu (DC4), Zachary Watkins (DC4), Gilbert Manso MD, Bruce Milliman ND, William Groskopp DC, Robert Silverman DC, Matthew Breske (DC4), Dean Neary ND, Thomas Walton DC, Fraser Smith ND, Ladd Carlston DC, David Jones MD, Joshua Levitt ND
- 2004 Edition of *Integrative Orthopedics*: Peter Knight ND, Kent Littleton ND MS, Barry Morgan MD, Ron Hobbs ND, Joshua Levitt ND, John Neustadt (Bastyr ND4), Allison Gandre BS (Bastyr ND4), Peter Kimble ND, Jack Powell III MD, Chad Kessler MD, Mike Gruber MD, Deirdre O'Neill ND, Mary Webb ND, Leslie Charles ND, Amy Neuzil ND

[1] Ames BN, et al. High-dose vitamin therapy stimulates variant enzymes with decreased coenzyme binding affinity (increased K(m). *Am J Clin Nutr*. 2002 Apr;75:616-58
[2] Williams RJ. Biochemical Individuality: The Basis for the Genetotrophic Concept. Austin and London: University of Texas Press; 1956
[3] Wilk CA. Medicine, Monopolies, and Malice: How the Medical Establishment Tried to Destroy Chiropractic. Garden City Park: Avery, 1996
[4] Getzendanner S. Permanent injunction order against AMA. *JAMA*. 1988 Jan 1;259(1):81-2
[5] Carter JP. Racketeering in Medicine: The Suppression of Alternatives. Norfolk: Hampton Roads Pub; 1993
[6] Morley J, Rosner AL, Redwood D. A case study of misrepresentation of the scientific literature: recent reviews of chiropractic. *J Altern Complement Med*. 2001;7:65-78
[7] Terrett AG. Misuse of the literature by medical authors in discussing spinal manipulative therapy injury. *J Manipulative Physiol Ther*. 1995 May;18(4):203-10

Format and Layout: The format/layout of this book is designed to efficiently take the reader though the clinically relevant spectrum of considerations for each condition that is detailed. Important topics are given their own section within each chapter, while other less important or less common conditions are only described briefly in terms of the four "clinical essentials" of 1) definition/pathophysiology, 2) clinical presentation, 3) assessment/diagnosis, and 4) treatment/management. Each expanded section which details the more important/common conditions maintains a consistent format, taking the reader through the spectrum of primary clinical considerations: definition/pathophysiology, clinical presentations, differential diagnoses, assessments (physical examination, laboratory, imaging), complications, management, and treatment. As my books have progressed, I am increasingly using an article-by-article review format (especially in the sections on management and treatment) so that readers have more direct access to the information so as to understand and *incorporate* more deeply what the research actually states; the goal and general approach here is to use a *representative sampling* of the research literature.

References and Citations: Citations to articles, abstracts, texts, and personal communications are footnoted throughout the text to provide supporting information and to provide interested readers the resources to find additional information. Many of the cited articles are available on-line for free, and often I have included the website addresses so that readers can easily access the complete article.

Peer-review and Quality Control: Peer-review is essential to help ensure accuracy and clinical applicability of health-related information. Consistent with the importance of these goals, I have employed several "checks and balances" to increase the accuracy and applicability of the information within my textbooks:

- Reliance upon authoritative references: Nearly all important statements are referenced to peer-reviewed biomedical journals or authoritative texts, examples of the latter include *The Merck Manual*, *Current Medical Diagnosis and Treatment*, and *5-Minute Clinical Consult*. Each citation is provided by a footnote at the bottom of each page so that readers will know quickly and easily exactly where the information was obtained.
- Extensive cross-referencing: Readers will notice, if not be overwhelmed by, the number of references and citations. Many important statements have several references. Many references (especially textbooks) are referenced several times even on the same page. The purpose of this extensive referencing is three-fold: 1) to guide you to additional information, 2) to help me (as writer) stay organized, and 3) to help you and me (the practicing physicians) employ this information with confidence.
- Periodic revision: Any significant errors that are discovered will be posted at InflammationMastery.com; please check this page periodically to ensure that you are working with the most accurate information of which I am aware.
- Peer-review: The peer-review process for my books takes several forms. First, colleagues and students are invited to review new and revised sections of the text before publication; every section of the book that you are holding has been independently reviewed by health science students and/or practicing clinicians from various backgrounds: allopathic, chiropractic, osteopathic, naturopathic. Second, you - the reader - are invited to provide feedback about the information in the book, typographical errors, syntax, case reports, new research, etc. If your ideas truly change the nature of the material, I will be glad to acknowledge you in the text (with your permission, of course). If your contribution is hugely significant, such as reviewing three or more chapters or helping in some important way, I will be glad to not only acknowledge you, but to also send you the next edition at a discount or courtesy when your ideas take effect. Third, I keep abreast of new literature by constantly perusing new research and advancements in the health sciences. Having been successful in three separate doctoral programs in the health sciences, I have learned not only to master large amounts of material but to also separate and integrate different viewpoints as appropriate. I also "field test" my protocols with patients in the various clinical arenas in which I work and also with professionals and academicians via presentations and critical dialogue. By implementing these quality control steps, I hope to create a useful text and advance our professions and our practices by improving the quality of care that we deliver to our patients.

How to Use This Book Safely and Most Effectively: Ideally, these books should be read cover-to-cover within a context of coursework that is supervised by a clinically experienced professor. For post-graduate professionals, they might consider forming a local or virtual "book club" and meeting for weekly or monthly discussions to check their understandings and share their clinical experiences to refine the application of clinical knowledge, perceptions, and skills. Virtual groups and internet forums—such as those hosted by International College of Human Nutrition and Functional Medicine at ICHNFM.ORG—can provide access to an assembly of international professional peers wherein sharing of clinical questions and experiences are synergistic. This book is not intended to extensively cover all aspects of clinical medicine, such as clinical pharmacology and prescribing (for which I recommend the clinical resource *Epocrates.com* and its associated app) and medical management (for which I recommend *5-Minute Clinical Consult* via book, website, and app).

Notice: The intention and scope of this text are to provide health science students and doctorate-level clinicians with useful information and a familiarity with available research and resources pertinent to the management of patients in integrative primary care and specialty care settings. Specifically, the information in this book is intended to be used by licensed healthcare professionals who have received hands-on/residential clinical training and supervision at accredited health science colleges. Additionally, information in this book should be used in conjunction with other resources, texts, and in combination with the clinician's best

> ### Purpose, scope, recommended companion resources
>
> The purpose of this book is not to serve as a stand-alone "recipe book" for the complete management of all reviewed conditions; rather the focus of this book is the delivery of clinically important concepts and facts to enhance the management of various clinical disorders, in particular by documenting and explicating this author's naturopathic, medical, integrative and functional medicine approach. Readers and instructors using this book are encouraged to use whichever additional resources they choose, including but not limited to the supporting videos at Vimeo.com/DrVasquez and Vimeo.com/ICHNFM; in particular, *5-Minute Clinical Consult* and *Epocrates* are excellent and strongly advised companion guides for overall medical diagnosis/management and clinical pharmacology/prescribing, respectively. Clinicians need to have a good understanding of clinical medicine before applying many of the approaches described in this book; cross-referencing and double-checking management strategies and drug doses are essential components of quality care. Both *5-Minute Clinical Consult* and *Epocrates* are available as point-of-care references, and their use is advised.

judgment and intention to "*first, do no harm*" and second to provide effective healthcare. Information and treatments applicable to a specific *condition* may not be appropriate for or applicable to a specific *patient* in your office; this is especially true for patients with multiple comorbidities and those taking pharmaceutical medications with multiple adverse effects and drug/nutrient/herb interactions. In my books and articles, I describe treatments—manual, dietary, nutritional, botanical, pharmacologic, and occasionally surgical—and their research support for the clinical condition being discussed; each practitioner must determine appropriateness of these treatments for his/her individual patient and with consideration of the doctor's scope of practice, education, training, skill, and—occasionally—the appropriateness of "off label" use of medications and treatments. This book has been carefully written and checked for accuracy by the author and professional colleagues. However, in view of the possibility of human error and new discoveries in the biomedical sciences, neither the author nor any party associated in any way with this text warrants that this text is perfect, accurate, or complete in every way, and we disclaim responsibility for harm or loss associated with the application of the material herein. With all conditions/treatments described herein, each physician must be sure to consider the balance between what is best for the patient and the physician's own level of ability, expertise, and experience. When in doubt, or if the physician is not a specialist in the treatment of a given severe condition, referral is appropriate. These notes are written with the routine "outpatient" in mind and are not tailored to severely injured patients or "playing field" or "emergency response" situations; consult your First Aid and Emergency Response texts and course materials for appropriate information. These notes represent the author's perspective based on academic education, experience, and post-graduate continuing education and are not inclusive of every fact that a clinician may need to know. This is not an "entry level" book except when used in an academic setting with a knowledgeable professor who can explain the concepts, tests, physical exam procedures, and treatments; this book requires a certain level of knowledge from the reader and familiarity with clinical concepts, laboratory assessments, and physical examination procedures.

Updates, Corrections, and Newsletter: When and if omissions, errata, and the need for important updates become clear, I will post these at the website InflammationMastery.com. A reader might access this page periodically to ensure staying informed of any corrections that might have clinical relevance. This book consists not only of the text in the printed pages you are holding, but also the footnotes and any updates at the website. Be alerted to new integrative clinical research, updates to this textbook and other news/publications/conferences/videos by signing-up for the free newsletter at InflammationMastery.com.

Language, Semantics, and Perspective: As a diligent student who previously aspired to be an English professor, I have written this text with great (though inevitably imperfect) attention to detail. Individual words were chosen with care. I confess to knowing, pushing, and creatively breaking several rules of grammar and punctuation. With regard to the he/she and him/her debacle of the English language, I've occasionally mixed singular and plural pronouns for the sake of being efficient and so that the images remain gender-neutral to the extent reasonable. In several previous publications, the subtitle *The art of creating wellness while effectively managing acute and chronic musculoskeletal/health disorders* was chosen to emphasize the intentional creation of wellness rather than a limited focus on disease treatment and symptom suppression; for the 2009 printing of *Chiropractic and Naturopathic Mastery of Common Clinical Disorders*, this subtitle was slightly modified from "creating" to "co-creating" to emphasize the team effort required between physician and patient. *Managing* was chosen to emphasize the importance of treating-monitoring-referring-reassessing, rather than merely *treating*. *Disorders* was chosen to reflect the fact that a distinguishing characteristic of *life* is the ability to regularly create *organized structure* and *higher order* from chaos and *disorder*. For example, plants organize the randomly moving molecules of air and water into the organized structure of biomolecules which eventually take shape as plant structure—fiber, leaves, flowers, petals. Similarly, the human body creates organized structure of increased complexity from consumed plants and other foods; molecules ingested and inhaled from the environment are organized into specific biochemicals and tissue structures with distinct characteristics and definite functions. Injury and disease *result in* or *result from* a lack of order, hence my use of the word "disorders" to characterize human illness and disease. For example, a motor vehicle accident that results in bodily injury, for example, is an example of an external chaotic force, which, when imparted upon human body tissues, results in a disruption (disorder) of the normal structure and organization that previously defined and characterized the now-damaged tissues of the body; likewise, an autoimmune disease process that results in tissue destruction is an *anti-evolutionary* process that takes molecules of higher complexity and reverts them to simpler, fragmented, and non-functional forms. From the perspective of "health" as *organized structure and meaningful function* and "disease" as *the reversion to chaos, destruction of structure, and the loss of function*, the task of healthcare providers is essentially to restore order, and to acutely reduce and proactively prevent/eliminate clinical-biochemical-biomechanical-emotional chaos insofar as it adversely affects the patient's life experience as an individual and our collective experience as an interdependent society. What is required of clinicians then is the ability *first* to create conceptual order from what appears to be chaotic phenomena, and then *second* to materialize—make real and practically applied for patients/people seeking improved health—that conceptual order into our physical world; this is our task, and no small task it is.

> **Authentic learning is life integration**
>
> "Ultimately, no one can extract from things—*books included*—more than he already knows. What one has no access to through experience, one has no ear for."
>
> Nietzsche FW [translated by RJ Hollingdale]. *Ecce Homo: How One Becomes What One Is*. New York & London: Penguin; 1979, page 70

Integrity and Creativity: I have endeavored to accurately represent the facts as they have been presented in texts and research, and to specifically resist any temptation to embellish or misrepresent data as others have done.[8,9] Conversely, I have not endeavored to make this book appeal to the "average" student or reader; my goal is to write and teach to the students at the top of the class, thereby affirming them and pulling the other students forward and upward. While I offer *explanations*, I intentionally resist *simplifications*, except when one

---

[8] **Vasquez A**. Zinc treatment for reduction of hyperplasia of prostate. *Townsend Letter for Doctors and Patients* 1996; January: 100
[9] Broad W, Wade N. Betrayers of the Truth: Fraud and Deceit in the Halls of Science. New York: Simon and Schuster; 1982

simplification might facilitate the comprehension of a more complex phenomenon, or when such a simplification might facilitation the conveyance of information from clinician to patient. I have allowed this text to be unique in format, content, and style, so that the personality of this text can be contrasted with that of the instructor and reader, thus enabling the learner to at least benefit from an intentionally different – and intentionally honest – perspective and approach. Students using this text with the guidance of a qualified professor will benefit from the experience of "two teachers" rather than just one.

Linearity, Nonlinearity, Redundancy, Asynchronicity: Although the overall flow of the text is highly linear and sequential, occasionally I place a conclusion before its introduction for the sake of foreshadowing and therefore for preparing the reader for what is to come. The purpose of this is not simply one of preparation for the sake of allowing the reader to know what is already lying ahead on the path, but more to begin creating new "shelf space" in the reader's intellectual-neuronal "library" so that when the new—particularly if *neoparadigmatic*—information is encountered, a space will already exist for it; it other words: the intent is to make learning easier. Likewise, for the sake of *information retention*—or what is better understood as synaptogenesis—important points are presented more than once, either identically or variantly. Given that *"No one ever reads the same book twice"*[10] (because the "person who starts" the reading of a meaningful book is changed into the "person who finishes" the reading of that book (assuming proper intentionality and application of one's "self"), the person reading these words might consider a second glace after the first.

Bon Voyage: All artists and scientists—regardless of genre—grapple with the divergent goals of *perfecting* their work and *presenting* their work; the former is impossible in the ultimate sense, while the latter is the only means by which the effort can create the desired effect in the world, whether that is pleasure, progress, or both. At some point, we must all agree that it is "good enough" and that it contains the essence of what needs to be communicated. While neither this nor any future edition of this book is likely to be "perfect", I am content with the literature reviewed, presented, and the new conclusions and implications which are described—many for the first time ever—in this text. Most notable in my *Integrative Rheumatology* (first published in 2006), each chapter achieved a paradigm shift which distanced/distances us farther from the simplistic pharmacocentric model and toward one which authentically empowers both practitioners and patients. With time, I will make future editions more complete, consistently passionate, and either more or less polemical. I hope you are able to implement these conclusions and research findings *into your own life* and into the treatment plans for your patients. In short time, I believe that we will see many of these concepts more broadly implemented. Hopefully this work's value and veracity will promote patients' vitality via the vigilant and virtuous clinicians viewing this volume; to the more attentive and thoroughgoing reader, more is revealed.

Perspectival note written in the latter part of 2013: Following the completion of the admittedly and surprisingly herculean task of orchestrating the 2013 International Conference of Human Nutrition and Functional Medicine — described and sampled at ICHNFM.ORG and Vimeo.com/ICHNFM, respectively— and a different obfuscating academic conundrum, I personally took the

---

Relevant philosophical perspectives for progressive changes and updates that will take effect starting in works published in 2014

"For the purpose of knowledge, one must know how to use that inner current that draws us to a thing, and then the one that, after a time, draws us away from it." *Nietzsche FW. Human, All Too Human #500*

"One has to be very light to drive one's will to knowledge into such a distance and, as it were, beyond one's time, to create for oneself eyes to survey millennia and, moreover, clear skies in these eyes. One must have liberated oneself from many things that oppress, inhibit, hold down, and make heavy precisely us Europeans today." *Nietzsche FW. Joyful Knowledge #380*

"My principle article of faith is that one can flourish only among people who share the identical ideas and the identical will." *Friedrich Nietzsche in a letter to his sister*

"The highest state a philosopher can attain is to stand in a Dionysian relationship to existence—my formula for this is amor fati— the love of fate. It is part of this state to perceive not merely the necessity of those sides of existence hitherto denied, but their desirability…" *Nietzsche FW. Will to Power #1041*

---

[10] Davies R. Reading and Writing. Salt Lake City: University of Utah Press; 1992, page 23

advice that I've often and easily given to patients and friends: at times we have to liberate ourselves from our duties and affiliations/relationships in order to be *more* true to ourselves, to flourish, to *live/write/think/experience* more broadly and profoundly. For those of us who continuously grow and learn, we often (and rather quickly and predictably) outgrow our relationships and affiliations, so that –except in rare situations of either maintained mutual loyalty and/or parallel growth– departure becomes inevitable, as it should. The relevance of these changes and events to the current work may be obvious from the Nietzschean perspective (#6 in *Beyond Good and Evil*), "Gradually it has become clear to me what every great philosophy so far has been: namely, the personal confession of its author and a kind of involuntary and unconscious memoir." What I quickly appreciated after the resignation of two of my long-held and previously-cherished positions is that they had come to have a limiting influence on my clarity and breadth of vision: in seeking to affirm and affiliate with these groups, I had compromised myself—at times unconsciously and at times knowingly—in order to be agreeable, for the sake of "teamwork", and to manifest the reverence which I held for these groups. Immediately following my resignations (and also due largely to the ultimate reasons for my resignations), I experienced an increase in clarity and perspective that has called for the reviewing, updating, and revisioning of all of my work, of which this current volume is the first to be bathed by the refreshing wave of these new *more liberated/free/clear/precise* perspectives. I already know that these changes will improve the quality of my writings and presentations and –thereby– the success and health of the clinicians and patients who are the ultimate recipients of these words and images, concepts and possibilities.

Note about the first version of the Third Edition—January 2014: The Third Edition published in early 2014 as *Integrative Rheumatology and Inflammation Mastery* is deserving of being called a new edition since it contains many updates, extensions, and much "brand new" information; however, the work won't be complete in my eyes until later in 2014 and into 2015 as I change the title to *Inflammation Mastery* and progressively publish volumes as they are truly complete "in all the perfection of their highest bloom" which will take weeks and months per chapter. With my current publisher, books are limited to 630 pages per volume, and for this work to be fully complete and manifested in paper as it exists in my mind, I anticipate that several volumes will be required. Thus, *Integrative Rheumatology and Inflammation Mastery* as published in early 2014 is a very reasonable summary of key points, but is not the highest manifestation of the work, for which I have simply not had sufficient time relative to academic schedules, international travel/relocation, and other logistical imperatives; Chapter 4 contains many urgent updates—the new information on mitochondrial dysfunction and nutritional immunomodulation is "must know" for today's students and clinicians. The chapter on Fibromyalgia is completely revised and expanded from previous publications; some of the latter chapters are still consistent with the 2007 edition and will need to be intermixed with the new information in Chapter 4— again, especially the sections on immunomodulation and mitochondriopathy—to be consistent with the way that I currently practice. This work is best used with the accompanying/relevant new videos available online for rental at https://vimeo.com/ondemand/ichnfm2013drv and a 426-page printed book of all slides available https://www.createspace.com/4478800.

Thank you for engaging with this work, and I wish you and your patients the best of success and health.

Alex Vasquez

Alex Vasquez, D.C., N.D., D.O., F.A.C.N.
Barcelona, Spain
January 3, 2014

Examples of commonly used abbreviations:

- **25-OH-D** = serum 25-hydroxy-vitamin D(3)
- **ACEi** = angiotensin-2 converting enzyme inhibitor
- **Alpha-blocker** = alpha-adrenergic antagonist
- **ARB** = angiotensin-2 receptor blocker/antagonist
- **ARF** = acute renal failure
- **BB** = beta blocker or beta-adrenergic antagonist
- **BMP** = basic metabolic panel, includes serum Na, K, Cl, CO2, BUN, creatinine, and glucose
- **BP** = blood pressure, **HBP** = high blood pressure
- **BUN** = blood urea nitrogen
- **C and S** = culture and sensitivity
- **CAD** = coronary artery disease
- **CBC** = complete blood count
- **CCB** = calcium channel blocker/antagonist
- **CE** = cardiac enzymes, generally including creatine kinase (CK), creatine kinase myocardial band (CKMB), and troponin-1, with the latter being the most specific serologic marker for acute myocardial injury; for the evaluation of acute MI, these are generally tested 2-3 times at 6-hour intervals with ECG performed at least as often.
- **CHF** = congestive heart failure
- **CHO** = carbohydrate
- **CK** = creatine kinase, historically named creatine phosphokinase (CPK)
- **CKD** = chronic kidney disease, generally stratified into five stages based on GFR of roughly <90, 90-60, 60-30, 30-15, and >15, respectively
- **CMP** = comprehensive metabolic panel, also called a chemistry panel, includes the BMP along with markers of hepatic status albumin, protein, ALT, AST, may also include alkaline phosphatase and rarely GGT; panels vary per laboratory and hospital.
- **CNS** = central nervous system
- **COPD** = chronic obstructive pulmonary disease
- **CRF, CRI** = chronic renal failure/insufficiency
- **CRP** = c-reactive protein, **hsCRP** = high-sensitivity c-reactive protein
- **CT** = computed tomography
- **CVD** = cardiovascular disease
- **CXR** = chest X-ray
- **DM** = diabetes mellitus
- **ECG or EKG** = electrocardiograph
- **Echo** = echocardiography
- **GFR** = glomerular filtration rate
- **HDL** = high density lipoprotein cholesterol
- **HTN** = hypertension
- **Ig** = immune globulin = antibodies of the G, A, M, E, or D classes.
- **IHD** = ischemic heart disease
- **I and D** = incision and drainage
- **IV** = intravenous
- **MCV** = mean cell volume
- **MI** = myocardial infarction
- **MRI** = magnetic resonance imaging, **MRI** = magnetic resonance angiography
- **PNS** = peripheral nervous system
- **PRN** = from the Latin "pro re nata" meaning "on occasion" or "when necessary"
- **PTH** = parathyroid hormone, **iPTH** = intact parathyroid hormone
- **PVD** = peripheral vascular disease
- **RA** = rheumatoid arthritis
- **RAD** = reactive airway disease, similar to asthma
- **SIBO** = small intestine bacterial overgrowth
- **SLE** = systemic lupus erythematosus
- **TRIG(s)** = serum triglycerides
- **UA** = urinalysis
- **US** = ultrasound

Dosing shorthand (mostly Latin abbreviations): q = each; qd = each day; bid = twice daily; tid = thrice daily; qid = four times per day; po = per os = by mouth; prn = as needed.

Begin at the beginning

"He who wishes one day to *fly*, must first learn *standing*
   and *walking*
      and *running*
         and *climbing*
            and *dancing*.
One does not *fly* into *flying*."

Nietzsche FW. *Thus Spoke Zarathustra—A Book for All and None*. 1883-1885

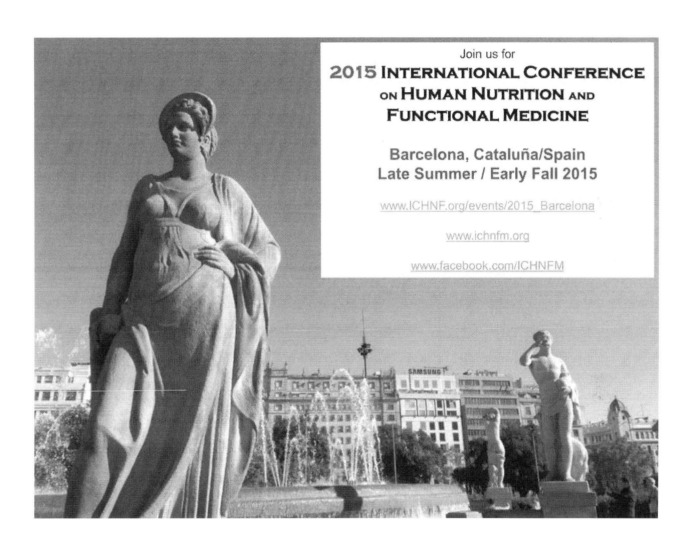

Join us for
2015 INTERNATIONAL CONFERENCE ON HUMAN NUTRITION AND FUNCTIONAL MEDICINE

Barcelona, Cataluña/Spain
Late Summer / Early Fall 2015

www.ICHNF.org/events/2015_Barcelona

www.ichnfm.org

www.facebook.com/ICHNFM

Work as love made tangible

"You work that you may keep pace with
  the earth and the soul of the earth.
For to be idle is to become a stranger unto
  the seasons, and to step out of life's
  procession. ...
Work is love made visible."

Kahlil Gibran (1883-1930). *The Prophet*.
Publisher Alfred A. Knopf, 1973

Reviews of previous and recent works:

- "I just wanted to tell you how much I appreciate the information I have received from you. I am still digesting most of it. I feel I have learned quite a bit already yet also feel I have barely scratched the surface." *Doctor and Graduate student under Dr Vasquez, 2013*

- "Dr. Vasquez, Thank you for all you do. **Your conference was simply amazing**. No one wanted to leave the room. I met medical professionals and very interesting lay people who were stimulated and invigorated to change their lives and the lives of others. **I am in awe at your intellectual integrity and veracity.** Best of luck to you in all of your future endeavors." *Medical physician and ICHNFM 2013 Conference Attendee*

- "Thanks for a fantastic conference!" *ICHNFM 2013 Conference Attendee*

- "I was so refreshed by the 'unfiltered excellence.' What humanness. Breaths of fresh air." *ICHNFM 2013 Conference Attendee*

- "Just got back to Guam. Great experience at the International Conference on Human Nutrition and Functional Medicine. Exciting concepts on functional medicine. Thanks Dr. Alex Vasquez and team!" *ICHNFM 2013 Conference Attendee*

- "Already waiting in line to buy next year's ticket! **Dr. Vasquez you crushed it!** The future is looking fun already ☺" *ICHNFM 2013 Conference Attendee*

- "Had an incredible time at the 2013 International Conference on Human Nutrition and Functional Medicine. Got to meet some amazing people and hear from some of the top researchers/health professionals about human nutrition and functional medicine approaches. It was definitely worth every penny and can't wait to go back next year!" *ICHNFM 2013 Conference Attendee*

- "Wonderful conference! Thanks so much." *ICHNFM 2013 Conference Attendee*

- "Really wonderful conference! Lots of material ready to implement Monday morning! **Congrats to Alex Vasquez on a herculean job very well done!**" *ICHNFM 2013 Conference Attendee*

- "Thanks for a great conference. I really enjoyed all of the speakers, but your lectures were by far the most useful for implementing ideas into my clinical practice. And the most entertaining." *ICHNFM 2013 Conference Attendee*

- "Thank you for your life-changing work." *Physician, 2011*

- "I want Dr. Vasquez to know that I have just received his book, Chiropractic and Naturopathic Mastery of Common Clinical Disorders. **It is a treasure. The best book in my library.** Thank you for the contribution that you are giving to the world of health care." *Clinician, 2010*

- "I appreciate the resources you offer the profession. I use your books and articles regularly." *Doctor, 2011*

- "Dr. Vasquez, I greatly appreciate your efforts. I am a student at ___, 8th trimester, and would like to express my gratitude for your research and works. After coming across your texts in the library, **I quickly found your insight and explanations of the current health care crisis, and in depth coverage and algorithms for inflammatory diseases as a profound inspiration and call to action. I appreciate your attention to detail, and have been taken back several times by the potency and meaning of your sentences. Thank you for your hard work, I will enjoy these books and will surely share with those that have the same drive for true and competent patient care.**" *Health Sciences Student, 2008*

- "I never told you this, but whenever I need to research a particular disease, **besides going on Pubmed and checking some classic Pathophysiology and Clinical Nutrition books, I use your books and I find them extremely well organized, concise, and up-to-date and with the functional/integrative medicine thinking I enjoy and believe it is the future of Health Care.**" *Nutrition Research Consultant and University Faculty in Europe, 2009*

- "Thanks so much. You are a great asset to our profession." *Doctor, 2010*

- "As a 7th trimester student quickly approaching 8th trimester and student clinic, I know I will be utilizing your books often. **Your "Chiropractic and Naturopathic Mastery of Common Clinical Disorders" book is referenced very frequently by many clinicians and faculty members at [our university]. Your work is highly regarded**, and I look forward to clinically utilizing the information I will obtain from your writings." *Health Sciences Student, 2011*

- "I am a chiropractic student at ___ Chiropractic College. I just wanted to drop a quick line thanking you for your thorough and accessible textbook Integrative Orthopedics. We are using it in our Differential Diagnosis class, and **it is the best book I've come across in Chiropractic College bar none. The writing is concise, informative and refreshingly eloquent. The material is super practical. I hope you continue putting out great resources.**" *Health Sciences Student, 2011*
- "I appreciate the resources you offer the profession. **I use your books and articles regularly**." *Doctor, 2011*
- "**Your Integrated Orthopedics book is magnificent**. I wish all textbooks were structured and as thoughtful as that one." *Health Sciences Student, 2008*
- "By reading the introduction I realize that calling it an orthopedics book; does not do it justice. **It is far more than that. It looks to me that you have created, or are creating, the bible of Integrative Orthopedics and physical medicine**. *Physician, 2007*
- "First of all let me say how honored I am that you have allowed me to review this work. You have done an amazing job! In my opinion **every healthcare provider SHOULD have this on their bookshelf**." *Physician, 2007*
- "Your work on Chapter 12: Hip and Thigh is very good. The chapter is inclusive of the typical pathologies seen in private practice and I particularly liked the separation of juvenile from adult pathologies. Your choice of tests to assess hip and thigh pathology on page 320 is very nice and inclusive. I appreciate your use of algorithms and find them very useful in teaching and in practice. In general, **I thought this chapter represents a quality, state of the art presentation**!" *Clinician and Professor in Clinical Sciences, 2007*
- "I saw your books in a colleague's office and was really impressed. Really appreciate the thoroughness you've put into them." *Doctor, 2010*
- "**It is with great interest and fascination that I have been reading your material both in your two books (Integrative Orthopedics and Integrative Rheumatology) and online. I consider myself very fortunate to have come across your work**, as many of the basic elements of health which you discuss I never learnt or even heard about while in chiropractic college." *Doctor, 2010*
- "I appreciate the resources you offer the profession. I use your books and articles regularly." *Doctor, 2011*
- "**I'm so pleased with your books and was inspired to let you know they have already been incredibly useful! Good index; well organized algorithms. Sometimes I buy educational material and it just sort of sits there... Your books now live on my main desk. Thanks**." *Physician and Journal Editor, 2009*
- "I just wanted to let you know how much I am enjoying reading **your book Integrative Rheumatology. It is having an extremely positive impact in the way I view health and am having a tough time putting it down. It is very inspirational.** I have long felt that it is very important to set a good example for your patients and now try my best to be one for my future patients. I like how you stress this in your book. In order to be the best example for my patients I am going to need to address some problems with my own health. I look healthy from the outside but I have been suffering from fatigue for about 4 years. It has a very negative impact on my health. People say that doing the same thing and expecting different results is the definition of insanity so I think it is time that I attempt to make some changes. ... **Thanks again for writing such a great book. I feel it is a must have for anyone in a musculoskeletal practice**." *Health Sciences Student, 2010*
- "My name is [recent graduate], and I've been a fan of your books since I was in chiropractic college at [university] campus. Dr. [Author, Presenter] made your book, Integrative Rheumatology, required reading for his 9th quarter nutrition class. I never looked back, and have since purchased Chiropractic & Naturopathic Mastery of Common Clinical Disorders as well as Chiropractic Management of Chronic Hypertension." *Doctor, 2010*
- "I saw your books in a colleague's office and was really impressed. Really appreciate the thoroughness you've put into them." *Doctor, 2010*

- "Reading the new integrative management of high blood pressure book and I am thoroughly enjoying it; excellent job. **I am feeling so empowered I'm opening another office focusing on 'restoring the foundations of health' for the community** that I open it in. I am looking for a location and networking to find an internist and cardiologist that are forward thinking; I'm very excited!" *Doctor, 2011*
- "Thank you for the presentation at [the university] this past weekend. **My horizons about what can be done to help people were greatly expanded. I am now still studying the notes from the seminar and am looking forward to more study and learning on how to** *correctly* **manage diabetes and hypertension.**" *Doctor, 2011*
- "Thank you for exposing so many people to the results of our research on the treatment of hypertension. I hope you can pay us a visit during your next trip to our area so we can give you the tour of our new 50+ bed inpatient facility." Dr Alan Goldhamer, Chief of Health Promoting Clinic, 2010
- "**I always enjoy reading your work.** I personally gain a lot of knowledge through being a peer-reviewer for you and am better because of it!" *Doctor, Faculty Member, and Postgraduate Instructor, 2011*
- "**I attended your seminar at [University] in June and have been utilizing your hypertension protocols. In that short time, I have seen some marked progress with various patients.**" *Doctor, 2010*

2013 INTERNATIONAL CONFERENCE ON HUMAN NUTRITION AND FUNCTIONAL MEDICINE

PORTLAND OREGON CONVENTION CENTER • SEPTEMBER 25-29, 2013

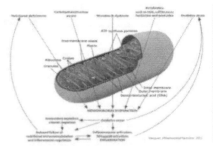
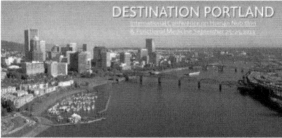
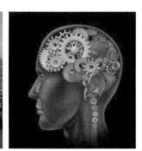

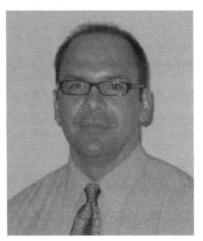

DrV's "Functional Inflammology Protocol":

Deciphering/Decoding/Deconstructing the Common Disorders of Chronic/Sustained Inflammation

Alex Vasquez D.C., N.D., D.O., F.A.C.N.

This work is best understood and clinically applied when assimilated in conjunction with Dr Vasquez's live lectures from the 2013 International Conference on Human Nutrition and Functional Medicine: All of Dr Vasquez's recorded lectures (8 hours) from this conference are available https://vimeo.com/ondemand/ichnfm2013drv and a 426-page printed book of all slides is available https://www.createspace.com/4478800.

Chapter 1:
Initial Considerations in Patient Assessment and Management:
An Overview of Key Concepts and Facts in Patient History,
Physical Examination, Laboratory Interpretation,
Risk Management and Clinical Approach,
Common Clinical Considerations

Overview of this chapter

Reviewed herein are the three essential components of patient assessment:

1. History,
2. Physical examination, and
3. Laboratory assessment.

Additional concepts and perspectives are provided that will help facilitate risk management and promote and contextualize optimal patient care.

This chapter concludes with two new additions titled "Common Clinical Considerations" for hemochromatosis and hypothyroidism, both of which are commonly encountered in clinical practice and which need to be considered "core" material in the routine evaluation of essentially all patients who present with disorders such as diabetes, depression, fatigue, and musculoskeletal pain. Previously, I had published these as separate chapters in various books, but—again—at this time I think these need to be integrated into basic/daily/routine clinical consideration.

Topics:

- **Moving past disease- and drug-centered medicine toward patient-centered health optimization: the goal is *wellness***
- **Acute Care and Musculoskeletal Care as Opportunities for Health Optimization**
- **Clinical Assessments**
  - History taking & physical examination
  - Orthopedic/musculoskeletal examination: Concepts and goals
  - Neurologic assessment: Review
  - Laboratory assessments: General considerations of commonly used tests
    - i. *Routine tests*: Chemistry/metabolic panel, lipid panel, CBC, 25(OH)-vitamin D, ferritin, thyroid stimulating hormone, CRP, ESR
    - ii. *Rheumatology/inflammation*: ANA (antinuclear antibodies), ANCA (antineutrophilic cytoplasmic antibodies), RF (rheumatoid factor), CCP (cyclic citrullinated protein antibodies), complement proteins, HLA-B27, additional tests for various immune/inflammatory disorders, tests for chronic infections/dysbiosis
    - iii. *Functional assessments*: Lactulose-mannitol assay, comprehensive stool analysis and comprehensive parasitology
- **High-Risk Pain Patients**
- **Clinical Concepts**
  - Not all injury-related problems are injury-related problems
  - Safe patient + safe treatment = safe outcome
  - Four clues to underlying problems
  - Special considerations in the evaluation of children
  - No errors allowed: Differences between primary healthcare and spectator sports
  - "Disease treatment" is different from "patient management"
  - Clinical practice involves much more than "diagnosis and treatment"
  - Clinical Management of Patients with Systemic Inflammatory/Autoimmune Diseases
  - Risk Management, Charting, and Avoiding Medical Errors: Useful Reminders and Acronyms
  - Risk Management: A note especially to students and recent licensees
- **Musculoskeletal Emergencies**
  - Acute compartment syndrome
  - Acute red eye, including acute iritis and scleritis
  - Atlantoaxial subluxation and instability
  - Cauda equina syndrome
  - Giant cell arteritis, temporal arteritis
  - Myelopathy, spinal cord compression
  - Neuropsychiatric lupus
  - Osteomyelitis
  - Septic arthritis, acute nontraumatic monoarthritis
- **Brief Overview of Integrative Healthcare Disciplines**
  - Chiropractic
  - Naturopathic Medicine
  - Osteopathic Medicine
  - Functional Medicine
- **Common Clinical Considerations**
  - Hemochromatosis and Iron Overload
  - Hypothyroidism, particularly Functional/Metabolic/Peripheral Hypothyroidism

Moving past "diagnosis/disease/drug"-centered medicine toward patient-centered health optimization: the goal is *wellness*

Written for students and experienced clinicians, this chapter introduces and reviews many new and common terms, procedures, and concepts relevant to the management of patients with musculoskeletal disorders. Especially for students, the reading of this chapter is essential to understanding the extensive material in this book and will facilitate the clinical assessment and management of patients with various clinical presentations.

Healthcare is currently in a time of significant fluctuation and is ready for changes in the balance of power and the paradigms which direct our therapeutic interventions. For nearly a century, allopathic medicine has hailed itself as "the gold standard", and other professions have either submitted to or been crushed by their ongoing political/scientific manipulations and their continual proclamation of intellectual and therapeutic superiority[1,2,3,4,5,6,7,8,9,10,11,12,13] despite 180,000-220,000 iatrogenic *medically-induced* deaths per year (500-600 iatrogenic deaths per day)[14,15] and consistent documentation that most medical/allopathic physicians are unable to provide accurate musculoskeletal diagnoses due to pervasive inadequacies in medical training.[16,17,18,19] Increasing disenchantment with allopathic *heroic medicine* and its adverse outcomes of inefficacy, exorbitant expenses, and unnecessary death are fostering change, such that allopathic medicine has been dethroned as the leading paradigm among American patients, who spend the majority of their discretionary healthcare dollars on consultations and treatments provided by "alternative" healthcare providers.[20,21] With the ever-increasing utilization of chiropractic, naturopathic, and osteopathic medical services,

> **Medical iatrogenesis kills 493 Americans per day**
> "Recent estimates suggest that each year more than 1 million patients are injured while in the hospital and approximately 180,000 die because of these injuries. Furthermore, drug-related morbidity and mortality are common and are estimated to cost more than $136 billion a year."
>
> Holland EG, Degruy FV. Drug-induced disorders. *Am Fam Physician*. 1997;56(7):1781-8, 1791-2

we must see that our paradigms and interventions keep pace with the evolving research literature and our increasing professional responsibilities so that we can deliver the highest possible quality of care.

While we all readily acknowledge the importance of emergency care for emergency situations, those of us who advocate and practice a more complete approach to healthcare and life readily see the shortcomings of a limited and mechanical approach to healthcare, and we aspire to do more than simply fix problems. The implementation of *multidimensional* (i.e., *comprehensive* and *multifaceted*) treatment plans that address many aspects

[1] Wilk CA. Medicine, Monopolies, and Malice: How the Medical Establishment Tried to Destroy Chiropractic. Garden City Park: Avery, 1996

[2] Getzendanner S. Permanent injunction order against AMA. *JAMA*. 1988 Jan 1;259(1):81-2 http://InflammationMastery.com/archives/wilk.html

[3] Carter JP. Racketeering in Medicine: The Suppression of Alternatives. Norfolk: Hampton Roads Pub; 1993

[4] Morley J, Rosner AL, Redwood D. A case study of misrepresentation of the scientific literature: recent reviews of chiropractic. *J Altern Complement Med*. 2001 Feb;7:65-78

[5] Terrett AG. Misuse of the literature by medical authors in discussing spinal manipulative therapy injury. *J Manipulative Physiol Ther*. 1995;18(4):203-10

[6] National Alliance of Professional Psychology Providers. AMA Seeks To Control and Restrict Psychologist's Scope of Practice. www.nappp.org/scope.pdf Accessed Nov 2006

[7] "In an effort to marshal the medical community's resources against the growing threat of expanding scope of practice for allied health professionals, the AMA has formed a national partnership to confront such initiatives nationwide… The committee will use $25,000…" Daly R, American Psychiatric Association. AMA Forms Coalition to Thwart Non-M.D. Practice Expansion. *Psychiatric News* 2006 March; 41: 17 http://pn.psychiatryonline.org/cgi/content/full/41/5/17-a?eaf Accessed November 25, 2006

[8] Spivak JL. The Medical Trust Unmasked. Louis S. Siegfried Publishers; New York: 1961

[9] Trever W. In the Public Interest. Los Angeles; Scriptures Unlimited; 1972. This is probably the most authoritative documentation of the illegal actions of the AMA up to 1972; contains numerous photocopies of actual AMA documents and minutes of official meetings with overt intentionality of destroying Americans' healthcare options so that the AMA and related organizations would have a monopoly in national healthcare.

[10] Wenban AB. Inappropriate use of the title 'chiropractor' and term 'chiropractic manipulation' in the peer-reviewed biomedical literature. *Chiropr Osteopat*. 2006;14:16 http://chiroandosteo.com/content/14/1/16

[11] Orme-Johnson DW, Herron RE. An innovative approach to reducing medical care utilization and expenditures. *Am J Manag Care*. 1997 Jan;3:135-44 http://www.ajmc.com/Article.cfm?Menu=1&ID=2154

[12] van der Steen WJ, Ho VK. Drugs versus diets: disillusions with Dutch health care. *Acta Biotheor*. 2001;49(2):125-40

[13] Texas Medical Association. Physicians Ask Court to Protect Patients From Illegal Chiropractic Activities. http://www.texmed.org/Template.aspx?id=5259 Accessed Feb 2007

[14] Starfield B. Is US health really the best in the world? *JAMA*. 2000 Jul 26;284(4):483-5

[15] "Recent estimates suggest that each year more than 1 million patients are injured while in the hospital and approximately 180,000 die because of these injuries. Furthermore, drug-related morbidity and mortality are common and are estimated to cost more than $136 billion a year." Holland EG, Degruy FV. Drug-induced disorders. *Am Fam Physician*. 1997;56(7):1781-8, 1791-2

[16] Freedman KB, Bernstein J. The adequacy of medical school education in musculoskeletal medicine. *J Bone Joint Surg Am*. 1998;80(10):1421-7

[17] Freedman KB, Bernstein J. Educational deficiencies in musculoskeletal medicine. *J Bone Joint Surg Am*. 2002;84-A(4):604-8

[18] Matzkin E, Smith ME, Freccero CD, Richardson AB. Adequacy of education in musculoskeletal medicine. *J Bone Joint Surg Am*. 2005;87-A(2):310-4

[19] Schmale GA. More evidence of educational inadequacies in musculoskeletal medicine. *Clin Orthop Relat Res*. 2005 Aug;(437):251-9

[20] "…Americans made an estimated 425 million visits to providers of unconventional therapy. This number exceeds the number of visits to all U.S. primary care physicians (388 million)." Eisenberg DM, Kessler RC, Foster C, Norlock FE, Calkins DR, Delbanco TL. Unconventional medicine in the United States. Prevalence, costs, and patterns of use. *N Engl J Med*. 1993 Jan 28;328(4):246-52

[21] "Estimated expenditures for alternative medicine professional services increased 45.2% between 1990 and 1997 and were conservatively estimated at $21.2 billion in 1997, with at least $12.2 billion paid out-of-pocket. This exceeds the 1997 out-of-pocket expenditures for all US hospitalizations." Eisenberg DM, Davis RB, Ettner SL, Appel S, Wilkey S, Van Rompay M, Kessler RC. Trends in alternative medicine use in the United States, 1990-1997: results of a follow-up national survey. *JAMA* 1998 Nov 11;280(18):1569-75

of pathophysiologic phenomena is a huge step forward in creating improved health and preventing future illness in the patients who seek our professional assistance. However, even complete multidimensional treatment plans still fall short of the goal of creating wellness, if for no other reasons than 1) they are still disease- and problem-oriented, rather than health-oriented, 2) they are prescribed from outside ("The doctor told me to do it.") rather than originating internally and spontaneously by the patient's own direction and affirmation ("I *do* this because I *am* this."), and, finally and most difficult to relay, 3) they are mechanistic

Ever-increasing popularity of nonallopathic medicine

"...Americans made an estimated 425 million visits to providers of unconventional therapy. This number exceeds the number of visits to all U.S. primary care physicians (388 million)."

Eisenberg DM, et al. Unconventional medicine in the United States. Prevalence, costs, and patterns of use. *N Engl J Med* 1993 Jan

rather than organic, they can do no better than the sum of their parts, they flow exclusively from the mind ("do") and not also from the body-soul ("am"). The art of creating wellness takes time to understand, longer to implement clinically, and even longer to apply to one's own life. Wellness is a state of being rather than a checklist of activities in a "preventive health program." The subtle differences that distinguish "wellness" from any "program" or "prescription" are the differences between *leading* versus *following* and *flowing* versus *performing*. Wellness transcends mere health (e.g., vitality and absence of disease) and health (e.g., beyond physical, mental, and psychosocial wellbeing). **True and fully developed authentic wellness is the embodiment of multidimensional health; it is as-complete-as-possible (e.g., asymptotic) self-actualization, full integration of one's life—present, past, and future; it must ultimately be and manifest in physical, mental, emotional, spiritual, sociopolitical, transpersonal and multigenerational dimensions, inclusive of one's shadow[22], work[23], feelings, thoughts, and goals into a cohesive living whole – "a wheel rolling from its own center"[24] and beyond itself, beyond— ultimately—its own place and time.**

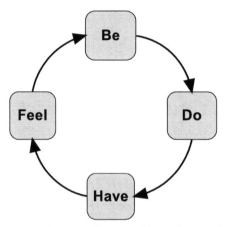

Self-reinforcing cycles of perception, manifestation, action, actualization, and reflection which reinforces (or changes) perception: "Reciprocal causality" is the term popularized by psychologist Nathaniel Branden in his excellent works such as *Psychology of Self-Esteem*. Relatedly, "reciprocal determinism" is the psychosocial theory set forth by psychologist Albert Bandura that a person's behavior both influences and is influenced by personal factors and the social environment.

Authentic Selfhood, Internal Locus of Control, Creativity, Self-Direction

"Innocence is the child, and forgetfulness, a new beginning, a game, a self-rolling wheel, a first movement, a holy "Yea". Surely, for the game of creating, my brethren, there is needed a holy "Yea" unto life."

Nietzsche FW. *Thus Spoke Zarathustra*. Part 1—The Three Metamorphoses.

---

[22] Robert Bly. The Human Shadow. Sound Horizons 1991 [ISBN: 1879323001] and Bly R. A Little Book on the Human Shadow. [ISBN: 0062548476]

[23] Rick Jarow. Creating the Work You Love: Courage, Commitment and Career; Inner Traditions Intl Ltd; (December 1995) [ISBN: 0892815426]

[24] Friedrich Wilhelm Nietzsche. Walter Kaufmann (Translator). Thus Spoke Zarathustra: A Book for None and All. Penguin USA; 1978, page 27

Acute Care and Musculoskeletal Care: Opportunities for Health Optimization

Clinicians should appreciate that every patient encounter is an opportunity for comprehensive care, disease prevention, and health optimization. This is true whether the presenting complaint is acne, psoriasis, a respiratory infection, or musculoskeletal pain. Given the relatively high frequency of musculoskeletal complaints in clinical practice in general and chiropractic and osteopathic practices in particular, the following section will emphasize the clinical presentation of musculoskeletal complaints as an underappreciated opportunity for wellness care.

Since **approximately 1 of every 7 (14% of total) visits to a primary healthcare provider is for the treatment of musculoskeletal pain or dysfunction**[25], every healthcare provider needs to have 1) knowledge of important concepts related to musculoskeletal medicine, 2) the ability to recognize urgent and emergency conditions, 3) the ability to competently perform orthopedic examination procedures and interpret laboratory assessments, and 4) the knowledge and ability to design and implement effective treatment plans and to coordinate patient management.

In pharmacosurgical allopathic medicine, the goal of musculoskeletal treatment is to address the patient's injury or disorder by alleviating pain with the use of drugs, preventing further injury, and returning the patient to his/her previous status and activities. The most commonly employed interventions are 1) rest and "watchful waiting", 2) non-steroidal anti-inflammatory drugs (NSAIDS) and cyclooxygenase-2-inhibitors (COX-2 inhibitors, or "coxibs"), and 3) surgery. The more action-oriented approaches used by many chiropractic, naturopathic, and osteopathic physicians differs from the allopathic approach because, although avoidance of and "rest" from damaging activities is reasonable and valuable, too much rest without an emphasis on active preventive rehabilitation ❶ encourages patient passivity and ❷ the assumption of the sick role, and it ❸ fails to actively promote tissue healing and ❹ fails to address the underlying proprioceptive deficits that are common in patients with chronic musculoskeletal pain and recurrent injuries.[26,27,28] **NSAIDs are considered "first line" therapy for musculoskeletal disorders by allopaths** despite the data showing that "**There is no evidence that widely used NSAIDs have any long-term benefit on osteoarthritis.**"[29] What is worse than this lack of efficacy is the evidence showing that NSAIDs *exacerbate* musculoskeletal disease (rather than *cure* it). **NSAIDs are known to inhibit cartilage formation and to promote bone necrosis and joint degradation with long-term use**[30,31,32,33] and **NSAIDs are responsible for more than 16,000 gastrohemorrhagic deaths and 100,000 hospitalizations each year.**[34] The "coxibs" were supposed to provide anti-inflammatory benefits with an enhanced safety profile, but the gastrocentric focus of the drug developers failed to appreciate that COX-2 is necessary for the formation of prostacyclin, a prostaglandin created from arachidonic acid via COX-2 that plays an important role in vasodilation and antithrombosis; not surprisingly therefore, use of COX-2-inhibiting drugs has consistently been associated with increased risk for adverse cardiovascular effects including myocardial infarction,

> **Allopathic medicine has been described (ie, has described itself) as "scientific" since a time when this was clearly not the case**
>
> "…only about 15% of medical interventions are supported by solid scientific evidence…"
>
> Smith R. Where is the wisdom…? The poverty of medical evidence. *BMJ.* 1991 Oct 5;303:798-9

unstable angina, cardiac thrombus, resuscitated cardiac arrest, sudden or unexplained death, ischemic stroke, and transient ischemic attacks.[35] Additionally, the use of a COX-2 inhibiting treatment in patients who overconsume

---

[25] American College of Rheumatology Ad Hoc Committee on Clinical Guidelines. Guidelines for the initial evaluation of the adult patient with acute musculoskeletal symptoms. *Arthritis Rheum.* 1996 Jan; 39(1):1-8 See also: Vasquez A. Musculoskeletal disorders and iron overload disease: comment on the American College of Rheumatology guidelines. *Arthritis Rheum* 1996;39: 1767-8

[26] McPartland JM, Brodeur RR, Hallgren RC. Chronic neck pain, standing balance, and suboccipital muscle atrophy--a pilot study. *J Manipulative Physiol Ther.* 1997;20:24-9

[27] Bullock-Saxton JE, Janda V, Bullock MI. Reflex activation of gluteal muscles in walking. An approach to restoration of muscle function for patients with low-back pain. *Spine* 1993 May;18(6):704-8

[28] Sinaki M, Brey RH, Hughes CA, Larson DR, Kaufman KR. Significant reduction in risk of falls and back pain in osteoporotic-kyphotic women through a Spinal Proprioceptive Extension Exercise Dynamic (SPEED) program. *Mayo Clin Proc.* 2005 Jul;80(7):849-55

[29] Beers MH, Berkow R (Eds). *The Merck Manual. 17th Edition.* Whitehouse Station; Merck Research Laboratories 1999 page 451

[30] "At…concentrations comparable to those… in the synovial fluid of patients treated with the drug, several NSAIDs suppress proteoglycan synthesis… These NSAID-related effects on chondrocyte metabolism … are much more profound in osteoarthritic cartilage than in normal cartilage, due to enhanced uptake of NSAIDs by the osteoarthritic cartilage." Brandt KD. Effects of nonsteroidal anti-inflammatory drugs on chondrocyte metabolism in vitro and in vivo. *Am J Med.* 1987 Nov 20; 83(5A): 29-34

[31] "The case of a young healthy man, who developed avascular necrosis of head of femur after prolonged administration of indomethacin, is reported here." Prathapkumar KR, Smith I, Attara GA. Indomethacin induced avascular necrosis of head of femur. *Postgrad Med J.* 2000 Sep; 76(899): 574-5

[32] "This highly significant association between NSAID use and acetabular destruction gives cause for concern, not least because of the difficulty in achieving satisfactory hip replacements in patients with severely damaged acetabula."Newman NM,Ling RS.Acetabular bone destruction related to non-steroidal anti-inflammatory drugs.*Lancet*1985;2:11-4

[33] Vidal y Plana RR, Bizzarri D, Rovati AL. Articular cartilage pharmacology: I. In vitro studies on glucosamine and non steroidal antiinflammatory drugs. *Pharmacol Res Commun.* 1978 Jun;10(6):557-69

[34] Singh G. Recent considerations in nonsteroidal anti-inflammatory drug gastropathy. *Am J Med.* 1998;105(1B):31S-38S

[35] Mukherjee D, Nissen SE, Topol EJ. Risk of cardiovascular events associated with selective COX-2 inhibitors. *JAMA.* 2001 Aug 22-29;286(8):954-9

arachidonic acid (i.e., most people in America and other industrialized nations[36]) would be expected to shunt bioavailable arachidonate into the formation of leukotrienes, a group of inflammatory mediators known to promote atherogenesis.[37] Thus, the outcome was entirely predictable: overuse of COX-2 inhibitors should have been expected to create a catastrophe of iatrogenic cardiovascular death, and this is exactly what was allowed to occur—clearly indicating independent but synergistic failures on the part of pharmaceutical companies, the FDA, and the medical profession.[38,39,40,41] According to statements by David J. Graham, MD, MPH, (Associate Director for Science, Office of Drug Safety, FDA) in 2005, an estimated 139,000 Americans who took Vioxx suffered serious complications including stroke or myocardial infarction; between 26,000 and 55,000 Americans died as a result of their doctors' prescribing Vioxx.[42] Additionally, the surgical procedures employed by allopaths for the treatment of musculoskeletal pain do not consistently show evidence of efficacy, safety, or cost-effectiveness. Arthroscopic surgery for osteoarthritis of the knee, for example, costs thousands of dollars to each individual and billions of dollars to the American healthcare system but is no more effective than placebo.[43,44,45] In a review which also noted that only 15% of medical procedures are supported by literature references and that only 1% of such references are deemed scientifically valid, Rosner[46] showed that the risks of serious injury (i.e., cauda equina syndrome or vertebral artery dissection) associated with spinal manipulation are "*400 times **lower*** than the death rates observed from gastrointestinal bleeding due to the use of nonsteroidal anti-inflammatory drugs and *700 times **lower*** than the overall mortality rate for spinal surgery."

In chiropractic, osteopathic, and naturopathic medicine, the goal and means of musculoskeletal treatment is to address the patient's injury or disorder by simultaneously alleviating pain with the use of natural, noninvasive, low-cost, and low-risk interventions while improving the patient's overall health, preventing future health problems, and "upgrading" the patient's overall paradigm of health maintenance and disease prevention from one that is passive and reactive to one that is empowered and pro-active. Commonly employed therapeutics include spinal manipulation[47,48,49], exercise[50] and the use of nutritional supplements and botanical medicines[51,52] which have been demonstrated in peer-reviewed clinical trials to be safe and effective for the alleviation of musculoskeletal pain. More specifically, chiropractic and naturopathic physicians are particularly well-versed in the clinical utilization of such treatments as niacinamide[53], glucosamine and chondroitin sulfates[54], vitamin D[55], vitamin B-12[56],

[36] Seaman DR. The diet-induced proinflammatory state: a cause of chronic pain and other degenerative diseases? *J Manipulative Physiol Ther.* 2002;25(3):168-79

[37] Dwyer JH, Allayee H, Dwyer KM, Fan J, Wu H, Mar R, Lusis AJ, Mehrabian M. Arachidonate 5-lipoxygenase promoter genotype, dietary arachidonic acid, and atherosclerosis. *N Engl J Med.* 2004 Jan 1;350(1):29-37

[38] Topol EJ. Arthritis medicines and cardiovascular events--"house of coxibs". *JAMA.* 2005 Jan 19;293(3):366-8. Epub 2004 Dec 28

[39] Ray WA, Griffin MR, Stein CM. Cardiovascular toxicity of valdecoxib. *N Engl J Med.* 2004 Dec 23;351(26):2767. Epub 2004 Dec 17

[40] Topol EJ. Failing the public health--rofecoxib, Merck, and the FDA. *N Engl J Med.* 2004 Oct 21;351(17):1707-9

[41] Horton R. Vioxx, the implosion of Merck, and aftershocks at the FDA. *Lancet.* 2004 Dec 4-10;364(9450):1995-6

[42] David J. Graham, MD, MPH, (Associate Director for Science, Office of Drug Safety, US FDA) estimated that 139,000 Americans who took Vioxx suffered serious side effects; he estimated that the drug killed between 26,000 and 55,000 people. http://www.commondreams.org/views05/0223-35.htm http://www.fda.gov/cder/drug/infopage/vioxx/vioxxgraham.pdf Accessed November 25, 2006

[43] Gina Kolata. A Knee Surgery for Arthritis Is Called Sham. *The New York Times*, July 11, 2002

[44] Moseley JB, O'Malley K, Petersen NJ, Menke TJ, Brody BA, Kuykendall DH, Hollingsworth JC, Ashton CM, Wray NP. A controlled trial of arthroscopic surgery for osteoarthritis of the knee. *N Engl J Med.* 2002;347:81-8

[45] Bernstein J, Quach T. A perspective on the study of Moseley: questioning the value of arthroscopic knee surgery for osteoarthritis. *Cleve Clin J Med* 2003;70:401, 405-6, 408-10

[46] Rosner AL. Evidence-based clinical guidelines for the management of acute low-back pain: response to the guidelines prepared for the Australian Medical Health and Research Council. *J Manipulative Physiol Ther.* 2001;24(3):214-20

[47] Manga P, Angus D, Papadopoulos C, et al. *The Effectiveness and Cost-Effectiveness of Chiropractic Management of Low-Back Pain.* Richmond Hill, Ontario: Kenilworth; 1993

[48] Meade TW, Dyer S, Browne W, Townsend J, Frank AO. Low-back pain of mechanical origin: randomised comparison of chiropractic and hospital outpatient treatment. *BMJ.* 1990;300(6737):1431-7

[49] Meade TW, Dyer S, Browne W, Frank AO. Randomised comparison of chiropractic and hospital outpatient management for low-back pain: results from extended follow up. *BMJ.* 1995;311(7001):349-5

[50] Harold Elrick, MD. Exercise is Medicine. *The Physician and Sportsmedicine* - Volume 24 - No. 2 - February 1996

[51] Vasquez A. Revisiting the Five-Part Nutritional Wellness Protocol: The Supplemented Paleo-Mediterranean Diet. *Nutritional Perspectives* 2011 January http://InflammationMastery.com/part8.html

[52] Vasquez A. Reducing pain and inflammation naturally - Part 3: Improving overall health while safely and effectively treating musculoskeletal pain. *Nutritional Perspectives* 2005; 28: 34-38, 40-42 http://InflammationMastery.com/part3.html

[53] Kaufman W. Niacinamide therapy for joint mobility. Therapeutic reversal of a common clinical manifestation of the "normal" aging process. *Conn State Med J* 1953;17:584-591

[54] Reginster JY, Deroisy R, Rovati LC, Lee RL, Lejeune E, Bruyere O, Giacovelli G, Henrotin Y, Dacre JE, Gossett C. Long-term effects of glucosamine sulphate on osteoarthritis progression: a randomised, placebo-controlled clinical trial. *Lancet.* 2001;357(9252):251-6

[55] Vasquez A, Manso G, Cannell J. The clinical importance of vitamin D: a paradigm shift with implications for all healthcare providers. *Altern Ther Health Med* 2004;10:28-36 http://InflammationMastery.com/monograph04.html

[56] Mauro GL, Martorana U, Cataldo P, Brancato G, Letizia G. Vitamin B12 in low back pain: a randomised, double-blind, placebo-controlled study. *Eur Rev Med Pharmacol Sci.* 2000 May-Jun;4(3):53-8

balanced and complete fatty acid therapy[57,58], anti-inflammatory diets[59,60,61], proteolytic/pancreatic enzymes[62], and botanical medicines such as *Boswellia*[63], *Harpagophytum*[64], *Uncaria*, and willow bark[65,66]—each of these interventions has been validated in peer-reviewed research for safety and effectiveness.[67] Furthermore, from the perspective of integrative chiropractic and naturopathic medicine, aiming for such a limited accomplishment as mere "returning the patient to previous status and activities" would be considered substandard, since the patient's overall health was neither addressed nor improved and since returning the patient to his/her previous status and activities would be a direct invitation for the problem to recur indefinitely. Chiropractic and naturopathic physicians appreciate that, especially regarding chronic health problems, any treatment plan that allows the patient to resume his/her previous lifestyle is by definition doomed to fail because a return to the patient's previous lifestyle and activities that allowed the onset of the disease/disorder in the first place will most certainly result in the perpetuation and recurrence of the illness or disorder. **Stated more directly: for *healing* to truly be effective, the comprehensive treatment plan must generally result in a permanent and profound change in the patient's lifestyle and emotional climate, which are the primary modifiable determinants of either health or disease.**

[57] Vasquez A. Reducing Pain and Inflammation Naturally. Part 1: New Insights into Fatty Acid Biochemistry and the Influence of Diet. *Nutritional Perspectives* 2004; Oct: 5, 7-10,12,14 http://InflammationMastery.com/part1.html

[58] Vasquez A. Reducing Pain and Inflammation Naturally. Part 2: New Insights into Fatty Acid Supplementation and Its Effect on Eicosanoid Production and Genetic Expression. *Nutritional Perspectives* 2005; January: 5-16 http://InflammationMastery.com/part2.html

[59] Seaman DR. The diet-induced proinflammatory state: a cause of chronic pain and other degenerative diseases? *J Manipulative Physiol Ther.* 2002 Mar-Apr;25(3):168-7

[60] Vasquez A. *Integrative Orthopedics*. http://InflammationMastery.com/orthopedics.html

[61] Vasquez A. Reducing Pain and Inflammation Naturally. Part 1: New Insights into Fatty Acid Biochemistry and the Influence of Diet. *Nutritional Perspectives* 2004; October: 5, 7-10, 12, 14 http://InflammationMastery.com/part1.html

[62] Trickett P. Proteolytic enzymes in treatment of athletic injuries. *Appl Ther.* 1964;30:647-52

[63] Kimmatkar N, Thawani V, Hingorani L, Khiyani R. Efficacy and tolerability of Boswellia serrata extract in treatment of osteoarthritis of knee--a randomized double blind placebo controlled trial. *Phytomedicine.* 2003 Jan;10(1):3-7

[64] Chrubasik S, Junck H, Breitschwerdt H, Conradt C, Zappe H. Effectiveness of Harpagophytum extract WS 1531 in the treatment of exacerbation of low-back pain: a randomized, placebo-controlled, double-blind study. *Eur J Anaesthesiol* 1999 Feb;16(2):118-29

[65] Chrubasik S, Eisenberg E, Balan E, Weinberger T, Luzzati R, Conradt C. Treatment of low-back pain exacerbations with willow bark extract: a randomized double-blind study. *Am J Med.* 2000;109:9-14

[66] Vasquez A, Muanza DN. Comment: Evaluation of Presence of Aspirin-Related Warnings with Willow Bark. *Ann Pharmacotherapy* 2005 Oct;39(10):1763

[67] Vasquez A. Reducing pain and inflammation naturally. Part 3: Improving overall health while safely and effectively treating musculoskeletal pain. *Nutritional Perspectives* 2005;28:34-42 http://InflammationMastery.com/part3.html

Clinical Assessments

The clinical assessments reviewed in the following sections are history-taking, orthopedic/musculoskeletal, and neurologic examinations, and commonly used laboratory tests. **History taking is the art of conducting an *informative* and *collaborative* patient interview.**

The role of the doctor during the interview process is not merely that of a data-collecting machine, spewing out questions and receiving responses. Patient interviews can be a creative, enjoyable, comforting opportunity to build rapport and to establish meaningful connection with another human being. Patients are not simply people with health problems – they are first and foremost our fellow human beings, not so dissimilar from ourselves perhaps, and always full of complexity. Our task is not to fully understand their complexity nor to solve all of their mysteries, but rather to help orchestrate these dynamics into a coordinated if not unified direction that promotes health and healing.

Beyond its diagnostic value, the interview process also provides a key opportunity to gain insight into the patient's psychoepistimology—the patient's operating system for interacting with data and the world and internalizing and metabolizing external inputs in such a way as to merge these with internal experiences (i.e., emotions, feelings, preferences, responses). Epistemology is the branch of philosophy concerned with the nature and scope of knowledge. Per Rand[68], psychoepistimology is a person's "method of awareness"; a person's psychoepistimology creates a "corollary view of existence" and in turn, "A man's method of using his consciousness determines his method of survival." By understanding how the patient views him/herself in the world, understanding his/her goals, and—in essence—what "drives" the patient and what "makes him/her tick", clinicians can shape the nuances of the conversation and the treatment plan to promote the desired cognitive-conceptual-behavioral changes in behavior that are prerequisite for the attainment of optimized health outcomes.

History & Assessment

History of the primary complaint: "D.O.P.P. Q.R.S.T."
- Description/location
- Onset
- Provocation: exacerbates
- Palliation: alleviates
- Quality
- Radiation of pain
- Severity
- Timing

Associated complaints
- Additional manifestations
- Concomitant diseases

Review of systems
- Head-to-toe inventory of health status, associated health problems, and complications

Past health history
- Surgeries
- Hospitalizations
- Traumas
- Vaccinations and medications
- Successful and failed treatments for the current complaint(s)

Family health history
- Genotropic illnesses and predispositions
- Lifestyle patterns
- Emotional expectations

Social history
- Hobbies, work, exposures
- Relationships and emotional experiences
- Interpersonal support
- Malpractice litigation

Health Habits
- Diet: appropriate intake of protein, fruits, vegetables, fats, sugars
- Sleep
- Stress management
- Exercise / Sedentary Lifestyle
- Spirituality / Centeredness
- Caffeine and tobacco
- Ethanol and recreational drugs

Medication and supplements
- Reason, doses, duration, cost
- Side-effects
- Interactions

Responsibility and Compliance
- Ability and willingness to comply with prescribed treatment plan and to incorporate the necessary diet-exercise-relationship-emotional-lifestyle modifications
- *Internal* versus *external* locus of control

---

[68] Rand A. For the New Intellectual. New York; Signet:1961, page 16

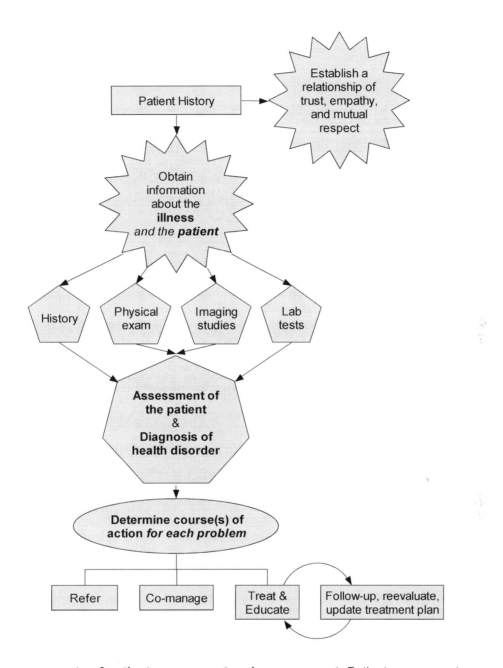

Key components of patient assessment and management: Patient assessment and management is an on-going process that begins with the initial history taken at the first clinical encounter and continues through the physical examination and laboratory assessments and thereafter by monitoring the patient's implementation of and response to the treatment plan. The plan is complete when the desired outcome of health optimization is achieved and sustained.

Components of a Complete Patient History: "D.O.P.P. Q.R.S.T."

Category	Patient history questions and implications
Description, Location: Always start with open-ended questions	• *What is it like for you?* • *What do you experience?* • *What are you feeling?* • *Where is the pain/sensation/problem?* • Ask about specifics: **Pain, numbness, weakness, tingling**, fatigue, recent or chronic infections, burning, aching, dull, sharp, cramping, stretching, pins and needles, weakness, changes in function (i.e., bowel and bladder continence).
Onset	• *When did it begin? Have you ever had anything like this before?* • *Was there a specific event associated with the onset of the problem, such as an injury or an illness, or did the problem start gradually or insidiously?* • *How has it changed over time?* • *Prior injuries to site?* • *Why are you seeking care for this now (rather than last week or last month)?* • *What has changed? How is the pain/problem developing over time—getting worse or getting better?*
Palliation	• *How have you tried treating it? Does anything make it go away?* • *What makes it better? What relieves the pain?* • Ask about prior and current treatments, radiographs, medications, supplements (herbs, vitamins, minerals), injections, surgery, massage, manipulation, and counseling. • Knowing response/resistance to previous treatments can provide clinical insight.
Provocation	• *Are your symptoms constant, or does the problem come and go?* • *What makes it worse? What makes the pain worse?* • *When during the day/week/month/year are your symptoms the worst?*
Quality	• *Can you describe the pain to me?* • *What does it feel like?* • *What do you experience?* • Get a clear understanding of the type of sensation(s): stabbing, shooting pain, pins and needles, sharp pain, electric sensation, numbness, burning, aching, throbbing, weakness, tingling, gel phenomenon (stiffness worsened by inactivity), dizziness, confusion, fatigue, shortness of breath.
Radiation	• *Does the pain stay localized or does it move to your arm/leg/head/face?* • *Do you feel pain in other areas of your body?*
Severity	• *How bad is it? How would you rate it on a scale of one to ten if one were almost no pain and ten was the worst pain you could imagine?* Use the validated VAS—visual analog scale—to quantify the level of pain and impairment. • *Does this problem prevent you from engaging in your daily activities, such as work, exercise, or hobbies?* This is a very important question for determining functional impairment and internal consistency; if the patient is "too injured to work" yet is still able to fully participate in recreational activities that are physically challenging, then malingering is likely.
Timing	• *When do you notice this problem?* • *Is it constant, or does it come and go? Where are you when you notice it the most?* • *Is it worse in the morning, or worse in the evening?* • *Does anyone else in your [home/office/worksite] have this same problem?* • *What times of the day or what days of the week is it the worst?*

Components of a Complete Patient History: "D.O.P.P. Q.R.S.T." —*continued*

Category	Patient history questions and implications
Associated manifestations and constitutional symptoms	• *Have you noticed any other problems associated with this problem?* • **Fatigue?** • **Fever?** • **Weight loss?** *Weight gain?* • *Night* **sweats?** • **Diarrhea? Constipation?** • **Weakness?** • *Nausea?* • *Bowel or bladder difficulties or changes? Difficulty with sexual function?* These could be related to hormonal imbalances, drug side-effects, relationship problems, nutritional deficiencies, nerve compression, and/or depression. • *Change in sensation near your anus/genitals?* Cauda equina syndrome is an important consideration in patients with low-back pain. • *Loss of appetite?* • *Difficulty sleeping?* • *Skin rash or change in pigmentation?*
ROS: review of systems	• <u>General constitution</u>: fatigue, malaise, fever, chills, weight gain/loss… • *"Now we are going to conduct a head-to-toe inventory just to make sure that we have covered everything."* • <u>Head</u>: headaches, head pain, pressure inside head, difficulty concentrating, difficulty remembering, mental function • <u>Ears:</u> ringing in ears, dizziness, hearing loss, hypersensitivity to noise, ear pain, discharge from ear, pressure in ears • <u>Eyes:</u> eye pain, loss of vision or decreased vision or ability to focus, redness or irritation, seeing flashing lights or spots, double vision • <u>Nose</u>: sinus problems, chronically stuffy nose, difficulty smelling things, nose bleeds, change or decrease in sense of smell or taste • <u>Mouth</u>, teeth, TMJ, pain or sores in mouth, difficulty chewing, sensitive teeth, bleeding gums, pain in jaw joint, change or decrease in sense of taste • <u>Neck:</u> pain at the base of skull, pain in neck, stiffness • <u>Throat:</u> difficulty swallowing, pain in throat, feeling like things get stuck in throat, change in voice, difficulty getting air or food in or out • <u>Chest and breasts</u>: any chest pain, difficult breathing, wheezing, coughing, pain, lumps, or discharge from nipple • <u>Shoulders:</u> pain or aching in your shoulders, restricted motion or stiffness • <u>Arms, elbows, hands:</u> pain or problems with your arms, elbows, hands …in the joints or the muscles…, numbness, tingling, weakness, swelling, changes in fingernails, cold hands? • <u>Stomach, abdomen, pelvis, genitals, urinary tract, rectum, :</u> pain in stomach or abdomen, difficulty with digestion, gas, bloating, regurgitation, ulcer, any problems lower down in your abdomen—near your lower intestines? Pain, lumps, swelling, difficulty passing stool, pain or itching near your anus, genitalia; any genital pain, burning, discharge, redness, irritation, sexual dysfunction or impotence, loss of bowel or bladder control? Diarrhea or constipation? How often do you have a bowel movement? • <u>Hips, legs, knees, ankles, feet:</u> numbness, weakness, pain or tingling in the hips, knees, ankles, or feet; pain in calves with walking, swelling of ankles, cold feet • *Is there anything else that you think I should know in order to help you?*

Components of a Complete Patient History: "D.O.P.P. Q.R.S.T." —*continued*

Category	Patient history questions and implications

Medical history	• *Are you taking any* **medications**? *What medications have you taken in the past few years?* Finding out that your new patient recently discontinued his 20-year regimen of valproic acid, lithium, and risperidone may significantly change your interpretation of the clinical interview. Likewise, a patient may not be taking immunosuppressive drugs on the day of your first clinical encounter—he or she may have discontinued such drugs against medical advice (AMA) the week prior to consulting with you.
	• *Have you been* **treated for any medical conditions** *or health problems?*
	• *Have you ever been* **hospitalized**?
	• *Have you ever had* **surgery**?
	• *Have you ever been* **diagnosed with any health problems** *such as high blood pressure or diabetes?*
	• Investigate for specific problems in the past health history that would be a major oversight to miss:
	   o Current or past diseases: cancer, diabetes, psychosis, infections, immune disorders
	   o Hypertension or high cholesterol
	   o Medications, especially corticosteroids
	   o Surgeries, hospitalizations, trauma or previous injuries

Social history	• **Work**—*What do you do for work? Are you exposed to chemicals or fumes at your workplace?* • **Hobbies**—*What do you do for recreation or hobbies? Are you exposed to chemicals or fumes at home or with your hobbies (e.g., painting, gardening)?* • **Eat**—*Tell me about your breakfast, lunch, dinner, snacks… Do you consume foods or drinks that contain aspartame* (linked to increased incidence of brain tumors[69]) *or carrageenan* (possibly linked to increased risk of breast cancer and inflammatory bowel disease[70,71])? • **Exercise**—*What do you do for exercise or physical activity?* • **Drink**—*Do you* **drink alcohol**? *Coffee/caffeine? Water?* • **Drugs**—*Do you use recreational* **drugs**? **Now or in the past?** • **Smoke**—*Do you* **smoke**? *Have you ever smoked on a regular basis?* • **Sex**—*Are you* **sex***ually active? If so, do you practice safer sex practices?* For all women: *Is there any chance you could be pregnant right now? A "yes" reply may contraindicate radiographic assessment and the use of certain nutrients, botanicals, and/or drugs.* • **Emotional support, family contact, relationships**: The typical American has no-one in whom to confide and has a social network of two people[72]; in all; Americans are the most medicated/drugged and most socially isolated society that has ever existed.
Family health history	• *Does anyone in your family have any health problems, especially your parents and siblings?* • *Do you have any children? Do they have any health problems?* • *Do any diseases "run in the family" such as cancer, diabetes, arthritis, heart disease?*
Additional questions	• *Do you have any other information for me? Is there anything that I did not ask?* • *What is your opinion as to why you are having this health problem?* • *Are you in litigation for your illness or injuries?*

---

[69] "In the past two decades brain tumor rates have risen in several industrialized countries, including the United States... Compared to other environmental factors putatively linked to brain tumors, the artificial sweetener aspartame is a promising candidate to explain the recent increase in incidence and degree of malignancy of brain tumors." Olney JW, Farber NB, Spitznagel E, Robins LN. Increasing brain tumor rates: is there a link to aspartame? *J Neuropathol Exp Neurol* 1996 Nov;55(11):1115-23

[70] Tobacman JK. Review of harmful gastrointestinal effects of carrageenan in animal experiments. *Environ Health Perspect.* 2001 Oct;109(10):983-94

[71] "However, the gum carrageenan which is comprised of linked, sulfated galactose residues has potent biological activity and undergoes acid hydrolysis to poligeenan, an acknowledged carcinogen." Tobacman JK, Wallace RB, Zimmerman MB. Consumption of carrageenan and other water-soluble polymers used as food additives and incidence of mammary carcinoma. *Med Hypotheses.* 2001 May;56(5):589-98

[72] "Discussion networks are smaller in 2004 than in 1985. The number of people saying there is no one with whom they discuss important matters nearly tripled. The mean network size decreases by about a third (one confidant), from 2.94 in 1985 to 2.08 in 2004. The modal respondent now reports having no confidant; the modal respondent in 1985 had three confidants." McPherson M, Smith-Lovin L, Brashears ME. Social Isolation in America: Changes in Core Discussion Networks over Two Decades. *American Sociological Review* June 2006 71: 353-375

Physical Examination: Goals and purpose of the orthopedic/musculoskeletal examination:

1. To establish an accurate diagnosis (or diagnoses),
2. To assess the patient's **functional status** and current condition,
   a. Range of motion,
   b. Muscle strength,
   c. Ability to perform activities/actions of daily living such as standing, walking, climbing stairs, reaching for overhead objects, etc.
3. To assess for concomitant and/or underlying and preexisting problems,
4. To rule out emergency situations
- *Example*: If your patient presents with low back and leg pain, and you determine that his fall off a horse resulted in ischial bursitis, have you also excluded a lumbar compression fracture? You can send the patient home with anti-inflammatory treatments and icepacks for the bursitis; but if you missed the spinal fracture, your patient could suffer neurologic injury resultant from your "failure to diagnose." Don't assume that the patient has only one problem until you have proven with your history and examination that other likely problems do not exist.

Functional assessment: When working with patients with acute injuries and systemic diseases, take a wider view of the patient than simply diagnosing the problem.

- Will she be able to return to work?
- Will he be able to drive home safely?
- Will she need help with activities of daily living?
- Is there an occult disease, infection, malignancy, or toxic exposure that is causing these problems?
- Is this an acute presentation of a new problem, or an acute exacerbation of a chronic problem?

Neurologic examination: One of the most important areas to assess when a patient presents with a musculoskeletal complaint is the neurologic system, especially if the complaint is related to a recent traumatic injury. Blood circulation is essential for life; but lack of circulation is only a major consideration in a small number of injuries, and it is usually readily apparent when severe because the problem will become acute quickly. Nerve injuries, however, can be subtle. All patients with spine (neck, thoracic, low back) pain must be questioned thoroughly for evidence of neurologic compromise. Neurologic insults—such as cauda equina syndrome and transverse myelitis— can be painless, can progress rapidly, and can lead to permanent functional disability from muscle weakness or paralysis. Every patient with pain, weakness, or recent trauma must be evaluated for neurologic deficits before the patient is treated and released from care. Neurologic examinations are briefly reviewed in the pages that follow; citations can be used for sources of additional information.

Resources for students on neurologic assessment:

- Goldberg S. The Four-Minute Neurologic Exam. Medmaster http://www.medmaster.net/
- http://www.neuroexam.com/neuroexam/ Information and free videos of a neurologic exam.
- Excellent interactive simulation of assessment of extraocular muscles in a neurologic examination: http://rad.usuhs.mil/rad/eye_simulator/eyesimulator.html
- Excellent review, noteworthy for its description of a "+5" level of reflex grading denoting sustained clonus: http://emedicine.medscape.com/article/1147993-overview

Orthopedic Musculoskeletal Examination: Concepts and Goals

Orthopedic tests are detailed or reviewed in each respective chapter of *Integrative Orthopedics*[73] (i.e., shoulder exams are in the chapter on shoulders, knee exams in the chapter on knees). This section reviews the concepts and goals that provide the rationale for performing these tests. Orthopedic tests are designed to place particular types of stress on specific body tissues. Types of stress include tension/distraction, compression/pressure, shear force, vibration, friction, and percussion. Each type of stress is applied to elicit specific information about the exact tissue or structure that is being tested. *If you understand the reason for the type of stress that you are applying, and you are aware of the tissue/structure that you are testing, then you will find it much easier to perform the dozens of tests that are required in clinical practice. If you understand the "how" and the "why" then you won't be overwhelmed with named tests that otherwise appear illogical or superfluous.*

The tests that are described in *Integrative Orthopedics* meet at least one of the following two criteria: 1) it is a common test that all doctors know and which is needed for the sake of communication and for passing academic and licensing examinations, or 2) it is going to be a useful test in clinical practice.

Always remember that abnormalities found during the physical examination—particularly the neurologic examination—are often indicative of an underlying *nonmusculoskeletal* problem that must be identified or—at the very least—considered and then excluded by additional testing. For example, a patient shoulder pain and neurologic deficits found during the neuromusculoskeletal portion of your examination could have a herniated cervical disc as the underlying cause; but the cause could also be syringomyelia, or an apical lung tumor that is invading local bone and destroying the nerves of the brachial plexus.[74]

Types of stress applied during the physical examination for specific purposes

- **Tension, traction**: To provoke pain from injured/compromised tissues: tendons, muscles, ligaments, and nerves
- **Compression, pressure**: To provoke pain from inflamed tissues; also used to assess for swelling and fluid accumulation in subcutaneous tissue, bursa, and joint spaces such as the knee
- **Shearing force**: To test the integrity of ligaments and intervertebral discs
- **Vibration (using ultrasound or 128 Hz tuning fork)**: To assess vibration sense (neurologic: peripheral nerves and dorsal columns) and screen for broken bones (orthopedic)
- **Friction, grinding**: To elicit pain from injured tissues (cross-fiber friction) and articular surfaces (grinding tests)
- **Percussion, over bone and discs**: To assess for bone fractures, bone infections, and acute disc injuries
- **Percussion, over peripheral nerves**: To assess hypesthesia/tingling suggesting reduced threshold for depolarization secondary to nerve irritation or compression, i.e., Tinel's sign
- **Fulcrum tests**: To assess for bone fractures: commonly the doctor's arm or a firm object is placed centrally under the bone in question and increasingly firm downward stress is applied to both ends of the bone to test for occult fracture
- **Torque, twisting**: To test joint integrity (restriction or laxity) or for occult bone fracture (particularly of the digits)

As a clinician, the successful management and treatment of your patients depends in large part on the following: ❶ knowledge: your ability to conceptualize broadly and to consider many *functional* and *pathologic* causes of your patient's complaints, ❷ tact: the efficiency and accuracy with which you assess, accept, and exclude the various differential diagnoses into your final working diagnosis from which your treatment, management, referral, and co-management decisions are made, ❸ art: your ability to create the changes in your patient's outlook, lifestyle, biochemistry, biomechanics/anatomy, and physiology to effect the desired outcome.

---

[73] Vasquez A. Integrative Orthopedics: Concepts, Algorithms, and Therapeutics. www.InflammationMastery.com
[74] "Pancoast tumor has long been implicated as a cause of brachial plexopathy...The possibility of Pancoast lesion should be considered not only in the presence of brachial plexopathy, but also when C8 or T1 radiculopathy is found." Vargo MM, Flood KM. Pancoast tumor presenting as cervical radiculopathy. *Arch Phys Med Rehabil.* 1990 Jul;71(8):606-9

Neurologic Assessment

Clinical neurology is a complex area of study. However, for most doctors, knowledge of clinical neurology hinges on answering three questions:

- Is this patient's presentation normal or abnormal?
- If it is abnormal, does it indicate a specific disease or lesion?
- Does this condition require referral to a specialist or emergency care?

Every clinician needs thorough training in anatomy and clinical neurology to be competent in the management of patients, because even common problems such as "pain" and "fatigue" and "headache" may herald devastating neurologic illness that must be assessed accurately and managed skillfully. While a complete review of clinical neurology is beyond the scope of this text, the following section provides a basic review of the clinical essentials. Clinicians needing a refresher course in clinical neurology are encouraged to read the concise reviews by Goldberg.[75,76]

Reliable indicators of organic (real) neurologic disease:
These cannot be feigned and must be assumed to reveal organic neurologic illness that must be evaluated by a neurologist:
• Significant asymmetry of pupillary light reflex,
• Ocular divergence,
• Papilledema,
• Marked nystagmus,
• Muscle atrophy and fasciculation,
• Muscle weakness with neurologic deficit; upper motor neuron lesions (UMNL) indicate a central nervous system (CNS) lesion and need to be fully evaluated by a specialist; the need for referral is less necessary in cases of peripheral neuropathy of known cause.

Purpose of Neurologic Examination and *Principle of Neurologic Localization*:

The purpose of the neurologic examination is to qualify ("yes" or "no") the presence of a neurologic deficit, and—if present—to localize the lesion so that it can be further assessed with the proper laboratory, imaging, electrodiagnostic, or biopsy techniques. The following 9-point summary of localized lesions does not supplant independent studies of neurology and neuroanatomy but is useful for a quick clinically-relevant review:

1. **Cerebral cortex and internal capsule**: Neurologic deficit depends on location of lesion but is typically a combination of sensory/motor deficit and impaired higher neurologic function such as comprehension (superior temporal gyrus) or socially appropriate behavior (frontal lobe, ventral frontal gyri).
2. **Basal ganglia and striatal system**: Athetosis (lentiform nucleus: putamen and globus pallidus), (hemi)ballism (subthalamic nucleus), chorea (putamen), akinesia, bradykinesia, hypokinesia (lack of nigrostriatal dopamine).
3. **Cerebellum**: Ataxia, awkward clumsy execution of *intentional* motions; may have nystagmus, hypotonia.
4. **Brainstem**: Cranial nerve deficit(s) with contralateral distal sensory and/or UMN motor deficits.
5. **Spinal cord**: Cranial nerves and higher cortical functions are intact; lesion can be a combination of sensory and motor (UMN and LMN) deficits and the pattern distal to lesion may be a complete or incomplete pattern of sensory and motor deficits on one or both sides of body depending on area of spinal cord affected.
6. **Nerve root**: Segmental unilateral motor deficit; dermatomal distribution pain or sensory disturbance.
7. **Peripheral nerve**: Localized combination of sensory and motor deficits; may be bilateral or unilateral.
8. **Neuromuscular junction**: Painless weakness and "fatigable weakness": weakness that *worsens* with repeated testing; typically involves cranial nerves first in myasthenia gravis; also consider Lambert-Eaton Syndrome (LES: autoimmune neuromuscular junction disorder associated with occult malignancy; contrasts with myasthenia gravis in that in LES strength *increases* with repeated testing).
9. **Muscle disease**: Painless weakness, typically involving proximal hip/shoulder muscles first; test for elevated serum aldolase and (phospho)creatine kinase (aka, creatine phosphokinase, CK, CPK).

---

[75] Goldberg S. Clinical Neuroanatomy Made Ridiculously Simple. Miami, Medimaster, Inc, 1990. Now in a third edition with interactive CD.
[76] Goldberg S. The Four-Minute Neurologic Exam. Miami, Medimaster, Inc, 1992

Clinical assessments of neurologic function and structures

Cortex	Cerebellum
<ul><li>Orientation: Person, place, time, situation</li><li>Mood and cooperation: E.g., calm vs agitated, cooperative vs noncooperative.</li><li>Level of consciousness: Alert, lethargic, stupor, coma (indirect assessment of reticular system in brainstem)</li><li>Memory: Remember objects or numbers; *recent* memory is most commonly affected by brain lesions: *What day of the month is it? How did you get here?*</li><li>Mentation: *Count backward from 100 by 7's.*</li><li>Spelling: *Spell the word "hand" backwards.*</li><li>Stereognosis: Identify by touch a familiar object such as a key or coin.</li><li>Hoffman's reflex: Doctor rapidly extends distal joint of patient's middle finger and watches for patient's hand to perform grasp reflex; this test is performed for motor tract lesions involving the cerebral cortex, cerebellum, and upper motor neurons of the spinal cord.</li><li>Pronator drift: Supinated hands and arms outstretched forward for 30 seconds; doctor taps on palms; falling of hands and arms into pronation suggests UMNL.</li><li>Babinski reflex: Scraping the bottom of the foot results in splaying and flexing of the toes and extension (dorsiflexion) of the big toe; normal in infants.</li></ul>	<ul><li>Gait (lesion: ataxia)</li><li>Heel-to-toe walk</li><li>Tandem gait</li><li>Hand flip, foot tap (lesion: dysdiadochokinesia)</li><li>Finger-to-nose: Patient reaches out to doctor's finger, then patient touches patient nose, then back to new location of doctor's finger.</li><li>Heel-to-shin: Slide heel along shin.</li><li>Walk in circle around chair</li><li>Move eyes in a rapid "figure 8": Technique for provoking latent nystagmus</li><li>Rhomberg's test: Patient stands with feet close together and eyes closed; tests proprioception (peripheral nerves, dorsal columns, spinocerebellar tracts); vision (eyes open tests optic righting reflex) and coordinated motor activity (cerebellum).</li></ul>

Several of the above '"cerebral" deficits may also result from intoxicative, nutritional, or metabolic disorders rather than an organic irreversible physical lesion. Likewise "cerebellar" deficits may also result from lesion of the brainstem tracts/nuclei and cerebellar peduncles, rather than the cerebellum itself.

Brainstem and Cranial Nerves	Spinal Cord, Roots, Nerves
1. Olfactory: **smell**	Motor and reflex
• Smell: Test with strong and common odors such as coffee; do not use ammonia or other irritants which are perceived via trigeminal nerve (cranial nerve 5)	• Strength: Specific muscles are tested and rated 0-5
	• Plantar (Babinski) reflex: Signifies UMNL
• This is a worthwhile test in patients with recent head trauma (direct or indirect) such as from motor vehicle accidents (MVA); any violent motion of the head may result in injury to the olfactory fibers passing through the cribiform plate; patients may have associated anosmia or altered sense of flavor; frontal lobe disorders such as altered social behavior may be noted in lesioned patients	• Abdominal reflexes: "Present" or "absent" (not rated 0-4); superficial reflexes are lost (rather than hyperactive) with UMNL
	o Upper abdominal: T8-10
	o Lower abdominal: T10-12
	• Anal reflex: Cauda equina and sacral nerve roots
2. Ophthalmic: **reading, peripheral vision, fundoscopic**	• Reflexes: Rate 0-4; asymmetric reflexes are more significant than finding absent or hyperactive (+3) reflexes; +4 reflex with sustained clonus is almost always pathologic and requires neurologist referral. Deep tendon reflexes with main spinal root levels are as follows:
• Snellen chart for far vision, Rosenbaum card for near vision	
• Peripheral vision	
• Fundoscopic examination	
3. Oculomotor: **move eyes and constrict pupils**	o Biceps: C5
• Eye motion in cardinal fields of gaze	o Brachioradialis: C6
• Pupil contraction to light	o Triceps: C7
• Pupil contraction to accommodation	o Patellar: L3-L4
4. Trochlear: **motor to superior oblique**	o Hamstring: L5
• Look "down and in" toward nose	o Achilles: S1
5. Trigeminal: **bite, sensory to face and eyes**	Sensory
• Bite (motor to muscles of mastication)	• Light touch
• Feel (sensory to face, eyes, and tongue)	• Two-point discrimination
6. Abducens: **motor to lateral rectus**	• Vibration (use 128 Hz tuning fork)
• Looks laterally to the ear	• Joint position sense and proprioception (eyes closed, locate position of joint)
7. Facial: **face muscles and taste to anterior tongue**	• Sharp and dull
• Furrow forehead, close eyes forcefully, smile and frown	• Hot and cold
	• Sensory loss mapping (if deficits are found)
• Taste to anterior tongue	• Romberg (peripheral nerves, dorsal columns, vestibular, cerebellar)
8. Vestibulocochlear: **hearing and balance**	
• Hearing, Rinne-Weber tests[77]	• Nerve root tension tests such as straight leg raising
• Balance: observe gait and Romberg test	• **Subjective pain and discomfort can be indicated on pain diagrams and VAS (visual analog scale) as shown on the following page**
9. Glossopharyngeal: **swallowing, and gag reflex**	
• Swallow	
• Gag reflex (sensory component)	
10. Vagus: **motor to palate**	
• Say "ahh" to raise uvula	
• Gag reflex (motor component)	
11. Spinal accessory: **motor to SCM and trapezius**	
• Raise your shoulders (against resistance)	
• Turn your head (against resistance)	
12. Hypoglossal: **motor to tongue**	
• Stick out tongue to front	

---

[77] "The Rinne and Weber tuning fork tests are the most important tools in distinguishing between conductive and sensorineural hearing loss." Ruckenstein MJ. Hearing loss. A plan for individualized management. *Postgrad Med.* 1995 Oct;98(4):197-200, 203, 206

Deep tendon reflexes are summarized below and on the following page. Hyperreflexia is noted with upper motor neuron lesions (UMNL) in the cortex, subcortical nuclei, brainstem, or corticospinal tracts of the spinal cord, whereas hyporeflexia can result from lesions of lower motor neurons (LMNL) in spinal cord, peripheral nerves, as well as from sensory/afferent defects including diabetic neuropathy, vitamin B-12 deficiency, and Guillain-Barre disorder. Muscle strength should always be "five over five" to be considered normal, whereas in the testing of reflexes, symmetry/asymmetry is generally more important than the grade of response (except with sustained clonus). **Asymmetry of reflex or strength (especially when seen together) is never normal and requires clinical correlation and investigation.** Reflexes and strength are evaluated as follows in the following table.

Deep tendon reflexes	Muscle strength
+5 <u>Hyperreflexia with sustained clonus</u>: Sustained clonus strongly suggests UMNL and requires investigation; most textbooks use a 0-4 scale, yet this 0-5 scale facilitates clear communication of observed lesions.[78]	5/5 <u>Normal</u>: **Full strength: able to withstand gravity and full resistance.**
+4 <u>Marked hyperreflexia</u>: Up to 4 beats of unsustained clonus may be normal[79]; suggests UMNL but may be caused by medications, electrolyte disturbances, etc.	4/5 <u>Partial strength</u>: Able to withstand gravity and partial resistance.
+3 <u>Hyperreflexia</u>: More than normal.	3/5 <u>Partial strength</u>: Only able to resist gravity.
+2 <u>Normal</u>: Neither hyporeflexia nor hyperreflexia.	2/5 <u>Partial strength</u>: Able to contract muscle but unable to resist gravity.
+1 <u>Hyporeflexia</u>: Less than normal	1/5 <u>Slight flicker of muscle contraction</u>: Does not result in joint movement.
0 <u>No reflex</u>: Requires clinical correlation for lesion of sensory receptors, peripheral nerve, spinal cord, anterior horn, or neuromuscular junction; this is a common finding in normal individuals.	0/5 <u>No clinically detectable contraction</u>: Correlate with lesion of peripheral nerve, cord, cerebrum, anterior horn, or neuromuscular junction.

---

[78] Oommen K, edited by Berman SA, et al. Neurological History and Physical Examination. Last Updated: October 4, 2006. *eMedicine* emedicine.com/neuro/topic632.htm
[79] "…three to four beats of clonus can be elicited at the ankles in some normal individuals." Waxman SG. <u>Clinical Neuroanatomy 25th Edition</u>. McGraw Hill Medical, New York, 2003, p 325

Patients can be asked to <u>localize</u> and <u>describe</u> their pain/discomfort on drawings such as these. *Examples of descriptions*:

- Numb
- Hypersensitive
- Tingling

- Shooting pain
- Electrical pain
- Stabbing pain

- Burning pain
- Dull ache
- Muscle weakness

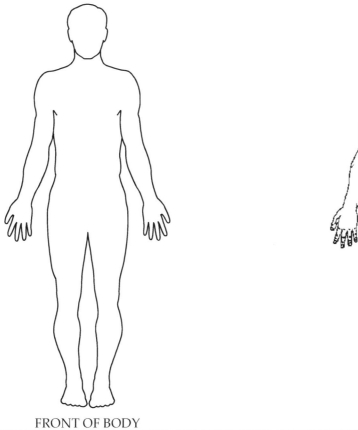 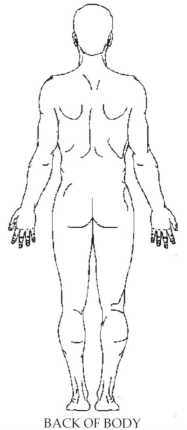

FRONT OF BODY   BACK OF BODY

On the lines below, indicate which pain/discomfort you are referring to and then quantify it by placing an "X" on the line.

Location of pain:_____

|——|

No pain at all   Worst pain imaginable

Location of pain:_____

|——|

No pain at all   Worst pain imaginable

Laboratory Assessments: General Considerations of Commonly Used Tests

"The laboratory evaluation of patients with rheumatic disease is often informative but rarely definitive."[80]

Laboratory tests are immensely important in evaluating patients with musculoskeletal pain, as these tests allow the clinician to 1) assess for infection (e.g., subacute osteomyelitis), 2) quantify the degree of inflammation (i.e., with CRP or ESR), 3) assess or exclude other disease processes that may be the cause of pain or dysfunction, and 4) assess for concomitant diseases (e.g., septic arthritis complicating rheumatoid arthritis). Additionally, 5) these tests open the door to more complete patient care and holistic management of the whole person because they allow for a more comprehensive and complete understanding of the patient's underlying physiology. **The recommended routine is to use the following panel of tests when assessing patients with musculoskeletal pain: 1) CBC, 2) CRP, 3) chemistry/metabolic panel, and preferably also 4) ferritin, 5) 25(OH)-vitamin D, and 6) thyroid assessment, minimally including TSH** and optimally including free T4, total T3, reverse T3 and anti-thyroid antibodies. The use of a screening evaluation on a routine basis helps identify patients with occult diseases and also allows for more comprehensive management of the patient's overall health. Other tests are indicated in specific situations. *Orthopedics* relies heavily upon physical examination and imaging, whereas *Rheumatology* relies more heavily upon laboratory analysis. In Orthopedics, laboratory tests are used mainly for the purposes of discovering or excluding rheumatic and systemic diseases. In Rheumatology, lab tests are used to specifically identify the type of illness, quantify the severity of the condition, and to assess for concomitant illnesses and complications.

Essential Tests: These Tests are Required for Basic Patient Assessment

Test	Purpose	Clinical application
CRP (or ESR)	Screening for infection, inflammation, and possibly cancer; if inflammation is present, then these tests allow for a generalized quantification of severity.	Useful in all new patients for helping to differentiate systemic/inflammatory disorders from those which are noninflammatory and mechanical. Also very helpful as a general "barometer" of health since higher values correlate with increased risk for diabetes mellitus and cardiovascular disease; thus this test helps bridge the gap between acute care and wellness promotion.
CBC	Screening for anemia, infection, certain cancers (namely leukemia).	Useful in any patient with nontraumatic musculoskeletal pain or systemic manifestations, especially fever or weight loss; occasionally detects occult B-12 and folate deficiencies.
Chemistry panel	Screening for diabetes, liver disease, kidney failure, bone lesions (alkaline phosphatase), electrolyte disturbances, adrenal insufficiency (hyponatremia with hyperkalemia), hyperparathyroidism, and hypercalcemia.	Use this panel in any patient with nontraumatic musculoskeletal pain or systemic manifestations; all patients with hypertension, diabetes, or who use medications that cause hepatotoxicity, nephrotoxicity, etc.
Thyroid assessments	Hypothyroidism is a common problem and is an often overlooked cause of musculoskeletal pain.[81]	This is a reasonable test panel for any patient with fatigue, cold extremities, depression, "arthritis", muscle pain, hypercholesterolemia, or other manifestations of hypothyroidism.

---

[80] Klippel JH (ed). Primer on the Rheumatic Diseases. 11th Edition. Atlanta: Arthritis Foundation. 1997 page 94
[81] "Hypothyroidism is frequently accompanied by musculoskeletal manifestations ranging from myalgias and arthralgias to true myopathy and arthritis." McLean RM, Podell DN. Bone and joint manifestations of hypothyroidism. *Semin Arthritis Rheum*. 1995 Feb;24(4):282-90

Overview of Important Tests: Additional Components of Routine Evaluation

Test	Purpose	Clinical Application
Ferritin	Important for assessing for iron overload (e.g., hemochromatoic polyarthropathy), and iron deficiency (e.g., low back pain due to colon cancer metastasis). Ferritin values less than 20 in adults (e.g., iron deficiency) or greater than 200 in women and 300 in men (e.g., iron overload) necessitate evaluation and effective treatment.	*Ferritin is the ideal test for both iron overload and iron deficiency.* All patients should be screened for hemochromatosis and other hereditary forms of iron overload regardless of age, gender, or ethnicity.[82] Iron deficiency—particularly in adults—may be the first clue to gastric/colon cancer and generally necessitates referral to gastroenterologist.
Serum 25-hydroxy-vitamin D, 25(OH)D	Vitamin D deficiency is a common cause of musculoskeletal pain and inflammation[83,84], and vitamin D deficiency is a significant risk factor for cancer and other serious health problems.[85,86,87]	Measurement of serum 25(OH) vitamin D (or empiric treatment with 2,000 – 4,000 IU vitamin D3 per day for adults) is indicated in patients with chronic musculoskeletal pain.[88,89] Optimal vitamin D status correlates with serum 25(OH)D levels of 50 – 100 ng/mL.[90]
Antinuclear antibodies (ANA)	Sensitive (but not specific) for the detection of several autoimmune diseases, especially systemic lupus erythematosus (SLE).	This test is particularly valuable for assessing patients with polyarthropathy, facial rash, and/or fatigue.
Rheumatoid factor (RF)	The primary value of this test is in supporting a diagnosis of rheumatoid arthritis; specificity is low.	RF may be positive in normal health, iron overload, chronic infections, hepatitis, sarcoidosis, and bacterial endocarditis.
Cyclic citrullinated protein (CCP) antibodies	Cyclic citrullinated protein (CCP) antibodies are currently the single best laboratory test for rheumatoid arthritis (RA) and have largely replaced RF.	Citrullinated protein antibodies are rapidly becoming *the* test for diagnosing and confirming RA; used with RF for highly specific "conjugate seropositivity."
Lactulose-mannitol assay	Assesses for malabsorption and excess intestinal permeability—"leaky gut."	Diagnostic test for intestinal damage; excellent nonspecific screening test for pathology or pathophysiology such as celiac and Crohn's disease.
Comprehensive parasitology, stool analysis	Identification and quantification of intestinal yeast, bacteria, and other microbes.	Extremely valuable test when working with patients with chronic fatigue syndromes, fibromyalgia, or autoimmunity; see chapter 4 of *Integrative Rheumatology.*

[82] Vasquez A. Musculoskeletal disorders and iron overload disease: comment on the American College of Rheumatology guidelines for the initial evaluation of the adult patient with acute musculoskeletal symptoms. *Arthritis Rheum* 1996;39: 1767-8   http://InflammationMastery.com/hemochromatosis.html

[83] Masood H, Narang AP, Bhat IA, Shah GN. Persistent limb pain and raised serum alkaline phosphatase the earliest markers of subclinical hypovitaminosis D in Kashmir. *Indian J Physiol Pharmacol.* 1989 Oct-Dec;33(4):259-61

[84] Al Faraj S, Al Mutairi K. Vitamin D deficiency and chronic low back pain in Saudi Arabia. *Spine.* 2003 Jan 15;28(2):177-9

[85] Grant WB. An estimate of premature cancer mortality in the U.S. due to inadequate doses of solar ultraviolet-B radiation. *Cancer.* 2002;94(6):1867-75

[86] Zittermannn A. Vitamin D in preventive medicine: are we ignoring the evidence? *Br J Nutr.* 2003 May;89(5):552-72

[87] Holick MF. Vitamin D: importance in the prevention of cancers, type 1 diabetes, heart disease, and osteoporosis. *Am J Clin Nutr.* 2004;79(3):362-71

[88] Plotnikoff GA, Quigley JM. Prevalence of severe hypovitaminosis D in patients with persistent, nonspecific musculoskeletal pain. *Mayo Clin Proc.* 2003 Dec;78(12):1463-70

[89] Al Faraj S, Al Mutairi K. Vitamin D deficiency and chronic low back pain in Saudi Arabia. *Spine.* 2003 Jan 15;28(2):177-9

[90] Vasquez A, Manso G, Cannell J. The Clinical Importance of Vitamin D (Cholecalciferol): A Paradigm Shift with Implications for All Healthcare Providers. *Alternative Therapies in Health and Medicine* 2004;10:28-37 and *Integrative Medicine* 2004;3:44-54 http://InflammationMastery.com/cholecalciferol.html

Chemistry/metabolic panel	
Overview and interpretation:	▪ Accurate interpretation requires knowledge and pattern-recognition by the doctor to translate numbers into differential diagnoses that are correlated with the clinical presentation, examination, and imaging findings to arrive at probable diagnoses. ▪ Variation exists in the components and ranges offered by different laboratories.
Advantages:	▪ Inexpensive and easy to perform—venipuncture + serum separator tube. ▪ Provides a quick screen for diabetes, hepatitis, renal insufficiency, suggestions of alcohol abuse, hyperparathyroidism, electrolyte imbalances, etc.

Limitation and considerations:	▪ Individual tests and the most common clinical considerations for low and high values are listed in the following section. These values and considerations are provided with the routine adult outpatient in mind and are not inclusive of every possible differential diagnosis and therapeutic consideration. Consult your laboratory texts and reference manuals as needed per patient.
	▪ Abnormal laboratory results are always due to one of four problems:
	    1. <u>Technical error</u>: Error with the laboratory analysis, improper patient identification correlating with the sample, alteration of the sample before delivery to the laboratory (e.g., too much time, too much heat, lysis of cells). Given the importance of laboratory accuracy and the life-and-death decisions that are based upon such reports, this type of error is inexcusable, however, it does occur, occasionally producing results that defy physiologic possibility or which contradict the clinical picture. Repeating the test is appropriate. *Example*: Hypercalcemia (elevated serum calcium) may be reported in error by the laboratory due to problems with the analyzing machinery.
	    2. <u>Drug effect</u>: An otherwise healthy patient may develop a laboratory abnormality due to a drug effect. *Example*: Hypercalcemia can be secondary to the effect of a calcium-sparing diuretic, such as hydrochlorothiazide (HCTZ).
	    3. <u>Pathology</u>: The patient has a diagnosable disease causing the laboratory abnormality. *Example*: Hypercalcemia can be secondary to a parathyroid adenoma which secretes abnormally high amounts of parathyroid hormone; hypercalcemia can also be a presentation of malignancy such as breast cancer or prostate cancer, or from a granulomatous disease such as sarcoidosis.
	    4. <u>Physiologic abnormality</u>: The patient has a physiologic abnormality causing the laboratory abnormality. *Example*: Hypercalcemia can be secondary to excess intake of vitamin D. In practice, hypercalcemia from hypervitaminosis D is very rare because vitamin D has a wide safety margin; but for the sake of this discussion, vitamin D toxicity will be listed as a possible cause of hypercalcemia.

Comments:	▪ All abnormalities require follow-up—repeat test within 2-4 weeks as part of routine follow-up along with additional investigation and clinical re-assessment. Extraordinary abnormalities and those with life-threatening implications should of course be retested immediately; often, the laboratory will hold the blood sample for 7 days and the repeat analysis can be performed on the same blood sample to exclude technical error. ▪ Many ill patients (such as those with chronic fatigue syndrome, fibromyalgia, etc) will have normal results with the metabolic panel and other basic routine laboratory assessments. Therefore, normal results do not ensure that the patient is healthy nor without life-threatening illness. ▪ Generally, laboratory tests are performed in the morning under fasting conditions; such is the standard but is not necessarily required depending on the nature of the test, convenience, and the clinical situation.

Practical overview of common abnormalities on the chemistry/metabolic panel

Low values—considerations	*Analyte*[91]	*High values*—considerations
Technical error due to faulty processing of sample (i.e., hemolysis); insulinoma, exogenous insulin administration (test serum C-peptide), overdose of anti-hyperglycemic drugs, hypopituitarism and adrenal insufficiency.	**Glucose**: 65-99 mg/dL *Clinical pearl*: *Fasting glucose levels can miss mild type-2 diabetes mellitus; a better test for long-term glucose status is hemoglobin A1c.*	Postprandial sample, diabetes mellitus type-1 or type-2, Cushing disease or syndrome, acromegaly, pheochromocytoma, glucagonoma, hyperthyroidism. Fasting glucose >126 mg/dL on two or more occasions is consistent with the diagnosis of diabetes mellitus, as is the finding of nonfasting glucose >200 mg/dL on any one occasion. If glucose is >300 mg/dL and patient is unstable (e.g., tachypnic or stuporous), evaluate for diabetic ketoacidosis or hyperosmolar state. Optimal fasting serum glucose is in the range of 70-75 up to 85 mg/dL, since levels >85 mg/dL have been associated with increased mortality.
Hyponatremia[92,93] is potentially fatal and is also a cause of permanent neurologic injury (e.g., pontine myelinolysis). Clinicians should be particularly concerned when the sodium level drops below 125 mmol/L. Symptomatic hyponatremia is worthy of treatment in hospital setting; mild cases due to a recent event such as excess diaphoresis (e.g., prolonged sweating and exercise) or excess fluid intake (e.g., beer potomania [i.e., binge drinking], overhydration with unmineralized water) might be managed with sodium replacement and water restriction. Adrenal insufficiency classically presents with fatigue, hypotension, and hyponatremia with hyperkalemia; ACTH challenge test is the most sensitive and specific laboratory assessment. Older patients, patients with pulmonary disease, and patients taking certain drugs such as serotonin-reuptake inhibitors may develop a chronic and relatively benign mild hyponatremia associated with "reset osmostat syndrome." Sodium levels can be altered downward by conditions that introduce osmotically active substances into the serum, such as immunoglobulins (e.g., multiple myeloma), hyperglycemia, and hypertriglyceridemia; corrective equations are available for such situations.	**Sodium**: 136 to 144 mEq/L (mmol/L)	Hypernatremia in outpatients is rare; assess for drug effect and dehydration with hemoconcentration. Some clinicians will determine the free water deficit, while others will treat with oral or IV hydration with plain water or half-normal saline, respectively. Electrolyte abnormalities—particularly involving sodium—should generally be corrected slowly and with close supervision.

---

[91] The reference range for this table and some provisional information was derived from Medline Plus provided by the U.S. Department of Health and Human Services and National Institutes of Health. http://www.nlm.nih.gov/medlineplus/ency/article/003468.htm Accessed June 28, 2011. However, the majority of the information in this table comes from the author's (Dr Vasquez's) clinical training and experience. Editorial and peer reviews were provided by colleagues Barry Morgan MD, William J Beakey DOM, et al.

[92] Goh KP. Management of hyponatremia. *Am Fam Physician*. 2004;69:2387-94 http://www.aafp.org/afp/2004/0515/p2387.html Accessed June 2011.

[93] Decaux G, Musch W. Clinical laboratory evaluation of the syndrome of inappropriate secretion of antidiuretic hormone. *Clin J Am Soc Nephrol*. 2008 Jul;3(4):1175-84 http://cjasn.asnjournals.org/content/3/4/1175.full.pdf Accessed June 29, 2011.

Practical overview of common abnormalities on the chemistry/metabolic panel—*continued*

Low values—considerations	Analyte	High values—considerations
Hypokalemia can cause fatal cardiac arrhythmias and needs to be taken seriously. Replacement is generally via oral administration of potassium-rich foods, juices, or supplements such as potassium citrate (best option) or potassium chloride (KCl, inexpensive and therefore commonly used in medical settings even though KCl is clearly not optimal therapy due to the acidifying effect of the chloride anion). Recalcitrant hypokalemia is often a sign of magnesium depletion.[94] Causes of hypokalemia include diarrhea, vomiting, diuretics, Cushing disease/syndrome, dietary insufficiency, overhydration with mineral-free fluids, hyperaldosteronism and renal artery stenosis. Acute metabolic acidosis should cause relative or absolute elevations in serum K; the finding of normal or low serum K in a patient with acidosis (e.g., diabetic ketoacidosis) indicates (severe) potassium depletion.	**Potassium**: 3.6 to 5.2 mEq/L (mmol/L)	**Hyperkalemia is defined as a potassium level greater than 5.5 mmol/L. Severe hyperkalemia (>7 mmol/L) can be fatal and needs to be taken seriously.** In severe hyperkalemia, treatment and emergency management should be implemented before a complete evaluation and differential diagnosis are performed.[95] ❶ Ensure that blood sample was not hemolyzed. Repeat test if patient is stable and time allows. ❷ If hyperkalemia is severe or patient is symptomatic or has electrocardiographic changes, treat hyperkalemia with intravenous calcium, beta-adrenergic agonists (e.g., albuterol), bicarbonate, insulin and glucose; magnesium sulfate may also help alleviate arrhythmias; oral sodium polystyrene sulfonate (SPS, also known as Kayexalate) is a frequently used potassium-binding agent. ❸ DDX includes adrenal insufficiency, potassium-sparing diuretics, ACE-inhibitors and ARBs, NSAIDs, rhabdomyolysis, renal failure, and massive cell necrosis such as with tumor lysis syndrome.
Evaluate hypocalcemia clinically with Chvostek's sign (~30% sensitive) and Trousseau sign (~90% sensitive) which may also be present in hypomagnesemia; evaluate clinically for arrhythmia, muscle spasm/hypertonicity, and hyperreflexia. Measure serum albumin and perform equation for "corrected calcium" if albumin is low. DDX includes renal failure, hypoparathyroidism, malabsorption, and drug effect (e.g., rarely a loop diuretic such as furosemide). Chronic mild hypocalcemia is treated with oral vitamin D and calcium supplementation; subacute symptomatic hypocalcemia can be treated with intravenous calcium gluconate especially if cardiac arrhythmias are present.	**Calcium**: 8.6 to 10.2 mg/dL	Outpatient hypercalcemia is potentially serious and needs to be evaluated in a stepwise manner: ❶ repeat the test to rule out lab error unless you are confident in the performance of the laboratory and stability of the submitted sample, ❷ review drug list for adverse effect, such as from hydrochlorothiazide (HCTZ) or rarely from excess cholecalciferol intake, ❸ test intact parathyroid hormone (iPTH) to evaluate for hyperparathyroidism, ❹ evaluate for possible granulomatous disease such as sarcoidosis, tuberculosis, Crohn's disease, and possible leukemia or lymphoma, ❺ consider metabolic bone disease such as Paget disease of bone or metastatic bone disease, ❻ evaluate for cancer, ❼ test urine calcium for familial hypocalciuric hypercalcemia, ❽ refer to specialist such as internist or endocrinologist if hypercalcemia persists and answer is not forthcoming.

Corrected calcium (cCa) equations: Used when both serum calcium and albumin are low
American units: cCa (mg/dL) = serum Ca (mg/dL) + 0.8 (4.0 - serum albumin [g/dL])
International units: cCa (mmol/L) = measured total Ca (mmol/L) + 0.02 (40 - serum albumin [g/L])

---

[94] "Herein is reviewed literature suggesting that magnesium deficiency exacerbates potassium wasting by increasing distal potassium secretion." Huang CL, Kuo E. Mechanism of hypokalemia in magnesium deficiency. *J Am Soc Nephrol*. 2007;18:2649-52 jasn.asnjournals.org/content/18/10/2649

[95] "If the hyperkalemia is severe (potassium >7.0 mEq/L) or if the patient is symptomatic, begin treatment before diagnostic investigation of the underlying cause." Garth D. Hyperkalemia in emergency medicine treatment and management. *Medscape Reference* http://emedicine.medscape.com/article/766479-treatment#a1126 Accessed June 2011

Practical overview of common abnormalities on the chemistry/metabolic panel—*continued*

Low values—considerations	Analyte	High values—considerations
Clinically meaningful hypochloremia is rare among outpatients. Hypochloremic metabolic alkalosis is commonly seen after persistent vomiting. Consider syndrome of inappropriate diuretic hormone (SIADH) secretion, cardiopulmonary disease, and adrenal insufficiency.	**Chloride:** 97 to 111 mmol/L	Hyperchloremia in outpatients is rare; assess for drug effect and dehydration with hemoconcentration; assess for acid-base disturbance, especially acidosis.
Reduced CO_2 correlates with hyperventilation; consider acid-base disturbance, salicylate overdose, asthma. Slight decrements in healthy outpatients are probably due to anxious hyperventilation at time of venipuncture.	**CO_2 (carbon dioxide):** 20 - 30 mmol/L	Elevated CO_2 can suggest cardiopulmonary compromise and/or acid-base disturbance; assess clinically. Slight elevations in otherwise healthy outpatients are probably due to breath-holding at time of venipuncture.
Reduced total protein with normal albumin suggests hypogammaglobulinemia; evaluate for nephrotic syndrome, liver disease, protein deficiency and malabsorption/enteropathy, immunosuppressive syndromes and consider intravenous gammaglobulin therapy.	**Total protein (albumin + globulins):** 6.3 - 8.0 g/dL	Elevated total protein with normal albumin suggests hypergammaglobulinemia, such as due to infection or plasma cell dyscrasia (e.g., multiple myeloma and Waldenstrom's disease). Evaluate within the clinical context; order serum protein electrophoresis if cause remains elusive, especially if patient has immune complex disease, neuropathy, or nephropathy.
Assess for liver disease, nephrotic syndrome, protein deficiency, malabsorption (consider celiac disease).	**Albumin:** 3.9 - 5.0 g/dL	Assess for dehydration/hemoconcentration.
Loss of hepatic mass due to cirrhosis, possible pyridoxine deficiency.	**ALT (alanine aminotransferase):** 10 - 40 IU/L	Hepatocellular liver injury due to chemical toxicity, viral hepatitis, hemochromatosis, metastatic or infectious disease, muscle injury. ALT is preferentially elevated over AST in viral hepatitis.
Loss of hepatic mass due to cirrhosis, possible pyridoxine deficiency.	**AST (aspartate aminotransferase):** 10 - 40 IU/L	Hepatocellular liver injury due to chemical toxicity, viral hepatitis, hemochromatosis, metastatic or infectious liver disease, myocardial infarct, muscle injury. AST is preferentially elevated over ALT in alcoholic hepatitis and rhabdomyolysis.
Consider zinc deficiency, malnutrition.	**Alkaline phosphatase (abbreviated as ALK PHOS or ALP):** 44 - 147 IU/L	Metabolic bone disease, metastatic bone disease, vitamin D deficiency, congestive liver disease. Test isoenzymes to differentiate bone versus hepatic origin if cause of elevation remains unclear.

Practical overview of common abnormalities on the chemistry/metabolic panel — *continued*

Low values—considerations	Analyte	High values—considerations
GGT levels are reduced in hypothyroidism, likely as a reflection of total reduction in protein synthesis. Oral contraceptive agents and clofibrate may also reduce levels. **GGT as a possible marker of oxidative stress and xenobiotic exposure** "It is possible that recently reported associations between serum GGT and various health outcomes may be explained by increases in serum GGT due to the exposure to various environmental pollutants." Lim et al. *Clin Chem* 2007 Jun	**GGT (Gamma-glutamyl transpeptidase):** 0 to 51 IU/L Discussion of HgbA1c and serum insulin is discussed in the chapters and presentations on diabetes, hypertension, and metabolic syndrome.	Because the GGT enzyme is highly represented in cells of the hepatobiliary tract, it is especially elevated in disorders of this region, especially obstructive jaundice, intrahepatic cholestasis, cholestasis of pregnancy, pancreatitis, liver metastases, alcohol/toxin/drug-induced liver disease, infectious mononucleosis, congestive heart failure, primary biliary cirrhosis, or biliary atresia. Clinicians should search for—when assessing a patient with possible/confirmed hepatobiliary obstruction—a triad of elevated GGT, ALP, and (conjugated) bilirubin. Combined elevations of GGT reflecting hepatic congestion and of MCV suggesting folate-cobalamin deficiency and/or bone marrow toxicity may suggest alcohol abuse. Milder elevations of GGT may be seen with systemic lupus erythematosus (SLE) or hyperthyroidism. GGT is considered the most sensitive laboratory marker for hepatobiliary obstruction; leucine aminopeptidase (LAP) or 5' nucleotidase are additional/confirmatory tests. Unlike ALP which can be elevated in disorders of either liver or bone (thus possibly contributing to a diagnostic dilemma), GGT has no origin in bone. The correlation between elevated GGT and insulin resistance / diabetes mellitus type-2 / metabolic syndrome[96] may be mediated via increased activity of the glutathione and detoxification systems[97] appropriately upregulated in response to the increased body burden of persistent organic pollutants.[98]
Low values are rare but might be noted with severe chronic anemia.	**Total bilirubin:** 0.2 to 1.5 mg/dL Direct (conjugated) bilirubin: 0 to 0.3 mg/dL Indirect (unconjugated) bilirubin: Determined by subtracting the *direct* from the *total* bilirubin.	Indirect/unconjugated bilirubin is elevated with hemolysis (e.g., hemolytic anemia) and impaired enzymatic conjugation (e.g., Gilbert's syndrome) or both (e.g., neonates). Direct/conjugated bilirubin has been enzymatically conjugated with glucuronic acid but is blocked from hepatobiliary excretion; consider performing liver and gall bladder sonogram (or CT or MRI) to evaluate for causes of biliary obstruction in addition to a careful abdominal exam. In patients with advanced liver disease, perform the Model for End-Stage Liver Disease (MELD) score and/or the MELD-Na score to predict 3-month mortality.[99] Fluoridated water inhibits glucuronidation in some patients with Gilbert's syndrome; biochemical improvement follows avoidance of fluoridated water.[100]

[96] Grundy SM. Gamma-glutamyl transferase: another biomarker for metabolic syndrome and cardiovascular risk. *Arterioscler Thromb Vasc Biol.* 2007 Jan;27(1):4-7
[97] McLennan SV et al .Changes in hepatic glutathione metabolism in diabetes. *Diabetes.* 1991 Mar;40(3):344-8
[98] Lim et al. A strong interaction between serum gamma-glutamyltransferase and obesity on the risk of prevalent type 2 diabetes. *Clin Chem* 2007;53:1092-8
[99] MELD calculations are best performed electronically, such as with http://www.mayoclinic.org/meld/mayomodel8.html or other medical calculator.
[100] Lee J. Gilbert's disease and fluoride intake. *Fluoride* 1983; 16: 139-45

Practical overview of common abnormalities on the chemistry/metabolic panel—*continued*

Low values—considerations	Analyte	High values—considerations
Liver disease, nephrotic syndrome, protein deficiency and malabsorption.	**BUN (blood urea nitrogen)**: 7 to 20 mg/dL	Consider renal underperfusion (e.g., due to heart failure, GI bleeding, renal artery stenosis, and dehydration), intrinsic renal failure, post-renal urinary tract obstruction. When renal disease is initially considered, order a urinalysis with microscopic analysis—see following section on urinalysis (UA).

BUN-to-creatinine ratio (normal = ~10)
>10-20: Renal underperfusion, post-renal obstruction
≤10: Suggests intrinsic renal disease

Low values—considerations	Analyte	High values—considerations
Sarcopenia (insufficient muscle mass), protein deficiency and malabsorption.	**Creatinine**: 0.8 to 1.3 mg/dL	Excess dietary protein, creatine supplementation, renal hypoperfusion; the most important consideration is intrinsic renal failure. Creatinine production (from arginine and creatine) is proportional to muscle mass. A rise in creatinine does not become evident until renal function (measured by glomerular filtration rate [GFR]) has fallen by approximately 50%. Creatinine levels indicative of impaired renal function to such an extent that modifications in diet, medications, and co-management become relevant are 1.4 mg/dL in women and 1.5 mg/dL in men. In the evaluation of renal function, the patient's age is a crucial determinant of how the serum creatinine is interpreted for the estimation of renal function (via GFR—see the Cockcroft-Gault equation). Cystatin C is more sensitive than are singular or conjugate interpretations of BUN and creatinine. If drug-induced nephritis is suspected, test urine eosinophils.

Methods for estimating creatinine clearance, glomerular filtration rate (GFR)

1. Modification of Diet in Renal Disease (MDRD) equation*,
2. 24-hour urine creatinine measurement,
3. Serum cystatin-C measurement,
4. Cockcroft-Gault equation (below):

$$GFR = \frac{(140 - \text{age years}) \times \text{wt kg} \times (0.85 \text{ if female})}{72 \times \text{serum creatinine in mg/dL}}$$

Clinical pearls for managing the chronic kidney disease (CKD) patient with declining renal function:

- When the GFR ≤ 60 (CKD stage 3): Modify dosages or withdraw certain drugs. Treat the causative problem and/or begin specialist co-management.
- When the GFR ≤ 30 (CKD stage 4): The patient needs to consult a nephrologist.
- When the GFR ≤ 15 (CKD stage 5): The patient needs a transplant or dialysis.

*National Institute of Diabetes and Digestive and Kidney Diseases (NIDDK). GFR MDRD Calculator for Adults (Conventional units). Accessed June 2011 nkdep.nih.gov/professionals/gfr_calculators/idms_con.htm

Cystatin C	

Overview and interpretation:	• Cystatin C is gaining acceptance as studies confirm and define its usefulness, especially as an early, sensitive marker for chronic kidney disease. Concentrations of cystatin C are not affected by gender, age, or race, and cystatin C is not affected by most drugs (prednisone increases; cyclosporine decreases), infections, diet, or inflammation.[101]
	• Produced at a constant rate by all nucleated cells.
	• Freely filtered by the glomerulus.
	• Elevated in: renal disorders.
	   o Cystatin C rises more rapidly than creatinine (Cr) in early renal impairment.
	   o Good predictor of the severity of ATN (acute tubular necrosis).
	   o The cystatin C concentration is an independent risk factor for heart failure, mortality, CVD and non-CVD outcomes in older adults and appears to provide a better measure of risk assessment than the serum Cr concentration.

Advantages:	• More accurate assessment of renal function than creatinine-based assessments. • Can be used to accurately assess renal function when creatinine-based assessments suggest impending renal impairment inconsistent with clinical presentation.
Limitations:	• Cost is approximately US $80. • False "non-renal" elevations may occur with cancer and/or rheumatic disease.

Presentation: 40yo male presenting for follow-up on abnormal renal function assessment—use of cystatin C to confirm normal kidney function: This apperantly healthy and athletic 40yo man displays consistently elevated creatinine and an estimated glomerular filtration rate (eGFR) that is close enough at 62 to warrant concern. Clinicians must appreciate that eGFR <60 is consistent with stage 3 chronic kidney disease (CKD) which warrants monitoring and which often necessitates changes in drug dosing (e.g., to avoid metformin-induced lactic acidosis) and diet (e.g., to avoid hyperkalemia).

Date and Time Collected	Date Entered	Date and Time Reported	Physician Name	NPI	Physician ID
12/07/11 11:10	12/08/11	12/13/11 04:07ET	VASQUEZ , A		

Tests Ordered
Comp. Metabolic Panel (14); FSH+TestT+LH+DHEA S+Prog+E2...; Chlamydia pneumoniae(IgG/M); Venipuncture

TESTS	RESULT	FLAG	UNITS	REFERENCE INTERVAL	LAB
Comp. Metabolic Panel (14)					
Glucose, Serum	89		mg/dL	65 – 99	01
BUN	18		mg/dL	6 – 24	01
Creatinine, Serum	**1.41**	**High**	mg/dL	0.76 – 1.27	01
eGFR If NonAfricn Am	62		mL/min/1.73	>59	
eGFR If Africn Am	72		mL/min/1.73	>59	
Note: A persistent eGFR <60 mL/min/1.73 m2 (3 months or more) may indicate chronic kidney disease. An eGFR >59 mL/min/1.73 m2 with an elevated urine protein also may indicate chronic kidney disease. Calculated using CKD-EPI formula.					
BUN/Creatinine Ratio	13			9 – 20	

In this situation, cystatin C was performed and confirmed normal renal function despite persistently elevated creatinine, which is probably attributable to this patient's athleticism and muscle mass.[102]

Date and Time Collected	Date Entered	Date and Time Reported	Physician Name	NPI	Physician ID
12/07/11 11:10	12/12/11	12/15/11 07:14ET	VASQUEZ , A		

Tests Ordered
Cystatin C; Written Authorization

TESTS	RESULT	FLAG	UNITS	REFERENCE INTERVAL	LAB
Cystatin C	0.71		mg/L	0.53 – 0.95	01

[101] http://labtestsonline.org/understanding/analytes/cystatin-c/tab/test Accessed April 2012
[102] Thank you, Bill Beakey DOM of Professional Co-op Services, Inc. professionalco-op.com for provision of these laboratory services.

Presentation: 69yo asymptomatic female presenting for routine health assessment found to have life-threatening hyperkalemia: Review the following labs and outline your treatment plan before reading the discussion below.

PATIENT NAME	PATIENT ID	ROOM NUMBER	AGE	SEX	PHYSICIAN
			69 Y 1941	F	*Vasquez*

REQUISITION NO	ACCESSION NO	ID.NO.	COLLECTION DATE & TIME	LOG-IN-DATE	REPORT DATE & TIME
			09/22/10 08:00 AM	09/22/10 06:37 PM	09/23/10 03:36AM

NOTES:
PT FASTING

TEST	RESULTS OUT OF RANGE	RESULTS WITHIN RANGE	UNITS	EXPECTED RANGE	LAB
BASIC METABOLIC PROFILE					
GLUCOSE		98	MG/DL	65-100	
BUN		19	MG/DL	8-25	
CREATININE		1.2	MG/DL	0.6-1.3	
EGFR AFRICAN AMER.	54		ML/MIN/1.73	>60	
EGFR NON-AFRICAN AMER.	45		ML/MIN/1.73	>60	
SODIUM		136	MEQ/L	133-146	
POTASSIUM	8.5		MEQ/L	3.5-5.3	

RESULTS RECHECKED AND VERIFIED
NOTE: NO VISIBLE HEMOLYSIS OBSERVED.

TEST	OUT OF RANGE	WITHIN RANGE	UNITS	EXPECTED RANGE	
CHLORIDE		100	MEQ/L	97-110	
CARBON DIOXIDE		27	MEQ/L	18-30	
CALCIUM		10.0	MG/DL	8.5-10.5	
LIPID PANEL					
CHOLESTEROL		193	MG/DL	<200	
TRIGLYCERIDES		129	MG/DL	<150	
HDL CHOLESTEROL		52	MG/DL	>39	
CALCULATED LDL CHOL	115		MG/DL	<100	
RISK RATIO LDL/HDL		2.22	RATIO	<3.22	
HEMOGLOBIN A1C	7.0		%	4.0-5.6	

AMERICAN DIABETES ASSOCIATION GUIDELINES FOR HGB A1C:
GLYCEMIC GOAL IN DIABETES . . . . . . <7.0%
DIAGNOSIS OF DIABETES . . . . >/=6.5%
CONFIRMED ON REPEAT ANALYSIS OR
WITH APPROPRIATE SYMPTOMS.
INCREASED RISK FOR DIABETES 5.7-6.4%

| TSH | 10.6 | | UIU/ML | 0.3-5.1 | |

PERFORMING LAB(S) LEGEND:

> **Chemistry/metabolic panels should be performed on all new patients prior to the initiation of treatment and periodically on all established patients to monitor for disease emergence, disease progression, and response to treatment**
>
> Treating this diabetic patient with a potassium-rich diet emphasizing low-carbohydrate fruits and vegetables would exacerbate her already life-threatening hyperkalemia. Note also that her hypothyroidism would be expected to contribute to her obesity which is exacerbating her diabetes and that (somewhat theoretically since we don't have her vital signs here) hypothyroid bradycardia could also reduce renal perfusion and contribute to her low GFR and hyperkalemia.

Assessments and plan: ❶ Life-threatening hyperkalemia: The clinician must focus on the emergency issue(s). Many books quote a potassium of 6 mEq/L as a panic value; note that the laboratory already excluded technical error and checked for hemolysis, which are the two most common causes of spurious hyperkalemia. This patient should be called at home and advised to immediately seek transportation by a secondary driver (e.g., taxi, ambulance, friend, neighbor, or relative) to the nearest hospital. If the patient is demented or otherwise incompetent, the clinician should contact the patient's caretaker or call directly for an ambulance. Attention must be given to the reliability of the driver, the urgency of the situation, and the speed by which the driver can get the patient to the hospital; failure by the clinician to ensure proper patient care—which in this case and most situations is best ensured by enrolling the ambulance service—could easily result in medicolegal complications. Hospital treatment for hyperkalemia will include assessment for electrocardiographic changes and treatment of hyperkalemia with intravenous calcium to stabilize cardioelectroconductivity, beta-adrenergic agonists, bicarbonate, diuretics, insulin and glucose; magnesium may also help alleviate arrhythmias; oral sodium polystyrene sulfonate (Kayexalate) is a potassium-binding agent. ❷ Diabetes mellitus: Notice that this patient's fasting glucose level is "normal" and yet the patient is clearly diabetic per the hemoglobin A1c value >6.5%. This patient needs a comprehensive nutritional plan for diabetes management. Promoting dependence on drugs at this early point should be considered inappropriate. ❸ Hypothyroidism: The TSH >10 indicates primary hypothyroidism by any standard; in all probability, unless major contraindications exist (of which very few exist), this patient should be started on a thyroid hormone combination as discussed in the section on thyroid assessment. ❹ Renal insufficiency: This patient has stage-3 chronic kidney disease and should begin a renoprotective and renorestorative program—beyond the basics of hypertension and hyperglycemia control—as discussed in *Chiropractic and Naturopathic Mastery of Common Clinical Disorders*. Use of ACE-inhibitor or ARB is contraindicated due to hyperkalemia. ❺ Dyslipidemia: The elevated LDL cholesterol and triglycerides should both be below 100 mg/dL. Diet is key, followed by fatty acid therapy, niacin, and berberine.

Lipid panel:	
Overview and interpretation:	• "High cholesterol" was a buzz phrase many years ago indicating an unfavorable lipid profile causally associated with accelerated atherogenesis and the resultant CVD in its myriad forms. The next step was to identify low-density lipoprotein (LDL) cholesterol as the most obvious kingpin of vascular villains. Advances over the past decade include: 1. Appreciation that other non-lipid molecules such as homocysteine and c-reactive protein (CRP) are important contributors to the atherogenic process, 2. Renewed interest in the beneficial effects of high-density lipoprotein (HDL) cholesterol in mediating vasculoprotection, 3. "Non-standard" CVD risk factors such as very-low-density lipoprotein (VLDL), β-VLDL, intermediate-density lipoprotein (IDL) cholesterol, and lipoprotein-a (Lp-a) are also clinically important. For the sake of this introductory section on the basics of laboratory interpretation, the discussion will be limited to the components of the standard lipid panel; additional tests and details are provided in disease-specific chapters on metabolic/inflammatory disorders.

Lipids: Goals	*Clinical notes:*
Total cholesterol: < 200 mg/dL	• Higher cholesterol levels correlate with increased risk for CVD. Except in very rare cases of genotropic disease, the vast majority of humans should be able to achieve a total cholesterol <200 mg/dL via nutritional optimization, exercise, and proper endocrine (especially thyroid) status. The so-called "statin" drugs which block HMG-CoA reductase (3-hydroxy-3-methyl-glutaryl-CoA reductase, the rate-limiting enzyme for the endogenous production of cholesterol) would and should be *orphan drugs*. Reducing serum levels of insulin—the primary inducer of HMG-CoA reductase—is the most rational means by which to reduce total cholesterol levels. Thyroid hormone downregulates HMG-CoA reductase; this explains the well-established association of hypothyroidism with dyslipidemia and hypercholesterolemia.
LDL: <100 mg/dL	• O'Keefe and Cordain and colleagues[103] have noted that optimal LDL is 50-70 mg/dl and that lower is better and is physiologically normal for humans who eat appropriate diets and who are physically active.
HDL: >50-60 mg/dL	• Per the American Heart Association[104], "An HDL of 60 mg/dL and above is considered protective against heart disease." Of note, a recent report linked accumulation of persistent organic pollutants (POP) with elevated HDL levels.[105]
Triglycerides: <100 mg/dL	• Elevated serum triglycerides—except in rare cases of genotropic disease—are indicators of dietary carbohydrate excess and/or alcohol excess and/or insulin resistance. Hypertriglyceridemia is associated with increased CVD risk, higher body mass index (BMI), vitamin D deficiency, and increased risks of breast cancer and prostate cancer. Extreme hypertriglyceridemia (500 mg/dL or more) can cause pancreatitis; administration of omega-3 fatty acids from fish oil is protective.
Advantages	• Allows for the monitoring of established cardiovascular risk factors and a surrogate marker for dietary compliance and lifestyle optimization.
Limitations:	• Other non-lipid risk factors should also be monitored and optimized.
Comments:	• Important panel for overall patient management and disease prevention.

---

[103] O'Keefe JH Jr, Cordain L, Harris WH, Moe RM, Vogel R. Optimal low-density lipoprotein is 50 to 70 mg/dl: lower is better and physiologically normal. *J Am Coll Cardiol.* 2004 Jun 2;43(11):2142-6

[104] American Heart Association. heart.org/HEARTORG/Conditions/What-Your-Cholesterol-Levels-Mean_UCM_305562_Article.jsp Accessed June 2011

[105] "However, unlike the findings with p,p'-DDE, after the initial decrease of HDL-cholesterol from the 1st to 2nd quartile, HDL-cholesterol increased from the 2nd to 4th quartile of these PCBs." Lee DH, Steffes MW, Sjödin A, Jones RS, Needham LL, Jacobs DR Jr. Low dose organochlorine pesticides and polychlorinated biphenyls predict obesity, dyslipidemia, and insulin resistance among people free of diabetes. *PLoS One.* 2011 Jan 26;6(1):e15977

CBC: complete blood count

Overview and interpretation:

This test measures numbers and indices of white and red blood cells and platelets. A routine "CBC with differential" is affordable, practical, and thus preferred for the vast majority of situations (step 1); the next step when the clinical picture remains unclear is—generally—to order a peripheral blood smear (step 2) before proceeding to a hematologist referral (step 3). Additional tests—more components of step 2—are listed below per topic. If all three blood cell populations are reduced (pancytopenia) consider nutritional anemia, hypersplenism (especially secondary to hepatic cirrhosis), autoimmunity (especially systemic lupus erythematosus), or bone marrow disorder such as myelofibrosis or aplastic anemia.

- WBC (white blood cells): The three most commonly encountered disorders that cause an abnormal WBC count are ❶ bone marrow suppression (causing low WBC count) and conditions associated with elevated WBC count including ❷ leukemia/lymphoma and ❸ response to infection. An elevated WBC count suggests the possibility of infection (especially bacterial infection) or leukemia/lymphoma and therefore requires the clinician's attention. However, relying on the WBC count for the assessment of serious infection is potentially misleading, particularly since, for example, it is elevated in less than 50% of patients with acute and chronic musculoskeletal infections; per Shaw et al[106] "Therefore, it [the WBC count] is helpful when it is high, but potentially misleading when it is normal." Clinicians can gain additional information by assessing percentage and quantitative indices of neutrophils, lymphocytes, and eosinophils, elevations of which may suggest bacterial infections, viral infections, or allergic or parasitic conditions, respectively. Primary care clinicians may also choose to perform lymphocyte immunophenotyping by flow cytometry in patients with unexplained lymphocytosis prior to hematologist consult.

  - Neutropenia: Severe suppression of WBC count resulting in neutropenia can occur in liver disease, viral infections (including but not limited to HIV), autoimmune disorders, bone marrow infiltration/failure, and toxin/alcohol exposure. For severe neutropenia, hospitalization, isolation precautions, prophylactic antibiotics, and marrow-stimulating agents are often indicated. Neutropenia is defined by an absolute

Absolute neutrophil count (ANC) = Total WBC x (% "Segs" + % "Bands")		
• Normal value: ≥ 1500 cells/mm3,
• Mild neutropenia: 1000-1500/mm3,
• Moderate neutropenia: 500-1000/mm3,
• Severe neutropenia: ≤ 500/mm3; hospitalization is generally advised

    neutrophil count (ANC) less than 1500 neutrophilic cells per mm3. Neutropenia is most commonly due to use of anti-cancer cytotoxic agents; other drugs that can cause neutropenia include anticonvulsants (e.g., carbamazepine, valproic acid, diphenylhydantoin), thyroid inhibitors (carbimazole, methimazole, propylthiouracil), antibacterial drugs (penicillins, cephalosporins, sulfonamides, chloramphenicol, vancomycin, trimethoprim-sulfamethoxazole), antipsychotic drugs (clozapine), antiarrhythmics (procainamide), antirheumatic drugs (penicillamine, gold salts, hydroxychloroquine), and NSAIDs.[107] The ANC is calculated with "segs" (segmented neutrophils) and "bands" (band neutrophils) reported on CBC with differential: ANC = Total WBC x (% Segs + % Bands).

---

[106] Shaw BA, Gerardi JA, Hennrikus WL. How to avoid orthopedic pitfalls in children. *Patient Care* 1999; Feb 28: 95-116

[107] Tefferi A, Hanson CA, Inwards DJ. How to interpret and pursue an abnormal complete blood cell count in adults. *Mayo Clin Proc.* 2005 Jul;80(7):923-36 www.mayoclinicproceedings.com/content/80/7/923.long This article serves as the main review for this section on CBC interpretation.

Overview and interpretation —continued:	▪ **RBC (red blood cells and associated indices):** Since polycythemia is relatively rare, in most situations the clinician is looking for anemia, most often related to the categories in the subsections that follow this paragraph. The first step is to classify the anemia based on the mean corpuscular volume (MCV) as microcytic (MCV, <80 fL), normocytic (MCV, 80-95 fL), or macrocytic (MCV, >95 fL)—details on following page.

▪ Clinical notes on the most common anemias:

- ○ Nutritional deficiency of B-12 or folate: My approach is to critique the mean corpuscular volume (MCV) and to interpret MCV values greater than 90 with an increased suspicion for folate and/or B-12 deficiency. Clinical experience has shown that MCV values greater than 95 correlate with increased homocysteine levels, and a clinical response (improvement in mood, energy, and a reduction in MCV) is commonly seen following three months of nutritional supplementation. Deficiency of vitamin B-12 can easily be treated with oral administration of 2,000 mcg per day of vitamin B-12.[108] I generally use 5 mg (rarely up to 20 mg) per day of oral folate for the treatment of probable or documented folic acid deficiency; this is safe for most patients, excluding those on antiepileptic drugs.[109] Vitamin B-12 and folic acid *function together* and should be *administered together*. Cyanocobalamin should be avoided due to its cyanide; hydroxocobalamin, methylcobalamin, adenosylcobalamin are better.

- ○ Iron deficiency (confirmed with assessment of serum ferritin): While inadequate intake, malabsorption, or menstrual bleeding may cause iron deficiency, **adult patients with iron deficiency are at higher probability for gastrointestinal pathology and should therefore be evaluated with endoscopy or other comprehensive assessment** *beyond fecal occult-blood testing* **to rule out gastrointestinal disease.**[110,111] **The standard of care for all healthcare professionals is that adult patients with inexplicable iron deficiency are referred for gastroenteroscopic evaluation to assess for occult gastrointestinal pathology; the major concerns are gastric/colon carcinoma, but malabsorptive conditions and bleeding noncancerous polyps are also worthy of diagnosis.** Iron supplementation should be administered and can reasonably be withheld during acute viral and bacterial infections as it promotes bacterial and viral replication and pathogenicity.

- ○ The anemia of chronic disease: Generally associated with a corresponding disease history such as long-term RA or renal insufficiency and often associated with increased ESR, CRP, and ferritin. **Do not assume that an anemic patient has iron deficiency until proven with measurement of serum ferritin.** Anemia of chronic kidney disease (CKD) is associated with reduced renal production of erythropoietin, thereby resulting in understimulation of bone marrow.

- ○ Anemia caused by hemolysis or splenic sequestration: Autoimmune hemolytic anemia most commonly occurs in patients with systemic lupus erythematosus (SLE). Pancytopenia—reduced numbers of RBC, WBC, and platelets—is seen with chronic liver disease that has progressed to cirrhosis and has resulted in hemolysis and splenic sequestration of blood cells; such patients are at risk for esophageal varicies, encephalopathy, and ascites with spontaneous bacterial peritonitis and should be screened and treated appropriately.

[108] Kuzminski AM, et al. Effective treatment of cobalamin deficiency with oral cobalamin. *Blood* 1998 Aug 15;92(4):1191-8

[109] "PGA administered in doses up to 1,000 mg orally a day... The folate was well absorbed, as reflected by marked increases in the serum and erythrocyte folate concentrations... There was no evidence of clinical or laboratory toxicity at these high doses of folate." Boss GR, Ragsdale RA, Zettner A, Seegmiller JE. Failure of folic acid (pteroylglutamic acid) to affect hyperuricemia. *J Lab Clin Med* 1980 Nov;96(5):783-9

[110] Rockey DC, Cello JP. Evaluation of the gastrointestinal tract in patients with iron-deficiency anemia. *N Engl J Med.* 1993;329(23):1691-5

[111] "Endoscopy revealed a clinically important lesion in 23 (12%) of 186 patients. ... CONCLUSIONS: Endoscopy yields important findings in premenopausal women with iron deficiency anemia, which should not be attributed solely to menstrual blood loss." Bini EJ, Micale PL, Weinshel EH. Evaluation of the gastrointestinal tract in premenopausal women with iron deficiency anemia. *Am J Med.* 1998 Oct;105(4):281-6

Anemia—the most common considerations in outpatient practice: Always assess patient for tachycardia, hypovolemia, orthostasis, and adequate perfusion; always test serum ferritin during the initial evaluation then perform peripheral blood smear (PBS) if diagnosis remains unclear

- Microcytic anemia:
  - Iron deficiency anemia (IDA)—Test serum ferritin. The confirmation of iron deficiency in adults generally requires gastroenterologic consultation to assess for occult gastrointestinal blood loss; this is especially true for all men and post-menopausal women but also applies to premenopausal women.* Testing for celiac disease and hematuria is advised.**
  - Thalassemia—Check for polycythemia, test Hgb electrophoresis; because the diagnosis of the various thalassemias can be complex, consider consulting a hematologist,
  - Anemia of chronic disease (ACD)—Assess patient, inflammatory markers, and renal function. The most common causes of ACD are temporal (giant cell) arteritis and polymyalgia rheumatica, rheumatoid arthritis, chronic infection, Hodgkin lymphoma, renal cell carcinoma, myelofibrosis, and Castleman disease (a noncancerous lymphoproliferative disorder).
- Normocytic anemia:
  - Nutritional anemia: Iron deficiency and vitamin B-12 deficiency can both cause normocytic anemia.
  - Bleeding—Assess patient for tachycardia, hypovolemia, and shock; consider transfusion and/or volume repletion as needed. Assess serum ferritin and the reticulocyte count.
  - Chronic renal failure (CRF): Anemia associated with elevated BUN and creatinine.
  - Hypersplenism: Assess for chronic hepatitis and cirrhosis. Cirrhotic patients are at increased risk for gastroesophageal hemorrhage and ascites with spontaneous bacterial peritonitis.
  - Hemolysis: Expect to see elevated reticulocytes (chronic) and lactate dehydrogenase (acute); expect high indirect bilirubin and low serum haptoglobin with intravascular hemolysis; assess for autoimmunity (ANA, direct Coombs test [direct antiglobulin test]), glucose-6-phosphate dehydrogenase (G6PD) deficiency, drug-induced hemolysis, and other causes as case warrants.
  - Bone marrow disorder: Correlate lab findings with patient presentation; consult hematologist if solution is not forthcoming.
- Macrocytosis:
  - Induced by toxins, drugs, alcohol—Assess per patient history and other findings; the most notorious offenders are hydroxyurea, zidovudine, and alcohol.
  - Vitamin B-12 and/or folate deficiency: Consider testing serum methylmalonate and homocysteine followed by empiric supplementation with B-12 at 2,000 or more micrograms per day and folate at 1-5 milligrams per day; determine cause of problem and strongly consider autoimmune gastritis, bacterial overgrowth, and celiac disease. Test serum ferritin because nutritional deficiencies commonly occur together. Administration of vitamin B-12 is advised in all patients suspected of having B-12 deficiency.*** Regarding the clinical presentation of vitamin B-12 deficiency, clinicians should remember the adage that one-third of patients will present with anemia, one-third with peripheral neuropathy, and one-third with central neurologic problems such as depression, psychosis, and/or other disturbances of mood, memory, or personality. Failure to diagnose and treat vitamin B-12 deficiency in a timely manner will result in permanent neurologic damage.
  - Hypothyroidism: Measure TSH and free T4 at a minimum; assess basal body temperature, and speed of Achilles reflex return.

* "A gastrointestinal source of chronic blood loss was identified in a substantial proportion of premenopausal women with iron deficiency anemia." Green BT, Rockey DC. Gastrointestinal endoscopic evaluation of premenopausal women with iron deficiency anemia. *J Clin Gastroenterol.* 2004 Feb;38(2):104-9

** Goddard AF, James MW, McIntyre AS, Scott BB; on behalf of the British Society of Gastroenterology. Guidelines for the management of iron deficiency anaemia. *Gut.* 2011 Jun http://www.epocrates.com/dacc/1106/irondefbmj1106.pdf

*** "Thus, therapeutic trials of Cbl are warranted when clinical findings consistent with Cbl deficiency are present..." Solomon LR. Cobalamin-responsive disorders in the ambulatory care setting: unreliability of cobalamin, methylmalonic acid, and homocysteine testing. *Blood* 2005 Feb:978-85 bloodjournal.hematologylibrary.org/content/105/3/978.full.pdf

Overview and interpretation —continued:	• <u>Platelets</u>: Elevated platelet count (thrombocytosis) can be due to malignant primary thrombocytosis, iron-deficiency anemia, hemolysis, asplenia, and reactive thrombocytosis due to cancer, infection, or chronic inflammation. Low platelet count (thrombocytopenia, fewer than 150,000 platelets per microliter) increases risk for spontaneous bleeding and can—rarely but importantly—be associated with serious and potentially life-threatening disorders such as thrombotic thrombocytopenic purpura/hemolytic uremic syndrome (TTP/HUS) and disseminated intravascular coagulation (DIC). In relatively asymptomatic and nonacute outpatients, the most common causes of thrombocytopenia are hypersplenism due to liver cirrhosis, idiopathic thrombocytopenic purpura (ITP), and drug reaction, most notoriously secondary to trimethoprim-sulfamethoxazole ("Bactrim"), cardiac medications (e.g., quinidine, procainamide, thiazide diuretics), antirheumatic drugs (gold salts [rarely used these days]), and heparin. Heparin-induced thrombocytopenia (HIT, type-2) is potentially fatal and requires immediate cessation of heparin administration. Patients with unexplained persistent thrombocytopenia should be tested for HIV, autoimmunity (ANA), and lymphoproliferative disorders (PBS, immunophenotyping, serum protein electrophoresis, and serum immunofixation). Isolated mild to moderate thrombocytopenia (75,000 – 150,000 platelets per microliter) during pregnancy generally is considered nonpathologic.
Advantages:	• The **CBC with differential** is inexpensive and easy to perform and is appropriate for asymptomatic patients. The "CBC with diff" is an appropriate first test for patients who are symptomatic (e.g., fatigue, fever) or have an ongoing history of health problems. In certain healthcare settings where cost containment is a major priority, CBC *without* differential is commonly ordered; however, in outpatient private practice, the additional expenditure of $2 for the CBC *with* differential is the preferred evaluation. It provides a quick screen for anemia, leukemia, infection, and for provisional evidence of B-12/folate and iron deficiencies. The CBC can also identify more complex conditions such as pancytopenia and thereby promote comprehensive patient management; for example, pancytopenia may unmask hepatic cirrhosis which may necessitate use of nadolol for prophylaxis against gastroesophageal variceal hemorrhage as well as use of prophylactic antibiotics against spontaneous bacterial peritonitis. • The **peripheral blood smear (PBS)** is used to further evaluate leukocytosis, anemias, and other abnormalities. In the investigation of persistent leukocytosis, the PBS is of limited value and therefore, while the PBS should certainly be performed, it is generally followed by **immunophenotyping by flow cytometry** if not a direct referral to a hematologist. An excellent review by Tefferi et al[112] concluded, "In general, it is prudent to perform a PBS in most instances of abnormal CBC, along with basic tests that are dictated by the type of CBC abnormalities. The latter may include, for example, serum ferritin in patients with microcytic anemia or lymphocyte immunophenotyping by flow cytometry in patients with lymphocytosis..."
Limitations:	• WBC count may be normal even in patients with serious infections. • RBC indices may be normal in people with severe iron deficiency. o **Dr Vasquez's experience**—*Many outpatients with no evidence of anemia on the CBC will be grossly iron deficient with ferritin values less than 6 mcg/L, clearly indicating iron deficiency. Nonanemic iron deficiency contributes to fatigue, depression, RLS, attention deficit.*
Comments:	• The **CBC** is a foundational part of the assessment for all new patients. Generally, "CBC *with* differential" should be ordered.

---

[112] Tefferi A, Hanson CA, Inwards DJ. How to interpret and pursue an abnormal complete blood cell count in adults. *Mayo Clin Proc* 2005;80(7):923-3

Presentation: Classic iron insufficiency in a healthy 32yo athletic female: This limited laboratory report is from a 32yo athletic female whose primary complaint is that of "less endurance than expected" given her healthy lifestyle and frequent participation in physical exercise of various types such as running, biking, hiking, and kayaking. Her TSH is on the low end of normal consistent with her taking 17 mcg daily of liothyroinine (T3); note however that the total T3 level remains on the low end of the normal range, suggesting that she may benefit from additional T3 supplementation. The RBC parameters Hgb and Hct are on the low end of the normal range consistent with recent menstruation; the response of the bone marrow to recent blood loss is noted with the RDW being toward the high end of normal, refecting increased marrow production of reticulocytes. Ferritin is suboptimal at 25 ng/mL, given that the optimal range is approximately 40-70 ng/mL.[113] Altough various iron supplements are available on the market and high-iron foods such as beef and blackstrap molasis can be used, typical treatment is with iron 18 mg per day often provided as ferrous sulfate 90 mg; note that 5 mg ferrous sulfate = 1 mg elemental iron. Other forms of iron such as ferrous aspartate may be better tolerated. Daily iron supplementation for 2-3 months should elevate the ferritin level and improve the feeling of energy not simply by ❶ improving oxygen delivery to tissues but also by ❷ improving function of the electron transport chain where iron is a required cofactor, ❸ improving the conversion of thyroid hormone (T4) into the active form of T3, and by ❹ improving the production of dopamine and norepinephrine, since iron is a required cofactor for the enzyme tyrosine hydroxylase which converts the amino acid tyrosine into L-DOPA which is converted to dopamine and then partially to norepinephrine. Given that this patient menstruates monthly and has no significant medical history and—specifically—no gastrointestinal complaints; the probability is high that her state of iron insufficiency is due to physiologic blood loss; however, a case could be made for endoscopic evaluation[114], and in the event that the patient suffered from an diagnosed intestinal lesion such as colon cancer, the practitioner who did not refer for gastroenterologic evaluation would be challenged to produce effective medicolegal defense. Guidelines[115] published in 2011 support testing for celiac disease, *H. pylori* infection, and hematuria while reserving endoscopy in premenopausal women to those aged 50 years or older, or with symptoms of gastrointestinal disease, or those with a strong family history of colorectal cancer.

Reported: 07/07/2011 / 06:02 CDT

Test Name	In Range	Out Of Range	Reference Range
TSH, 3RD GENERATION	0.54		mIU/L
	Reference Range		
	> or = 20 Years 0.40-4.50		
	Pregnancy Ranges		
	First trimester 0.20-4.70		
	Second trimester 0.30-4.10		
	Third trimester 0.40-2.70		
T3, TOTAL	97		76-181 ng/dL
CBC (INCLUDES DIFF/PLT)			
WHITE BLOOD CELL COUNT	7.1		3.8-10.8 Thousand/uL
RED BLOOD CELL COUNT	4.28		3.80-5.10 Million/uL
HEMOGLOBIN	12.1		11.7-15.5 g/dL
HEMATOCRIT	36.2		35.0-45.0 %
MCV	84.5		80.0-100.0 fL
MCH	28.4		27.0-33.0 pg
MCHC	33.6		32.0-36.0 g/dL
RDW	14.8		11.0-15.0 %
PLATELET COUNT	248		140-400 Thousand/uL
ABSOLUTE NEUTROPHILS	3586		1500-7800 cells/uL
ABSOLUTE LYMPHOCYTES	2854		850-3900 cells/uL
ABSOLUTE MONOCYTES	525		200-950 cells/uL
ABSOLUTE EOSINOPHILS	107		15-500 cells/uL
ABSOLUTE BASOPHILS	28		0-200 cells/uL
NEUTROPHILS	50.5		%
LYMPHOCYTES	40.2		%
MONOCYTES	7.4		%
EOSINOPHILS	1.5		%
BASOPHILS	0.4		%
FERRITIN	25		10-154 ng/mL

---

[113] See excerpt from Vasquez A. *Integrative Rheumatology*. http://InflammationMastery.com/hemochromatosis.html
[114] "A gastrointestinal source of chronic blood loss was identified in a substantial proportion of premenopausal women with iron deficiency anemia." Green BT, Rockey DC. Gastrointestinal endoscopic evaluation of premenopausal women with iron deficiency anemia. *J Clin Gastroenterol*. 2004 Feb;38(2):104-9
[115] Goddard AF, James MW, McIntyre AS, Scott BB; on behalf of the British Society of Gastroenterology. Guidelines for the management of iron deficiency anaemia. *Gut*. 2011 Jun 6. [Epub ahead of print] http://www.epocrates.com/dacc/1106/irondefbmj1106.pdf

Presentation: Vitamin B-12 deficiency without hematologic abnormality—report and discussion: This elderly patient shows no signs of anemia; note also that the MCV is perfectly normal. Given that the psychiatric literature supports a minimal serum vitamin B-12 level of 600 pg/ml, the advocation by medical reference laboratories of a lower "normal" limit of 200 pg/ml is scientifically absurd and ethically indefensible; this is yet another example of the importance of clinicians' knowledge of the literature overriding the laboratory's reference range. The consistent documentation of the rapid reversibility of severe neuropsychiatric illness with vitamin B-12 therapy as the only intervention[116,117] provides additional justification for empiric vitamin B-12 administration in patients with clinical symptoms consistent with vitamin B-12 deficiency regardless of hematologic and serologic findings.[118] Vitamin B-12 deficiency is very serious because it can lead to permanent brain damage, resulting in personality changes, memory impairment, and overt psychotic disorders, including catatonia; mechanisms of neurologic injury may include homocysteine toxicity, autoimmune neuronal demyelinization, and axonal degeneration and nerve-sheath demyelination especially in the median forebrain bundle.[119]

HEMATOLOGY

----- CBC - WBC STUDIES -----

Procedure:	WBC 10E3
Reference:	[4.50-11.00]
Units:	/CMM
07DEC06 0926 THU	7.32

----- CBC - RBC STUDIES -----

Procedure:	RBC 10E6	HEMOGLOBIN	HEMATOCRIT	MCV	MCH	MCHC	RDW-CV
Reference:	[4.50-5.90]	[13.5-17.5]	[41.0-53.0]	[80.0-94.0]	[27.0-31.0]	[32.0-36.0]	[11.0-16.0]
Units:	/CMM	G/DL	%	FL	PG	%	%
07DEC06 0926 THU	5.16	15.7	46.3	89.7	30.4	33.9	14.1

----- CBC - PLATELET STUDIES -----

Procedure:	PLATELET 10E3	MPV
Reference:	[150-500]	[9.0-13.0]
Units:	/CMM	FL
07DEC06 0926 THU	308	11.2

CHEMISTRY PROFILES

----- ROUTINE CHEMISTRY PROFILES -----

Procedure:	SODIUM	POTASSIUM	CHLORIDE	CO2	GLUCOSE	BUN	CREATININE	CALCIUM
Reference:	[133-145]	[3.5-5.3]	[100-110]	[22.0-29.0]	[70-110]	[5-25]	[0.5-1.4]	[8.3-10.3]
Units:	MMOL/L	MEQ/L	MMOL/L	MMOL/L	MG/DL	MG/DL	MG/DL	MG/DL
07DEC06 0926 THU	137	4.3	101	27.0	90	16	0.9	9.9

Procedure:	ANION GAP	OSMOLARITY	BUN/CREAT
Reference:	[6-14]	[272-305]	
Units:	MEQ/L	MOSM/K	MG/DL
07DEC06 0926 THU	13	275	17.8

SPECIAL CHEMISTRY

----- CHEMISTRY SPECIAL/MISCELLANEOUS -----

Procedure:	FOLATE	VITAMIN B-12
Reference:	[2.0-18.0]	[193-982]
Units:	NG/ML	PG/ML
07DEC06 0926 THU	14.7	182 L

---

[116] Berry N, Sagar R, Tripathi BM. Catatonia and other psychiatric symptoms with vitamin B12 deficiency. *Acta Psychiatr Scand.* 2003 ;108(2):156-9
[117] Newbold HL. Vitamin B-12: placebo or neglected therapeutic tool? *Med Hypotheses.* 1989 Mar;28(3):155-64
[118] Solomon LR. Cobalamin-responsive disorders in the ambulatory care setting: unreliability of cobalamin, methylmalonic acid, and homocysteine testing. *Blood.* 2005 Feb 1;105(3):978-85. This is a very important article supporting empiric vitamin B12 supplementation rather than unnecessary reliance on unreliable (and expensive) laboratory tests.
[119] Catalano G, Catalano MC, Rosenberg EI, Embi PJ, Embi CS. Catatonia. Another neuropsychiatric presentation of vitamin B12 deficiency? *Psychosomatics.* 1998 Sep-Oct;39(5):456-60 http://psy.psychiatryonline.org/cgi/reprint/39/5/456

Nutritional deficiency, diet-responsive disorders, and the allopathic medical paradigm: Review and commentary with emphases on diabetes mellitus and vitamins D and B-12

Consequences of vitamin B-12 deficiency:
Initially the manifestations are mild and reversible, but over time they become more severe and strongly refractory to treatment to the point that permanent damage (particularly in the CNS) is anticipated:

- "Bipolar disorder"—a condition indistinguishable from a bipolar disorder,
- Organic brain syndrome, delirium, confusion, poor memory, impaired cognition,
- Dementia and erroneous diagnosis of "Alzheimer's disease",
- Mood disorders, depression, catatonia, paranoia, paranoid psychosis, violent behavior,
- Peripheral neuropathy, "combined degeneration" of anterior and posterior columns of the spinal cord,
- As a result of the above problems, patients who are mismanaged by doctors unknowledgeable about basic nutrition often suffer directly from these effects but also suffer from the medical management from these problems. Mood disorders and psychosis may result from B-12 deficiency, and the medical management of mood disorders and psychosis includes medicalization, electroconvulsive therapy (ECT), and institutionalization.

The medical profession's failure to train its students and doctors in nutrition is widely and consistently documented; given that such a profession-wide policy can do nothing other than result in patient harm and/or drug dependency under the guise of "healthcare", it is—borrowing a phrase from Nietzsche—"the highest of all conceivable corruptions."

- Nutritional deficiencies and the medical paradigm (*J Clin Endocrinol Metab* 2003 Nov): "But public health measures in the first half of the 20th century eradicated the most extreme of the vitamin deficiencies in the industrialized nations, and the physician's actual experience of [obvious] deficiency disease dropped to near zero. Perhaps as a result, the medical profession's approach to nutrition today is still dominated by the external agent paradigm, as witnessed in the national campaigns for cholesterol, saturated fat, and salt. Those who think more seriously in terms of the continuing importance of deficiency per se are often derogated or relegated to the quackery fringe. The result, at the very least, is inattention to the real deficiencies that may masquerade as other disorders, or that may simply be ignored altogether."
- Failure of surgical treatment for low-back pain caused by vitamin D deficiency (*J Am Board Fam Med* 2009 Jan): The author of this case series describes six cases of chronic debilitating back pain—three of which "required surgery"—which were greatly relieved or completely cured by correction of vitamin D deficiency. The author notes, "Chronic low back pain and failed back surgery may improve with repletion of vitamin D from a state of deficiency/insufficiency to sufficiency. Vitamin D insufficiency is common; repletion of vitamin D to normal levels in patients who have chronic low back pain or have had failed back surgery may improve quality of life or, in some cases, result in complete resolution of symptoms."

That nutritional deficiencies can cause mood disorders and mental disease is well-known; in contrast to what patients actually need, the general allopathic approach to these clinical presentations is founded upon the administration of drugs, followed by ECT, institutionalization, and psychosurgery and—lately, instead of scalpel-induced brain damage—radiofrequency heating (thermocapsulotomy) or gamma radiation (radiosurgery, gammacapsulotomy) for the destruction of brain structures, and the surgical implantation of brain electrostimulators. Meanwhile, thousands of these psychiatrically-labeled patients simply need nutritional supplementation. Minor exceptions noted, the medical profession as a whole chooses to remain blind to the value of nutrition so that the pharmacosurgical paradigm can remain dominant by continuing to *appear* omnipotent. The dual illusions that are maintained are "Drugs and surgery are the answers to all major health problems" and "If no drug exists for a condition, then it is idiopathic and no curative treatment is available."

As an example, type-2 diabetes mellitus (T2DM) has burgeoned into an epidemic under the dominance of the allopathic disease model, and patients are told that the condition is genetic, progressive and incurable; a review published in the May 2011 issue of *Journal of the American Osteopathic Association* admonished physicians to (mis)educate their patients as follows, with Dr Vasquez's comments in brackets: "Be absolutely clear that T2DM is a lifelong disease [false statement] that will require lifelong treatment [false statement fostering dependency]. Success in controlling the disease and preventing future complications will depend on the patient and physician working together [creation of dependency under the guise of "working together"]. There is often a fatalistic attitude in patients with T2DM [perhaps because they have been lied to and disempowered], so it is important to establish a relationship that on one hand offers hope [creating the illusion of hope while enforcing drug dependency] and on the other does not suggest that the disease will be cured [although the diseases is generally curable with appropriate nutritional intervention]. Be up front with the patient from the first visit and make it clear that T2DM is a chronic illness [enforce drug dependency starting at the first visit]…" This babble was published in a peer-reviewed medical journal despite clear multi-decade evidence showing that T2DM is reversible with nutritional intervention.

Nutritional deficiency, diet-responsive disorders, and the allopathic medical paradigm: Review and commentary with emphases on diabetes mellitus and vitamins D and B-12

Recent examples of the safety and efficacy of diet intervention for T2DM are provided here with many more examples and details in *Nutritional, Integrative and Functional Medicine Mastery of Common Clinical Disorders*.

- T2DM is rapidly reversible with diet (*Diabetologia* 2011 Jun): "Normalization of both beta cell function and hepatic insulin sensitivity in type 2 diabetes was achieved by dietary energy restriction alone. This was associated with decreased pancreatic and liver triacylglycerol stores. **The abnormalities underlying type 2 diabetes are reversible by reducing dietary energy intake.**"
- Diet therapy effective, safe, and is at least as effective as injected insulin for reducing chronic hyperglycemia in T2DM (*Nutr Metab* 2009 May): "The number of patients on sulfonylureas decreased from 7 at baseline to 2 at 6 months. No patient required inpatient care or insulin therapy. In summary, the 30%-carbohydrate diet over 6 months led to a remarkable reduction in HbA1c levels, even among outpatients with severe type 2 diabetes, without any insulin therapy, hospital care or increase in sulfonylureas. **The effectiveness of the [low-carbohydrate] diet may be comparable to that of insulin therapy.**"

Ironically (or not), the first-line drug for T2DM—metformin—causes vitamin B-12 (cobalamin, Cbl) deficiency and exacerbation of the often debilitating peripheral neuropathy of T2DM which is often treated with the drugs gabapentin/Neurontin or pregabalin/Lyrica, which exacerbates obesity and T2DM, thereby promoting a vicious cycle.

- Pregabalin/Lyrica and gabapentin/Neurontin promote fat-weight gain, thereby exacerbating T2DM (*Prescrire Int* 2005 Dec): "Pregabalin, like gabapentin, can lead to weight gain and peripheral edema especially in elderly patients."
- Metformin causes vitamin B-12 deficiency and exacerbates diabetic peripheral neuropathy (*Diabetes Care* 2010 Jan): "Metformin-treated patients had depressed Cbl levels and elevated fasting MMA and Hcy levels. Clinical and electrophysiological measures identified more severe peripheral neuropathy in these patients; the cumulative metformin dose correlated strongly with these clinical and paraclinical group differences. CONCLUSIONS: Metformin exposure may be an iatrogenic cause for exacerbation of peripheral neuropathy in patients with type 2 diabetes."
- Vitamin B-12 deficiency secondary to metformin prescription (*Rev Assoc Med Bras* 2011 Jan): "The present findings suggest a high prevalence of vitamin B12 deficiency in metformin-treated diabetic patients [n=144]. Older patients, patients in long term treatment with metformin and low vitamin B12 intake are probably more prone to this deficiency."
- Metformin-induced vitamin B12 deficiency presenting as a peripheral neuropathy (*South Med J* 2010 Mar): "Chronic metformin use results in vitamin B12 deficiency in 30% of patients. ... **Vitamin B12 deficiency, which may present without anemia and as a peripheral neuropathy, is often misdiagnosed as diabetic neuropathy, although the clinical findings are usually different. Failure to diagnose the cause of the neuropathy will result in progression of central and/or peripheral neuronal damage which can be arrested but not reversed with vitamin B12 replacement.**"
- Low vitamin B-12 status correlates with expedited brain atrophy (*Neurology* 2008 Sep): "The decrease in brain volume was greater among those with lower vitamin B(12) and holoTC levels and higher plasma tHcy and MMA levels at baseline. ... Using the upper (for the vitamins) or lower tertile (for the metabolites) as reference in logistic regression analysis and adjusting for the above covariates, vitamin B(12) in the bottom tertile (<308 pmol/L) was associated with increased rate of brain volume loss (odds ratio 6.17, 95% CI 1.25-30.47)."

Consequences for the clinician:
Given that the evidence in favor of early and empiric treatment for possible vitamin B-12 deficiency is stronger than evidence in favor of allowing vitamin B-12 deficiency or dependency to persist with potentially catastrophic outcomes, no scientific argument can be made in favor of failing to diagnose and treat vitamin B-12 deficiency/dependency. However, since, in general, the allopathic and osteopathic medical professions have failed to educate their students and doctors about nutrition, these professions have established ignorance as their defense and therefore no standard of care exists for the treatment or failure of treatment of chronic nutritional deficiencies. Ethically, the results are failure to achieve beneficence via failure to diagnose and treat, and the widespread implementation of malfeasance via diagnostic/therapeutic failure complicated by the unnecessary expenses and adverse effects of drugs/surgeries/interventions used in place of nutritional supplementation. The enforcement of a standard of care is meaningless when nutritional incompetence is the standard. Fortunately for patients, the biomedical literature uses increasingly strong language in favor of mandating standards for nutritional evaluation and treatment:

- Nutritional deficiencies and the medical paradigm (*J Clin Endocrinol Metab* 2003 Nov): "J. Cannell (submitted for publication) has written that measures such as this editorial will not change the situation, and that only tort litigation will work. One can only hope that he is wrong. Either way, something needs to change"
- Physicians should routinely use vitamin supplementation as treatment for patients (*JAMA* 2002 Jun): "Physicians should make specific efforts to ensure that patients are taking vitamins they should..."

Nutritional deficiency, diet-responsive disorders, and the allopathic medical paradigm: Review and commentary with emphases on diabetes mellitus and vitamins D and B-12

- Testing and treating for vitamin D deficiency among patients with chronic nonspecific musculoskeletal pain should be the standard of care (*Mayo Clin Proc* 2003 Dec): "Because osteomalacia is a known cause of persistent, nonspecific musculoskeletal pain, screening all outpatients with such pain for hypovitaminosis D should be standard practice in clinical care."
- Testing and treating for vitamin D deficiency among patients with chronic low-back pain should be the standard of care (*Spine* 2003 Jan): "Screening for vitamin D deficiency and treatment with supplements should be mandatory in this setting."

Citations for this section:
1. Catalano G, Catalano MC, Rosenberg EI, Embi PJ, Embi CS. Catatonia. Another neuropsychiatric presentation of vitamin B12 deficiency? *Psychosomatics*. 1998 Sep-Oct;39(5):456-60
2. Newbold HL. Vitamin B-12: placebo or neglected therapeutic tool? *Med Hypotheses*. 1989 Mar;28(3):155-64
3. Solomon LR. Cobalamin-responsive disorders in the ambulatory care setting: unreliability of cobalamin, methylmalonic acid, and homocysteine testing. *Blood*. 2005 Feb 1;105(3):978-85
4. Christmas D, Eljamel MS, Butler S, et al. Long term outcome of thermal anterior capsulotomy for chronic, treatment refractory depression. *J Neurol Neurosurg Psychiatry*. 2011 Jun;82(6):594-600
5. Malone DA Jr. Use of deep brain stimulation in treatment-resistant depression. *Cleve Clin J Med*. 2010 Jul;77 Suppl 3:S77-80
6. Heaney RP. Vitamin D, nutritional deficiency, and the medical paradigm. *J Clin Endocrinol Metab*. 2003;88:5107-8
7. Schwalfenberg G. Improvement of chronic back pain or failed back surgery with vitamin D repletion: a case series. *J Am Board Fam Med*. 2009 Jan-Feb;22(1):69-74
8. Gavin JR 3rd, Freeman JS, Shubrook JH Jr, Lavernia F. Type 2 diabetes mellitus: practical approaches for primary care physicians. *J Am Osteopath Assoc*. 2011 May;111(5 Suppl 4):S3-S12
9. Lim EL, Hollingsworth KG, Aribisala BS, et al. Reversal of type 2 diabetes: normalisation of beta cell function in association with decreased pancreas and liver triacylglycerol. *Diabetologia*. 2011 Jun 9. Published on-line.
10. Haimoto H, Sasakabe T, Wakai K, Umegaki H. Effects of a low-carbohydrate diet on glycemic control in outpatients with severe type 2 diabetes. *Nutr Metab* 2009:6;21
11. Gabapentin/Neurontin causes "Gains of up to 15 kg (33lbs) during 3 months of treatment." http://pacmedweightloss.com/docs/medications_that_cause_weight_gain.pdf Accessed July 2011.
12. Vogiatzoglou A, Refsum H, Johnston C, Smith SM, Bradley KM, de Jager C, Budge MM, Smith AD. Vitamin B12 status and rate of brain volume loss in community-dwelling elderly. *Neurology*. 2008 Sep 9;71(11):826-32
13. Wile DJ, Toth C. Association of metformin, elevated homocysteine, and methylmalonic acid levels and clinically worsened diabetic peripheral neuropathy. *Diabetes Care*. 2010 Jan;33(1):156-61
14. Nervo M, Lubini A, Raimundo FV, Faulhaber GA, Leite C, Fischer LM, Furlanetto TW. Vitamin B12 in metformin-treated diabetic patients: a cross-sectional study in Brazil. *Rev Assoc Med Bras*. 2011 Jan-Feb;57(1):46-9
15. Bell DS. Metformin-induced vitamin B12 deficiency presenting as a peripheral neuropathy. *South Med J*. 2010 Mar;103(3):265-7
16. [No authors listed] Pregabalin: new drug. Very similar to gabapentin. *Prescrire Int*. 2005 Dec;14(80):203-6
17. Fletcher RH, Fairfield KM. Harvard Medical School. Vitamins for chronic disease prevention in adults: clinical applications. *JAMA*. 2002;287:3127-9
18. Plotnikoff GA, Quigley JM. Prevalence of severe hypovitaminosis D in patients with persistent, nonspecific musculoskeletal pain. *Mayo Clin Proc*. 2003;78:1463-70
19. Al Faraj S, Al Mutairi K. Vitamin D deficiency and chronic low back pain in Saudi Arabia. *Spine* 2003 ;28:177-9

UA: Urinalysis

Overview and interpretation:

- <u>Collection</u>: Unless catheterized, patients are advised to pass approximately one-third of their available urine into the toilet, then pass approximately the middle-third of their urine into the specimen container. Use of an antiseptic to clean the urethral meatus was once advocated to avoid/reduce specimen contamination, but this step is ineffective and therefore unnecessary because contamination rates remain similar at 32% and 29% whether or not, respectively, urethral meatus cleansing is performed.[120]

- <u>Analysis</u>: Analysis should be performed on fresh urine, preferably within 1-2 hours; in outpatient clinical practice this two-hour timeframe is consistently possible only if the clinician performs in-office dipstick analysis (and perhaps microscopic visualization). Samples that cannot be analyzed within 1-2 hours or those which are destined for a reference laboratory should be refrigerated. Dipstick UA can be performed in office and is simple, inexpensive, and—when performed and interpreted with a modicum of competence—sufficiently accurate. Per Klatt[121], "The color change occurring on each segment of the strip is compared to a color chart to obtain results. However, a careless doctor, nurse, or assistant is entirely capable of misreading or misinterpreting the results." Urine samples can be sent to a reference laboratory for more accurate chemical analysis as well as microscopic analysis, culture and sensitivity. Whether infection is clinically suspected or not, clinicians might chose to order "UA with reflex to microscopy and culture" to ensure that urine samples are appropriately processed if the laboratory finds suspicion of UTI upon dipstick analysis.

- <u>Scope of this review</u>: The purpose of this brief review is to concisely refresh clinicians' appreciation of the components of the routine urinalysis, one that is generally performed in-office with a dipstick reagent stick or that is performed by a reference laboratory. This is not an exhaustive review, and microscopic findings have not been detailed here because most clinicians do not perform microscopy in their offices; additional details on UA and microscopic assessment is available in articles such as the excellent review by Simerville, Maxted, and Pahira published in *American Family Physician* 2005 and available on-line at http://www.aafp.org/afp/2005/0315/p1153.html as of July 2011.

- <u>Components of routine urinalysis</u>:
  - <u>Visual inspection</u>: Urine should be clear with a color ranging from faint yellow (well hydrated, dilute urine) to bright yellow (especially with B-vitamin supplementation). An amber-brown hue might be due to dehydration or a pathologic process resulting in myoglobinuria (i.e., rhabdomyolysis) or the presence of bile pigments (i.e., biliary tract obstruction). A red color to urine suggests hematuria, recent beet consumption, or use of certain drugs or food dyes; the antibiotic rifampin/rifampicin is notorious for adding a red-orange color to the urine (and to a lesser extent to sweat and tears). The urine of patients with porphyria cutanea tarda will be red-brown in natural light and pink-red in fluorescent light.[122] Cloudy urine is due to pyuria (infection), proteinuria, or precipitated phosphate crystals in alkaline urine.
  - <u>Strong odor</u>: Odiferous or malodorous urine suggests infection, recent ingestion of foods such as asparagus or nutritional supplements such as lipoic acid, certain medications, concentrated urine due to dehydration or underperfusion of the kidneys.
  - <u>Specific gravity</u>: Specific gravity is a measure of solute concentration and thus is proportional to urine osmolality; as such it reflects renal perfusion, hydration, and the ability of the kidneys to perform their critical function of concentrating filtrate. Dilute urine has a specific gravity <1.010 and is seen with adequate/excessive hydration, diuretic use, diabetes insipidus, adrenal insufficiency, hyperaldosteronism, and

---

[120] Simerville JA, Maxted WC, Pahira JJ. Urinalysis: a comprehensive review. *Am Fam Physician*. 2005 Mar 15;71(6):1153-62 http://www.aafp.org/afp/2005/0315/p1153.html
[121] Klatt EC. WebPath. Savannah, Georgia, USA. http://library.med.utah.edu/WebPath/tutorial/urine/urine.html Accessed July 1, 2011
[122] Rich MW. Porphyria cutanea tarda. Don't forget to look at the urine. *Postgrad Med*. 1999 Apr;105(4):208-10, 213-4

UA: Urinalysis

impaired renal function (i.e., failure of the kidneys to concentrate urine). Concentrated urine has a specific gravity >1.020 and correlates with dehydration, renal artery stenosis, hypoperfusion/shock, glucosuria, and syndrome of inappropriate anti-diuretic hormone secretion (SIADH), which is often associated with hyponatremia.

o   pH: Urine pH may range from 4.5 (very acidic) to as high as 8.5 (very alkaline). Urine pH correlates with serum pH except in patients with renal tubular acidosis (RTA type-1, a condition associated with chronically alkaline urine). Therefore, urine pH can be used to screen for various conditions of systemic alkalosis and acidosis. The Western diet—also called the standard American diet or S.A.D.—causes mild diet-induced metabolic acidosis[123] which promotes degenerative diseases; in contrast, a diet rich in fruits and vegetables such as the Paleo-Mediterranean diet[124] promotes mild systemic and urinary alkalinization.[125] From a wellness perspective, urine pH should be 7.5 up to 8.0 because urinary alkalinization facilitates xenobiotic excretion[126], promotes urinary retention of minerals such as potassium, magnesium, and calcium, and causes a reduction in serum cortisol.[127] Urine pH—like urine sodium:potassium ratio—can be used as a marker of compliance for intake of fruits, vegetables, and alkalinizing supplements such as potassium citrate. For some patients (mostly female), urine alkalinization may encourage urinary tract infection, especially if gastrointestinal dysbiosis[128] is present; in such situations, the often causative GI dysbiosis should be treated, and consistent or transient urinary acidification can be achieved with oral ascorbic acid. Urea-splitting bacteria can cause the urine to be alkaline, and such bacteria can also promote development of magnesium-ammonium phosphate crystals and so-called staghorn nephrolithiasis. Acidic urine promotes development of uric acid nephrolithiasis; therapeutic urinary alkalinization such as by use of supplemental potassium citrate or an alkalinizing diet is preventive and therapeutic. On this topic, Cicerello et al[129] wrote, "In conclusion urinary alkalization with maintaining continuously high urinary pH values, could be the treatment of choice for stone dissolution and prevention of uric acid stones."

o   Bilirubin in urine: If present, bilirubin in urine is of the direct/conjugated fraction (rather than indirect/unconjugated, which is nonhydrosoluble) and indicates the need to evaluate for biliary tract obstruction.

o   Urobilinogen: Urobilinogen is (direct) bilirubin that has been conjugated in the liver, passed through the biliary system into the intestine, partially metabolized by bacteria, then reabsorbed via the portal circulation and filtered by the kidney. Elevated urobilinogen is associated with liver disease and hemolytic diseases.

o   Glucose: Glucose is found in the urine when the serum glucose exceeds approximately 190 mg/dL and overwhelms the reabsorptive/resorptive capacity of the proximal tubule. Glucose in the urine is presumptive evidence supporting the diagnosis of diabetes mellitus. Rare non-diabetic causes of glucosuria/glycosuria include liver disease,

[123] "The modern Western-type diet is deficient in fruits and vegetables and contains excessive animal products, generating the accumulation of non-metabolizable anions and a lifespan state of overlooked metabolic acidosis, whose magnitude increases progressively with aging due to the physiological decline in kidney function." Adeva MM, Souto G. Diet-induced metabolic acidosis. *Clin Nutr*. 2011 Aug;30(4):416-21. Epub 2011 Apr 9.

[124] Vasquez A. Revisiting the Five-Part Nutritional Wellness Protocol: The Supplemented Paleo-Mediterranean Diet. *Nutritional Perspectives* 2011 January This article is available at http://InflammationMastery.com/part8.html and is also included in this textbook.

[125] Cordain L, Eaton SB, Sebastian A, Mann N, Lindeberg S, Watkins BA, O'Keefe JH, Brand-Miller J. Origins and evolution of the Western diet: health implications for the 21st century. *Am J Clin Nutr*. 2005 Feb;81(2):341-54

[126] Proudfoot AT, Krenzelok EP, Vale JA. Position Paper on urine alkalinization. *J Toxicol Clin Toxicol*. 2004;42(1):1-26

[127] Maurer M, Riesen W, Muser J, Hulter HN, Krapf R. Neutralization of Western diet inhibits bone resorption independently of K intake and reduces cortisol secretion in humans. *Am J Physiol Renal Physiol*. 2003 Jan;284(1):F32-40

[128] Vasquez A. Reducing Pain and Inflammation Naturally - Part 6: Nutritional and Botanical Treatments Against "Silent Infections" and Gastrointestinal Dysbiosis, Commonly Overlooked Causes of Neuromusculoskeletal Inflammation and Chronic Health Problems. *Nutritional Perspectives* 2006; January. For a more extensive review, see the most recent edition of Integrative Rheumatology: http://InflammationMastery.com/rheumatology.html

[129] Cicerello E, Merlo F, Maccatrozzo L. Urinary alkalization for the treatment of uric acid nephrolithiasis. *Arch Ital Urol Androl*. 2010 Sep;82(3):145-8

pancreatic disease, and Fanconi's syndrome (characterized by a failure of the proximal renal tubules to reabsorb glucose, amino acids, uric acid, phosphate and bicarbonate).

o Ketones: Most UA dipsticks detect acetic acid; other products of fatty acid metabolism found in urine include acetone and beta-hydroxybutyric acid. Ketonuria indicates either metabolic disturbance such as diabetes mellitus or normal physiology in the fasting or lipolytic state. Many clinicians—particularly medical students and physicians[note 130]—have been taught to view ketonuria as synonymous with ketoacidosis; this is obviously inaccurate since lipolysis and the resulting ketonuria are normal *and quite desirable* physiologic states. Ketonuria can be measured with ketone-specific dipsticks as a marker of weight-loss efficacy and compliance with diet and exercise programs.

o Protein: Urine should not contain measurable protein on routine urinalysis. Any finding of protein in the urine—even a "trace" amount—requires follow-up; specifically, the test should be repeated within 2-4 weeks and consistently positive results require more detailed testing including serum BUN and creatinine. Urine protein can also be measured in 24-hour urine collections and should not exceed 150 mg/day; greater than this amount is diagnostic of proteinuria, while ≥ 3.5 gm/day is consistent with nephrotic syndrome, mandating a much more comprehensive *and urgent* patient evaluation. Testing for "protein" with a routine urinalysis will not detect all forms of clinically relevant proteinuria; specifically and classically, routine UA is insensitive for the microalbuminuria of diabetes mellitus (detected with the urinary albumin:creatinine ratio) and also the Bence-Jones proteinuria seen with multiple myeloma.

Evaluation of persistent proteinuria
1. Comprehensive evaluation of patient history, physical exam, and overall clinical impression,
2. Measurement of serum BUN, creatinine, albumin, and lipids; consider measuring cystatin c,
3. Microscopic examination of urinary sediment,
4. Assessment for conditions that commonly cause proteinuria, especially hypertension (sphygmomanometry), diabetes (hemoglobin A1c), autoimmune conditions (screen with ANA);
5. Measurement of 24-hour urinary creatinine excretion (or spot urinary albumin-creatinine ratio),
6. Urinary protein electrophoresis,
7. If the above measures are pathoetiologically unfruitful, refer to an internist or nephrologist.

---

[130] One of the arguments most commonly leveled against the ketogenic diet—in particular the Atkins diet—is that the induction of ketosis, as measured by ketonuria, is a potentially problematic state that should be avoided. This is an example of selective medical ignorance since mild ketosis is physiologically normal is clinically advantageous for weight loss and seizure control. In our osteopathic medical school, one lecturer advised our student body of 170 that ketosis was evidence of the "danger from diet therapies." On the contrary, given that most of my medical school professors were obese, they should have more carefully considered the benefits of rational dietary therapy, including low-carbohydrate versions of the Paleo-Mediterranean diet (described in this text) which can produce mild ketosis en route to alleviating diabetes mellitus and hypertension. Examples of selective medical ignorance and bias against low-carbohydrate ketogenic diets abound from allopathic institutions. "One diet that has raised safety concerns among the scientific community is the low-carbohydrate, high-protein diet." Tapper-Gardzina Y, Cotugna N, Vickery CE. Should you recommend a low-carb, high-protein diet? *Nurse Pract.* 2002 Apr;27(4):52-3, 55-6, 58-9. "High Protein / Low Carb (Carbohydrate) Diets. Long term, these fad diets can be harmful. Many of the health claims about these diets are not based on scientific proof. Low carb diets are still just that – a diet. Most people find maintaining a low carb diet difficult if not impossible long term. Even if weight is lost, 90% of fad dieters gain all or most of the weight back in five years." Ohio State University. http://medicalcenter.osu.edu/PatientEd/Materials/PDFDocs/nut-diet/nut-other/high-pro.pdf Accessed July 2011.

UA: Urinalysis—*continued*	
Overview and interpretation:	○ <u>Nitrite</u>: Urinary nit<u>ri</u>te is most often the result of bacterial action on excreted urinary nit<u>ra</u>te; students and clinicians can remember this by recalling that nit<u>ra</u>te is consumed in foods via the <u>a</u>limentary tract, while nit<u>ri</u>te in the urine generally indicates urinary tract <u>i</u>nfection (UTI). A small amount of nitrate is naturally present in some foods, including tap water, beer, some cheese products, cured meats and bacon. Additional environmental sources of nitrate include the nitrates that are intentionally added to foods as preservatives, those which are contaminants from nitrate-containing fertilizers, and those which are present in our polluted environment from pesticides and the manufacture of rubber and latex. Not all bacteria can convert nitrate to nitrite; generally, this reaction indicates the presence of Gram-negative rods such as *Escherichia coli*, the causative agent in the vast majority of UTIs in both men and women. Much less commonly, Gram-positive bacteria may also cause nitrite-positive UTI. A negative urine nitrite does not exclude UTI as it may be due to either a low-nitrate diet, diuretic use, or infection with bacteria that are incapable of reducing nitrate to nitrite. **UTI management** Finding evidence of a UTI requires the clinician to determine the nature of that UTI—urethritis, prostatitis/vaginitis, cystitis, pyelonephritis—and to evaluate the severity of the infection in the context of the patient's age and comorbidities. ○ <u>Leukocyte esterase</u>: Leukocyte esterase—as its name suggests—is an enzyme produced by white blood cells and is therefore associated with urinary tract infection. Up to five minutes is required for the enzyme to fully react with the dipstick reagent. Obviously, a positive dipstick leukocyte esterase does not itself distinguish between benign infectious cystitis and life-threatening pyelonephritis. ○ <u>Red blood cells (RBC)</u>: On a dipstick urinalysis (in contrast to a legitimate microscopic exam), "RBC" are reported not because of the presence of cells but because of the peroxidase activity of erythrocytes, which is also noted with myoglobinuria or hemoglobinuria. Thus, a dipstick analysis "positive for RBC" could indicate legitimate hematuria, or the presence of hemoglobin or myoglobin such as from marked intravascular hemolysis or rhabdomyolysis, respectively. Red blood cells in urine are not "normal" per se, but are not necessarily pathologic. Microhematuria can be induced by many benign events, including sexual intercourse, exercise, and sample contamination from menstruation. Conversely, pathologic causes of hematuria include urinary tract infections, glomerulonephritis, IgA nephropathy, and nephrolithiasis; overt hematuria **Overt hematuria and cancer** "Up to 20 percent of patients with gross hematuria have urinary tract malignancy; a full work-up with cystoscopy and upper-tract imaging is indicated in patients with this condition." Simerville JA, Maxted WC, Pahira JJ. Urinalysis: a comprehensive review. *Am Fam Physician*. 2005 Mar 15;71(6):1153-62 aafp.org/afp/2005/0315/p1153.html is often the first sign of renal or bladder carcinoma. Thus, when consistently present over 2-3 samples, overt or microscopic hematuria—just like any degree of proteinuria—always requires the clinician's attention.
Advantages:	▪ Allows point-of-care testing and thereby facilitates assessment and treatment.
Limitations:	▪ Noted above, e.g., insensitivity to microalbuminuria and mild Bence-Jones proteinuria
Comments:	▪ For additional information, please see any of several excellent clinically-oriented reviews such as Simerville JA, Maxted WC, Pahira JJ. Urinalysis: a comprehensive review. *Am Fam Physician* 2005 Mar http://www.aafp.org/afp/2005/0315/p1153.html

Presentation: Routine lab evaluation in an asymptomatic elderly female—part 1: Whereas a healthy young adult might be treated nonpharmacologically such as with fluid loading and cranberry juice for a routine UTI, clinicians should appreciate several nuances of this case that add to the complexity of appropriate management. This female patient presented for a routine annual examination. Note the patient's date of birth and the date of examination in the lower right-hand corner of the report. Because of the patient's advanced age, additional considerations are warranted. This patient was also noted to be vitamin D deficient and diabetic at the time of the exam—how does this change the overall management? Clinicians must appreciate that elderly patients are less likely to mount a symptomatic and febrile response to advanced urinary tract infections; therefore consideration to the possiblity of pyelonephritis (life-threatening) in contrast to a simple cystitis (benign) must be considered. If the patient has dementia or clinically significant forgetfulness (both of which are easily tested during the office visit), compliance with treatment is much less likely, particularly if the patient does not have access to home nursing and/or does not have a spouse, relative, friend or neighbor who can aid with the supervision of care. Urinary tract infections tend to be more aggressive in elderly patients, especially those who are diabetic, especially those with micronutrient deficiencies.

Questions:
1.   What additional assessments are warranted?
2.   Would fluid-loading and use of cranberry juice be appropriate treatment for this patient's UTI?
3.   What follow-up is recommended?

```
URINALYSIS              01/06/10
                        11:21
U COLOR                 YELLOW
U CLARITY               CLOUDY**
U GLUCOSE               NEGATIVE
U BILE                  NEGATIVE
U KETONES               NEGATIVE
U SPEC GRAVITY           1.012
U BLOOD                 NEGATIVE
U PH                     6.0
                        (NOTE06)
U PROTEIN QUAL           20**
U UROBILINOGEN           0.2
U NITRITE               NEGATIVE
U LEUK ESTERASE         MODERATE**
U WBC                   53*H
U WBCC                  RARE**
U RBC                    5*H
U SQUAM EPITH           13
U HYALINE CAST           2
U MUCOUS                RARE
(NOTE06)
URINE SAMPLES SUBMITTED FOR TESTING MORE THAN 2 HOURS AFTER COLLECTION MAY
YIELD UNRELIABLE RESULTS WHICH INCLUDE INCREASED pH, INCREASED CRYSTAL
FORMATION AND BACTERIAL CONTENT, AND DEGRADATION OF CELLULAR ELEMENTS.
```

          BDATE: 03/20/1926 SEX: F RACE:
          13:59 01/29/10

Answers:
1.   Assessments: Clinical examination must include cardiac auscultatory exam, careful pulmonary auscultation for basilar crackles, distal extremity examination for edema and peripheral vascular disease, assessment for tenderness of the flanks, abdomen, and back. Vital signs are assessed: ❶ temperature, ❷ pulse, ❸ blood pressure, ❹ respiratory rate, and ❺ pain. A chemistry panel, CBC with differential, and CRP or ESR should be performed. The urinalysis is sent for microbial culture and sensitivity. Review patient's current drug regimen. If WBC casts were noted on the microscopic exam, then suspected pyelonephritis would warrant hospitalization.
2.   Treatments: Fluid-loading would not be appropriate in an elderly patient who might have cardiopulmonary failure, renal insufficiency, or plasma electrolyte imbalance. Cranberry juice is not universally effective and is generally used for UTIs in younger patients who have evidence of *E coli* infection as evidenced by positive urinary nitrite; because this patient's nitrite is negative, a more likely probability exists that the UTI is due to Gram-positive bacteria and thus cranberry juice is less likely to be effective. A clinician could reasonably label this a complicated UTI due to the patient's advanced age and diabetes; thus, either an extended course of Bactrim DS (po b.i.d. for 7-10 days), or Ciprofloxacin (250-500 mg po b.i.d. for 3 days), or Nitrofurantoin (50-100 mg po q6h x7 days or 100 mg ER po q12h x7 days; give w/ food) would be considered. Drug choice depends on patient's tolerance, recent exposure, renal status, drugs, and results of culture and sensitivity.
3.   Follow-up: Review laboratory results as soon as possible; if this visit is occurring at the end of the week, the lab should be alerted to phone the clinician with results over the weekend because concomitant leukocytosis or severe acute phase response (suggesting possible pyelonephritis or urosepsis) would change the management on an urgent basis. Patient should return to the office within 24-48 hours for reassessment and repeat UA. Patient is advised to return to office or go to hospital if symptoms develop— especially fever, chills, dizziness, or persistent nausea.

Presentation: Routine laboratory evaluation in an asymptomatic elderly female—part 2: Readers should review the lab report in the left side of the page before reading the discussion on the right side of the page. *Write the appropriate interpretation and intervention before looking at the answers in the column on the right.* Normal ranges were not provided with the original report.

CBC	01/06/10
	11:21
WBC 10E3	7.50
NRBC %	0.0
NRBC 10E3	0.00
RBC 10E6	4.08*L
HGB	11.7*L
HCT	35.1*L
MCV	86.0
MCH	28.7
MCHC	33.3
RDW-CV	13.7
RDW-SD	43.1
PLATELET 10E3	175
MPV	12.3

CHEM PANEL	01/06/10
	11:21
SODIUM	140
POTASSIUM	4.2
CHLORIDE	102
CO2 VENOUS	27.0
GLUCOSE	248*H
BUN	22
SER CREATININE	1.2
CALCIUM	9.5
GLOBULIN	3.2
TOTAL PROTEIN	7.3
ALBUMIN TOT	4.1
BILI TOTAL	0.5
ALKALINE PHOSPHA	63
SGOT (AST)	15
CHOLESTEROL	186
	(NOTE01)
TRIGLYCERIDES	122
SGPT (ALT)	11
ANION GAP	11
OSMOLRTY CALC	291
BUN/CREAT	18.3
ALB/GLOB RATIO	1.30
HDL	31
	(NOTE02)
LDL CALC	131*H
	(NOTE03)

(NOTE01)
BORDERLINE HIGH RISK = 200-239
HIGH RISK = 240 AND ABOVE.
(NOTE02)
12-16 HR FASTING:
(NOTE03)
NORMAL = LESS THAN 130 MG/DL
130-159 BORDERLINE/HIGH RISK
>/= 160 HIGH RISK

CHEM SPECIAL	01/06/10
	11:21
HEMOGLOBIN A1C	7.6*H
	(NOTE04)
25-OHD TOTAL	29

BDATE: 03/20/1926 SEX: F
13:59 01/29/10 FROM E585

This patient is anemic. The anemia is not of a severity that would be expected to cause cardiopulmonary/perfusion deficits, but the patient should be assessed, particularly if he/she has history of heart failure or lung disease such as emphysema. The MCV is not elevated, nor is it low. This could be due to combined B-12/folate and iron deficiencies; the patient should be tested and treated appropriately. Assuming that the ferritin is low, what is the next mandatory step in the management of this patient? [Answer: Treat the iron deficiency with iron supplementation but be sure to refer the patient for gastrointestinal endoscopy because of the increased probability of intestinal lesion, especially colon cancer.]

This patient is diagnosed with diabetes mellitus because the glucose is above 200. Cardioprotective measures must be implemented, ophthalmologist eye exam initiated, and foot exam performed. An integrative anti-diabetes plan[131] should be implemented.

Clinicians must appreciate the importance of the MDRD equation in this case. The answer is provided below. Perform the Cockcroft-Gault equation on paper (with use of a calculator if necessary), then perform the MDRD equation. Does this change the management of this patient's UTI? Does this change the overall management of this patient? [Answer: This patient has renal insufficiency (GFR 48-55 if African-American and 42-45 if "other race") and therefore some drugs are now contraindicated. Patient is at increased risk of hyperkalemia, especially if taking ACEi or ARB medications. The wise clinician would consider referral to an internist or nephrologist in order to ensure that the patient receives proper monitoring; for example, if the diabetes and renal insufficiency progress, the patient may require dialysis and—possibly—renal transplant, although transplant is unlikely in a patient of this advanced age.][Note 132]

Triglycerides and LDL are higher than optimal. Diet therapy and combination fatty acid supplementation (described later in this text) is indicated. Berberine might be considered as an adjunct.

HgbA1c greater than 6.5% diagnoses diabetes mellitus.

The vitamin D level is low and should be supported with oral administration of 2,000 - 10,000 IU/d and retested at 2-6 months. Serum calcium should be tested after 2-4 weeks of therapy—sooner if the patient is taking a calcium-sparing drug such as hydrochlorothiazide—and again at about 6 and 12 months.

---

[131] Vasquez A. *Chiropractic and Naturopathic Mastery of Common Clinical Disorders*. http://InflammationMastery.com/clinical_mastery.html
[132] Review of this case by Dr Barry Morgan (MD, emergency medicine) is acknowledged and appreciated.

Presentation: 45yo HLA-B27+ woman with recurrent UTIs and a 7-year history of ankylosing spondylitis treated with anti-TNF drugs: Positive urine culture and positive stool culture demonstrating bacteria (*Escherichia coli* and *Klebsiella pneumoniae*) known to share molecular mimicry and cross-reactivity with HLA-B27: The Gram-negative bacterium *E. coli* produces a protein named "hypothetical protein 168" (Protein Identification Resource [PIR] data bank access code #jp0612) which shares the amino acid sequence "**RRYLE**" with HLA-B27, which contains the sequence "EWL**RRYLE**IGKETLQRVDP."[133] Per the same citation, *Klebsiella pneumoniae*'s protein (PIR s01840) nitrogenase (reductase) molybdenum-iron protein NifN contains the sequence "EWLRR." This amino acid homology confers validation to the phenomenon of molecular mimicry and thus that immune system components such as immunoglobulins and activated T-cells can cross-react between microbial peptides and human tissue antigens.[134] This patient was treated with the combination pharmaceutical antibiotic trimethoprim and sulfamethoxazole commonly referred to as "Bactrim DS" in addition to dietary optimization, hormonal optimization, and nutritional supplementation. Antimicrobial treatment with amoxicillin-clavulanate would have been reasonable, too, except for this patient's prior allergic reaction to the drug.

Urine Culture, Routine

Urine Culture, Routine   Final Report
Result 1
      Escherichia coli
      50,000-100,000 colony forming units per mL
Antimicrobial Susceptibility
      ***** S = Susceptible; I = Intermediate; R = Resistant *****
                P = Positive; N = Negative
            MICS are expressed in micrograms per mL

Antibiotic	RSLT#1
Amoxicillin/Clavulanic Acid	S
Ampicillin	S
Cefazolin	S
Cefepime	S
Ceftriaxone	S
Cefuroxime	S
Cephalothin	I
Ciprofloxacin	R
ESBL	N
Ertapenem	S
Gentamicin	S
Imipenem	S
Levofloxacin	R
Nitrofurantoin	S
Piperacillin	S
Tetracycline	S
Tobramycin	S
Trimethoprim/Sulfa	S

Comprehensive Stool Analysis / Parasitology x3

BACTERIOLOGY CULTURE

Expected/Beneficial flora	Commensal (Imbalanced) flora	Dysbiotic flora
4+ Bacteroides fragilis group	3+ Alpha hemolytic strep	3+ Klebsiella pneumoniae ssp pneumoniae
3+ Bifidobacterium spp.		
4+ Escherichia coli		
3+ Lactobacillus spp.		
NG Enterococcus spp.		
2+ Clostridium spp.		
NG = No Growth		

PRESCRIPTIVE AGENTS

	Resistant	Intermediate	Susceptible
Amoxicillin-Clavulanic Acid			S
Ampicillin	R		
Cefazolin			S
Ceftazidime			S
Ciprofloxacin			S
Trimeth-sulfa			S

Susceptible results imply that an infection due to the bacteria may be appropriately treated when the recommended dosage of the tested antimicrobial agent is used.
Intermediate results imply that response rates may be lower than for susceptible bacteria when the tested antimicrobial agent is used.
Resistant results imply that the bacteria will not be inhibited by normal dosage levels of the tested antimicrobial agent.

[133] Scofield RH, Warren WL, Koelsch G, Harley JB. A hypothesis for the HLA-B27 immune dysregulation in spondyloarthropathy: contributions from enteric organisms, B27 structure, peptides bound by B27, and convergent evolution. *Proc Natl Acad Sci U S A*. 1993 Oct 15;90(20):9330-4
[134] Rashid T, Ebringer A. Ankylosing spondylitis is linked to Klebsiella--the evidence. *Clin Rheumatol*. 2007 Jun;26(6):858-64

CRP: C-reactive protein	

Overview and interpretation:	▪ CRP is a protein made by the liver in response to the immunologic activation characteristic of infectious and inflammatory conditions. Generally, any tissue injury or inflammatory process especially that involves the immune system's increased production of IL-6 will result in increased production of CRP.[135] High sensitivity CRP (hsCRP) is preferred over regular CRP due to its greater sensitivity and use in assessing cardiovascular risk.
	
	▪ Elevated values are seen with:
	    ▪ <u>Infections</u>: Bacterial, fungal, parasitic, viral diseases; some patients with dysbiosis[136] will have mildly-moderately elevated CRP,
	    ▪ <u>Inflammatory bowel disease</u>: Crohn's disease and ulcerative colitis (higher in CD than UC),
	    ▪ <u>Autoimmune disease</u>: Rheumatoid arthritis, polymyalgia rheumatica, giant cell arteritis, polyarteritis nodosa, (not always SLE),
	    ▪ <u>Acute myocardial infarction or other tissue ischemia</u>
	    ▪ <u>Organ transplant rejection</u>: Renal, (not cardiac),
	    ▪ <u>Trauma</u>: Burns, surgery,
	    ▪ <u>Obesity</u>: Leads to modest elevations in CRP.

Advantages:	▪ This is an excellent screening test for differentiating "serious problems" (e.g., inflammatory and infectious arthropathy) from "benign problems" such as osteoarthritis. ▪ Since higher values of CRP are a well-recognized risk factor for cardiovascular disease, screening "musculoskeletal patients" with hsCRP provides data for cardiovascular risk assessment and a more comprehensive and holistic treatment approach, thus bridging the gap between acute care and preventive care.
Limitations:	▪ Elevations in CRP are completely nonspecific, requiring clinical investigation to determine the underlying cause of the immune activation. ▪ CRP may be normal in some patients with severe systemic diseases (such as lupus or cancer), and therefore a normal CRP does not entirely exclude the presence of significant illness.
Comments:	▪ Writing in *The New England Journal of Medicine*, authors Gabay and Kushner[137] note that measurements of plasma or serum **C-reactive protein can help differentiate inflammatory from non-inflammatory conditions and are useful in managing the patient's disease, since "the concentration often reflects the response to and the need for therapeutic intervention."** Additionally, they note, "Most normal subjects have plasma C-reactive protein concentrations of 2 mg per liter or less, but some have concentrations as high as 10 mg per liter." Deodhar[138] noted that **"Any clinical disease characterized by tissue injury and/or inflammation is accompanied by significant elevation of serum CRP…"** and that **CRP should replace ESR as a method of laboratory evaluation.** Deodhar also noted that **some patients with severe SLE will have normal CRP levels.**

[135] Deodhar SD. C-reactive protein: the best laboratory indicator available for monitoring disease activity. *Cleve Clin J Med* 1989 Mar-Apr;56(2):126-30

[136] See chapter 4 of *Integrative Rheumatology* and Vasquez A. Reducing Pain and Inflammation Naturally. Part 6: Nutritional and Botanical Treatments Against "Silent Infections" and Gastrointestinal Dysbiosis, Commonly Overlooked Causes of Neuromusculoskeletal Inflammation and Chronic Health Problems. *Nutr Perspect* 2006; Jan http://InflammationMastery.com/part6.html

[137] Gabay C, Kushner I. Acute-phase proteins and other systemic responses to inflammation. *N Engl J Med.* 1999 Feb 11;340(6):448-54

[138] Deodhar SD. C-reactive protein: the best laboratory indicator available for monitoring disease activity. *Cleve Clin J Med* 1989 Mar-Apr;56(2):126-30

Presentation: Elevated hsCRP (high-sensitivity c-reactive protein) in a male patient with metabolic syndrome and rheumatoid arthritis—response to treatment protocol in *Integrative Rheumatology*: This 52-year-old male patient presented with a 4-year history of rheumatoid arthritis which was unresponsive to prednisone and anti-TNF (tumor necrosis factor alpha) drugs, ie, "biologics." As expected, the prednisone exacerbated the patient's insulin resistance and hypertension; the drug failed to produce an anti-inflammatory benefit for this patient. At a cost of several thousand dollars per treatment, the anti-TNF "biologic" drugs failed to provide any benefit. At the intial visit in July 2005, the hsCRP level was 124 mg/L (normal range 0-3 mg/L), as shown in these lab results.

DATE OF SPECIMEN	TIME	DATE RECEIVED	DATE REPORTED	TIME		Houston	TX	77036-0000
7/08/2005	16:19	7/08/2005	7/11/2005	7:38	419	ACCOUNT NUMBER: 42407150		

TEST	RESULT	LIMITS	LAB
C-Reactive Protein, Cardiac			
> C-Reactive Protein, Cardiac	124.00H mg/L	0.00 - 3.00	HD

Relative Risk for Future Cardiovascular Event
Low	<1.00
Average	1.00 - 3.00
High	>3.00

The patient was treated with the protocol outlined in Chapter 4 of *Integrative Rheumatology*.[139] Stool testing showed *Citrobacter freundii* (renamed *Citrobacter rodentium*) which was addressed with botanical medicines; the insufficiency dysbiosis was also corrected per the five-part protocol. Slightly low testosterone and slightly elevated estradiol was optimized with a pharmaceutical aromatase inhibitor (Arimidex) given twice weekly. The five-part nutritional wellness protocol (supplemented Paleo-Mediterranean diet [SPMD]) was implemented.[140]

Comprehensive Parasitology, stool, x2

MICROBIOLOGY

Bacteriology Culture

Beneficial flora		Imbalances		Dysbiotic flora	
Bifidobacter	0+	Gamma strep	1+	Citrobacter freundii	1+
E. coli	2+	Enterobacter sp.	1+		
Lactobacillus	0+				

Mycology (Yeast) Culture

Normal flora	Dysbiotic flora
No yeast isolated	

PARASITOLOGY

	Sample 1		Sample 2
No	Ova or Parasites	No	Ova or Parasites

No anti-inflammatory drugs or botanicals were used. Within five weeks of treatment, the patient's hsCRP dropped from 124 mg/L to 7.58 mg/L—a reduction of approximately 95%—far superior to any previoius response to corticosteroid and biologic drugs. Patient experienced significant alleviation of pain and improved mobility.

8/17/2005	11:06	8/18/2005	8/18/2005	12:32	738	ACCOUNT NUMBER: 42407150

TEST	RESULT	LIMITS	LAB
C-Reactive Protein, Cardiac			
C-Reactive Protein, Cardiac	7.58H mg/L	0.00 - 3.00	HD

[139] Vasquez A. *Integrative Rheumatology*. http://InflammationMastery.com/textbooks/rheumatology.html
[140] Vasquez A. Revisiting the Five-Part Nutritional Wellness Protocol. *Nutritional Perspectives* 2011 January http://InflammationMastery.com/spmd.html

ESR: erythrocyte sedimentation rate	

Overview and interpretation:	• Values may be elevated even when no pathology is present because ESR increases with anemia and with age.
	• Much more sensitive than WBC count when screening for infection.[141]
	• May be normal in about 10% of patients who have pathology such as **giant cell arteritis** and **polymyalgia rheumatica** (conditions where it is generally the only lab abnormality, besides anemia); may also be normal in several other diseases.
	• **May be normal in patients with septic arthritis and patients with crystal-induced arthritis: joint aspiration for synovial fluid analysis is indicated if septic arthritis is suspected.**[142]
	• Increased with age, anemia, inflammation; higher in women than men. Age-adjusted normal ranges: any value over 25 is considered high in young people, or 40 in elderly women.
	• Age-related adjustments for men and women are as follows:
	    • Men: age divided by 2
	    • Women: (age + 10) divided by 2

Advantages:	• Inexpensive and easy to perform—use the same lavender-topped tube that you use for CBC. • Provides a quick screen for infection, inflammation, and multiple myeloma—the most common primary bone tumor in adults. • In patients with elevated levels, ESR can be used to monitor progression of disease and response to treatment.[143] However, a negative/normal test result does not exclude the presence of significant disease; some noteworthy examples include the following: 1) elderly—due to diminished ability to mount an inflammatory response, 2) patients taking anti-inflammatory drugs and immunosuppressants, 3) a significant proportion of patients with lupus will have normal ESR despite aggressive disease, and 4) some cancer patients with clinically significant tumor burden will not show signs of systemic inflammation. • ESR may be more reliable than CRP for multiple myeloma.[144]
Limitations:	• ESR may be normal in a subset of patients with clinically significant infection or inflammation. • Values are elevated in the elderly and patients with anemia and are thus not necessarily indicative of disease in these populations.
Comments:	• This test is generally considered *outdated* and has been replaced in most circumstances by CRP for the evaluation of inflammation and infection. • The only time I use this test clinically is when I am highly suspicious of inflammation and the CRP is normal. Further, this test may be preferred when assessing for temporal arteritis and for multiple myeloma, two conditions which are classically associated with elevated ESR.

[141] Shaw BA, Gerardi JA, Hennrikus WL. How to avoid orthopedic pitfalls in children. *Patient Care* 1999; Feb 28: 95-116

[142] Klippel JH (ed). Primer on the Rheumatic Diseases. 11th Edition. Atlanta: Arthritis Foundation. 1997 page 94

[143] Shojania K. Rheumatology: 2. What laboratory tests are needed? *CMAJ.* 2000 Apr 18;162(8):1157-63 http://www.cmaj.ca/cgi/content/full/162/8/1157

[144] "We conclude that ESR, a simple and easily performed marker, was found to be an independent prognostic factor for survival in patients with multiple myeloma." Alexandrakis MG, Passam FH, Ganotakis ES, Sfiridaki K, Xilouri I, Perisinakis K, Kyriakou DS. The clinical and prognostic significance of erythrocyte sedimentation rate (ESR), serum interleukin-6 (IL-6) and acute phase protein levels in multiple myeloma. *Clin Lab Haematol.* 2003;25:41-6

Ferritin	
Overview and interpretation:	▪ Ferritin levels are directly proportional to body iron stores, except in patients with inflammation, infection, hepatitis, or cancer. Therefore, measuring ferritin allows assessment for iron deficiency (a cause of fatigue, or early manifestation of GI cancer) and allows for assessment of iron overload (as a cause of joint pain and arthropathy). This test should be performed in all African Americans[145,146], white men over age 30 years[147], diabetics[148], and patients with peripheral arthropathy[149], and exercise-associated joint pain[150,151] The research also justifies testing children[152], women[153], young adults[154] and the general asymptomatic public.[155] ▪ Low ferritin = iron deficiency ▪ High ferritin = iron overload, cancer, inflammation, infection, and/or hepatitis (viral, alcoholic, or toxic)
Advantages:	▪ Reliable screening test for iron overload when used in conjunction with patient assessment and evidence (e.g., normal CRP) of no infection or acute phase response. ▪ This is the blood test of choice for iron deficiency *and* iron overload.
Limitations:	▪ Iron-deficient patients with an acute phase response may have a falsely normal level of ferritin since ferritin is an acute phase reactant and will be elevated *disproportionate to iron status* during inflammation. ▪ Elevations of ferritin (i.e., >200 mcg/L in women and >300 mcg/L in men) need to be retested along with CRP (to rule out false elevation due to excessive inflammation) before making the presumptive diagnosis of iron overload. **In the absence of significant inflammation, ferritin values >200 mcg/L in women and >300 mcg/L in men indicate iron overload and the need for treatment regardless of the absence of symptoms or end-stage complications.**[156]
Comments:	▪ Note that since ferritin is an acute-phase reactant, a high level of serum ferritin by itself does not allow differentiation between iron overload, infection, and the inflammation associated with tissue injury or metastatic disease. Ferritin must be evaluated within the context of the patient's clinical condition and the assessment of at least one other marker for inflammation such as CRP. If the patient is not acutely ill or has not recently suffered tissue injury (e.g., myocardial infarction) and the CRP is normal, then an elevated ferritin value indicates iron overload until proven otherwise with diagnostic phlebotomy, which is safer and less expensive than liver biopsy or MRI. Transferrin saturation can also be measured when the interpretation of ferritin is unclear. By itself, serum iron is unreliable.

[145] Barton JC, Edwards CQ, Bertoli LF, Shroyer TW, Hudson SL. Iron overload in African Americans. *Am J Med.* 1995 Dec;99(6):616-23

[146] Wurapa RK, Gordeuk VR, Brittenham GM, et al. Primary iron overload in African Americans. *Am J Med.* 1996;101(1):9-18

[147] Baer DM, Simons JL, et al. Hemochromatosis screening in asymptomatic ambulatory men 30 years of age and older. *Am J Med.* 1995 May;98:464-8

[148] Phelps G, Chapman I, Hall P, Braund W, Mackinnon M. Prevalence of genetic haemochromatosis among diabetic patients. *Lancet* 1989; 2: 233-4

[149] Olynyk J, Hall P, Ahern M, KwiatekR, MackinnonM. Screening for hemochromatosis in a rheumatology clinic. *Aust NZ J Med* 1994; 24: 22-5

[150] McCurdie I, Perry JD. Haemochromatosis and exercise related joint pains. *BMJ.* 1999 Feb 13;318(7181):449-5

[151] "RESULTS: Our findings indicate a high prevalence of HFE gene mutations in this population (49.2%) compared with sedentary controls (33.5%). No association was detected in the athletes between mutations and blood iron markers. CONCLUSIONS: The findings support the need to assess regularly iron stores in elite endurance athletes." Chicharro JL, Hoyos J, Gomez-Gallego F, et al. Mutations in the hereditary haemochromatosis gene HFE in professional endurance athletes. *Br J Sports Med.* 2004 Aug;38(4):418-21. Erratum in: *Br J Sports Med.* 2004 Dec;38(6):793 http://bjsm.bmjjournals.com/cgi/content/full/38/4/418 Accessed September 12, 2005

[152] Kaikov Y, Wadsworth LD, Hassall E, Dimmick JE, Rogers PCJ. Primary hemochromatosis in children: report of three newly diagnosed cases and review of the pediatric literature. *Pediatrics* 1992; 90: 37-42

[153] Edwards CQ, Kushner JP. Screening for hemochromatosis. *N Engl J Med* 1993; 328: 1616-20

[154] Gushusrt TP, Triest WE. Diagnosis and management of precirrhotic hemochromatosis. *W Virginia Med J* 1990; 86: 91-5

[155] Balan V, et al. Screening for hemochromatosis: a cost-effectiveness study based on 12, 258 patients. *Gastroenterology* 1994; 107: 453-9

[156] Barton JC, McDonnell SM, Adams PC, Brissot P, Powell LW, Edwards CQ, Cook JD, Kowdley K V. Management of hemochromatosis. Hemochromatosis Management Working Group. *Ann Intern Med.* 1998 Dec 1;129(11):932-9—one of the best papers ever written on this topic.

Ferritin—*Interpretation of serum levels*

Ferritin	Categorization and management
≥ 800 mcg/L	<u>Practically diagnostic of iron overload</u>[157]: Repeat tests; rule out inflammation or occult pathology. Initiate phlebotomy and consider liver biopsy or MRI.
≥ 300 mcg/L	<u>Probable iron overload</u>[158]: Repeat tests; rule out inflammation or occult pathology. In men, initiate phlebotomy and consider liver biopsy or MRI.[159]
≥ 200 mcg/L	*In women*: <u>Suggestive of iron overload</u>[160]: Repeat tests, rule out inflammation or occult pathology. In women, initiate phlebotomy and consider liver biopsy or MRI.[161] *In men*: <u>High-normal *unhealthy* iron status with increased risk of myocardial infarction</u>[162]: Rule out inflammation or occult pathology. No follow-up is mandated, yet blood donation and/or abstention from dietary iron are recommended preventative healthcare measures.
≥ 160 mcg/L	*In women*: <u>Abnormal iron status</u>[163]: Repeat tests, rule out inflammation or occult pathology. Consider phlebotomy and liver biopsy or MRI.
≥80-120 mcg/L	<u>High-normal unhealthy iron status</u>[164,165]: No follow-up is mandated; blood donation and abstention from dietary iron are suggested preventative healthcare measures. A subset of patients with restless leg syndrome (RLS, a condition also causally associated with intestinal bacterial overgrowth dysbiosis) have impaired transport of iron into the brain and therefore require slightly elevated ferritin/iron levels (up to 120) to enhance cerebral iron uptake.
40-70 mcg/L	**Optimal iron status for most people**[166,167]
< 20 mcg/L	<u>Iron deficiency</u>: Search for occult gastrointestinal blood loss with endoscopy or imaging assessments in adults; refer to gastroenterologist.[168,169]

Ferritin is an acute-phase reactant, which means that its production is increased during the acute phase of inflammatory and/or infectious disorders. Therefore the numeric value and hence its clinical meaning can be interpreted only within a context that also includes assessment of the patient's inflammatory status, which is best assessed with either ESR or CRP. If CRP/ESR is high, then the physician might assume that the ferritin value is "falsely elevated"—disproportionately elevated with respect to body iron stores. *Common clinical examples requiring use and skillful interpretation of ferritin*:

- **Elderly or arthritic patient with iron deficiency despite normal serum ferritin**: An elderly patient with normal ferritin and elevated CRP/ESR is probably iron deficient; retesting of ferritin and measurement of transferrin saturation and CBC should be performed promptly. If iron deficiency is confirmed or cannot be excluded, referral for endoscopic examination must be implemented. In a patient with known inflammatory arthropathy, the ferritin may appear normal even though the patient is iron deficient and in need of supplementation and endoscopy.
- **Non-anemic iron deficiency**: A middle-aged patient (commonly a premenopausal woman) presents with fatigue and during the course of evaluation is found to have a normal CBC. **Do not let a normal CBC prevent you from assessing ferritin; many of these patients are completely iron deficient with ferritin values of 2-6 mcg/L and are in need of iron replacement as well as evaluation for celiac disease, *H. pylori* infection, hematuria, and—as is often warranted—gastrointestinal bleeding/lesions.**

[157] Milman N, Albeck MJ. Distinction between homozygous and heterozygous subjects with hemochromatosis using iron status markers and receiver operating characteristic (ROC) analysis. *Eur J Clin Biochem* 1995; 33: 95-8. See also Milman N. Iron status markers in hereditary hemochromatosis: distinction between individuals being homozygous and heterozygous for the hemochromatosis allele. *Eur J Haematol* 1991;47:292-8

[158] Olynyk JK, Bacon BR. Hereditary hemochromatosis: detecting and correcting iron overload. *Postgrad Med* 1994;96: 151-65

[159] "Therapeutic phlebotomy is used to remove excess iron and maintain low normal body iron stores, ... initiated in men with serum ferritin levels of 300 microg/L or more and in women with serum ferritin levels of 200 microg/L or more, regardless of the presence or absence of symptoms." Barton JC, McDonnell SM, Adams PC, Brissot P, Powell LW, Edwards CQ, Cook JD, Kowdley KV. Management of hemochromatosis. Hemochromatosis Management Working Group. *Ann Intern Med*. 1998 Dec 1;129(11):932-9

[160] Barton JC, Edwards CQ, Bertoli LF, Shroyer TW, Hudson SL. Iron overload in African Americans. *Am J Med* 1995; 99: 616-23

[161] Barton JC, McDonnell SM, Adams PC, et al. Management of hemochromatosis. *Ann Intern Med*. 1998 Dec 1;129(11):932-9

[162] Salonen JT, Nyyssonen K, Korpela H,et al. High stored iron levels are associated with excess risk of myocardial infarction in eastern Finnish men. *Circulation* 1992; 86: 803-11

[163] Nicoll D. Therapeutic drug monitoring and laboratory reference ranges. In: Tierney LM, McPhee SJ, Papadakis MA. *Current Medical Diagnosis and Treatment 1996 (35th Edition)*. Stamford: Appleton and Lange, 1996: 1442

[164] Lauffer, RB. *Iron and Your Heart*. New York: St. Martin's Press, 1991: 79-8, 83-88, 162

[165] Sullivan JL. Iron and the sex difference in heart disease risk. *Lancet*. 1981 Jun 13;1(8233):1293-4

[166] Lauffer, RB. *Iron and Your Heart*. New York: St. Martin's Press, 1991: 79-8, 83-88, 162

[167] Vasquez A. High body iron stores: causes, effects, diagnosis, and treatment. *Nutritional Perspectives* 1994; 17: 13, 15-7, 19, 21, 28 and Vasquez A. Men's Health: Iron in men: why men store this nutrient in their bodies and the harm that it does. *MEN Magazine* 1997; Jan:11,21-23 vix.com/menmag/alexiron.htm

[168] Rockey DC, Cello JP. Evaluation of the gastrointestinal tract in patients with iron-deficiency anemia. *N Engl J Med*. 1993;329(23):1691-5

[169] "Endoscopy revealed a clinically important lesion in 23 (12%) of 186 patients. ... CONCLUSIONS: Endoscopy yields important findings in premenopausal women with iron deficiency anemia, which should not be attributed solely to menstrual blood loss." Bini EJ, Micale PL, Weinshel EH. Evaluation of the gastrointestinal tract in premenopausal women with iron deficiency anemia. *Am J Med*. 1998 Oct;105(4):281-6

Arthritis & Rheumatism

Official Journal of the American College of Rheumatology

VOLUME 39   OCTOBER 1996   NO. 10

1767   1768

Musculoskeletal disorders and iron overload disease: comment on the American College of Rheumatology guidelines for the initial evaluation of the adult patient with acute musculoskeletal symptoms

To the Editor:

The recent clinical guidelines for the initial evaluation of the adult patient with acute musculoskeletal symptoms, proposed by the American College of Rheumatology (1), provide useful information and a good review for clinicians. However, there is one important omission in these guidelines. Nowhere in the guidelines is hemochromatosis mentioned. Such a prevalent and potentially life-threatening disease certainly deserves to be considered in the evaluation of patients with musculoskeletal disorders.

Hereditary hemochromatosis is now thought to be the most common genetic disorder in the white population (2). Approximately 1 in 250 persons is homozygous for this disorder and will develop the characteristic clinical manifestations such as diabetes, cardiomyopathy, liver disease, endocrine dysfunction, and, most notable for this discussion, arthropathy or other musculoskeletal disorders (2). Although hereditary iron overload disorders have traditionally been thought of as occurring exclusively in whites, recent research by Barton et al (3) indicates that approximately 1 in 67 African-Americans is affected by an etiologically distinct and severe form of iron overload. Hereditary iron overload disorders have been detected in persons of every ethnic background.

Arthropathy affects up to 80% of iron-overloaded patients and is often the only manifestation of this disease (4). Joint pain is a common and early symptom of iron overload, and "bone pain" has also been described as a common initial complaint (5). Clinically and radiographically, hemochromatoic arthropathy can resemble osteoarthritis, calcium pyrophosphate dihydrate deposition disease, pseudogout, rheumatoid arthritis, ankylosing spondylitis, or generalized osteopenia with osteoporotic fractures (4,6,7). Since iron overload can cause such a wide array of musculoskeletal manifestations and because definitive clinical differentiation of iron overload from other arthropathies is very difficult, patients with peripheral arthropathy should be screened for iron overload. Indeed, recent research by Olynyk et al (8) indicates that the prevalence of iron overload is 5 times higher in patients with peripheral arthropathy than in the general population. Therefore, screening of patients with peripheral arthropathy for the possible presence of iron overload is justified.

Thus, since iron overload affects such a large portion of the population and arthropathy is a common manifestation of this disorder, patients with musculoskeletal symptoms should be screened for iron overload (4,8). The current literature suggests that everyone should be screened for iron overload even if there are no symptoms (8–10).

Alex Vasquez, DC
Seattle, WA

1. American College of Rheumatology Ad Hoc Committee on Clinical Guidelines: Guidelines for the initial evaluation of the adult patient with acute musculoskeletal symptoms. Arthritis Rheum 39:1–8, 1996
2. Olynyk JK, Bacon BR: Hereditary hemochromatosis: detecting and correcting iron overload. Postgrad Med 96:151–165, 1994
3. Barton JC, Edwards CQ, Bertoli LF, Shroyer TW, Hudson SL: Iron overload in African Americans. Am J Med 99:616–623, 1995
4. Faraawi R, Harth M, Kertesz A, Bell D: Arthritis in hemochromatosis. J Rheumatol 20:448–452, 1993
5. Adams PC, Kertesz AE, Valberg LS: Clinical presentation of hemochromatosis: a changing scene. Am J Med 90:445–449, 1991
6. Bywaters EGL, Hamilton EBD, Williams R: The spine in idiopathic hemochromatosis. Ann Rheum Dis 30:453–465, 1971
7. Eyres KS, McCloskey EV, Fern ED, Rogers S, Beneton M, Aaron JE, Kanis JA: Osteoporotic fractures: an unusual presentation of hemochromatosis. Bone 13:431–433, 1992
8. Olynyk J, Hall P, Ahern M, Kwiatek R, Mackinnon M: Screening for hemochromatosis in a rheumatology clinic. Aust N Z J Med 24:22–25, 1994
9. Baer DM, Simmons JL, Staples RL, Runmore GJ, Morton CJ: Hemochromatosis screening in asymptomatic ambulatory men 30 years of age and older. Am J Med 98:464–468, 1995
10. Adams PC, Gregor JC, Kertesz AE, Valberg LS: Screening blood donors for hereditary hemochromatosis: decision analysis model based on a 30-year database. Gastroenterology 109:177–188, 1995

Vasquez A. Musculoskeletal disorders and iron overload disease: comment on the American College of Rheumatology guidelines for the initial evaluation of the adult patient with acute musculoskeletal symptoms. *Arthritis Rheum*. 1996 Oct;39(10):1767-8 http://www.ncbi.nlm.nih.gov/pubmed/8843875

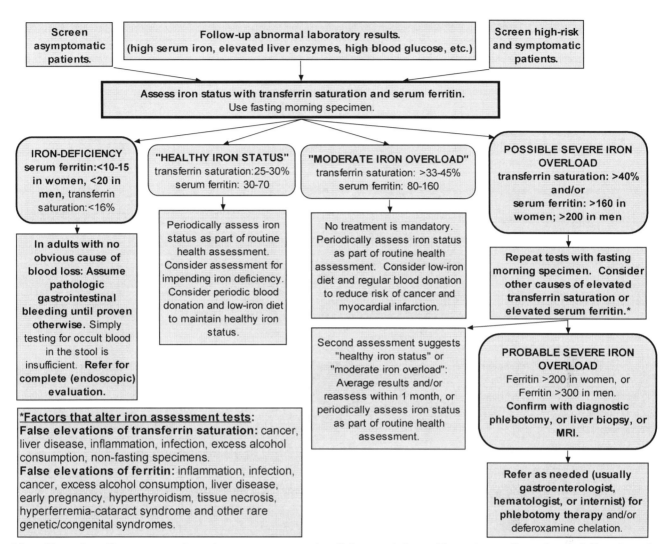

Algorithm for the comprehensive management of iron status: The above flow-chart delineates the management of high-moderate-healthy-low iron status.

Basic treatments for severe iron overload:

- **Iron-removal therapy is mandatory**: Phlebotomy therapy is generally performed weekly or twice-weekly; deferoxamine chelation is reserved for patients who do not withstand phlebotomy (due to cardiomyopathy, severe anemia, or hypoproteinemia) or may be used concurrently with phlebotomy in some patients. Periodically assess hematologic and iron indexes. Continue with weekly iron removal therapy until patient reaches mild iron-deficiency anemia, then decrease frequency and continue phlebotomy as needed (e.g., 4 times per year).
- **Laboratory tests and physical examination**: Assess general physical condition and hepatic, cardiac, endocrine, and general health status.
- **Confirm diagnosis**: Liver biopsy ("gold standard") or diagnostic phlebotomy; perhaps MRI.
- **Assess liver status**: Liver biopsy or perhaps MRI. Cirrhosis indicates increased risk of hepatocellular carcinoma and reduced life expectancy. Consider liver ultrasound, serum liver enzyme measurement, and serum alpha-fetoprotein to screen for hepatocellular carcinoma every 6 months. Hepatoma surveillance is mandatory in cirrhotic patients.
- **Implement dietary modifications and nutritional therapies**: Avoid iron supplements, multivitamin supplements with iron, iron-fortified foods, liver, beef, pork, alcohol, and excess vitamin C. Ensure adequate protein intake to replace protein lost during phlebotomy. Diet modifications are not substitutes for iron removal therapy. Consider antioxidant therapy.
- **Screen all blood relatives of patients with primary iron overload**. *Mandatory!*
- **Monitor patient condition, and compliance** with lifelong phlebotomy therapy
- **Assess and address psychoemotional issues/concerns**

25(OH)D: serum 25(OH) vitamin D

Overview and interpretation:	▪ **Vitamin D deficiency is a common cause of musculoskeletal pain**[170,171,172], and vitamin D deficiency is a significant risk factor for cancer, autoimmunity, diabetes, mental illness, chronic pain and physical disability.[173,174,175] ▪ Measurement of serum 25(OH) vitamin D (or empiric treatment with 2,000 – 10,000 IU vitamin D3 per day for adults) is indicated in patients with chronic musculoskeletal pain, particularly low-back pain.[176] Optimal vitamin D status correlates with serum 25(OH)D levels of 50 – 100 ng/mL (125 - 250 nmol/L)—see our review article for more details[177]; levels greater than 100 ng/mL are unnecessary and increase the risk of hypercalcemia. 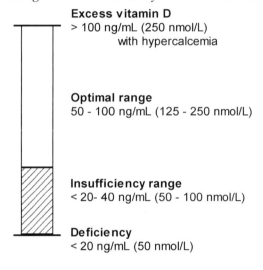 **Interpretation of serum 25(OH) vitamin D levels**. Modified from Vasquez et al, *Alternative Therapies in Health and Medicine* 2004 and Vasquez A. <u>*Musculoskeletal Pain: Expanded Clinical Strategies*</u> (Institute for Functional Medicine) 2008.
Advantages:	▪ Accurate assessment of vitamin D status.
Limitations:	▪ Patients with certain granulomatous conditions such as sarcoidosis or Crohn's disease and patients taking certain drugs such as thiazide diuretics (hydrochlorothiazide) can develop hypercalcemia due to "vitamin D hypersensitivity" or drug side effects—these patients require frequent monitoring of serum calcium while taking vitamin D supplements.
Comments:	▪ **Routine measurement and/or empiric treatment with vitamin D3 needs to become a routine component of patient care.**[178] ▪ Periodic assessment of 25(OH)D and serum calcium are required to ensure effectiveness and safety of treatment, respectively. ▪ I'm increasingly convinced of the merit of measuring 1,25-dihydroxyvitamin D3, at least for the initial assessment of patients with inflammatory/autoimmune/dysbiotic conditions.

[170] Masood H, Narang AP, Bhat IA, Shah GN. Persistent limb pain and raised serum alkaline phosphatase the earliest markers of subclinical hypovitaminosis D in Kashmir. *Indian J Physiol Pharmacol.* 1989 Oct-Dec;33(4):259-61

[171] Al Faraj S, Al Mutairi K. Vitamin D deficiency and chronic low back pain in Saudi Arabia. *Spine.* 2003 Jan 15;28(2):177-9

[172] Plotnikoff GA, Quigley JM. Prevalence of severe hypovitaminosis D in patients with persistent, nonspecific musculoskeletal pain. *Mayo Clin Proc.* 2003 Dec;78(12):1463-70

[173] Grant WB. An estimate of premature cancer mortality in the U.S. due to inadequate doses of solar ultraviolet-B radiation. *Cancer* 2002;94(6):1867-75

[174] Zittermannn A. Vitamin D in preventive medicine: are we ignoring the evidence? *Br J Nutr.* 2003 May;89(5):552-72

[175] Holick MF. Vitamin D: importance in the prevention of cancers, type 1 diabetes, heart disease, and osteoporosis. *Am J Clin Nutr.* 2004;79(3):362-71

[176] Al Faraj S, Al Mutairi K. Vitamin D deficiency and chronic low back pain in Saudi Arabia. *Spine.* 2003 Jan 15;28(2):177-9

[177] Vasquez A, Manso G, Cannell J. The Clinical Importance of Vitamin D (Cholecalciferol): A Paradigm Shift with Implications for All Healthcare Providers. *Alternative Therapies in Health and Medicine* 2004; 10: 28-37 http://InflammationMastery.com/cholecalciferol.html

[178] Heaney RP. Vitamin D, nutritional deficiency, and the medical paradigm. *J Clin Endocrinol Metab.* 2003;88:5107-8 http://jcem.endojournals.org/cgi/content/full/88/11/5107

CME
CONTINUING MEDICAL EDUCATION

THE CLINICAL IMPORTANCE OF VITAMIN D (CHOLECALCIFEROL): A PARADIGM SHIFT WITH IMPLICATIONS FOR ALL HEALTHCARE PROVIDERS

Alex Vasquez, DC, ND, Gilbert Manso, MD, John Cannell, MD

Alex Vasquez, DC, ND is a licensed naturopathic physician in Washington and Oregon, and licensed chiropractic doctor in Texas, where he maintains a private practice and is a member of the Research Team at Biotics Research Corporation. He is a former Adjunct Professor of Orthopedics and Rheumatology for the Naturopathic Medicine Program at Bastyr University. **Gilbert Manso**, MD, is a medical doctor practicing integrative medicine in Houston, Texas. In prac-tice for more than 35 years, he is Board Certified in Family Practice and is Associate Professor of Family Medicine at University of Texas Medical School in Houston. **John Cannell**, MD, is a medical physician practicing in Atascadero, California, and is president of the Vitamin D Council (Cholecalciferol-Council.com), a non-profit, tax-exempt organization working to promote awareness of the manifold adverse effects of vitamin D deficiency.

InnoVision Communications is accredited by the Accreditation Council for Continuing Medical Education to provide continuing medical education for physicians. The learner should study the article and its figures or tables, if any, then complete the self-evaluation at the end of the activity. The activity and self-evaluation are expected to take a maximum of 2 hours.

OBJECTIVES

Upon completion of this article, participants should be able to do the following:

1. Appreciate and identify the manifold clinical presentations and consequences of vitamin D deficiency
2. Identify patient groups that are predisposed to vitamin D hypersensitivity
3. Know how to implement vitamin D supplementation in proper doses and with appropriate laboratory monitoring

Reprint requests: InnoVision Communications, 169 Saxony Rd. Suite 103, Encinitas, CA 92024; phone, (760) 633-3910 or (866) 828-2962; fax, (760) 633-3918; e-mail, alternative.therapies@ innerdoorway.com. Or visit our online CME Web site by going to http://www.alternative -therapies.com and selecting the Continuing Education option.

While we are all familiar with the important role of vitamin D in calcium absorption and bone metabolism, many doctors and patients are not aware of the recent research on vitamin D and the widening range of therapeutic applications available for cholecalciferol, which can be classified as both a vitamin and a pro-hormone. Additionally, we also now realize that the Food and Nutrition Board's previously defined Upper Limit (UL) for safe intake at 2,000 IU/day was set far too low and that the physiologic requirement for vitamin D in adults may be as high as 5,000 IU/day, which is less than half of the >10,000 IU that can be produced endogenously with full-body sun exposure.[1,2] With the discovery of vitamin D receptors in tissues other than the gut and bone—especially the brain, breast, prostate, and lymphocytes—and the recent research suggesting that higher vitamin D levels provide protection from diabetes mellitus, osteoporosis, osteoarthritis, hypertension, cardiovascular disease, metabolic syndrome, depression, several autoimmune diseases, and cancers of the breast, prostate, and colon, we can now utilize vitamin D for a wider range of preventive and therapeutic applications to maintain and improve our patients' health.[3] Based on the research reviewed in this article, the current authors believe that assessment of vitamin D status and treatment of vita-

Vasquez A, Manso G, Cannell J. The clinical importance of vitamin D (cholecalciferol): a paradigm shift with implications for all healthcare providers. *Altern Ther Health Med* 2004 Sep-Oct;10:28-36: This article indexed on Medline at http://www.ncbi.nlm.nih.gov/pubmed/15478784 and is available widely on the internet, specifically www.ICHNFM.ORG/faculty/vasquez/profile.html

Proof of the cause-and-effect relationship between vitamin D deficiency and chronic musculoskeletal pain comes from clinical trials among deficient patients showing that vitamin D monotherapy alleviates pain. The exemplary study by Al Faraj and Al Mutairi[35] showed that among patients with "idiopathic chronic low back pain," 83% (n = 299) were vitamin D deficient, and supplementation with 5000 to 10 000 IU/d of cholecalciferol for 3 months alleviated or cured the low back pain in more than 95% of patients. The authors concluded that, in the evaluation of chronic musculoskeletal pain among populations with a sufficiently high prevalence of vitamin D deficiency, "Screening for vitamin D deficiency and treatment with supplements should be mandatory in this setting."

Vitamin D has a wide range of safety according to an extensive review of the literature performed by Vieth.[228] Doses of 2000 IU/d of vitamin D3 have been given to children starting at 1 year of age and were not associated with toxicity but led to a reduction in the incidence of type 1 diabetes by 80%, consistent with the vitamin's anti-infective and immunomodulatory roles.[229] A 2004 review[36] on the clinical importance of vitamin D proposed that optimal vitamin D status is defined as 40 ng/mL to 65 ng/mL (100–160 nmol/L) and that "until proven otherwise, the balance of the research indicates that oral supplementation in the range of 1000 IU per day for infants, 2000 IU per day for children and 4000 IU per day for adults is safe and reasonable to meet physiological requirements, to promote optimal health, and to reduce the risk of several serious diseases. Safety and effectiveness of supplementation are assured by periodic monitoring of serum 25(OH)D and serum calcium." Current data and laboratory reference ranges support a higher top limit for serum 25(OH)D of approximately 100 ng/mL (250 nmol/L). Vitamin D hypersensitivity is seen with primary hyperparathyroidism, granulomatous diseases (such as sarcoidosis, Crohn's disease, and tuberculosis), adrenal insufficiency, hyperthyroidism, hypothyroidism, and various forms of cancer, as well as adverse drug effects, particularly with thiazide diuretics. Thiazide diuretics are known to potentiate hypercalcemia.

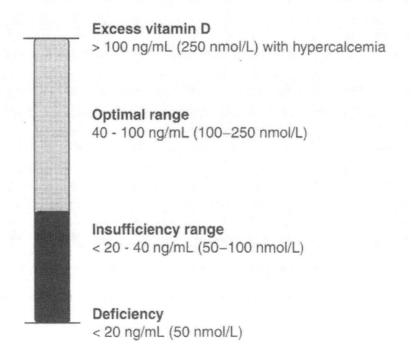

Excess vitamin D
> 100 ng/mL (250 nmol/L) with hypercalcemia

Optimal range
40 - 100 ng/mL (100–250 nmol/L)

Insufficiency range
< 20 - 40 ng/mL (50–100 nmol/L)

Deficiency
< 20 ng/mL (50 nmol/L)

Figure 2.1—Interpretation of Serum 25(OH)D Levels
Adapted from Vasquez A, Manso G, Cannell J. *Altern Ther Health Med.* 2004;10:28-37.36

35

Vasquez A. Musculoskeletal Pain: Expanded Clinical Strategies. Institute for Functional Medicine, 2008: This peer-reviewed monograph on common pain syndromes was approved for continuing medical education (CME).

THE LANCET.com

May 6, 2005

Subphysiologic Doses of Vitamin D are Subtherapeutic:
Comment on the Study by The Record Trial Group

Dear Editor,

Based on recently published research, it is clear that the study by The Record Trial Group [1] on vitamin D and calcium in the prevention of fractures suffered from at least four important shortcomings which negatively skewed their results.

First, and most important, the dose of vitamin D used in their study (800 IU/d) is subphysiologic and would therefore not be expected to produce a clinically meaningful effect. The physiologic requirement for vitamin D was determined scientifically in a recent study by Heaney and colleagues [2], who showed that healthy men utilize 3,000 to 5,000 IU of cholecalciferol per day, and several recent clinical trials have been published documenting the safety and effectiveness of administering vitamin D in physiologic doses of at least 4,000 IU per day.[3-5] In fact, studies have shown a dose-response relationship with vitamin D supplementation [6], and low doses (e.g., 600 IU) are clearly less effective than higher doses in the physiologic range (e.g., 4,000 IU).[5] It is important to note that the commonly used dose of vitamin D at 800 IU per day was not determined scientifically; rather this amount was determined arbitrarily before sufficient scientific methodology was available.[2,7] Given that the commonly recommended daily intake of vitamin D in the range of 200-800 IU is not sufficient for maintaining adequate serum levels of vitamin D [8], it is therefore incumbent upon modern researchers and clinicians to use doses of vitamin D that are consistent with the physiologic requirement as established in current research.

Second, the authors recognize that patient compliance in their study population was quite poor. This poor compliance obviously contributed to the purported lack of treatment efficacy.

Third, and consistent with recent data published elsewhere [8], virtually all of their patients were still vitamin D deficient at the end of one year of treatment, thereby affirming the inadequacy of the treatment dose. Vitamin D deficiency is common in industrialized nations, particularly those of northern latitudes [9-11], including the UK, where this study was performed. By modern criteria for serum vitamin D levels [12], virtually all of the patients in this study were vitamin D deficient at the beginning of the study, and the insufficient treatment dose of 800 IU/d failed to correct this deficiency even after 1 year of treatment. Given that vitamin D levels must be raised to approximately 40 ng/mL (100 nmol/L) in order to maximally reduce parathyroid hormone levels and bone resorption [13,14], supplementation that does not accomplish the goal of raising serum vitamin D levels into the optimal physiologic range cannot be considered adequate therapy.[12]

Fourth, and finally, there is reason to question the bioavailability of their vitamin D3 supplement, as the authors note that their dose-response was generally lower than that seen in other studies. Bioavailability is a prerequisite for treatment efficacy, and the elderly have higher likeliness of comorbid conditions that impair digestion and absorption of nutrients. Specifically, it is well documented that vitamin D absorption is decreased in elderly patients compared to younger controls [15,16], and this is complicated by an age-related reduction in renal calcitriol production [17,18] and intestinal vitamin D receptors [19], thereby further impairing vitamin D metabolism and calcium absorption. Since emulsification of fat soluble vitamins is required for their absorption [20], and since pre-emulsification of nutrients has been shown to increase absorption and dose-responsiveness of the fat-soluble nutrient coenzyme Q [21, 22], it seems apparent that attention to the form (not merely the dose) of nutrient supplementation is clinically important, particularly when working with elderly patients.

These shortcomings, when combined, could have lead to an additive or synergistic reduction in treatment potency that skewed their results toward a conclusion of inefficacy. In order to produce more meaningful results in clinical trials, our group published guidelines [12] recommending that future studies 1) ensure patient compliance, 2) use physiologic doses of vitamin D (e.g., 4,000 IU per day), and 3) ensure that serum levels are raised to a minimum of 40 ng/mL (100 nmol/L), since levels below this threshold are associated with increased parathyroid hormone levels, increased bone resorption, and recalcitrance to bone-building interventions.[23,24]

Alex Vasquez
Biotics Research Corporation
Rosenberg, Texas, USA 77471

Competing Interests: Dr. Vasquez is a researcher at Biotics Research Corporation, an FDA-licensed drug manufacturing facility in the USA.

References:
1. Record Trial Group. Oral vitamin D3 and calcium for secondary prevention of low-trauma fractures in elderly people (Randomised Evaluation of Calcium Or vitamin D, RECORD): a randomised placebo-controlled trial. *Lancet* (Early Online Publication), 28 April 2005
2. Heaney RP, Davies KM, Chen TC, Holick MF, Barger-Lux MJ. Human serum 25-hydroxycholecalciferol response to extended oral dosing with cholecalciferol. *Am J Clin Nutr* 2003;77:204-10
3. Vieth R, Chan PC, MacFarlane GD. Efficacy and safety of vitamin D3 intake exceeding the lowest observed adverse effect level. *Am J Clin Nutr*. 2001;73:288-94
4. Al Faraj S, Al Mutairi K. Vitamin D deficiency and chronic low back pain in Saudi Arabia. *Spine*. 2003;28:177-9
5. Vieth R, Kimball S, Hu A, Walfish PG. Randomized comparison of the effects of the vitamin D3 adequate intake versus 100 mcg (4000 IU) per day on biochemical responses and the wellbeing of patients. *Nutr J*. 2004 Jul 19;3(1):8 http://www.nutritionj.com/content/pdf/1475-2891-3-8.pdf
6. Van den Berghe G, Van Roosbroeck D, Vanhove P, Wouters PJ, De Pourcq L, Bouillon R. Bone turnover in prolonged critical illness: effect of vitamin D. *J Clin Endocrinol Metab*. 2003;88:4623-32
7. Vieth R. Vitamin D supplementation, 25-hydroxyvitamin D concentrations, and safety. *Am J Clin Nutr*. 1999;69:842-56 http://www.ajcn.org/cgi/reprint/69/5/842.pdf
8. Glerup H, Mikkelsen K, Poulsen L, Hass E, Overbeck S, Thomsen J, Charles P, Eriksen EF. Commonly recommended daily intake of vitamin D is not sufficient if sunlight exposure is limited. *J Intern Med*. 2000;247:260-8
9. Thomas MK, Lloyd-Jones DM, Thadhani RI, Shaw AC, Deraska DJ, Kitch BT, Vamvakas EC, Dick IM, Prince RL, Finkelstein JS. Hypovitaminosis D in medical inpatients. *N Engl J Med* 1998;338:777-83
10. Dubbelman R, Jonxis JH, Muskiet FA, Saleh AE. Age-dependent vitamin D status and vertebral condition of white women living in Curacao (The Netherlands Antilles) as compared with their counterparts in The Netherlands. *Am J Clin Nutr* 1993;58:106-9
11. Kauppinen-Makelin R, Tahtela R, Loyttyniemi E, Karkkainen J, Valimaki MJ. A high prevalence of hypovitaminosis D in Finnish medical in- and outpatients. *J Intern Med*. 2001;249:559-63
12. Vasquez A, Manso G, Cannell J. The clinical importance of vitamin D (cholecalciferol): a paradigm shift with implications for all healthcare providers. *Altern Ther Health Med*. 2004;10:28-36; quiz 37, 94
13. Kinyamu HK, Gallagher JC, Rafferty KA, Balhorn KE. Dietary calcium and vitamin D intake in elderly women: effect on serum parathyroid hormone and vitamin D metabolites. *Am J Clin Nutr* 1998;67:342-8
14. Dawson-Hughes B, Harris SS, Dallal GE. Plasma calcidiol, season, and serum parathyroid hormone concentrations in healthy elderly men and women. *Am J Clin Nutr* 1997;65:67-71
15. Harris SS, Dawson-Hughes B, Perrone GA. Plasma 25-hydroxyvitamin D responses of younger and older men to three weeks of supplementation with 1800 IU/day of vitamin D. *J Am Coll Nutr*. 1999;18:470-4
16. Barragry JM, France MW, Corless D, Gupta SP, Switala S, Boucher BJ, Cohen RD. Intestinal cholecalciferol absorption in the elderly and in younger adults. *Clin Sci Mol Med*. 1978;55:213-20
17. Tsai KS, Heath H 3rd, Kumar R, Riggs BL. Impaired vitamin D metabolism with aging in women. Possible role in pathogenesis of senile osteoporosis. *J Clin Invest*. 1984;73:1668-72
18. Gallagher JC, Riggs BL, Eisman J, Hamstra A, Arnaud SB, DeLuca HF. Intestinal calcium absorption and serum vitamin D metabolites in normal subjects and osteoporotic patients: effect of age and dietary calcium.*J Clin Invest* 1979;64:729-36
19. Ebeling PR, Sandgren ME, DiMagno EP, Lane AW, DeLuca HF, Riggs BL. Evidence of an age-related decrease in intestinal responsiveness to vitamin D: relationship between serum 1,25-dihydroxyvitamin D3 and intestinal vitamin D receptor concentrations in normal women. *J Clin Endocrinol Metab*. 1992;75:176-82
20. Gallo-Torres HE. Obligatory role of bile for the intestinal absorption of vitamin E. *Lipids*. 1970;5:379-84
21. Bucci LR, Pillors M, Medlin R, Henderson R, Stiles JC, Robol HJ, Sparks WS. Enhanced uptake in humans of coenzyme Q10 from an emulsified form. *Third International Congress of Biomedical Gerontology*; Acapulco, Mexico: June 1989
22. Bucci LR, Pillors M, Medlin R, Klenda B, Robol H, Stiles JC, Sparks WS. Enhanced blood levels of coenzyme Q-10 from an emulsified oral form. In Faruqui SR and Ansari MS (editors). *Second Symposium on Nutrition and Chiropractic Proceedings*. April 15-16, 1989 in Davenport, Iowa
23. Stepan JJ, Burckhardt P, Hana V. The effects of three-month intravenous ibandronate on bone mineral density and bone remodeling in Klinefelter's syndrome: the influence of vitamin D deficiency and hormonal status. *Bone* 2003;33:589-596
24. Vasquez A. Health care for our bones: a practical nutritional approach to preventing osteoporosis. [letter] *J Manipulative Physiol Ther*. 2005;28:213

Citation: Vasquez A. Subphysiologic Doses of Vitamin D are Subtherapeutic: Comment on the Study by The Record Trial Group. *Lancet* 2005 published online May 6

Internet: Originally posted at http://www.thelancet.com/journals/lancet/article/PIIS0140673605630139/comments and now available at http://InflammationMastery.com/cholecalciferol.html

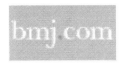

Calcium and vitamin D in preventing fractures

Data are not sufficient to show inefficacy

EDITOR—The study by Porthouse et al had two major design flaws.[1] Firstly, the dose of vitamin D (800 IU per day) is subphysiological and therefore subtherapeutic. Secondly, their use of "self report" as a measure of compliance is unreliable.

The dose of vitamin D at 800 IU daily was not determined scientifically but determined arbitrarily before sufficient scientific methodology was available.[2-4] Heaney et al determined the physiological requirement of vitamin D by showing that healthy men use 4000 IU cholecalciferol daily,[2] an amount that is safely attainable with supplementation[3] and often exceeded with exposure of the total body to equatorial sun.[4]

We provided six guidelines for interventional studies with vitamin D.[5] Dosages of vitamin D must reflect physiological requirements and natural endogenous production and should therefore be in the range of 3000-10 000 IU daily. Vitamin D supplementation must be continued for at least five to nine months. The form of vitamin D should be D_3 rather than D_2. Supplements should be assayed for potency. Effectiveness of supplementation must include measurement of serum 25-hydroxyvitamin D. Serum 25(OH)D concentrations must enter the optimal range, which is 40-65 ng/ml (100-160 nmol/l).

Since the study by Porthouse et al met only the second and third of these six criteria, their data cannot be viewed as reliable for documenting the inefficacy of vitamin D supplementation.

Alex Vasquez, *researcher*

Biotics Research Corporation, 6801 Biotics Research Drive, Rosenberg, TX 77471, USA avasquez@bioticsresearch.com

John Cannell, *president*

Vitamin D Council, 9100 San Gregorio Road, Atascadero, CA 93422, USA

Competing interests: AV is a researcher at Biotics Research Corporation, a drug manufacturing facility in the United States that has approval from the Food and Drug Administration.

References

1. Porthouse J, Cockayne S, King C, Saxon L, Steele E, Aspray T, et al. Randomised controlled trial of calcium and supplementation with cholecalciferol (vitamin D3) for prevention of fractures in primary care. *BMJ* 2005;330: 1003. (30 April.)[Abstract/Free Full Text]
2. Heaney RP, Davies KM, Chen TC, Holick MF, Barger-Lux MJ. Human serum 25-hydroxycholecalciferol response to extended oral dosing with cholecalciferol. *Am J Clin Nutr* 2003;77: 204-10.[Abstract/Free Full Text]
3. Vieth R, Chan PC, MacFarlane GD. Efficacy and safety of vitamin D3 intake exceeding the lowest observed adverse effect level. *Am J Clin Nutr* 2001;73: 288-94.[Abstract/Free Full Text]
4. Vieth R. Vitamin D supplementation, 25-hydroxyvitamin D concentrations, and safety. *Am J Clin Nutr* 1999;69: 842-56.[Abstract/Free Full Text]
5. Vasquez A, Manso G, Cannell J. The clinical importance of vitamin D (cholecalciferol): a paradigm shift with implications for all healthcare providers. *Altern Ther Health Med* 2004;10: 28-36.[ISI][Medline]

Related Article

Randomised controlled trial of calcium and supplementation with cholecalciferol (vitamin D$_3$) for prevention of fractures in primary care
Jill Porthouse, Sarah Cockayne, Christine King, Lucy Saxon, Elizabeth Steele, Terry Aspray, Mike Baverstock, Yvonne Birks, Jo Dumville, Roger Francis, Cynthia Iglesias, Suezann Puffer, Anne Sutcliffe, Ian Watt, and David J Torgerson
BMJ 2005 330: 1003. [Abstract] [Full Text]

Vasquez A, Cannell J. Calcium and vitamin D in preventing fractures: Data are not sufficient to show inefficacy. *BMJ*. 2005 Jul 9;331(7508):108-9 http://www.ncbi.nlm.nih.gov/pubmed/16002891

Thyroid status—laboratory assessments

Overview and interpretation:

- Context: Thyroid disorders are common in clinical practice and thus all clinicians need to have a clear understanding of the clinical presentations and laboratory assessments. Although various aspects of thyroid dysfunction, laboratory tests and clinical presentations will be reviewed here, the primary emphasis will be upon hypothyroidism, which is the most common and *unnecessarily* enigmatic of the thyroid disorders.

- Controversy: In the allopathic medical paradigm, much confusion exists regarding a common but "mysterious" and "enigmatic" condition known as hypothyroidism—low thyroid function. Its converse—**hyper**thyroidism and Graves disease—is well understood, easily diagnosed, and readily treated. Because the medical treatment for **hyper**thyroidism often leaves patients in a **hypo**thyroid state, affected patients thus transition from *clarity* (hyperthyroidism) wherein they feel ill due to the disease process into *"mystery"* (hypothyroidism) wherein they feel ill due to incomplete/inaccurate treatment. The basis for the confusion within the allopathic medical community about hypothyroidism is primarily two-fold: ❶ first, they rely on the wrong test (TSH) as the main basis for laboratory assessment, ❷ second, they use incomplete treatment (T4 without T3) which defies the known physiology of the thyroid gland, which makes at least two hormones rather than one. One might get the impression that perpetual confusion is at times the goal of the medical profession; we certainly see this with the management of hypertension, depression, diabetes mellitus, psoriasis and other inflammatory/autoimmune conditions. For people who seek clarity, it is available.

- Basic physiology: The hypothalamus produces thyrotropin-releasing hormone (TRH) which stimulates the anterior pituitary gland to make thyroid-stimulating hormone (TSH), which stimulates the thyroid gland to produce thyroxine (T4, approximately 85% of thyroid gland hormone production) and triiodothyronine (T3, approximately 15% of thyroid gland hormone production). In the periphery, the prohormone T4 is converted to active T3 by deiodinase enzymes. Stress, glucagon, and environmental toxins (halogenated phenolics, plastic monomers, flame retardants[179]) impair production of T3 and/or increase production of reverse T3, which is either inert or inhibitory to the action of T3. If the thyroid gland begins to fail, then TSH levels increase as the body attempts to stimulate production of thyroid hormones from a failing gland, which typically fails due to autoimmune attack (Hashimoto's thyroiditis); hence the association of elevated blood TSH levels with "primary hypothyroidism." Thyroid hormones have many different functions in the body, and one of the chief effects is contributing to maintenance of the basal metabolic rate, or the speed of reactions within and the temperature of the body. An insufficiency of thyroid hormone adversely effects numerous biochemical reactions and body/organ functions; hence the myriad of clinical presentations reflecting variations in biochemical and physiologic individuality. Conversely yet similarly, excess thyroid hormone (whether endogenously produced or exogenously administered) also affects numerous body systems.

- Clinical presentation of *hyper*thyroidism: The clinical pattern of thyroid excess is more narrowly-focused and thus more predictable and consistent than is the presentation of low thyroid function. The clinical manifestations of hyperthyroidism generally fall into three categories: hyper-adrenergic, hypermetabolic, and ophthalmologic/ocular. ❶ hyper-adrenergic: tachycardia, tremor, diaphoresis, insomnia and a feeling of nervousness and psychomotor agitation due to upregulation of adrenergic tone and generally some degree of relative or absolute hyperthermia; increased dopaminergic and noradrenergic tone in the brain accounts for the neuropsychiatric manifestations, such as mania, psychosis, and hypersexuality, ❷ hyper-metabolic: fecal frequency often described as "diarrhea" due to

---

[179] "All studied contaminants inhibited DI activity in a dose-response manner... This study suggests that some halogenated phenolics, including current use compounds such as plastic monomers, flame retardants and their metabolites, may disrupt thyroid hormone homeostasis through the inhibition of DI activity in vivo." Butt CM, Wang D, Stapleton HM. Halogenated Phenolic Contaminants Inhibit the In Vitro Activity of the Thyroid Regulating Deiodinases in Human Liver. *Toxicol Sci.* 2011 May 11. [Epub ahead of print]

Thyroid status—laboratory assessments

expedited intestinal transit, elevated temperature, and weight loss due to increased overall metabolic rate, ❸ ophthalmologic/ocular: in chronic cases particularly of the autoimmune variety, exophthalmos develops secondary to retro-orbital connective tissue proliferation and autoimmunity directed toward the extraocular muscles; the histologic abnormalities are chiefly characterized by increased accumulation of collagen (behind the eye and within the extraocular muscles, leading to muscle weakness), accumulation of glycosaminoglycans (GAGs), and the attendant edema.

- Clinical presentation of *hypo*thyroidism: In his classic book *Biochemical Individuality*, Williams[180] noted that "a wide variation in thyroid activity exists among 'normal' human beings." Clearly, some patients do not make enough thyroid hormone to function optimally[181]; or, perhaps more precisely, they make enough thyroid hormone (T4) but do not efficiently convert it to the active form (T3) in the periphery. Further complicating the picture is that some patients make appropriate amounts of TSH, T4, and T3 but they make excess of inactive reverse T3 (rT3) which puts them into a physiologic state of hypothyroidism despite adequate glandular function. Patients may have one or more of the following: fatigue, depression, **cold hands and feet** (excluding Raynaud's syndrome, peripheral vascular disease)**,** dry skin, menstrual irregularities, infertility, premenstrual syndrome (PMS), uterine fibroids, excess menstrual bleeding, **low basal body temperature,** weak fingernails, sleep apnea and increased need for sleep (hypersomnia), slow heart rate (relative or absolute **bradycardia**), easy weight gain and difficult weight loss (thus, predisposition to overweight and obesity), hypercholesterolemia, slow healing, decreased memory and concentration, frog-like husky voice, low libido, recurrent infections, hypertension especially diastolic hypertension, poor digestion (due to insufficient gastric production of hydrochloric acid), **delayed Achilles return** (due to delayed muscle relaxation), carotenodermia, vitamin A deficiency, and gastroesophageal acid reflux, constipation, and predisposition to small intestine bacterial overgrowth (SIBO) due to slow intestinal transit. Of these manifestations, cold hands and feet, low basal body temperature, bradycardia, and delayed Achilles return are the most specific; some very competent physicians will—following proper patient evaluation—treat with thyroid hormone based on the clinical presentation of the patient and *with proper consideration of* and *without dependency upon* laboratory findings.

- Overview of thyroid tests:
  - Thyrotropin-releasing hormone (TRH): The hypothalamus releases TRH to stimulate pituitary production of TSH. TRH is not routinely tested in clinical practice, although abnormalities of TRH secretion are noted in patients with mental "depression."
  - Thyroid-stimulating hormone (TSH: 0.4 - 5.0 mIU/L [milli-international units per liter]): TSH is the most commonly performed test for evaluating thyroid status; its frequent (over)use owes more to habit and inexpensiveness than to aspirations for clinical excellence. TSH values greater than 2 mIU/L represent a disturbance of the thyroid-pituitary axis and an increased risk for future thyroid problems[182], and the American Association of Clinical Endocrinologists states, "The target TSH level should be between 0.3 and 3.0 µIU/mL."[183] Clinical rationale is available to support implementation of a therapeutic trial of thyroid hormone treatment in patients who are clinically hypothyroid even if they are biochemically euthyroid (per TSH) provided that treatment is implemented cautiously, in appropriately selected

---

[180] Williams RJ. *Biochemical Individuality: The Basis for the Genetotrophic Concept*. Austin and London: University of Texas Press, 1956 page 82

[181] Broda Barnes MD, Lawrence Galton, *Hypothyroidism: The Unsuspected Illness*. Ty Crowell Co; 1976

[182] Weetman AP. Fortnightly review: Hypothyroidism: screening and subclinical disease. *BMJ: British Medical Journal* 1997;314: 1175

[183] American Association of Clinical Endocrinologists. "The target TSH level should be between 0.3 and 3.0 µIU/mL." AACE Medical Guidelines for Clinical Practice for Evaluation and Treatment of Hyperthyroidism and Hypothyroidism. 2002, 2006 Amended Version. https://www.aace.com/sites/default/files/hypo_hyper.pdf Accessed Aug 2011

patients, and patients are appropriately informed.[184,185] If the clinical world were as perfect as it is portrayed in basic physiology textbooks, then a clinician might fancifully rely on TSH to perform the diagnosis *prima facie*, with reduced TSH values correlating with glandular overperformance and negative feedback suppressing TSH secretion, whilst an underperforming gland would require greater stimulation with elevated TSH levels; however, TSH has never been thus vested with infallible reliability, which explains in part why doctors need brains of their own and why better clinicians have developed the capacity for independent thought.

o Free thyroxine (free T4: 4.5 - 11.2 mcg/dL): Unbound T4 is tested to provide evidence of glandular production of thyroid hormone(s). Because T4 is the major thyroid hormone produced by the thyroid gland it serves as an excellent marker for glandular productivity but it reveals nothing about peripheral conversion of T4 to the active thyroid hormone triiodothyronine (T3); in the practice of medicine, conversion of T4 to the active T3 is assumed to reliably occur unabated despite evidence to the contrary, especially among symptomatic patients.

o Triiodothyronine (T3: 100 - 200 ng/dL[186]): In textbook-perfect physiology, T4 is converted by deiodinase enzymes type-1 and type-2 to the active thyroid hormone T3; in reality, this is only part of the story. Because T3 is the active form of the hormone responsible for the physiologic functions of thyroid physiology, a clinician desiring to assess a patient's thyroid status might reasonably ask the proper question by performing the proper test. T3 is tested as "total T3" or "free T3" in large part based on the clinician's preference; the current author prefers total T3 because it can be compared to the total level of reverse T3 (rT3) in a ratio, the optimal range of which is generally considered to be 10-14 as originally presented by McDaniel[187] and reviewed in the following pages. Patients with psychiatric depression have lower levels of T3 than do healthy controls and have been described as having "low T3 syndrome"[188]; very obviously—whether cause or effect—the low T3 levels in these patients would serve to promote and perpetuate their state of mental depression. Although the focus of this review within the subject of laboratory evaluation is not to describe the implementation of thyroid hormone treatment, clinicians should be aware that T3 administration increases hepatic production of sex hormone binding globulin (SHBG) and that therefore T3 administration can reduce cellular bioavailability of protein-bound hormones. Many authoritative and clinically-experienced sources recommend using a time-released (e.g., sustained-release) form of T3 due to its shorter half-life compared with T4. However, obtaining time-released T3 via a compounding pharmacy can be cumbersome and expensive for the patient; clearly some patients respond to once daily dosing of *non*-time-released preparations with good effects and without adverse effects. Some patients can divide the immediate-release dose into two servings per day for enhanced effect and lessened physiologic fluctuations, if necessary. Per Drugs.com[189] in August 2011, "Since liothyronine sodium (T3) is not firmly bound to serum protein, it is readily available to body tissues. The onset of activity of liothyronine sodium is rapid, occurring within a few hours. Maximum pharmacologic response occurs within 2 or 3 days, providing early clinical response. The biological half-life is about 2.5 days." Very

[184] Skinner GR, Thomas R, Taylor M, Sellarajah M, Bolt S, Krett S, Wright A. Thyroxine should be tried in clinically hypothyroid but biochemically euthyroid patients. *BMJ: British Medical Journal* 1997 Jun 14; 314(7096): 1764

[185] McLaren EH, Kelly CJ, Pollack MA. Trial of thyroxine treatment for biochemically euthyroid patients has been approved. *BMJ* 1997; 315: 1463

[186] U.S. National Library of Medicine (NLM) and National Institutes of Health (NIH) http://www.nlm.nih.gov/medlineplus/ency/article/003687.htm Accessed August 2011

[187] McDaniel AB. Thyroid Assessment: Controversies and Conundrums. Institute for Functional Medicine 14th International Symposium. Tucson, Arizona. May 23-26, 2007

[188] "Out of 250 subjects with major psychiatric depression, 6.4% exhibited low T3 syndrome (mean serum T3 concentration 0.94 nmol/l vs normal mean serum concentration of 1.77 nmol/l)." Premachandra BN, Kabir MA, Williams IK. Low T3 syndrome in psychiatric depression. *J Endocrinol Invest*. 2006 Jun;29(6):568-72

[189] http://www.drugs.com/pro/cytomel.html Accessed August 2011.

Thyroid status—laboratory assessments

clearly, a significant portion of hypothyroid patients respond to T3 alone (either time-released, divided-dosing, or once-daily dosing) or a combination of T4 and T3 when other treatments have failed.[190,191]

o <u>Reverse triiodothyronine (rT3: 90 - 320 pg/mL[192])</u>: T4 is converted by deiodinase enzymes type-1 and type-3 to the inactive thyroid hormone rT3; per a standard endocrinology textbook, "Approximately 70–80% of released T4 is converted by deiodinases to the biologically active T3, the remainder to reverse-T3 (rT3) which has no significant biological activity."[193] Clinicians must know that, "The prohormone T4 must be converted to T3 in the body before it can exert biological effects. **During periods of illness or stress, this conversion is often inhibited and can be diverted to the inactive reverse T3 (rT3) moiety.**"[194] Furthermore and very importantly, clinicians should appreciate that rT3 is not simply inactive but that it may actually impair production/utilization of normal T3; "T4-T3 and T4-rT3 conversion are provoked by different enzymes. **The <u>elevation of rT3</u> might be a cause of the observed decrease in peripheral T3 generation** in old [elderly] subjects, acting by an **<u>inhibition of the T4-T3 conversion</u>**."[195] During times of psychologic/physiologic stress and specific types of pharmacologic stress (e.g., propanolol[196] and corticosteroids), T4 metabolism is preferentially shunted away from T3 toward rT3; an anthropocentric explanation holds that by making less of the active T3 and more of the inactive rT3, the body is better able to conserve energy during times of stress by reducing overall metabolic rate, particularly resting energy expenditure and protein utilization. For example, caloric restriction and fasting result in a decrease in resting metabolic rate (RMR), and the reduced RMR persists for months after the fasting has ended and a normal diet is resumed.[197] This author (AV) terms this stress-induced impairment of thyroid hormone conversion "**metabolic hypothyroidism**" or "**functional hypothyroidism**" because the defect is in the metabolism (not the production) of thyroid hormone into its most active form; "**peripheral hypothyroidism**" might also be used to distinguish the fact that the defect is in the peripheral metabolism rather than located more centrally, within the thyroid gland itself. Because psychologic stress and certain pharmacologic exposures—as well as the thyro-metabolic stress of fasting and caloric restriction in which the counterregulatory hormone glucagon appears to trigger enhanced rT3 production—reduce T3 while simultaneously increasing rT3 levels, clinicians can appreciate that calculation of the T3/rT3 ratio will be more significantly altered (and thus a more sensitive indicator of metabolic disruption) than will be the isolated measurements of T3 or rT3 alone. Functional medicine clinicians[198] note the importance of the ratio of total T3 to reverse T3 (tT3:rT3 ratio) and consider the optimal range to be 10-14 with lower ratios indicating impaired formation or T3 and/or excess production of rT3.[199]

[190] Bunevicius R, Kazanavicius G, Zalinkevicius R, Prange AJ Jr. Effects of thyroxine as compared with thyroxine plus triiodothyronine in patients with hypothyroidism. *N Engl J Med.* 1999 Feb 11;340(6):424-9

[191] Kelly T, Lieberman DZ. The use of triiodothyronine as an augmentation agent in treatment-resistant bipolar II and bipolar disorder NOS. *J Affect Disord.* 2009;116(3):222-6

[192] The reference range provided here for rT3 is a compilation from the laboratory reference ranges from the sample reports on the following pages, each of which is performed by either Quest Diagnostics or LabCorp, the two largest medical laboratories in the United States.

[193] Nussey S, Whitehead S. *Endocrinology: An Integrated Approach.* Oxford: BIOS Scientific Publishers; 2001. See also Box 3.29 Metabolism of thyroid hormones. http://www.ncbi.nlm.nih.gov/books/NBK28/box/A270/?report=objectonly Accessed July 2011

[194] *1998 Mosby's GenRX. Sixth Edition.* St. Louis Missouri; Mosby-Year Book, Inc., 1998

[195] Szabolcs I, Weber M, Kovács Z, Irsy G, Góth M, Halász T, Szilágyi G. The possible reason for serum 3,3'5'-(reverse) triiodothyronine increase in old people. *Acta Med Acad Sci Hung.* 1982;39(1-2):11-7

[196] "Propranolol administration (40 mg t.i.d. for a week) caused a similar rT3 elevation in old persons (n = 18) as in 12 young ones." Szabolcs I, Weber M, Kovács Z, Irsy G, Góth M, Halász T, Szilágyi G. The possible reason for serum 3,3'5'-(reverse) triiodothyronine increase in old people. *Acta Med Acad Sci Hung.* 1982;39(1-2):11-7

[197] Elliot DL, Goldberg L, Kuehl KS, Bennett WM. Sustained depression of the resting metabolic rate after massive weight loss. *Am J Clin Nutr* 1989 Jan;49(1):93-96

[198] The conclusion of this paragraph is derived from Vasquez A. *Musculoskeletal Pain: Expanded Clinical Strategies.* Published 2008 by The Institute for Functional Medicine. http://www.functionalmedicine.org/ifm_ecommerce/ProductDetails.aspx?ProductID=127

[199] McDaniel AB. Thyroid Assessment: Controversies and Conundrums. Institute for Functional Medicine 14th International Symposium. Tucson, Arizona. May 23-26, 2007

Contrary to the previous view which held that rT3 was simply inactive, we now appreciate that rT3 actually impairs normal thyroid hormone metabolism thus functioning as an thyrometabolic monkeywrench or "brake" on normal metabolism. Elevated rT3 levels predict mortality among critically ill patients.[200] Aberrancies in thyroid hormone levels may reflect organic disease, psychoemotional stress, or nutritional deficiency[201], and therefore such serologic abnormalities warrant consideration of underlying problems and direct treatment when possible. If no underlying cause is apparent, then a trial of thyroid hormone/hormones is reasonable in appropriately selected patients. Beyond stress reduction, allergen/gluten avoidance, and nutritional supplementation with iodine, selenium, and zinc (as indicated per patient), correction of overt, subclinical, and functional hypothyroidism generally centers on the administration of natural or synthetic thyroid hormones in the form of T4 and T3. Correction of functional hypothyroidism (relatively reduced total T3 and increased rT3) is accomplished with either time-released or twice-daily dosing of T3 *without T4* to suppress endogenous T4 conversion to T3, thereby allowing rT3 levels to fall precipitously. T3 administration allows temporary downregulation of transforming enzymes so that rT3 production is reduced following withdrawal of T3 replacement; thus, short-term and/or periodic T3 administration helps normalize or "reset" peripheral thyroid metabolism so that, following withdrawal of T3 administration, T4 can be converted to T3 without excess production of rT3. The safety and effectiveness of this approach—using T3 administration (often twice daily or in a sustained-release compounded tablet or capsule) to recalibrate peripheral thyroid hormone metabolism—has documented safety and effectiveness.[202] Alleviation of symptoms, restoration of morning body temperature to 98.6° F (oral or axillary) and other clinical objective improvements achieved by the judicious and safe administration of T3 are the criteria of success; physiologic improvement following T3 administration retrospectively confirms the diagnosis.

- Antithyroid antibodies—antithyroglobulin (anti-TG) and anti-thyroid peroxidase (anti-TPO): Autoimmune thyroiditis (also called Hashimoto's disease or chronic lymphocytic thyroiditis) or is the most common cause of overt primary hypothyroidism. The diagnosis of autoimmune thyroiditis can be made clinically (i.e., without biopsy) upon detection of elevated blood levels of antibodies against thyroglobulin (anti-thyroglobulin antibodies) and anti-thyroid peroxidase (anti-TPO) antibodies. Autoimmune thyroiditis may present asymptomatically and with normal thyroid hormone levels; classically, patients may have a slightly hyperthyroid presentation as the inflamed gland releases extra thyroid hormone before becoming atrophic and hypofunctional.

Advantages:	• Thyroid disorders are quite common in general practice and are often undiagnosed, undertreated, or inappropriately treated.
	• Consistent with the principle of beneficence, patients and doctors benefit when thyroid disorders are diagnosed and treated appropriately.
Limitations:	• A properly interpreted TSH may overlook problems of T4 production or conversion to active T3. Additionally, in some patients, all of these tests are normal but they may have thyroid autoimmunity (i.e., thyroid peroxidase antibodies, anti-TPO) and should receive

---

[200] Peeters RP, Wouters PJ, van Toor H, Kaptein E, Visser TJ, Van den Berghe G. Serum 3,3',5'-triiodothyronine (rT3) and 3,5,3'-triiodothyronine/rT3 are prognostic markers in critically ill patients and are associated with postmortem tissue deiodinase activities. *J Clin Endocrinol Metab.* 2005 Aug;90(8):4559-65

[201] Kelly GS. Peripheral metabolism of thyroid hormones: a review. Altern Med Rev. 2000 Aug;5(4):306-33

[202] Friedman M, Miranda-Massari JR, Gonzalez MJ. Supraphysiological cyclic dosing of sustained release T3 in order to reset low basal body temperature. *P R Health Sci J.* 2006 Mar;25(1):23-9

Thyroid status—laboratory assessments	
	treatment with thyroid hormone[203] or some other corrective treatment (e.g., selenium supplementation[204,205] and a gluten-free diet[206]) to normalize thyroid status.
Comments:	▪ Comprehensive thyroid laboratory testing includes ❶ history, ❷ TSH, ❸ free T4, ❹ total T3, ❺ rT3, ❻ antithyroid antibodies, should be evaluated alongside the ❼ heart rate,❽ cold extremities and basal body temperature, ❾ Achilles' return speed, and ❿ response to treatment.
	▪ The combination of T3 and T4 (as in the prescription Liotrix/Thyrolar or Armour thyroid) appears to have similar safety to T4 alone (Levothyroxine, Synthroid) and may result in greater improvements in mood and neuropsychological function.[207]
	▪ Glandular thyroid supplements and Armour thyroid generally should ***not*** be used in patients with thyroid autoimmunity (Hashimoto's thyroiditis) because the bovine/porcine antigens will exacerbate the anti-thyroid immune response as evidenced by increased anti-TPO antibodies.

Optimal thyroid status

Concept by Dr Vasquez: Optimal thyroid status is not defined by basic laboratory testing with TSH and free T4. It is defined *per patient* based on the levels and ratios of all major thyroid-related hormones and antibodies—in association with other hormonal, psychologic, dysbiotic, nutritional and environmental factors— that work best for that particular unique biochemically-individual patient.

Laboratory interpretation by Dr McDaniel: "Optimal hormone balance is debatable. My observations: A few "well" people and patients treated successfully with T4 and T3 seem best with:
- TSH around 0.7–0.9μIU/mL
- fT4 around 0.7–0.8ng/dL
- fT3 optimally 3.4–3.8pg/mL
- **Total T3-RT3 ratio 12 +/-2**"

McDaniel AB. Thyroid Assessment: Controversies and Conundrums. Institute for Functional Medicine Fourteenth International Symposium. Tucson, Arizona. May 23-26, 2007

[203] Beers MH, Berkow R (eds). The Merck Manual. 17th Edition. Whitehouse Station; Merck Research Laboratories 1999 page 96
[204] Duntas LH, Mantzou E, Koutras DA. Effects of a six month treatment with selenomethionine in patients with autoimmune thyroiditis. *Eur J Endocrinol.* 2003 Apr;148(4):389-93 http://eje-online.org/cgi/reprint/148/4/389
[205] Gartner R, Gasnier BC. Selenium in the treatment of autoimmune thyroiditis. *Biofactors.* 2003;19(3-4):165-70
[206] Sategna-Guidetti C, Volta U, Ciacci C, Usai P, Carlino A, De Franceschi L, Camera A, Pelli A, Brossa C. Prevalence of thyroid disorders in untreated adult celiac disease patients and effect of gluten withdrawal: an Italian multicenter study. *Am J Gastroenterol.* 2001 Mar;96(3):751-7
[207] "CONCLUSIONS: In patients with hypothyroidism, partial substitution of triiodothyronine for thyroxine may improve mood and neuropsychological function; this finding suggests a specific effect of the triiodothyronine normally secreted by the thyroid gland." Bunevicius R, Kazanavicius G, Zalinkevicius R, Prange AJ Jr. Effects of thyroxine as compared with thyroxine plus triiodothyronine in patients with hypothyroidism. *N Engl J Med.* 1999 Feb 11;340(6):424-9

Presentation: 31yo female with fatigue, a recent history of extreme emotional stress (death of first-degree family member), maternal history of Hashimotos thyroiditis, and a personal history of presumed gluten intolerance—testing performed in May 2010 by Quest Diagnostics: Outline your treatment plan before reading discussion.

Test Name	In Range	Out of Range	Reference Range
THYROGLOBULIN ANTIBODIES	<20		<20 IU/mL
THYROID PEROXIDASE ANTIBODIES		38 H	<35 IU/mL
T3, TOTAL	89		76-181 ng/dL
T3 UPTAKE		37 H	22-35 %
T4, FREE	1.6		0.8-1.8 ng/dL
T4 (THYROXINE), TOTAL			
T4 (THYROXINE), TOTAL	10.9		4.5-12.5 mcg/dL
FREE T4 INDEX (T7)		4.0 H	1.4-3.8
TSH, 3RD GENERATION	0.82		mIU/L

Reference Range

> or = 20 Years   0.40-4.50

Pregnancy Ranges
First trimester   0.20-4.70
Second trimester   0.30-4.10
Third trimester   0.40-2.70

T3, FREE	318		230-420 pg/dL
T3, REVERSE		43 H	11-32 ng/dL

This test was performed using a kit that has not been approved or cleared by the FDA. The analytical performance characteristics of this test have been determined by Quest Diagnostics Nichols Institute, San Juan Capistrano. This test should not be used for diagnosis without confirmation by other medically established means.

Discussion: Note that the TSH is completely normal and thus would give the impression of normalcy and "health" if the clinician had not ordered the additional tests. Thyroid peroxidase antibodies are minimally elevated; this is consistent with thyroid autoimmunity but titers this low are of limited clinical importance. Note that the rT3 level is abnormally elevated. Note that because the units provided for total T3 (89 ng/dL) and rT3 (43 ng/dL) are identical, no unit conversion is required, thereby making the calculation of the ideal ratio (range: 10-14) very simple. In this patient's case, the ratio comes to 2.06 which is obviously significantly lower than the proposed optimal of 10-14; the patient responded well to liothyronine/Cytomel supplementation with 15 mcg/d. Patients with thyroid autoimmunity often benefit from a gluten-free diet[208] and supplementation with selenium 200 mcg/d.[209] Finally, note that the reference range for total T3 provided by this laboratory is 76-181 ng/dL which contrasts significantly from the range recommended by the US National Institutes of Health (NIH) 100 to 200 ng/dL[210]; using the NIH's reference range, this patient's T3 production is inadequate.

---

[208] "Hypothyroidism, diagnosed in 31 patients (12.9%) and nine controls (4.2%), was subclinical in 29 patients and of nonautoimmune origin in 21. ... In most patients who strictly followed a 1-yr gluten withdrawal (as confirmed by intestinal mucosa recovery), there was a normalization of subclinical hypothyroidism. The greater frequency of thyroid disease among celiac disease patients justifies a thyroid functional assessment. In distinct cases, gluten withdrawal may single-handedly reverse the abnormality." Sategna-Guidetti C, Volta U, Ciacci C, et al. Prevalence of thyroid disorders in untreated adult celiac disease patients and effect of gluten withdrawal: an Italian multicenter study. *Am J Gastroenterol.* 2001 Mar;96(3):751-7

[209] "Patients with HT assigned to Se supplementation for 3 months demonstrated significantly lower thyroid peroxidase autoantibodies (TPOab) titers (four studies, random effects weighted mean difference: −271.09, 95% confidence interval: −421.98 to −120.19, p< 10⁻⁴) and a significantly higher chance of reporting an improvement in well-being and/or mood (three studies, random effects risk ratio: 2.79, 95% confidence interval: 1.21-6.47, p= 0.016) when compared with controls. .. On the basis of the best available evidence, Se supplementation is associated with a significant decrease in TPOab titers at 3 months and with improvement in mood and/or general well-being."Toulis KA, Anastasilakis AD, Tzellos TG, Goulis DG, Kouvelas D. Selenium supplementation in the treatment of Hashimoto's thyroiditis: a systematic review and a meta-analysis. *Thyroid.* 2010 Oct;20(10):1163-73

[210] U.S. National Library of Medicine and NIH www.nlm.nih.gov/medlineplus/ency/article/003687.htm Accessed Aug 2011

Toxic metal testing—emphasis on lead and mercury	
Overview and application:	• <u>Introduction</u>: Per the US Department of Labor's Occupational Safety and Health Administration (OSHA)[211], toxic metals, including "heavy metals", are individual metals and metal compounds that negatively affect people's health. While lists of toxic metals can vary per source, OSHA names the following: arsenic, beryllium, cadmium, hexavalent chromium, lead, and mercury; of these, lead and mercury are the most commonly observed problematic toxic metals in outpatient practice. The three most important clinical concepts with regard to testing for "heavy metals" or "toxic metals" are as follows: 1. <u>Heavy metal toxicity/accumulation is not uncommon in clinical practice</u>: Toxic/heavy metal accumulation is clinically important due both to its frequency and its pathophysiologic consequences. An article published in *Journal of the American Medical Association (JAMA)*[212] showed that approximately 8% of [1,709 American] women had [blood mercury] concentrations higher than the US Environmental Protection Agency's recommended reference dose (5.8 µg/L), below which exposures are considered to be without adverse effects; stated more plainly, 8% of American women have (potentially) toxic levels of mercury *even when evaluated by the least sensitive of laboratory methods—blood mercury*, which represents only 5% of total body mercury. Another study, also published in *JAMA*[213], showed a positive relationship between blood lead levels and hypertension, even at blood lead levels considered within the normal range; the authors wrote, "At levels well below the current US occupational exposure limit guidelines (40 µg/dL), blood lead level is positively associated with both systolic and diastolic blood pressure and risks of both systolic and diastolic hypertension among women aged 40 to 59 years." 2. <u>The clinical presentation of heavy metal toxicity/accumulation is generally diverse and nonspecific</u>: Clinical presentations due to or associated with toxic metal accumulation can include dyscognition, fatigue, anemia, chronic pain from myalgia or neuropathy, hypertension, autism, and immune disorders including autoimmunity and allergy. In particular, autism[214,215,216] and hypertension[217,218] are noteworthy for their consistent associations with mercury and with mercury and lead, respectively. 3. <u>(Therefore), clinicians should test for and treat toxic metal accumulation</u>: When problems are clinically significant and not extremely unlikely, clinicians have an obligation to test for and treat such problems for the benefit of the patient. Therefore, because toxic metal accumulation is common, clinically significant, and because it is a reversible cause of numerous symptoms, syndromes, and a contributing factor in the development/perpetuation of many other diagnosable conditions commonly labeled as "idiopathic" (e.g., hypertension, immune disorders, mood disorders), clinicians have an obligation to consider and test for toxic metals among their patients.

[211] http://www.osha.gov/SLTC/metalsheavy/index.html Accessed July 2011.

[212] Schober SE, Sinks TH, Jones RL, Bolger PM, McDowell M, Osterloh J, Garrett ES, Canady RA, Dillon CF, Sun Y, Joseph CB, Mahaffey KR. Blood mercury levels in US children and women of childbearing age, 1999-2000. *JAMA* 2003;289:1667-74 http://jama.ama-assn.org/content/289/13/1667.long

[213] Nash D, Magder L, Lustberg M, Sherwin RW, Rubin RJ, Kaufmann RB, Silbergeld EK. Blood lead, blood pressure, and hypertension in perimenopausal and postmenopausal women. *JAMA*. 2003 Mar 26;289(12):1523-32. See also Muntner P, He J, Vupputuri S, Coresh J, Batuman V. Blood lead and chronic kidney disease in the general United States population: results from NHANES III. *Kidney Int*. 2003 Mar;63(3):1044-50 http://www.nature.com/ki/journal/v63/n3/pdf/4493526a.pdf

[214] Stamova B, Green PG, Tian Y, Hertz-Picciotto I, Pessah IN, Hansen R, Yang X, Teng J, Gregg JP, Ashwood P, Van de Water J, Sharp FR. Correlations between gene expression and mercury levels in blood of boys with and without autism. *Neurotox Res*. 2011;19:31-48. Epub 2009 Nov 24.

[215] "The results of the study indicated that the participants' overall ATEC scores and their scores on each of the ATEC subscales (Speech/Language, Sociability, Sensory/Cognitive Awareness, and Health/Physical/Behavior) were linearly related to urinary porphyrins associated with mercury toxicity. The results show an association between the apparent level of mercury toxicity as measured by recognized urinary porphyrin biomarkers of mercury toxicity and the magnitude of the specific hallmark features of autism as assessed by ATEC." Kern JK, Geier DA, Adams JB, Geier MR. A biomarker of mercury body-burden correlated with diagnostic domain specific clinical symptoms of autism spectrum disorder. *Biometals*. 2010 Dec;23(6):1043-51

[216] Kempuraj D, Asadi S, Zhang B, Manola A, Hogan J, Peterson E, Theoharides TC. Mercury induces inflammatory mediator release from human mast cells. *J Neuroinflammation*. 2010 Mar 11;7:20 http://www.jneuroinflammation.com/content/7/1/20

[217] Schober SE, Sinks TH, Jones RL, Bolger PM, McDowell M, Osterloh J, Garrett ES, Canady RA, Dillon CF, Sun Y, Joseph CB, Mahaffey KR. Blood mercury levels in US children and women of childbearing age, 1999-2000. *JAMA* 2003;289:1667-74 http://jama.ama-assn.org/content/289/13/1667.long

[218] Nash D, Magder L, Lustberg M, Sherwin RW, Rubin RJ, Kaufmann RB, Silbergeld EK. Blood lead, blood pressure, and hypertension in perimenopausal and postmenopausal women. *JAMA*. 2003 Mar 26;289(12):1523-32

- **Additional details—mercury:** Mercury is an established neurotoxin, immunotoxin, and nephrotoxin. Because pathophysiologic effects are noted even with very small doses of exposure, one could reasonably argue that no safe amount exists and therefore that any detected mercury is an indication for therapeutic intervention to remove this toxicant. According to an article by Schober et al[219] published in *JAMA—Journal of the American Medical Association* in 2003, "Approximately 8% of [1,709 American] women had [blood mercury] concentrations higher than the US Environmental Protection Agency's recommended reference dose (5.8 µg/L), below which exposures are considered to be without adverse effects." Sources of exposure include dental amalgams, vaccinations, airborne pollution, deep-water fish such as tuna, some cosmetics[220], and selected herbicides, fungicides, and germicides; recently, high-fructose corn syrup was shown to contain mercury in clinically meaningful amounts.[221] Mercury impairs catecholamine degradation and can thereby cause a clinical syndrome that can include hypertension, tremor, tachycardia, diaphoresis, and neurocognitive changes.[222] Per Shih and Gartner[223], "Mercury combines with the sulfhydryl group of S-adenosylmethionine, which is a cofactor for catecholamine-O-methyltransferase (COMT), and this inhibition of COMT allows accumulation of norepinephrine, epinephrine, and dopamine." The clinical presentation of mercury toxicity can include any of the following: diffuse erythematosus rash, dermatitis (acrodynia), anorexia, malaise, fatigue, muscle pain, proximal and/or distal muscle weakness, tremor, weight loss, insomnia, night sweats, burning peripheral neuropathy (axonal neuropathy), renal insufficiency/failure, inattention, neurocognitive compromise, personality changes, depression, diaphoresis, tachycardia, and hypertension. Mercury poisoning/accumulation can occur in humans as a result of consumption of contaminated foods—especially seafood such as shark, swordfish, king mackerel, tilefish, and albacore ("white") tuna.[224] The immunologic effects of organic and/or inorganic mercury include immunosuppression, immunostimulation, formation of antinucleolar antibodies targeting fibrillarin, and formation and deposition of immune-complexes, resulting in a syndrome called "mercury-induced autoimmunity" which can be induced by exposure of susceptible animals to mercury.[225] Mercury/"silver" amalgam dental fillings rank highly among the most significant source of mercury exposure in humans, and implantation of mercury-silver dental amalgams in susceptible animals causes chronic stimulation of the immune system with induction of systemic autoimmunity.[226] Besides being a neurotoxin with no safe exposure limit[227], mercury is known to modify/antigenize/haptenize endogenous proteins to promote autoimmunity[228], and mercury may also promote autoimmunity by contributing to a pro-inflammatory environment that

---

[219] Schober SE, Sinks TH, Jones RL, et al. Blood mercury levels in US children and women of childbearing age, 1999-2000. *JAMA.* 2003 Apr 2;289(13):1667-74 http://jama.ama-assn.org/content/289/13/1667.long

[220] "Most makeup manufacturers have phased out the use of mercury, but it's still added legally to some eye products as a preservative and germ-killer, said John Bailey, chief scientist with the Personal Care Products Council in Washington." Associated Press. Minnesota Bans Adding Mercury To Cosmetics. February 11, 2009. http://www.cbsnews.com/stories/2007/12/14/health/main3618048.shtml Accessed August 2011

[221] "Average daily consumption of high fructose corn syrup is about 50 grams per person in the United States. With respect to total mercury exposure, it may be necessary to account for this source of mercury in the diet of children and sensitive populations." Dufault R, LeBlanc B, Schnoll R, Cornett C, Schweitzer L, Wallinga D, Hightower J, Patrick L, Lukiw WJ. Mercury from chlor-alkali plants: measured concentrations in food product sugar. *Environ Health.* 2009 Jan 26;8:2. See also: "High fructose corn syrup has been shown to contain trace amounts of mercury as a result of some manufacturing processes, and its consumption can also lead to zinc loss." Dufault R, Schnoll R, Lukiw WJ, Leblanc B, Cornett C, Patrick L, Wallinga D, Gilbert SG, Crider R. Mercury exposure, nutritional deficiencies and metabolic disruptions may affect learning in children. *Behav Brain Funct.* 2009 Oct 27;5:44.

[222] Wössmann W, Kohl M, Grüning G, Bucsky P. Mercury intoxication presenting with hypertension and tachycardia. *Arch Dis Child.* 1999 Jun;80(6):556-7 http://www.ncbi.nlm.nih.gov/pmc/articles/PMC1717944/pdf/v080p00556.pdf

[223] Shih H, Gartner JC Jr. Weight loss, hypertension, weakness, and limb pain in an 11-year-old boy. *J Pediatr.* 2001 Apr;138(4):566-9

[224] See http://www.fda.gov/Food/FoodSafety/Product-SpecificInformation/Seafood/FoodbornePathogensContaminants/Methylmercury/ucm115662.htm for the white-washed version; see http://www.ewg.org/news/bamboozled-fish for a more accurate and complete perspective.

[225] Havarinasab S, Hultman P. Organic mercury compounds and autoimmunity. *Autoimmun Rev.* 2005;4(5):270-5 www.generationrescue.org/pdf/havarinasab.pdf Dec 2005

[226] "We hypothesize that under appropriate conditions of genetic susceptibility and adequate body burden, heavy metal exposure from dental amalgam may contribute to immunological aberrations, which could lead to overt autoimmunity." Hultman P, Johansson U, Turley SJ, Lindh U, Enestrom S, Pollard KM. Adverse immunological effects and autoimmunity induced by dental amalgam and alloy in mice. *FASEB J.* 1994 Nov;8(14):1183-90

[227] University of Calgary Faculty of Medicine. How Mercury Causes Brain Neuron Degeneration.http://commons.ucalgary.ca/mercury/ Current Aug 2011

[228] Havarinasab S, Hultman P. Organic mercury compounds and autoimmunity. *Autoimmun Rev.* 2005 Jun;4(5):270-5. www.generationrescue.org/pdf/havarinasab.pdf Dec 2005

| **Toxic metal testing**—emphasis on lead and mercury |

awakens quiescent autoreactive immunocytes via bystander activation.[229] For example, administration of mercury to "susceptible" mice induces autoimmunity via modification of the nucleolar protein *fibrillarin*[230]; noteworthy in this regard is the fact that antifibrillarin antibodies are characteristic of the human autoimmune disease scleroderma.[231] The mercury-based preservative thimerosol is a type-IV (delayed hypersensitivity) sensitizing agent[232], and recent research implicates mercury as a contributor to autism[233,234] and eczema.[235] A review and clinical report published by Bains et al[236], stated, "Eczematous eruptions may be produced through topical contact with mercury and by systemic absorption in mercury sensitive individuals. Mercury…may cause hypersensitivity leading to contact dermatitis or Coomb's Type IV hypersensitivity reactions. The typical manifestation is an urticarial or erythematous rash, and pruritus on the face and flexural aspects of limbs, followed by progression to dermatitis." Thus, this survey of the literature supports the notions that mercury toxicity—i.e., a level of mercury in human patients sufficient to cause adverse health effects—is ❶ common (e.g., 8% of American women), ❷ problematic via causation of or contribution to various health problems commonly encountered in clinical practice, ❸ diagnosable via laboratory testing followed by monitoring response to treatment, and ❹ treatable, most notably with DMSA but also to a lesser extent with potassium citrate, selenium, and phytochelatins.

- Additional details—lead: The International Agency for Research on Cancer (IARC, part of the World Health Organization [WHO]) classified lead as a "possible human carcinogen" in 1987. A 2003 review published in *British Medical Bulletin* by Järup[237] noted that lead exposure (which comes equally from air and food, particularly food served via lead-contaminated ceramics) should be avoided as much as possible because physiologic toxicity occurs with low-level exposure; "Blood levels in children should be reduced below the levels so far considered acceptable, recent data indicating that there may be neurotoxic effects of lead at lower levels of exposure than previously anticipated." Occupational exposure to lead occurs in mines, smelting plants, glass-manufacturing facilities, battery plants, and among workers who weld metals already painted with lead-containing paints; air emissions near such facilities and activities may also contaminate nonworkers. Air contamination frequently leads to water contamination, threatening wildlife and humans who are exposed to contaminated water. Children are particularly vulnerable to lead exposure due to very efficient (compared with adults) gastrointestinal absorption and a more permeable ("leaky") blood-brain barrier. Organic lead compounds such as tetramethyl-lead and tetraethyl lead easily penetrate skin and blood-brain barrier of children as well as adults. Classic, large-dose, acute and subacute lead poisoning manifests as anemia, renal tubular damage, and dark blue line of lead sulphide at the gingival margin; clinicians awaiting this classic presentation prior

[229] "It is therefore theoretically possible that compounds present in vaccines such as thiomersal or aluminium hydroxyde can trigger autoimmune reactions through bystander effects." Fournie GJ, Mas M, Cautain B, et al. Induction of autoimmunity through bystander effects. Lessons from immunological disorders induced by heavy metals. *J Autoimmun*. 2001 May;16(3):319-26

[230] Nielsen JB, Hultman P. Mercury-induced autoimmunity in mice. *Environ Health Perspect*. 2002 Oct;110 Suppl 5:877-81 http://ehp.niehs.nih.gov/docs/2002/suppl-5/877-881nielsen/abstract.html

[231] "Since anti-fibrillarin antibodies are specific markers of scleroderma, the present animal model may be valuable for studies of the immunological aberrations which are likely to induce this autoimmune response." Hultman P, Enestrom S, Pollard KM, Tan EM. Anti-fibrillarin autoantibodies in mercury-treated mice. *Clin Exp Immunol*. 1989;78(3):470-7

[232] "Thimerosal is an important preservative in vaccines and ophthalmologic preparations. The substance is known to be a type IV sensitizing agent. High sensitization rates were observed in contact-allergic patients and in health care workers who had been exposed to thimerosal-preserved vaccines." Westphal GA, Schnuch A, Schulz TG, Reich K, Aberer W, Brasch J, Koch P, Wessbecher R, Szliska C, Bauer A, Hallier E. Homozygous gene deletions of the glutathione S-transferases M1 and T1 are associated with thimerosal sensitization. *Int Arch Occup Environ Health*. 2000 Aug;73(6):384-8

[233] Vojdani A, Pangborn JB, Vojdani E, Cooper EL. Infections, toxic chemicals and dietary peptides binding to lymphocyte receptors and tissue enzymes are major instigators of autoimmunity in autism. *Int J Immunopathol Pharmacol*. 2003 Sep-Dec;16(3):189-99

[234] Geier DA, Geier MR. A comparative evaluation of the effects of MMR immunization and mercury doses from thimerosal-containing childhood vaccines on the population prevalence of autism. *Med Sci Monit*. 2004 Mar;10(3):PI33-9. http://www.medscimonit.com/pub/vol_10/no_3/3986.pdf

[235] Weidinger S, Kramer U, Dunemann L, Mohrenschlager M, Ring J, Behrendt H. Body burden of mercury is associated with acute atopic eczema and total IgE in children from southern Germany. *J Allergy Clin Immunol*. 2004 Aug;114(2):457-9

[236] Bains VK, Loomba K, Loomba A, Bains R. Mercury sensitisation: review, relevance and a clinical report. *Br Dent J*. 2008 Oct 11;205(7):373-8 http://www.intolsante.com/documents/publications/-mercury-sensitisation-review-relevance-and-clinical-report-22.pdf Accessed August 2011

[237] Järup L. Hazards of heavy metal contamination. *Br Med Bull*. 2003;68:167-82

	to considering lead toxicity should fortify their knowledge of and reconsider their perspective on this topic. Other symptoms of acute lead poisoning are headache, irritability, abdominal pain and various neurologic-psychiatric symptoms generally referred to as "lead encephalopathy" characterized by sleeplessness, restlessness, confusion/dyscognition, behavioral disturbances, particularly learning and concentration difficulties in children; more extreme manifestations can include acute psychosis and stupor. Per the previously cited review by Järup, "Individuals [chronically exposed to lead] with average blood lead levels under 3 μmol/l may show signs of peripheral nerve symptoms with reduced nerve conduction velocity and reduced dermal sensibility."
Overview and application:	▪ No universally accepted consensus exists for the most accurate testing methodology. However, from the science-based perspectives that toxic metals have been proven to cause harm at levels previously believed to be "acceptable" and that—very importantly—toxic metals are exponentially more toxic when in combination than when present alone, reasonable clinicians can therefore conclude that the best test for clinical use is the one that is most sensitive, along with being reasonably convenient for the patient as well as affordable. For these reasons, the current author and many other clinicians chose DMSA-provoked urine toxic metal testing. Hair and nails can also be tested for chronic exposure, as can blood which is generally only useful for recent and relatively high-level exposure. Our clinical concern in general outpatient practice is not with recent and relatively high-level exposure, and therefore blood is not necessarily optimal. Our clinical concern in general outpatient practice is with chronic low-level exposure which leads to adverse cellular effects despite the failure to "spike" the serum level into the detectable toxic range. Arguments in favor of allowing symptomatic patients to persist untreated in a state of toxic metal accumulation would be difficult to justify scientifically and ethically.
Advantages:	▪ Toxic metal accumulation is ❶ <u>sufficiently common to warrant testing in selected patients— such testing should be used frequently with a low threshold for implementation</u>, ❷ <u>problematic</u> via causation of or contribution to various health problems commonly encountered in clinical practice, ❸ <u>diagnosable</u> via laboratory testing followed by monitoring response to treatment, and ❹ <u>treatable</u>. Therefore, clinicians should establish pathways for the assessment and treatment of metal toxicity.
Limitations:	▪ Patients with toxic metal accumulation frequently have accumulation of chemical xenobiotics as well; thus testing for and treating toxicity due to metals only relieves one type of toxicity.
Comments:	▪ Clinicians should establish pathways for the assessment and treatment of toxic metal accumulation.

Presentation: Widespread musculoskeletal pain resembling fibromyalgia secondary to lead and mercury accumulation: This 54yo athletic female with healthy diet, lifestyle, and supportive relationship presented with chronic diffuse musculoskeletal pain. Health history was sigificant for decades of environmental illness/intolerance (EI) also known as multiple chemical sensitivity (MCS). Family history was positive for maternal temporal (giant cell) arteritis. Physical examination revealed numerous tender points consistent with fibromyalgia; yet the history and stool analysis with comprehensive bacteriology and parasitology were unsupportive of gastrointestinal dysbiosis, particularly of the subtype small intestine bacterial overgrowth, which is causal for fibromyalgia.[238] Laboratory investigations revealed normal results for hsCRP (high-sensitity c-reactive protein), CK (creatine kinase, a marker of muscle damage and myositis), ANA (anti-nuclear antibodies), vitamin D, calcium, phosphorus, and comprehensive thyroid evaluation. The patient was then (defensively) referred to an osteopathic internist who diagnosed fibromyalgia.

Date Completed: 10/22/2005

| Lead | 30 | < | 5 |
| Mercury | 21 | < | 3 |

Discussion: The patient, unsatisfied with the diagnosis of fibromyalgia, returned to the current author, who then performed urine heavy metal testing provoked with 10 mg per kilogram of dimercaptosuccinic acid (DMSA). Results revealed the highest levels of lead and mercury encountered in the author's practice at that time. As shown above, lead levels were 6x above the reference range and mercury levels were 7x above the reference range. The patient was commenced on DMSA 10 mg/kg/d on alternating weeks to avoid toxicity in general and bone marrow toxicity (neutropenia) in particular, selenium 800 mcg/d to promote excretion of toxic metals and to support renal and antoxidant protection, vegetable juices to provide potassium and citrate for urinary alkalinization and enhanced excretion of xenobiotics[239], and a proprietary phytochelatin (metal-binding peptides from plants[240]) concetrate to bind toxic metals in the gut and thereby promote their fecal excretion by blocking enterohepatic recycling/recirculation. The use of DMSA for children and adults is supported by peer-reviewed literature.[241,242,243,244,245] DMSA chelation is approved by the US Food and Drug Administration (FDA) for the treatment of marked lead toxicity in children.[246] After approximately 8 months of treatment, the patient was completely free of pain, and the clinical improvement was associated with a reduction in both lead and mercury of approximately 50% as demonstrated by follow-up laboratory testing. Testing was performed by Doctors Data. This case was published in peer-reviewed literature for continuing education credits.[247]

Date Completed: 6/30/2006

| Lead | 15 | < | 5 |
| Mercury | 8.2 | < | 4 |

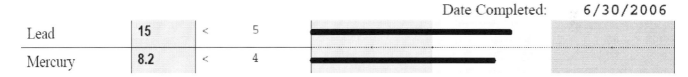

[238] Vasquez A. Musculoskeletal Pain: Expanded Clinical Strategies. Institute for Functional Medicine. 2008
[239] Crinnion WJ. Environmental medicine, part three: long-term effects of chronic low-dose mercury exposure. *Altern Med Rev.* 2000 Jun;5(3):209-23 http://www.thorne.com/altmedrev/.fulltext/5/3/209.pdf
[240] Cobbett CS. Phytochelatins and their roles in heavy metal detoxification. *Plant Physiol.* 2000;123:825-32 plantphysiol.org/content/123/3/825
[241] Bradstreet J, Geier DA, Kartzinel JJ, Adams JB, Geier MR. A case-control study of mercury burden in children with autistic spectrum disorders. *Journal of American Physicians and Surgeons* 2003; 8: 76-79 http://www.jpands.org/vol8no3/geier.pdf
[242] Crinnion WJ. Environmental medicine, part three: long-term effects of chronic low-dose mercury exposure. *Altern Med Rev.* 2000 Jun;5(3):209-23
[243] Forman J, Moline J, Cernichiari E, Sayegh S, Torres JC, Landrigan MM, Hudson J, Adel HN, Landrigan PJ. A cluster of pediatric metallic mercury exposure cases treated with meso-2,3-dimercaptosuccinic acid (DMSA). *Environ Health Perspect.* 2000 Jun;108(6):575-7 http://ehp.niehs.nih.gov/docs/2000/108p575-577forman/abstract.html
[244] Miller AL. Dimercaptosuccinic acid (DMSA), a non-toxic, water-soluble treatment for heavy metal toxicity. *Altern Med Rev.* 1998 Jun;3(3):199-207 http://www.thorne.com/altmedrev/.fulltext/3/3/199.pdf
[245] DMSA. *Altern Med Rev.* 2000 Jun;5(3):264-7 http://thorne.com/altmedrev/.fulltext/5/3/264.pdf
[246] "The Food and Drug Administration has recently licensed the drug DMSA (succimer) for reduction of blood lead levels >/= 45 micrograms/dl. This decision was based on the demonstrated ability of DMSA to reduce blood lead levels. An advantage of this drug is that it can be given orally." Goyer RA, Cherian MG, Jones MM, Reigart JR. Role of chelating agents for prevention, intervention, and treatment of exposures to toxic metals. *Environ Health Perspect.* 1995 Nov;103(11):1048-52 Http://ehp.niehs.nih.gov/docs/1995/103-11/meetingreport.html
[247] Vasquez A. Musculoskeletal Pain: Expanded Clinical Strategies. Institute for Functional Medicine. 2008

Presentation: Chronic "idiopathic" hypertension associated with lead and mercury accumulation (per DMSA-provoked urine testing): This 43yo male presents with recalcitrant stage-1 hypertension. His cardiologist prescribed drugs to "treat" (some would say "mask") his elevated blood pressure. Since hypertension always has an underlying cause, the ethical and appropriate course of action is to determine the cause of the problem rather than silencing the alarm that is alerting to an underlying dysfunction. While this case is currently in progress at the time of this writing (the patient's medical records arrived in July 2011), it does offer a model case for clinical decision-making. Clinicians should be aware that, per animal studies, the toxicity of lead and mercury are greatly enhanced when both toxins are present at the same time.

Date Collected: 6/3/2010

Lead	8.5	<	2	
Mercury	17	<	3	

Mercury and hypertension: Mercury is an established neurotoxin, immunotoxin, and nephrotoxin. Because pathophysiologic effects are noted even with very small doses of exposure, one could reasonably argue that no safe amount exists and therefore that any detected mercury is an indication for therapeutic intervention to remove this toxicant. Sources of exposure include dental amalgams, vaccinations, airborne pollution, and fish; recently, high-fructose corn syrup was shown to contain mercury.[248] Mercury impairs catecholamine degradation and can thereby cause a clinical syndrome that can include hypertension, tremor, tachycardia, diaphoresis, and neurocognitive changes.[249] Per Shih and Gartner[250], "Mercury combines with the sulfhydryl group of S-adenosylmethionine, which is a cofactor for catecholamine-O-methyltransferase (COMT), and this inhibition of COMT allows accumulation of norepinephrine, epinephrine, and dopamine."

Lead and hypertension: In the United States, a consistent correlation has been found between body burden of lead and HTN, even when blood lead levels are well below the current US occupational exposure limit guidelines (40 microg/dl).[251] Harlan et al[252] analyzed data from the second National Health and Nutrition Examination Survey (1976-1980) and thereby found a direct relationship between blood lead levels and systolic and diastolic pressures for men and women and for white and black persons aged 12 to 74 years; they concluded, "Blood lead levels were significantly higher in younger men and women (aged 21 to 55 years) with high blood pressure, but not in older men or women (aged 56 to 74 years)." Schwartz and Stewart[253] found that blood lead was the assessment that most strongly correlated with HTN; they concluded, "Systolic blood pressure was elevated by blood lead levels as low as 5 microg/dl." Thus, clinicians might first measure blood lead levels, which do not measure total body burden but rather the lead that is mobile or *in transit* within the body and which appears to have the best correlation with HTN; the finding of normal blood lead results could then be followed with the more sensitive DMSA-provoked heavy metal testing before concluding that heavy metals are noncontributory to that particular patient's HTN. For heavy metal testing in various clinical scenarios, this author's preference is to use DMSA-provoked measurement of urine toxic metals. After a minimal test dose of DMSA (e.g., in the range of 50-100 mg) to screen for hypersensitivity, patients take oral DMSA 10 mg/kg as a single oral dose in the morning on an empty stomach after emptying the bladder and send a sample from the next urination for laboratory analysis; follow laboratory protocol if different from these instructions. Use of DMSA for lead and mercury chelation/detoxification and for diagnostic purposes is generally safe and effective.[254,255,256]

[248] "Average daily consumption of high fructose corn syrup is about 50 grams per person in the United States. With respect to total mercury exposure, it may be necessary to account for this source of mercury in the diet of children and sensitive populations." Dufault R, LeBlanc B, Schnoll R, Cornett C, Schweitzer L, Wallinga D, Hightower J, Patrick L, Lukiw WJ. Mercury from chlor-alkali plants: measured concentrations in food product sugar. *Environ Health*. 2009 Jan 26;8:2. See also: "High fructose corn syrup has been shown to contain trace amounts of mercury as a result of some manufacturing processes, and its consumption can also lead to zinc loss." Dufault R, Schnoll R, Lukiw WJ, Leblanc B, Cornett C, Patrick L, Wallinga D, Gilbert SG, Crider R. Mercury exposure, nutritional deficiencies and metabolic disruptions may affect learning in children. *Behav Brain Funct*. 2009 Oct 27;5:44.
[249] Wössmann W, Kohl M, Grüning G, Bucsky P. Mercury intoxication presenting with hypertension and tachycardia. *Arch Dis Child*. 1999 Jun;80(6):556-7 http://www.ncbi.nlm.nih.gov/pmc/articles/PMC1717944/pdf/v080p00556.pdf
[250] Shih H, Gartner JC Jr. Weight loss, hypertension, weakness, and limb pain in an 11-year-old boy. *J Pediatr*. 2001 Apr;138(4):566-9
[251] Nash D, Magder L, Lustberg M, Sherwin RW, Rubin RJ, Kaufmann RB, Silbergeld EK. Blood lead, blood pressure, and hypertension in perimenopausal and postmenopausal women. *JAMA*. 2003 Mar 26;289(12):1523-32 http://jama.ama-assn.org/cgi/content/full/289/12/1523
[252] Harlan WR, Landis JR, Schmouder RL, Goldstein NG, Harlan LC. Blood lead and blood pressure. Relationship in the adolescent and adult US population. *JAMA*. 1985 Jan 25;253(4):530-4
[253] "Systolic blood pressure was elevated by blood lead levels as low as 5 microg/dl." Schwartz BS, Stewart WF. Different associations of blood lead, meso 2,3-dimercaptosuccinic acid (DMSA)-chelatable lead, and tibial lead levels with blood pressure in 543 former organolead manufacturing workers. *Arch Environ Health*. 2000 Mar-Apr;55(2):85-92
[254] Bradstreet J, Geier DA, Kartzinel JJ, Adams JB, Geier MR. A case-control study of mercury burden in children with autistic spectrum disorders. *Journal of American Physicians and Surgeons* 2003; 8: 76-79 http://www.jpands.org/vol8no3/geier.pdf
[255] Miller AL. Dimercaptosuccinic acid (DMSA), a non-toxic, water-soluble treatment for heavy metal toxicity. *Altern Med Rev*. 1998 Jun;3(3):199-207
[256] DMSA. *Altern Med Rev*. 2000 Jun;5(3):264-7 http://thorne.com/altmedrev/.fulltext/5/3/264.pdf

Antinuclear antibody: ANA

Overview and interpretation:	• Good screening test for autoimmune conditions: SLE, Sjogren's syndrome, and various other "connective tissue" inflammatory/rheumatic/autoimmune diseases. • Good and "highly sensitive" for initial assessment of SLE; positive in 95-98% of SLE patients; negative result strongly suggests against diagnosis of SLE.[257] Only 2% of patients with SLE have a negative ANA test—these patients may be identified by testing with anti-RO antibodies and CH50 (complement levels). • This test measures for the presence of antibodies that react to nucleoproteins. Some labs report titers of 1:20 or 1:40 as "positive"; however, low levels of ANA are common (5-15%) in the general population. Thus, ANA is not specific for any one disease; may be positive in SLE, RA, scleroderma, Sjogren's, also seen with elderly, infected patients, cancer, and with certain medications. Titers less than 1:160 may not indicate the presence of *clinical* autoimmunity[258]; titers >=1:160 usually indicate the presence of active SLE, or other autoimmunity.[259] Titers greater than 1:320 are considered indicative of clinically significant autoimmunity. • Methodologies (indirect immunofluorescence is most popular), subtypes, and patterns reported for ANA results may be irrelevant or clinically meaningful; the most common descriptors are provided in the table below. Clinicians should order quantitative ANA with reflex to FANA staining patterns

ANA patterns and descriptions[260,261]	*Clinical correlation*
Homogeneous, diffuse nuclear staining	SLE, lupus nephritis, and other autoimmunity
Speckled	SLE, scleroderma, Sjogren's, other autoimmunity
Rim or peripheral staining	Correlates with SLE and lupus nephritis
Anti-centromere: selective staining of the centromeres of nuclei in metaphase	Highly specific for the limited scleroderma subtype associated with **CREST** syndrome
Nucleolar	Correlated with diffuse scleroderma (systemic sclerosis), Sjogren's syndrome, SLE
FANA: fluorescent ANA	The standard ANA test in the US
Anti-Sm: anti-Smith[262]	**Highly specific for SLE**; insensitive: positive in 20-30% of SLE patients
Anti-dsDNA: anti-double stranded DNA	**Highly specific for SLE** and indicative of an increased likelihood of poor prognosis with major organ involvement[263] especially active renal disease
Anti-Ro (anti-SS-A)	Correlates with SLE, Sjögren's syndrome, and neonatal SLE
Anti-La (anti-SS-B)	Sjögren's syndrome or low risk of SLE nephritis
Anti-RNP	SLE and/or mixed connective tissue disease (MCTD)
Anti-Jo-1	Specific but not sensitive for polymyositis/dermatomyositis
Antihistone	SLE and especially drug-induced SLE
Antitopoisomerase (Scl-70)	**Correlates with diffuse scleroderma, especially with interstitial lung disease**

---

[257] Shojania K. Rheumatology: 2. What laboratory tests are needed? *CMAJ.* 2000 Apr 18;162(8):1157-63 http://www.cmaj.ca/cgi/content/full/162/8/1157

[258] Hardin JG, Waterman J, Labson LH. Rheumatic disease: Which diagnostic tests are useful? *Patient Care* 1999; March 15: 83-102

[259] Antinuclear Antibodies (ANA), Synonyms: FANA, Test Number: 164947, CPT Code: 86038. https://www.labcorp.com March 2013

[260] Shojania K. Rheumatology: 2. What laboratory tests are needed? *CMAJ.* 2000 Apr 18;162(8):1157-63 http://www.cmaj.ca/cgi/content/full/162/8/1157

[261] Ward MM. Laboratory testing for systemic rheumatic diseases. *Postgrad Med.* 1998 Feb;103(2):93-100.

[262] Lane SK, Gravel JW Jr. Clinical utility of common serum rheumatologic tests. *Am Fam Physician.* 2002;65:1073-80 http://www.aafp.org/afp/20020315/1073.html

[263] Shojania K. Rheumatology: 2. What laboratory tests are needed? *CMAJ.* 2000 Apr 18;162(8):1157-63 http://www.cmaj.ca/cgi/content/full/162/8/1157

Antinuclear antibody: ANA—*continued*	
Advantages:	▪ ANA has 98% sensitivity and 90% specificity for SLE in an unselected population. ▪ The negative predictive value in an unselected population is greater than 99%. ANA is therefore an excellent test for *excluding* the diagnosis of SLE.
Limitations:	▪ The positive predictive value in an unselected population is about 30%; only 30% of unselected people with a positive result will have SLE—this fact underscores the importance of patient selection and judicious interpretation of this test. ▪ Positive ANA is seen in patients with conditions other than SLE, including rheumatoid arthritis, Sjogren's syndrome, scleroderma, polymyositis, vasculitis, juvenile rheumatoid arthritis (JRA), and infectious diseases.
Comments:	▪ ANA is most often used to support the diagnosis of SLE in a patient with multisystemic illness and a clinical picture compatible with SLE. Nearly all patients with SLE will have positive ANA. **A positive ANA does not mean that the patient necessarily has SLE; be weary of paraneoplastic syndromes and viral hepatitis as underlying causative processes in patients with an unclear clinical picture.** ▪ I view any "positive ANA" as an indicator of poor health in general and immune dysfunction in particular. The goal, then, is to restore health. I have seen ANA show a trend toward normalization or completely normalize with effective health restoration as detailed in <u>Integrative Rheumatology</u> (chapter 4). I realize that my experience in this regard contrasts sharply with the allopathic view that serial measurements of ANA are worthless because the result never normalizes once a patient is ANA-positive[264]; I consider this evidence of the effectiveness of my integrative-functional approach and the comparable failure of the allopathic approach.

Antineutrophilic cytoplasmic antibodies: ANCA	
Overview:	▪ ANCA are autoantibodies to the cytoplasmic constituents of granulocytes and are characteristically found in vasculitic syndromes and also in (Chinese) patients with inflammatory bowel disease[265] and nearly all patients with hepatic amebiasis due to *Entamoeba histolytica.*[266] Two types: ▪ <u>Cytoplasmic ANCA (C-ANCA)</u>: classically seen in Wegener's granulomatosis; also seen in some types of glomerulonephritis and vasculitis; this test is highly sensitive and specific for these conditions. In fact, a positive C-ANCA result can replace biopsy in a patient with a clinical picture of Wegener's granulomatosis.[267] ▪ <u>Perinuclear ANCA (P-ANCA)</u>: considered a nonspecific finding[268] that correlates with SLE, drug induced lupus, and some types of glomerulonephritis and vasculitis. Shojania[269] stated that this test must be confirmed with antimyeloperoxidase antibodies to evaluate for Churg–Strauss syndrome, crescentic glomerulonephritis, and microscopic polyarteritis.
Advantages, limitations, and comments	▪ Not to be used as a screening test, except in patients with idiopathic vasculitis or glomerulonephritis. ▪ The fact that hepatic amebiasis due to *Entamoeba histolytica* induces production of C-ANCA antibodies in nearly 100% of infected patients may support the hypothesis that autoimmunity can be induced or exacerbated by parasitic infections.

[264] Shojania K. Rheumatology: 2. What laboratory tests are needed? *CMAJ.* 2000 Apr 18;162(8):1157-63 http://www.cmaj.ca/cgi/content/full/162/8/1157
[265] "Fourteen patients (73.5%) were positive, of which six (31.5%) showed a perinuclear staining pattern and eight (42%) demonstrated a cytoplasmic pattern." Sung JY, Chan KL, Hsu R, Liew CT, Lawton JW. Ulcerative colitis and antineutrophil cytoplasmic antibodies in Hong Kong Chinese. *Am J Gastroenterol.* 1993 Jun;88(6):864-9
[266] "ANCA was detected in 97.4% of amoebic sera; the pattern of staining was cytoplasmic, homogeneous, without central accentuation (C-ANCA)." Pudifin DJ, Duursma J, Gathiram V, Jackson TF. Invasive amoebiasis is associated with the development of anti-neutrophil cytoplasmic antibody. *Clin Exp Immunol.* 1994 Jul;97(1):48-5
[267] Shojania K. Rheumatology: 2. What laboratory tests are needed? *CMAJ.* 2000 Apr 18;162(8):1157-63 http://www.cmaj.ca/cgi/content/full/162/8/1157
[268] Shojania K. Rheumatology: 2. What laboratory tests are needed? *CMAJ.* 2000 Apr 18;162(8):1157-63 http://www.cmaj.ca/cgi/content/full/162/8/1157
[269] Shojania K. Rheumatology: 2. What laboratory tests are needed? *CMAJ.* 2000 Apr 18;162(8):1157-63 http://www.cmaj.ca/cgi/content/full/162/8/1157

RF: Rheumatoid Factor	
Overview and application:	▪ Rheumatoid factor — "anti-IgG antibodies" — are antibodies directed to the Fc portion of the patient's own IgG. Rheumatoid factors are anti-immunoglobulin antibodies, classically anti-IgG IgM. RF are found in low levels in most patients, and despite the "rheumatoid" name, RF is not specific for rheumatoid arthritis.[270] Current tests (latex fixation or nephelometry) detect IgM anti-immunoglobulin antibodies; however Ig<u>A</u>-RF appears to have clinical superiority over other forms of RF because it correlates more strongly with clinical status.[271] ▪ This test is most commonly used to support the diagnosis of rheumatoid arthritis in a patient with a compelling clinical picture: peripheral polyarthritis lasting >6 weeks.[272] A negative result with a compelling clinical presentation of RA is termed "seronegative rheumatoid arthritis" by allopathic textbooks whereas a more appropriate term might be oligoarthritis, a condition described as "idiopathic" by allopathic text books despite the clear evidence that the majority of patients have one or more subsets of dysbiosis.[273] ▪ Titers (latex fixation) of 1:160 are considered clinically significant, favoring the diagnosis of RA.[274] However the positive predictive value is low — only 20-34% of people in an unselected population with a positive test result actually have RA.[275,276]
Advantages:	▪ Supports the diagnosis of rheumatoid arthritis: about 60-85% positive/sensitive in patients with rheumatoid arthritis (RA).[277,278] Quantitative titers of RF correlate with prognosis: a very high RF value portends a poor prognosis.
Limitations:	▪ Positive findings are common in the following conditions: rheumatoid arthritis, viral hepatitis, Sjögren's syndrome, endocarditis, scleroderma, mycobacteria diseases, polymyositis and dermatomyositis, syphilis, systemic lupus erythematosus, old age, mixed connective tissue disease, sarcoidosis; positive results may also been noted in: cryoglobulinemia, parasitic infection, interstitial lung disease, asymptomatic relatives of people with autoimmune diseases. ▪ Febrile patients with arthralgia are more likely to have endocarditis than RA.[279] ▪ Patients with iron overload present with a similar clinical picture (i.e., polyarthropathy with systemic complaints) and may have a positive RF. Thus, patients with positive RF and polyarthropathy should be tested for iron overload; use serum ferritin.[280,281]
Comments:	▪ This test should only be used to confirm the diagnosis of rheumatoid arthritis in patients with a compelling clinical picture of the disease: inflammatory peripheral polyarthropathy with systemic complaints for > 6 weeks. A negative result does not mean that the patient *does not* have rheumatoid arthritis; a positive result does not mean that the patient *does* have rheumatoid arthritis.[282] ▪ CCP (cyclic citrullinated protein) antibodies appear to be more specific and sensitive for RA and is becoming the test of choice for RA as described on the following page.

[270] Shojania K. Rheumatology: 2. What laboratory tests are needed? *CMAJ.* 2000 Apr 18;162(8):1157-63 http://www.cmaj.ca/cgi/content/full/162/8/1157
[271] Jonsson T, Valdimarsson H. What about IgA rheumatoid factor in rheumatoid arthritis? *Ann Rheum Dis.* 1998 Jan;57(1):63-4
[272] Shojania K. Rheumatology: 2. What laboratory tests are needed? *CMAJ.* 2000 Apr 18;162(8):1157-63 http://www.cmaj.ca/cgi/content/full/162/8/1157
[273] See chapter 4 of *Integrative Rheumatology* and Vasquez A. Reducing Pain and Inflammation Naturally. Part 6: Nutritional and Botanical Treatments Against "Silent Infections" and Gastrointestinal Dysbiosis, Commonly Overlooked Causes of Neuromusculoskeletal Inflammation and Chronic Health Problems. *Nutr Perspect* 2006; Jan http://InflammationMastery.com/part6.html
[274] Beers MH, Berkow R (eds). The Merck Manual. Seventeenth Edition. Whitehouse Station; Merck Research Laboratories 1999 Page 417
[275] Ward MM. Laboratory testing for systemic rheumatic diseases. *Postgrad Med.* 1998 Feb;103(2):93-100.
[276] Shojania K. Rheumatology: 2. What laboratory tests are needed? *CMAJ.* 2000 Apr 18;162(8):1157-63 http://www.cmaj.ca/cgi/content/full/162/8/1157
[277] Tierney ML. McPhee SJ, Papadakis MA (eds). Current Medical Diagnosis and Treatment 2002, 41st Edition. New York: Lange Medical, 2002 p854
[278] Shojania K. Rheumatology: 2. What laboratory tests are needed? *CMAJ.* 2000 Apr 18;162(8):1157-63 http://www.cmaj.ca/cgi/content/full/162/8/1157
[279] Klippel JH (ed). Primer on the Rheumatic Diseases. 11th Edition. Atlanta: Arthritis Foundation. 1997 page 96
[280] Bensen WG, Laskin CA, Little HA, Fam AG. Hemochromatoic arthropathy mimicking rheumatoid arthritis. A case with subcutaneous nodules, tenosynovitis, and bursitis. *Arthritis Rheum* 1978; 21: 844-8
[281] Vasquez A. Musculoskeletal disorders and iron overload disease: comment on the American College of Rheumatology guidelines for the initial evaluation of the adult patient with acute musculoskeletal symptoms. *Arthritis Rheum* 1996;39: 1767-8
[282] Shojania K. Rheumatology: 2. What laboratory tests are needed? *CMAJ.* 2000 Apr 18;162(8):1157-63 http://www.cmaj.ca/cgi/content/full/162/8/1157

CCP: Cyclic citrullinated protein antibody; Citrullinated protein antibodies (CPA); anti-CCP antibodies	
Overview and use:	▪ CCP—cyclic citrullinated protein antibodies; anticitrullinated protein antibodies: this is a relatively new auto-antibody marker that shows great promise and specificity for the early diagnosis of rheumatoid arthritis (RA). The test often becomes positive/present in asymptomatic patients years before the onset of clinical manifestations of RA. ▪ As of the first inclusion of this information in my books in December 2006, the information on anti-CCP antibodies is so new that it is not even included in most 2006-edition medical and rheumatology reference textbooks; nonetheless, doctors nationwide are already starting to use this test for the early diagnosis of RA. This may be particularly important because some research has shown that *early* and *aggressive* treatment of RA has an important impact on long-term prognosis[283]; however, the importance of early intervention is debatable.[284] ▪ Anti-CCP antibodies are directed toward several native proteins (e.g., filaggrin, fibrinogen, and vimentin) that have become posttranslationally modified by an uncharged citrulline in contrast to the normal positively charged arginine. This "citrullination" is catalyzed by a calcium-dependent enzyme, peptidylarginine deiminase (PAD). These changes in protein charge and sequence make the native protein a target of auto-antibody attack by IgG antibodies in RA.[285] However, this does not necessarily imply that citrullination of native proteins is "the cause" of RA because citrullination of native proteins can also occur *de novo* in inflamed joints, which are then further targeted for inflammatory destruction. Until more information is available, we should withhold final judgment as to the ultimate role and origin of anti-CCP antibodies and in the meanwhile view them as a very strong and sensitive association with RA that facilitates the early diagnosis of this disease.
Advantages:	▪ Anti-CCP antibodies have 98% specificity for RA[286] and is likely to become the future laboratory standard in the diagnosis and prognosis of RA.[287] Anti-CCP antibodies with a positive rheumatoid factor (RF) is termed "composite seropositivity" and appears to be more specific than isolated anti-CCP antibodies or RF.[288]
Limitations:	▪ The best current data indicates that anti-CCP antibodies are sensitive and specific for RA[289], and clinicians should use this test to diagnose and confirm RA.
Comments:	▪ Healthy people do not generally have anti-CCP antibodies. Asymptomatic patients with anti-CCP antibodies are at increased risk for clinical RA and are probably *en route* to the manifestation of clinical autoimmunity—RA, Sjogren's disease, or SLE. *Holistically intervene.* ▪ I hypothesize that PAD may become upregulated in synovial joints exposed to allergens, xenobiotics, bacterial debris/toxins/lipopolysaccharides and that the subsequent citrullination of joint proteins may lead to an autoimmune arthropathy that persists, perhaps despite removal of the inciting immunogen. More obviously (or perhaps more theoretically), given that PAD is calcium-dependent, it may be upregulated secondary to intracellular hypercalcinosis secondary to vitamin D deficiency, magnesium deficiency, or fatty acid imbalance.[290]

[283] "CONCLUSION: An initial 6-month cycle of intensive combination treatment that includes high-dose corticosteroids results in sustained suppression of the rate of radiologic progression in patients with early RA, independent of subsequent antirheumatic therapy." Landewe RB, et al. COBRA combination therapy in patients with early rheumatoid arthritis: long-term structural benefits of a brief intervention. *Arthritis Rheum*. 2002 Feb;46:347-56

[284] "By 5 years patients receiving early DMARDs had similar disease activity and comparable health assessment questionnaire scores to patients who received DMARDs later in their disease course." Scott DL. Evidence for early disease-modifying drugs in rheumatoid arthritis. *Arthritis Res Ther*. 2004;6(1):15-18 http://arthritis-research.com/content/6/1/15

[285] Hill J, Cairns E, Bell DA. The joy of citrulline. *J Rheumatol*. 2004 Aug;31(8):1471-3 http://www.jrheum.com/subscribers/04/08/1471.html

[286] Hill J, Cairns E, Bell DA. The joy of citrulline. *J Rheumatol*. 2004 Aug;31(8):1471-3

[287] "We conclude that, at present, the antibody response directed to citrullinated antigens has the most valuable diagnostic and prognostic potential for RA." van Boekel MA, Vossenaar ER, van den Hoogen FH, van Venrooij WJ. Autoantibody systems in rheumatoid arthritis: specificity, sensitivity and diagnostic value. *Arthritis Res*. 2002;4(2):87-93 http://arthritis-research.com/content/4/2/87

[288] "…our findings suggest that a positive anti-CCP antibody result does not necessarily exclude SLE in African American patients presenting with inflammatory arthritis. In such patients, the additional assessment of IgA-RF or IgM-RF isotypes may be of added value since composite seropositivity appears to be nearly exclusive to patients with RA." Mikuls TR, Holers VM, Parrish L, et al. Anti-cyclic citrullinated peptide antibody and rheumatoid factor isotypes in African Americans with early rheumatoid arthritis. *Arthritis Rheum*. 2006 Sep;54(9):3057-9

[289] "Serum antibodies reactive with citrullinated proteins/peptides are a very sensitive and specific marker for rheumatoid arthritis." Migliorini P, Pratesi F, Tommasi C, Anzilotti C. The immune response to citrullinated antigens in autoimmune diseases. *Autoimmun Rev*. 2005 Nov;4(8):561-4

[290] See InflammationMastery.com/archives/intracellular-hypercalcinosis and naturopathydigest.com/archives/2006/sep/vasquez.php for discussion

Exemplary case of clinical and laboratory evidence of reversal of "severe, aggressive, drug-resistant" rheumatoid arthritis in a 51yoWF following implementation of the Functional Inflammology Protocol: This summarizes the 13-month clinical outcome of the first patient treated with the updated functional inflammology protocol after its revision and expansion in March 2012.[291] After being diagnosed accurately by a rheumatologist—for this patient very clearly met diagnostic criteria—this patient presented for care following notably inefficacious treatment with the full medicopharmaceutical antirheumatic protocol comprised of NSAIDs, prednisone (she had only minimal response to prednisone >60mg/d), methotrexate, hydroxychloroquine, and "biologics" including etanercept/Enbrel; she was now being recommended to start newer "experimental" drugs. Following the failure of medical treatment, the patient was treated at the teaching clinic of a naturopathic college where her treatments included a clinician-supervised 26-day water-only fast, which resulted in the loss of 30 pounds (13.6 kilograms) but provided no clinical benefit for the rheumatoid arthritis. [Note: I/Dr Vasquez treat this patient at no charge. Dr William J Beakey of Professional Co-Op Services (Professionalco-op.com) generously donated these laboratory tests for collaborative/research purposes. Biotics Research Corporation (BioticsResearch.com) generously donates nutritional supplements for this patient.

March 2012: Patient reports suffering significantly with joint pain and lower extremity edema; foundational nutritional protocol[292] is implemented with antidysbiotic/antimicrobial intervention limited to emulsified oregano oil 600mg/d, mitochondrial support and the nutritional immunomodulation protocol. CCP level at this time is beyond laboratory testing limits, measured simply as "greater than" 250 units.

```
CCP Antibodies IgG/IgA            >250   High    units             0 - 19
                                                  Negative            <20
                                                  Weak positive     20 - 39
                                                  Moderate positive 40 - 59
                                                  Strong positive     >59
```

January 2013: Few modifications are made for the first 9 months and patient feels progressively better, but wants to "move to the next level of improvement" because—despite feeling and functioning significantly better solely with dietary and nutritional interventions—patient still notes exacerbations of pain, particularly following extended manual farm labor. At this time, labs are drawn showing an impressive reduction in CCP levels from "greater than" 250 units to 195 units, correlating with a reduction of at least 22%. At this time, patient was commenced on additional treatments including cabergoline, oral vancomycin, and azithromycin.

```
CCP Antibodies IgG/IgA            195    High    units             0 - 19
                                                  Negative            <20
                                                  Weak positive     20 - 39
                                                  Moderate positive 40 - 59
                                                  Strong positive     >59
```

April 2013: Patient continues to improve clinically; her subjective and objective clinical improvements (including additional loss of 30 pounds [13.6 kilograms] and reduction in hand swelling necessitating resizing of wedding ring) correlate nicely with the reduction in CCP levels, which have reduced from >250 units to 54 units, for a reduction of more than 78%. Thus, by objective physical and laboratory criteria, this patient appears to be experiencing authentic reversal—cure—of her disease due to the functional inflammology protocol.

```
CCP Antibodies IgG/IgA            54     High    units             0 - 19
                                                  Negative            <20
                                                  Weak positive     20 - 39
                                                  Moderate positive 40 - 59
                                                  Strong positive     >59
```

---

[291] Vasquez A. Functional Immunology and Nutritional Immunomodulation. 2012 https://www.createspace.com/3899760 and updated as "F.I.N.D. S.E.X®" The Easily Remembered Acronym for the Functional Inflammology Protocol. 2013 https://www.createspace.com/4234627
[292] Vasquez A. Revisiting the Five-Part Nutritional Wellness Protocol: The Supplemented Paleo-Mediterranean Diet. *Nutritional Perspectives* 2011 January http://www.ichnfm.org/faculty/vasquez/profile.html

HLA-B27: Human leukocyte antigen B-27	
Overview and interpretation:	▪ A common (5-10% of general population) genetic marker strongly associated with seronegative* spondyloarthropathy (all of which occur more commonly in men[293]): <ul><li>Ankylosing spondylitis (90-95% of 'whites' and 50% of 'blacks')[294]</li><li>Reactive arthritis [formerly called Reiter's syndrome] (85%)</li><li>Enteropathic spondyloarthropathy</li><li>Psoriatic spondylitis (<60%)</li></ul> * Recall that "seronegative" in this context implies that the *rheumatoid factor is negative*, even though *the HLA-B27 may be positive.*
Advantages: *Limitations:* *Comments:*	▪ *From a diagnostic perspective*: The clinical application and significance of this test is of limited value. All of the above-listed conditions are better assessed with the combination of clinical assessment and radiographs. In a patient with early and mild disease, this test may add evidence either supporting or refuting the diagnosis; but the test itself is not diagnostic of anything other than a genetic/histologic marker associated with various types of infection-induced arthropathy and autoimmunity (dysbiotic arthropathy[295]). ▪ *From an integrative/functional medicine perspective*: This test can be of some value if the result is positive and the patient has evidence of a systemic inflammatory/autoimmune disorder since it therefore more strongly suggests that a dysbiotic locus is the cause of disease.[296] A consistent theme in the rheumatology literature is that of "molecular mimicry"—the phenomenon by which structural similarities between human and microbial structures lead to targeting of human tissues by immune responses aimed at microbial antigens. This topic is explored in considerable detail in the section on multifocal dysbiosis in *Integrative Rheumatology*. The important link between microbe-induced autoimmunity and HLA-B27 is that many dysbiotic bacteria produce an HLA-B27-like molecule that appears to trigger an immune response which then erroneously affects human tissues, leading to the clinical picture of autoimmune inflammation. Many of these HLA-B27-producing bacteria colonize the gastrointestinal and genitourinary tracts, promoting musculoskeletal inflammation via molecular mimicry and other mechanisms.[297,298] A strong and growing body of research shows that HLA-B27 is a risk factor for microbe-induced autoimmunity. "Autoimmune" patients positive for HLA-B27 are presumed to have an occult infection—especially gastrointestinal, genitourinary, or sinorespiratory—until proven otherwise. ▪ Keep in mind that HLA-B27 itself is not a "disease" and therefore a "positive" result merely means that the patient has this particular human leukocyte antigen; this test is not and will never be diagnostic of a specific disease—it simply correlates with increased propensity toward dysbiotic arthropathy and suggests the need for dysbiosis testing and the (re)establishment of eubiosis.[299]

[293] "The major diseases associated with HLA-B27 (Reiter's disease, ankylosing spondylitis, acute anterior uveitis, and psoriatic arthritis) all occur much more commonly in men." James WH. Sex ratios and hormones in HLA related rheumatic diseases. *Ann Rheum Dis*. 1991 Jun;50(6):401-4

[294] Shojania K. Rheumatology: 2. What laboratory tests are needed? *CMAJ*. 2000 Apr 18;162(8):1157-63 http://www.cmaj.ca/cgi/content/full/162/8/1157

[295] See chapter 4 of *Integrative Rheumatology* and Vasquez A. Reducing Pain and Inflammation Naturally. Part 6: Nutritional and Botanical Treatments Against "Silent Infections" and Gastrointestinal Dysbiosis, Commonly Overlooked Causes of Neuromusculoskeletal Inflammation and Chronic Health Problems. *Nutr Perspect* 2006; Jan http://InflammationMastery.com/part6.html

[296] "The association between HLA-B27 and reactive arthritis (ReA) has also been well established... In a similar way, microbiological and immunological studies have revealed an association between Klebsiella pneumoniae in AS and Proteus mirabilis in RA." Ebringer A, Wilson C. HLA molecules, bacteria and autoimmunity. *J Med Microbiol*. 2000 Apr;49(4):305-11

[297] Inman RD. Antigens, the gastrointestinal tract, and arthritis. *Rheum Dis Clin North Am*. 1991 May;17(2):309-21

[298] Hunter JO. Food allergy--or enterometabolic disorder? *Lancet*. 1991 Aug 24;338(8765):495-6

[299] Dysbiotic arthropathy—joint inflammation and destruction as a result of a neuroimmune inflammatory response to microorganisms. Phrase coined by Alex Vasquez on December 15, 2005. No matching term on Medline or Google search. See chapter 4 of *Integrative Rheumatology* and Vasquez A. Reducing Pain and Inflammation Naturally. Part 6: Nutritional and Botanical Treatments Against "Silent Infections" and Gastrointestinal Dysbiosis, Commonly Overlooked Causes of Neuromusculoskeletal Inflammation and Chronic Health Problems. *Nutr Perspect* 2006; Jan http://InflammationMastery.com/part6.html

Complement levels: CH50, C3, and C4	
Overview and interpretation:	• Complement proteins are consumed in the complement cascades (typically activated by immune complexes) and thus low levels of complement proteins provide indirect evidence of extensive consumption due to immune complex-mediated inflammation. *Low* levels of complement are seen with *increased* disease activity in immune complex disorders (such as SLE, vasculitis, mixed cryoglobulinemia, rheumatoid vasculitis, glomerulonephritis). As expected, low levels of complement are also seen with inherited complement deficiencies; 10%–15% of Caucasian patients with SLE have an inherited complement deficiency.[300] • "CH50" is a screening test for complement levels whereas "C3" and "C4" are more specific for the monitoring of disease activity in autoimmune diseases hallmarked by immune complex deposition, most typically systemic lupus erythematosus (SLE) but also chronic active hepatitis, some chronic infections, poststreptococcal and membranoproliferative glomerulonephritis, and others. Given the wide range of diseases that can cause alterations in complement levels, clinical correlation and differential diagnosis are essential.
Advantages:	• Low complement levels—if not due to genotropic deficiency—provide indirect evidence of immune complex-mediated inflammation. • Elevated levels of complement are seen in conditions of infection or inflammation.
Limitations:	• Some patients have a hereditary absence of complement proteins and thus their levels are always abnormally low; obviously the test cannot be used in these patients for monitoring inflammatory disease.

CIC: Circulating immune complexes	
Overview: 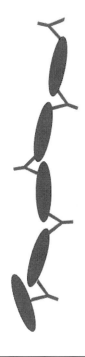	• Antibodies/immunoglobulins are produced in several different "classes": IgG, IgA, IgM, IgE, IgD. IgA antibodies are produced mostly in response to mucosal infections, such as from gastrointestinal dysbiosis or overt infections. When antibodies (in the shape of the letter "Y" with 2 antigen-binding sites on one end and the immuno-reactive site on the other) combine with the target antigen (depicted here in the shape of an oval, such as a bacteria or globular protein), "immune complexes" are formed which are chain-like links of antigens and antibodies. • Although formed in small amounts in healthy persons, in certain disease states, immune complexes may accumulate and initiate complement-dependent injury in various organs and tissues. This activation of complement may begin a series of potentially destructive events in the host, including anaphylatoxin production, cell lysis, leukocyte stimulation, and activation of macrophages and other cells. When immune complexes become fixed to vessel walls, destruction of normal tissue can occur, as in some types of glomerulonephritis and vasculitis. Predisposed to deposition in joints, vessels, and kidneys, immune complexes contribute directly to tissue injury in several autoimmune-inflammatory diseases.[301] **Immune Complexes, (Raji Cell), Quantitative** Reference Range: (Enzyme immunoassay [EIA]; cost $130) • Normal: ≤ 15.0 µg Eq/mL • Equivocal: 15.1-19.9 µg Eq/mL • **Positive: ≥20.0 µg Eq/mL**
Advantages:	• This test allows for direct quantification of immune-complex production.
Limitations:	• This test has only recently become available to practicing clinicians; however, it is very well supported by many publications in peer-reviewed research.[302]

[300] Shojania K. Rheumatology: 2. What laboratory tests are needed? *CMAJ.* 2000 Apr 18;162(8):1157-63 http://www.cmaj.ca/cgi/content/full/162/8/1157
[301] Jancar S, Sánchez Crespo M. Immune complex-mediated tissue injury: a multistep paradigm. *Trends Immunol.* 2005 Jan;26(1):48-55
[302] Davies KA,etal. Immune complex processing in patients with systemic lupus erythematosus. *J Clin Invest* 1992;90:2075-83 jci.org/articles/view/116090

Other tests for autoimmunity and immune dysfunction

Overview and interpretation:	▪ The table below is a quick reference guide to additional clinical disorders and *additional* laboratory tests; diagnostic criteria and lab tests change from time to time. Evaluation should always include history, physical exam, and basic labs such as CBC, UA, and chemistry panel.

Clinical consideration	Laboratory (or other) assessment
Autoimmune thyroid disease	• Anti(TPO) thyroid peroxidase antibodies: Hashimoto's thyroiditis • Antithyroglobulin antibodies: Hashimoto's thyroiditis • Thyroid stimulating immunoglobulins (TSI, 78%) and thyrotropin receptor antibodies (90%) are noted in Grave's disease
Latent autoimmune diabetes in adults (LADA), diabetes mellitus type 1.5	• Islet cell antibodies (ICA, also known as antipancreatic islet antibodies) and glutamic acid decarboxylase (GAD) antibodies • LADA/DM1.5 accounts for roughly 10 percent of cases of adult diabetes mellitus; has characteristics of type-1 (autoantibodies) and type-2 (insulin resistance); progresses to insulin-dependence within 6 years of diagnosis; assess beta-cell failure with C-peptide • Consider also tyrosine phosphatase (IA2) antibodies—positive in DM type-1 if this diagnosis is suspected
Autoimmune hepatitis	• Serum antinuclear antibodies (ANA) • Anti–smooth muscle antibodies (SMA) • Liver-kidney microsomal (type-1 [LKM-1]) antibodies • Anti–liver cytosol-1 (anti-LC1) antibodies • Consider also serum protein electrophoresis (SPEP) and quantitative immunoglobulin analysis; confirm with biopsy
Primary sclerosing cholangitis (PSC)	• ANA (53%), (p)ANCA (87%), anticardiolipin (66%) and anti-smooth muscle antibodies • Imaging of the bile duct, usually endoscopic retrograde cholangiopancreatography (ERCP)
Primary biliary cirrhosis (PBC)	• Anti-mitochondrial antibodies (AMA): 93% sensitivity, 98% specificity • ANA: positive in 20-50% of PBC patients • Imaging and biopsy; consider autoimmune cholangitis
Celiac disease	• IgA Anti-tissue Transglutaminase antibodies (anti-tTG) • IgG and IgA Anti-Gliadin antibodies (AGA) • IgA Deamidated Gliadin Peptide (DGP) antibodies • Quantitative immunoglobulin A (IgA)—performed to exclude selective sIgA deficiency, one of the most common immune deficiency disorders • > 95% of celiac patients have HLA-DQ2 or HLA-DQ8
Inflammatory bowel disease (IBD)	• IgA and IgG antibodies for *Saccharomyces cerevisiae*—nearly 80% of Crohn's disease patients are positive for either IgA or IgG. "In ulcerative colitis, <15% are positive for IgG, and <2% are positive for IgA. Fewer than 5% of healthy controls are positive for either IgG or IgA antibody, and no healthy controls had antibody for both."[303] • "Atypical ANCA"—positive in a significant percentage of patients with ulcerative colitis, primary sclerosing cholangitis, autoimmune hepatitis • P-ANCA antibodies—"found in 50-70% of ulcerative colitis (UC) patients, but in only 20% of Crohn disease (CD) patients"[304]
Antiphospholipid/ anticardiolipin/ Hughes syndrome	• IgA, IgG, IgM cardiolipin antibody and IgG, IgM (preferably with IgA) Beta-2 glycoprotein-I antibodies; lupus anticoagulant(s) • Clinical correlation is essential to determine significance

Advantages:	▪ Labs always provide additional data, some of which may be diagnostic.
Limitations:	▪ Laboratory data must be interpreted within a clinical context in order to properly inform clinical decision-making, diagnostic criteria, and therapeutic intervention.

---

[303] Inflammatory Bowel Disease (IBD) Profile. https://www.labcorp.com   March 2013
[304] Inflammatory Bowel Disease Differentiation Profile . http://www.aruplab.com/guides/ug/tests/0050567.jsp March 2013

Testing for Occult Infections and Dysbiosis—A Practical Introduction and Clinical Approach	

Conceptual overview, advantages and limitations:	• With the publication of my *Integrative Rheumatology* textbook in 2006/2007, I was the first to promote the ideas that patients with systemic inflammation in general and autoimmunity in particular <u>***always***</u> have occult "infections" or microbial colonization—dysbiosis—and that this dysbiotic foci is general not singular, nor due to only one offending microbe; rather, inflammatory dysbiosis tends to be multifocal and polymicrobial—what I have termed "multifocal polydysbiosis." In the ensuing years, additional research has consistently proven this model to be correct. I have further defined dysbiosis as "a relationship of non-acute host-microorganism interaction that adversely affects the human host" (*Integrative Rheumatology*[305]), and I have more recently subdivided the general effects of dysbiosis on the human host as either inflammatory/immunogenic ("inflammatory dysbiosis") or metabolic ("metabolic dysbiosis") although clearly overlap exists. • Microbial colonization is *necessary but not sufficient* for the existence of the host-microbe relationship that characterizes dysbiosis; the host must be susceptible to the effects of the microbes, and the hosts defense system must be sufficiently impaired to allow the microbial biomass to become qualitatively sufficient (and diverse) to surpass the host's threshold of immunologic and metabolic tolerance.

> **Terminology**
>
> **Dysbiosis**: A relationship of non-acute non-infectious host-microorganism interaction that adversely affects the human host.
>
> **Dysbiosis subtypes (based on location):**
> 1. Orodental
> 2. Sinorespiratory
> 3. Gastrointestinal
> 4. Parenchymal
> 5. Genitourinary
> 6. Cutaneous
> 7. Environmental
> 8. Microbial
>
> **Multifocal dysbiosis**: A clinical condition characterized by a patient's having more than one foci/location of dysbiosis; generally the adverse physiologic and clinical consequences are additive and synergistic.
>
> **Polydysbiosis**: Concurrent dysbiosis with microbes of different species.
>
> **Main treatment approaches for dysbiosis**: ❶ antimicrobial, ❷ immunorestorative, ❸ tolerogenic.
>
> These concepts were initially detailed in Vasquez A. *Integrative Rheumatology* (2006, 2007) and the *Inflammation Mastery* series starting in 2014.

Nevertheless, despite the tripartite requirements for the establishment of dysbiosis—microbes, immunoincompetence, and intolerance—the fact remains clear that dysbiosis requires microbes. Equally clear is the fact that microbes alone are insufficient for dysbiotic inflammation.

• One of the first questions that arises for clinicians that of choosing methodology for the detection of the offending microbe(s). Briefly, the quest for the identification of the offending microbe(s) is simultaneously wise and sophomoric (soph-, "wise," and moros, "fool"). This approach is wise because the quest for identification and thereafter targeted eradication of the offending microbe is intellectually "clean", clinically efficient, and—most legitimately—allows for precise use of antimicrobial therapy; in reality, this approach is based on numerous erroneous presuppositions including:

- <u>Presumed physiologic reliability</u>: A common error is that of using antibody assays for the detection of current "infections", especially of the dysbiotic type. Antigen detection is preferable to antibody measurement, given that antibodies may be present even when an infection is presently absent, and that infection/colonization may be present even when antibodies are absent.
- <u>Presumed equivalence of tests for acute infections and tests for chronic dysbiotic colonizations</u>: Another common error is that of using testing methods developed for the detection of acute infections (e.g., the rapid strep test for acute [extracellular] streptococcal pharyngitis) when seeking to detect dysbiotic infections (e.g., chronic [intracellular] streptococcal pharyngeal colonization of psoriasis).

---

[305] Vasquez A. *Integrative Rheumatology*. 2006 and 2007. http://InflammationMastery.com/textbooks/rheumatology.html

- Concept: Microbial phenotype varies per type and chronicity of infection/colonization—example of streptococci in chronic psoriasis (*Clinical and Experimental Immunology* 2004 Jan[306]): "Although streptococci have traditionally been viewed as *extracellular* pathogens, they are able to *invade several eukaryotic cell types* [i.e., manifest an intracellular phenotype] including squamous epithelium and macrophages, and this has been associated with persistent streptococcal carriage and recurrent infections."
- Presumed performance reliability: Culture-based methodology is notoriously insensitive for anaerobic bacteria, and it is impractical for the detection and identification of complex microbial quorums and biosystems. DNA-based tests exist as numerous methodologies—many of which are patented for research use and are therefore not commercially available; DNA-based testing is impractical for the detection and identification of complex microbial quorums and biosystems with thousands of different microbes.
- Presumed stability of identity of microbes: Microbes have historically been presumed to have stable identities and microbe-disease associations; what we now know is that microbes readily exchange genetic material and that microbial phenotype and metabolic and inflammatory/immunogenic properties can change for example in response to the host's diet or psychoemotional state (the latter described as the study of "microbial endocrinology"[307]).
  - Concept: The emerging irrelevance of microbial identification (*Autoimmune Reviews* 2009 Jul[308]): "These [human-colonizing] bacteria rapidly and frequently share their DNA with their fellow species – even distantly related species – through horizontal gene transfer. … Some argue that the number of microbes created through genetic recombination is so high that the concept of distinct bacterial species may become obsolete."
- Identification and eradication of a singular offending microbe is noted in the research literature and in clinical practice to occasionally produce brilliant and stunning clinical responses; more commonly—and even more powerfully supported by major trends in the research literature—what we find is a positive clinical response to the combination of ❶ nonspecific antimicrobial therapy (e.g., drugs or botanicals, often and preferably both synthetic and natural agents at the same time), ❷ immunorestorative interventions such as stress reduction and immunonutrition, and ❸ nutritional immunomodulation[309] to induce immunotolerance. Therefore, the expense and pursuit of identifying the offending microbe(s) is not necessary for a therapeutic response; indeed, the expense and pursuit of identifying the offending microbe(s) may actually deter or delay implementation of effective therapy. However—and finally, the use of testing to determine the presence and persistence of dysbiotic microbial infections/colonizations is occasionally helpful to direct antimicrobial drug therapy especially when more dangerous antimicrobial agents are being employed and/or when previous empiric approaches have not been useful; clinicians can use these and other tests with consideration of the discussion provided above as well as in detailed to much greater extents in my books starting with *Integrative Rheumatology*. For the sake of organization, this author's more common test considerations will be listed here by location, with the appreciation that the concept of location is itself somewhat misleading, given that microbes may apparently affect/infect one location (e.g., herpes simplex virus infection of the oral mucosa and associated cranial nerve body) while occultly affecting/infecting a distant location (e.g., the hippocampus).[310]

---

[306] Gudjonsson JE, Johnston A, Sigmundsdottir H, Valdimarsson H. Immunopathogenic mechanisms in psoriasis. *Clin Exp Immunol*. 2004 Jan;135(1):1-8

[307] Freestone PP, Sandrini SM, Haigh RD, Lyte M. Microbial endocrinology: how stress influences susceptibility to infection. *Trends Microbiol*. 2008 Feb;16(2):55-64

[308] Proal AD, Albert PJ, Marshall T. Autoimmune disease in the era of the metagenome. *Autoimmun Rev*. 2009 Jul;8(8):677-81

[309] Vasquez A. *Functional Immunology and Nutritional Immunomodulation*. 2012. https://www.createspace.com/3899760

[310] "HSV-1, for example, can infect oral and nasal mucosa and then travels through retrograde axonal transport to the trigeminal ganglion or the olfactory bulb, respectively, where it establishes a latent infection or may rapidly enter the CNS. … Periodic reactivations from latency are followed by axonal transport of newly produced HSV-1 virions either back to the site of primary infection, where they cause new skin vesicles or mucosal ulcers, or onward to the CNS, where they can cause a productive, but usually mild infection, which may later become latent, as described for rodents. In particular, newly produced virions may target the limbic system, which includes the hippocampus, thalamus and amygdala." De Chiara G, Marcocci ME, Sgarbanti R, et al. Infectious agents and neurodegeneration. *Mol Neurobiol*. 2012 Dec;46(3):614-38

Laboratory tests per location of dysbiotic microbial colonization:	▪ Per the above discussion and context, some of the more common and/or more useful laboratory tests are listed here; these are listed per location for organizational purposes only, with the full appreciation that the location itself is mostly irrelevant, with the possible exception of the gastrointestinal tract which harbors the greatest quantity and diversity of microbes and which harbors these microbes in intimate contact with the bulk of the human immune system—the gut-associated lymphoid tissue (GALT) possesses the largest mass of lymphoid tissue in the human body. In sum, testing for microbes provides either direct and specific evidence of microbes or indirect evidence (both with varying levels of sensitivity), or—at the opposite extreme—empiric evidence (i.e., monitoring response to antimicrobial or immunorestorative interventions) which is completely nonspecific yet much more clinically meaningful. ❶ <u>Direct testing—culture/DNA/antigen</u>: Swab for culture and sensitivity (C-S), DNA-based testing such as polymerase chain reaction (PCR), or antigen detection, ❷ <u>Indirect testing—most commonly antibody assays</u>: Various antibody tests against microbes are available and clinically meaningful, ❸ <u>Empiric testing</u>: Monitoring response to therapeutic-diagnostic intervention with antimicrobial therapy.

	▪ <u>Orodental dysbiosis/colonization—introduction to assessment</u>:
	  ❶ <u>Direct testing—culture/DNA/antigen</u>: Swabs of mucosa, gingiva, teeth, and dentures can be used for culture, DNA, and antigen testing.
	  ❷ <u>Indirect testing—antibody assays</u>: Antibody titers specific for oral/dental/periodontal microbes correlate with numerous inflammatory disorders, ranging from insulin resistance to rheumatoid arthritis (RA).
	  ❸ <u>Empiric observation</u>: Oral exam may reveal tooth and gum disease. *Example*—rheumatoid arthritis: "Control of periodontal infection and gingival inflammation by scaling/root planing and plaque control in subjects with periodontal disease may reduce the severity of RA."[311]

	▪ <u>Sinorespiratory dysbiosis/colonization—introduction to assessment</u>:
	  ❶ <u>Direct testing—culture/DNA/antigen</u>: Swabs of nasal and pharyngeal mucosa can be used for culture, DNA, and antigen testing. Sputum can be submitted for culture and direct microscopic analysis. *Example*—atopic dermatitis: In eczema, skin cultures yielded *Staphylococcus aureus* from lesional skin in 87.1% of patients and from the nares in 80.6% of patients.
	  ❷ <u>Indirect testing—antibody assays</u>: Antibody titers specific for respiratory microbes correlate with numerous inflammatory disorders, ranging from cardiovascular disease to oligoarthritis.
	  ❸ <u>Empiric observation</u>: *Example*—Wegener's granulomatosis/vasculitis: Treatment with trimethoprim-sulfamethoxazole (co-trimoxazole, a broad-spectrum antibiotic) reduces the incidence of relapses in patients with Wegener's granulomatosis in remission.[312,313]

	▪ <u>Gastrointestinal dysbiosis/colonization—introduction to assessment</u>: ❶ <u>Direct testing—culture/DNA/antigen</u>: Jejunal aspiration is the gold standard for diagnosis of SIBO—small intestinal bacterial overgrowth; similarly, aspiration with or without biopsy followed by direct microscopy or culture is generally the gold standard for the identification of most infections. Stool tests are available using culture, DNA, and antigen-detecting methodology; routine pathogens such as

---

[311] Al-Katma MK, Bissada NF, Bordeaux JM, et al. Control of periodontal infection reduces the severity of active rheumatoid arthritis. *J Clin Rheumatol*. 2007 Jun;13(3):134-7
[312] Zycinska K, et al. Co-trimoxazole and prevention of relapses of PR3-ANCA positive vasculitis with pulmonary involvement. *Eur J Med Res*. 2009 Dec 7;14 Suppl 4:265-7
[313] Stegeman CA, et al. Trimethoprim-sulfamethoxazole (co-trimoxazole) for the prevention of relapses of Wegener's granulomatosis. *N Engl J Med*. 1996 Jul 4;335(1):16-20

Salmonella, Shigella, Campylobacter, and enterohemorrhagic *E coli* (EHEC) can be detected by routine (i.e., standard, hospital-based) medical reference laboratories. When testing for dysbiotic-type colonizations, clinicians should utilize a specialty laboratory that presents the results within a context of additional markers for clinical decision-making as discussed in a following section on stool testing.

❷ <u>Indirect testing—antibody assays, lactulose:mannitol assay, inflammatory markers, sIgA, breath hydrogen and methane</u>: Antibody assays specific for gastrointestinal yeast, bacteria, and protozoans are available. In specific situations, very indirect testing such as the lactulose:mannitol assay can be used to determine increased intestinal permeability which can provide indirect evidence of intestinal dysbiosis; likewise, inflammatory markers such as calprotectin, lactoferrin, and lysozyme can also indicate intestinal inflammation which is commonly caused by intestinal microbial overgrowth/colonization. Secretory IgA is also measured in fecal samples and can be interpreted in clinical context; elevated levels suggest immunologic response to intraluminal antigens, the most offensive of which are microbial/dysbiotic. Exhaled hydrogen and methane can be measured following a carbohydrate challenge to assess for nonspecific SIBO. *Example*—fibromyalgia: "3/15 (20%) controls had an abnormal breath test compared with 93/111 (84%) subjects with IBS (p<0.01) and 42/42 (100%) with fibromyalgia (p<0.0001 v controls, p<0.05 v IBS). ... The degree of somatic pain in fibromyalgia correlated significantly with the hydrogen level seen on the breath test. An abnormal lactulose breath test is more common in fibromyalgia than IBS. In contrast with IBS, the degree of abnormality on breath test is greater in subjects with fibromyalgia and correlates with somatic pain."[314]

❸ <u>Empiric observation</u>: Response to antimicrobial therapy confirms intestinal microbial overgrowth/dysbiosis/parasitosis; the retrospective diagnosis is made most clearly with observation of a positive clinical response following treatment with orally-administered nonabsorbed antimicrobial agents, such as oregano oil, berberine, nystatin, rifaximin, and vancomycin. *Example*—empiric diagnosis and treatment of small intestinal bacterial overgrowth: "For cases in which a firm diagnosis cannot be made, but clinical symptoms favor SIBO, empirical antibiotic use may be a more cautious approach to prevent delay of treatment and to prevent increases in symptom severity."[315]

- <u>Genitourinary dysbiosis/colonization—introduction to assessment</u>:
  - ❶ <u>Direct testing—culture/DNA/antigen</u>: Reactive/inflammatory arthritis secondary to genitourinary infection is well known, formerly called Reiter's syndrome; a similar association is established in chronic oligoarthritis. *Example*—reactive arthritis: "Urogenital swab cultures showed a microbial infection in 44% of the patients with oligoarthritis (15% *Chlamydia*, 14% *Mycoplasma*, 28% *Ureaplasma*), whereas in the control group only 26% had a positive result (4% *Chlamydia*, 7% *Mycoplasma*, 21% *Ureaplasma*) (P < 0.001). ... Urogenital swab culture is the only useful diagnostic method for the detection of the arthritogenic infection in extra-articularly asymptomatic patients with undifferentiated oligoarthritis."[316]
  - ❷ <u>Indirect testing—antibody assays</u>: Antibody assays specific for genitourinary microbes are available. *Example*—oligoarthritis: "A Chlamydia IgG-antibody titer > or = 1:256 was found in 22% of the patients in the oligoarthritis group and in 9% of the controls (P <

[314] Pimentel M, Wallace D, Hallegua D, Chow E, Kong Y, Park S, Lin HC. A link between irritable bowel syndrome and fibromyalgia may be related to findings on lactulose breath testing. *Ann Rheum Dis*. 2004 Apr;63(4):450-2

[315] Malik BA, Xie YY, Wine E, Huynh HQ. Diagnosis and pharmacological management of small intestinal bacterial overgrowth in children with intestinal failure. *Can J Gastroenterol*. 2011 Jan;25(1):41-5. This is a very excellent article—highly recommended.

[316] Erlacher L, Wintersberger W, Menschik M, et al. Reactive arthritis: urogenital swab culture is the only useful diagnostic method for the detection of the arthritogenic infection in extra-articularly asymptomatic patients with undifferentiated oligoarthritis. *Br J Rheumatol*. 1995 Sep;34(9):838-42

0.01). However, for only half of *Chlamydia* IgG-positive patients could a *Chlamydia* infection be confirmed by urogenital swab culture."[317]

❸ Empiric observation: Response to antimicrobial and immunorestorative interventions. *Example*—rheumatoid arthritis: "We propose that sub-clinical *Proteus* urinary tract infections are the main triggering factors and that the presence of molecular mimicry and cross-reactivity between these bacteria and RA-targeted tissue antigens assists in the perpetuation of the disease process through production of cytopathic auto-antibodies. Patients with RA especially during the early stages of the disease could benefit from *Proteus* anti-bacterial measures involving the use of antibiotics, vegetarian diets and high intake of water and fruit juices such as cranberry juice in addition to the currently employed treatments."[318]

- Cutaneous dysbiosis/colonization—introduction to assessment:
  - ❶ Direct testing—culture/DNA/antigen: For bacterial infections/colonizations, culture and DNA methods can be used; for fungi, skin scraping followed by KOH wet-mount and microscopic examination is commonly used. *Example*—atopic dermatitis: In eczema, skin cultures yielded *Staphylococcus aureus* from lesional skin in 87.1% of patients and from the nares in 80.6% of patients.[319]
  - ❷ Indirect testing—antibody assays: Antibodies to dermal microbes can be measured. *Example*—atopic dermatitis: Eczema patients commonly have serum IgE antibodies specific for *Malassezia sympodialis*, *Candida albicans*, and *Staphylococcus aureus*, and these antibody levels correlate with disease severity.[320]
  - ❸ Empiric observation: *Example*—atopic dermatitis: "Patients with AD can have sudden exacerbations of AD attributable to overgrowth of *S aureus* that can be independent of true secondary bacterial infection, a notion supported by the clinical response of patients with severe AD to anti- staphylococcal antibiotics [*Dr Vasquez*: and other antimicrobial measures]."

- Environmental dysbiosis/colonization—introduction to assessment:
  - ❶ Direct testing—culture/DNA/antigen: Home, work, and recreational environments can be surveyed for microbial contamination, particularly mold. Pier-and-beam homes should be inspected for mold and water in the crawlspace; likewise, attics should be inspected for occult leaks and mold. Mold plates, Petri dishes, and filter cartridges can be used to identify airborne microbes. *Fusarium*, *Trichoderma*, and *Stachybotrys* produce mycotoxins.[321]
  - ❷ Indirect testing—antibody assays: Tests can be performed for evidence of microbial exposure and immune response (e.g., antibodies specific for microbes); correlative tests can also be performed to assess the clinical and immunological significance of the exposure (e.g., RF, ANA, CCP, and other autoantibodies). *Example*—inflammatory disease associated with working/living in moisture-damaged building: *Chlamydophila pneumoniae* antibodies may be elevated in correlation with clinical symptoms and environmental exposure to microbes.[322] *Example*—biochemical changes noted in persons exposed to microbial contamination: An article co-authored by Vojdani[323] noted,

[317] Erlacher L, Wintersberger W, Menschik M, et al. Reactive arthritis: urogenital swab culture is the only useful diagnostic method for the detection of the arthritogenic infection in extra-articularly asymptomatic patients with undifferentiated oligoarthritis. *Br J Rheumatol*. 1995 Sep;34(9):838-42

[318] Ebringer A, Rashid T. Rheumatoid arthritis is an autoimmune disease triggered by Proteus urinary tract infection. *Clin Dev Immunol*. 2006 Mar;13(1):41-8

[319] Huang JT, Abrams M, Tlougan B, Rademaker A, Paller AS. Treatment of Staphylococcus aureus colonization in atopic dermatitis decreases disease severity. *Pediatrics*. 2009 May;123(5):e808-14

[320] Sonesson A, Bartosik J, Christiansen J, et al. Sensitization to Skin-associated Microorganisms in Adult Patients with Atopic Dermatitis is of Importance for Disease Severity. *Acta Derm Venereol*. 2012 Oct 16. doi: 10.2340/00015555-1465. http://www.medicaljournals.se/acta/content/?doi=10.2340/00015555-1465

[321] Am Acad Pediatrics. Toxic effects of indoor molds. Committee on Environ Health. *Pediatrics* 1998;101(4 Pt1):712-4 http://aappolicy.aappublications.org/cgi/content/full/pediatrics;101/4/712

[322] Seuri M, Paldanius M, Leinonen M, Roponen M, Hirvonen MR, Saikku P. Chlamydophila pneumoniae antibodies in office workers with and without inflammatory rheumatic diseases in a moisture-damaged building. *Eur J Clin Microbiol Infect Dis*. 2005 Mar;24(3):236-7

[323] Anyanwu E, Campbell AW, Vojdani A, Ehiri JE, Akpan AI. Biochemical changes in the serum of patients with chronic toxigenic mold exposures: a risk factor for multiple renal dysfunctions. *ScientificWorldJournal*. 2003 Nov 3;3:1058-64

"biochemical abnormal concentrations in creatinine, uric acid, phosphorus, alkaline phosphatase, cholesterol, LDH [*Dr Vasquez*: LDH here is corrected from "HDH" per data in Table 1 of the full-text article], SGOT/AST, segmented neutrophils, lymphocytes, total T3, IgG and IgA immunoglobulins with significant differences between patients and controls."; the authors note an increased prevalence of renal disorders among such patients. *Example*—increased serum autoantibodies in patients exposed to environmental molds: "Abnormally high levels of ANA, ASM, and CNS myelin (immunoglobulins [Ig]G, IgM, IgA) and PNS myelin (IgG, IgM, IgA) were found; odds ratios for each were significant at 95% confidence intervals, showing an increased risk for autoimmunity."[324] *Example*—elevated mold counts, and elevations of non-IgE antibodies in mold-exposed persons: "Detection of high levels (colony-forming units per cubic meter) of molds—which, in this study, strongly suggested that there existed a reservoir of spores in the building at the time of sampling—along with a significant elevation in IgG, IgM, or IgA antibodies against molds and mycotoxins, could be used in future epidemiologic investigations of fungal exposure. In addition to IgE, measurements of IgG, IgM, and IgA antibodies should be considered in mold-exposed individuals."
- ❸ Empiric observation: Alleviation of clinical symptoms and signs following building evacuation or remediation substantiates the exposure-immunopathology link.

- Parenchymal dysbiosis/colonization—introduction to assessment: Many different "internal" infections/colonizations can contribute to chronic inflammatory disease and—at its most extreme—autoimmunity. Some of these situations are perhaps best described/characterized as true "infections" such as noted with hepatitis C infection contributing to immune-complex-mediated dermatitis and arthritis; infection in this context is noted to have the classic pathologic manifestations of histologic observability and tissue damage (e.g., viral hepatitis and cirrhosis). In other situations, the microbe is neither consistently observable in tissue nor does microbe-induced tissue damage characterize the clinical condition; these situations are perhaps better defined as "parenchymal dysbiosis"—a state of microbe-induced inflammation lacking the classic pathological findings of histologic observability and microbe-induced tissue damage. An example of the latter includes chronic systemic inflammation and—occasionally—inflammatory arthritis (but not septic arthritis) triggered by *Chlamydia/Chlamydophila pneumoniae*. See the following tables for microbe-specific assessments and disease associations.
  - ❶ Direct testing—culture/DNA/antigen: *Example*—hepatitis C: Hepatitis C virus RNA detected by quantitative or qualitative PCR.
  - ❷ Indirect testing—antibody assays: *Example*—chronic fatigue, chronic oligoarthritis: IgG antibodies specific for *Chlamydia/Chlamydophila pneumonia*.
  - ❸ Empiric observation: *Example*—psoriasis: Beneficial response to empiric antimicrobial treatment with penicillin[325] or azithromycin[326] confirms the microbial basis of the disease.

[324] Gray MR, Thrasher JD, Crago R, Madison RA, Arnold L, Campbell AW, Vojdani A. Mixed mold mycotoxicosis: immunological changes in humans following exposure in water-damaged buildings. *Arch Environ Health*. 2003 Jul;58(7):410-20
[325] Saxena VN, Dogra J. Long-term use of penicillin for the treatment of chronic plaque psoriasis. *Eur J Dermatol*. 2005 Sep-Oct;15(5):359-62
[326] Saxena VN, Dogra J. Long-term oral azithromycin in chronic plaque psoriasis: a controlled trial. *Eur J Dermatol*. 2010 May-Jun;20(3):329-33

Parenchymal/internal/occult dysbiotic microbes and/or occult infections that can contribute to chronic inflammation, metabolic impairment, or autoimmunity

Viruses	Laboratory assessment	Disease association(s)
Cytomegalovirus (CMV)	IgM antibodies may not peak until 4-7 weeks after onset; IgG antibodies increase by 4x during acute infection; in immunosuppressed patients, PCR and antigen testing is preferred over antibody testing	Fatigue, mononucleosis-like illness, retinopathy in immunosuppressed
Epstein-Barr virus (EBV)	IgG and IgM antibodies to viral antigens are specific and include EBV-early antigen (EA) IgG, EBV-viral capsid antigen (VCA) IgG; EBV-VCA IgM; Epstein-Barr nuclear antigen antibodies (EBNA); IgG titers >1:640 appear to correlate with increased fatigue and clinical response to antiviral treatment in patients with chronic fatigue syndrome[327]	Fatigue, chronic fatigue syndrome, mononucleosis
Hepatitis B virus (HepB, HBV)	HepB surface antigen and DNA are most specific	Liver disease, immune complex (IC)-mediated vasculitis and arthritis
Hepatitis C virus (HepC, HCV)	HCV RNA becomes positive 1-3 weeks postexposure	Liver disease, immune complex (IC)-mediated vasculitis and arthritis
Human herpes virus type-6 (HHV-6)	IgG antibody titers >1:320 correlate with increased fatigue and clinical response to antiviral treatment in patients with chronic fatigue syndrome[328]; IgM and viral DNA levels are elevated in patients with multiple sclerosis[329]	Fatigue, chronic fatigue syndrome, multiple sclerosis
Human immunodeficiency virus (HIV)	Typical protocol is ELISA antibody testing (and/or Western blot) followed by PCR for viral load; for acute infection (prior to [antibody] seroconversion) and severe immunosuppression, DNA-based testing is preferred	Fatigue, peripheral neuropathy, opportunistic infections, severe acute psoriasis
Herpes simplex virus types 1 and 2 (HSV1, HSV2)	Measured by chemiluminescence (CI) or enzyme immunoassay (EIA), IgG antibody titers correlate with exposure/infection and level of viral replication (i.e., higher titers indicate higher viral replication); Western blot methodology is considered the epidemiologic gold standard[330] but IgG measurements by CI/EIA are clinically very reliable and are more widely available.	Fatigue, acute encephalitis, Alzheimer's disease, multiple sclerosis

---

[327] "Nine out of 12 (75%) patients experienced near resolution of their symptoms, allowing them all to return to the workforce or full time activities. In the nine patients with a symptomatic response to treatment, EBV VCA IgG titers dropped from 1:2560 to 1:640 (p = 0.008) and HHV-6 IgG titers dropped from a median value of 1:1280 to 1:320 (p = 0.271)." Kogelnik AM, Loomis K, Hoegh-Petersen M, et al. Use of valganciclovir in patients with elevated antibody titers against Human Herpesvirus-6 (HHV-6) and Epstein-Barr Virus (EBV) who were experiencing central nervous system dysfunction including long-standing fatigue. *J Clin Virol*. 2006 Dec;37 Suppl 1:S33-8

[328] "Nine out of 12 (75%) patients experienced near resolution of their symptoms, allowing them all to return to the workforce or full time activites. In the nine patients with a symptomatic response to treatment, EBV VCA IgG titers dropped from 1:2560 to 1:640 (p = 0.008) and HHV-6 IgG titers dropped from a median value of 1:1280 to 1:320 (p = 0.271)." Kogelnik AM, Loomis K, Hoegh-Petersen M, et al. Use of valganciclovir in patients with elevated antibody titers against Human Herpesvirus-6 (HHV-6) and Epstein-Barr Virus (EBV) who were experiencing central nervous system dysfunction including long-standing fatigue. *J Clin Virol*. 2006 Dec;37 Suppl 1:S33-8

[329] "Results demonstrate increased levels of anti-HHV6-IgG (78.2% versus 76.4% in controls; P = NS), and IgM (34.6% versus 6.5% in controls; P < 0.05) in MS patients. ... Moreover, load of cell-free viral DNA was higher in RRMS and SPMS patients and detected in 60.2% (47/78) of MS patients, compared with 14.6% (18/123) of healthy controls (P < 0.001)." Ramroodi N, Sanadgol N, Ganjali Z, Niazi AA, Sarabandi V, Moghtaderi A. Monitoring of active human herpes virus 6 infection in Iranian patients with different subtypes of multiple sclerosis. *J Pathog*. 2013;2013:194932

[330] Accessed in March 2013. "The Western Blot, the most accurate of these blood tests, is done at the University of Washington." http://depts.washington.edu/herpes/faq.php#faqCat-3. "The Western blot assay is the most validated method for identifying type-specific antibodies and is considered the gold standard. ... The Western blot assay is conducted exclusively at the University of Washington where clinical specimens can be sent and processed. Two type-specific glycoprotein G serological tests are commercially available in the United States. Sensitivity and specificity of these tests are comparable to the Western blot assay. These tests cost $10 to $40 (U.S. dollars)." http://www.uspreventiveservicestaskforce.org/uspstf05/herpes/herpesup.htm

Parenchymal/internal/occult dysbiotic microbes and/or occult infections that can contribute to chronic inflammation, metabolic impairment, or autoimmunity —*continued*

Viruses	*Laboratory assessment*	*Disease association(s)*
Parvovirus B19	IgG and IgM antibodies are commonly used; however, "high-level viremia in acutely infected persons may cause virus-antibody complexes, which will result in a false-negative IgM test result. In this setting, polymerase chain reaction (PCR) may be a better diagnostic modality."[331]	Arthritis/arthralgia, which can mimic rheumatoid arthritis[332]
Bacteria, protozoa, etc.	*Assessment*	*Disease association(s)*
Infectious agents well-known to cause reactive/inflammatory arthritis: *Chlamydia trachomatis* and various species in the genera *Salmonella, Shigella, Campylobacter,* and *Yersinia*	Direct microscopy, culture, DNA-based testing; antibody testing is less commonly used for these acute and subacute infections; empiric antimicrobial treatment without laboratory testing is reasonable with a compelling clinical picture of infection and associated inflammopathy/arthropathy	Reactive arthritis, chronic arthritis, autoimmune thyroiditis (especially *Yersinia*, in which case anti-*Yersinia* antibodies are strongly correlated with thyroid disease[333])
Borrelia burgdorferi, Babesia species including *microti, divergens,* MO1, *duncani* (WA-1)	IgG and IgM antibodies, Western blot, PCR; many experienced clinicians prefer IGeneX testing; much controversy exists about the "best" testing method(s)	Fatigue, Lyme disease (erythema chronicum migrans, myocarditis, arthritis, meningitis, neuropathies)
Chlamydia/Chlamydophila pneumoniae	IgG titers > 1:64 correlate with chronic/persistent infection/colonization[334]; likewise, IgA titers > 1:20 correlate with chronic/persistent infection/colonization; IgA positivity and/or PCR positivity correlate with myocardial infarction[335]; as expected PCR is considered best evidence of current active infection, since antibody levels do not always correlate with active infection whereas nuclear material is rapidly degraded by human restriction endonucleases and therefore when present provides clear proof of current infection/colonization	Chronic fatigue, chronic inflammatory arthritis (responds to prolonged combination therapy with azithromycin and rifampin[336]), multiple sclerosis[337], myocardial infarction

[331] Cennimo DJ, Steele RW. Parvovirus B19 Infection Workup. http://emedicine.medscape.com/article/961063-workup Accessed March 2013

[332] Sabella C, Goldfarb J. Parvovirus B19 infections. *Am Fam Physician*. 1999 Oct 1;60(5):1455-60

[333] "In contrast to the low prevalence of antibodies in controls (less than 8%), 48 of 67 patients (75%) with a variety of thyroid disorders had titers greater than 1:8. Antibodies were found in 24 of 36 patients with Graves' disease, five of six with autonomous adenoma, seven of seven with Hashimoto's thyroiditis, three of five with idiopathic primary hypothyroidism, four of 11 with nontoxic nodular goiter, and one of two with thyroid carcinoma." Shenkman L, Bottone EJ. Antibodies to Yersinia enterocolitica in thyroid disease. *Ann Intern Med*. 1976 Dec;85(6):735-9

[334] "Because there is as yet no standardisation of serological criteria for persistent infection, we considered antibody titres of > 1/20 in the IgA fraction, together with IgG titres of 1/64 to 1/256, to be indicative of persistent infection." Ben-Yaakov M, Eshel G, Zaksonski L, Lazarovich Z, Boldur I. Prevalence of antibodies to Chlamydia pneumoniae in an Israeli population without clinical evidence of respiratory infection. *J Clin Pathol*. 2002 May;55(5):355-8

[335] Haider M, et al. Acute and chronic Chlamydia pneumoniae infection and inflammatory markers in coronary artery disease patients. *J Infect Dev Ctries*. 2011 Aug;5:580-6

[336] Carter JD, Espinoza LR, Inman RD, Sneed KB, Ricca LR, Vasey FB, Valeriano J, Stanich JA, Oszust C, Gerard HC, Hudson AP. Combination antibiotics as a treatment for chronic Chlamydia-induced reactive arthritis: a double-blind, placebo-controlled, prospective trial. *Arthritis Rheum*. 2010 May;62(5):1298-307

[337] "In clinically definite MS patients, the VUMC and USF detection rates were 72 and 61%, respectively, and in patients with monosymptomatic MS, the VUMC and USF detection rates were 41 and 54%, respectively. The PCR signal was positive for 7% of the OND controls at VUMC and for 16% at USF. These studies confirm our previous reports concerning the high prevalence of C. pneumoniae in the CSF of MS patients." Sriram S, Yao SY, Stratton C, et al. Comparative study of the presence of Chlamydia pneumoniae in cerebrospinal fluid of Patients with clinically definite and monosymptomatic multiple sclerosis. *Clin Diagn Lab Immunol*. 2002 Nov;9(6):1332-7.

Parenchymal/internal/occult dysbiotic microbes and/or occult infections that can contribute to chronic inflammation, metabolic impairment, or autoimmunity—*continued*

Bacteria, protozoa, etc.	Assessment	Disease association(s)
Helicobacter pylori	Serum IgA, IgM, IgG antibodies—IgG antibodies are the most useful *serologic* test (>90% sensitive and specific) for monitoring response to eradication therapy despite the fact that antibody titer may remain elevated for a long time after *H pylori* eradication; urea breath test (gives false-negative results with coccoid forms of *H pylori* that do not produce urease, use of antibiotics, bismuth, histamine-2 blockers, or proton pump inhibitors), stool antigen shows excellent specificity (98%) and sensitivity (94%) and is highly responsive to the presence or absence of the infection[338]	Chronic gastritis and gastroduodenal ulceration, hypochlorhydria and subsequent maldigestion and small intestine bacterial overgrowth (SIBO), Sjogren syndrome, GI lymphoma, migraine, reactive/chronic arthritis, Raynaud's phenomenon
Mycoplasma species including *pneumoniae, fermentans, hominis, penetrans, genitalium*	IgG and IgM antibodies to various subspecies; PCR showed positivity in patients with fatigue/fibromyalgia: *M. pneumoniae* (54/91), *M. fermentans* (44/91), *M. hominis* (28/91) and *M. penetrans* (18/91)[339]	Chronic fatigue syndrome and fibromyalgia, Gulf War Illness[340], autoimmunity
Pseudomonas aeruginosa, Acinetobacter spp	Culture of site (urine, stool, sputum, wounds, cerebrospinal fluid) as indicated, otherwise, use stool culture and urine culture if investigating neuronal autoimmunity; serum IgA and IgG antibodies against *Pseudomonas aeruginosa* and *Acinetobacter* spp antigens are elevated in patients with multiple sclerosis[341,342], however such testing is not widely commercially available for routine clinical use; the current author has found stool testing and culture for *Pseudomonas aeruginosa* to be valuable in the treatment of neuronal autoimmunity	Neuronal autoimmunity including peripheral neuropathy and multiple sclerosis
Streptococcal infections: *Streptococcus pyogenes,* streptococci hemolytic groups A, B, D, and G	Acute pharyngeal infections are generally diagnosed clinically, with or without the use of "rapid Strep tests" or throat culture and treated with short-term penicillin-based antibiotic. However, with chronic infections/colonizations, the microbiologic phenotype of the bacteria changes from the extracellular form prototypical of acute infections to that of an intracellular form; as a general guideline, acute/extracelluar infections respond more rapidly to treatment than do chronic/intracellular infections. Standard laboratory testing includes culture, and serum measurements of antistreptolysin-O (ASO), antihyaluronidase, anti-DNase-B, and Streptozyme; diagnosis can also be supported by response to treatment.	Psoriasis, rheumatoid arthritis, polymyositis, dermatomyositis, rheumatic fever, and many other chronic inflammatory disorders

[338] Santacroce L, Katz J. Helicobacter Pylori Infection Workup. http://emedicine.medscape.com/article/176938-workup#a0719 Updated: Feb 15, 2013

[339] Nasralla M, Haier J, Nicolson GL. Multiple mycoplasmal infections detected in blood of patients with chronic fatigue syndrome and/or fibromyalgia syndrome. *Eur J Clin Microbiol Infect Dis.* 1999 Dec;18(12):859-65

[340] "In studies on hundreds of U.S. and British veterans with Gulf War Illness, approximately 40-50% of Gulf War Illness patients show evidence of mycoplasmal infections compared to 6-9% in non- deployed, healthy subjects." Nicolson GL, Nasralla MY, Nicolson NL, Haier J. High Prevalence of Mycoplasmal Infections in Symptomatic (Chronic Fatigue Syndrome) Family Members of Mycoplasma-Positive Gulf War Illness Patients. *J Chronic Fatigue Syndrome* 2003; 11(2): 21-36

[341] Hughes LE, Smith PA, Bonell S, et al. Cross-reactivity between related sequences found in Acinetobacter sp., Pseudomonas aeruginosa, myelin basic protein and myelin oligodendrocyte glycoprotein in multiple sclerosis. *J Neuroimmunol.* 2003 Nov;144(1-2):105-15

[342] Hughes LE, Bonell S, Natt RS, et al. Antibody responses to Acinetobacter spp. and Pseudomonas aeruginosa in multiple sclerosis: prospects for diagnosis using the myelin-acinetobacter-neurofilament antibody index. *Clin Diagn Lab Immunol.* 2001 Nov;8(6):1181-8

Polymicrobial positivity in a patient diagnosed with systemic lupus erythematosus (SLE), mixed connective tissue disease (MCTD), Raynaud's syndrome, and secondary amyloidosis (inaccurately diagnosed as bilateral carpal tunnel syndrome and peripheral edema)—positivity toward *Mycoplasma*, *Chlamydia/Chlamydophila*, and parvovirus: Of these three results, the positivity against *Chlamydia/Chlamydophila pneumoniae* is the most actionable per published research; antibody titers against *Mycoplasma* and parvovirus are may indicate past "extinguished" or current "smouldering" infection/colonization—only a clinical trial with antibacterial and antiviral interventions (respectively) followed by monitoring 1) clinical response to treatment, 2) reduction in other markers of autoimmune disease activity, such as Sjogren's antibodies and anti-double-stranded DNA antibodies in this case, and 3) reduction in microbe-specific antibody titers would be able to prove or refute the microbe-autoimmunity links in this particular case. Negative results for anti-dsANA and CCP not shown.

DATE OF COLLECTION TIME		DATE RECEIVED	DATE REPORTED	TIME	
11/02/2012	13:15	11/03/2012	11/05/2012	14:11	

TEST	RESULT		LIMITS
Antiextractable Nuclear Ag			
> RNP Antibodies	5.6H	AI	0.0 - 0.9
> Smith Antibodies	1.8H	AI	0.0 - 0.9

Test	Result	Units	Flag	Reference Range
Sjorgren's Ant-SS-A	2.0	AI	H	0.0-0.9
Sjorgren's Ant-SS-B	<0.2			-

Account Number	Patient ID	Control Number	Date and Time Collected	Date Reported	Sex	Age(Y/M/D)	Date of Birth
		0	04/26/13 09:46	04/30/13	F	69	

TESTS	RESULT	FLAG	UNITS	REFERENCE INTERVAL	LAB
Mycoplasma pneu. IgG/IgM Abs					
M pneumoniae IgG Abs	203	High	U/mL	0 - 99	
			Negative:	<100	
			Indeterminate:	100 - 320	
			Positive:	>320	

The reference interval established is intended as a baseline only. Values >100 may indicate a recent infection with Mycoplasma pneumoniae and need to be confirmed either by a positive IgM result and/or an additional specimen drawn 2-4 weeks later showing a significant increase in antibody levels.

M pneumoniae IgM Abs	<770		U/mL	0 - 769	
			Negative	<770	

Clinically significant amount of M. pneumoniae antibody not detected.

Chl. pneumoniae (IgG/IgM/IgA)				
Chlamydia pneumoniae IgG	>1:256	High		Neg:<1:16
Chlamydia pneumoniae IgM	<1:10			Neg:<1:10
Chlamydia pneumoniae IgA	>1:256	High		Neg:<1:16

Parvovirus, Antibody   Stage: Final   **Resulted:** 11/2/2012

Test	Result	Units	Flag	Reference Range
Parvo IgG 163303	5.7	index	H	0.0-0.8
Negative <0.9				
Equivocal 0.9 - 1.1				
Positive >1.1				
Parvo IgM 163303	0.1	index		0.0-0.8
Negative <0.9				
Equivocal 0.9 - 1.1				
Positive >1.1				

Multiple laboratory abnormalities and multifocal polydysbiosis in a patient diagnosed with RA, psoriasis, and Hashimoto's thyroiditis—positivity toward *Proteus* (most likely urogenital), inflammatory gastrointestinal dysbiosis (markedly elevated lysozyme and lactoferrin with no obviously dysbiotic microbes detected), and high-"normal" titers against ASO (most likely pharyngeal): Patient has three different autoimmune diseases, HTN, and severe obesity.

Date and Time Collected	Date Entered	Date and Time Reported	Physician Name	NPI	Physician ID
05/24/12 14:42	05/24/12	05/30/12 15:39ET	VASQUEZ , A		

Tests Ordered
Testosterone, F Eqlib+T LC/MS; Thyroid Antibodies; Hemoglobin A1c; Thyroxine (T4) Free, Direct, S; DHEA-Sulfate; TSH; Prolactin; Estradiol; Reverse T3, Serum; Vitamin D, 25-Hydroxy; t-Transglutaminase (tTG) IgA; Triiodothyronine (T3); Ferritin, Serum; Venipuncture

TESTS	RESULT	FLAG	UNITS	REFERENCE INTERVAL	LAB
Testosterone, F Eqlib+T LC/MS					
Testosterone, Total, LC/MS	**334.1**	**Low**	ng/dL	348.0 - 1197.0	
Testosterone, Free	7.85		ng/dL	5.00 - 21.00	
% Free Testosterone	2.35		%	1.50 - 4.20	
Thyroid Antibodies					
Thyroid Peroxidase (TPO) Ab	**235**	**High**	IU/mL	0 - 34	
	Please note reference interval change				
Antithyroglobulin Ab	<20		IU/mL	0 - 40	
Siemens (DPC) ICMA Methodology					
Hemoglobin A1c	5.4		%	4.8 - 5.6	

Increased risk for diabetes: 5.7 - 6.4
Diabetes: >6.4
Glycemic control for adults with diabetes: <7.0

TESTS	RESULT	FLAG	UNITS	REFERENCE INTERVAL	LAB
Thyroxine (T4) Free, Direct, S					
T4, Free(Direct)	1.12		ng/dL	0.82 - 1.77	
DHEA-Sulfate	267.7		ug/dL	160.0 - 449.0	
TSH	3.510		uIU/mL	0.450 - 4.500	
Prolactin	5.6		ng/mL	4.0 - 15.2	
Estradiol	28.4		pg/mL	7.6 - 42.6	
Roche ECLIA methodology					
Reverse T3, Serum	25.5		ng/dL	13.5 - 34.2	
Vitamin D, 25-Hydroxy	**19.4**	**Low**	ng/mL	30.0 - 100.0	

Date and Time Collected	Date Entered	Date and Time Reported	Physician Name	NPI	Physician ID
08/27/12 14:06	08/27/12	08/29/12 15:09ET	VASQUEZ , A		679

Tests Ordered
Anticardiolipin Ab, IgG/M, Qn; Immunoglobulin A, Qn, Serum; Antistreptolysin O Ab; Venipuncture

TESTS	RESULT	FLAG	UNITS	REFERENCE INTERVAL	LAB
Antistreptolysin O Ab	199.5		IU/mL	0.0 - 200.0	

PROTEUS OX - 19	**POSITIVO 1:80**	(This appears to be an antibody titer.)		
ESTUDIO	**RESULTADO**		**UNIDAD**	**REFERENCIA**
Acs. ANTI PEPTIDO CICLICO CITRULINADO (Ac. CCP) IgG	***200.0**		U/mL	0.00-5.00
Ac. ANTI-NUCLEARES	**NEGATIVOS**			NEGATIVOS

RHEUMATOID FACTOR	183 (H)	0 - 14 IU/mL
SED RATE WESTERGREN	28 (H)	0 - 15
C-REACTIVE PROTEIN	1.3 (H)	0 - 0.8 mg/dL
ANA TITER	1:80 (Abnl)	Negative
ANA PATTERN	Homogeneous (Abnl)	Negative
Result Narrative		
ANA TITER 2	1:160 (Abnl)	Negative
ANA PATTERN 2	Speckled (Abnl)	Negative

Multiple laboratory abnormalities and multifocal polydysbiosis in a patient diagnosed with RA, psoriasis, and Hashimoto's thyroiditis (continued): Inflammatory gastrointestinal dysbiosis, presumably due to low-level *Klebsiella* and nonculturable yeast

Comprehensive Stool Analysis / Parasitology x3

BACTERIOLOGY CULTURE		
Expected/Beneficial flora	**Commensal (Imbalanced) flora**	**Dysbiotic flora**
2+ Bacteroides fragilis group	1+ Klebsiella pneumoniae ssp pneumoniae	
3+ Bifidobacterium spp.		
4+ Escherichia coli		
3+ Lactobacillus spp.		
4+ Enterococcus spp.		
NG Clostridium spp.		
NG = No Growth		

BACTERIA INFORMATION
Expected /Beneficial bacteria make up a significant portion of the total microflora in a healthy & balanced GI tract. These beneficial bacteria have many health-protecting effects in the GI tract including manufacturing vitamins, fermenting fibers, digesting proteins and carbohydrates, and propagating anti-tumor and anti-inflammatory factors.
Clostridia are prevalent flora in a healthy intestine. Clostridium spp. should be considered in the context of balance with other expected/beneficial flora. Absence of clostridia or over abundance relative to other expected/beneficial flora indicates bacterial imbalance. If *C. difficile* associated disease is suspected, a Comprehensive Clostridium culture or toxigenic *C. difficile* DNA test is recommended.
Commensal (Imbalanced) bacteria are usually neither pathogenic nor beneficial to the host GI tract. Imbalances can occur when there are insufficient levels of beneficial bacteria and increased levels of commensal bacteria. Certain commensal bacteria are reported as dysbiotic at higher levels.
Dysbiotic bacteria consist of known pathogenic bacteria and those that have the potential to cause disease in the GI tract. They can be present due to a number of factors including: consumption of contaminated water or food, exposure to chemicals that are toxic to beneficial bacteria; the use of antibiotics, oral contraceptives or other medications; poor fiber intake and high stress levels.

YEAST CULTURE	
Normal flora	**Dysbiotic flora**
No yeast isolated	

MICROSCOPIC YEAST		YEAST INFORMATION
Result:	**Expected:**	Yeast normally can be found in small quantities in the skin, mouth, intestine and mucocutaneous junctions. Overgrowth of yeast can infect virtually every organ system, leading to an extensive array of clinical manifestations. Fungal diarrhea is associated with broad-spectrum antibiotics or alterations of the patient's immune status. Symptoms may include abdominal pain, cramping and irritation. When investigating the presence of yeast, disparity may exist between culturing and microscopic examination. Yeast are not uniformly dispersed throughout the stool, this may lead to undetectable or low levels of yeast identified by microscopy, despite a cultured amount of yeast. Conversely, microscopic examination may reveal a significant amount of yeast present, but no yeast cultured. Yeast does not always survive transit through the intestines rendering it unviable.
Many	None - Rare	
The microscopic finding of yeast in the stool is helpful in identifying whether there is proliferation of yeast. Rare yeast may be normal; however, yeast observed in higher amounts (few, moderate, or many) is abnormal.		

Despite lackluster results in the microbiologic section of this comprehensive stool/microbiology text, results show markedly elevated lysozyme and lactoferrin, most likely attributable to exaggerated "dysbiotic" immune response against *Klebsiella pneumoniae* and nonculturable yeast. This case exemplifies the importance of interpreting microbiologic tests in patient-specific context.

INFLAMMATION				
	Within	**Outside**	**Reference Range**	
Lysozyme*		1280	<= 600 ng/mL	**Lysozyme*** is an enzyme secreted at the site of inflammation in the GI tract and elevated levels have been identified in IBD patients. **Lactoferrin** is a quantitative GI specific marker of inflammation used to diagnose and differentiate IBD from IBS and to monitor patient inflammation levels during active and remission phases of IBD. **White Blood Cells** (WBC): in the stool are an indication of an inflammatory process resulting in the infiltration of leukocytes within the intestinal lumen. WBCs are often accompanied by mucus and blood in the stool. **Mucus** in the stool may result from prolonged mucosal irritation or in a response to parasympathetic excitability such as spastic constipation or mucous colitis.
Lactoferrin		29.2	< 7.3 µg/mL	
White Blood Cells	**None**		None - Rare	
Mucus	**Neg**		Neg	

Multiple laboratory abnormalities and multifocal polydysbiosis in a patient diagnosed with RA, psoriasis, and Hashimoto's thyroiditis (continued): Urinalysis showing mild metabolic acidosis along with asymptomatic bacteruria/bacteriuria; urinary leukocytes (not normal) is noted.

FECHA   20/08/2011   # 200037

EXAMEN GENERAL DE ORINA

EDAD   33 AÑOS   **Sexo** M

PRUEBA	RESULTADO		REFERENCIA	
Densidad	+1.030		1.01 - 1.03	
pH	5.5		5.00 8.00	
Proteinas	0	mg/dl	0	mg/dl
Glucosa	0	mg/dl	0	mg/dl
Cetonas	0	mg/dl	0	mg/dl
Bilirrubinas	0		0	
Urobilinogeno	NORMAL		0.2	E.U./dl.
Hemoglobina	0		0	
Nitritos	NEGATIVO		Negativo	

Examen Microscopico 40x

Leucocitos:	0 A 1 POR 3 CAMPOS	Piocitos:	0
Eritrocitos:	0	Cilindros:	0
Cristales:	0	Bacterias:	MODERADAS
Filamento Moco:	MODERADO	Levaduras:	0

Multiple laboratory abnormalities in a patient diagnosed with multiple sclerosis: Elevated IgE corresponding with food allergies and immune dysfunction/activation; oxidative stress clearly indicated by low levels of glutathione.

Test Name	In Range	Out Of Range	Reference Range
HOMOCYSTEINE, CARDIOVASCULAR	5.2		<10.4 umol/L
IMMUNOGLOBULIN E		862 H	<OR=114 kU/L
GLUTATHIONE		526 L	544-1228 umol

Immune reactivity suggesting chronic *Chlamydia/Chlamydophila pneumoniae* colonization; the particular relevance of this finding in this case is the correlation between *Chlamydia/Chlamydophila pneumoniae* infection and multiple sclerosis.[343]

```
CHLAMYDIA/CHLAMYDOPHILA
  ANTIBODY PANEL 1 (IGG)
  C. TRACHOMATIS IGG          <1:64
  C. PNEUMONIAE IGG                        1:256 H
  C. PSITTACI IGG             <1:64
     REFERENCE RANGE:  <1:64
```

Elevated IL-6 at 5.85 pg/ml (range 0.31-5.0) indicating immune activation; one might question the value of this test (ordered by another physician) except possibly for use in monitoring responsiveness to treatment.

```
INTERLEUKIN 6, HIGHLY
   SENSITIVE, ELISA          5.85 H        0.31-5.00 pg/mL
```

Low intracellular red blood cell magnesium at 3.9 mg/dl (range 4.0-6.4) correlates with 1) insufficient magnesium intake, 2) increased renal loss and metabolic acidosis, and 3) oxidative stress in general and gluathone depletion in particular.

```
MAGNESIUM, RBC               3.9 L         4.0-6.4 mg/dL
```

Normalization of antibody titers against *Streptococcus* following antibiotic-immunorestorative treatment in a patient with difficult-to-treat rheumatoid arthritis: Elevated anti-Streptococcal antibodies showing reduction/normalization following nutritional supplementation with immunorestorative vitamins, minerals and fatty acids and administration of azithromycin, emulsified oregano oil, and oral vancomycin. Patient also positive for *Chlamydia/Chlamydophila pneumoniae* at a titer of 1:256 (data not shown). Streptococcal bacteria can be involved in acute and chronic infections; typically the acute infection phenotype is extracellular while the chronic "dysbiotic" phenotype can be either/both extracellular and intracellular. Streptococcal bacteria are associated with numerous inflammatory and autoimmune diseases, particularly psoriasis, rheumatoid arthritis, and dermatomyositis. In brilliant research publshed by Svartz[344] rheumatoid arthritis was induced in animals by innoculating them with group B streptococci isolated from the nasopharynx of RA patients. Note also in the example below that in the intial testing, only 1 of the 3 tests was positive.

Account Number	Patient ID	Control Number	Date and Time Collected	Date Reported	Sex	Age(Y/M/D)	Date of Birth
			12/22/12 09:22	12/26/12	F		

TESTS	RESULT	FLAG	UNITS	REFERENCE INTERVAL	LAB
Anti-DNase B Strep Antibodies	134	High	U/mL	0 - 120	
Streptozyme	Negative			Neg:<1:100	
Antistreptolysin O Ab	63.3		IU/mL	0.0 - 200.0	

Date and Time Collected	Date Entered	Date and Time Reported	Physician Name	NPI	Physician ID
07/13/13 00:00	07/17/13	07/22/13 04:05ET			

Tests Ordered
Anti-DNase B Strep Antibodies; Written Authorization

TESTS	RESULT	FLAG	UNITS	REFERENCE INTERVAL	LAB
Anti-DNase B Strep Antibodies	99		U/mL	0 - 120	

```
**Results verified by repeat testing**
```

---

[343] Sriram S, et al. Comparative study of the presence of Chlamydia pneumoniae in cerebrospinal fluid of Patients with clinically definite and monosymptomatic multiple sclerosis. *Clin Diagn Lab Immunol.* 2002 Nov;9(6):1332-7 http://cvi.asm.org/content/9/6/1332.long

[344] "In experimental arthritis, produced by streptococci group B (Svartz), there appears in rats the same type of joint disease as in human RA and, besides, a rheumatoid factor (RF)-like macroglobulin, which cannot be distinguished by available methods from human RF macroglobulin. ...The streptococci B used in our investigations were mostly isolated from the nasopharynx of RA patients. Svartz N. The origin of rheumatoid arthritis. *Rheumatology.* 1975;6:322-8

Dr V's perspective on the relativity of microbial activity—herpes simplex virus (HSV) as an example: Too often, doctors and clinicians seem to misunderstand the complexity and relativity of human microbial colonization, which—in this conversation—very clearly includes occult viral activity, even and specifically that which is not clinically manifest, that which is nonacute, and/or which is commonplace. Distinctions will be presented in the following table with clinical examples of HSV infection to follow.

Common (mis)perceptions	*More accurate perceptions*
• Patients either have infections that are clinically apperant or they are unaffected by microbes.	• In the human metaorganism/superorganism, microbial cells outnumber human cells by a ratio of 10 to 1, meaning that for each human cell, the body harbors ~10 microbes, allowing the statement that "humans" are really 90% microbes/bacteria.[345] • "Each person is host to some 100 trillion microbes, predominantly bacteria."[346] Thus, the total microbial load (TML) and total antigenic immunostimulatory load (TAIL) is quite considerable, whether or not a patient has an obvious "infection".
• If a patient has had a common infection such as HSV-1 or *Chlamydophila/Chlamydia pneumoniae*, then —when the infection is not appearant even though it might be persistent— it is considered to be irrelevant.	• Just because an infection is common does not mean that it is benign; HSV-1 is an example of a common infection (seen in approximately 50% of people worldwide) which has been correlated with several chronic health problems ranging from multiple sclerosis to Alzheimer's disease. • Just because the infection is not clinically *appearant* does not mean that the infection is "cleared" or clinically *irrelevant*; many chronic and persistent infections/colonizations remain subclinically active despite —or perhaps because of— the absense of an obvious vigorous immunological response.
• Chronic infections are seen quantitatively (ie, "you either had/have it or you don't").	• Chronic infections are both quantitative (ie, present or absent) and qualitative with respect to the impact that they have on metabolic processes and immunological/inflammatory reponses. Thus, the degree of the microbal load and microbial activity/replication is important, not simply the presence or absense of the microbe(s).
• Chronic inflammatory disorders are idiopathic; they result from "a combination of genetic predisposition with unidentified environmental triggers."	• Total microbial load (TML) and total antigenic immunostimulatory load (TAIL) contribute to activation of the innate immune response and the subsequent development of inflammatory diseases, the pattern of which will depend on other pro- and anti-inflammatory and immuno-regulatory and –dysregulatory balances.
• Microbial colonizations—like nutritional defiencies—are primarily singular.	• Microbial colonizations—like nutritional defiencies—are nearly always multiple—not singular. • The patterns of inflammatory responses are primarily secondary to the TML and TAIL of the patient's genetic, nutritional, microbial, immunological, mitochondrial, psychosocial, hormonal and xenobiotic statuses.

Lower antibody titers correlate with less viral activity: Here we see evidence of HSV seropositivity with a relatively low titer in a patient who has never experienced a clinical herpetic outbreak.

```
HSV I/II, IgG/Rfx Type II IgG
   HSV I/II IgG                  21.6    High      index        0.0 - 0.8
```

Higher antibody titers correlate with more viral activity: Here we see evidence of HSV seropositivity with a relatively high titer in a patient who experiences frequent clinical (oral) herpetic outbreaks.

```
HSV I/II, IgG/Rfx Type II IgG
   HSV I/II IgG                  36.5    High      index        0.0 - 0.8
                                                   Negative         <0.9
                                                   Equivocal  0.9 - 1.0
                                                   Positive         >1.0
```

---

[345] Dizikes C. 'We are 90% bacteria,' says researcher for Hospital Microbiome Project. *Chicago Tribune* 2013, Jan 02 http://articles.chicagotribune.com/2013-01-02/news/ct-met-microbiome-20130102_1_human-microbiome-bacteria-human-life
[346] Betts KS. A study in balance: how microbiomes are changing the shape of environmental health. *Environ Health Perspect.* 2011 Aug;119(8):A340-6

Lactulose-mannitol assay: assessment for intestinal hyperpermeability and malabsorption	
Overview and interpretation:	▪ The lactulose-mannitol assay is a highly validated assessment for the accurate determination of small intestine permeability. This test is used to diagnose "leaky gut", which is a common problem and contributor to systemic inflammation in patients with inflammation and immune dysfunction—see chapter 4 of *Integrative Rheumatology*. Intestinal hyperpermeability reflects inflammation of and damage to the small intestine mucosa and is seen in patients with parasite infections, food allergies, celiac disease, malnutrition, bacterial infections, systemic ischemia or inflammation, ankylosing spondylitis, Crohn's disease, eczema, psoriasis, and those who consume enterotoxins such as NSAIDs and excess ethanol.[347] ▪ Elevations of **lactulose** indicate increased **paracellular** permeability caused by intestinal damage and are diagnostic of "leaky gut." *Clinical pearl*: remember that the "L" in *lactulose* rhymes with *leaky*. ▪ Decrements in **mannitol** suggest impaired **transcellular** absorption and suggest malabsorption in general and villous atrophy in particular. *Clinical pearl*: remember that the "M" in *mannitol* rhymes with *malabsorption*. ▪ Classically, in patients with damaged intestinal mucosa, we generally see a combined ***increase in*** ***paracellular*** permeability (measured with lactulose) and a ***reduction in transcellular*** transport (measured with mannitol); these divergent effects result in an increased lactulose-to-mannitol ratio.

Advantages:	▪ This test is safe and affordable for the assessment of small intestine mucosal integrity. Abnormal results—"leaky gut" and/or malabsorption—generally indicate one or more of following, which can be recalled by the acronym M.E.D. F.I.T. [348]
	   1. <u>Malnutrition</u>: Such as due to poor intake, catabolism, or malabsorption; we might also consider in particular: zinc, glutamine, and vitamin D3.
	   2. <u>Enterotoxins</u>: Such as NSAIDs or ethanol.
	   3. <u>Dysbiosis</u>: including yeast, bacteria, protozoa, amebas, worms, etc. [349]**
	   4. <u>Food allergies</u>: Including celiac disease, but also with milder food allergies.**
	   5. <u>Inflammatory bowel disease</u>: Crohn's disease, ulcerative colitis, or family history of IBD.
	   6. <u>Trauma or major injury/inflammation (sufficient to induce a catabolic response)</u>: Tissue hypoxia, trauma, recent surgery, etc.
	**Note that of these six items, all but two can be excluded by history and patient assessment; therefore, a clinician could very reasonably perform specialized stool testing to assess for dysbiosis since negative results in a patient with increased intestinal permeability would then point toward food allergy.

Limitations:	▪ Abnormalities and the identification of "leaky gut" are nonspecific and do not point to a specific or single diagnosis or treatment.
Comments:	▪ The value of this test is two-fold: 1) as a screening test for the above-mentioned disorders, and 2) as a method for determining the efficacy of treatment once the cause of the problem has been putatively identified and treated. ▪ This test can be used to promote compliance and to encourage the use of additional testing in patients who are otherwise prone to noncompliance or who resist other tests, such as stool testing. In other words, the clinician can gain an advantage by showing the patient an objective abnormality which then validates the need for treatment and additional testing. ▪ I only use this test on rare occasions because I more commonly either assume that a patient has leaky gut if he/she has one of the aforementioned conditions or we move directly to stool testing and comprehensive parasitology—clearly one of the most valuable tests in the management and treatment of systemic inflammation and immune dysfunction—otherwise known as "autoimmunity" and "allergy."

[347] Miller AL. The Pathogenesis, Clinical Implications, and Treatment of Intestinal Hyperpermeability. *Alt Med Rev 1997*:2(5):330-345 http://www.thorne.com/pdf/journal/2-5/intestinalhyperpermiability.pdf

[348] Credit to Angelique Marquez for the MEDFIT acronym and proving that great teachers inspire genious in their students ☺

[349] See chapter 4 of *Integrative Rheumatology* and Vasquez A. Reducing Pain and Inflammation Naturally. Part 6: Nutritional and Botanical Treatments Against "Silent Infections" and Gastrointestinal Dysbiosis, Commonly Overlooked Causes of Neuromusculoskeletal Inflammation and Chronic Health Problems. *Nutr Perspect* 2006; Jan

Presentation: Highly abnormal lactulose-mannitol ratio in a patient with idiopathic peripheral neuropathy prior to comprehensive stool analysis and parasitology showing intestinal dysbiosis: This 40-yo man presented with a multiyear history of periodic febrile exacerbations of peripheral neuropathy that would cause severe paresthesias and motor deficits. Patient had been evaluated by several board-certified medical neurologists to no avail. Laboratory, imaging, electrodiagnostic studies, and cerebrospinal fluid (CSF) analysis revealed nonspecific abnormalities that did not lead to an established diagnosis. From an integrative naturopathic and functional medicine perspective, food allergy and intestinal dysbiosis are the most obvious probable etiologies; these clinical suspicions were confirmed with laboratory testing showing increased intestinal permeability and gastrointestinal dysbiosis.

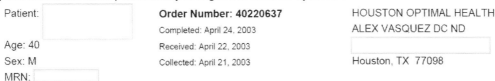

Patient:	**Order Number: 40220637**	HOUSTON OPTIMAL HEALTH
	Completed: April 24, 2003	ALEX VASQUEZ DC ND
Age: 40	Received: April 22, 2003	
Sex: M	Collected: April 21, 2003	Houston, TX 77098
MRN:		

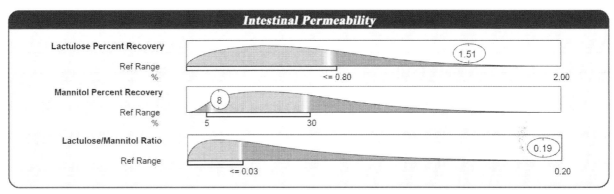

As expected, comprehensive parasitology showed intestinal dysbiosis, including insufficiency of *Lactobacillus* and presence of *Psuedomonas* and abnormal yeast species. Of particular note, *Psuedomonas aeruginosa* shows cross-reactivity with human neuronal tissues.[350,351] Eradication of the dysbiotic condition with a combination of dietary improvement, nutritional supplementation, hormonal optimization, and antimicrobial drugs and herbs lead to rapid and sustained remission of this "idiopathic peripheral neuropathy" which had defied standard medical diagnosis and treatment for many years.

Comprehensive Stool Analysis / Parasitology x3

MICROBIOLOGY

Bacteriology Culture

Beneficial flora		Imbalances		Dysbiotic flora	
Bifidobacter	4+	Haemolytic E. coli	4+	Pseudomonas sp.	4+
E. coli	4+	Gamma strep	2+		
Lactobacillus	2+				

Mycology (Yeast) Culture

Normal flora		Dysbiotic flora
Candida glabrata	1+	
Rhodotorula sp.	1+	

---

[350] Hughes LE, Bonell S, Natt RS, et al. Antibody responses to Acinetobacter spp. and Pseudomonas aeruginosa in multiple sclerosis: prospects for diagnosis using the myelin-acinetobacter-neurofilament antibody index. *Clin Diagn Lab Immunol*. 2001 Nov;8(6):1181-8 http://cvi.asm.org/content/8/6/1181.full.pdf

[351] Hughes LE, Smith PA, Bonell S, Natt RS, Wilson C, Rashid T, Amor S, Thompson EJ, Croker J, Ebringer A. Cross-reactivity between related sequences found in Acinetobacter sp., Pseudomonas aeruginosa, myelin basic protein and myelin oligodendrocyte glycoprotein in multiple sclerosis. *J Neuroimmunol*. 2003 Nov;144(1-2):105-15

Comprehensive stool analysis and comprehensive parasitology	

Overview and interpretation:	• **This is clearly one of the most valuable tests in clinical practice when working with patients with chronic fatigue, systemic inflammation, and autoimmunity. Second only to routine laboratory assessments such as CBC, chemistry panel, and CRP, the importance of stool testing and comprehensive parasitology assessments must be appreciated by progressive clinicians of all disciplines.**
	
	▪ Stool testing must be performed by a specialty laboratory because the quality of testing provided by most standard "medical labs" and hospitals is completely inadequate. Initial samples should be collected on three separate occasions by the patient and each sample should be analyzed separately by the laboratory.
	
	▪ Important qualitative and quantitative markers include the following:
	
	   ▫ **Beneficial bacteria ("probiotics")**: Microbiological testing should quantify and identify various beneficial bacteria, which should be present at "+4" levels on a 0-4 scale.
	
	   ▫ **Harmful and potentially harmful bacteria, protozoans, amebas, etc.**: Questionable or harmful microbes should be eradicated even if they are not identified as true pathogens in the Paleo-classic Pasteurian/Kochian sense.[352]
	
	   ▫ **Yeast and mycology**: At least two tests must be performed for a complete assessment: 1) yeast culture, and 2) microscopic examination for yeast elements. Both tests are necessary because some patients—perhaps those with the most severe symptomatology and the most favorable response to anti-yeast treatment—will have a negative yeast culture and positive findings on the microscopic examination. In other words, these patients have intestinal yeast that contributes to their disease/symptomatology but which does not grow on culture despite being clearly visible with microscopy; a similar pattern (using a swab of the rectal mucosa rather than microscopy) is referred to as "negative culture with positive smear."[353]
	
	   ▫ **Microbial sensitivity testing**: An important component to parasitology testing is the determination of which anti-microbial agents (natural and synthetic) the microbe is sensitive to. This helps to guide and enhance the effectiveness of anti-microbial therapy.
	
	   ▫ **Secretory IgA**: SIgA levels are elevated in patients who are having an immune response to either food or microbial antigens.[354] Thus, in a patient with minimal dysbiosis, say for example with *Candida albicans*, an elevated sIgA can indicate that the patient is having a hypersensitivity reaction to an otherwise benign microbe—in this case, eradication of the microbe is warranted and may result in a positive clinical response. Low sIgA suggests either primary or secondary immune defect such as selective sIgA deficiency[355] or malnutrition, stress, prednisone/corticosteroids, or possibly mycotoxicosis (immunosuppression due to fungal immunotoxins). In addition to addressing any systemic causative factors, a low sIgA may be addressed with the administration of bovine colostrum, glutamine, vitamin A, and *Saccharomyces boulardii*; the following doses may be considered for use in adults with proportionately smaller doses for children:
	
	      ◆ Bovine colostrum: 2.4 – 3.6 grams per day in divided doses for adults. No drug interactions are known. Side effects may include increased energy, insomnia, and stimulation. One study in particular used very large doses of 10 grams per

---

[352] Vasquez A. Reducing Pain and Inflammation Naturally. Part 6: Nutritional and Botanical Treatments Against "Silent Infections" and Gastrointestinal Dysbiosis, Commonly Overlooked Causes of Neuromusculoskeletal Inflammation and Chronic Health Problems. *Nutr Perspect* 2006; Jan

[353] "According to Galland, the best predictor of who will respond to anticandida medication is a negative stool culture combined with a positive smear of the rectal mucosa (for the identification of intracellular hyphal forms of the organism); however, even that test is not 100% reliable." Gaby AR. Before you order that lab test: part 2. *Townsend Letter for Doctors and Patients*. 2004; January findarticles.com/p/articles/mi_m0ISW/is_246/ai_112728028

[354] Quig DW, Higley M. Noninvasive assessment of intestinal inflammation: inflammatory bowel disease vs. irritable bowel syndrome. *Townsend Letter for Doctors and Patients* 2006;Jan:74-5

[355] "Selective IgA deficiency is the most common form of immunodeficiency. Certain select populations, including allergic individuals, patients with autoimmune and gastrointestinal tract disease and patients with recurrent upper respiratory tract illnesses, have an increased incidence of this disorder." Burks AW Jr, Steele RW. Selective IgA deficiency. *Ann Allergy*. 1986;57:3-13

Comprehensive stool analysis and comprehensive parasitology

day for four days in children and found no adverse effects[356]; another case report of a child involved the use of 50 grams per day for at least two weeks and showed no adverse effects.[357]

- ◆ Glutamine: 6 grams 3 times per day (18 grams per day) is a common dosage with significant literature support.
- ◆ Vitamin A: Correction of subclinical vitamin A deficiency improves mucosal integrity and increases sIgA production in humans.[358] Common doses used by integrative clinicians are in the range of 200,000 IU to 300,000 for a limited amount of time, generally 1-4 weeks; thereafter the dose is tapered. Patients are educated as to manifestations of toxicity (see the chapter on *Therapeutics* toward the end of this book) and the importance of limited duration of treatment.
- ◆ *Saccharomyces boulardii*: Common dose for adults is 250 mg thrice daily; ability of this treatment to increase sIgA levels and its anti-infective efficacy have been documented in human and animal studies.

- □ **Short-chain fatty acids**: These are produced by intestinal bacteria. Quantitative excess indicates bacterial overgrowth of the intestines, while insufficiency indicates a lack of probiotics or an insufficiency of dietary substrate, i.e., soluble fiber. Abnormal patterns of individual short-chain fatty acids indicate qualitative/quantitative abnormalities in gastrointestinal microflora, particularly anaerobic bacteria that cannot be identified with routine bacterial cultures.

- □ **Beta-glucuronidase**: This is an enzyme produced by several different intestinal bacteria. High levels of beta-glucuronidase in the intestinal lumen serve to nullify the benefits of detoxification (specifically glucuronidation) by cleaving the toxicant from its glucuronide conjugate. This can result in re-absorption of the toxicant through the intestinal mucosa which then re-exposes the patient to the toxin that was previously detoxified ("enterohepatic recirculation" or "enterohepatic recycling"[359]). This is an exemplary aspect of "auto-intoxication" that results in chronic fatigue and upregulation of Phase 1 detoxification systems (chapter 4 of *Integrative Rheumatology*).

- □ **Lactoferrin**: The iron-binding glycoprotein lactoferrin is an inflammatory marker that helps distinguish functional disorders (i.e., IBS) from more serious diseases (i.e., IBD). Approximate values are as follows:
  - ◆ Healthy and IBS: 2 mcg/ml
  - ◆ Severe dysbiosis: up to 120 mcg/ml
  - ◆ Inactive IBD: 60-250 mcg/ml
  - ◆ Active IBD: > 400 mcg/ml.

- □ **Lysozyme**: Elevated in proportion to intestinal inflammation in dysbiosis and IBD.

- □ **Other markers**: Other markers of digestion, inflammation, and absorption are reported with the more comprehensive panels performed on stool samples. These tests are not always necessary, but such additional information is always helpful when working with

---

[356] "In this double blind placebo-controlled trial, 80 children with rotavirus diarrhea were randomly assigned to receive orally either 10 g of IIBC (containing 3.6 g of antirotavirus antibodies) daily for 4 days or the same amount of a placebo preparation." Sarker SA, Casswall TH, Mahalanabis D, Alam NH, Albert MJ, Brussow H, Fuchs GJ, Hammerstrom L. Successful treatment of rotavirus diarrhea in children with immunoglobulin from immunized bovine colostrum. *Pediatr Infect Dis J.* 1998 Dec;17(12):1149-54

[357] Lactobin-R is a commercial hyperimmune bovine colostrum with some specificity for cryptosporidiosis; administration to a 4 year old child with AIDS and severe diarrhea resulted in significant clinical improvement in the diarrhea and "permanent elimination of the parasite from the gut as assessed through serial jejunal biopsy and stool specimens." Shield J, Melville C, Novelli V, Anderson G, Scheimberg I, Gibb D, Milla P. Bovine colostrum immunoglobulin concentrate for cryptosporidiosis in AIDS. *Arch Dis Child.* 1993 Oct;69(4):451-3

[358] "It can increase resistance to infection by increasing mucosal integrity, increasing surface immunoglobulin A (sIgA) and enhancing adequate neutrophil function. If infection occurs, vitamin A can act as an immune enhancer, increasing the adequacy of natural killer (NK) cells and increasing antibody production." Faisel H, Pittrof R. Vitamin A and causes of maternal mortality: association and biological plausibility. *Public Health Nutr.* 2000 Sep;3(3):321-7

[359] Parker RJ, Hirom PC, Millburn P.Enterohepatic recycling of phenolphthalein, morphine, lysergic acid diethylamide (LSD) and diphenylacetic acid in the rat. Hydrolysis of glucuronic acid conjugates in the gut lumen. *Xenobiotica.* 1980 Sep;10(9):689-70

Comprehensive stool analysis and comprehensive parasitology	
	complex patients. These markers are relatively self-explanatory and/or are described on the results of the test by the laboratory.
Advantages:	**• Stool analysis in general and parasitology assessments in particular provide supremely valuable information in the comprehensive assessment and treatment of patients with complex illnesses such as chronic fatigue, irritable bowel syndrome, fibromyalgia, and all of the autoimmune/rheumatic diseases.**
Limitations:	• Tests vary in price from $250-$400. • Anaerobic bacteria are difficult to culture. • Specialty examinations, such as for *Helicobacter pylori* antigen and enterohemorrhagic *E. coli* cytotoxin, must be requested specifically at additional cost.
Comments:	• I have found stool testing to be the single most powerful diagnostic tool for helping chronically ill patients to attain improved health. Insights from stool/parasitology testing can be used to implement powerfully effective treatments. The value of this test in the treatment of patients with rheumatic disease must be appreciated and is extensively detailed in ***Integrative Rheumatology***.

Concept: Not all "Injury-related Problems" are "Injury-related Problems"

In the case of most acute injuries, the underlying problem is often the injury itself. However, the physician must conduct a thorough history and examination to assess for possible underling pathologies that cause or contribute to the problem that "appears" to be injury-related. Congenital anomalies, underlying pathology, previous injury, occult infections, and psychoemotional disorders may have been present *before* the "injury."

> **"Pediatric infections and neoplasms are notorious for masquerading as sport injuries."**
>
> "…Take the relevant history directly from the patient, and keep tumors and infections high on your list of differential diagnoses… For example, about 15% of children with leukemia present with musculoskeletal complaints…"
>
> Shaw BA, Gerardi JA, Hennrikus WL. How to avoid orthopedic pitfalls in children. *Patient Care* 1999 Feb

Just because the patient reports a problem such as pain following an injury does not mean that the injury is the *sole* cause of the pain. *Do not let a biased history lead you down the wrong path.* **In children and young adults, 5% of "sports-related" injuries are associated with preexisting infection, anomalies, or other conditions.** In adult women, "…between 9% and 20% of women with breast cancer attribute their symptoms to previous trauma to the breast. In these cases, the association of the breast mass with a traumatic event resulted in a delay in diagnosis ranging from four months to one year."[360]

A group of German physicians describe a man who presented with a soft-tissue pain following a soccer game; he was later diagnosed with a malignant tumor—synovial sarcoma.[361] Similarly, Wakeshima and Ellen[362] describe a young athletic woman who presented with chronic hip pain. The woman's history was significant for ulcerative colitis, but otherwise her radiographs were normal and her history and examination lead to a diagnosis of trochanteric bursitis. However, the patient's condition did not respond to routine treatment, and additional investigation over several months lead to a diagnosis of giant cell carcinoma. The authors concluded, "This case shows **the importance of repeat radiographic studies in patients whose joint pain does not respond or responds slowly to conservative therapy, despite initial normal findings."**

What you expect to find and hear when taking a trauma-related history is that **1) a healthy patient** with no previous health concerns was **2) exposed to a traumatic event**, the history and consequences of which perfectly coincide with the injury you are assessing in your office, and that **3) your physical examination findings are all consistent** and lead to a specific diagnosis, which then **4) responds to your treatment. If you find discrepancies between the history of the injury and your physical examination findings (e.g., fever after a "sports-related" injury), if the patient appears unhealthy in disproportion to the presenting complaint, or if the patient does not respond to your treatment, then you must consider the possibility of preexisting or concomitant disease.**

When treating children, be very careful to get an accurate history—this is difficult since your two sources of information are not very reliable: parents often think that they already have the problem figured out, and so their history will be biased toward convincing you of what they think is the problem and solution; children are often not good historians and can form illogical relationships between events that can be misleading.

Astute doctors search for and rule-out/exclude preexisting and underlying pathology before ascribing the problem to the "obvious cause." Always assess for consistency between the history, examination findings, and response to treatment—inconsistencies suggest the need for additional investigation.

[360] Seifert S. Medical Illness Simulating Trauma (MIST) syndrome: case reports and discussion of syndrome. *Fam Med* 1993 Apr;25(4):273-6
[361] Engel C, Kelm J, Olinger A. Blunt trauma in soccer. The initial manifestation of synovial sarcoma. [Article in German] *Zentralbl Chir* 2001 Jan;126(1):68-71
[362] Wakeshima Y, Ellen MI. Atypical hip pain origin in a young athletic woman: a case report of giant cell carcinoma. *Arch Phys Med Rehabil* 2001 Oct;82(10):1472-5

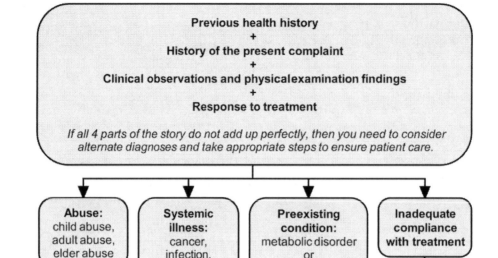

Previous health history
+
History of the present complaint
+
Clinical observations and physicalexamination findings
+
Response to treatment

If all 4 parts of the story do not add up perfectly, then you need to consider alternate diagnoses and take appropriate steps to ensure patient care.

| **Abuse:** child abuse, adult abuse, elder abuse | **Systemic illness:** cancer, infection, rheumatic | **Preexisting condition:** metabolic disorder or congenital anomaly | **Inadequate compliance with treatment** |

Assess and report to authorities as indicated

Discover and address cause of non-compliance

If you have a specific condition in mind, then test specifically for it. If you suspect preexisting/concomitant illness but are unsure of exact nature of the condition, gather additional information by:

1) taking a more detailed history,
2) ordering lab tests: CRP, CBC, chemistry panel, ferritin, ANA.
3) obtaining diagnostic imaging radiographs, bone scan, MRI, CT, US
4) reassessing patient within two weeks for progression of disease or crossing diagnostic threshold.
5) referral or co-management: if the patient does not respond to your treatment and/or you suspect an underlying serious pathology, refer the patient to another physician at least for co-management. Put your referral in writing and chart appropriately. "When in doubt, refer it out."

<u>**Clinical management**</u>: Inconsistencies between the history, exams, and response to treatment indicate the need for additional investigation and additional diagnostic considerations.

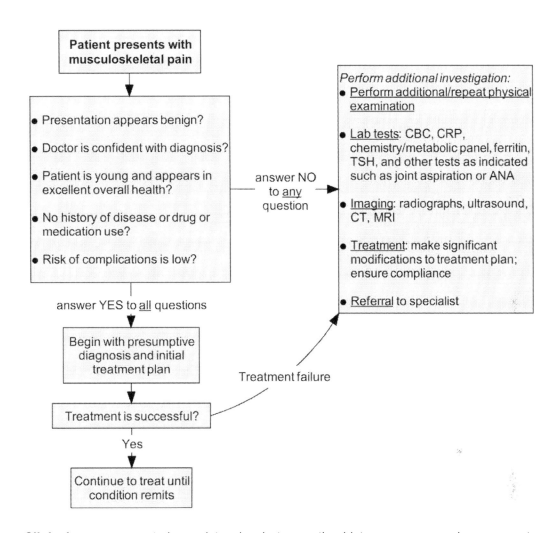

Clinical management: Inconsistencies between the history, exams, and response to treatment indicate the need for additional investigation and additional diagnostic considerations.

High-Risk Pain Patients

When a patient has musculoskeletal pain and any of the following characteristics, radiographs should be considered as an appropriate component of comprehensive evaluation. These considerations are particularly—though not exclusively—relevant for spine and low-back pain.[363]

1. More than 50 years of age
2. Physical trauma (accident, fall, etc.)
3. Pain at night
4. Back pain not relieved by lying supine
5. Neurologic deficits (motor or sensory)
6. Unexplained weight loss
7. Documentation or suspicion of inflammatory arthropathy[364]
    - Ankylosing spondylitis
    - Lupus
    - Rheumatoid arthritis
    - Juvenile rheumatoid arthritis
    - Psoriatic arthritis
8. Drug or alcohol abuse (increased risk of infection, nutritional deficiencies, anesthesia)
9. History of cancer
10. Intravenous drug use
11. Immunosuppression, due to illness (e.g., HIV) or medications (e.g., steroids or cyclosporine)
12. History of corticosteroid use (causes osteoporosis and increased risk for infection)
13. Fever above 100° F or suspicion of septic arthritis or osteomyelitis
14. Diabetes (increased risk of infection, nutritional deficiencies, anesthesia)
15. Hypertension (abdominal aneurysm: low back pain, nausea, pulsatile abdominal mass)
16. Recent visit for same problem and not improved
17. Patient seeking compensation for pain/ injury (increased need for documentation)
18. Skin lesion (psoriasis, melanoma, dermatomyositis, the butterfly rash of lupus, scars from previous surgery, accident, etc....)
19. Deformity or immobility
20. Lymphadenopathy (suggests cancer or infection)
21. Elevated ESR/CRP (cancer, infection, inflammatory disorder)
22. Elevated WBC count
23. Elevated alkaline phosphatase (bone lesions, metabolic bone disease, hepatopathy, vitamin D deficiency)
24. Elevated acid phosphatase (occasionally used to monitor prostate cancer)
25. Positive rheumatoid factor and/or CCP—cyclic citrullinated protein antibodies
26. Positive HLA-B27 (propensity for inflammatory arthropathies)
27. Serum gammopathy (multiple myeloma is the most common primary bone tumor)
28. "High-risk for disease" *examples:*
    - Long-term heavy smoking of cigarettes
    - Long-term exposure to radiation
    - Obesity
29. Strong family history of inflammatory, musculoskeletal, or malignant disease
30. Others:_____

_____

_____

_____

---

[363] Remember that metastasis often travel first from the primary site to bone, therefore bone pain may be an early manifestation of occult cancer. Most of the above are from "Table 1: The high-risk patient: clinical indications for radiography in low back pain patients." J Taylor, DC, DACBR, D Resnick, MD. Imaging decisions in the management of low back pain. Advances in Chiropractic. Mosby Year Book. 1994; 1-28

[364] Radiographs are often essential for diagnosis or to rule out complications of the disease. For example, in patients with inflammatory arthropathies such as these, spontaneous rupture of the transverse ligament (at the odontoid process) has been reported; although rare, this complication could be life-threatening if mismanaged or undiagnosed.

Concept: Safe Patient + Safe Treatment = Safe Outcome

The purpose of performing the history and physical examination on a new *or established* patient is to determine their current health status—including their mental and emotional health and their physical health, particularly as this relates to important and life-threatening possibilities such as cancer, infections, fractures, systemic diseases, and neurologic compromise. The questions that lead this investigation are: "**What is this patient's current status?**" "**Does this patient have a serious disease, neurologic injury, or are they at high risk for developing a serious complication in the near future that can be prevented with appropriate care** *now*?"

Is your patient safe?
- ♦ The question to ask yourself is, "Is this patient's health problem or current complaint/exacerbation a manifestation of an underlying condition that could result in a negative outcome?
- ♦ If a patient comes to you with a headache, and you neglect to find that their blood pressure is 230/130, then you missed the opportunity to help them avoid the stroke that they could have after leaving your office.
- ♦ If a patient comes to you with a complaint of low back pain, and you neglect to perform a neurologic examination to find that *the patient already has a neurologic deficit even before you treated them*, then you have lost the opportunity to defend yourself in court when the patient later claims that *your* treatment and *your* management of their case is the reason that they now have a permanent neurologic deficit.

Is your treatment safe?: Have you been perfectly clear with the patient about the risks and benefits of your treatment plan? **Have you obtained informed consent**? Have you charted **"PAR-B"** to indicate that you have discussed the **P**rocedures, **A**lternatives, **R**isks, and **B**enefits of your treatment plan? Have you been clear about the duration of treatment and the need for appropriate follow-up? If you are prescribing nutrition or botanical medicines, have you informed the patient about the duration of treatment? **Have you looked for contraindications to your otherwise brilliant treatment plan**? What about the fact that this patient was on corticosteroids for the past 15 years and only discontinued prednisone 2 months before arriving at your office? *The patient may have steroid-induced osteoporosis even though he is no longer on prednisone.* When you recommend that your patient take 100,000 IU of vitamin A to treat her throat infection, what happens when she presents to your office 8 months later with signs of vitamin A toxicity because she continued her treatment plan indefinitely rather than using it only for 7 days as you had intended? *Be sure to put a time limit on your*

> **Check your work**
> Double-check to ensure that your patient is safe (no forthcoming complications or predictable emergencies) and that your treatment is safe (appropriate, effective, clearly communicated, and time-limited with instructions to return for office visit).

treatment plans. Every treatment plan should be 1) given to the patient in legible print and clear statements, 2) be copied for the chart, 3) include "what to do if things get worse" in the event of adverse treatment effect or exacerbation of problem, and 4) include patient's responsibility for returning to office/clinic for follow-up and reassessment.

Informed consent: From a legal standpoint, doctors can only treat a patient after the patient has given *consent to treatment*. Patients can only authoritatively consent to treatment after they have been educated about the treatment—thereafter, they can provide *informed consent*. Educating the patient requires discussion (and documentation) of each of the following:
- Procedures—what may take place, what is required; duration, costs, follow-up,
- Alternatives—what options are available,
- Risks—what risks are involved,
- Benefits—what benefits can be reasonably expected,
- Questions—allow for the patient to ask questions and receive answers.

This is commonly charted as "**PARB—no questions**" or "**PARB—questions answered**" once the patient gives consent to treatment; alternatively and more humorously, this may be charted as "**PAR-B-Q**".

Concept: Four Clues to Discovering Underlying Problems

When I taught Orthopedics at Bastyr University I encouraged students to search for specific **sets of clues** when evaluating patients. These clues—often insignificant in isolation but meaningful in combination—were often the "red flags" that could help make the difference between an accurate diagnosis and a missed diagnosis. These four categories can be recalled with the mnemonic "*S.C.I.N.*" or "*S.C.I.M.*" These four areas of assessment/safety emphasis differ from the "vindicates" mnemonic which is used for differential diagnosis.

- **Systemic symptoms and signs**: Ask about systemic signs and symptoms such as fever, weight loss, lymphadenopathy, or skin rash in patients who present with pain because these "whole body" manifestations might indicate an underlying or concomitant disease that deserves attention, either independently from the musculoskeletal pain, or as a cause of the musculoskeletal pain. For example, "headache" may appear benign, whereas "headache with fever and skin rash" suggests meningitis—a medical emergency. "Low-back pain" is a common occurrence; yet "low-back pain with weight loss and fever" might suggest occult malignancy, osteomyelitis, or other systemic disease.

- **Complications:** We *ask about* and *look for* already existing complications, such as "numbness, weakness, tingling in the arms or hands, legs or feet" to rapidly screen for neurologic deficits and we follow this up with screening assessments such as "squat and rise", toe walk, heel walk, and reflexes for spinal cord and lower extremity neuromuscular integrity. Additionally, when dealing with patients with spine-related complaints or injuries, we also ask about changes or loss of function in bowel and bladder control and numbness near the anus or genitals, which may be the *only* clinical clues to cauda equina syndrome—a medical emergency. Ask about effects of the condition on ADL (activities of daily living) to attain a more comprehensive view of the condition and to ensure that the patient's story is consistent.

Vindicates: a popular mnemonic acronym for differential diagnosis	
V	Vascular
	Visceral referral
I	Infectious
	Inflammatory
	Immunologic
N	Neurologic
	Nutritional
	New growth: neoplasia or pregnancy
D	Deficiency
	Degenerative
I	Iatrogenic (drug related)
	Intoxication
	Idiosyncratic
C	Congenital
	Cardiac or circulatory
A	Allergy / Autoimmune
	Abuse: drugs, alcohol, physical
T	Trauma
	Toxicity
E	Endocrine
	Exposure
S	Subluxation
	Somatic dysfunction
	Structural
	Stress
	Secondary gain

- **Indicators from the history**: We look for specific "red flags" and "yellow flags" such as trauma, risk factors (such as smoking, prednisone, alcohol), or a positive history of chronic infections or cancer. Nonmechanical musculoskeletal pain in a patient with a history of or high risk for cancer is highly suspicious and mandates thorough investigation.

- **Non-Mechanical pain**: Non-mechanical pain suggests a pathologic etiology rather than simple joint dysfunction. Pain at night, pain that occurs without an inciting injury, pain that is not strongly affected by motion and is not powerfully provoked by your physical examination assessments suggests the possibility of underlying disorder such as cancer, neuropathy, or infection. However, the ability to elicit an exacerbation of pain with "mechanical" maneuvers does not indicate that the pain is "mechanical" and therefore "non-pathologic." Mechanical pain can still be pathologic pain, such as the exquisite pain felt by patients with spinal fractures—they may be neurologically intact, they do have pain worse with motion, but they are not safe to manipulate, and they require appropriate treatment and referral on an urgent basis.

Check your work
Keeping these four assessment categories in mind can serve as a useful "checkpoint" to ensure that your patient is safe, and that your treatment is appropriate and therefore safe, too.

Concept: Special Considerations in the Evaluation of Children

> "Pediatric infections and neoplasms are notorious for masquerading as sport injuries. … There is only one way to avoid this trap: Take the relevant history directly from the patient, and keep tumors and infections high on your list of differential diagnoses."[365]

- **Consider the possibility of child abuse when a child presents with an injury:** As a non-naïve physician, you always have to consider the possibility of child abuse when a child presents with an injury. Be detailed in your history taking, and be sure to search for discrepancies between 1) the child's version of the incident, 2) the adult's version of the incident, and 3) what is realistic (based on your practical life experience and clinical training). As a primary care physician, you are obligated to report your *suspicion* of child abuse to law enforcement agencies and/or child protective services.
- **Children heal quickly:** This rapid healing is good as long as tissues are approximated. But if a fractured bone is displaced and not correctly replaced, then problematic malunion deformities may result *within days*.
- **Children are more susceptible to rapidly progressing infections than are adults:** Soft tissue, joint, and bone infections need to be diagnosed expeditiously and treated aggressively.
- **Children are radiographically different from adults:** Make sure that your radiographs are interpreted by a competent radiologist with experience in the interpretation of *pediatric radiographs*. Radiographic considerations specific to children include:
  - **Epiphyseal growth plates**
  - **Secondary ossification centers**
  - **Variants in trabecular patterns and bone densities**
  - **Specific conditions that happen only in children, such as slipped capital femoral epiphysis**
  - **Congenital anomalies**
  - **Difficulty following directions with positioning** (applies to some adults, too!)
  - **Bone scans can be difficult to interpret in children:** Bone scans derive their value from the demonstration of a focal increase in uptake of radioactive isotopes, which demonstrates and localizes an area of increased metabolic activity. In adults, this increased and localized activity generally indicates pathology, especially malignant disease in bone (primary or metastatic) and recent fracture. In children, however, since their bones are already highly metabolically active due to the normal growth process, bone scans are difficult to interpret and are not highly reliable for the demonstration of focal lesions.

Playground injury or child abuse? Infection or cancer? Undiagnosed developmental disorder, congenital anomaly, or metabolic illness?
Always consider the possibility of abuse, cancer, infection, or congenital anomaly as a cause of musculoskeletal pain in children, even if the injury appears to be related to injury or trauma. Strongly consider lab tests, as well as radiographs (interpreted by a pediatric radiologist). When in doubt, refer for second opinion. If you suspect abuse, you have a legal and ethical obligation to report your _suspicion_.

---

[365] Shaw BA, Gerardi JA, Hennrikus WL. How to avoid orthopedic pitfalls in children. *Patient Care* 1999; Feb 28: 95-116

Concept: Differences between Primary Healthcare and Spectator Sports

In baseball, "errors" have been defined as "a defensive mistake that allows a batter to stay at the plate or reach first base, or that advances a base runner."[366] In baseball, a few errors can make the difference between winning and losing a particular game or season. However, a few errors in a game are to be expected, and ultimately the team can start over at the next game or season and try to do better.

Healthcare, however, is not a game, and even relatively minor errors such as the doctor's forgetting to ask a particular question or perform a specific test can result in a patient's catastrophic injury or death. In healthcare, when we are dealing with serious injuries and illnesses, even a single "error" is not allowed. "Failure to diagnose" is one of the biggest reasons for malpractice claims against doctors; such judgments often result in loss of licensure and awards of hundreds of thousands of dollars. "Failure to treat" results when the patient is injured because the doctor failed to

Don't be naïve
While your compassion for human suffering and your love of nutrition and exercise may have directed you into healthcare, your professional success and survival will depend in large part on your ability to manage the technical and defensive aspects of clinical practice. Neuromusculoskeletal disorders and autoimmune diseases are "big league" clinical problems, and they need to be taken seriously.

effectively treat the patient or when the doctor failed to provide the appropriate referral to a specialist in a timely manner. Such failures are not only capable of destroying a physician's career and forcing the liquidation of his/her possessions, but such cases can also greatly damage the integrity of whole professions, especially the naturopathic and chiropractic professions which are generally guilty until proven innocent due to the double standards imposed by those adherent to the "always right" dogma of the medical paradigm.[367] Stated differently, **if the doctor does not ask the right questions and perform the right tests, then the doctor may miss an emergency diagnosis. Missing an emergency diagnosis can result in patient death. Patient death may result in litigation, loss of license for the doctor, and irreparable harm to the profession.** The upcoming section on **Musculoskeletal Emergencies** represents ***core competencies*** that every clinician must keep present in his/her mind during each interaction with a patient with musculoskeletal complaints, especially patients who are elderly, on medications such as prednisone, and those with known autoimmune or immunosuppressive disorders.

Concept: "Disease Treatment" is Different from "Patient Management"

> "The key to successful intervention for orthopedic problems in a primary care practice is to know what conditions to refer and when and to whom to refer the refractory patient."[368]

Treating a problem is one thing, managing a patient is something different. "Problems" such as "low back pain" are abstract concepts, and we automatically form mental lists of treatments for problems that are irrespective of the patient who has the condition. However this list may be of only very limited applicability to the individual patient with whom you are working. Management of patients includes ❶ assessing and reassessing the differential diagnoses, ❷ monitoring compliance with treatments, including the treatments of other healthcare providers, ❸ co-treating with other healthcare providers, ❹ assessing for contraindications, ❺ monitoring patient status and effectiveness of treatments, and also ❻ the office-related tasks of charting, documentation, billing, and correspondence. The management of emergency conditions often involves transport to the nearest hospital. In some situations, the patient will be able to drive himself/herself without difficulty. In other situations, the patient should be driven by friend, family, or taxi. In the most extreme, the patient should be transported by ambulance. When in doubt about the mode of transport, do not hesitate to call 911 for an ambulance. If the taxi driver gets lost on the way to the hospital, or your patient goes into shock while being driven by a friend, the liability will come back to haunt the ***doctor***, not the *friend* or the *taxi driver*.

---

[366] http://www.nocryinginbaseball.com/glossary/glossary.html Accessed November 11, 2006
[367] Micozzi MS. Double standards and double jeopardy for CAM research. *J Altern Complement Med.* 2001 Feb;7(1):13-4
[368] Brier S. Primary Care Orthopedics. St. Louis: Mosby, 1999 page ix

Concept: Clinical Practice Involves Much More than "Diagnosis and Treatment"

Emergency room and hospital-based physicians are appropriately able to focus solely on diagnosis and treatment as their primary spheres of activity and interaction with patients. However, those of us in private practice learn that *healthcare* involves much more than simply being a "good doctor." From an integrative perspective we have to go beyond diagnosis and treatment *for each health disorder* with each patient. Beyond *diagnosis* and *treatment* are *understanding* and *integration*. Orchestrating all of this into a treatment plan that the patient can actually implement requires creativity, resourcefulness, and the ability to enroll patients in the process of *redesigning*—often *rebuilding*—their lives.

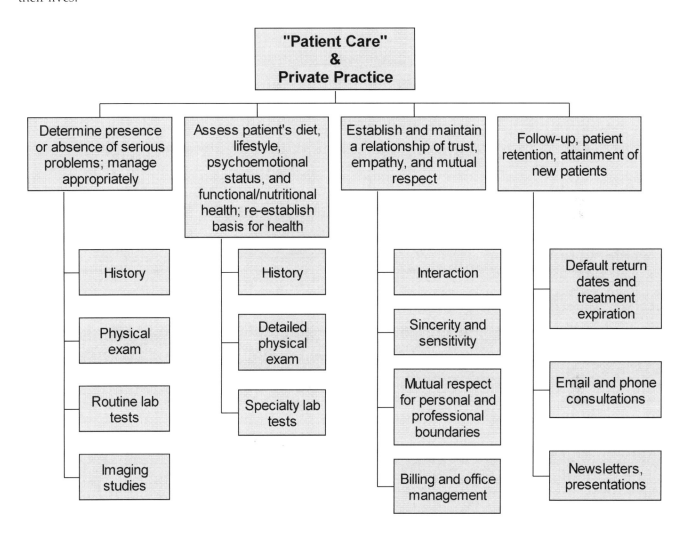

Components of Patient Care and Practice Management: Recall that **28% of malpractice claims involve mistakes made by medical office staff**; this includes unreturned phone calls which can culminate in malpractice by way of "patient abandonment." Similarly, inability to get a timely consultation may result in sufficient "sense of harm" that a patient may decide to sue; this is a factor in 10% of malpractice cases.[369]

---

[369] James R. Hall, Ph.D., L.Psych., FABMP, FGICPP. Departments of Internal Medicine and Psychology, UNT Health Science Center at Fort Worth. "Communication and Medico-Legal Issues." October 19, 2006

Clinical Management of Patients with Systemic Inflammatory/Autoimmune Diseases

In _Integrative Rheumatology_, I provide what—to the best of my knowledge—is an original conceptualization of rheumatic diseases. In the original Chapter 4 and the disease-specific chapters that follow, I provide additional scientific rationale for _theses_ that I originally presented elsewhere[370,371,372]:

1) Autoimmunity is a manifestation of immune dysfunction.

2) "Different" autoimmune diseases have much in common despite the different labels applied and manifestations observed. The commonalities in their etiologies and pathogenesis provides the rationale for the similarities in their treatments and a focus on identifying and ameliorating the underlying causes of autoimmunity as detailed: 1) food allergies/incompatibilities, 2) multifocal dysbiosis, 3) hormonal imbalances, 4) xenobiotic immunotoxicity, and 5) a pro-inflammatory diet and lifestyle. The new additions to this list in 2012[373] and 2013[374] are 6) mitochondrial dysfunction, and 7) nutritional immunomodulation.

3) Autoimmunity can be _ameliorated_ (not always eliminated) in the majority of patients with combined and coordinated effort on the part of the physician and the patient to address the most common cause**s** of immune dysfunction, which rarely operate in isolation and are generally found in synergistic combination.

4) Since the etiopathogenesis is generally complex and multifaceted, treatment must be assertive and likewise multifaceted. Only rarely will a simple "silver bullet" cure be effective and sustainable.

Of the four major healthcare paradigms in Western medicine—i.e., osteopathic, chiropractic, naturopathic, and allopathic—the naturopathic paradigm is uniquely—and perhaps _solitarily_—well-suited for the successful assessment of and intervention for most autoimmune diseases. For it is only in naturopathic medicine that we find the specific admonishment to _Treat the Cause_, and this is a critical differentiation from the allopathic model which codifies and compels the use of symptom-suppressing and immune-suppressing medications. The original chiropractic model acknowledges the multifaceted nature of health and disease but is too vague in this context to direct assessment and treatment. The original osteopathic model did not include an appreciation of biochemical/nutritional considerations and environmental contributions which are essential for the treatment of autoimmunity. It will be obvious to any student of rheumatology that the allopathic paradigm which turns to symptom-suppressing drugs as "first line treatment" for rheumatic disease is an abysmal failure except that it reduces symptomatology and protracts the disease while imposing an impressive array of medication side-effects and nearly unbearable financial burdens. The failure of the modern allopathic medical paradigm is evidenced in the increased utilization of high-dose chemotherapy and stem-cell transplantation for the treatment of autoimmune diseases[375], an action which seems to confess, "Since we were

---

The failure of long-term drug management of rheumatic disease

- Brigham Rheumatoid Arthritis Sequential Study (BRASS) cohort is a prospective, observational, single-center cohort with RA patients diagnosed by board-certified rheumatologists at the Brigham and Women's Hospital Arthritis Center. Patients are prospectively monitored, and their RA is managed according to the preference of the treating rheumatologist.

- Survival analysis performed separately for each remission criterion demonstrated that < 50% of subjects remained in remission 1 year later. Median remission survival time was 1 year.

- Other studies have described sustained remission in daily practice as uncommon, being reached by only 17% to 36% of RA patients for up to 6 months. These studies did not evaluate time in remission beyond 6 months. A recent study investigated the probability of remaining in remission up to 24 months, according to the ACR/EULAR, SDAI, and CDAI remission criteria in two different cohorts. They also concluded that long-term remission is rare, considering that the probability of a remission lasting 2 years was 6% to 14%

- Conclusions: This study shows that in clinical practice, a minority of RA patients are in sustained remission.

Prince FH, et al. Sustained rheumatoid arthritis remission is uncommon in clinical practice. _Arthritis Res Ther._ 2012 Mar http://arthritis-research.com/content/14/2/R68

---

[370] Vasquez A. "Inflammation and Autoimmunity: A Functional Medicine Approach." David S. Jones, MD (Editor-in-Chief). Textbook of Functional Medicine. Gig Harbor, WA; Institute for Functional Medicine (www.FunctionalMedicine.org): 2006, pages 409-417

[371] Vasquez A. Web-like Interconnections of Physiological Factors. _Integrative Medicine: A Clinician's Journal_ 2006, April/May, 32-37

[372] Vasquez A. Reducing Pain and Inflammation Naturally. Part 6: Nutritional and Botanical Treatments Against "Silent Infections" and Gastrointestinal Dysbiosis, Commonly Overlooked Causes of Neuromusculoskeletal Inflammation and Chronic Health Problems. _Nutritional Perspectives_ 2006; January http://www.InflammationMastery.com/part6

[373] Vasquez A. Functional Immunology and Nutritional Immunomodulation. 2012 https://www.createspace.com/3899760

[374] Vasquez A. Integrative Rheumatology, Nutritional Immunomodulation, and Functional Inflammology. 2013

[375] "Hematopoietic stem cell transplantation is an increasingly used therapy for treatment of autoimmune diseases and severe immune-mediated disorders." Burt RK, Verda L, Statkute L, Quigley K, Yaung K, Brush M, Oyama Y. Stem cell transplantation for autoimmune diseases. _Clin Adv Hematol Oncol._ 2004 May;2(5):313-9

unsuccessful with our first use of a hammer, instead of trying a different approach, we will just use a bigger hammer." It is thus with the firmly established scaffolding of the naturopathic paradigm that we begin our ascent to a vantage point high enough to allow a blurring of the rhetorical boundaries between diseases and from which we can ascertain the best path by which to traverse these complex and intricate labyrinths.

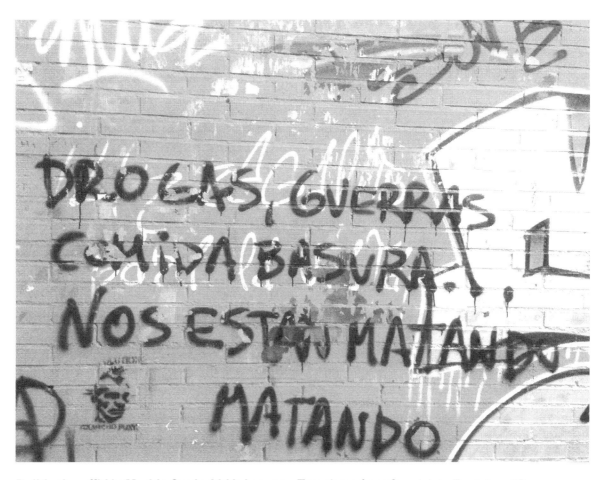

Political graffiti in Merida Spain 2013 January: Translates from Spanish to English as "Drugs, wars, and junk [garbage] food are killing us." One might wonder if "drogas/drugs" is meant to imply illegal recreational drugs or legal prescriptions drugs, the latter of which—in the form of "adverse drug effects" and other iatrogenesis—kill 3,500 patients per week in the United States alone; per the excellent clinical review published in *American Family Physician* (1997 Nov[376]): "Recent estimates suggest that each year more than 1 million patients are injured while in the hospital and approximately 180,000 die because of these injuries. Furthermore, drug-related morbidity and mortality are common and are estimated to cost more than $136 billion a year."

---

[376] Holland EG, Degruy FV. Drug-induced disorders. *Am Fam Physician.* 1997;56(7):1781-8,1791-2

Risk Management, Charting, and Avoiding Medical Errors: Useful Reminders & Acronyms

This page conveniently summarizes the most important acronyms for risk management, documentation, treatment, and patient education.

Acronym	Components	Exegesis
D.I.R.T.	Defensive mindset	Start with the conscious intention to practice defensively and effectively
	Duration of treatment	Define and limit the duration of each component of the treatment plan; define the next steps of care (e.g., continued care or laboratory tests) and the date of the return visit
	Interactions with disease and drugs	Double-check for interactions of the treatment plan with drugs and the patient's disease(s), especially renal insufficiency
	Referral	Determine the need for additional consultation
	Treatment plan, charted, dated, signed	Treatment plan must be archived in chart and should be given to patient; the clinician must sign and date the chart note and treatment plan
S.O.A.P.	Subjective	Patient's concerns, goals, changes in status
	Objective	Clinician's findings, including physical examination, reports from laboratory, imaging, biopsy, and consultations
	Assessments	Global assessments, firm diagnoses
	Plan	Treatments—definitions, durations for each concern, goal, assessment, diagnosis
F.I.N.D. S.E.X.® [377]	Food and nutrition	5-part nutritional wellness protocol—supplemented Paleo-Mediterranean diet: low-carbohydrate Paleo diet, multivitamin/mineral, physiologic doses of cholecalciferol, combination fatty acid therapy (CFAT), probiotics, allergy elimination-challenge, avoid genetically modified pseudofoods
	Infections and dysbiosis	Assess or treat empirically; components of treatment include antimicrobial, immunomodulation, immunorestoration
	Nutritional immunomodulation	See *Integrative Rheumatology, Inflammation Mastery* (2014 and beyond) for the latest update to the protocol—component #10 added in 2014 Jan.
	Dysfunctional mitochondria	Optimize mitochondrial function via mitophagy, resuscitation, and interventional disinhibition
	Stress, sleep, spinal health, sociology, sweat/exercise	Stress management and lifestyle/psychosocial optimization, sleep, spinal manipulation as indicated, sweat via daily exercise
	Endocrine/hormonal optimization	Especially assess and correct thyroid, prolactin, estradiol, insulin, DHEA, testosterone, and cortisol
	Xenobiotics and toxins	Toxicity is pandemic, therefore daily detoxification is mandatory and should target metals and organic/carbon-based toxins
P.A.R.B.Q.	Procedures	Explain the components of the treatment plan
	Alternatives	Explain what options and modifications exist
	Risks	Explain the risks of treatment, consider the aforementioned components of drug-interactions, disease-interactions, referral, and duration of treatment
	Benefits	Explain the anticipated benefits in realistic terms; never guarantee efficacy since "Each patient is different and each patient's response to treatment is unique."
	Questions answered	Document that questions—if any—were answered

---

[377] The FINDSEX acronym is a registered trademark by Dr Vasquez associated with <u>Functional Immunology and Nutritional Immunomodulation</u>. 2012 and updated as "<u>F.I.N.D. S.E.X®" The Easily Remembered Acronym for the Functional Inflammology Protocol.</u> 2013

Risk Management: A Note Especially to Students and Recent Licensees

Even if you are a board-certified rheumatologist and an assertive and astute clinician with years of experience, the consideration of these guidelines may help protect **you** from malpractice liability and **your patient** from harm. Practicing "good medicine" is inherently defensive and in the best interests of the patient and the doctor.

1. **Document the specifics of your treatment plan and the rationale behind it**.
2. **Do not tell your patient to discontinue their anti-rheumatic drugs unless these drugs are in your scope of practice *and* discontinuing such drugs is therapeutically appropriate**.
3. **Give your patient written instructions, and specifically delineate time parameters for the next visit to monitor for therapeutic effectiveness, adverse effects, and disease progression/regression**.
4. **Always have an internist or rheumatologist (or appropriate specialist) on-board as part of the clinical team in case the patient experiences an exacerbation and needs to be hospitalized or acutely immunosuppressed**.
5. **When working with patients that have potentially serious diseases such as most of the autoimmune diseases, you should have a back-up plan integrated into your treatment plan from day one.** You might consider having patients sign a consent form that includes language consistent with the following:
   - *"Due to the uniqueness of each disease and each individual, including his or her willingness and ability to implement the treatment plan, no guarantees of successful treatment can be offered."*
   - *"Dr.___ may not be available on a 24-hour basis at all times. If you have a serious health problem that requires immediate attention, you should call your other doctors(s), call 911, or have someone take you to the nearest hospital emergency room. If you notice an adverse effect from one of the components of your health plan, you should discontinue it then call Dr.___ and inform him/her of what occurred."*
   - *"Treatments with other physicians or healthcare providers are not necessarily to be discontinued. Please let Dr.___ know if you are being treated by other healthcare providers (physicians, counselors, therapists, etc.). Consult your prescribing doctor before discontinuing medications."*
6. **Test responsibly.**
7. **Treat responsibly.**
8. **Re-test to document effectiveness of your intervention.**
9. **When in doubt, refer the patient for co-management.** If you are working with a serious life-threatening disease, and *your plan* or *the patient's implementation of it* is unable to produce **documentable results**, then you should refer the patient for allopathic/osteopathic/specialist co-management for the sake of protecting the patient from harm and for protecting yourself from undue liability.
10. **Practice defensively.** You will thereby safeguard your patient and your livelihood.

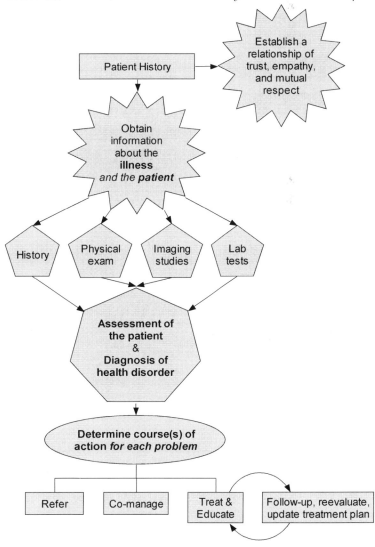

Musculoskeletal Emergencies

These are some of the "core competencies" that clinicians can never afford to miss, and these are pertinent to patients with musculoskeletal disorders, whether structural/orthopedic or metabolic/rheumatic. With these conditions, clinicians are wise to err on the side of caution— *"When in doubt, refer out"* —and implement the appropriate referral on an expedient basis. These are organized in a clinical/logical manner rather than listed alphabetically.

Neurovascular Disorders

Problem	Presentation	Assessment	Management
Neuropsychiatric lupus	▪ Psychosis ▪ Seizures ▪ Transient ischemic attacks ▪ Severe depression ▪ Delirium, confusion	▪ Neuropsychiatric manifestations with history of lupus	▪ Emergency or prompt referral as indicated
Giant cell arteritis, Temporal arteritis: Considered a medical emergency since it may rapidly progress to blindness due to associated involvement of the ophthalmic artery: *"Loss of vision is the most feared manifestation and occurs quite commonly."*[378]	Presentation typically includes the following: ▪ Headache, scalp tenderness ▪ Jaw claudication ▪ Changes in vision ▪ Systemic manifestations of rheumatic disease: fever, weight loss, muscle aches	▪ Palpation of the temporal artery may reveal a "cord-like" artery ▪ Elevated ESR ▪ CBC may show anemia ▪ Temporal artery biopsy is diagnostic	▪ Standard medical treatment is with immediate prednisone ▪ Implement treatment that is immediately effective or refer patient for medical treatment
Acute red eye: General term including acute iritis and scleritis; despite the name of this condition, redness may actually be rather minimal, and it is typically accompanied by cloudy changes in region of the iris and lens	▪ Eye pain and redness ▪ May have facial pain ▪ May be the presenting manifestation of rheumatic disease	▪ Red eye ▪ Photophobia ▪ Reduced vision ▪ May have fixed pupil ▪ Differential diagnosis includes acute glaucoma, bacterial/amebic/viral conjunctivitis or keratitis, allergy, and irritation due to contact lens	▪ "The **acute** onset of a **painful, red** eye, even in the absence of visual upset, should be regarded primarily as an ophthalmological emergency."[379] ▪ **Granulomatous uveitis** occurs in 15% of patients with sarcoidosis and can result in bilateral blindness—this must be managed as a medically urgent condition

[378] Tierney ML. McPhee SJ, Papadakis MA (eds). Current Medical Diagnosis and Treatment, 41st Edition. New York: Lange Medical ; 2002. P999-1005
[379] McInnes I, Sturrock R. Rheumatological emergencies. *Practitioner*. 1994 Mar;238(1536):220-4

Neural canal compression

Problem	Presentation	Assessment	Management
<u>Atlantoaxial instability</u>: Excess mobility between the atlas and axis (commonly due to lesion of the dens or transverse ligament) makes the spinal cord vulnerable to compressive injury when the atlas translates anteriorly on the axis especially during cervical flexion; may progress to neurologic compromise including respiratory and somatic paralysis	• Post-traumatic neck injury • Down's syndrome • May present spontaneously (without trauma) in patients with inflammatory rheumatic disease, especially rheumatoid arthritis and ankylosing spondylitis • May have gradual or sudden onset of myelopathy: upper motor neuron lesion (UMNL) signs (e.g., spastic weakness), changes in bowel-bladder function, numbness	• Clinical suspicion is followed by lateral cervical and APOM (anteroposterior open mouth) radiographs to assess ADI (atlantodental interval) and dens • MRI should be performed in patients with suspected myelopathy • Neurologic examination of the upper and lower extremities • Do not force neck flexion; do not perform the Soto Hall test	• **Urgent neurosurgical consultation is recommended; stabilizing surgery is the best option for the prevention of neurologic catastrophes**[380] • Onset of myelopathy mandates referral to ER and/or neurosurgeon; immobilize with spine board or hard cervical collar and transport appropriately • Asymptomatic and mild increases in ADI (< 5mm) might be managed conservatively with activity restriction, exercises, and bracing/collars) • PAR discussion and referral for surgical consultation is necessary for informed consent and safe management
<u>Myelopathy, spinal cord compression or lesion:</u> May occur due to infection, edema, tumor, spinal fracture, stenosis, or inflammatory disease	• **Spastic weakness** • Bowel-bladder dysfunction • Numbness • Problems are distal to cord lesion	• Hyperreflexia • Rigidity • Muscle weakness • MRI (with and without contrast) should be performed in patients with suspected myelopathy; CT may also be indicated	• Obtain MRI to confirm diagnosis • Immobilize spine and transport if necessary • Acute myelopathy is a medical emergency that can result in rapid-onset paralysis
<u>Cauda equina syndrome</u>: Compression of the sacral nerve roots due to lumbar disc herniation **Cauda equina syndrome is a surgical emergency.**	• History of sciatic low back pain • Urinary retention, perineal numbness, and fecal incontinence are common • May have lower extremity weakness	• Assess for bladder distention • Assess anal sphincter strength with rectal exam • Lower extremity neurologic examination	• Urgent referral for CT/MRI to confirm diagnosis • If diagnosis is confirmed or strongly suspected clinically, urgent referral for surgical decompression is mandatory

---

[380] "When atlantoaxial stability is lost...it is thought that surgical stabilisation of the atlantoaxial joint is more reasonable and beneficial than conservative management. Minimal trauma of an unstable atlantoaxial joint can lead to serious neurological injury." Moon MS, Choi WT, Moon YW, Moon JL, Kim SS. Brooks' posterior stabilization surgery for atlantoaxial instability: review of 54 cases. *J Orthop Surg* (Hong Kong). 2002 Dec;10(2):160-4. http://www.josonline.org/PDF/v10i2p160.pdf

Acute peripheral nerve compression

Problem	Presentation	Assessment	Management
Acute compartment syndrome: acute onset of *potentially irreversible* muscle and/or nerve compression injury due to inflammation, swelling, or bleeding within a fascial compartment **Acute compartment syndrome is a surgical emergency.**	▪ Most commonly occurs in the anterior leg; may also occur in the posterior leg as well as forearm—these are the areas most notable anatomically for the investment of muscle in tight and resilient fascial sheaths ▪ Onset generally follows strenuous exercise that leads to reactive hyperemia and secondary edema ▪ May occur following trauma or fracture	Assess for: ▪ Pulselessness ▪ Palor ▪ Painful passive stretch ▪ Weakness ▪ **Numbness** ▪ Assessment and treatment should be performed on an emergency basis since irreversible nerve damage begins within 6 hours of intracompartmental hypertension	▪ Decompressive fasciotomy is the standard treatment for acute compartment syndrome that could result in permanent muscle necrosis and/or permanent nerve death ▪ Acute compartment syndrome can be fatal if rhabdomyolysis precipitates renal failure[381]

Musculoskeletal infections

Problem	Presentation	Assessment	Management
Septic arthritis: intraarticular bacterial infection; complications of septic arthritis are 1) articular destruction and 2) **death in 5-10% of patients**[382] **Septic arthritis is a medical emergency**	▪ **Febrile** patient has **acute/subacute mono/oligo-arthritis** ▪ Some patients may not have fever ▪ Other possible findings: Immuno-suppression due to medications, concomitant disease (RA, DM), elderly ▪ In some patients with concomitant disease or medications, the clinical picture can be blurred.	▪ **Warm, swollen, tender joint** ▪ Clinical assessment with **immediate referral for joint aspiration**, which reveals manifestations of infection such as WBC's and bacteria ▪ Differential diagnosis includes trauma, gout, CPPD, hemochromatosis	▪ **Immediate referral for joint aspiration** ▪ **An aggressive and prolonged course of IV and oral antimicrobials** ▪ "Immune support" such as vitamin A and glutamine and general measures to improve health and prevent recurrence
Osteomyelitis, infectious discitis: considered a medical emergency[383] **Osteomyelitis—especially vertebral osteomyelitis—is a medical emergency**	▪ Febrile patient with bone pain ▪ Assess for constitutional manifestations such as weight loss, night sweats, and malaise	▪ Exacerbation of bone pain when stress/percussion is applied to the bone ▪ Lab: CRP & WBC may be elevated ▪ MRI is more sensitive than CT, bone scan, or radiography[384]	▪ Emergency referral for vertebral osteomyelitis, since **up to 15% of patients will develop nerve lesions or cord compression**[385] ▪ Urgent referral for other types of osteomyelitis

[381] Paula R. Compartment Syndrome, Extremity. *eMedicine* June 22, 2006 http://www.emedicine.com/emerg/topic739.htm Accessed November 26, 2006
[382] Tierney ML. McPhee SJ, Papadakis MA. <u>Current Medical Diagnosis and Treatment. 35th edition</u>. Stamford: Appleton & Lange, 1996 page 759
[383] American College of Rheumatology Ad Hoc Committee on Clinical Guidelines. Guidelines for the initial evaluation of the adult patient with acute musculoskeletal symptoms. *Arthritis Rheum*. 1996;39(1):1-8
[384] Tierney ML. McPhee SJ, Papadakis MA (eds). <u>Current Medical Diagnosis and Treatment 2002, 41st Edition</u>. New York: Lange Medical; 2002. p 883
[385] King RW, Johnson D. Osteomyelitis. Updated July 13, 2006. *eMedicine* http://www.emedicine.com/emerg/topic349.htm Accessed Dec 24, 2006

Acute Nontraumatic Monoarthritis and Septic Arthritis

- "Acute monoarthritis is a potential medical emergency that must be investigated and treated promptly."[386]
- "Monoarthropathies should initially be investigated to exclude sepsis. ... Diagnostic joint aspiration ... should be carried out immediately."[387]
- "In acute monoarthritis, it is essential that infection of a joint be diagnosed or excluded, and this can only be done by joint aspiration and synovial fluid culture."[388]
- "Acute monoarthritis should be considered infectious until proven otherwise."[389]

Clinical presentations:

- Patient presents with acute joint pain in one joint (occasionally more than one joint may be involved).
- May or may not have fever and other systemic manifestations of infection.

Clinical Pearl
The primary goal of this section is to solidify your awareness of septic arthritis, its differential diagnoses, and the method and importance of assertive diagnosis and management.
Septic arthritis is a medical emergency, and some authoritative textbooks report a mortality rate of 5-10%.
Septic arthritis must be diagnosed urgently with joint aspiration, and it must be treated with antibiotics in order to preserve the joint and prevent spread of the infection.

Major Differential Diagnoses for Nontraumatic Monoarthritis

Problem	Presentation	Assessment & Management
<u>Septic arthritis</u>: intraarticular bacterial infection; complications of septic arthritis are 1) articular destruction and 2) **death in 5-10% of patients**[390]	▪ **Febrile** patient has **acute/subacute mono/oligo-arthritis** ▪ **Onset over hours or days** Other possible findings: ▪ Immuno-suppression due to medications, concomitant disease (RA, DM), elderly ▪ Some patients may not have fever ▪ In some patients with a previous or concomitant disease process, the clinical picture can be blurred	▪ **Warm, swollen, red, painful joint** ▪ Clinical assessment with **immediate referral for <u>joint aspiration</u>, which reveals characteristic manifestations of infection such as WBCs and bacteria** ▪ **Immediate joint aspiration** ▪ An aggressive and prolonged course of IV and oral antimicrobials ▪ "Immune support" and general measures to improve health and prevent recurrence
		Septic arthritis is life-threatening "Septic arthritis is still a life-threatening disease with a mortality of 2–5% and high morbidity." Zacher J, Gursche A. Regional musculoskeletal conditions: 'hip' pain. *Best Practice & Research Clinical Rheumatology.* 2003 Feb;17:71-85

---

[386] Cibere J. Rheumatology: 4. Acute monoarthritis. CMAJ (*Canadian Medical Association Journal*). 2000;162(11):1577-83 www.cmaj.ca/cgi/content/full/162/11/1577 Jan 2004

[387] McInnes I, Sturrock R. Rheumatological emergencies. Practitioner. 1994 Mar;238(1536):220-4

[388] American College of Rheumatology Ad Hoc Committee on Clinical Guidelines. Guidelines for the initial evaluation of the adult patient with acute musculoskeletal symptoms. *Arthritis Rheum.* 1996 Jan;39(1):1-8

[389] Cibere J. Rheumatology: 4. Acute monoarthritis. CMAJ (*Canadian Medical Association Journal*). 2000;162(11):1577-83 www.cmaj.ca/cgi/content/full/162/11/1577 Jan 2004

[390] Tierney ML. McPhee SJ, Papadakis MA. <u>Current Medical Diagnosis and Treatment. 35th edition</u>. Stamford: Appleton and Lange, 1996 page 759

Major differential diagnoses for non-traumatic monoarthritis—*continued*

Problem	Presentation	Assessment & Management
Osteochondritis dissecans: A disorder of unclear etiology (trauma and/or avascular necrosis) which results in the death and subsequent fragmentation of subchondral bone[391]	▪ Primarily affects ages 10-30 years ▪ **Most common in the knees and elbows** ▪ Locking and crepitus due to intraarticular loose bodies ("joint mice") ▪ Some patients are almost asymptomatic, while others have acute pain ▪ Swelling of the affected joint	▪ Radiographs—consider to assess both knees as the condition is bilateral in 30% ▪ MRI is used to assess severity and need for surgical intervention ▪ Stable and nondisplaced lesions may be managed nonsurgically; larger and displaced fragments require surgical repair to reduce long-term complications[392]
Transient synovitis, irritable hip: Non-specific short-term inflammation and effusion of the hip joint	▪ Acute onset of painful hip and limp ▪ Decreased pain with hip in flexion and abduction ▪ Considered the most common cause of hip pain in children[393] ▪ More common in boys, age 3-6 years and generally younger than 10 years ▪ May have recent history of viral infection, and some children (1.5-10%) eventually manifest RA or AVN[394]	▪ May have slight elevation of ESR ▪ Normal WBC ▪ No fever; the child appears healthy ▪ "…radiography is indicated to exclude osseous pathological conditions…"[395] ▪ **Joint aspiration is indicated if septic arthritis is suspected**[396] ▪ Conservative treatment, restricted exertion and weight-bearing for several weeks
Legg-Calve-Perthe's disease: Idiopathic ischemic necrosis of the femoral head occurring in children **Avascular necrosis (AVN) of the femoral head, osteonecrosis**: Ischemic necrosis of the femoral head	Perthe's disease: ▪ 80% occur in children generally between ages of 4-9 years; more common in boys; may present with hip pain or knee pain AVN: ▪ Ages 20-40 years ▪ Unilateral hip pain ▪ May have knee pain ▪ History of trauma is common AVN associations: ▪ Steroid use, prednisone ▪ Hyperlipidemia ▪ Alcoholism ▪ Pancreatitis ▪ Hemoglobinopathies ▪ Smoking ▪ Fatty liver disease: "fat globules from the liver"[397]	▪ Limited ROM ▪ **Radiographs**; if normal and clinical suspicion is high order MRI or bone scan ▪ **Crutches** ▪ **Orthopedic referral is recommended** although not all patients will require surgery and some may be managed conservatively[398]

[391] Tatum R. Osteochondritis dissecans of the knee: a radiology case report. *J Manipulative Physiol Ther* 2000 Jun;23(5):347-51

[392] Browne RF, Murphy SM, Torreggiani WC, Munk PL, Marchinkow LO. Radiology for the surgeon: musculoskeletal case 30. Osteochondritis dissecans of the medial femoral condyle. *Can J Surg.* 2003;46(5):361-3 cma.ca/multimedia/staticContent/HTML/N0/l2/cjs/vol-46/issue-5/pdf/pg361.pdf

[393] Maroo S. Diagnosis of hip pain in children. *Hosp Med* 1999 Nov;60(11):788-93

[394] Souza TA. Differential Diagnosis for the Chiropractor: Protocols and Algorithms. Gaithersberg, Maryland: Aspen Publications. 1997 page 265

[395] Maroo S. Diagnosis of hip pain in children. *Hosp Med* 1999 Nov;60(11):788-93

[396] Maroo S. Diagnosis of hip pain in children. *Hosp Med* 1999 Nov;60(11):788-93

[397] Skinner HB, Scherger JE. Identifying structural hip and knee problems. *Postgrad Med* 1999;106(7):51-2, 55-6, 61-4

[398] Souza TA. Differential Diagnosis for the Chiropractor: Protocols and Algorithms. Gaithersberg, Maryland: Aspen Publications. 1997 page 263

Major differential diagnoses for non-traumatic monoarthritis—*continued*

Problem	Presentation	Assessment & Management
<u>Gout</u>	<ul><li>**Febrile** patient has **acute/subacute mono/oligo-arthritis**</li><li>**Onset over hours or days**</li><li>"A history of discreet attacks, usually affecting one joint, that precede the onset of fixed symmetric arthritis is the major clue."[399]</li><li>May have fever, chills, tachycardia, leukocytosis—just like septic arthritis</li></ul>	<ul><li>Clinical presentation may be sufficient for DX; however septic arthritis should be excluded</li><li>Serum uric acid is generally meaningless for the diagnosis of gout since many gout patients will have normal serum uric acid</li><li>Medical treatment is rest, NSAID's, and allopurinol</li><li>Fluid loading: >3 liters per day; monitor for electrolyte imbalances and hyponatremia as needed</li><li>Integrative assessment and treatment for insulin resistance, hormonal imbalances, and nutritional deficiencies</li></ul>
<u>**CPPD**</u>: Calcium pyrophosphate dihydrate deposition disease	<ul><li>Idiopathic</li><li>May be caused by iron overload in some patients</li><li>Presentation may be acute or subacute</li></ul>	<ul><li>Medical diagnosis is by synovial biopsy</li><li>Radiographs reveal chondrocalcinosis</li><li>Allopathic treatment is NSAIDs; phytonutritional anti-inflammatory treatments may also be used (see chapter 3 of *Integrative Orthopedics/Rheumatology*)</li><li>Oral colchicine 0.5 to 1.5 mg per day prevents attacks[400]</li></ul>
<u>**Hemarthrosis**</u>: Generally associated with trauma, anticoagulation (i.e., coumadin), leukemia, hemophilia	<ul><li>Monoarthralgia with limited motion</li><li>May follow direct trauma</li><li>Nontraumatic hemarthrosis may be due to anticoagulation, leukemia, hemophilia</li></ul>	<ul><li>Synovial fluid analysis reveals blood</li><li>Treatment of underlying disorder; refer as indicated</li></ul>
<u>**Slipped capital femoral epiphysis (SCFE)**</u>: The most common cause of hip pain in adolescents[401]	<ul><li>Seen in adolescents generally 8-17 years of age</li><li>Classic presentation is a tall overweight boy with **hip pain**, knee pain, and/or a painful limp: "*Slipped femoral capital epiphysis is a developmental injury that must be considered in any adolescent who presents with hip pain.*"[402]</li></ul>	<ul><li>**Radiographs** of both hips (bilateral SCFE in 40%): "<u>**AP and frog lateral views are recommended in all children over age of 9 years with hip pain**</u>."[403]</li><li>Orthopedic referral—"*…the patient should be referred immediately to an orthopedist for surgical stabilization.*" [404]</li></ul>

---

[399] Hardin JG, Waterman J, Labson LH. Rheumatic disease: Which diagnostic tests are useful? *Patient Care* 1999; March 15: 83-102
[400] Beers MH, Berkow R (eds). <u>The Merck Manual. Seventeenth Edition</u>. Whitehouse Station; Merck Research Laboratories 1999 Page
[401] Maroo S. Diagnosis of hip pain in children. *Hosp Med* 1999 Nov;60(11):788-93
[402] O'Kane JW. Anterior hip pain. *Am Fam Physician* 1999 Oct 15;60(6):1687-96
[403] Maroo S. Diagnosis of hip pain in children. *Hosp Med* 1999 Nov;60(11):788-93
[404] O'Kane JW. Anterior hip pain. *Am Fam Physician* 1999 Oct 15;60(6):1687-96

Clinical assessment of non-traumatic monoarthritis:
- History and orthopedic assessment of the joint
- Laboratory tests must be performed if you have a suspicion of infection

History/subjective:
- Acute or subacute joint pain with or without systemic manifestations and fever.
- History or may not be significant; other than the obvious risk factor of immunosuppression, septic arthritis can occur with impressive spontaneity and randomness

Differential physical examination and objective findings:
- **Septic arthritis**: pain and limitation of motion, swelling, redness; patient may have systemic symptoms of fever and malaise
- **Gout**: pain and limitation of motion, swelling, redness; patient may have systemic symptoms of fever and malaise
- **Pseudogout and calcium pyrophosphate dihydrate deposition disease (CPDD/CPPD)**: pain and limitation of motion, swelling, redness; patient may have systemic symptoms of fever and malaise
- **Ischemic necrosis**: pain and limitation of motion; swelling, redness and systemic symptoms are less likely.
- **Hemarthrosis**: pain and limitation of motion; often associated with trauma, use of anticoagulant medications[405], or hemophilia and other hematologic abnormalities[406]
- **Tumor**: assess with history, imaging, and biopsy if possible
- **Injury**: Meniscal injury, fracture, ligament injury; physical examination procedures are described in the chapters that follow

Imaging and laboratory assessments:
- **Septic arthritis**: joint aspiration; STAT CBC (for WBC count) and CRP
- **Gout**: joint aspiration; CBC (for WBC count) and CRP
- **Pseudogout and PPDD**: rule out septic arthritis with joint aspiration, CBC, and CRP; radiographs often show chondrocalcinosis
- **Ischemic necrosis**: radiographs are diagnostic
- **Hemarthrosis**: joint aspiration and assessment for underlying disease or medication, especially if the condition was not trauma-induced
- **Tumor**: assess with radiographs
- **Injury**: rule out infection; consider imaging with radiography or MRI.

Establishing the diagnosis:
- The aforementioned examinations and lab assessments should establish the exact diagnosis. **The priorities are 1) first exclude life-threatening illness (i.e., septic arthritis), then 2) to exclude serious injury or illness,** and finally 3) to help manage the exact problem.

Complications:
- **Septic arthritis can result in death in 5-10% of patients. "Five to 10 percent of patients with an infected joint die, chiefly from respiratory complications of sepsis. The mortality rate is 30% for patients with polyarticular sepsis. Bony ankylosis and articular destruction commonly also occur if the treatment is delayed or inadequate."**[407] Complications vary per location, infecting organism, severity, and patient.

---

[405] Riley SA, Spencer GE. Destructive monarticular arthritis secondary to anticoagulant therapy. *Clin Orthop.* 1987 Oct;(223):247-51

[406] Jean-Baptiste G, De Ceulaer K. Osteoarticular disorders of haematological origin. *Baillieres Best Pract Res Clin Rheumatol.* 2000 Jun;14(2):307-23

[407] Tierney ML. McPhee SJ, Papadakis MA. Current Medical Diagnosis and Treatment. 35th edition. Stamford: Appleton & Lange, 1996 page 759

Clinical management of non-traumatic monoarthritis:

- **Suspected septic arthritis requires referral for joint aspiration and antimicrobial drugs.**
- Referral if clinical outcome is unsatisfactory or if serious complications are evident.
- Treatment of other conditions that cause acute monoarthritis (such as gout and calcium pyrophosphate dihydrate deposition disease) is based on the problem and individual patient.

Treatments:

- <u>**Septic arthritis requires IV/oral antimicrobial drugs**</u>: Intravenous antibiotics are generally started before culture results are available. After results and culture from synovial fluid analysis have been considered, the dose, combination, and administration of antibiotics can be fine-tuned. Frequently, antibiotics are administered intravenously for at least 3-4 weeks. Surgical/endoscopic drainage/debridement and immobilization during the acute phase may also be implemented.[408]
- **Immunonutrition considerations:** Immunonutritional considerations are listed below; doses listed are for adults. Although studies have not been performed specifically in patients with bone/joint infections, general benefits derived from the use of immunonutrition are reductions in severity/frequency/duration of major infections, abbreviated hospitalization (i.e., early discharge due to expedited healing and recovery), reductions in the need for medications, significant improvements in survival, and hospital savings.[409,410,411,412,413,414,415]
  - <u>Paleo-Mediterranean diet</u>: as detailed later in this text and elsewhere[416,417]
  - <u>Vitamin and mineral supplementation</u>: anti-infective benefits shown in elderly diabetics[418]
  - <u>High-dose vitamin A</u>: Vitamin A shows potent immunosupportive benefits, and vitamin A stores are depleted by the stress of infection and injury. Consider 200,000-300,000 IU per day of retinol palmitate for 1-4 weeks, then taper; reduce dose or discontinue with onset of toxicity symptoms such as skin problems (dry skin, flaking skin, chapped or split lips, red skin rash, hair loss), joint pain, bone pain, headaches, anorexia (loss of appetite), edema (water retention, weight gain, swollen ankles, difficulty breathing), fatigue, and/or liver damage.
  - <u>Arginine</u>: Dose for adults is in the range of 5-10 grams daily

---

[408] Brusch JL. Septic Arthritis (Last Updated: October 18, 2005). *eMedicine*. http://www.emedicine.com/med/topic3394.htm Accessed Nov 25, 2006

[409] "To evaluate the metabolic and immune effects of dietary arginine, glutamine and omega-3 fatty acids (fish oil) supplementation, we performed a prospective study... CONCLUSIONS: The feeding of Neomune in critically injured patients was well tolerated as Traumacal and significant improvement was observed in serum protein. Shorten ICU stay and wean-off respirator day may benefit from using the immunonutrient formula." Chuntrasakul C, Siltham S, Sarasombath S, Sittapairochana C, Leowattana W, Chockvivatanavanit S, Bunnak A. Comparison of a immunonutrition formula enriched arginine, glutamine and omega-3 fatty acid, with a currently high-enriched enteral nutrition for trauma patients. *J Med Assoc Thai*. 2003 Jun;86(6):552-6

[410] "CONCLUSIONS: In conclusion, arginine-enhanced formula improves fistula rates in postoperative head and neck cancer patients and decreases length of stay." de Luis DA, Izaola O, Cuellar L, Terroba MC, Aller R. Randomized clinical trial with an enteral arginine-enhanced formula in early postsurgical head and neck cancer patients. *Eur J Clin Nutr*. 2004;58(11):1505-8

[411] "In this prospective, randomised, double-blind, placebo-controlled study, we randomly assigned 50 patients who were scheduled to undergo coronary artery bypass to receive either an oral immune-enhancing nutritional supplement containing L-arginine, omega3 polyunsaturated fatty acids, and yeast RNA (n=25), or a control (n=25) for a minimum of 5 days... Intake of an oral immune-enhancing nutritional supplement for a minimum of 5 days before surgery can improve outlook in high-risk patients who are undergoing elective cardiac surgery." Tepaske R, Velthuis H, Oudemans-van Straaten HM, Heisterkamp SH, van Deventer SJ, Ince C, Eysman L, Kesecioglu J. Effect of preoperative oral immune-enhancing nutritional supplement on patients at high risk of infection after cardiac surgery: a randomised placebo-controlled trial. *Lancet*. 2001 Sep 1;358(9283):696-701

[412] "The feeding of IMMUNE FORMULA was well tolerated and significant improvement was observed in nutritional and immunologic parameters as in other immunoenhancing diets. Further clinical trials of prospective double-blind randomized design are necessary to address the so that the necessity of using immunonutrition in critically ill patients will be clarified." Chuntrasakul C, Siltharm S, Sarasombath S, Sittapairochana C, Leowattana W, Chockvivatanavanit S, Bunnak A. Metabolic and immune effects of dietary arginine, glutamine and omega-3 fatty acids supplementation in immunocompromised patients. *J Med Assoc Thai*. 1998 May;81(5):334-43

[413] "enteral diet supplemented with arginine, dietary nucleotides, and omega-3 fatty acids (IMPACT, Sandoz Nutrition, Bern, Switzerland)" Senkal M, Mumme A, Eickhoff U, Geier B, Spath G, Wulfert D, Joosten U, Frei A, Kemen M. Early postoperative enteral immunonutrition: clinical outcome and cost-comparison analysis in surgical patients. *Crit Care Med* 1997;25(9):1489-96

[414] "supplemented diet with glutamine, arginine and omega-3-fatty acids... It was clearly established in this trial that early postoperative enteral feeding is safe in patients who have undergone major operations for gastrointestinal cancer. Supplementation of enteral nutrition with glutamine, arginine, and omega-3-fatty acids positively modulated postsurgical immunosuppressive and inflammatory responses." Wu GH, Zhang YW, Wu ZH. Modulation of postoperative immune and inflammatory response by immune-enhancing enteral diet in gastrointestinal cancer patients. *World J Gastroenterol*. 2001 Jun;7(3):357-62 http://www.wjgnet.com/1007-9327/7/357.pdf

[415] "using a formula supplemented with arginine, mRNA, and omega-3 fatty acids from fish oil (Impact)... CONCLUSIONS: Immune-enhancing enteral nutrition resulted in a significant reduction in the mortality rate and infection rate in septic patients admitted to the ICU. These reductions were greater for patients with less severe illness." Galban C, Montejo JC, Mesejo A, Marco P, Celaya S, Sanchez-Segura JM, Farre M, Bryg DJ. An immune-enhancing enteral diet reduces mortality rate and episodes of bacteremia in septic intensive care unit patients. *Crit Care Med*. 2000 Mar;28(3):643-8

[416] Vasquez A. A Five-Part Nutritional Protocol that Produces Consistently Positive Results. *Nutritional Wellness* 2005 September http://InflammationMastery.com/protocol

[417] Vasquez A. Implementing the Five-Part Nutritional Wellness Protocol for the Treatment of Various Health Problems. *Nutritional Wellness* 2005 November. http://InflammationMastery.com/protocol

[418] "CONCLUSIONS: A multivitamin and mineral supplement reduced the incidence of participant-reported infection and related absenteeism in a sample of participants with type 2 diabetes mellitus and a high prevalence of subclinical micronutrient deficiency." Barringer TA, Kirk JK, Santaniello AC, Foley KL, Michielutte R. Effect of a multivitamin and mineral supplement on infection and quality of life. A randomized, double-blind, placebo-controlled trial. *Ann Intern Med*. 2003 Mar 4;138(5):365-71 http://www.annals.org/cgi/reprint/138/5/365

- o <u>Fatty acid supplementation</u>: In contrast to the higher doses used to provide an anti-inflammatory effect in patients with autoimmune/inflammatory disorders, doses used for immunosupportive treatments should be kept rather modest to avoid the *relative* immunosuppression that has been controversially reported in patients treated with EPA and DHA. Reasonable doses are in the following ranges for adults: EPA+DHA: 500-1,500, and GLA: 300-500 mg.
- o <u>Glutamine</u>: Glutamine enhances bacterial killing by neutrophils[419], and administration of 18 grams per day in divided doses to patients in intensive care units was shown to improve survival, expedite hospital discharge, and reduce total healthcare costs.[420] Another study using glutamine 12-18 grams per day showed no benefit in overall mortality but significant benefits in terms of reduced healthcare costs (-30%) and significantly reduced need for medical interventions.[421] After administering glutamine 26 grams/d to severely burned patients, Garrel et al[422] concluded that glutamine reduced the risk of infection by 3-fold and that oral glutamine "may be a life-saving intervention" in patients with severe burns. A dose of 30 grams/d was used in a recent clinical trial showing hemodynamic benefit in patients with sickle cell anemia.[423] The highest glutamine dose that the current author is aware of is the study by Scheltinga et al[424] who used 0.57 gm/kg/day in cancer patients following chemotherapy administration; for a 220-lb-pt, this would be approximately 57 grams of glutamine per day.
- o <u>Melatonin</u>: 20-40 mg hs (*hora somni*—Latin: sleep time). Immunostimulatory anti-infective action of melatonin was demonstrated in a small clinical trial wherein septic newborns administered 20 mg melatonin showed significantly increased survival over nontreated controls.[425]

[419] Furukawa S, Saito H, Fukatsu K, Hashiguchi Y, Inaba T, Lin MT, Inoue T, Han I, Matsuda T, Muto T. Glutamine-enhanced bacterial killing by neutrophils from postoperative patients. *Nutrition* 1997;13(10):863-9. *In vitro* study.

[420] Griffiths RD, Jones C, Palmer TE. Six-month outcome of critically ill patients given glutamine-supplemented parenteral nutrition. *Nutrition* 1997;13(4):295-302

[421] "There was no mortality difference between those patients receiving glutamine-containing enteral feed and the controls. However, there was a significant reduction in the median postintervention ICU and hospital patient costs in the glutamine recipients $23 000 versus $30 900 in the control patients." Jones C, Palmer TE, Griffiths RD. Randomized clinical outcome study of critically ill patients given glutamine-supplemented enteral nutrition. *Nutrition.* 1999 Feb;15(2):108-15

[422] The glutamine dose in this study was "a total of 26 g/day" administered in four divided doses. CONCLUSION: "The results of this prospective randomized clinical trial show that enteral G reduces blood culture positivity, particularly with P. aeruginosa, in adults with severe burns and may be a life-saving intervention." Garrel D, Patenaude J, Nedelec B, et al. Decreased mortality and infectious morbidity in adult burn patients given enteral glutamine supplements: a prospective, controlled, randomized clinical trial. *Crit Care Med.* 2003 Oct;31(10):2444-9

[423] Niihara Y, Matsui NM, Shen YM, et al. L-glutamine therapy reduces endothelial adhesion of sickle red blood cells to human umbilical vein endothelial cells. *BMC Blood Disord.* 2005 Jul 25;5:4 http://www.biomedcentral.com.proxy.hsc.unt.edu/1471-2326/5/4

[424] "Subjects with hematologic malignancies in remission underwent a standard treatment of high-dose chemotherapy and total body irradiation before bone marrow transplantation. After completion of this regimen, they were randomized to receive either standard parenteral nutrition (STD, n = 10) or an isocaloric, isonitrogenous nutrient solution enriched with crystalline L-glutamine (0.57 g/kg/day, GLN, n = 10)." Scheltinga MR, Young LS, Benfell K, Bye RL, Ziegler TR, Santos AA, Antin JH, Schloerb PR, Wilmore DW. Glutamine-enriched intravenous feedings attenuate extracellular fluid expansion after a standard stress. *Ann Surg.* 1991 Oct;214(4):385-93; discussion 393-5 pubmedcentral.nih.gov/articlerender.fcgi?tool=pubmed&pubmedid=1953094 For additional review, see Ziegler TR. Glutamine supplementation in cancer patients receiving bone marrow transplantation and high dose chemotherapy. J Nutr. 2001 Sep;131(9 Suppl):2578S-84S http://jn.nutrition.org/cgi/content/full/131/9/2578S

[425] Gitto E, et al. Effects of melatonin treatment in septic newborns. *Pediatr Res.* 2001;50:756-60 pedresearch.org/cgi/content/full/50/6/756

Brief Overview of Integrative Healthcare Disciplines

Chiropractic

"The human body represents the actions of three laws—spiritual, mechanical, and chemical—united as one triune. As long as there is perfect union of these three, there is health." *Daniel David Palmer, founder of the modern chiropractic profession*[426]

The basic philosophical model which is taught in many chiropractic colleges is to envision health, disease, and patient care from a conceptual model named the "triad of health" which gives its attention to the three fundamental foundations for well-being: namely, the physical/structural, mental/emotional, and biochemical/nutritional aspects of health. Revolutionary at the time of its inception in the early 1900's, this model now forms the foundation for the increasingly dominant and very popular paradigm of "holistic medicine." It remains a powerful contrast and an attractive alternative to the reductionistic allopathic approach, which generally approaches the human body as if it were simply a conglomerate of independent organ systems that have little or no functional relationship to each other.[427]

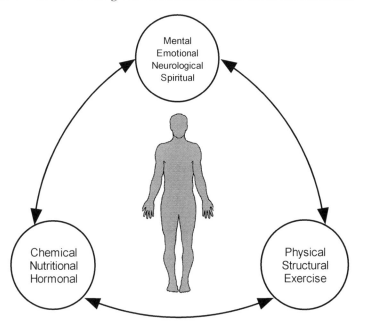

The chiropractic "triad of health"

Using the state of the sciences before the year 1910, chiropractic was founded with a profound appreciation of the integrated nature of health, and the therapeutic focus was on spinal manipulation. In describing the chiropractic model of health, DD Palmer[428] wrote, "The human body represents the actions of three laws—spiritual, mechanical, and chemical—united as one triune. As long as there is perfect union of these three, there is health." While the therapeutic focus of the profession has been spinal manipulation, from its inception the chiropractic profession has emphasized a holistic, integrative model of therapeutic intervention, health, and disease, and chiropractic was the first healthcare profession in America to specifically claim that the optimization of health requires attention to spiritual-emotional-psychological, mechanical-physical-structural, and biochemical-nutritional-hormonal-chemical considerations.

From its inception, chiropractic was a philosophy of healing that considered the entire health of the patient by addressing the interconnected aspects of our chemical-spiritual-physical being. Later, intraprofessional factions polarized between holistic and vitalistic paradigms; the latter has been presumed to be the philosophy of the entire profession by organizations such as the American Medical Association[429] that have sought to contain and eliminate chiropractic and other forms of natural healthcare[430] by falsifying research[431,432], intentionally misleading the public

---

[426] Palmer DD. The Science, Art, and Phiosophy, of Chiropractic. Portland, OR; Portland Printing House Company, 1910: 107
[427] Beckman JF, Fernandez CE, Coulter ID. A systems model of health care: a proposal. *J Manipulative Physiol Ther.* 1996 Mar-Apr; 19(3): 208-15
[428] Palmer DD. The Science, Art, and Phiosophy, of Chiropractic. Portland, OR; Portland Printing House Company, 1910: 107
[429] American Medical Association. Report 12 of the Council on Scientific Affairs (A-97) Full Text. http://www.ama-assn.org/ama/pub/category/13638.html Accessed Sep 10, 2005
[430] Getzendanner S. Permanent injunction order against AMA. *JAMA.* 1988 Jan 1;259(1):81-2
[431] Terrett AG. Misuse of the literature by medical authors in discussing spinal manipulative therapy injury. *J Manipulative Physiol Ther.* 1995 May;18(4):203-10
[432] Morley J, Rosner AL, Redwood D. A case study of misrepresentation of the scientific literature: recent reviews of chiropractic. *J Altern Complement Med.* 2001 Feb;7(1):65-78

and manipulating politicians[433,434,435], arriving at illogical conclusions which support the medical paradigm and refute the value of manual therapies[436], and exploiting weaknesses within the profession for its own financial profitability and political advantage.[437] Intentional misrepresentation and defamation of chiropractic continues to occur to current times, as documented by the 2006 review by Wenban.[438]

In accord with the comprehensive chiropractic training in musculoskeletal management, numerous sources of evidence demonstrate that chiropractic management of the most common spinal pain syndromes is safer and less expensive than allopathic medical treatment, particularly for the treatment of low-back pain. In their extensive review of the literature, Manga et al[439] published in 1993 that chiropractic management of low-back pain is superior to allopathic medical management in terms of greater safety, greater effectiveness, and reduced cost; they concluded, "There is an overwhelming body of evidence indicating that chiropractic management of low-back pain is more cost-effective than medical management" and "There would be highly significant cost savings if more management of LBP [low-back pain] was transferred from medical physicians to chiropractors." In a randomized trial involving 741 patients, Meade et al[440] showed, "Chiropractic treatment was more effective than hospital outpatient management, mainly for patients with chronic or severe back pain... The benefit of chiropractic treatment became more evident throughout the follow up period. Secondary outcome measures also showed that chiropractic was more beneficial." A 3-year follow-up study by these same authors[441] in 1995 showed, "At three years the results confirm the findings of an earlier report that when chiropractic or hospital therapists treat patients with low-back pain as they would in day to day practice, those treated by chiropractic derive more benefit and long term satisfaction than those treated by hospitals." In 2004 Legorreta et al[442] reported that the availability of chiropractic care was associated with significant cost savings among 700,000 patients with chiropractic coverage compared to 1 million patients whose insurance coverage was limited to allopathic medical treatments. Simple extrapolation of the average savings per patient in this study ($208 annual savings associated with chiropractic coverage) to the US population (295 million citizens in 2005[443]) suggests that, if fully implemented in a nation-wide basis, America could save $61,360,000,000 (more than $61 billion per year) in annual healthcare expenses by ensuring chiropractic for all citizens in contrast to failing to provide such coverage; obviously extrapolations such as this should consider other variables, such as the relatively higher prevalence of injury and death among patients treated with drugs and surgery.[444,445] Furthermore, whether the cost savings associated with chiropractic availability are due to 1) improved overall health and reduced need for pharmacosurgical intervention, 2) greater safety and lower cost of chiropractic treatment versus pharmacosurgical treatment, and/or 3) self-selection by wellness-oriented, perhaps healthier, and higher-income patients, remains to be determined.

A literature review by Dabbs and Lauretti[446] showed that spinal manipulation is safer than the use of NSAIDs in the treatment of neck pain. Contrasting the rates of manipulation-associated cerebrovascular accidents to the dangers of medical and surgical treatments for spinal disorders, Rosner[447] noted, "These rates are 400 times lower than the death rates observed from gastrointestinal bleeding due to the use of nonsteroidal anti-inflammatory drugs and 700 times lower than the overall mortality rate for spinal surgery." Similarly, in his review of the

[433] Spivak JL. The Medical Trust Unmasked. Louis S. Siegfried Publishers; New York: 1961

[434] Trever W. In the Public Interest. Los Angeles; Scriptures Unlimited; 1972. This is probably the most authoritative documentation of the illegal actions of the AMA up to 1972; contains numerous photocopies of actual AMA documents and minutes of official meetings with overt intentionality of destroying Americans' healthcare options so that the AMA and related organizations would have a monopoly in healthcare.

[435] Wolinsky H, Brune T. The Serpent on the Staff: The Unhealthy Politics of the American Medical Association. GP Putnam and Sons, New York, 1994

[436] Mein EA, Greenman PE, McMillin DL, Richards DG, Nelson CD. Manual medicine diversity: research pitfalls and the emerging medical paradigm. J Am Osteopath Assoc. 2001 Aug;101(8):441-4

[437] Wilk CA. Medicine, Monopolies, and Malice: How the Medical Establishment Tried to Destroy Chiropractic. Garden City Park: Avery, 1996

[438] Wenban AB. Inappropriate use of the title 'chiropractor' and term 'chiropractic manipulation' in the peer-reviewed biomedical literature. Chiropr Osteopat. 2006;14:16 http://chiroandosteo.com/content/14/1/16

[439] Manga P, Angus D, Papadopoulos C, et al. The Effectiveness and Cost-Effectiveness of Chiropractic Management of Low-Back Pain. Richmond Hill, Ontario: Kenilworth Publishing; 1993

[440] Meade TW, Dyer S, Browne W, Townsend J, Frank AO. Low-back pain of mechanical origin: randomised comparison of chiropractic and hospital outpatient treatment. BMJ. 1990;300(6737):1431-7

[441] Meade TW, Dyer S, Browne W, Frank AO. Randomised comparison of chiropractic and hospital outpatient management for low-back pain: results from extended follow up. BMJ. 1995;311(7001):349-5

[442] Legorreta AP, Metz RD, Nelson CF, Ray S, Chernicoff HO, Dinubile NA. Comparative analysis of individuals with and without chiropractic coverage: patient characteristics, utilization, and costs. Arch Intern Med. 2004;164:1985-92

[443] US Census Bureau http://factfinder.census.gov/home/saff/main.html?_lang=en Accessed January 12, 2005

[444] Rosner AL. Evidence-based clinical guidelines for the management of acute low-back pain: response to the guidelines prepared for the Australian Medical Health and Research Council. J Manipulative Physiol Ther. 2001;24(3):214-20

[445] Topol EJ. Failing the public health--rofecoxib, Merck, and the FDA. N Engl J Med. 2004 Oct 21;351(17):1707-9

[446] Dabbs V, Lauretti WJ. A risk assessment of cervical manipulation vs. NSAIDs for the treatment of neck pain. J Manipulative Physiol Ther. 1995;18:530-6

[447] Rosner AL. Evidence-based clinical guidelines for the management of acute low-back pain: response to the guidelines prepared for the Australian Medical Health and Research Council. J Manipulative Physiol Ther. 2001;24(3):214-20

literature comparing the safety of chiropractic manipulation in patients with low-back pain associated with lumbar disc herniation, Oliphant[448] showed that, "The apparent safety of spinal manipulation, especially when compared with other [medically] accepted treatments for [lumbar disk herniation], should stimulate its use in the conservative treatment plan of [lumbar disk herniation]."

The clinical benefits and cost-effectiveness of chiropractic management of musculoskeletal conditions is extensively documented, and that spinal manipulation generally shows superior safety to drug and surgical treatment of back and neck pain is also well established.[449,450,451,452,453,454,455]

Osteopathic medicine, discussed in a following section, shares a few features in common with chiropractic. Osteopathic medicine and chiropractic are American-born healthcare professions and paradigms that started at nearly the same time in history and from many of the same foundational principles. Both professions were started in the late 1800's and early 1900's and were founded upon the philosophical premise that the body functioned as a whole and that therefore medicine in general and therapeutic interventions in particular needed to be comprehensive in scope and multifaceted in their application. Further, both professions emphasized the importance of structural integrity as a foundational component of health and thus embraced manual manipulative therapy and spinal manipulation. From their common origins, subtle differences and chance historic events shaped and further separated these professions from each other.

Wilk vs American Medical Association: The successful antitrust case against an attempt at medical monopolization

The following two pages provide the transcript of the judgment in 1987 that was intended to end the American Medical Association's antitrust violations and attempt to destroy the chiropractic profession.

A PDF copy of this document is available online:
http://ICHNFM.org/library/WilkAMAjudgement.pdf

---

[448] Oliphant D. Safety of spinal manipulation in the treatment of lumbar disk herniations: a systematic review and risk assessment. *J Manipulative Physiol Ther*. 2004;27:197-210

[449] Dabbs V, Lauretti WJ. A risk assessment of cervical manipulation vs. NSAIDs for the treatment of neck pain. *J Manipulative Physiol Ther*. 1995;18:530-6

[450] Rosner AL. Evidence-based clinical guidelines for the management of acute low-back pain: response to the guidelines prepared for the Australian Medical Health and Research Council. *J Manipulative Physiol Ther*. 2001 Mar-Apr;24(3):214-20

[451] Oliphant D. Safety of spinal manipulation in the treatment of lumbar disk herniations: a systematic review and risk assessment. *J Manipulative Physiol Ther*. 2004;27:197-210

[452] Meade TW, Dyer S, Browne W, Townsend J, Frank AO. Low-back pain of mechanical origin: randomised comparison of chiropractic and hospital outpatient treatment. *BMJ*. 1990;300(6737):1431-7

[453] Meade TW, Dyer S, Browne W, Frank AO. Randomised comparison of chiropractic and hospital outpatient management for low-back pain: results from extended follow up. *BMJ*. 1995;311(7001):349-5

[454] Manga P, Angus D, Papadopoulos C, et al. *The Effectiveness and Cost-Effectiveness of Chiropractic Management of Low-Back Pain*. Richmond Hill, Ontario: Kenilworth Publishing; 1993

[455] Legorreta AP, Metz RD, Nelson CF, Ray S, Chernicoff HO, Dinubile NA. Comparative analysis of individuals with and without chiropractic coverage: patient characteristics, utilization, and costs. *Arch Intern Med*. 2004;164:1985-92

Special Communication

IN THE UNITED STATES DISTRICT COURT
FOR THE NORTHERN DISTRICT OF ILLINOIS
EASTERN DIVISION

CHESTER A. WILK, et al.,   )
)
                         Plaintiffs,   )
)
        v.   )   No. 76 C
)   3777
AMERICAN MEDICAL ASSOCIATION,   )
et al.,   )
)
                         Defendants.   )

PERMANENT INJUNCTION ORDER AGAINST AMA

Susan Getzendanner, District Judge

The court conducted a lengthy trial of this case in May and June of 1987 and on August 27, 1987, issued a 101 page opinion finding that the American Medical Association ("AMA") and its members participated in a conspiracy against chiropractors in violation of the nation's antitrust laws. Thereafter an opinion dated September 25, 1987 was substituted for the August 27, 1987 opinion. The question now before the court is the form of injunctive relief that the court will order.

See also p 83.

As part of the injunctive relief to be ordered by the court against the AMA, the AMA shall be required to send a copy of this Permanent Injunction Order to each of its current members. The members of the AMA are bound by the terms of the Permanent Injunction Order if they act in concert with the AMA to violate the terms of the order. Accordingly, it is important that the AMA members understand the order and the reasons why the order has been entered.

The AMA's Boycott and Conspiracy

In the early 1960s, the AMA decided to contain and eliminate chiropractic as a profession. In 1963 the AMA's Committee on Quackery was formed. The committee worked aggressively—both overtly and covertly—to eliminate chiropractic. One of the principal means used by the AMA to achieve its goal was to make it unethical for medical physicians to professionally associate with chiropractors. Under Principle 3 of the AMA's Principles of Medical Ethics, it was unethical for a physician to associate with an "unscientific practitioner," and in 1966 the AMA's House of Delegates passed a resolution calling chiropractic an unscientific cult. To complete the circle, in 1967 the AMA's Judicial Council issued an opinion under Principle 3 holding that it was unethical for a physician to associate professionally with chiropractors.

The AMA's purpose was to prevent medical physicians from referring patients to chiropractors and accepting referrals of patients from chiropractors, to prevent chiropractors from obtaining access to hospital diagnostic services and membership on hospital medical staffs, to prevent medical physicians from teaching at chiropractic colleges or engaging in any joint research, and to prevent any cooperation between the two groups in the delivery of health care services.

Published by order of Susan Getzendanner, US District Judge, Sept 25, 1987.

The AMA believed that the boycott worked—that chiropractic would have achieved greater gains in the absence of the boycott. Since no medical physician would want to be considered unethical by his peers, the success of the boycott is not surprising. However, chiropractic achieved licensing in all 50 states during the existence of the Committee on Quackery.

The Committee on Quackery was disbanded in 1975 and some of the committee's activities became publicly known. Several lawsuits were filed by or on behalf of chiropractors and this case was filed in 1976.

Change in AMA's Position on Chiropractic

In 1977, the AMA began to change its position on chiropractic. The AMA's Judicial Council adopted new opinions under which medical physicians could refer patients to chiropractors, but there was still the proviso that the medical physician should be confident that the services to be provided on referral would be performed in accordance with accepted scientific standards. In 1979, the AMA's House of Delegates adopted Report UU which said that not everything that a chiropractor may do is without therapeutic value, but it stopped short of saying that such things were based on scientific standards. It was not until 1980 that the AMA revised its Principles of Medical Ethics to eliminate Principle 3. Until Principle 3 was formally eliminated, there was considerable ambiguity about the AMA's position. The ethics code adopted in 1980 provided that a medical physician "shall be free to choose whom to serve, with whom to associate, and the environment in which to provide medical services."

The AMA settled three chiropractic lawsuits by stipulating and agreeing that under the current opinions of the Judicial Council a physician may, without fear of discipline or sanction by the AMA, refer a patient to a duly licensed chiropractor when he believes that referral may benefit the patient. The AMA confirmed that a physician may also choose to accept or to decline patients sent to him by a duly licensed chiropractor. Finally, the AMA confirmed that a physician may teach at a chiropractic college or seminar. These settlements were entered into in 1978, 1980, and 1986.

The AMA's present position on chiropractic, as stated to the court, is that it is ethical for a medical physician to professionally associate with chiropractors provided the physician believes that such association is in the best interests of his patient. This position has not previously been communicated by the AMA to its members.

Antitrust Laws

Under the Sherman Act, every combination or conspiracy in restraint of trade is illegal. The court has held that the conduct of the AMA and its members constituted a conspiracy in restraint of trade based on the following facts: the purpose of the boycott was to eliminate chiropractic; chiropractors are in competition with some medical physicians; the boycott had substantial anti-competitive effects; there were no pro-competitive effects of the boycott; and the plaintiffs were injured as a result of the conduct. These facts add up to a violation of the Sherman Act.

In this case, however, the court allowed the defendants the opportunity to establish a "patient care defense" which has the following elements:

(1) that they genuinely entertained a concern for what they perceive as scientific method in the care of each person with whom they have entered into a doctor-patient relationship; (2) that this concern is objectively reasonable; (3) that this concern has been the dominant motivating factor in defendants' promulgation of Principle 3 and in the

conduct intended to implement it; and (4) that this concern for scientific method in patient care could not have been adequately satisfied in a manner less restrictive of competition.

The court concluded that the AMA had a genuine concern for scientific methods in patient care, and that this concern was the dominant factor in motivating the AMA's conduct. However, the AMA failed to establish that throughout the entire period of the boycott, from 1966 to 1980, this concern was objectively reasonable. The court reached that conclusion on the basis of extensive testimony from both witnesses for the plaintiffs and the AMA that some forms of chiropractic treatment are effective and the fact that the AMA recognized that chiropractic began to change in the early 1970s. Since the boycott was not formally over until Principle 3 was eliminated in 1980, the court found that the AMA was unable to establish that during the entire period of the conspiracy its position was objectively reasonable. Finally, the court ruled that the AMA's concern for scientific method in patient care could have been adequately satisfied in a manner less restrictive of competition and that a nationwide conspiracy to eliminate a licensed profession was not justified by the concern for scientific method. On the basis of these findings, the court concluded that the AMA had failed to establish the patient care defense.

None of the court's findings constituted a judicial endorsement of chiropractic. All of the parties to the case, including the plaintiffs and the AMA, agreed that chiropractic treatment of diseases such as diabetes, high blood pressure, cancer, heart disease and infectious disease is not proper, and that the historic theory of chiropractic, that there is a single cause and cure of disease is wrong. There was disagreement between the parties as to whether chiropractors should engage in diagnosis. There was evidence that the chiropractic theory of subluxations was unscientific, and evidence that some chiropractors engaged in unscientific practices. The court did not reach the question of whether chiropractic theory was in fact scientific. However, the evidence in the case was that some forms of chiropractic manipulation of the spine and joints was therapeutic. AMA witnesses, including the present Chairman of the Board of Trustees of the AMA, testified that some forms of treatment by chiropractors, including manipulation, can be therapeutic in the treatment of conditions such as back pain syndrome.

Need for Injunctive Relief

Although the conspiracy ended in 1980, there are lingering effects of the illegal boycott and conspiracy which require an injunction. Some medical physicians' individual decisions on whether or not to professionally associate with chiropractors are still affected by the boycott. The injury to chiropractors' reputations which resulted from the boycott has not been repaired. Chiropractors suffer current economic injury as a result of the boycott. The AMA has never affirmatively acknowledged that there are and should be no collective impediments to professional association and cooperation between chiropractors and medical physicians, except as provided by law. Instead, the AMA has consistently argued that its conduct has not violated the antitrust laws.

Most importantly, the court believes that it is important that the AMA members be made aware of the present AMA position that it is ethical for a medical physician to professionally associate with a chiropractor if the physician believes it is in the best interests of his patient, so that the lingering effects of the illegal group boycott against chiropractors finally can be dissipated.

Under the law, every medical physician, institution, and hospital has the right to make an individual decision as to whether or not that physician, institution, or hospital shall associate professionally with chiropractors. Individual choice by a medical physician voluntarily to associate professionally with chiropractors should be governed only by restrictions under state law, if any, and by the individual medical physician's personal judgment as to what is in the best interest of a patient or patients. Professional association includes referrals, consultations, group practice in partnerships, Health Maintenance Organizations, Preferred Provider Organizations, and other alternative health care delivery systems; the provision of treatment privileges and diagnostic services (including radiological and other laboratory facilities) in or through hospital facilities; association and cooperation in educational programs for students in chiropractic colleges; and cooperation in research, health care seminars, and continuing education programs.

An injunction is necessary to assure that the AMA does not interfere with the right of a physician, hospital, or other institution to make an individual decision on the question of professional association.

Form of Injunction

1. The AMA, its officers, agents and employees, and all persons who act in active concert with any of them and who receive actual notice of this order are hereby permanently enjoined from restricting, regulating or impeding, or aiding and abetting others from restricting, regulating or impeding, the freedom of any AMA member or any institution or hospital to make an individual decision as to whether or not that AMA member, institution, or hospital shall professionally associate with chiropractors, chiropractic students, or chiropractic institutions.

2. This Permanent Injunction does not and shall not be construed to restrict or otherwise interfere with the AMA's right to take positions on any issue, including chiropractic, and to express or publicize those positions, either alone or in conjunction with others. Nor does this Permanent Injunction restrict or otherwise interfere with the AMA's right to petition or testify before any public body on any legislative or regulatory measure or to join or cooperate with any other entity in so petitioning or testifying. The AMA's membership in a recognized accrediting association or society shall not constitute a violation of this Permanent Injunction.

3. The AMA is directed to send a copy of this order to each AMA member and employee, first class mail, postage prepaid, within thirty days of the entry of this order. In the alternative, the AMA shall provide the Clerk of the Court with mailing labels so that the court may send this order to AMA members and employees.

4. The AMA shall cause the publication of this order in JAMA and the indexing of the order under "Chiropractic" so that persons desiring to find the order in the future will be able to do so.

5. The AMA shall prepare a statement of the AMA's present position on chiropractic for inclusion in the current reports and opinions of the Judicial Council with an appropriate heading that refers to professional association between medical physicians and chiropractors, and indexed in the same manner that other reports and opinions are indexed. The court imposes no restrictions on the AMA's statement but only requires that it be consistent with the AMA's statements of its present position to the court.

6. The AMA shall file a report with the court evidencing compliance with this order on or before January 10, 1988.

It is so ordered.

Susan Getzendanner
United States District Judge

Naturopathic Medicine

"The work of the naturopathic physician is to elicit healing by helping patients to create or recreate conditions for health to exist within them. Health will occur where the conditions for health exist. Disease is the product of conditions which allow for it."

Jared Zeff, ND[456]

The diagram on this page is derived from the review by Zeff published in 1997 in *Journal of Naturopathic Medicine* entitled "The process of healing: a unifying theory of naturopathic medicine." By my interpretation, the diagram is important for at least three reasons.

First, whereas the allopathic profession describes the genesis of most diseases as *idiopathic* and therefore [somehow] exclusively serviceable by drugs and surgery, the naturopathic profession describes disease processes as *multifactorial* and *logical* and therefore treatable by the skilled discovery and treatment of the underlying causes. Such underlying causes, which nearly always occur as a plurality, may vary mildly or significantly even within a group of patients with the same diagnosis.

Second, the diagram shows that the development of disease and the restoration of health are both *processes*. The restoration and retention of health requires *intentionality* and *tenacity* in lieu of the simplistic *miracle medicines* and *passive treatments* proffered by the pharmaceutical industry. Generally, disease does not arrive from outside; it is the result of one or more internal imbalances. Chronic illness is generally the result of manifold internal imbalances that culminate in numerous physiologic insults which compromise essential functions to the point that one or more organ systems begin to fail; we as patients and doctors generally label this as some specific "disease" or other, and the general—often erroneous—assumption has been that each *specific disease* (i.e., label, ...abstraction, ...conceptual entity) requires a *specific treatment* rather than a generalized health-restorative approach. Health is restored through a progressive and stepwise program that addresses as many facets of the illness as possible while vigorously supporting optimal physiologic function.

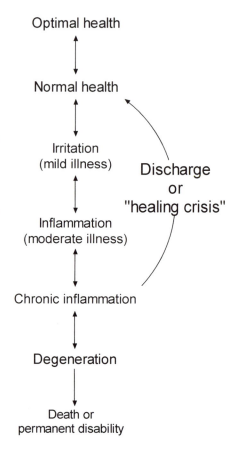

Third, the fact that Zeff considered the discharge or "healing crisis" so important that it merited inclusion in this diagram shows, indirectly, the naturopathic emphasis on detoxification and the eradication of dysbiosis. Both in the treatment of toxic metal/chemical exposure and in the treatment of chronic infections, patients often go through an acute or subacute phase of feeling ill before experiencing a dramatic alleviation of symptoms; the fact that symptoms may temporarily "get worse before getting better" has been referred to as the "healing crisis." This can occur for at least three reasons. First, in the elimination of chemicals and metals from the body, they must first be released from the tissues; the transition from tissues to blood is similar to a subacute re-exposure which triggers symptoms of toxicity until the toxin is excreted via sweat, urine, bile, or breath. Similarly, improvement in nutritional status—a cornerstone of all naturopathic interventions—expedites/facilitates/restores physiologic processes that have been relatively dormant due to lack of enzymatic cofactors such as vitamins and minerals[457]; optimization of nutritional status provides an opportunity for these pathways (such as detoxification of stored xenobiotics) to function again at which time they must "catch up" on work that has not been performed during the time of nutritional deficiency. The activation of these pathways is an essential step toward health restoration but results in an initial upregulation of hepatic phase-1/oxidative biotransformation which often results in the formation of reactive intermediates that temporarily impair physiologic processes and cause an initial exacerbation

[456] Zeff JL. The process of healing: a unifying theory of naturopathic medicine. *Journal of Naturopathic Medicine* 1997; 7: 122-5
[457] Ames BN. The metabolic tune-up: metabolic harmony and disease prevention. *J Nutr.* 2003 May;133(5 Suppl 1):1544S-8S

of symptoms. Third, whether through immunorestoration or the use of botanical/pharmacologic antimicrobial agents, the symptom-exacerbating "die off" reaction—classically called the Jarisch-Herxheimer reaction in the context of treating syphilis—is a result of increased (endo)toxin production/release by bacteria/microbes in response effective antimicrobial processes, whether physiologic or pharmacologic.

Modern naturopathic medicine has grown from deeply rooted European healing traditions reaching back several centuries. Naturopathic physicians have unwaveringly demonstrated respect, love, and appreciation for the healing powers of nature and the process of life itself.[458] Following their coursework in the basic biomedical sciences, naturopathic physicians are trained in urology, oncology, neurology, pediatrics, obstetrics and gynecology, urology, manual physical manipulation (including spinal manipulation), minor surgery, medical procedures, professional ethics, therapeutic diets, clinical and interventional nutrition, botanical medicines, psychological counseling, environmental medicine, and other modalities. Licensed naturopathic physicians commonly practice as generalists and family doctors.[459,460,461,462]

Naturopathic Principles, Concepts, & the *Vis Medicatrix Naturae*

"The healing power of nature is the inherent self-organizing and healing process of living systems… It is the naturopathic physician's role to support, facilitate and augment this process by identifying and removing obstacles to health and recovery, and by supporting the creation of a healthy internal and external environment."[463]

1. **First, Do No Harm *(Primum Non Nocere)*:** Naturopathic physicians use good judgment and compassion to ensure that the treatment does not cause harm to the patient. This contrasts with the effects of allopathic treatment, which collectively kill more than 180,000-220,000 patients per year, at least 493 American patients per day.[464]

2. **Identify and Treat the Causes *(Tolle Causam)*:** *"Illness does not occur without cause."* Naturopathic physicians focus on identifying and addressing the underlying deficiency, toxicity, impairment, or imbalance that is the cause of the health problem or disease.

3. **Treat the Whole Person**: *"The multifactorial nature of health and disease requires a personalized and comprehensive approach to diagnosis and treatment."* On some occasions the illness does take precedence over the person who has it—such in emergency situations like septic arthritis, acute ischemia, and pulmonary edema. In these cases, the situation must be managed appropriately, and these situations are not immediately amenable to long-term lifestyle changes—they require immediate treatment. However, the vast majority of cases in routine outpatient clinical practice will require detailed and bipartite attention to the facets of both **the disease process** and **the person who has the illness**. Our focus as naturopathic physicians on the individual patient is what sets our healing profession apart from others that focus exclusively on the disease and do not consider the manifold intricacies of the individual patient.

4. **The Healing Power of Nature: *Vis Medicatrix Naturae***: Naturopathic medicine recognizes an inherent self-healing process in the person that is ordered and intelligent. The body has many highly efficient mechanisms for sustaining and regaining health. These mechanisms have their specific and necessary components (e.g., nutrients) and means by which they can be impaired (e.g., xenobiotic immunosuppression). Poor health and disease can result from impairment of these self-healing processes

[458] Kirchfeld F, Boyle W. Nature Doctors: Pioneers in Naturopathic Medicine. Portland, Oregon; Medicina Biologica (Buckeye Naturopathic Press, East Palestine, Ohio), 1994

[459] Boon HS, Cherkin DC, Erro J, Sherman KJ, Milliman B, Booker J, Cramer EH, Smith MJ, Deyo RA, Eisenberg DM. Practice patterns of naturopathic physicians: results from a random survey of licensed practitioners in two US States. *BMC Complement Altern Med.* 2004;4(1):14

[460] Smith MJ, Logan AC. Naturopathy. *Med Clin North Am.* 2002 Jan;86(1):173-84

[461] Cherkin DC, Deyo RA, Sherman KJ, et al. Characteristics of visits to licensed acupuncturists, chiropractors, massage therapists, and naturopathic physicians. *J Am Board Fam Pract.* 2002 Nov-Dec;15(6):463-72

[462] Cherkin DC, Deyo RA, Sherman KJ, et al. Characteristics of licensed acupuncturists, chiropractors, massage therapists, and naturopathic physicians *J Am Board Fam Pract.* 2002 Sep-Oct;15(5):378-90

[463] Quoted from the American Association of Naturopathic Physicians website http://aanp.net/Basics/h.naturo.philo.html on February 4, 2001. Other italicized quotes in this section are from the same source. This website has since been replaced by http://naturopathic.org/

[464] "Recent estimates suggest that each year more than 1 million patients are injured while in the hospital and approximately 180,000 die because of these injuries. Furthermore, drug-related morbidity and mortality are common and are estimated to cost more than $136 billion a year." Holland EG, Degruy FV. Drug-induced disorders. *Am Fam Physician.* 1997;56(7):1781-8, 1791-2

and biologic mechanisms, and thus the body's inherent, natural, self-healing mechanisms—the "healing power of nature"—can be diminished to the state of ineffectiveness or harm (e.g., autoimmunity). Recognizing that the body has this inherent goal of and movement toward self-healing, naturopathic physicians start by identifying and removing "obstacles to cure" rather than ignoring these factors and masking the manifestations of dysfunction with symptom-suppressing drugs.

5. **Prevention**: Healthy lifestyle, proper nutrition, and emotional hygiene go a long way toward preventing (and treating) most conditions. Specific conditions have specific risk factors and causes that have to be considered per patient and condition.

6. **Doctor as Teacher** (*Docere*): Naturopathic physicians explain the situation and the proposed solution to the patient so that the patient is empowered with understanding and with the comfort of knowing what has happened, what is happening, and the proposed course of upcoming events. Naturopathic physicians strive to let their own lives serve as a models for our patients. This does not mean that naturopathic doctors have to feign perfection; the task is to live the best and most conscious life that we can, to be present with our emotions, qualities, and faults and to treat ourselves

> **"Physician, heal thyself.**
>
> Thus you help your patient, too.
> Let this be his best medicine that he beholds with his eyes: the doctor who heals himself."
>
> Nietzsche FW. Thus Spoke Zarathustra (1892). [Kaufmann W, translator]. Viking Penguin: 1954, page 77

with respect and acceptance. We can exemplify health (rather than perfection) to our patients by being who we authentically are and by so doing we can facilitate their own acceptance of their current health situation, which is a prerequisite to self-initiated change.

7. **Re-Establish the Foundation for Health**: An overview of this important naturopathic concept is provided throughout this chapter.

8. **Removing "obstacles to cure"**: *examples*

Obstacle to the optimization of health	*Example of possible intervention*
o Toxic exposures, medication side-effects	▪ Reduce drug use and dependency
o Toxic relationships, emotional obstacles, past events, unfulfilling occupation,	▪ Improve self-esteem, develop conflict resolution skills, determine life goals and values and a plan for their pursuit
o Social isolation: the typical American has only two friends no-one in whom to confide[465]	▪ Encourage social interaction
o Diet with excess fat, arachidonate, sugar, additives, colorants, and insufficiency of protein, fiber, phytonutrients, and health-promoting fatty acids: ALA, GLA, EPA, DHA, and oleic acid	▪ Diet improvement and nutritional supplementation
o Sedentary lifestyle, lack of exercise	▪ Encourage exercise
o Weight gain/loss as necessary for weight optimization	▪ Encourage self-valuing
o Epidemic exposure to mercury, lead, and xenobiotics	▪ Support detoxification process as a lifestyle

Hierarchy of Therapeutics: This naturopathic concept articulates the importance of addressing *the underlying cause* rather than simply focusing on *the presenting problem*, which is the *symptom of the cause*. Further, interventions are **prioritized**, *for example*:

- Patient-implemented *before* doctor-implemented.

---

[465] McPherson M, Smith-Lovin L, Brashears ME. Social Isolation in America: Changes in Core Discussion Networks over Two Decades. *American Sociological Review* 2006; 71: 353-75 http://www.asanet.org/galleries/default-file/June06ASRFeature.pdf

- Removal of harming agent *before* addition of a therapeutic agent: e.g., stop smoking *before* investing in respiratory therapy; implement healthy diet and exercise before higher-risk and higher-cost drugs for hypertension and hypercholesterolemia.
- Low-force interventions *before* high-force interventions.
- Diet *before* nutritional supplements; nutrients *before* botanicals; botanicals *before* drugs; modulatory drugs *before* suppressive/inhibitory drugs; integrative care *before* surgery.
- *See examples below*.

Hierarchy of Therapeutics (specifically sequential)	Example of possible intervention
1. Reestablishing the foundation for health	<ul><li>Mental/emotional/spiritual health</li><li>Meditation, freeze-frame, "time out"</li><li>Relaxation</li><li>Positive visualization, positive expectation, affirmation</li><li>Counseling, social contact, group work[466]</li><li>Family contact and resolution</li><li>Dietary intake and nutritional health which addresses the patient's biochemical individuality[467] and correction of deficiencies or excesses</li><li>Identification and elimination of food allergies and food sensitivities</li><li>Reduce toxin exposure, promote detoxification</li><li>Identification and elimination of exposure to gastrointestinal and inhalant xenobiotics</li><li>Remove or reduce specific "obstacles to cure"</li></ul>
2. Stimulation of the "healing power of nature" and the "vital force"	<ul><li>Constitutional hydrotherapy</li><li>Homeopathy</li><li>Exercise</li><li>Acupuncture, Spinal manipulation</li><li>Meditation, rest</li><li>Tai Chi, Qigong: "energy-cultivation"</li><li>Botanical adaptogens</li></ul>
3. Tonification of weakened systems:	<ul><li>Botanical medicines and other supplements to help restore normal tissue function</li><li>Spinal manipulation to address the primary somatovisceral dysfunction and/or secondary musculoskeletal disorders</li><li>Hormonal supplementation</li><li>Nutritional supplementation</li><li>Exercise</li><li>Physiotherapy</li></ul>
4. Correction of structural integrity:	<ul><li>Spinal manipulation, deep tissue massage, visceral manipulation, lymphatic pump to promote immune surveillance[468]</li><li>Stretching, balancing, muscle strengthening, and proprioceptive retraining</li><li>Surgery, as a last resort</li></ul>

---

[466] See http://www.mkp.org and www.WomanWithin.org for examples.
[467] Williams RJ. Biochemical Individuality: The Basis for the Genetotrophic Concept. Austin and London: University of Texas Press, 1956
[468] "Lymph flow in the thoracic duct increased from 1.57±0.20 mL·min-1 to a peak TDF of 4.80±1.73 mL·min-1 during abdominal pump, and from 1.20±0.41 mL·min-1 to 3.45±1.61 mL·min-1 during thoracic pump." Knott EM, Tune JD, Stoll ST, Downey HF. Increased lymphatic flow in the thoracic duct during manipulative intervention. *J Am Osteopath Assoc.* 2005 Oct;105(10):447-56 http://www.jaoa.org/cgi/content/full/105/10/447

Osteopathic Medicine

Osteopathy was founded by Andrew Taylor Still, a medical doctor who sought to reform what was then called the "Heroic" paradigm of medicine, which embraced bloodletting and the administration of leeches, purgatives, emetics, and poisons such as mercury as means for "rebalancing" what were perceived to be internal causes of disease, namely the "four humours" of the body which were thought to be blood, phlegm, black bile, and yellow bile. In part because of his training within and identification with the medical profession, Still sought to *reform* rather than *directly oppose* the "mainstream medicine" of his day; in contrast, chiropractic's founder Daniel David Palmer was more strongly opposed to the horrific medicine of his time and thus was more *revolutionary* than *evolutionary* in his approach to forging a new paradigm of health and healthcare. Still's willingness to align with the medical profession and the increasingly powerful and influential pharmaceutical industry unquestionably helped his fledgling profession survive the extinction that otherwise would have been swift at the hands of allopathic groups such as the American Medical Association (AMA), which labeled osteopathic physicians as "cultists" and systematically restricted inclusion of the osteopathic profession into mainstream healthcare by proclamation in 1953 that "…all voluntary associations with osteopaths are unethical." When osteopathic resistance mounted, the AMA and its co-conspirators, who were later found guilty of violating the nation's antitrust laws by illegally suppressing competition and attempting to build a medical monopoly[469], acquiesced and accepted osteopaths into its ranks—a strategy which the medical profession believed would eventually destroy the osteopathic profession by forcing it to resign its ideals and identity. In his review of osteopathic history, Gevitz[470] writes, "…the M.D.'s gradually came to believe that the only way to destroy osteopathy was through the absorption of D.O.'s, much as the homeopaths and eclectics [naturopaths] had been swallowed up early in the century." Even recently, the AMA has listed osteopathic medicine under "alternative medicine"[471] although several osteopathic medical colleges have consistently provided training that is superior to most "conventional" allopathic medical schools.[472] Today, osteopathic physicians practice in most ways similarly to allopaths—i.e., with unlimited scope of practice in all 50 states, full access to the use of drugs and surgery, and with a very pharmacosurgical paradigm of disease and healthcare. Osteopathic medicine is one of the fastest growing healthcare professions in America.

Osteopathic Manipulative Medicine:

Osteopathic manipulative medicine (OMM) is similar to and yet distinct from chiropractic manipulation; the naturopathic profession—true to its eclectic roots—incorporates techniques from all professions. In contrast to chiropractic, OMM terminology and therapeutics focus much more on soft tissues, and the osteopathic lesion—"somatic dysfunction"—is clearly originated from soft tissues in contrast to the chiropractic lesion—the "vertebral subluxation"—which obviously originates from spinal articulations. Whereas the chiropractic intent of correcting or "adjusting" the "subluxation" was historically to improve function of the nervous system, the osteopathic lesion is addressed to more fully improve not only function of the nervous system but also of the vascular, lymphatic, and myofascial systems, too.[473] With regard to the latter, the osteopathic profession has always emphasized the importance of fascia in the genesis of "somatic dysfunction." Indeed, fascia appears to play an important and dynamic (not passive) role in neuromusculoskeletal health, particularly as it is a major contributor to proprioception and may also have a more direct effect through the recently described ability of fascia to actively contract in a smooth-muscle-like manner.[474]

From this author's perspective, two of the most widely used osteopathic texts—*Osteopathic Principles in Practice* (1994) by Kuchera and Kuchera[475], and *Outline of Osteopathic Manipulative Procedures* (2006) by Kimberly[476]—both leave very much to be desired with respect to their clarity, terminology, clinical applicability, and referencing to the scientific literature. *Manipulation of the Spine, Thorax and Pelvis: An Osteopathic Perspective* (2006) by Gibbons

[469] Getzendanner S. Permanent injunction order against AMA. *JAMA*. 1988 Jan 1;259(1):81-2

[470] Gevitz N. The D.O.'s: Osteopathic Medicine in America. Johns Hopkins University Press; 1991; pages 100-103

[471] American Medical Association. Report 12 of the Council on Scientific Affairs (A-97) Full Text http://www.ama-assn.org/ama/pub/category/13638.html November 23, 2006

[472] Special report. America's best graduate schools. Schools of Medicine. The top schools: primary care. *US News World Rep*. 2004 Apr 12;136(12):74

[473] Williams N. Managing back pain in general practice--is osteopathy the new paradigm? *Br J Gen Pract*. 1997 Oct;47(423):653-5

[474] "…the existence of an active fascial contractility could have interesting implications for the understanding of musculoskeletal pathologies with an increased or decreased myofascial tonus. It may also offer new insights and a deeper understanding of treatments directed at fascia, such as manual myofascial release therapies or acupuncture." Schleip R, Klingler W, Lehmann-Horn F. Active fascial contractility: Fascia may be able to contract in a smooth muscle-like manner and thereby influence musculoskeletal dynamics. *Med Hypotheses*. 2005;65(2):273-7

[475] Kuchera WA, Kuchera ML. *Osteopathic Principles In Practice, revised second edition*. Kirksville, MO, KCOM Press; 1994

[476] Kimberly PE. *Outline of Osteopathic Manipulative Procedures.The Kimberly Manual 2006*. Kirksville College Osteopathic Medicine. Walsworth Publish. Co., Marceline, Mo

and Tehan[477] is much more accessible and clinically applicable; however the text focuses exclusively on high-velocity low-amplitude (HVLA) techniques and therefore does not provide sufficient background and training for students in the very techniques that distinguish osteopathic from chiropractic techniques, namely heightened attention to the myofascial dysfunction that (appropriately) underlies the osteopathic lesion.

Ironically, the very growth and "allopathicization" of the profession that has threatened the profession's adherence to its holistic tenets has caused a reflexive re-affirmation of these tenets, and the profession has responded with a well-funded and intentional directive to scientifically investigate the mechanisms and efficacy of osteopathic manipulative medicine.[478,479] Recent findings include improved function and reduced pain in patients treated with a comprehensive manipulative technique for the shoulder[480], as well as the significant efficacy of ankle manipulation for patients with recent ankle injuries.[481]

Further, OMM treatment of patients medicated for depression was found to triple the effectiveness of drug monotherapy.[482] Other studies have shown benefit of OMM in the treatment of geriatric pneumonia[483], pediatric asthma[484], pediatric dysfunctional voiding[485], carpal tunnel syndrome[486], low-back pain[487], and recovery from cardiac bypass surgery.[488] Replication and validation of these studies—many of which are small or of nonrigorous design (e.g., open clinical trials with no control group)—is important to further define and establish the value of osteopathic manipulation in clinical care.

> ## Osteopathic Interventions need to be Consistent with Osteopathic Philosophy
>
> "In contrast to the description of the osteopathic medical profession by the American Osteopathic Association, namely, "doctors of osteopathic medicine, or D.O.s, apply the philosophy of treating the whole person to the prevention, diagnosis and treatment of illness, disease and injury," [the authors of the article in question] essentially reviewed only pharmacologic treatment. ...It is hoped that future reviews in this journal can include a more balanced survey of the literature, inclusive of non-pharmacologic and "holistic" interventions that are consistent with osteopathic philosophy."
>
> **Vasquez A**. Interventions need to be Consistent with Osteopathic Philosophy. [Letter] *JAOA: Journal of the American Osteopathic Association* 2006 Sep http://www.jaoa.org/cgi/content/full/106/9/528

---

[477] Gibbons P, Tehan P. Manipulation of the Spine, Thorax and Pelvis: An Osteopathic Perspective. Churchill Livingstone; 2006. Isbn: 044310039X

[478] Wisnioski SW 3rd. "Circle Turns Round" to "Allopathic Osteopathy." *J Am Osteopath Assoc* 2006; 106: 423-4 http://www.jaoa.org/cgi/content/full/106/7/423

[479] Teitelbaum HS, et al. Osteopathic medical education: renaissance or rhetoric? *J Am Osteopath Assoc.* 2003 Oct;103(10):489-90 http://www.jaoa.org/cgi/reprint/103/10/489

[480] Knebl JA, Shores JH, Gamber RG, Gray WT, Herron KM. Improving functional ability in the elderly via the Spencer technique, an osteopathic manipulative treatment: a randomized, controlled trial. *J Am Osteopath Assoc.* 2002 Jul;102(7):387-96 http://www.jaoa.org/cgi/reprint/102/7/387

[481] This study shows the rapid onset and benefit of manipulative medicine for the treatment of acute ankle sprains: Eisenhart AW, Gaeta TJ, Yens DP. Osteopathic manipulative treatment in the emergency department for patients with acute ankle injuries. *J Am Osteopath Assoc.* 2003 Sep;103(9):417-21 http://www.jaoa.org/cgi/reprint/103/9/417

[482] This study impressively showed that musculoskeletal manipulation improved treatment effectiveness for depression from 33% to 100%. "After 8 weeks, 100% of the OMT treatment group and 33% of the control group tested normal by psychometric evaluation. ... The findings of this pilot study indicate that OMT may be a useful adjunctive treatment for alleviating depression in women." Plotkin BJ, Rodos JJ, Kappler R, Schrage M, Freydl K, Hasegawa S, Hennegan E, Hilchie-Schmidt C, Hines D, Iwata J, Mok C, Raffaelli D. Adjunctive osteopathic manipulative treatment in women with depression: a pilot study. *J Am Osteopath Assoc.* 2001 Sep;101(9):517-23 http://www.jaoa.org/cgi/reprint/101/9/517

[483] This study showed improved clinical outcomes and reduced antibiotic use in elderly patients with pneumonia when treated with manipulative medicine: "The treatment group had a significantly shorter duration of intravenous antibiotic treatment and a shorter hospital stay." Noll DR, Shores JH, Gamber RG, Herron KM, Swift J Jr. Benefits of osteopathic manipulative treatment for hospitalized elderly patients with pneumonia. *J Am Osteopath Assoc.* 2000 Dec;100(12):776-82 http://www.jaoa.org/cgi/reprint/100/12/776

[484] Osteopathic manipulation improved pulmonary function in pediatric patients with asthma: "With a confidence level of 95%, results for the OMT group showed a statistically significant improvement of 7 L per minute to 9 L per minute for peak expiratory flow rates. These results suggest that OMT has a therapeutic effect among this patient population." Guiney PA, Chou R, Vianna A, Lovenheim J. Effects of osteopathic manipulative treatment on pediatric patients with asthma: a randomized controlled trial. *J Am Osteopath Assoc.* 2005 Jan;105(1):7-12 http://www.jaoa.org/cgi/content/full/105/1/7

[485] Nemett DR, Fivush BA, Mathews R, Camirand N, Eldridge MA, Finney K, Gerson AC. A randomized controlled trial of the effectiveness of osteopathy-based manual physical therapy in treating pediatric dysfunctional voiding. *J Pediatr Urol.* 2008 Apr;4(2):100-6

[486] Sucher BM, Hinrichs RN, Welcher RL, Quiroz LD, St Laurent BF, Morrison BJ. Manipulative treatment of carpal tunnel syndrome: biomechanical and osteopathic intervention to increase the length of the transverse carpal ligament: part 2. Effect of sex differences and manipulative "priming". *J Am Osteopath Assoc.* 2005 Mar;105(3):135-43. Erratum in: *J Am Osteopath Assoc.* 2005 May;105(5):238 http://www.jaoa.org/cgi/content/full/105/3/135

[487] "CONCLUSION: OMT significantly reduces low back pain. The level of pain reduction is greater than expected from placebo effects alone and persists for at least three months." Licciardone JC, Brimhall AK, King LN. Osteopathic manipulative treatment for low back pain: a systematic review and meta-analysis of randomized controlled trials. *BMC Musculoskelet Disord.* 2005 Aug 4;6:43 http://www.biomedcentral.com/1471-2474/6/43

[488] This study showed benefit from osteopathic manipulation administered immediately after coronary artery bypass graft surgery: "The observed changes in cardiac function and perfusion indicated that OMT had a beneficial effect on the recovery of patients after CABG surgery. The authors conclude that OMT has immediate, beneficial hemodynamic effects after CABG surgery when administered while the patient is sedated and pharmacologically paralyzed." O-Yurvati AH, Carnes MS, Clearfield MB, Stoll ST, McConathy WJ. Hemodynamic effects of osteopathic manipulative treatment immediately after coronary artery bypass graft surgery. *J Am Osteopath Assoc.* 2005 Oct;105(10):475-81 http://www.jaoa.org/cgi/content/full/105/10/475

Functional Medicine

<u>Note</u>: This section is from the final pre-edited draft which introduces functional medicine in *Vasquez A. Musculoskeletal Pain: Expanded Clinical Strategies (2008)*, published by the Institute for Functional Medicine; used here with permission. Slight modifications were made to this section during revisions in 2011.

<u>Introduction</u>: The purpose of this monograph is to provide healthcare professionals with an overview of the "functional medicine" assessment and management strategies that are applicable to painful neuromusculoskeletal disorders. A comprehensive description of functional medicine from the Institute for Functional Medicine (IFM) is provided later in this section, while a more comprehensive explication is provided in *The Textbook of Functional Medicine*.[489] In recognition of the diversity of this document's readership (inclusive of students, recent graduates, experienced professionals, academicians, and policymakers) and the pervasive deficiencies in musculoskeletal knowledge among healthcare providers[490,491,492,493,494,495], this monograph on pain will necessarily review some basic concepts; however, this document alone cannot replace professional training in musculoskeletal medicine nor does it include protocols for patient management and differential diagnosis for each of the neuromusculoskeletal problems seen in clinical practice. This

A Functional Medicine Monograph

MUSCULOSKELETAL PAIN:
Expanded Clinical Strategies

Alex Vasquez, DC, ND

THE INSTITUTE FOR FUNCTIONAL MEDICINE

The information in this section on functional medicine is derived from the final pre-edited draft of chapter 1 from Vasquez A. *Musculoskeletal Pain: Expanded Clinical Strategies*, published by the Institute for Functional Medicine in 2008.

text should be used in conjunction with the reader's professional training and other reference texts. Clinicians utilizing a functional medicine approach to patient care must be knowledgeable in the details of integrative physiology and nutritional biochemistry and must also possess the clinical acumen necessary to ensure safe and expedient patient care. These traits and skills are of particular necessity when a serious condition is presented. Life-threatening and limb-threatening neuromusculoskeletal problems are notorious for presenting under the guise of an apparently benign complaint such as fatigue, headache, or simple joint pain.

Since approximately 1 of every 7 (14% of total) visits to a primary healthcare provider is for the treatment of musculoskeletal pain or dysfunction[496], every healthcare provider needs to have: 1) knowledge of important concepts related to musculoskeletal medicine, 2) the ability to recognize urgent and emergency conditions, 3) the ability to competently perform orthopedic examination procedures and interpret laboratory assessments, and 4) the knowledge and ability to design and implement effective treatment plans and to coordinate patient management. While this monograph will be thorough in its review of topics discussed, like any other textbook it cannot contain every nuance and examination procedure that clinicians should have in their clinical toolkits. This text should be used in conjunction with the clinician's previous professional training, other textbooks, and best judgment for the delivery of personalized care for each individual patient, including those who present with similar or identical diagnoses. Supportive texts include *Current Medical Diagnosis and Treatment* edited by Tierney et al[497],

[489] Jones DS (Editor-in-Chief). *Textbook of Functional Medicine*. Institute for Functional Medicine, Gig Harbor, WA 2005

[490] Freedman KB, Bernstein J. The adequacy of medical school education in musculoskeletal medicine. *J Bone Joint Surg Am*. 1998;80(10):1421-7

[491] Freedman KB, Bernstein J. Educational deficiencies in musculoskeletal medicine. *J Bone Joint Surg Am*. 2002;84-A(4):604-8

[492] Joy EA, Hala SV. Musculoskeletal Curricula in Medical Education: Filling In the Missing Pieces. *The Physician and Sportsmedicine*. 2004; 32: 42-45

[493] Matzkin E, Smith ME, Freccero CD, Richardson AB. Adequacy of education in musculoskeletal medicine. *J Bone Joint Surg Am*. 2005 Feb;87-A(2):310-4

[494] Schmale GA. More evidence of educational inadequacies in musculoskeletal medicine. *Clin Orthop Relat Res*. 2005 Aug;(437):251-9

[495] Stockard AR, Allen TW. Competence levels in musculoskeletal medicine: comparison of osteopathic and allopathic medical graduates. *J Am Osteopath Assoc*. 2006 Jun;106(6):350-5

[496] American College of Rheumatology Ad Hoc Committee on Clinical Guidelines. Guidelines for the initial evaluation of the adult patient with acute musculoskeletal symptoms. *Arthritis Rheum*. 1996 Jan;39(1):1-8 See also: Vasquez A. Musculoskeletal disorders and iron overload disease: comment on the American College of Rheumatology guidelines. *Arthritis Rheum* 1996;39: 1767-8

[497] Tierney ML. McPhee SJ, Papadakis MA (eds). Current Medical Diagnosis and Treatment. New York: Lange Medical Books. Updated annually

Orthopedic Physical Assessment by Magee[498], and *Integrative Orthopedics* and *Integrative Rheumatology* by Vasquez.[499,500] Further, clinicians can note that this monograph is written primarily for routine outpatient management rather than emergency department management or "playing field" situations.

Musculoskeletal disorders are extremely prevalent and represent a major cause of human suffering, healthcare expenses, and lost productivity. Additionally, many standard medical interventions show high rates of inefficacy and iatrogenesis in addition to their high costs.[501,502,503] The vast majority of painful neuromusculoskeletal disorders can be alleviated and often effectively treated with nutritional interventions, but physicians trained only in standard medicine receive little to no training in nutrition and are therefore generally unable or unwilling to use these science-based interventions to help their patients.[504,505] Further, distain toward nutritional and other nonsurgical and nonpharmacologic interventions is represented in many standard medical textbooks despite proof of efficacy shown in replicable high-quality clinical trials published in top-tier medical journals. For example, despite the more than 800 articles documenting the role of nutritional interventions in the direct or adjunctive treatment of rheumatoid arthritis, the seventeenth edition of *The Merck Manual* published in 1999 wrote that, "Food and diet quackery is common and should be discouraged."[506] Combining these factors with the aforementioned pervasive lack of competence in musculoskeletal knowledge among healthcare providers (exceptions noted[507]), we see that patients with musculoskeletal disorders often face a series of difficult and insurmountable obstacles between their present condition of suffering and the relief that they seek and deserve. Clearly, the field of musculoskeletal medicine is in need of pervasive paradigm shifts in both physician training and patient management to improve patient care.

Background: Historically, prevailing views of disorders of pain and inflammation were conceptually similar to those of most other diseases and premodern accounts of life in general. Our clinical predecessors did the best they could to understand, describe, and treat the health problems with which their patients presented, and the paradigm from which these clinical entities were viewed and addressed was shaped by the social, religious, and scientific views and limitations of their time. Lacking a molecular and physiologic understanding of disease origination, and restrained by metaphysical and simplistic models of "cause and effect", premodern clinicians devised models for the understanding and treatment of disease that generally appear unsatisfactory today in light of the advances in our understanding in disparate yet interrelated fields such as psychoneuroimmunology, molecular biology, nutrigenomics, environmental medicine and toxicology. Despite these advances, we as a human society and as healthcare providers still carry many of these previous conceptualizations and misconceptualizations with us as we move forward toward a future wherein our views and interventions will be much more precise and "objective" in contrast to the generalized and phenomenalistic approaches that typified premodern medicine and which still permeate certain aspects of clinical care today. For example, we still use the term "stroke" to describe acute cerebrovascular insufficiency, although the term originated from the view that affected patients had been "struck" by the gods or fates perhaps as a form of punishment for some ethical or religious transgression. Even today, patients and clinicians commonly interpret disease as some form of punishment or as an extension of spiritual or intrapersonal shortcoming. Advancing science allows us to disassemble complex events that were previously experienced as ***phenomena***, that is, as undecipherable and enigmatic events that overwhelmed comprehension. The **Functional Medicine Matrix** provides an extremely useful tool for helping clinicians grasp a multidimensional decipherable view of disease and its corresponding treatment which facilitates the achievement of higher clinical efficacy, improved patient outcomes, and more favorable safety and cost-effectiveness profiles.

[498] Magee DJ. Orthopedic Physical Assessment. Third edition. Philadelphia: WB Saunders, 1997. Newer editions have been published.

[499] Vasquez A. *Integrative Orthopedics: Second Edition*. Fort Worth, Texas; Integrative and Biological Medicine Research and Consulting, 2007 InflammationMastery.com

[500] Vasquez A. *Integrative Rheumatology: Second Edition*. Fort Worth, Texas; Integrative and Biological Medicine Research and Consulting, 2007 InflammationMastery.com

[501] Moseley JB, O'Malley K, Petersen NJ, Menke TJ, Brody BA, Kuykendall DH, Hollingsworth JC, Ashton CM, Wray NP. A controlled trial of arthroscopic surgery for osteoarthritis of the knee. *N Engl J Med* 2002 Jul 11;347(2):81-8

[502] Kolata G. A Knee Surgery for Arthritis Is Called Sham. *The New York Times*, July 11, 2002

[503] Rosner AL. Evidence-based clinical guidelines for the management of acute low-back pain: response to the guidelines prepared for the Australian Medical Health and Research Council. *J Manipulative Physiol Ther*. 2001;24(3):214-20

[504] Lo C. Integrating nutrition as a theme throughout the medical school curriculum. *Am J Clin Nutr*. 2000 Sep;72(3 Suppl):882S-9S

[505] Adams KM, Lindell KC, Kohlmeier M, Zeisel SH. Status of nutrition education in medical schools. *Am J Clin Nutr*. 2006 Apr;83(4):941S-944S

[506] Beers MH, Berkow R (eds). The Merck Manual. Seventeenth Edition. Whitehouse Station; Merck Research Laboratories; 1999, page 419

[507] Humphreys BK, Sulkowski A, McIntyre K, Kasiban M, Patrick AN. An examination of musculoskeletal cognitive competency in chiropractic interns. *J Manipulative Physiol Ther*. 2007;30(1):44-9

Whereas the advancement of our scientific knowledge often leads us to discard previous models and interventions, occasionally modern science helps us to understand and revisit previous interventions that may have been prematurely or unduly discarded. For example, Hippocrates' admonition to "Let thy food be thy medicine, and thy medicine be thy food" experienced decades of devaluation when dietary, nutritional, and other natural interventions were misbranded as "quackery." On the contrary to these premature and unsubstantiated condemnations, simple natural interventions such as therapeutic fasting and augmentation of vitamin D3 status (via nutritional supplementation or exposure to ultraviolet-B radiation) have shown remarkable safety and efficacy in the mitigation of chronic hypertension, musculoskeletal pain, and autoimmunity.[508,509,510,511,512,513,514,515,516] Furthermore, the appropriate use of vitamin supplements helps prevent chronic disease by numerous mechanisms including modulation of gene transcription, enhancement of DNA repair and stability, and enhancement of metabolic efficiency.[517,518,519] This document will provide a representative survey of current research in the use of dietary, nutritional, and integrative therapeutics commonly utilized in the clinical management of disorders characterized by pain and inflammation.

State of the Evidence: The bulk of information in this monograph is derived from and referenced to peer-reviewed publications indexed in the database known as Medline/Pubmed provided by the U.S. National Library of Medicine and the National Institutes of Health. For the sake of practicality and publishability, not all statements carry citations, but the most important ones do; citations are always provided when referenced to a particular intervention of importance so that clinicians can access the primary source when refining their clinical decisions. A "blanket statement" to cover all the different assessments and interventions described herein would be necessarily inaccurate and therefore each intervention will be considered on the merits of its own rationale, safety, effectiveness, and cost-effectiveness. Again, however, these considerations must ultimately be viewed within the context of the individual patient's condition and the overall cohesion and comprehensiveness of the treatment plan.

While all clinicians can appreciate the importance of protocols and clinical practice guidelines, we must also perpetually ratify the preeminence of patient individuality and therefore the importance of tailoring treatment to the patient's unique combination of biochemical individuality, comorbid conditions, drug use, personal goals, and willingness to participate in a health-promoting lifestyle. Standardized protocols and practice guidelines are founded on the fallacy of disease homogeneity and the irrelevance of physiologic, psychosocial, and biochemical individuality. As the advancement of biomedical science provides the means for and underscores the importance of customized treatments for each patient, so too has the standard of care begun to shift in the direction of requiring the consideration of these variables before and during the implementation of treatment. Failure to utilize nutritional interventions when such interventions are clinically indicated is inconsistent with the delivery of quality healthcare and may be considered malpractice.[520,521,522,523]

A clinician who is unaware of the political forces that shape healthcare policy and research is analogous to a captain of an oceangoing ship not knowing how to use a compass, sextant, or coastline map. Medical science and healthcare policy are influenced by a myriad of powerful private interests which are motivated by their own goals, at times different from the stated goals of medicine, which purports to hold paramount the patient's welfare. Scientific objectivity and the guiding ethical principles of informed consent, beneficence, autonomy, and non-

[508] Goldhamer A, et al. Medically supervised water-only fasting in the treatment of hypertension. *J Manipulative Physiol Ther* 2001 Jun;24(5):335-9

[509] Goldhamer AC, et al. Medically supervised water-only fasting in the treatment of borderline hypertension. *J Altern Complement Med*. 2002 Oct;8(5):643-50

[510] Goldhamer AC. Initial cost of care results in medically supervised water-only fasting for treating high blood pressure and diabetes. *J Altern Complement Med*. 2002 Dec;8(6):696-7

[511] Krause R, Bühring M, Hopfenmüller W, Holick MF, Sharma AM. Ultraviolet B and blood pressure. *Lancet*. 1998 Aug 29;352(9129):709-10

[512] Pfeifer M, Begerow B, Minne HW, Nachtigall D, Hansen C. Effects of a short-term vitamin D(3) and calcium supplementation on blood pressure and parathyroid hormone levels in elderly women. *J Clin Endocrinol Metab*. 2001 Apr;86(4):1633-7

[513] McCarty MF. A preliminary fast may potentiate response to a subsequent low-salt, low-fat vegan diet in the management of hypertension - fasting as a strategy for breaking metabolic vicious cycles. *Med Hypotheses*. 2003 May;60(5):624-33

[514] Hyppönen E, Läärä E, Reunanen A, Järvelin MR, Virtanen SM. Intake of vitamin D and risk of type 1 diabetes: a birth-cohort study. *Lancet*. 2001 Nov 3;358(9292):1500-3

[515] Fuhrman J, Sarter B, Calabro DJ. Brief case reports of medically supervised, water-only fasting associated with remission of autoimmune disease. *Altern Ther Health Med*. 2002 Jul-Aug;8(4):112, 110-1

[516] Holick MF. Vitamin D deficiency: what a pain it is. *Mayo Clin Proc*. 2003 Dec;78(12):1457-9

[517] Fletcher RH, Fairfield KM. Vitamins for chronic disease prevention in adults: clinical applications. *JAMA*. 2002 Jun 19;287(23):3127-9

[518] Heaney RP. Long-latency deficiency disease: insights from calcium and vitamin D. *Am J Clin Nutr*. 2003 Nov;78(5):912-9

[519] Ames BN. The metabolic tune-up: metabolic harmony and disease prevention. *J Nutr*. 2003 May;133(5 Suppl 1):1544S-8S

[520] Heaney RP. Vitamin D, nutritional deficiency, and the medical paradigm. *J Clin Endocrinol Metab*. 2003 Nov;88(11):5107-8

[521] Fletcher RH, Fairfield KM. Vitamins for chronic disease prevention in adults: clinical applications. *JAMA*. 2002 Jun 19;287(23):3127-9

[522] Berg A. Sliding toward nutrition malpractice: time to reconsider and redeploy. *Am J Clin Nutr*. 1993 Jan;57(1):3-7

[523] Cobb DK, Warner D. Avoiding malpractice: the role of proper nutrition and wound management. *J Am Med Dir Assoc*. 2004 Jul-Aug;5(4 Sup):H11-6

malfeasance are subject to different interpretations depending upon the lens through which a dilemma is viewed. When this "dilemma" is the whole of healthcare, what first appears as order and structure now appears as the disarrayed tug-of-war between factions and private interests, with paradigmatic victory often being awarded to those with the best marketing campaigns and political influence with less importance given to safety, efficacy, and the economic burden to consumers.[524,525,526,527,528,529,530,531,532,533,534,535,536,537,538,539,540,541,542,543,544,545,546,547,548,549,550,551,552,553,554,555] To be ignorant of such considerations is to be blind to the nature of research, policy, and our own biased inclinations for and against particular paradigms, assessments, and interventions. Research articles and sources of authority must be approached with an artist's delicacy, and with a willingness to receive new information as worthy of preeminence over deeply rooted and well ensconced institutionalized fallacies.

[524] Editorial. Drug-company influence on medical education in USA. *Lancet*. 2000 Sep 2;356(9232):781

[525] Horton R. Lotronex and the FDA: a fatal erosion of integrity. *Lancet*. 2001 May 19;357(9268):1544-5

[526] Editorial. Politics trumps science at the FDA. *Lancet*. 2005 Nov 26;366(9500):1827

[527] Topol EJ. Failing the public health--rofecoxib, Merck, and the FDA. *N Engl J Med*. 2004 Oct 21;351(17):1707-9

[528] Wolinsky H, Brune T. The Serpent on the Staff: The Unhealthy Politics of the American Medical Association. GP Putnam and Sons, New York, 1994

[529] Wilk CA. Medicine, Monopolies, and Malice: How the Medical Establishment Tried to Destroy Chiropractic. Garden City Park: Avery, 1996

[530] Carter JP. Racketeering in Medicine: The Suppression of Alternatives. Norfolk: Hampton Roads Pub; 1993

[531] National Alliance of Professional Psychology Providers. AMA Seeks To Control and Restrict Psychologist's Scope of Practice. http://www.nappp.org/scope.pdf Accessed November 25, 2006

[532] Daly R, American Psychiatric Association. AMA Forms Coalition to Thwart Non-M.D. Practice Expansion. *Psychiatric News* 2006 March; 41: 17

[533] Angell M. The Truth About the Drug Companies: How They Deceive Us and What to Do About it. Random House; August 2004

[534] Terrett AG. Misuse of the literature by medical authors in discussing spinal manipulative therapy injury. *J Manipulative Physiol Ther*. 1995 May;18(4):203-10

[535] Morley J, Rosner AL, Redwood D. A case study of misrepresentation of the scientific literature: recent reviews of chiropractic. *J Altern Complement Med*. 2001 Feb;7(1):65-78

[536] Wenban AB. Inappropriate use of the title 'chiropractor' and term 'chiropractic manipulation' in the peer-reviewed biomedical literature. *Chiropr Osteopat*. 2006 Aug 22;14:16

[537] Spivak JL. The Medical Trust Unmasked. Louis S. Siegfried Publishers; New York: 1961

[538] Trever W. In the Public Interest. Los Angeles; Scriptures Unlimited; 1972. This is probably the most authoritative documentation of the illegal actions of the AMA up to 1972; contains numerous photocopies of actual AMA documents and minutes of official meetings with overt intentionality of destroying Americans' healthcare options so that the AMA and related organizations would have a monopoly in healthcare.

[539] Getzendanner S. Permanent injunction order against AMA. *JAMA*. 1988 Jan 1;259(1):81-2

[540] "A national study released today reports 20 million American families — or one in seven families — faced hardships paying medical bills last year, which forced many to choose between getting medical attention or paying rent or buying food..." Freeman, Liz. 'Working poor' struggle to afford health care. *Naples Daily News*. Published in Naples, Florida and online at http://www.naplesnews.com/npdn/news/article/0,2071,NPDN_14940_3000546,00.html Accessed July 28, 2004

[541] "The USA's 5.8 million small companies... Health care costs are rising about 15% this year for those with fewer than 200 workers vs. 13.5% for those with 500 or more... But many small employers cite increases of 20% or more. That's made insurance the No. 1 small business problem..." Jim Hopkins. Health care tops taxes as small business cost drain. *USA TODAY*. http://www.usatoday.com/news/health/2003-04-20-small-business-costs_x.htm. Accessed July 28, 2004

[542] "Though the U.S. has slightly fewer doctors per capita than the typical developed nation, we have almost twice as many MRI machines and perform vastly more angioplasties. ...at least 31 percent of all the incremental income we'll earn between 1999 and 2010 will go to health care." Pat Regnier, *Money Magazine*. Healthcare myth: We spend too much. October 13, 2003: 11:29 AM EDT http://money.cnn.com/2003/10/08/pf/health_myths_1/ Accessed Monday, July 12, 2004

[543] "Although they spend more on health care than patients in any other industrialized nation, Americans receive the right treatment less than 60 percent of the time, resulting in unnecessary pain, expense and even death..." Ceci Connolly. U.S. Patients Spend More but Don't Get More, Study Finds: Even in Advantaged Areas, Americans Often Receive Inadequate Health Care. *Washington Post*, May 5, 2004; Page A15. On-line at http://www.washingtonpost.com/ac2/wp-dyn/A1875-2004May4 accessed on July 28, 2004

[544] McGlynn EA, Asch SM, Adams J, Keesey J, Hicks J, DeCristofaro A, Kerr EA. The quality of health care delivered to adults in the United States. *N Engl J Med*. 2003 Jun 26;348(26):2635-45

[545] Brennan TA, Leape LL, Laird NM, Hebert L, Localio AR, Lawthers AG, Newhouse JP, Weiler PC, Hiatt HH. Incidence of adverse events and negligence in hospitalized patients: results of the Harvard Medical Practice Study I. 1991. *Qual Saf Health Care*. 2004 Apr;13(2):145-51; discuss 151-2

[546] "Basically, you die earlier and spend more time disabled if you're an American rather than a member of most other advanced countries." Christopher Murray MD PhD, Director of World Health Organization's Global Program on Evidence for Health Policy http://www.who.int/inf-pr-2000/en/pr2000-life.html Accessed July 12, 2004

[547] Shi L. Health care spending, delivery, and outcome in developed countries: a cross-national comparison. *Am J Med Qual* 1997;12(2):83-93

[548] Holland EG, Degruy FV. Drug-induced disorders. *Am Fam Physician*. 1997 Nov 1;56(7):1781-8, 1791-2

[549] Brennan TA, Leape LL, Laird NM, Hebert L, Localio AR, Lawthers AG, Newhouse JP, Weiler PC, Hiatt HH. Incidence of adverse events and negligence in hospitalized patients: results of the Harvard Medical Practice Study I. 1991. *Qual Saf Health Care*. 2004 Apr;13(2):145-51; discuss 151-2

[550] Whitaker R. The case against antipsychotic drugs: a 50-year record of doing more harm than good. *Med Hypotheses*. 2004;62(1):5-13

[551] The relevance of these citations is to show that the misuse of horse estrogens in humans as "hormone replacement therapy" exemplified the application of a strong carcinogen to millions of unsuspecting women: Zhang F, Chen Y, Pisha E, Shen L, Xiong Y, van Breemen RB, Bolton JL. The major metabolite of equilin, 4-hydroxyequilin, autoxidizes to an o-quinone which isomerizes to the potent cytotoxin 4-hydroxyequilenin-o-quinone. *Chem Res Toxicol*. 1999 Feb;12(2):204-13; Pisha E, Lui X, Constantinou AI, Bolton JL. Evidence that a metabolite of equine estrogens, 4-hydroxyequilenin, induces cellular transformation in vitro. *Chem Res Toxicol*. 2001;14(1):82-90; Zhang F, Swanson SM, van Breemen RB, Liu X, Yang Y, Gu C, Bolton JL. Equine estrogen metabolite 4-hydroxyequilenin induces DNA damage in the rat mammary tissues: formation of single-strand breaks, apurinic sites, stable adducts, and oxidized bases. *Chem Res Toxicol*. 2001 Dec;14(12):1654-9

[552] Newman NM, Ling RS. Acetabular bone destruction related to non-steroidal anti-inflammatory drugs. *Lancet*. 1985 Jul 6; 2(8445): 11-4

[553] "In 1983, 2876 people died from medication errors. ... By 1993, this number had risen to 7,391 - a 2.57-fold increase." Phillips DP, Christenfeld N, Glynn LM. Increase in US medication-error deaths between 1983 and 1993. *Lancet*. 1998 Feb 28;351(9103):643-4

[554] Smith R. Medical journals are an extension of the marketing arm of pharmaceutical companies. *PLoS Med*. 2005 May;2(5):e138

[555] van der Steen WJ, Ho VK. Drugs versus diets: disillusions with Dutch health care. *Acta Biotheor*. 2001;49(2):125-40

Understanding the Multifaceted Nature of Disease Pathogenesis: The Functional Medicine Matrix as Paradigm and Clinical Tool: At its simplest and most practical level, the Functional Medicine Matrix is a teaching tool and clinical method that facilitates consideration of the different contributions of major intrinsic systems and extrinsic influences that are at play in a given disease process or individual patient. When viewed as a diagram, the web of influences can be appreciated to reveal the interconnected nature of influences and body systems and how imbalance or disruption in one area can lead to problems in another. Once homeostatic reserves and compensatory mechanisms are depleted, the patient experiences progressively worsening health (which may be asymptomatic) and the eventual manifestation of clinical disease.

Over the course of many years and discussions and reconsiderations, the faculty at IFM has elucidated eight preeminent systems or loci ("core clinical imbalances") for clinicians to consider when working with any chronic health disorder. These will be listed and described below with particular consideration of the topic of this monograph, which is neuromusculoskeletal pain and inflammation. Interested readers are directed to IFM's monograph series on topics such as "Depression" and "The Role of Gastrointestinal Inflammation in Systemic Disease" to see how this model is applied to disease states in different organ systems.

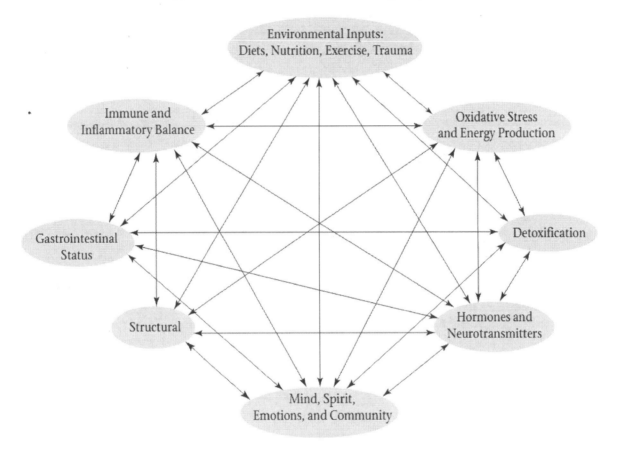

Functional Medicine Matrix illustrated by Alex Vasquez (2003): This version of "the Matrix" by Alex Vasquez provides an illustration of the interdependency of physiologic factors and organ systems; this version was published in *Textbook of Functional Medicine* (2005 and 2010 Editions) and as Vasquez, *Integrative Medicine* 2006 Apr/May.

Exploring the Different Aspects of the Functional Medicine Matrix

1. Hormonal and neurotransmitter imbalances: While most clinicians are aware that neurotransmitters can either transmit pain signals or dampen their reception, many clinicians are not aware that neurotransmitter status is somewhat malleable and can be modulated with nutritional supplementation and botanical medicines. The examples that will be considered here are the tryptophan-serotonin-melatonin and the phenylalanine-tyrosine-dopamine-norepinephrine-epinephrine and enkephalin pathways.

- Tryptophan and 5-hydroxytryptophan (5HTP) are prescription and nonprescription nutritional supplements that are the amino acid precursors for the formation of the neurotransmitter serotonin and, subsequently, the pineal hormone melatonin. Biochemically, these conversions are linear as follows: tryptophan → 5HTP → serotonin → melatonin. Tryptophan depletion and low levels of serotonin are consistently associated with depression, anxiety, exacerbation of eating disorders, and increased sensitivity to acute and chronic pain. Serotonergic pathways are impaired by chronic stress due to increased utilization of serotonin (e.g., serotonin-dependent cortisol release) and increased hepatic degradation of tryptophan by cortisol-stimulated tryptophan pyrrolase.[556] Therapeutically, supplementation with 5HTP augments serotonin and melatonin synthesis and has specific applicability in the alleviation of depression and pain syndromes such as fibromyalgia and headache, including migraine, tension headaches, and juvenile headaches.[557,558] Certainly part of the benefit from 5HTP supplementation is derived from the increased formation of melatonin, as the biological effects of melatonin extend beyond its sleep-promoting role to include powerful antioxidation, anti-infective immunostimulation[559], and preservation of mitochondrial function, a benefit which is of particular relevance to the treatment of fibromyalgia.[560]

- The conditionally essential fatty acids found in fish oil modulate serotonergic and adrenergic activity in the human brain[561], and given the role of serotonin and norepinephrine in the central processing of pain perception[562], a reasonable hypothesis holds that the pain-relieving activity of fish oil supplementation[563] is partly due to central modulation of pain perception and is not wholly due to modulation of eicosanoid production and inflammatory mediator transcription as previously believed.

- Vitamin D3 supplementation may also augment serotonergic activity[564], and this mechanism may partly explain the mood-enhancing and pain-relieving benefits of vitamin D3 supplementation. Attentive readers will note that this brief discussion has already begun to bridge the gaps between nutritional status, neurotransmitter synthesis, pain sensitivity, immune function, and mitochondrial bioenergetics.

- Supplementation with DL-phenylalanine (DLPA; racemic mixture of D- and L-forms of the amino acid phenylalanine derived from synthetic production) has long been used in the treatment of pain and depression.[565] The nutritional L-isomer is converted from phenylalanine to tyrosine to L-dopa to dopamine to norepinephrine and epinephrine. Augmentation of this pathway promotes resistance to fatigue, depression, and pain. The synthetic D-isomer augments pain-relieving enkephalin function by inhibiting enkephalin degradation by the enzyme carboxypeptidase A (enkephalinase); the resultant augmentation of enkephalin levels is generally believed to underlie the analgesic and mood-enhancing benefits of DLPA supplementation.

- Therapeutic massage is yet another means to modulate neurotransmitter synthesis for the alleviation of pain. In a study of patients with chronic back pain, massage increased serotonin and dopamine levels (measured in urine).[566]

Hormonal imbalances are particularly relevant to the discussion of chronic pain caused by inflammation characteristic of autoimmune diseases such as rheumatoid arthritis (RA). Often clinically subtle but nonetheless of extreme importance, these hormonal influences on painful inflammation are worthy of their own detailed discussion and thus will be reviewed later in this monograph in the context of the prototypic

[556] Sandyk R. Tryptophan availability and the susceptibility to stress in multiple sclerosis: a hypothesis. *Int J Neurosci.* 1996 Jul;86(1-2):47-53

[557] Turner EH, Loftis JM, Blackwell AD. Serotonin a la carte: supplementation with the serotonin precursor 5-hydroxytryptophan. *Pharmacol Ther.* 2006 Mar;109(3):325-38

[558] Birdsall TC. 5-Hydroxytryptophan: a clinically-effective serotonin precursor. *Altern Med Rev.* 1998 Aug;3(4):271-80

[559] Gitto E, Karbownik M, Reiter RJ, Tan DX, Cuzzocrea S, Chiurazzi P, Cordaro S, Corona G, Trimarchi G, Barberi I. Effects of melatonin treatment in septic newborns. *Pediatr Res.* 2001 Dec;50(6):756-60

[560] Acuna-Castroviejo D, Escames G, Reiter RJ. Melatonin therapy in fibromyalgia. *J Pineal Res.* 2006 Jan;40(1):98-9

[561] Hibbeln JR, Ferguson TA, Blasbalg TL. Omega-3 fatty acid deficiencies in neurodevelopment, aggression and autonomic dysregulation: opportunities for intervention. *Int Rev Psychiatry.* 2006 Apr;18(2):107-18

[562] Wise TN, Fishbain DA, Holder-Perkins V.Painful physical symptoms in depression: a clinical challenge. *Pain Med.* 2007 Sep;8 Suppl 2:S75-82

[563] Goldberg RJ, Katz J. A meta-analysis of the analgesic effects of omega-3 polyunsaturated fatty acid supplementation for inflammatory joint pain. *Pain.* 2007;129(1-2):210-23

[564] Lansdowne AT, Provost SC. Vitamin D3 enhances mood in healthy subjects during winter. *Psychopharmacology* (Berl). 1998 Feb;135(4):319-23

[565] Russell AL, McCarty MF. DL-phenylalanine markedly potentiates opiate analgesia - an example of nutrient/pharmaceutical up-regulation of the endogenous analgesia system. *Med Hypotheses.* 2000 Oct;55(4):283-8

[566] Hernandez-Reif M, Field T, Krasnegor J, Theakston H. Lower back pain is reduced and range of motion increased after massage therapy. *Int J Neurosci* 2001;106(3-4):131-45

inflammatory disease RA. Generally speaking and with a few noted exceptions (such as Sjogren's syndrome), the research literature points to a specific pattern of hormonal imbalances among patients with autoimmunity, and this pattern is consistent with the proinflammatory and immunodysregulatory effects of estrogens and prolactin and the anti-inflammatory and immunomodulatory effects of cortisol, dehydroepiandrosterone (DHEA), and testosterone. Patients with autoimmune neuromusculoskeletal inflammation generally display a complete or partial pattern of hormonal disturbances typified by elevated estrogen and prolactin and lowered testosterone, DHEA, and cortisol; appropriate therapeutic correction of these imbalances can safely result in disease amelioration. Rectification of endocrinologic imbalances ("orthoendocrinology") will be discussed in the section on RA and has been detailed with broader clinical applicability elsewhere by this author.[567]

2. Oxidation-reduction imbalances and mitochondriopathy: Oxidative stress results from the chronic systemic inflammation seen in painful inflammatory disorders such as RA, and oxidative stress contributes to the perpetuation and exacerbation of inflammatory diseases via expedited tissue destruction and alterations in gene transcription and resultant enhancement of inflammatory mediator production.[568] Immune activation increases production of reactive oxygen species (ROS; "free radicals"), and oxidant stress increases activation of pro-inflammatory transcription factors (such as nuclear factor KappaB, NFkB) and also increases spontaneous oxidative modification of endogenous proteins such as cartilage matrix which then undergoes expedited degradation or immunologic attack; thus a vicious cycle of oxidation and inflammation exacerbates and perpetuates various inflammation-associated diseases, resulting in therapeutic recalcitrance and autonomous disease progression.[569,570] A rational clinical approach to breaking this vicious pathogenic cycle can include simultaneous antioxidation and immunomodulation, the former with diet optimization and nutritional supplementation and the latter with allergen avoidance, hormonal correction, xenobiotic detoxification, and specific phytonutritional modulation of pro-inflammatory pathways. Severe and acute inflammation can and often should be suppressed pharmacologically, but sole reliance on pharmacologic immunosuppression leaves the patient vulnerable to iatrogenic immunosuppression and the well-known increased risk for cardiovascular disease, infection, and clinical malignancy while failing to address the underlying biochemical and immunologic imbalances which lie at the bottom of all chronic inflammatory and autoimmune diseases. The contribution of mitochondrial dysfunction to chronic recurrent or persistent pain is most plainly demonstrated in migraine and fibromyalgia (discussed later in this monograph). An important characteristic of migraine is mitochondrial dysfunction, the severity of which correlates positively with the severity of the headache syndrome.[571] In fibromyalgia, numerous abnormalities in cellular bioenergetics are noted, which correlate clinically with the lowered lactate threshold, persistent muscle pain, reduced functional capacity, and the subjective fatigue that characterize the disorder.[572] Nutritional preservation and enhancement of mitochondrial function was termed "mitochondrial resuscitation" by Jeffrey Bland PhD in the 1990s, and clinical implementation of such an approach generally includes, in addition to diet and lifestyle modification, supplementation with coenzyme Q-10, niacin, riboflavin, thiamin, lipoic acid, magnesium, and other nutrients and botanical medicines which enhance production of adenosine triphosphate (ATP).[573]

3. Detoxification and biotransformational imbalances: As our environment becomes increasingly polluted and as researchers and clinicians mature and expand their appreciation and knowledge of the adverse effects of xenobiotics (toxic metals and chemicals), healthcare providers will need to attend to their patients' detoxification capacity and xenobiotic load as a component of the prevention and treatment of disease. By now, senior students and practicing clinicians should be aware of the association of xenobiotics in

[567] Vasquez A. *Integrative Rheumatology*. Fort Worth, Texas; Integrative & Biological Medicine Research & Consulting, 2007 InflammationMastery.com
[568] Hitchon CA, El-Gabalawy HS. Oxidation in rheumatoid arthritis. *Arthritis Res Ther*. 2004;6(6):265-78
[569] Tak PP, Zvaifler NJ, Green DR, Firestein GS. Rheumatoid arthritis and p53: how oxidative stress might alter the course of inflammatory diseases. *Immunol Today*. 2000 Feb;21(2):78-82
[570] Kurien BT, Hensley K, Bachmann M, Scofield RH. Oxidatively modified autoantigens in autoimmune diseases. *Free Radic Biol Med*. 2006 Aug 15;41(4):549-56
[571] Lodi R, Kemp GJ, Montagna P, Pierangeli G, Cortelli P, Iotti S, Radda GK, Barbiroli B. Quantitative analysis of skeletal muscle bioenergetics and proton efflux in migraine and cluster headache. *J Neurol Sci*. 1997 Feb 27;146(1):73-80
[572] Park JH, Phothimat P, Oates CT, Hernanz-Schulman M, Olsen NJ. Use of P-31 magnetic resonance spectroscopy to detect metabolic abnormalities in muscles of patients with fibromyalgia. *Arthritis Rheum*. 1998 Mar;41(3):406-13
[573] Pieczenik SR, Neustadt J. Mitochondrial dysfunction and molecular pathways of disease. *Exp Mol Pathol*. 2007 Aug;83(1):84-92

prototypic diseases such as Parkinson's disease[574,575], adult-onset diabetes mellitus[576,577,578,579], and attention-deficit hyperactivity disorder.[580,581,582] The role of xenobiotic exposure and impaired detoxification in neuromusculoskeletal pain and inflammatory disorders is more subtle and is generally mediated through the resultant immunotoxicity that manifests as autoimmunity. Occasionally, clinicians will encounter patients with musculoskeletal symptomatology that defies standard diagnosis and treatment but which responds remarkably and permanently to empiric clinical detoxification treatment; such a case will be presented in the Case Reports later in this monograph. The numerous roles of xenobiotic exposure in the genesis and perpetuation of chronic health problems and the role of clinical detoxification in the treatment of such problems has been detailed elsewhere by Crinnion[583,584,585,586,587], Rea[588], Bland[589,590], Vasquez[591,592], and others.[593,594]

4. <u>Immune imbalances</u>: Immune imbalances have an obvious role in musculoskeletal inflammation when discussed in the context of autoimmune diseases such as rheumatoid arthritis, ankylosing spondylitis, and systemic lupus erythematosus. While the standard medical approach to this pathophysiology has focused almost exclusively on the pharmacologic suppression of resultant inflammation and tissue destruction, other disciplines such as naturopathic medicine and functional medicine have emphasized the importance of determining and addressing the underlying causes of such immune imbalance. While clinicians of all disciplines must appreciate the important role of pharmacologic immunosuppression in the treatment of inflammatory exacerbations as seen with giant cell arteritis or neuropsychiatric lupus, they should also appreciate that sole reliance on immunosuppression for long-term management of inflammatory disorders is destined to therapeutic failure insofar as it does not correct the underlying cause of the disease and creates dependency upon perpetual immunosuppression with its attendant costs (not uncommonly in the range of $20,000 - 50,000 per year) and adverse effects including infection and increased risk for cancer. Rather than presuming that immune dysfunction and the resultant inflammation and autoimmunity are results of spontaneous generation, astute clinicians seek to identify and correct the causes of these immune imbalances. By identifying and correcting the underlying causes of immune imbalance (when possible), clinicians can lessen or obviate the need for chronic polypharmaceutical treatment with anti-inflammatory and immunosuppressive agents. Vasquez[595] proposed that secondary immune imbalances (distinguished from primary congenital disorders) generally arise from one or more of five main problems: ❶ habitual consumption of a pro-inflammatory diet, ❷ food allergies and intolerances, ❸ microbial dysbiosis, including multifocal polydysbiosis, ❹ hormonal imbalances, and ❺ xenobiotic exposure and accumulation resulting in immunotoxicity via bystander activation and enhanced processing of autoantigens as well as

[574] Corrigan FM, Wienburg CL, Shore RF, Daniel SE, Mann D. Organochlorine insecticides in substantia nigra in Parkinson's disease. *J Toxicol Environ Health A.* 2000 Feb 25;59(4):229-34

[575] Fleming L, Mann JB, Bean J, Briggle T, Sanchez-Ramos JR. Parkinson's disease and brain levels of organochlorine pesticides. *Ann Neurol.* 1994 Jul;36(1):100-3

[576] Fujiyoshi PT, Michalek JE, Matsumura F. Molecular epidemiologic evidence for diabetogenic effects of dioxin exposure in U.S. Air force veterans of the Vietnam war. *Environ Health Perspect*, 2006 Nov;114(11):1677-83

[577] Lee DH, Lee IK, Song K, Steffes M, Toscano W, Baker BA, Jacobs DR Jr. A strong dose-response relation between serum concentrations of persistent organic pollutants and diabetes: results from the National Health and Examination Survey 1999-2002. *Diabetes Care* 2006 Jul;29(7):1638-44

[578] Lee DH, Lee IK, Jin SH, Steffes M, Jacobs DR Jr. Association between serum concentrations of persistent organic pollutants and insulin resistance among nondiabetic adults: results from the National Health and Nutrition Examination Survey 1999-2002. *Diabetes Care*, 2007 Mar;30(3):622-8

[579] Remillard RB, Bunce NJ. Linking dioxins to diabetes: epidemiology and biologic plausibility. *Environ Health Perspect*, 2002 Sep;110(9):853-8

[580] Rauh VA, Garfinkel R, Perera FP, Andrews HF, Hoepner L, Barr DB, Whitehead R, Tang D, Whyatt RW. Impact of prenatal chlorpyrifos exposure on neurodevelopment in the first 3 years of life among inner-city children. *Pediatrics.* 2006 Dec;118(6):e1845-59

[581] Cheuk DK, Wong V. Attention-deficit hyperactivity disorder and blood mercury level: a case-control study in Chinese children. *Neuropediatrics.* 2006 Aug;37(4):234-40

[582] Nigg JT, Knottnerus GM, Martel MM, Nikolas M, Cavanagh K, Karmaus W, Rappley MD. Low blood lead levels associated with clinically diagnosed attention-deficit/hyperactivity disorder and mediated by weak cognitive control. *Biol Psychiatry.* 2008 Feb 1;63(3):325-31

[583] Crinnion W. Results of a Decade of Naturopathic Treatment for Environmental Illnesses: A Review of Clinical Records. *J Naturopathic Medicine* vol. 7; 2, 21-27

[584] Crinnion WJ. Environmental medicine, part 1: the human burden of environmental toxins and their common health effects. *Altern Med Rev.* 2000 Feb;5(1):52-63

[585] Crinnion WJ. Environmental medicine, part 2 - health effects of and protection from ubiquitous airborne solvent exposure. *Altern Med Rev.* 2000 Apr;5(2):133-43

[586] Crinnion WJ. Environmental medicine, part 3: long-term effects of chronic low-dose mercury exposure. *Altern Med Rev.* 2000 Jun;5(3):209-23

[587] Crinnion WJ. Environmental medicine, part 4: pesticides - biologically persistent and ubiquitous toxins. *Altern Med Rev.* 2000 Oct;5(5):432-47

[588] Rea WJ, Pan Y, Johnson AR. Clearing of toxic volatile hydrocarbons from humans. *Bol Asoc Med P R.* 1991 Jul;83(7):321-4

[589] Bland JS, Barrager E, Reedy RG, Bland K. A Medical Food-Supplemented Detoxification Program in the Management of Chronic Health Problems. *Altern Ther Health Med.* 1995 Nov 1;1(5):62-71

[590] Minich DM, Bland JS. Acid-alkaline balance: role in chronic disease and detoxification. *Altern Ther Health Med.* 2007 Jul-Aug;13(4):62-5

[591] Vasquez A. *Integrative Rheumatology: Second Edition*. Fort Worth, Texas; Integrative and Biological Medicine Research and Consulting, 2007 InflammationMastery.com

[592] Vasquez A. Diabetes: Are Toxins to Blame? *Naturopathy Digest* 2007; April

[593] Kilburn KH, Warsaw RH, Shields MG. Neurobehavioral dysfunction in firemen exposed to polycholorinated biphenyls (PCBs): possible improvement after detoxification. *Arch Environ Health.* 1989 Nov-Dec;44(6):345-50

[594] Cecchini M, LoPresti V. Drug residues store in the body following cessation of use: impacts on neuroendocrine balance and behavior--use of the Hubbard sauna regimen to remove toxins and restore health. *Med Hypotheses.* 2007;68(4):868-79

[595] Vasquez A. *Integrative Rheumatology: Second Edition*. Fort Worth, Texas; Integrative and Biological Medicine Research and Consulting, 2007 InflammationMastery.com

haptenization and neoantigen formation. These influences may act singularly or when combined may be additive and synergistic. While it is beyond the scope of this monograph to detail each of these here, they will be sufficiently reviewed in later sections dealing with assessment and interventions as well as in the clinical focus subsections, particularly the section on rheumatoid arthritis.

5. Inflammatory imbalances: Inflammatory imbalances may be distinguished from immune imbalances insofar as inflammatory imbalances connote disorders of inflammatory mediator production in the absence of the immunodysfunction that typifies allergy, autoimmunity, or immunosuppression. Here again, long-term consumption of a pro-inflammatory diet[596] is a primary consideration because such a diet typically oversupplies inflammatory precursors such as arachidonate and undersupplies anti-inflammatory phytonutrients such as vitamin D, zinc, selenium, and the numerous phytochemicals that reduce activation of inflammatory pathways.[597,598,599,600] Three of the best examples of correctable inflammatory imbalances are those due to vitamin D deficiency, fatty acid imbalances, and overconsumption of simple sugars and saturated fats. Vitamin D deficiency is a widespread and serious health problem that spans nearly all geographic regions and socioeconomic strata with several important adverse effects. Vitamin D deficiency results in systemic inflammation[601] and chronic musculoskeletal pain[602] which both resolve quickly upon correction of the nutritional deficiency. Similarly and consistent with the Western/American pattern of dietary intake, overconsumption of alpha-linoleic acid and arachidonate along with underconsumption of alpha-linolenic acid (ALA), gamma-linolenic acid (GLA), eicosapentaenoic acid (EPA), docosahexaenoic acid (DHA), and oleic acid subtly yet powerfully shift nutrigenomic tendency and precursor availability in favor of enhanced systemic inflammation. Correction of this imbalance such as with reduced consumption of arachidonate and increased consumption of EPA and DHA has consistently proven to be of significant clinical value in the management of chronic inflammatory disorders.[603,604] Measurable increases in systemic inflammation and oxidative stress follow glucose challenge[605], consumption of saturated fatty acids as found in cream[606], and consumption of a "fast food" breakfast, which triggers the prototypic inflammatory activator NF-kappaB for enhanced production of inflammatory mediators.[607] This triad (vitamin D deficiency, fatty acid imbalance, and overconsumption of sugars and saturated fats) is typical of the Western/American pattern of dietary intake, and the molecular means and clinical consequences of such dietary choices is quite clear, evidenced by burgeoning epidemics of metabolic and inflammatory diseases.

6. Digestive, absorptive, and microbiological imbalances: The grouping of digestive and absorptive considerations suggests that the alimentary tract and its accessory organs of the liver, gall bladder and pancreas will be the focus of these core clinical imbalances, and the addition of microbiological imbalances should remind current clinicians that gastrointestinal dysbiosis is an important and frequent clinical consideration. Impaired digestion begins neither in the stomach nor in the mouth, but it stems rather from any socioeconomic milieu which deprives people of the means to prepare wholesome health-promoting meals and the time to consume those meals in a relaxed parasympathetic-dominant mode, preferably among good company, stimulating conversation, and appropriate ambiance. Poor dentition, xerostomia, hypochlorhydria, cholestasis or cholecystectomy, pancreatic insufficiency, mucosal atrophy, altered gut

[596] Seaman DR. The diet-induced proinflammatory state: a cause of chronic pain and other degenerative diseases? *J Manipulative Physiol Ther.* 2002 Mar-Apr;25(3):168-79

[597] Vasquez A. Reducing Pain and Inflammation Naturally. Part 1: New Insights into Fatty Acid Biochemistry and the Influence of Diet. *Nutritional Perspectives* 2004; October: 5, 7-10, 12, 14

[598] Vasquez A. Reducing Pain and Inflammation Naturally. Part 2: New Insights into Fatty Acid Supplementation and Its Effect on Eicosanoid Production and Genetic Expression. *Nutritional Perspectives* 2005; January: 5-16

[599] Vasquez A. Reducing pain and inflammation naturally - Part 3: Improving overall health while safely and effectively treating musculoskeletal pain. *Nutritional Perspectives* 2005; 28: 34-38, 40-42

[600] Vasquez A. Reducing pain and inflammation naturally - Part 4: Nutritional and Botanical Inhibition of NF-kappaB, the Major Intracellular Amplifier of the Inflammatory Cascade. A Practical Clinical Strategy Exemplifying Anti-Inflammatory Nutrigenomics. *Nutritional Perspectives* 2005;July: 5-12

[601] Timms PM, Mannan N, Hitman GA, Noonan K, Mills PG, Syndercombe-Court D, Aganna E, Price CP, Boucher BJ. Circulating MMP9, vitamin D and variation in the TIMP-1 response with VDR genotype: mechanisms for inflammatory damage in chronic disorders? *QJM.* 2002 Dec;95(12):787-96

[602] Al Faraj S, Al Mutairi K. Vitamin D deficiency and chronic low back pain in Saudi Arabia. *Spine.* 2003 Jan 15;28(2):177-9

[603] James MJ, Gibson RA, Cleland LG. Dietary polyunsaturated fatty acids and inflammatory mediator production. *Am J Clin Nutr.* 2000 Jan;71(1 Suppl):343S-8S

[604] James MJ, Proudman SM, Cleland LG. Dietary n-3 fats as adjunctive therapy in a prototypic inflammatory disease: issues and obstacles for use in rheumatoid arthritis. Prostaglandins *Leukot Essent Fatty Acids.* 2003 Jun;68(6):399-405

[605] Mohanty P, Hamouda W, Garg R, Aljada A, Ghanim H, Dandona P. Glucose challenge stimulates reactive oxygen species (ROS) generation by leucocytes. *J Clin Endocrinol Metab.* 2000 Aug;85(8):2970-3

[606] Mohanty P, Ghanim H, Hamouda W, Aljada A, Garg R, Dandona P. Both lipid and protein intakes stimulate increased generation of reactive oxygen species by polymorphonuclear leukocytes and mononuclear cells. *Am J Clin Nutr.* 2002 Apr;75(4):767-72

[607] Aljada A, Mohanty P, Ghanim H, Abdo T, Tripathy D, Chaudhuri A, Dandona P. Increase in intranuclear nuclear factor kappaB and decrease in inhibitor kappaB in mononuclear cells after a mixed meal: evidence for a proinflammatory effect. *Am J Clin Nutr.* 2004 Apr;79(4):682-90

motility, and bacterial overgrowth of the small bowel are important and common contributors to impaired digestion and absorption; clinicians should consider these frequently and implement treatment with a low threshold for intervention. The relevance of these problems to pain and the musculoskeletal system is generally that of malnutrition and its macro- and micronutrient consequences. Sunlight-deprived individuals must rely on dietary sources of vitamin D, which are hardly adequate for the prevention of overt deficiency; any impairment in digestion, emulsification, or absorption of this fat-soluble vitamin can readily lead to hypovitaminosis D and its resultant musculoskeletal consequences of osteomalacia and unremitting pain.[608] Consumption of foods to which the individual is sensitized ("food allergies") can trigger migraine and other chronic headaches[609,610] as well as generalized musculoskeletal pain and arthritis.[611,612,613] Avoidance of the offending foods often results in amelioration or complete remission of the painful syndrome at low cost and high efficacy without reliance on expensive or potentially harmful or addictive pain-reliving drugs. Occasionally, gluten enteropathy (celiac disease) presents with arthritic pain and chronic synovitis; the pain and inflammation remit on a gluten-free diet.[614] Alterations in intestinal microbial balance or an individual's unique response to endogenous bacteria (i.e., dysbiosis) can lead to systemic inflammation, arthritis, vasculitis, and musculoskeletal pain; clinical nuances and molecular mechanisms of gastrointestinal dysbiosis will be surveyed later in this monograph based on a previous review by Vasquez.[615] Clinicians should appreciate that dysbiosis can occur at sites other than the gastrointestinal tract, most importantly the nasopharynx and genitourinary tracts. Eradication of the occult infection or mucosal colonization often results in marked reductions in systemic inflammation and its clinical complications. Interested readers are directed to the excellent review by Noah[616] on the relevance of dysbiosis and its treatment relative to psoriasis; additional citations and clinical applications will be discussed later in this monograph.

7. <u>Structural imbalances from cellular membrane function to the musculoskeletal system</u>: Molecular structural imbalances lie at the heart of the concept of "biochemical individuality" originated by Roger J. Williams[617] in 1956, and this concept was soon thereafter expanded into the theory and practice of "orthomolecular medicine" pioneered by Linus Pauling and colleagues.[618,619] Pauling is considered by many authorities to be the original source of the concept of molecular medicine because he coined the phrase "molecular disease" after his team's discovery in 1949 that sickle cell anemia resulted from a single amino acid substitution that caused physical deformation of the hemoglobin molecule in hypoxic conditions.[620] (One of Pauling's students, Jeffery Bland, continued this legacy with the organization of "functional medicine" which now lives on as the Institute for Functional Medicine.[621]) Single nucleotide polymorphisms (SNP; pronounced "snip") are DNA sequence variations that can result in amino acid substitutions that render the final protein (e.g., structural protein or enzyme) abnormal in structure and therefore function. This aberrancy may or may not cause clinical disease (depending on the severity and importance of the variation), and consequences of the dysfunction may be occult, subtle, or obvious. One of the most powerful and effective means for treating diseases resultant from SNPs that result in enzyme defects is the use of high-dose vitamin supplementation, and this forms the scientific basis for "mega-vitamin therapy" as elegantly and authoritatively reviewed by Bruce Ames, et al.[622] SNP-induced

[608] Basha B, Rao DS, Han ZH, Parfitt AM. Osteomalacia due to vitamin D depletion: a neglected consequence of intestinal malabsorption. *Am J Med*. 2000 Mar;108(4):296-300

[609] Grant EC. Food allergies and migraine. *Lancet*. 1979 May 5;1(8123):966-9

[610] Millichap JG, Yee MM. The diet factor in pediatric and adolescent migraine. *Pediatr Neurol*. 2003 Jan;28(1):9-15

[611] van de Laar MA, Aalbers M, Bruins FG, et al. Food intolerance in rheumatoid arthritis. II. Clinical and histological aspects. *Ann Rheum Dis*. 1992 ;51(3):303-6

[612] Golding DN. Is there an allergic synovitis? *J R Soc Med*. 1990 May;83(5):312-4

[613] Hvatum M, Kanerud L, Hällgren R, Brandtzaeg P. The gut-joint axis: cross reactive food antibodies in rheumatoid arthritis. *Gut*. 2006 Sep;55:1240-7

[614] Bourne JT, Kumar P, Huskisson EC, Mageed R, Unsworth DJ, Wojtulewski JA. Arthritis and coeliac disease. *Ann Rheum Dis*. 1985 Sep;44(9):592-8

[615] Vasquez A. Reducing Pain and Inflammation Naturally. Part 6: Nutritional and Botanical Treatments Against "Silent Infections" and Gastrointestinal Dysbiosis, Commonly Overlooked Causes of Neuromusculoskeletal Inflammation and Chronic Health Problems. *Nutr Perspect* 2006; Jan: 5-21

[616] Noah PW. The role of microorganisms in psoriasis. *Semin Dermatol*. 1990 Dec;9(4):269-76

[617] Williams RJ. <u>Biochemical Individuality : The Basis for the Genetotrophic Concept</u>. Austin and London: University of Texas Press, 1956. Page x

[618] Pauling L. On the Orthomolecular Environment of the Mind: Orthomolecular Theory. In: Williams RJ, Kalita DK. <u>A Physician's Handbook on Orthomolecular Medicine</u>. New Cannan; Keats Publishing; 1977. Page 76

[619] Pauling L, Robinson AB, Teranishi R, Cary P. Quantitative analysis of urine vapor and breath by gas-liquid partition chromatography. *Proc Natl Acad Sci* 1971 Oct;68:2374-6

[620] Pauling L, Itano HA, Singer SJ, Wells IC. Sickle cell anemia, a molecular disease. *Science*. 1949 Nov 25;110(2865):543-8

[621] Bland JS. Jeffrey S. Bland, PhD, FACN, CNS: functional medicine pioneer. *Altern Ther Health Med*. 2004 Sep-Oct;10(5):74-81

[622] Ames BN, Elson-Schwab I, Silver EA. High-dose vitamin therapy stimulates variant enzymes with decreased coenzyme binding affinity (increased K(m)): relevance to genetic disease and polymorphisms. *Am J Clin Nutr*. 2002 Apr;75(4):616-58

alterations in enzyme structure reduce affinity for vitamin-derived coenzyme binding; this reduced affinity can be "overpowered" by administration of high doses of the required vitamin cofactor to increase tissue concentrations of the nutrient to promote binding of the enzyme with its ligand for the performance of enzymatic function. Thus, the scientific rationale for nutritional therapy is derived in part from the recognition that altered enzymatic function due to altered enzyme structure can often be corrected by administration of supradietary doses of nutrients. Relatedly, the structure and function of cell membranes is determined by their composition, which is influenced by dietary intake of fatty acids, and which influences production prostaglandins and leukotrienes. This is an important aspect of the scientific rationale for the use of specific fatty acid supplements in the prevention and treatment of painful inflammatory musculoskeletal disease. Cell membrane structure and function can also be altered by systemic oxidative stress; the concomitant alterations in intracellular ions (e.g., calcium) and receptor function along with activation of transcription factors such as NF-kappaB contribute to widespread physiologic impairment which creates a vicious cycle of inflammation, metabolic disturbance, and additional free radical generation.[623,624] Somatic dysfunction, musculoskeletal disorders, and inefficient biomechanics contribute to pain, increased production of inflammatory mediators, and the expedited degeneration of tissues such as collagen and cartilage matrix. Physicians trained in clinical biomechanics and physical medicine appreciate the subtle nuances of musculoskeletal structure-function relationships and address these problems directly with physical and manual means rather than ignoring the physical problem and only treating its biochemical sequelae. While biomechanics, palpatory diagnosis, and manual therapeutics takes years of diligent study for the achievement of proficiency, some of these concepts will be reviewed later in this monograph, particularly in the section on chronic low back pain.

8. <u>Psychological and Spiritual Equilibrium</u>: The connections between physical pain and psychoemotional status and events is worthy of thorough discussion and not merely for the sake of improving upon outdated clinical practices which have typically marginalized these ethereal considerations or considered them only long enough to substantiate psychopharmaceutical intervention. A survey of the literature makes clear the interconnected nature of pain, inflammation, psychoemotional stress, depression, social isolation, and nutritional status; due to space limitations in this monograph, a brief overview must necessarily suffice for the exemplification of representative concepts. Stressful and depressive life events promote the development, persistence, and exacerbation of disorders of pain and inflammation through nutritional, hormonal, immunologic, oxidative, and microbiologic mechanisms. Stated most simply, the perception of stressful events and the resultant neurohormonal cascade results in expedited metabolic utilization and increased urinary excretion of nutrients (e.g., tryptophan , and zinc, magnesium, retinol, respectively) which sum to effect nutritional imbalances and depletion, particularly when the stress response is severe and prolonged.[625,626,627] Specific to the consideration of pain, the depletion of tryptophan (and thus serotonin and melatonin) leaves the patient vulnerable to increased pain from lack of antinociceptive serotonin and to increased inflammation due to impaired endogenous production of anti-inflammatory cortisol, the adrenal release of which requires serotonin-dependent stimulation.[628] Severe stress, inflammation, and drugs used to suppress immune-mediated tissue damage (e.g., cyclosporine) increase urinary excretion of magnesium[629], and the eventual magnesium depletion renders the patient more vulnerable to hyperalgesia, depression, and other central nervous system and psychiatric disorders.[630,631] Furthermore, experimental and clinical data have shown that magnesium deficiency leads to a systemic pro-inflammatory state associated with oxidative stress and increased levels of the nociceptive and proinflammatory

[623] Evans JL, Maddux BA, Goldfine ID. The molecular basis for oxidative stress-induced insulin resistance. *Antioxid Redox Signal*. 2005 Jul-Aug;7(7-8):1040-52

[624] Joseph JA, Denisova N, Fisher D, Shukitt-Hale B, Bickford P, Prior R, Cao G. Membrane and receptor modifications of oxidative stress vulnerability in aging. Nutritional considerations. *Ann N Y Acad Sci*. 1998 Nov 20;854:268-76

[625] Stephensen CB, Alvarez JO, Kohatsu J, Hardmeier R, Kennedy JI Jr, Gammon RB Jr. Vitamin A is excreted in the urine during acute infection. *Am J Clin Nutr*. 1994 Sep;60(3):388-92

[626] Ingenbleek Y, Bernstein L. The stressful condition as a nutritionally dependent adaptive dichotomy. *Nutrition*. 1999 Apr;15(4):305-20

[627] Henrotte JG, Plouin PF, Lévy-Leboyer C, Moser G, Sidoroff-Girault N, Franck G, Santarromana M, Pineau M. Blood and urinary magnesium, zinc, calcium, free fatty acids, and catecholamines in type A and type B subjects. *J Am Coll Nutr*. 1985;4(2):165-72

[628] Sandyk R. Tryptophan availability and the susceptibility to stress in multiple sclerosis: a hypothesis. *Int J Neurosci*. 1996 Jul;86(1-2):47-53

[629] DiPalma JR. Magnesium replacement therapy. *Am Fam Physician*. 1990 Jul;42(1):173-6

[630] Murck H. Magnesium and affective disorders. *Nutr Neurosci*. 2002 Dec;5(6):375-89

[631] Hashizume N, Mori M. An analysis of hypermagnesemia and hypomagnesemia. *Jpn J Med*. 1990 Jul-Aug;29(4):368-72

neurotransmitter substance P.[632] Stress increases secretion of prolactin, a hormone which plays an important pathogenic role in chronic inflammation and autoimmunity.[633,634] An abundance of experimental and clinical research supports the model that chronic psychoemotional stress reduces mucosal immunity, increases intestinal permeability, and allows for increased intestinal colonization by microbes that then stimulate immune responses that cross-react with musculoskeletal tissues and result in the clinical manifestation of autoimmunity and painful rheumatic syndromes which appear clinically as variants of acute and chronic reactive arthritis (formerly Reiter' syndrome[635]) in susceptible patients.[636,637,638,639,640,641,642,643] Very interestingly, certain intestinal bacteria can sense when their human host is stressed, and they take advantage of the situation by becoming more virulent whereas previously these same bacteria may have been incapable of causing disease.[644,645] Psychoemotional stress also reduces mucosal immunity and increases colonization in locations other than the gastrointestinal tract. Microbial colonization of the genitourinary tract ("genitourinary dysbiosis"[646]) appears highly relevant in the genesis and perpetuation of rheumatoid arthritis.[647,648,649,650] Stressful life events also lower testosterone in men and the resultant lack of hormonal immunomodulation can increase the frequency and severity of exacerbations of rheumatoid arthritis[651]; resultant inflammation further suppresses testosterone production and bioavailability[652] leading to a self-perpetuating cycle of hypogonadism and inflammation. Thus, by numerous routes and mechanisms, psychoemotional stress increases the prevalence, persistence, and severity of musculoskeletal inflammation and pain.

Psychiatric codiagnoses are common among patients with painful neuromusculoskeletal disorders, and when the prevailing medical logic cannot solve the musculoskeletal riddle, the disorder is often ascribed to its accompanying mental disorder. The "appropriate" treatment from this perspective is the prescription of psychoactive drugs, generally of the "antidepressant" class. Science-based explanations are needed to expand clinicians' consideration of new possibilities which may someday prevail over commonplace suppositions that leave both clinician and patient trapped within a paradigm of futilely cyclical reasoning and its resultant simplistic symptom-targeting interventions. The following subsections provide alternatives to the "idiopathic pain is caused by its associated depression and both should be treated with antidepressant drugs" hypothesis.

    a.   <u>Pain, inflammation, and mental depression are final common pathways for nutritional deficiencies and imbalances</u>: As a scientific community we now know that the epidemic problem of vitamin D

---

[632] Weglicki W, Quamme G, Tucker K, Haigney M, Resnick L. Potassium, magnesium, and electrolyte imbalance and complications in disease management. *Clin Exp Hypertens.* 2005 Jan;27(1):95-112

[633] Imrich R. The role of neuroendocrine system in the pathogenesis of rheumatic diseases (minireview). *Endocr Regul.* 2002 Jun;36(2):95-106

[634] Orbach H, Shoenfeld Y. Hyperprolactinemia and autoimmune diseases. Autoimmun Rev. 2007 Sep;6(8):537-42

[635] Panush RS, Wallace DJ, Dorff RE, Engleman EP. Retraction of the suggestion to use the term "Reiter's syndrome" sixty-five years later: the legacy of Reiter, a war criminal, should not be eponymic honor but rather condemnation. *Arthritis Rheum.* 2007 Feb;56(2):693-4

[636] Tlaskalová-Hogenová H, Stepánková R, Hudcovic T, Tucková L, Cukrowska B, Lodinová-Zádníková R, Kozáková H, Rossmann P, Bártová J, Sokol D, Funda DP, Borovská D, Reháková Z, Sinkora J, Hofman J, Drastich P, Kokesová A. Commensal bacteria (normal microflora), mucosal immunity and chronic inflammatory and autoimmune diseases. *Immunol Lett.* 2004 May 15;93(2-3):97-108

[637] Collins SM. Stress and the Gastrointestinal Tract IV. Modulation of intestinal inflammation by stress: basic mechanisms and clinical relevance. *Am J Physiol Gastrointest Liver Physiol.* 2001 Mar;280(3):G315-8

[638] Hart A, Kamm MA. Review article: mechanisms of initiation and perpetuation of gut inflammation by stress. *Aliment Pharmacol Ther.* 2002 Dec;16(12):2017-28

[639] Farhadi A, Fields JZ, Keshavarzian A. Mucosal mast cells are pivotal elements in inflammatory bowel disease that connect the dots: stress, intestinal hyperpermeability and inflammation. *World J Gastroenterol.* 2007 Jun 14;13(22):3027-30

[640] Yang PC, Jury J, Söderholm JD, Sherman PM, McKay DM, Perdue MH. Chronic psychological stress in rats induces intestinal sensitization to luminal antigens. *Am J Pathol.* 2006 Jan;168(1):104-14

[641] Rashid T, Ebringer A. Ankylosing spondylitis is linked to Klebsiella--the evidence. *Clin Rheumatol.* 2007 Jun;26(6):858-64

[642] Vasquez A. *Integrative Rheumatology.* Fort Worth, Texas; Integrative and Biological Medicine Research and Consulting, 2007 InflammationMastery.com

[643] Samarkos M, Vaiopoulos G. The role of infections in the pathogenesis of autoimmune diseases. *Curr Drug Targets Inflamm Allergy.* 2005 Feb;4(1):99-103

[644] Alverdy J, Holbrook C, Rocha F, Seiden L, Wu RL, Musch M, Chang E, Ohman D, Suh S. Gut-derived sepsis occurs when the right pathogen with the right virulence genes meets the right host: evidence for in vivo virulence expression in Pseudomonas aeruginosa. *Ann Surg.* 2000 Oct;232(4):480-9

[645] Wu L, Holbrook C, Zaborina O, Ploplys E, Rocha F, Pelham D, Chang E, Musch M, Alverdy J. Pseudomonas aeruginosa expresses a lethal virulence determinant, the PA-I lectin/adhesin, in the intestinal tract of a stressed host: the role of epithelia cell contact and molecules of the Quorum Sensing Signaling System. *Ann Surg.* 2003;238(5):754-64

[646] Vasquez A. *Integrative Rheumatology: Second Edition.* Fort Worth, Texas; Integrative and Biological Medicine Research and Consulting, 2007 InflammationMastery.com

[647] Ebringer A, Rashid T. Rheumatoid arthritis is an autoimmune disease triggered by Proteus urinary tract infection. *Clin Dev Immunol.* 2006 Mar;13(1):41-8

[648] Erlacher L, Wintersberger W, Menschik M, Benke-Studnicka A, Machold K, Stanek G, Söltz-Szöts J, Smolen J, Graninger W. Reactive arthritis: urogenital swab culture is the only useful diagnostic method for the detection of the arthritogenic infection in extra-articularly asymptomatic patients with undifferentiated oligoarthritis *Br J Rheumatol.* 1995 Sep;34(9):838-42

[649] Rashid T, Ebringer A. Rheumatoid arthritis is linked to Proteus--the evidence. *Clin Rheumatol.* 2007 Jul;26(7):1036-43

[650] Ebringer A, Rashid T, Wilson C. Rheumatoid arthritis: proposal for the use of anti-microbial therapy in early cases. *Scand J Rheumatol.* 2003;32:2-11

[651] James WH. Further evidence that low androgen values are a cause of rheumatoid arthritis: the response of rheumatoid arthritis to seriously stressful life events. *Ann Rheum Dis* 1997;56:566

[652] Karagiannis A, Harsoulis F. Gonadal dysfunction in systemic diseases. *Eur J Endocrinol.* 2005 Apr;152(4):501-13

deficiency leads to both musculoskeletal pain[653] as well as depression[654], and that supplementation with physiologic doses of vitamin D results in an enhanced sense of well-being[655] and high-efficacy alleviation of musculoskeletal pain and depression while providing other major collateral benefits.[656] Since the existence of vitamin D deficiency is more probable than that of antidepressant deficiency, the appropriate intervention for the former is more scientific and rational than that of the latter. Relatedly, research in various fields has shown that Western/American lifestyle and diet patterns diverge radically from human physiologic expectations and human nutritional requirements.[657] With regard to fatty acid intake and the resultant effects on inflammation and neurotransmission, modernized diets are a "set up" for musculoskeletal pain and mental depression, which frequently occur concomitantly and which are both alleviated by corrective fatty acid intervention such as fish oil supplementation as a source of EPA and DHA.[658,659] Correction of fatty acid imbalance is therefore more rational in the comanagement of pain and depression than is sole reliance on antidepressant and anti-inflammatory drugs; the latter have their place in treatment but neither addresses the primary cause of the problem and both drug classes have important adverse effects and significant cost in contrast to the safety, affordability, and collateral benefits derived from fatty acid supplementation. Also relevant to this discussion of chronic pain triggered and perpetuated by nutritional imbalances are the pro-inflammatory nature of the Western/American diet[660] and the pain-sensitizing effects of epidemic magnesium deficiency.[661] Therefore, correction of nutritional deficiencies and optimization of nutritional status might supersede the prescription of drugs in patients with concomitant depression and pain.

b. <u>Pain, inflammation, and depression are final common pathways of physical inactivity</u>: Exercising muscle elaborates cytokines ("myokines") with anti-inflammatory activity; a sedentary lifestyle fails to stimulate this endogenous anti-inflammation and is therefore relatively pro-inflammatory.[662] Further, exercise has antidepressant benefits mediated by positive influences on neurotransmission, growth factor elaboration, endocrinologic function, self-image, and social contact.[663] Patients with musculoskeletal pain should be encouraged to exercise to the extent possible given the individual's capacity and type of injury and/or degree of disability. Thus, a prescription for exercise might supersede the prescription of drugs in patients with concomitant depression and pain. Exercise prescriptions must consider frequency, duration, intensity, variety, safety, enjoyment, accountability and objective measures of compliance and progress, as well as appropriate combinations of components which emphasize aerobic fitness, strengthening, flexibility, muscle balancing, and coordination.

c. <u>Pain and depression are final common pathways of inflammation</u>: Several pro-inflammatory cytokines are psychoactive and cause depression, social withdrawal, impaired cognition, and sickness behavior.[664] As an alternative to the use of antidepressant drugs, correction of the underlying inflammatory disorder by natural, pharmacologic, or integrative means may subsequently promote restoration of normal affect and cognitive function.

d. <u>Pain, inflammation, and mental depression are final common pathways for hormonal deficiencies and imbalances</u>: Deficiencies of thyroid hormones, estrogen (insufficiency or excess), testosterone,

---

[653] Plotnikoff GA, Quigley JM. Prevalence of severe hypovitaminosis D in patients with persistent, nonspecific musculoskeletal pain. *Mayo Clin Proc*. 2003 Dec;78(12):1463-70
[654] Wilkins CH, Sheline YI, Roe CM, Birge SJ, Morris JC. Vitamin D deficiency is associated with low mood and worse cognitive performance in older adults. *Am J Geriatr Psychiatry*. 2006 Dec;14(12):1032-40
[655] Vieth R, Kimball S, Hu A, Walfish PG. Randomized comparison of the effects of the vitamin D3 adequate intake versus 100 mcg (4000 IU) per day on biochemical responses and the wellbeing of patients. *Nutr J*. 2004 Jul 19;3:8
[656] Vasquez A, Manso G, Cannell J. The clinical importance of vitamin D (cholecalciferol): a paradigm shift with implications for all healthcare providers. *Altern Ther Health Med*. 2004 Sep-Oct;10(5):28-36
[657] O'Keefe JH Jr, Cordain L. Cardiovascular disease resulting from a diet and lifestyle at odds with our Paleolithic genome: how to become a 21st-century hunter-gatherer. *Mayo Clin Proc*. 2004 Jan;79(1):101-8
[658] Kiecolt-Glaser JK, Belury MA, Porter K, Beversdorf DQ, Lemeshow S, Glaser R. Depressive symptoms, omega-6:omega-3 fatty acids, and inflammation in older adults. *Psychosom Med*. 2007 Apr;69(3):217-24
[659] Simopoulos AP. Omega-3 fatty acids in inflammation and autoimmune diseases. *J Am Coll Nutr*. 2002 Dec;21(6):495-505
[660] Aljada A, Mohanty P, Ghanim H, Abdo T, Tripathy D, Chaudhuri A, Dandona P. Increase in intranuclear nuclear factor kappaB and decrease in inhibitor kappaB in mononuclear cells after a mixed meal: evidence for a proinflammatory effect. *Am J Clin Nutr*. 2004 Apr;79(4):682-90
[661] Park JH, Niermann KJ, Olsen N. Evidence for metabolic abnormalities in the muscles of patients with fibromyalgia. *Curr Rheumatol Rep*. 2000 Apr;2(2):131-40
[662] Petersen AM, Pedersen BK. The anti-inflammatory effect of exercise. *J Appl Physiol*. 2005 Apr;98(4):1154-62
[663] Cotman CW, Berchtold NC, Christie LA. Exercise builds brain health: key roles of growth factor cascades and inflammation. *Trends Neurosci*. 2007 Sep;30(9):464-72
[664] Wilson CJ, Finch CE, Cohen HJ. Cytokines and cognition--the case for a head-to-toe inflammatory paradigm. *J Am Geriatr Soc*. 2002 Dec;50(12):2041-56

cortisol, and DHEA can cause depression and impaired neuroemotional status. Hormonal aberrations are common in patients with chronic musculoskeletal pain, particularly of the inflammatory and autoimmune types. Clinical trials have shown that administration of thyroid hormones, testosterone, DHEA, cortisol and suppression prolactin can each provide anti-inflammatory, analgesic, and antidepressant benefits among appropriately selected patients. Thus, identification and correction of hormonal imbalances might supersede the prescription of antidepressant drugs in patients with concomitant depression, inflammation, and pain.

Our cultural and scientific advancements in the knowledge of how the brain and mind function have been paradoxically paralleled by social trends showing increasing depression and social isolation; the typical American has only two friends and no one in whom to confide.[665] In the United States, violent injuries are epidemic, and the level of firearm morbidity and mortality in the US is far higher than anywhere else in the industrialized world.[666] This does to some extent beg the question of the value of "scientific knowledge" of the brain and mind within a social structure that is increasingly violent and fragmented. Further, the mental depression resultant from pandemic social isolation would be better served by physicians' admonition for increased social contact than by the continued overuse of drugs which inhibit neurotransmitter reuptake.

Conclusion: The clinical employment of the functional medicine approach to chronic disease management and health promotion rests upon a foundation of competent patient management and then extends to consider the well documented contributions of the causative *core clinical imbalances* that have allowed the genesis and perpetuation of the problem(s) under consideration. The attainment of wellness, the success of preventive medicine, and the optimization of socioemotional health cannot be attained by pharmacological suppression of the manifestations of dysfunction that result from nutritional and neuroendocrine imbalances, xenobiotic accumulation, sedentary lifestyles, social isolation, and mucosal microbial colonization. Rather, these problems are addressed directly, and these and other causative considerations must remain foremost in the mind of the physician committed to the successful, ethical, and cost-effective long-term prevention and management of chronic health disturbances, particularly those characterized by inflammation and pain.

[665] McPherson M, Smith-Lovin L, Brashears ME. Social Isolation in America: Changes in Core Discussion Networks over Two Decades. *Am Sociological Rev* 2006; 71: 353-75
[666] Preventing firearm violence: a public health imperative. American College of Physicians. *Ann Intern Med*. 1995 Feb 15;122(4):311-3

Iron Overload and Genetic Hemochromatosis

Introduction to Iron Overload

In its "classic" form, homozygous genetic hemochromatosis is noted in about 1 per 200-250 Caucasian persons, with a similar incidence among Hispanics. The incidence among persons of African descent is notably higher, reported as high as 1 per 80 among hospitalized African Americans. The heterozygous form of iron overload which is phenotypically milder occurs in as many as 1 per 7 (14% of total) persons; any disorder that is common in the general population will be even more common in a clinical population of symptomatic care-seeking patients, especially those with musculoskeletal disorders and complaints.[667]

Testing serum ferritin on a routine basis in clinical practice allows for the detection of iron deficiency (very common, even among non-anemic patients) and iron overload (quite common, especially among patients with joint pain, diabetes, heart failure, and liver disease as well as many other clinical manifestations—most common of which is asymptomaticity.

---

[667] Vasquez A. Musculoskeletal disorders and iron overload disease: comment on the American College of Rheumatology guidelines for the initial evaluation of the adult patient with acute musculoskeletal symptoms. *Arthritis & Rheumatism*: Official Journal of the American College of Rheumatology 1996; 39:1767-8

Iron Overload
Primary/Genetic Hemochromatosis
Secondary Hemochromatosis

Description/pathophysiology:

- Hereditary iron overload disorders are now recognized as being among the most common genetic diseases in the human population.[668,669,670,671,672,673,674]

- Iron overload is a phenotypic state to which a patient arrives by either genetic or environmental/iatrogenic routes. The severity of iron overload can range from moderate to severe.

- Excess iron catalyzes oxidative stress which damages body tissues and structures in which the iron is stored. In patients with genetic hemochromatosis, two problems exist simultaneously: 1) a disproportionately large amount of iron is absorbed from the gastrointestinal tract (i.e., these patients' iron absorption is "too efficient"), and 2) iron is preferentially deposited in parenchymal tissues such as the heart, liver, pancreas, pituitary gland, and joints rather than being stored safely within the reticuloendothelial system. The deposition of excess iron in parenchymal tissues promotes destruction of these organs/tissues via oxidative mechanisms and subsequent tissue necrosis and fibrosis, leading to the protean manifestations of the disease dependent upon which organs are most affected in the individual patient: heart failure, hepatic fibrosis, hypoinsulinemic diabetes, hypopituarism, and hemochromatoic arthropathy.[675]

- Iron overload can be defined as a state of "iron toxicity" similar to mercury toxicity or poisoning with any other heavy metal or toxin, except that the mechanism is more related to the *quantity* of the iron rather than the unique characteristics or *quality* of iron itself. In other words, whereas the toxicity of mercury can be seen even when only small amounts of the metal are present, the toxicity of iron is directly related to the amount of the excess iron, rather than the inherent toxicity of the iron itself.

> **Iron overload disorders are common in all ethnic/racial populations**
>
> Genetic hemochromatosis is considered one of the most common hereditary disorders in the Caucasian population with a homozygote frequency of 1 per 200-250 (approx 0.5%) and a heterozygote frequency of about 1 in 7 (approx 14%); the condition is at least as common in other ethnic groups except that this predisposition toward iron overload is more common in Africans (as high as 1 in 20) and African-Americans (as high as about 1 in 80 in some series among hospitalized patients). Of course, the expected frequency would be even higher among symptomatic patients than among the general population. **Thus, for a clinician in full-time practice, the only reason for not appreciating this condition among one's patient population several times per year is because one is simply not sufficiently looking and testing for this condition.**

> **Rationale for screening all patients**
> 1. Hereditary iron-accumulation disorders occur in a large percentage of the population.
> 2. Persons with the disease usually have no symptoms.
> 3. Clinical manifestations are often indicative of irreversible organ damage or organ failure.
> 4. Iron overload can cause death if not treated early.
> 5. Early treatment ensures normal life expectancy.
> 6. **Therefore, early detection (before the onset of symptoms and organ damage) requires screening asymptomatic patients.**
>
> **Test of choice:** **Serum ferritin**, shows the best correlation with body iron stores and thus prognosis and need for treatment.

[668] Olynyk JK, Bacon BR. Hereditary hemochromatosis: detecting and correcting iron overload. *Postgrad Med* 1994; 96: 151-65

[669] Phatak PD, Cappuccio JD. Management of hereditary hemochromatosis. *Blood Rev* 1994; 8: 193-8

[670] Rouault TA. Hereditary hemochromatosis. *JAMA* 1993; 269: 3152-4

[671] Crosby WH. Hemochromatosis: current concepts and management. Hosp Pract 1987; 22:173-92

[672] Bloom PD, Gordeuk VR, MacPhail AP. HLA-linked hemochromatosis and other forms of iron overload. *Dermatol Clin* 1995; 13: 57-63

[673] Barton JC, Bertoli LF. Hemochromatosis: the genetic disorder of the twenty-first century. *Nat Med* 1996; 2: 394-5

[674] Lauffer, RB. Iron and Your Heart. New York: St. Martin's Press, 1991

[675] Vasquez A. Musculoskeletal disorders and iron overload disease: comment on the American College of Rheumatology guidelines for the initial evaluation of the adult patient with acute musculoskeletal symptoms. *Arthritis Rheum* 1996 Oct;39(10):1767-8

Clinical presentations:

- **Many patients are asymptomatic.**
- **Most patients eventually present with a problem that is attributed to another disorder:**
  - *Diabetes*: Patients may present with diabetes, which is erroneously attributed to metabolic syndrome or type-2 diabetes.[676]
  - *Musculoskeletal pain*: Patients may present with joint pain that is erroneously attributed to osteoarthritis[677], rheumatoid arthritis[678], or some other musculoskeletal syndrome.[679]
  - *Cardiomyopathy*: Patients may present with heart failure that is written off as "idiopathic cardiomyopathy."[680]
  - *Liver disease*: Hemochromatosis liver disease resembles and exacerbates viral hepatitis, alcoholic hepatitis, and porphyria.
- Fatigue, lethargy, weakness
- Chronic abdominal pain
- Liver damage: hepatomegaly, elevated serum levels of liver enzymes and alkaline phosphatase, fibrosis and cirrhosis, hepatocellular carcinoma, or other findings such as hematemesis and melena, ascites, hyperbilirubenemia and jaundice, hypoalbuminemia, hepatic encephalopathy, clotting dysfunction, anemia, liver abscess, increased incidence of esophageal carcinoma.
- Abnormal glucose metabolism or diabetes mellitus: elevated glucose levels. Usually asymptomatic, yet can cause weight loss, polyuria, polyphagia, polydypsia.
- Musculoskeletal disorders: arthritis and arthralgia, generalized osteoporosis, bone pain, myalgia. Especially arthropathy of the hands and wrists, hips, and knees.
- Cardiac dysfunction: cardiomyopathy, arrhythmia, fibrillation, congestive heart failure; shortness of breath or dyspnea on exertion, fatigue.
- Cutaneous manifestations: 'slate-gray' or ashen coloration, increased pigmentation ('tan') of the skin, atrophy of the skin, ichthyosis, koilonychia, loss of body hair, increased incidence of malignant melanoma.
- Endocrine disorders: hypogonadotrophic hypogonadism, (autoimmune) hypothyroidism, hyperthyroidism; manifest as decreased libido, impotence, testicular atrophy, or sterility in males, amenorrhea or difficulty conceiving in females, loss of body hair.
- Susceptibility to increased frequency and severity of infections, especially infections due to *Yersinia enterocolitica*, *Vibrio vulnificus*, HIV, and *Mycobacterium tuberculosis*.
- Neurologic symptoms: blurred vision, sensorineural hearing loss, hyperactivity, dementia, attention deficit disorder, ataxia, lightheadedness, dizziness, anxiety, depression, tinnitus, confusion, lethargy, memory loss,

---

Conditions causally associated with iron overload

Primary/genetic disorders
1. Homozygous genetic hemochromatosis
2. Heterozygous genetic hemochromatosis
3. African iron overload
4. African-American hemochromatosis (African-American iron overload)
5. Non-HLA-linked hemochromatosis
6. Juvenile hemochromatosis
7. Neonatal hemochromatosis

Secondary and metabolic disorders
8. Dietary excess of iron
9. Parenteral administration of iron in the form of iron injections and blood transfusions
10. Porphyria cutanea tarda
11. Portacaval shunt
12. Hepatic cirrhosis, portal hypertension, and splenomegally
13. AIDS
14. Sudden infant death syndrome
15. Alcoholism
16. Metabolic syndrome

Inherited red blood cell abnormalities ("iron-loading anemias", hemoglobinopathies)
17. Alpha-thalassemia
18. Beta-thalassemia
19. Thalassemia intermedia
20. Sideroblastic anemia
21. Aplastic anemia
22. Anemia associated with pyruvate kinase deficiency
23. AC hemoglobinopathy
24. AS hemoglobinopathy
25. X-linked hypochromic anemia
26. Pyridoxine-responsive anemia
27. Atransferrinemia

---

[676] "Most of the patients (95%) had one or more of the following conditions; obesity, hyperlipidaemia, abnormal glucose metabolism, or hypertension. INTERPRETATION: We have found a new non-HLA-linked iron-overload syndrome which suggests a link between iron excess and metabolic disorders." Moirand R, Mortaji AM, Loreal O, Paillard F, Brissot P, Deugnier Y. A new syndrome of liver iron overload with normal transferrin saturation. *Lancet*. 1997 Jan 11;349(9045):95-7

[677] Axford JS, Bomford A, Revell P, Watt I, Williams R, Hamilton EBD. Hip arthropathy in genetic hemochromatosis: radiographic and histologic features. *Arthritis Rheum* 1991; 34: 357-61

[678] Bensen WG, Laskin CA, Little HA, Fam AG. Hemochromatoic arthropathy mimicking rheumatoid arthritis. A case with subcutaneous nodules, tenosynovitis, and bursitis. *Arthritis Rheum* 1978; 21: 844-8

[679] Olynyk J, Hall P, Ahern M, Kwiatek R, Mackinnon M. Screening for genetic hemochromatosis in a rheumatology clinic. *Australian and New Zealand Journal of Medicine* 1994; 24: 22-25

[680] [No authors listed] Case records of the Massachusetts General Hospital. Weekly clinicopathological exercises. Case 31-1994. A 25-year-old man with the recent onset of diabetes mellitus and congestive heart failure. *N Engl J Med*. 1994 Aug 18;331(7):460-6

disorientation, headaches and migraine headaches, personality changes, hallucinations, paranoia, chronic treatment-resistant psychiatric illness such as schizophrenia, compulsive disorders, bipolar affective disorder.

- 'Alcoholism': Alcoholism can cause elevated liver enzymes and liver damage, and many iron overload patients are erroneously diagnosed as alcoholics despite their abstinence from alcohol when the clinician fails to consider iron overload as the cause for the hepatopathy.

- Any race, nationality, or ethnic background: Hereditary iron overload conditions have been identified in people of all ethnic backgrounds and nationalities. Secondary iron overload conditions can occur irrespective of genetic predisposition.

- Either gender: Iron overload conditions occur in both men and women

- A family history of, or suggestive of, a hereditary iron overload condition: family history of iron overload, hereditary anemia or iron-loading anemia, cardiac disorders or "heart disease", arthritis, diabetes, neurologic disorders, liver disease, impotence, amenorrhea, sterility.

Musculoskeletal manifestations of iron overload
Clinical findings may include:
▪ **Joint pain**
▪ **Bone pain**
▪ Joint swelling
▪ Loss of motion
▪ Bursitis
▪ Tendonitis
▪ Tenosynovitis
▪ Subcutaneous nodules
Sites of involvement
▪ **Metacarpophalangeal joints**
▪ **Wrist**
▪ **Hip**
▪ **Knee**
▪ Shoulder
▪ Ankle
▪ Metatarsophalangeal joints
▪ Elbow
▪ Spine
▪ Symphysis pubis
▪ Achilles tendon
▪ Plantar fascia
Radiographic findings
▪ **Joint space narrowing**
▪ **Sclerosis**
▪ Cysts
▪ Pseudocysts
▪ Osteophytes
▪ **Hook-like osteophytes at the metacarpal heads (high specificity)**
▪ Flattened or "squared-off" metacarpal heads
▪ Generalized osteopenia
▪ Generalized osteoporosis
▪ Chondrocalcinosis
▪ Subchondral cysts
▪ Carpal erosions
▪ Calcific tendonitis

Differential diagnoses:

- Diabetes mellitus: Remember that the classic presentation of hemochromatosis is "bronze diabetes with cirrhosis." **All patients with diabetes should be tested for iron overload.**[681,682]

- Cardiomyopathy:

- Hepatopathy: **Iron overload is one of the most important rule-outs in patients with liver disease.**[683] Liver biopsy is often indicated to assess condition and disease co-existence.

- Musculoskeletal disorders: **Patients with polyarthropathy should be tested for iron overload.**[684,685]
  - o Degenerative arthritis or osteoarthritis
  - o Pseudogout, calcium pyrophosphate dihydrate deposition disease
  - o Rheumatoid arthritis[686]
  - o Ankylosing spondylitis: The resemblance here is only superficial, related primarily to calcification of the intervertebral discs and ligaments.[687]

- Hypogonadotrophic hypogonadism: impotence in men, subfertility in women[688]

- Hyperthyroidism and hypothyroidism[689,690]

- Porphyria cutanea tarda: "Virtually all patients have increased iron stores; serum iron, iron saturation, and ferritin values."[691] **All patients with porphyria cutanea tarda must be tested for iron overload.**

---

[681] Czink E, Tamas G. Screening for idiopathic hemochromatosis among diabetic patients. *Diabetes Care* 1991; 14: 929-30

[682] Phelps G, Chapman I, Hall P, Braund W, Mackinnon M. Prevalence of genetic haemochromatosis among diabetic patients. *Lancet* 1989; 2: 233-4

[683] Herrera JL. Abnormal liver enzyme levels: clinical evaluation in asymptomatic patients. *Postgrad Med* 1993; 93: 119-32

[684] M'Seffar AM, Fornasier VL, Fox IH. Arthropathy as the major clinical indicator of occult iron storage disease. *JAMA* 1977; 238: 1825-8

[685] Vasquez A. Musculoskeletal disorders and iron overload disease: comment on the American College of Rheumatology guidelines for the initial evaluation of the adult patient with acute musculoskeletal symptoms [letter/ comment]. *Arthritis Rheum* 1996;39:1767-8

[686] Bensen WG, Laskin CA, Little HA, Fam AG. Hemochromatoic arthropathy mimicking rheumatoid arthritis. *Arthritis Rheum* 1978; 21: 844-8

[687] Bywaters EGL, Hamilton EBD, Williams R. The spine in idiopathic hemochromatosis. *Ann Rheum Dis* 1971; 30: 453-65

[688] Tweed MJ, Roland JM. Haemochromatosis as an endocrine cause of subfertility. *BMJ*. 1998 Mar 21;316(7135):915-6 http://bmj.bmjjournals.com/cgi/content/full/316/7135/915

[689] Edwards CQ, Kelly TM, Ellwein G, Kushner JP. Thyroid disease in hemochromatosis. Increased incidence in homozygous men. *Arch Intern Med* 1983 Oct;143(10):1890-3

[690] Phillips G Jr, Becker B, Keller VA, Hartman J 4th. Hypothyroidism in adults with sickle cell anemia. *Am J Med* 1992 May;92(5):567-70

[691] "Virtually all patients have increased iron stores; serum iron, iron saturation, and ferritin values." Rich MW. Porphyria cutanea tarda. Don't forget to look at the urine. *Postgrad Med.* 1999;105: 208-10, 213-4

Clinical assessment:

- **History/subjective**:
  - The manifestations of the condition are so protean that history is generally non-sensitive and non-specific for the disorder. Rarely, a patient will mention that a relative was diagnosed with iron overload or that a relative had an unusual heart or liver disease, and this clue may lead to a diagnosis of iron overload in unsuspecting family members.
- **Physical examination/objective**:
  - The classic presentation of the fully developed disease is "bronze diabetes with arthritis and cirrhosis."
  - Physical examination should be specific for the patient's complaint(s) of arthritis, cardiomyopathy, diabetes, etc.
- **Imaging & laboratory assessments**:
  - **Routine screening with serum ferritin for iron overload among all patients should be the standard of care in clinical practice**.
    - "In view of the high prevalence of hereditary hemochromatosis, its dire consequences when untreated, and its treatability, screening for the disorder should be performed routinely."[692]
    - "Screening for hemochromatosis is both feasible and cost-effective, and we recommend its use in patients seeking medical care."[693]
    - "The high gene frequency in the general population warrants routine screening tests in asymptomatic healthy young adults."[694]
    - "CONCLUSIONS: Primary iron overload occurs in African Americans… Clinicians should look for this condition."[695]
  - Imaging: The radiographic findings are nearly identical to those of osteoarthritis, except more joints are typically involved and that the distribution is typically symmetric (both due to the systemic/metabolic nature of the disease). Hook-like osteophytes at the metacarpal heads—with the "hooks" pointing proximally (rather than distally, as in rheumatoid arthritis) may be the only finding that could be called pathognomonic. Flattened or "squared-off" metacarpal heads are also seen. See previous table labeled *"Musculoskeletal manifestations of iron overload"* for more details.
  - Laboratory evaluation: Serum ferritin is the test of choice when looking for primary iron overload, secondary iron overload, and/or iron deficiency and should be a component of each new patient's evaluation, just as are CBC and the chemistry/metabolic panel. Transferrin saturation is a common test used for the detection of genetic hemochromatosis in research studies because it measures both iron levels but also disordered iron handling; this is why this test is best used in research screening of large populations. For clinicians, serum ferritin is very obviously the superior lab test for iron overload and deficiency.
    - Transferrin saturation: Good test for detecting genetic hemochromatosis before iron overload has occurred; values greater than 40% should be repeated *in conjunction with a measurement of serum ferritin*. Guidelines for screening for genetic hemochromatosis advocate the transferrin saturation test because it is a more sensitive assessment (compared to serum ferritin) for the hemochromatosis genotype which manifests phenotypically not simply as increased iron absorption and accumulation but also as an abnormality in iron handling which preferentially alters the transferrin saturation value, which is the ratio of serum iron to serum transferrin; the former rises due to increased iron absorption while the latter declines due to impaired hepatic synthetic function secondary to the preferential intraparenchymal deposition of iron in genetic hemochromatosis. Thus, genetic hemochromatosis is not simply a disorder characterized by increased iron absorption; it is also a disorder of iron handling/metabolism wherein iron is stored intracellularly in tissue parenchyma rather than (as in non-GH persons) in the reticuloendothelial system.

---

[692] Fairbanks VF. Laboratory testing for iron status. *Hosp Pract* (Off Ed) 1991 Suppl 3:17-24
[693] Balan V, Baldus W, Fairbanks V, Michels V, Burritt M, Klee G. Screening for hemochromatosis: a cost-effectiveness study based on 12, 258 patients. *Gastroenterology* 1994; 107: 453-9
[694] Gushusrt TP, Triest WE. Diagnosis and management of precirrhotic hemochromatosis. *W Virginia Med J* 1990; 86: 91-5
[695] Wurapa RK, Gordeuk VR, Brittenham GM, Khiyami A, Schechter GP, Edwards CQ. Primary iron overload in African Americans. *Am J Med.* 1996 Jul;101(1):9-18

- **Ferritin: Routine use of serum ferritin is the most reasonable and cost-effective means for diagnosing this condition in symptomatic and asymptomatic patients.** Elevations of ferritin (i.e., >200 mcg/L in women and >300 mcg/L in men) need to be retested along with CRP (to rule out false elevation due to excessive inflammation) before making the presumptive diagnosis of iron overload. **In the absence of significant inflammation, ferritin values >200 mcg/L in women and >300 mcg/L in men indicate iron overload and the need for treatment/phlebotomy regardless of the absence of symptoms or end-stage complications.**[696] Another benefit to the use of serum ferritin is the frequent detection of iron deficiency.

- **<u>Interpretation of iron status based on serum ferritin</u>**

Ferritin	Categorization and management
≥ 800 mcg/L	<u>Practically diagnostic of severe iron overload</u>[697]: Repeat tests; rule out inflammation or occult pathology. Initiate phlebotomy and consider liver biopsy or MRI.
≥ 300 mcg/L	<u>Probable iron overload; clear predisposition to iron accumulation</u>[698]: Repeat tests; rule out inflammation or occult pathology. In men, initiate phlebotomy and consider liver biopsy or MRI.[699]
≥ 200 mcg/L	*In women*: <u>Probable iron overload; clear predisposition to iron accumulation</u>[700]: Repeat tests, rule out inflammation or occult pathology. In women, initiate phlebotomy and consider liver biopsy or MRI.[701] *In men*: <u>High-normal *unhealthy* iron status with increased risk of myocardial infarction</u>[702]: Rule out inflammation or occult pathology. No follow-up is mandated, yet blood donation and/or abstention from dietary iron are recommended preventative healthcare measures.
≥ 160 mcg/L	*In women*: <u>Abnormal iron status</u>[703]: Repeat tests, rule out inflammation or occult pathology. Consider phlebotomy and liver biopsy or MRI.
≥80-120 mcg/L	<u>High-normal unhealthy iron status</u>[704,705]: No follow-up is mandated; blood donation and abstention from dietary iron are suggested preventative healthcare measures. A subset of patients with restless leg syndrome (RLS, a condition also causally associated with intestinal bacterial overgrowth dysbiosis) have impaired transport of iron into the brain and therefore require slightly elevated ferritin/iron levels (up to 120) to enhance cerebral iron uptake.
40-70 mcg/L	**Optimal iron status for most people**[706,707]
< 20 mcg/L	<u>Iron deficiency</u>: Search for occult gastrointestinal blood loss with endoscopy or imaging assessments in adults; refer to gastroenterologist.[708,709]

[696] Barton JC, McDonnell SM, Adams PC, Brissot P, Powell LW, Edwards CQ, Cook JD, Kowdley KV. Management of hemochromatosis. Hemochromatosis Management Working Group. *Ann Intern Med*. 1998 Dec 1;129(11):932-9

[697] Milman N, Albeck MJ. Distinction between homozygous and heterozygous subjects with hemochromatosis using iron status markers and receiver operating characteristic (ROC) analysis. *Eur J Clin Biochem* 1995; 33: 95-8. See also Milman N. Iron status markers in hereditary hemochromatosis: distinction between individuals being homozygous and heterozygous for the hemochromatosis allele. *Eur J Haematol* 1991;47:292-8

[698] Olynyk JK, Bacon BR. Hereditary hemochromatosis: detecting and correcting iron overload. *Postgrad Med* 1994;96: 151-65

[699] "Therapeutic phlebotomy is used to remove excess iron and maintain low normal body iron stores, ... initiated in men with serum ferritin levels of 300 microg/L or more and in women with serum ferritin levels of 200 microg/L or more, regardless of the presence or absence of symptoms." Barton JC, McDonnell SM, Adams PC, Brissot P, Powell LW, Edwards CQ, Cook JD, Kowdley KV. Management of hemochromatosis. Hemochromatosis Management Working Group. *Ann Intern Med*. 1998 Dec 1;129(11):932-9

[700] Barton JC, Edwards CQ, Bertoli LF, Shroyer TW, Hudson SL. Iron overload in African Americans. *Am J Med* 1995; 99: 616-23

[701] Barton JC, McDonnell SM, Adams PC, et al. Management of hemochromatosis. *Ann Intern Med*. 1998 Dec 1;129(11):932-9

[702] Salonen JT, Nyyssonen K, Korpela H,et al. High stored iron levels are associated with excess risk of myocardial infarction in eastern Finnish men. *Circulation* 1992; 86: 803-11

[703] Nicoll D. Therapeutic drug monitoring and laboratory reference ranges. In: Tierney LM, McPhee SJ, Papadakis MA. *Current Medical Diagnosis and Treatment 1996 (35th Edition)*. Stamford: Appleton and Lange, 1996: 1442

[704] Lauffer, RB. *Iron and Your Heart*. New York: St. Martin's Press, 1991: 79-8, 83-88, 162

[705] Sullivan JL. Iron and the sex difference in heart disease risk. *Lancet* 1981 Jun 13;1(8233):1293-4

[706] Lauffer, RB. *Iron and Your Heart*. New York: St. Martin's Press, 1991: 79-8, 83-88, 162

[707] Vasquez A. High body iron stores: causes, effects, diagnosis, and treatment. *Nutritional Perspectives* 1994; 17: 13, 15-7, 19, 21, 28 and Vasquez A. Men's Health: Iron in men: why men store this nutrient in their bodies and the harm that it does. *MEN Magazine* 1997; Jan:11,21-23 vix.com/menmag/alexiron.htm

[708] Rockey DC, Cello JP. Evaluation of the gastrointestinal tract in patients with iron-deficiency anemia. *N Engl J Med*. 1993;329(23):1691-5

[709] "Endoscopy revealed a clinically important lesion in 23 (12%) of 186 patients. ... CONCLUSIONS: Endoscopy yields important findings in premenopausal women with iron deficiency anemia, which should not be attributed solely to menstrual blood loss." Bini EJ, Micale PL, Weinshel EH. Evaluation of the gastrointestinal tract in premenopausal women with iron deficiency anemia. *Am J Med*. 1998 Oct;105(4):281-6

- **CRP**: Should be relatively normal as iron overload is not inflammatory, per se. If the ferritin is elevated and the CRP is markedly elevated, then inflammatory and hepatic diseases must be considered, namely advanced cancer, viral hepatitis or other hepatopathy, and alcoholic liver disease. If the ferritin is elevated and the CRP is normal, then the most likely diagnosis is iron overload, which should be confirmed either with liver biopsy or diagnostic/therapeutic phlebotomy.
- **CBC**: may show anemia, but the findings here are nonspecific
- **Chemistry panel**: may show evidence of diabetes and hepatopathy
- **Thyroid assessment**: may show hyperthyroidism or hypothyroidism, both of which are more common in patients with iron overload.
- **Bone marrow biopsy**: unnecessary and archaic in this setting, now that serum ferritin is widely available.
- **Liver biopsy**: traditionally considered the "gold standard" for diagnosing iron overload but is now clearly unnecessary for the diagnosis, which can be established by monitoring the response to therapeutic phlebotomy, which is the treatment of choice.[710] **Life-saving diagnostic and therapeutic phlebotomy should never be denied or delayed for lack of liver biopsy in patients with laboratory indicators of iron overload.**[711]
- **Genetic testing, such as for the HFE mutation**: This is a waste of time and money in most clinical situations; these tests should be reserved for research purposes and for evaluation of affected relatives—especially children—of index cases. The only value these tests may have in clinical practice is that of supporting a diagnosis in a patient with elevated serum ferritin who refuses biopsy, liver MRI, or phlebotomy; however, a negative result is meaningless if the ferritin is high and the clinical picture is compatible with iron overload. If the diagnosis is established, genetic relatives must be tested.

Establishing the diagnosis: Any *one* of the following three is sufficient:
- Diagnostic liver biopsy shows heavy iron deposits.
- Characteristic laboratory findings (ferritin >200 in women or >300 in men) *and* the ability to resist intractable anemia with serial/weekly phlebotomies.
- Characteristic MRI of liver *and* the ability to tolerate serial/weekly phlebotomies.

Complications:
- Patients diagnosed *and effectively treated* before the onset of signs and symptoms have normal life expectancy.
- The most common causes of premature mortality in undiagnosed and untreated patients are related to heart failure, liver failure, infections and/or complications of diabetes.

Clinical management:
- Treatment for severe iron overload is iron-removal therapy. Since blood is high in iron, the removal of blood—therapeutic phlebotomy—is the treatment of choice. Deferoxamine chelation can be administered to patients who refuse or cannot withstand phlebotomy (i.e., patients with cardiomyopathy, severe anemia, hypoproteinemia) but is much less effective, much more expensive, and with side effects such as neurotoxicity. Adjunctive nutritional and lifestyle modifications are no substitute for iron-removal therapy, and weekly phlebotomy is the treatment of choice.
- When a hereditary iron overload disorder is diagnosed, all (first-degree) blood relatives must be screened for iron overload.

Treatments:
- **Medical standard**: Iron-removal is accomplished by weekly phlebotomy of 1-2 units (250-500 mL of blood, each of which removes 250 mg of iron), and deferoxamine chelation is used in patients who cannot tolerate phlebotomy. Complications of the disease, such as arthritis, heart failure, hypogonadism, and diabetes are treated appropriately. Cirrhotic patients must be monitored for hepatoma with twice-yearly liver ultrasound

---

[710] "Therapeutic phlebotomy is used to remove excess iron and maintain low normal body iron stores, and it should be initiated in men with serum ferritin levels of 300 microg/L or more and in women with serum ferritin levels of 200 microg/L or more, regardless of the presence or absence of symptoms." Barton JC, McDonnell SM, Adams PC, Brissot P, Powell LW, Edwards CQ, Cook JD, Kowdley KV. Management of hemochromatosis. Hemochromatosis Management Working Group. *Ann Intern Med.* 1998 Dec 1;129:932-9
[711] Sullivan JL, as quoted in Crawford R, ed. "The debate." In: *Ironic Blood: information on iron overload.* West Palm Beach: Iron Overload Diseases Association. 1996; 16 (2)

and measurement of serum alpha-fetoprotein. Always, when a hereditary iron overload disorder is diagnosed, all (first-degree) blood relatives must be screened for iron overload.

- <u>Diet modifications</u>: These are no substitute for iron-removal therapy with phlebotomy and are weak in their effectiveness by comparison.
  - Decrease consumption of foods and nutritional supplements which are significant sources of iron: Iron supplements, iron-fortified foods and supplements, liver, beef, pork, lamb.
  - Increase consumption of foods that will decrease intestinal absorption of iron from ingested food: tannins in tea, phytates (in whole-grain products, bran, legumes, nuts, and seeds), soy protein, egg, calcium supplements.
  - Ensure adequate protein intake to replace protein lost during phlebotomy.
  - Decrease consumption of excess ascorbic acid (vitamin C); high-dose vitamin C supplementation is clearly contraindicated.[712]
  - Alcohol consumption should be avoided because ethanol exacerbates liver damage and increases iron absorption from the gut.
- <u>Silymarin</u>: Milk thistle has proved benefit in an animal model of iron overload[713] and is probably suitable for use in patients with iron overload, particularly given its ability to reverse cirrhosis.[714]
- <u>Antioxidant supplementation (excluding high-dose ascorbate)</u>: Oxidative stress is increased and antioxidant reserves are decreased in patients with iron overload.
- <u>Coenzyme Q10</u>: CoQ-10 probably has a role in the treatment of hemochromatoic cardiomyopathy given its safety and efficacy in other cardiomyopathies.[715,716,717,718,719,720,721,722]

---

[712] Mclarlan CJ, et al. Congestive cardiomyopathy and hemochromatosis: rapid progression possibly accelerated by excessive ingestion of ascorbic acid. *Aust NZ J Med* 1982; 12: 187-8

[713] "CONCLUSIONS: Oral administration of silybin protects against iron-induced hepatic toxicity in vivo. This effect seems to be caused by the prominent antioxidant activity of this compound." Pietrangelo A, Borella F, Casalgrandi G, et al. Antioxidant activity of silybin in vivo during long-term iron overload in rats. *Gastroenterology.* 1995 Dec;109(6):1941-9

[714] Salmi HA, Sarna S. Effect of silymarin and chemical, functional, and morphological alterations of the liver. A double-blind controlled study. *Scand J Gastroenterol* 1982; 17: 517-21

[715] Greenberg S, Frishman WH. Co-enzyme Q-10: a new drug for cardiovascular disease. *J Clin Pharmacol* 1990; 30: 596-608

[716] Langsjoen PH, Langsjoen PH, Folkers K. Long-term efficacy and safety of coenzyme Q-10 therapy for idiopathic dilated cardiomyopathy. *Am J Cardiol* 1990; 65: 521-3

[717] Manzoli U, Rossi E, Littarru GP, et al. Coenzyme Q-10 in dilated cardiomyopathy. *Int J Tiss Reac* 1990; 12: 173-8

[718] Langsjoen PH, Folkers K, Lyson K, Muratsu K, Lyson T, Langsjoen P. Pronounced increase of survival of patients with cardiomyopathy when treated with coenzyme Q-10 and conventional therapy. *Int J Tiss Reac* 1990; 12: 163-8

[719] Folkers K. Heart failure is a dominant deficiency of coenzyme Q-10 and challenges for future clinical research on CoQ-10. *Clin Investig* 1993; 71: s51-s54

[720] Folkers K, Langsjoen P, Langsjoen PH. Therapy with coenzyme Q-10 of patients in heart failure who are eligible or ineligible for a transplant. *Biochem Biophys Res Commun* 1992;182:247-53

[721] Mortensen SA, et al. Coenzyme Q-10: clinical benefits with biochemical correlates suggesting a scientific breakthrough.... *Int J Tiss Reac* 1990;12:155-62

[722] Langsjoen PH, Langsjoen PH, Folkers K. A six-year clinical study of therapy of cardiomyopathy with coenzyme Q-10. *Int J Tiss Reac* 1990; 12: 169-71

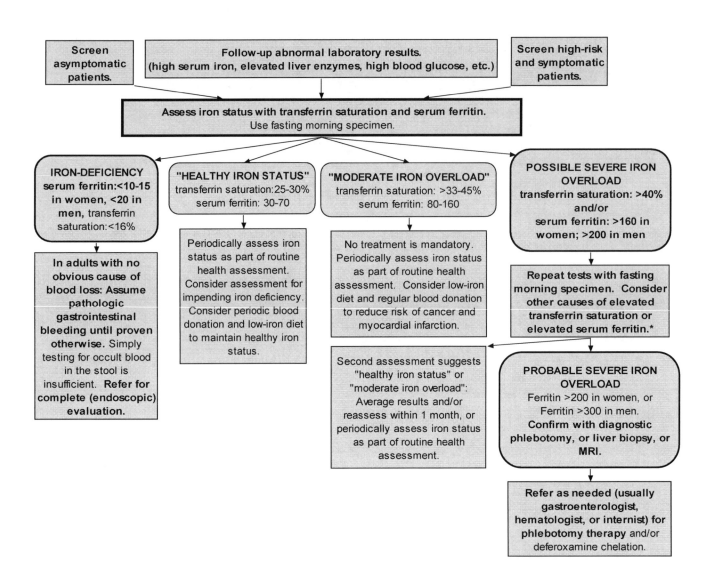

Guide to Patient Management Based on Iron Status: Adult patients with iron deficiency must generally be presumed to have occult gastrointestinal blood loss and should therefore be referred for gastrointestinal endoscopy; this is consistent with the standard of care in medicine. Ferritin levels between 40-70 mcg/L are generally optimal for most men and women; up to 120 mcg/L is reasonable for subsets of patients with restless leg syndrome, perhaps also those with recalcitrant depression and/or Parkinsonian features to allow sufficient iron entry into the brain for maximal dopamine production. Levels greater than 200 mcg/L in a woman or 300 mcg/L in a man are suggestive of iron overload and/or tendency toward accumulation and are physiologically unnecessary and medically unjustifiable, particularly as increased iron stores correlate with increased cancer mortality, increased cardiovascular mortality, and increased all-cause mortality. Diagnosis and treatment for iron overload can occur simultaneously with diagnostic/therapeutic phlebotomy. Genetic testing and liver biopsy are generally inefficient expenditures of financial and medial resources; genetic testing is irrelevant in the presence of the hemochromatosis phenotype (i.e., otherwise inexplicable iron accumulation) while liver biopsy exposes the patient to unnecessary treatment delays, risk, and expenses.

Arthritis & Rheumatism

Official Journal of the American College of Rheumatology

VOLUME 39   OCTOBER 1996   NO. 10

1767   1768

Musculoskeletal disorders and iron overload disease: comment on the American College of Rheumatology guidelines for the initial evaluation of the adult patient with acute musculoskeletal symptoms

To the Editor:

The recent clinical guidelines for the initial evaluation of the adult patient with acute musculoskeletal symptoms, proposed by the American College of Rheumatology (1), provide useful information and a good review for clinicians. However, there is one important omission in these guidelines. Nowhere in the guidelines is hemochromatosis mentioned. Such a prevalent and potentially life-threatening disease certainly deserves to be considered in the evaluation of patients with musculoskeletal disorders.

Hereditary hemochromatosis is now thought to be the most common genetic disorder in the white population (2). Approximately 1 in 250 persons is homozygous for this disorder and will develop the characteristic clinical manifestations such as diabetes, cardiomyopathy, liver disease, endocrine dysfunction, and, most notable for this discussion, arthropathy or other musculoskeletal disorders (2). Although hereditary iron overload disorders have traditionally been thought of as occurring exclusively in whites, recent research by Barton et al (3) indicates that approximately 1 in 67 African-Americans is affected by an etiologically distinct and severe form of iron overload. Hereditary iron overload disorders have been detected in persons of every ethnic background.

Arthropathy affects up to 80% of iron-overloaded patients and is often the only manifestation of this disease (4). Joint pain is a common and early symptom of iron overload, and "bone pain" has also been described as a common initial complaint (5). Clinically and radiographically, hemochromatoic arthropathy can resemble osteoarthritis, calcium pyrophosphate dihydrate deposition disease, pseudogout, rheumatoid arthritis, ankylosing spondylitis, or generalized osteopenia with osteoporotic fractures (4,6,7). Since iron overload can cause such a wide array of musculoskeletal manifestations and because definitive clinical differentiation of iron overload from other arthropathies is very difficult, patients with peripheral arthropathy should be screened for iron overload. Indeed, recent research by Olynyk et al (8) indicates that the prevalence of iron overload is 5 times higher in patients with peripheral arthropathy than in the general population. Therefore, screening of patients with peripheral arthropathy for the possible presence of iron overload is justified.

Thus, since iron overload affects such a large portion of the population and arthropathy is a common manifestation of this disorder, patients with musculoskeletal symptoms should be screened for iron overload (4,8). The current literature suggests that everyone should be screened for iron overload even if there are no symptoms (8–10).

Alex Vasquez, DC
Seattle, WA

1. American College of Rheumatology Ad Hoc Committee on Clinical Guidelines: Guidelines for the initial evaluation of the adult patient with acute musculoskeletal symptoms. Arthritis Rheum 39:1–8, 1996
2. Olynyk JK, Bacon BR: Hereditary hemochromatosis: detecting and correcting iron overload. Postgrad Med 96:151–165, 1994
3. Barton JC, Edwards CQ, Bertoli LF, Shroyer TW, Hudson SL: Iron overload in African Americans. Am J Med 99:616–623, 1995
4. Faraawi R, Harth M, Kertesz A, Bell D: Arthritis in hemochromatosis. J Rheumatol 20:448–452, 1993
5. Adams PC, Kertesz AE, Valberg LS: Clinical presentation of hemochromatosis: a changing scene. Am J Med 90:445–449, 1991
6. Bywaters EGL, Hamilton EBD, Williams R: The spine in idiopathic hemochromatosis. Ann Rheum Dis 30:453–465, 1971
7. Eyres KS, McCloskey EV, Fern ED, Rogers S, Beneton M, Aaron JE, Kanis JA: Osteoporotic fractures: an unusual presentation of hemochromatosis. Bone 13:431–433, 1992
8. Olynyk J, Hall P, Ahern M, Kwiatek R, Mackinnon M: Screening for hemochromatosis in a rheumatology clinic. Aust N Z J Med 24:22–25, 1994
9. Baer DM, Simmons JL, Staples RL, Runmore GJ, Morton CJ: Hemochromatosis screening in asymptomatic ambulatory men 30 years of age and older. Am J Med 98:464–468, 1995
10. Adams PC, Gregor JC, Kertesz AE, Valberg LS: Screening blood donors for hereditary hemochromatosis: decision analysis model based on a 30-year database. Gastroenterology 109:177–188, 1995

Useful redundancy. Musculoskeletal disorders and iron overload disease: comment on the American College of Rheumatology guidelines for the initial evaluation of the adult patient with acute musculoskeletal symptoms. *Arthritis Rheum.* 1996 Oct;39(10):1767-8 http://www.ncbi.nlm.nih.gov/pubmed/8843875

Hypothyroidism:
Clinical, Functional, and Practical Considerations

Introduction:

Due mostly to the allopathic medical profession's limited view of hypothyroidism, the condition has remained enigmatic, and both doctors and patients have been rendered ineffective in their ability to understand and treat this common clinical condition. In the following few pages, the illusion of complexity and incomprehensibility will be deflated.

This chapter details the most important considerations in the assessment and treatment of various types of low thyroid function. As with the other chapters of the book, information will be presented in an outlined format.

Hypothyroidism, particularly Functional/Metabolic/Peripheral Hypothyroidism

Description/pathophysiology:

- **Anatomy and normal physiology of thyroid hormone production and function**: The base of the brain contains a region called the hypothalamus, which coordinates many body functions and secretes thyrotropin releasing hormone (TRH) which stimulates the nearby pituitary gland to produce thyroid stimulating hormone (TSH). The TSH produced from the pituitary gland on the underside of the brain provides the stimulating signal to the thyroid gland, located at the front of the neck, for it to produce its hormones. The main hormones secreted by the thyroid gland are thyroxine (also called "T4" because it is the thyroid hormone made from the amino acid tyrosine [T] that has four [4] molecules of iodine) and triiodothyronine, also called "T3" because it has three molecules of iodine. Most of the hormone produced by the thyroid gland is in the form of T4, which is much less biologically active than T3. T4 is converted into T3 in the liver and in the peripheral tissues of the body. Although the thyroid gland's production of T3 is quantitatively less than that of T4, because T3 is the active form of the hormone, the direct production of T3 from the thyroid gland itself is important for peripheral tissues such as the brain which are unable to sufficiently convert T4 into T3.

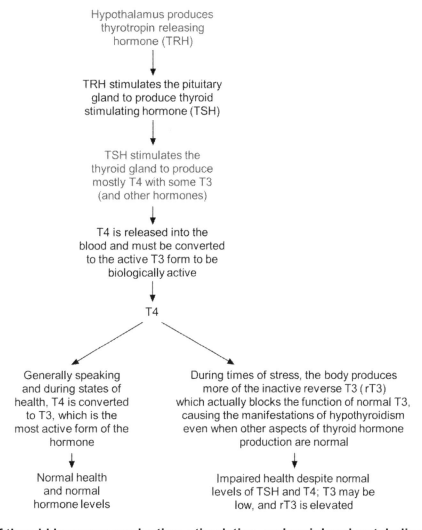

Illustration of thyroid hormone production, stimulation, and peripheral metabolism

- **Hormones and feedback mechanisms**: When thyroid hormone production is insufficient, receptors in the hypothalamus and pituitary sense the hormone deficiency and respond by increasing the production of TSH to stimulate hormone production from the thyroid gland; when thyroid hormone production increases, feedback to the hypothalamus and pituitary reduces TSH production to lower thyroid hormone production. In these ways, as with many other body systems and physiological processes, the body is able to maintain a steady state of thyroid hormone production; most people have heard of this phenomenon of self-regulation referred to as *homeostasis*, even though a more accurate term is *homeodynamics*, because it is an active (not static) process in constant fluctuation and regulation. If a patient is given too much thyroid hormone by prescription, then the TSH level will be reduced; if a patient has hypothyroidism and is undertreated with an insufficient amount of thyroid hormone, then the TSH will remain elevated. Lab tests and optimal hormone levels will be discussed later in this chapter.

- **Problems that may arise in thyroid hormone production and metabolism**: In this section, details will be provided about common problems that can arise in thyroid hormone production and metabolism:
  - Problems of the hypothalamus: Damage to the hypothalamus from an injury such as head trauma, cancer, or infection can result in an inability to produce TRH; these problems are very rare. Doctors do not generally test for TRH production; however, some abnormalities in TRH production have been noted in patients with chronic depression. "Hypothalamic hypothyroidism" is hypothyroidism resulting from a problem in the hypothalamus; this is also called *tertiary hypothyroidism*, because it is two "steps" away from the primary location of thyroid hormone production—the thyroid gland itself.
  - Problems of the pituitary gland: Rarely, the pituitary gland might overproduce TSH and function autonomously from TRH stimulation; this will result in excess thyroid hormone production. More commonly but still rare, damage to the pituitary gland—for example if a nearby tumor compresses the gland, or if the gland is damaged by a disease like iron overload (e.g., hemochromatosis) or by a stroke (e.g., Sheenan's syndrome)—can cause a reduction in TSH production. Problems localized to the pituitary gland resulting in either excess or deficient production of TSH are very rare and are not responsible for the majority of thyroid disorders. Hypothyroidism caused by problems in the pituitary gland is called *secondary hypothyroidism*.
  - Problems of the thyroid gland: Several problems can affect the thyroid gland and its ability to produce the proper amount of thyroid hormone. Some of the more relevant disorders are discussed in the following subsections:
    - Graves' disease: Graves' disease is a fairly common autoimmune disease wherein the body's immune system creates antibodies to the TSH receptor. These antibodies stimulate the TSH receptor just as would the normal TSH hormone, and thus the result is an increased production of thyroid hormones from the gland, causing excess thyroid gland function and the clinical manifestations of hyperthyroidism. Common manifestations of the disease are weight loss, excess body heat, diarrhea due to more rapid gastrointestinal transit, and tremor (shakiness) and tachycardia (fast heart rate) due to increased stimulation of the sympathetic nervous system. Another common trademark manifestation of Graves' disease is exophthalmos—"bulging of the eyes"—because excess fibrous tissue is deposited behind the eyes and because the muscles surrounding the outside of the eyes are weakened by immune (antibody) damage. Graves' disease is most commonly treated with drugs that block the metabolism of thyroid hormones, or with other drugs such as radioactive iodine which cause destruction of the thyroid gland, resulting in hypothyroidism which is then treated with prescription thyroid hormone. Graves' disease can be considered a form of primary hyperthyroidism because it is hyperthyroidism resulting from abnormal function of the gland itself, even though the cause of the problem is the antibodies that are interacting with the gland receptors. With Graves' disease or any other cause of primary hyperthyroidism, lab tests will show that TSH is low and T4 is high.
    - Viral infection: The thyroid gland can be infected by a viral infection, perhaps as a consequence of an upper respiratory infection; this is called "viral thyroiditis. (Keep in mind that the suffix "-itis" simply means inflammation, so "thyroiditis" just means inflammation of the thyroid gland, whether from infection, trauma [rare], or autoimmune disease [most common].) Classically, the patient has had a recent viral infection—such as a common cold—and the thyroid gland, located at the anterior lower neck just barely above the rib cage, is tender and slightly swollen. In these situations, infection of the gland causes release of thyroid hormone from the gland, temporarily resulting in hyperthyroidism. If the gland is damaged by the infection, then the period of transient *hyper*thyroidism may be followed

by *hypo*thyroidism due to failure of the gland to produce sufficient thyroid hormone. This resulting hypothyroidism may be mild or severe, temporary or permanent.

- Autoimmune thyroiditis: The most common cause of *primary hypothyroidism* is autoimmune destruction of the thyroid gland, also called Hashimoto's thyroiditis in recognition of the Japanese medical scientist Hashimoto Hakaru who first described the condition in 1912. The condition is also called lymphocytic thyroiditis because biopsy of the thyroid gland will show infiltration of immune cells called lymphocytes, which cause damage to the glandular tissue. In

If autoimmune hypothyroidism is the problem, then what is the cause of the problem.
Given that an autoimmune disease process (involving auto-antibodies and auto-reactive T-cells) can lead to destruction of the thyroid gland, a reasonable question becomes "What triggers the immune system to attack the thyroid gland?" The top four answers to this question are ❶ exposure to the dietary protein gluten, found in grains such as wheat, ❷ nutritional deficiency of selenium, iron, and possibly vitamins D and A, ❸ localized infection, ❹ infection with specific bacteria—such as *Yersinia enterocolitica*—anywhere in the body; a genetic predisposition atop any of these other four triggers will increase the probability of developing autoimmune thyroiditis but is by itself insufficient.

this condition, the body's own immune system—specifically the T-cells and the antibodies/immunoglobulins made by the B-cells or plasma cells—causes injury to and eventual destruction of the thyroid gland. Autoimmune destruction of the thyroid gland can occur as a solitary phenomenon, or it may occur as part of another autoimmune disorder, such as rheumatoid arthritis (RA), systemic lupus erythematosus (SLE, lupus), or Sjögren's Syndrome. If the thyroid gland itself is failing to produce sufficient amounts of thyroid hormone, then feedback mechanisms will cause TSH to increase; thus, what most doctors look for when screening for hypothyroidism is simply an elevated TSH. For many doctors, if they fail to find an elevated TSH, then they will exclude hypothyroidism as a diagnosis and will not treat the patient with thyroid hormone even if the patient is clinically hypothyroid, that is, showing all the manifestations expected with hypothyroidism. Blood levels of T4 may be normal due to compensatory stimulation by extra TSH; T4 levels might also be reduced. Most often, laboratory tests will also reveal elevated levels of antibodies which specifically target components of the thyroid gland. The two most common antibodies seen in Hashimoto/autoimmune thyroiditis are directed toward thyroglobulin, which is a protein found in the thyroid gland, and against the enzyme peroxidase; these are called anti-thyroglobulin antibodies and anti-thyroid peroxidase (anti-TPO) antibodies.

- Problems of peripheral metabolism: As reviewed above in the section on normal thyroid metabolism, the thyroid's production of thyroid hormone—mostly T4—is followed by conversion of T4 into the active form of thyroid hormone, which is T3. During times of stress, the body's ability to produce and utilize T3 is impaired because the enzymes that catalyze this conversion change in a way that produces a different hormone called "reverse T3" (rT3), which is certainly less active than normal T3 and which appears to actually block the function of the normal T3 that is produced. In these situations, TSH and T4 levels are generally normal, and since most doctors do not test the levels of T3 and rT3, the problem is never discovered. Reliable test for T3 and rT3 have been available for many years; the reason that most doctors do not use these tests is that they were not taught to do so in medical school.

- **Definitions and descriptions of hypothyroidism**: The American Thyroid Association has described hypothyroidism as follows in a 2003 publication—ATA Hypothyroidism Booklet[723]—available on their website in December 2011: "Hypothyroidism is an underactive thyroid gland ("hypo-"means *under* or below *normal*). Hypothyroidism means that the thyroid gland cannot make enough thyroid hormone to keep the body running normally. People are hypothyroid if they have too little thyroid hormone in their blood." Patients and clinicians should appreciate that while this definition is accurate, it is incomplete because hypothyroidism involves more than the state of insufficient hormone production from the gland; in some situations we see that patients make sufficient thyroid hormone from their thyroid gland, but that the peripheral metabolism of their thyroid hormone

---

[723] American Thyroid Association. ATA Hypothyroidism Booklet. 2003 Available at http://www.thyroid.org/patients/brochures/Hypothyroidism%20_web_booklet.pdf on December 2011. "This booklet was prepared by the American Thyroid Association (ATA), a professional society of physicians and researchers specializing in the thyroid gland. Founded in 1923, the ATA fosters excellence and innovation in patient care, research, education, and public advocacy. The recommendations given here are those of the ATA."

is impaired, thereby creating the paradox of hypothyroid manifestations despite normalcy of commonly performed lab tests. Hypothyroidism should therefore be at least partially defined as a clinical syndrome of health problems which are fully or partly reversible with proper replacement of thyroid hormones.

- **A new practical definition of hypothyroidism**: Rather than defining hypothyroidism by "hormone levels in the blood", a wiser and more accurate definition of hypothyroidism holds that the condition should be defined as "an adverse physiological state caused by insufficient function of thyroid hormone at the cellular level." This definition of hypothyroidism is based on physiology, i.e., the fact that the purpose of thyroid hormone is to effect action and changes at the cellular level. The purpose of the thyroid gland is to make sufficient thyroid hormone to effect normal healthy physiology; the purpose of the thyroid gland is not to produce a level of thyroid hormone that fits within a laboratory reference range defined by a small group of laboratories, researchers, and clinicians. Therefore, any accurate definition of hypothyroidism must be based on physiology rather than on blood tests; again, the purpose of the hormonal system is to create certain physiologic effects, not to produce an amount of hormone considered "normal."

- **One way to explain this to patients**: The way that I have often explained this to patients is so say something to the effect that, "Thyroid hormones have many different functions in the body, and their chief effect is contributing to the control of the basal metabolic rate, or the "speed" of reactions and the "temperature" of the body. For reasons that are not entirely clear, some people do not make enough thyroid hormone to function optimally.[724] Other people make enough to be considered "normal" but they do not feel well, and they often feel better when taking additional thyroid hormone as prescribed by their doctor.[725,726] Indeed, a famous physiology researcher at the University of Texas at Austin—Dr. Roger J Williams—noted in his classic book *Biochemical Individuality*, "a wide variation in thyroid activity exists among "normal" human beings."[727]

Clinical presentations:

- **Prevalence**: Hypothyroidism is common, affecting about 10% of the population. It is more commonly diagnosed in women than in men; this may be because autoimmune disorders (such as autoimmune thyroiditis) are generally more common in women.
  - Fatigue: Fatigue and "not enough energy" are among the most common complaints of patients with hypothyroidism. Fatigue and low energy are nonspecific subjective complaints that correlate with innumerable health conditions, including depression, existential crisis, anemia, hypothyroidism, infection, cancer, autoimmune diseases, cardiopulmonary disease, nutritional deficiency, and many others.
  - Depression: Depression is common among patients with hypothyroidism. The most direct explanations for this are ❶ reduced function of the adrenergic nervous system, specifically the reception of neurotransmitters norepinephrine and dopamine, which support energy/attention/vigilance and drive/direction/pleasure, respectively, ❷ reduced metabolic function overall due to lower body temperature (most enzymes function most efficiently within a narrow range of temperatures, ❸ nutritional deficiencies due to reduced stomach acid production (noted in patients with hypothyroidism) and/or bacterial overgrowth of the small bowel (SIBO) secondary to slow intestinal transit, which is well noted in patients with hypothyroidism. Additionally, patients with hypothyroidism often have weight gain, difficult weight loss, various health problems, and also the experience of being underdiagnosed, undertreated, and feeling misunderstood by their doctors and perhaps by friends, family, and intimate/romantic partners as well; these can all contribute to the psychological and social aspects of depression and feelings of sadness, despair, and isolation.
  - Low body temperature, cold hands and feet: Because T3 increases energy expenditure and therefore increases body heat, patients with an insufficiency of thyroid hormone commonly notice feeling cold—a phenomenon referred to as cold intolerance. This can be assessed simply by touching the skin and hands of a person with hypothyroidism; often the initial handshake at the start of the patient's office visit is the first clue to hypothyroidism. Many of these patients have low oral temperatures that never reach the

[724] Broda Barnes MD, Lawrence Galton, Hypothyroidism: The Unsuspected Illness. Ty Crowell Co; 1976
[725] Skinner GR, Thomas R, Taylor M, Sellarajah M, Bolt S, Krett S, Wright A. Thyroxine should be tried in clinically hypothyroid but biochemically euthyroid patients. *BMJ: British Medical Journal* 1997 Jun 14; 314(7096): 1764
[726] McLaren EH, Kelly CJ, Pollack MA. Trial of thyroxine treatment for biochemically euthyroid patients has been approved. *BMJ* 1997; 315: 1463
[727] Williams RJ. Biochemical Individuality : The Basis for the Genetotrophic Concept. Austin and London: University of Texas Press, 1956 page 82

normal temperature of 98.6° Fahrenheit (F) or 37° Celsius (C); often they report that the only time their oral temperature reaches the normal temperature is when they have a "fever" due to an infection. Very few conditions cause low body temperature; therefore, the finding of a consistently low body temperature is a clinical finding that is objective and significant and which warrants evaluation. Low body temperature is most consistent with hypothyroidism; to a lesser extent it is consistent with low testosterone levels and—in women and on a menstrual basis—low progesterone levels. Poor peripheral circulation to the extremities can also produce the feeling of localized coldness; the main conditions to consider in this regard are peripheral arterial disease and Raynaud's disorder.

o   <u>Dry skin</u>: Dry skin is commonly noted in patients with hypothyroidism. This may be due to a combination of impaired nutrient absorption and also impaired function of the oil-producing glands of the skin.

o   <u>Constipation, poor digestion, acid reflux</u>: Because hypothyroidism leads to a generalized slowing of the body's functions, it commonly leads to slower intestinal transit, which manifests as constipation. Impaired gastrointestinal motility can also promote acid reflux. Approximately 30% of patients with Hashimoto's/autoimmune thyroiditis also make antibodies to the acid-producing cells in the stomach, and this can eventually lead to damage to the stomach lining and reduced stomach acid production, thereby impairing protein digestion.

o   <u>Menstrual irregularities, premenstrual syndrome (PMS), uterine fibroids, excess menstrual bleeding, polycystic ovarian syndrome (PCOS)</u>: Women with hypothyroidism commonly have one or more menstrual or reproductive disorders[728]; these are generally reversible or at least partially treatable with normalization of thyroid hormone status and optimization of other health factors. Women with polycystic ovary syndrome have higher-than-normal rates of goiter and autoimmune hypothyroid disease.[729]

o   <u>Infertility and the feeling and experience of not having enough sex hormones</u>: Proper thyroid status is needed for the complexities of gonadal function and reproductive success. Male and female with hypothyroidism may have no symptoms or problems with regard to sexual function, desire, and reproduction; but infertility and subfertility are common among this patient population. Thyroid hormone is directly necessary for sex hormone production and for the successful maintenance of pregnancy. Primary hypothyroidism associated with elevated TSH levels commonly leads to elevated levels of a pituitary hormone called prolactin, which causes infertility either by direct mechanisms or by secondary mechanisms, such as increasing the liver's production of a protein called sex-hormone-binding globulin (SHBG) which binds to sex hormones (estrogen and testosterone) so tightly that they are unavailable to cells to complete their functions, such as supporting sex drive, sexual function, and reproductive capability. As a cause of low libido, hypothyroidism impairs neurotransmitters such as norepinephrine and dopamine which promote sex drive in men and women. Hypothyroidism also impairs internal production of testosterone, which is a necessary hormone for sex drive and sexual performance.

o   <u>Weak fingernails, hair loss</u>: The weak fingernails seen in hypothyroidism are almost certainly due to impaired protein digestion and amino acid and mineral absorption, as well as impairment of the cells in the nail matrix which produces the toenails and fingernails. Probably via similar mechanisms,

---

Hypothyroidism is a cause of sexual dysfunction and reproductive disorders in men and women

"Via its interaction in several pathways, normal thyroid function is important to maintain normal reproduction. ... Male reproduction is adversely affected by both thyrotoxicosis [hyperthyroidism] and hypothyroidism. Erectile abnormalities have been reported. ... In females, thyrotoxicosis and hypothyroidism can cause menstrual disturbances. Thyrotoxicosis is associated mainly with hypomenorrhea and polymenorrhea, whereas hypothyroidism is associated mainly with oligomenorrhea [reduced frequency of menstruation]. Thyroid dysfunction has also been linked to reduced fertility. ... Autoimmune thyroid disease is present in 5-20% of unselected pregnant women. ... Overt hypothyroidism has been associated with increased rates of spontaneous abortion, premature delivery and/or low birth weight, fetal distress in labor, and perhaps gestation-induced hypertension and placental abruption."

Krassas et al. Thyroid function and human reproductive health. *Endocr Rev.* 2010 Oct

---

[728] Weeks AD. Menorrhagia and hypothyroidism. Evidence supports association between hypothyroidism and menorrhagia. *BMJ.* 2000 Mar 4;320(7235):649
[729] "In this case-control study, anti-thyroid antibodies and goiter prevalence were significantly higher in PCOS patients. These data suggest that thyroid exam and evaluation of thyroid function and autoimmunity should be considered in such patients." Kachuei M, Jafari F, Kachuei A, Keshteli AH. Prevalence of autoimmune thyroiditis in patients with polycystic ovary syndrome. *Arch Gynecol Obstet.* 2011 Aug 25. [Epub ahead of print]

hypothyroidism also causes loss of head hair, which is particularly notable in women. The finding of weak fingernails is a relatively specific finding for a limited number of considerations; generally these are protein deficiency (due to insufficient intake, impaired digestion or absorption, or increased metabolic consumption or increased renal excretion), deficiency of minerals such as zinc, and hypothyroidism. Severe cases of skin diseases such as psoriasis can also affect the nails, but generally these conditions are evident upon observation of the patient; the clinical findings are also different from those seen in hypothyroidism (e.g., pitting of the nails with psoriasis).

o <u>Increased need for sleep</u>: An increased need for sleep—termed either hypersomnia or hypersomnolence— is sometimes noted among hypothyroid patients, who might have the experience of needing extra sleep (e.g., > 9 hours per night) and yet not feeling refreshed after a good night's sleep. Other causes of increased need for and/or reduced quality of sleep are heart failure and sleep apnea; these can generally be distinguished from hypothyroidism based on history, physical exam, laboratory tests, and—more accurately but not generally needed—special tests such as echocardiography and sleep tests (polysomnography).

o <u>Overweight, gain weight easily, difficulty losing weight</u>: Thyroid hormone is an important factor energy utilization and thus caloric expenditure and therefore calorie intake-expenditure balance. Any low thyroid condition will promote weight gain and reduced weight loss because the overall metabolic rate is lowered in states of low thyroid status. The caveat to this situation is that patients with hypothyroidism often have reduced appetite, and therefore food intake may be reduced and thereby mask reduced caloric expenditure because body weight may not change much. When present, the paradox of "weight gain despite reduced food intake" strongly suggests hypothyroidism.

o <u>High cholesterol</u>: Thyroid hormone suppresses the activity of the rate-limiting enzyme for endogenous cholesterol production, which is commonly called HMG-CoA reductase, an abbreviation for hydroxy-methyl-glutaryl-CoA reductase. If thyroid hormone is not present in sufficient amounts to act as a brake for the HMG-CoA reductase enzyme, then the activity of the enzyme will be increased and blood cholesterol levels will rise. Many patients noted to have high cholesterol levels are prescribed a lifetime of cholesterol-lowering drugs; this is unfortunate because what these patients often need is thyroid hormone.

o <u>Slow heart rate</u>: The average adult heart rate is approximately 72 beats per minute (b/m); abnormally slow heart rate (bradycardia) is defined as less than 60 b/m and excessively fast heart rate is greater than 100 b/m. In certain situations, a fast or slow heart rate might be normal for the situation at hand; for example, well-trained athletes may have a "normal" heart rate in the 50s, and an individual who is anxious, severely anemic, sick with an infection, or over-caffeinated might have an elevated heart rate that does not indicate a serious/real disease. If I see a patient with a heart rate <65 b/m and the patient is not athletic and does not have a heart condition or is not taking a medication that slows the heart rate, then I become suspicious of hypothyroidism and will look for other historical, physical, or laboratory evidence of hypothyroidism. Hypothyroidism can also cause a rare heart disorder called

o <u>High blood pressure</u>: Hypothyroidism is a well-known cause of high blood pressure, specifically a type of high blood pressure called diastolic hypertension.

o <u>Slow healing</u>: Reduced overall metabolic rate and impaired protein digestion and utilization—both of which are noted in patients with hypothyroidism—leads to impaired healing of wounds and injuries.

o <u>Decreased memory and concentration</u>: Reduced overall metabolic rate and impaired protein digestion and utilization—both of which are noted in patients with hypothyroidism—leads to impaired memory and cognition. Protein is the source of amino acids, which are used by the body to make neurotransmitters such as serotonin, dopamine, and norepinephrine. Low thyroid state also impairs the function of the nervous system, specifically the adrenergic aspect of the nervous system which uses dopamine and norepinephrine to promote attention, mood, and pleasure.

o <u>Muscle weakness</u>: In more severe cases, hypothyroidism can cause a muscle disease (hypothyroid myopathy); this can lead to muscle weakness.

o <u>Sleep apnea</u>: Hypothyroidism contributes to sleep apnea, which is impaired breathing during sleep.

o <u>Frog-like husky voice</u>: Changes in voice is commonly noted among patients with reduced thyroid function.

- o **Recurrent infections**: Hypothyroidism impairs immune function, resulting in more severe and more frequent infections.
- o **Many other manifestations**: Because thyroid hormone is necessary for every body system, its lack or insufficiency thereby also affects all body systems. Thus, *many* adverse health effects and symptoms may result from an insufficiency of thyroid hormone.

Major differential diagnoses for hypothyroidism:

- Because hypothyroidism can result in so many different health problems and subjective symptoms, the list of diagnostic considerations that share similarities with hypothyroidism is virtually endless. Each of the symptoms above has its own list of possible different diagnostic considerations. However, the pattern of symptoms in hypothyroidism is unique. The most specific symptoms and findings for hypothyroidism are
    - ❶ slow heart rate,
    - ❷ persistently low body temperature,
    - ❸ delayed Achilles reflex return (discussed below),
    - ❹ weight gain associated with reduced appetite.

Clinical assessment:

- **History/subjective**: Historical findings and clinical presentations are listed above.
- **Physical examination/objective**: The most relevant clinical findings are discussed here:
    - o **Low body temperature**: Very few conditions result in persistently low body temperature; clearly the most common and important of these conditions is hypothyroidism. Patients who are persistently uncomfortable with cold hands and feet and persistent cold intolerance are worthy of assessment and treatment. Objectively, the physician will note that upon the welcoming handshake, the patient's hands feel cold; this assessment will be invalidated if the patient recently washed hands in hot water, is wearing gloves, or if the physician also has hypothyroidism and is therefore just as cold. A persistently low first-morning oral temperature below 98.6° F warrants consideration for hypothyroidism. A persistently low first-morning axillary (underarm) temperature below 97.8-98.2° F warrants consideration for hypothyroidism.

How to measure first-morning axillary temperature
1. Shake down mercury thermometer before going to bed; leave thermometer near bedside (but obviously not in the bed where it could be warmed or broken)
2. Immediately upon wakening, before any other activity, place thermometer deep in axilla (armpit) and measure temperature for 7-10 minutes,
3. Normal is 97.8-98.2°F; less than this temperature warrants consideration of hypothyroidism, especially if other manifestations are present.

    - o **Delayed Achillies reflex return**: The deep tendon reflexes assessed by doctors during most clinical encounters contain two components: the contraction phase and the relaxation phase. Most of the time, we as doctors are primarily concerned with the contraction phase, which tells us about the integrity of the neuromuscular system. However, when we are looking for hypothyroidism, we are more concerned with the relaxation phase of the reflex; patients with hypothyroidism have reduced speed of muscular relaxation, and therefore the relaxation phase of the reflex cycle is prolonged. This finding is highly specific for hypothyroidism.
    - o **Slow heart rate—bradycardia**: A heart rate less than 65 b/m suggests the possibility of hypothyroidism unless the patient is a well-conditioned athlete, has heart conduction problems, or is taking a medication such as a beta-blocking drug which will slow the rate of heart contractions.
- **Imaging & laboratory assessments**:
    - o **Imaging**: Imaging is not routinely relevant in the assessment and monitoring of hypothyroidism. Ultrasound scans and radionucleotide scans can be used to assess for more serious thyroid diseases, such as thyroid cancer.

- o Laboratory evaluation: Laboratory evaluation of the patient with clinical manifestations of low thyroid function should be tertiary in importance to the physician's assessment, judgment, and experience and the patient's need for effective treatment for his/her complaints. As is stated with regard to the treatment of hypertension: the physician's judgment remains paramount.
  - Thyrotropin-releasing hormone (TRH): The hypothalamus releases TRH to stimulate pituitary production of TSH. TRH is not routinely tested in clinical practice, although abnormalities of TRH secretion are noted in patients with mental "depression."
  - Thyroid-stimulating hormone (TSH: 0.4 - 5.0 mIU/L [milli-international units per liter]): TSH is the most commonly performed test for evaluating thyroid status; its frequent (over)use owes more to habit and inexpensiveness than to aspirations for clinical excellence. TSH values greater than 2 mIU/L represent a disturbance of the thyroid-pituitary axis and an increased risk for future thyroid problems[730], and the American Association of Clinical Endocrinologists states, "The target TSH level should be between 0.3 and 3.0 µIU/mL."[731] Clinical rationale is available to support implementation of a therapeutic trial of thyroid hormone treatment in patients who are clinically hypothyroid even if they are biochemically euthyroid (per TSH) provided that treatment is implemented cautiously, in appropriately selected patients, and patients are appropriately informed.[732,733] If the clinical world were as perfect as it is portrayed in basic physiology textbooks, then a clinician might fancifully rely on TSH to perform the diagnosis *prima facie*, with reduced TSH values correlating with glandular overperformance and negative feedback suppressing TSH secretion, whilst an underperforming gland would require greater stimulation with elevated TSH levels; however, TSH has never been thus vested with infallible reliability, which explains in part why doctors need brains of their own and why better clinicians have developed the capacity for independent thought.
  - Free thyroxine (free T4: 4.5 - 11.2 mcg/dL): Unbound T4 is tested to provide evidence of glandular production of thyroid hormone(s). Because T4 is the major thyroid hormone produced by the thyroid gland it serves as an excellent marker for glandular productivity but it reveals nothing about peripheral conversion of T4 to the active thyroid hormone triiodothyronine (T3); in the practice of medicine, conversion of T4 to the active T3 is assumed to reliably occur unabated despite evidence to the contrary, especially among symptomatic patients.
  - Triiodothyronine (T3: 100 - 200 ng/dL[734]): In textbook-perfect physiology, T4 is converted by deiodinase enzymes type-1 and type-2 to the active thyroid hormone T3; in reality, this is only part of the story. Because T3 is the active form of the hormone responsible for the physiologic functions of thyroid physiology, a clinician desiring to assess a patient's thyroid status might reasonably ask the proper question by performing the proper test. T3 is tested as "total T3" or "free T3" in large part based on the clinician's preference; the current author prefers total T3 because it can be compared to the total level of reverse T3 (rT3) in a ratio, the optimal range of which is generally considered to be 10-14 as originally presented by McDaniel[735] and reviewed in the following pages. Patients with psychiatric depression

Optimal thyroid status
Concept by Dr Vasquez: Optimal thyroid status is not defined by basic laboratory testing with TSH and free T4. It is defined *per patient* based on the levels and ratios of all major thyroid-related hormones and antibodies—in association with other hormonal, psychologic, dysbiotic, nutritional and environmental factors— that work best for that particular unique biochemically-individual patient.
Laboratory interpretation by Dr McDaniel: "Optimal hormone balance is debatable. My observations: A few "well" people and patients treated successfully with T4 and T3 seem best with: <ul><li>TSH around 0.7–0.9 µIU/mL</li><li>fT4 around 0.7–0.8 ng/dL</li><li>fT3 optimally 3.4–3.8 pg/mL</li><li>**Total T3-RT3 ratio 12 +/-2**"</li></ul>
McDaniel AB. Thyroid Assessment: Controversies and Conundrums. Institute for Functional Medicine Fourteenth International Symposium. Tucson, Arizona. May 23-26, 2007

[730] Weetman AP. Fortnightly review: Hypothyroidism: screening and subclinical disease. *BMJ: British Medical Journal* 1997;314: 1175

[731] American Association of Clinical Endocrinologists. "The target TSH level should be between 0.3 and 3.0 µIU/mL." AACE Medical Guidelines for Clinical Practice for Evaluation and Treatment of Hyperthyroidism and Hypothyroidism. 2002, 2006 Amended Version. https://www.aace.com/sites/default/files/hypo_hyper.pdf Accessed Aug 2011

[732] Skinner GR, Thomas R, Taylor M, Sellarajah M, Bolt S, Krett S, Wright A. Thyroxine should be tried in clinically hypothyroid but biochemically euthyroid patients. *BMJ: British Medical Journal* 1997 Jun 14; 314(7096): 1764

[733] McLaren EH, Kelly CJ, Pollack MA. Trial of thyroxine treatment for biochemically euthyroid patients has been approved. *BMJ* 1997; 315: 1463

[734] U.S. National Library of Medicine (NLM) and National Institutes of Health (NIH) http://www.nlm.nih.gov/medlineplus/ency/article/003687.htm Accessed August 2011

[735] McDaniel AB. Thyroid Assessment: Controversies and Conundrums. Institute for Functional Medicine Fourteenth International Symposium. Tucson, Az. May 23-26, 2007

have lower levels of T3 than do healthy controls and have been described as having "low T3 syndrome"[736]; very obviously—whether cause or effect—the low T3 levels in these patients would serve to promote and perpetuate their state of mental depression. Although the focus of this review within the subject of laboratory evaluation is not to describe the implementation of thyroid hormone treatment, clinicians should be aware that T3 administration increases hepatic production of sex hormone binding globulin (SHBG) and that therefore T3 administration can reduce cellular bioavailability of protein-bound hormones. Many authoritative and clinically-experienced sources recommend using a time-released (e.g., sustained-release) form of T3 due to its shorter half-life compared with T4. However, obtaining time-released T3 via a compounding pharmacy can be cumbersome and expensive for the patient; clearly some patients respond to once daily dosing of *non*-*time*-released preparations with good effects and without adverse effects. Some patients can divide the immediate-release dose into two servings per day for enhanced effect and lessened physiologic fluctuations, if necessary. Per Drugs.com[737] in August 2011, "Since liothyronine sodium (T3) is not firmly bound to serum protein, it is readily available to body tissues. The onset of activity of liothyronine sodium is rapid, occurring within a few hours. Maximum pharmacologic response occurs within 2 or 3 days, providing early clinical response. The biological half-life is about 2.5 days." Very clearly, a significant portion of hypothyroid patients respond to T3 alone (either time-released, divided-dosing, or once-daily dosing) or a combination of T4 and T3 when other treatments have failed.[738,739]

- Reverse triiodothyronine (rT3: 90 - 320 pg/mL[740]): T4 is converted by deiodinase enzymes type-1 and type-3 to the inactive thyroid hormone rT3; per a standard endocrinology textbook, "Approximately 70–80% of released T4 is converted by deiodinases to the biologically active T3, the remainder to reverse-T3 (rT3) which has no significant biological activity."[741] Clinicians must know that, "The prohormone T4 must be converted to T3 in the body before it can exert biological effects. **During periods of illness or stress, this conversion is often inhibited and can be diverted to the inactive reverse T3 (rT3) moiety.**"[742] Furthermore and very importantly, clinicians should appreciate that rT3 is not simply inactive but that it may actually impair production/utilization of normal T3; "T4-T3 and T4-rT3 conversion are provoked by different enzymes. **The <u>elevation of rT3</u> might be a cause of the observed decrease in peripheral T3 generation** in old [elderly] subjects, acting by an <u>**inhibition of the T4-T3 conversion**</u>."[743] During times of psychologic/physiologic stress and specific types of pharmacologic stress (e.g., propanolol[744] and corticosteroids), T4 metabolism is preferentially shunted away from T3 toward rT3; an anthropocentric explanation holds that by making less of the active T3 and more of the inactive rT3, the body is better able to conserve energy during times of stress by reducing overall metabolic rate, particularly resting energy expenditure and protein utilization. For example, caloric restriction and fasting result in a decrease in resting metabolic rate (RMR), and the reduced RMR persists for months after the fasting has ended and a normal diet is resumed.[745] This author (AV) terms this stress-induced impairment of thyroid hormone conversion "**metabolic hypothyroidism**" or "**functional hypothyroidism**" because the defect is in the metabolism (not the production) of thyroid hormone into its most active form; "**peripheral hypothyroidism**" might also be used to distinguish the fact that the defect is in the peripheral metabolism rather than located more centrally, within the thyroid gland itself. Because psychologic stress and certain pharmacologic

[736] "Out of 250 subjects with major psychiatric depression, 6.4% exhibited low T3 syndrome (mean serum T3 concentration 0.94 nmol/l vs normal mean serum concentration of 1.77 nmol/l)." Premachandra BN, Kabir MA, Williams IK. Low T3 syndrome in psychiatric depression. *J Endocrinol Invest.* 2006 Jun;29(6):568-72

[737] http://www.drugs.com/pro/cytomel.html Accessed August 2011.

[738] Bunevicius R, Kazanavicius G, Zalinkevicius R, Prange AJ Jr. Effects of thyroxine as compared with thyroxine plus triiodothyronine in patients with hypothyroidism. *N Engl J Med.* 1999 Feb 11;340(6):424-9

[739] Kelly T, Lieberman DZ. The use of triiodothyronine as an augmentation agent in treatment-resistant bipolar II and bipolar disorder NOS. *J Affect Disord.* 2009;116(3):222-6

[740] The reference range provided here for rT3 is a compilation from the laboratory reference ranges from the sample reports on the following pages, each of which is performed by either Quest Diagnostics or LabCorp, the two largest medical laboratories in the United States.

[741] Nussey S, Whitehead S. *Endocrinology: An Integrated Approach*. Oxford: BIOS Scientific Publishers; 2001. See also Box 3.29 Metabolism of thyroid hormones. http://www.ncbi.nlm.nih.gov/books/NBK28/box/A270/?report=objectonly Accessed July 2011

[742] *1998 Mosby's GenRX. Sixth Edition*. St. Louis Missouri; Mosby-Year Book, Inc., 1998

[743] Szabolcs I, Weber M, Kovács Z, Irsy G, Góth M, Halász T, Szilágyi G. The possible reason for serum 3,3'5'-(reverse) triiodothyronine increase in old people. *Acta Med Acad Sci Hung.* 1982;39(1-2):11-7

[744] "Propranolol administration (40 mg t.i.d. for a week) caused a similar rT3 elevation in old persons (n = 18) as in 12 young ones." Szabolcs I, Weber M, Kovács Z, Irsy G, Góth M, Halász T, Szilágyi G. The possible reason for serum 3,3'5'-(reverse) triiodothyronine increase in old people. *Acta Med Acad Sci Hung.* 1982;39(1-2):11-7

[745] Elliot DL, Goldberg L, Kuehl KS, Bennett WM. Sustained depression of the resting metabolic rate after massive weight loss. *Am J Clin Nutr* 1989 Jan;49(1):93-96

exposures—as well as the thyro-metabolic stress of fasting and caloric restriction in which the counterregulatory hormone glucagon appears to trigger enhanced rT3 production—reduce T3 while simultaneously increasing rT3 levels, clinicians can appreciate that calculation of the T3/rT3 ratio will be more significantly altered (and thus a more sensitive indicator of metabolic disruption) than will be the isolated measurements of T3 or rT3 alone. Functional medicine clinicians[746] note the importance of the ratio of total T3 to reverse T3 (tT3:rT3 ratio) and consider the optimal range to be 10-14 with lower ratios indicating impaired formation or T3 and/or excess production of rT3.[747] Contrary to the previous view which held that rT3 was simply inactive, we now appreciate that rT3 actually impairs normal thyroid hormone metabolism thus functioning as an thyrometabolic monkeywrench or "brake" on normal metabolism. Elevated rT3 levels predict mortality among critically ill patients.[748] Aberrancies in thyroid hormone levels may reflect organic disease, psychoemotional stress, or nutritional deficiency[749], and therefore such serologic abnormalities warrant consideration of underlying problems and direct treatment when possible. If no underlying cause is apparent, then a trial of thyroid hormone/hormones is reasonable in appropriately selected patients. Beyond stress reduction, allergen/gluten avoidance, and nutritional supplementation with iodine, selenium, and zinc (as indicated per patient), correction of overt, subclinical, and functional hypothyroidism generally centers on the administration of natural or synthetic thyroid hormones in the form of T4 and T3. Correction of functional hypothyroidism (relatively reduced total T3 and increased rT3) is accomplished with either time-released or twice-daily dosing of T3 *without T4* to suppress endogenous T4 conversion to T3, thereby allowing rT3 levels to fall precipitously. T3 administration allows temporary downregulation of transforming enzymes so that rT3 production is reduced following withdrawal of T3 replacement; thus, short-term and/or periodic T3 administration helps normalize or "reset" peripheral thyroid metabolism so that, following withdrawal of T3 administration, T4 can be converted to T3 without excess production of rT3. The safety and effectiveness of this approach—using T3 administration (often twice daily or in a sustained-release compounded tablet or capsule) to recalibrate peripheral thyroid hormone metabolism—has documented safety and effectiveness.[750] Alleviation of symptoms, restoration of morning body temperature to 98.6° F (oral or axillary) and other clinical objective improvements achieved by the judicious and safe administration of T3 are the criteria of success; physiologic improvement following T3 administration retrospectively confirms the diagnosis.

- Antithyroid antibodies—antithyroglobulin (anti-TG) and anti-thyroid peroxidase (anti-TPO): Autoimmune thyroiditis (also called Hashimoto's disease or chronic lymphocytic thyroiditis) or is the most common cause of overt primary hypothyroidism. The diagnosis of autoimmune thyroiditis can be made clinically (i.e., without biopsy) upon detection of elevated blood levels of antibodies against thyroglobulin (anti-thyroglobulin antibodies) and anti-thyroid peroxidase (anti-TPO) antibodies. Autoimmune thyroiditis may present asymptomatically and with normal thyroid hormone levels; classically, patients may have a slightly hyperthyroid presentation as the inflamed gland releases extra thyroid hormone before becoming atrophic and hypofunctional.

- **Establishing the diagnosis**:
  - The diagnosis of hypothyroidism is supported by the constellation of ❶ the patient's history and subjective complaints, ❷ physical examination findings, ❸ laboratory findings, and ❹ response to a clinical trial of thyroid hormone, preferably in the combination of T4 and T3 which are consistent with the physiologic production of thyroid hormones from the thyroid gland. Treatment with T4 alone cannot
  - The diagnosis of Hashimoto's/autoimmune thyroiditis is strongly suggested by the finding of elevated antibody levels against thyroglobulin and/or TPO.

---

[746] The conclusion of this paragraph is derived from Vasquez A. *Musculoskeletal Pain: Expanded Clinical Strategies*. Published 2008 by The Institute for Functional Medicine.

[747] McDaniel AB. Thyroid Assessment: Controversies and Conundrums. Institute for Functional Medicine Fourteenth International Symposium. Tucson, Az. May 23-26, 2007

[748] Peeters RP, Wouters PJ, van Toor H, Kaptein E, Visser TJ, Van den Berghe G. Serum 3,3',5'-triiodothyronine (rT3) and 3,5,3'-triiodothyronine/rT3 are prognostic markers in critically ill patients and are associated with postmortem tissue deiodinase activities. *J Clin Endocrinol Metab*. 2005 Aug;90(8):4559-65

[749] Kelly GS. Peripheral metabolism of thyroid hormones: a review. *Altern Med Rev*. 2000 Aug;5(4):306-33

[750] Friedman M, Miranda-Massari JR, Gonzalez MJ. Supraphysiological cyclic dosing of sustained release T3 in order to reset low basal body temperature. *P R Health Sci J*. 2006 Mar;25(1):23-9

Complications:

- Complications of hypothyroidism: The complications of hypothyroidism are mainly continuations of the health problems previously mentioned in the sections on clinical presentations and clinical assessments. The "most important" problems from a clinical "medical" perspective are depression, hypertension, hypercholesterolemia, hormonal/reproductive/sexual problems, and increased susceptibility to infection. From a more personal perspective for the patients with *undiagnosed*, *untreated* or *insufficiently treated* hypothyroidism, the impaired quality of life, the chronic tiredness and fatigue, the lack of mental clarity and chronic low-grade depression, plus the feeling that "something is wrong with me" and the lack of understanding from doctors, friends, family, and intimate partners can be very distressing.

Clinical management:

- Implementation of effective treatment: Patients with laboratory evidence of hypothyroidism and/or a compelling clinical picture of hypothyroid deserve treatment with thyroid hormone if no important conditions contraindicate its use. Conditions such as mania, seizure disorder, cardiac arrhythmia, coronary artery disease, and adrenal insufficiency are the main contraindications.
- Consideration of other immune disorders: Patients with autoimmune thyroiditis have higher-than-normal rates of celiac disease (gluten intolerance) and other autoimmune disorders.
- Periodic monitoring: Patients should be monitored for safety with clinical assessment and laboratory tests at the initiation of treatment and at approximately 3-6 months after the initiation of treatment and then yearly thereafter.

Treatments:

- **Overall considerations**: Treatment of low thyroid function generally centers on the administration of thyroid hormone(s), although some patients are able to restore normal thyroid function with specific dietary modification (e.g., avoidance of allergens and gluten-containing grains) and nutritional supplementation (e.g., selenium). A few people are able to take thyroid hormone treatment for a few months or years, and then discontinue the medication and yet maintain normal function. Many people take the hormones for life.

Patients often feel better with combination T4 and T3 rather than T4 alone
"Twelve patients preferred combination treatment, 6 patients preferred the add-on combination treatment, 2 patients preferred standard treatment, and 6 patients had no preference."
Escobar-Morreale HF, et al. Thyroid hormone replacement therapy in primary hypothyroidism: a randomized trial comparing L-thyroxine plus liothyronine with L-thyroxine alone. *Ann Intern Med.* 2005 Mar

    - Thyroid hormone replacement—physiologically appropriate—with T4 and T3: Patients with insufficient function of thyroid hormone generally need more thyroid hormone, which is generally in the form of biologically identical synthetic thyroid hormones, T4 and/or T3. Unfortunately, most (allopathic) doctors have been trained to use T4 without T3; this is nonphysiologic and therefore neither intellectually nor scientifically valid. When patients are hypothyroid, they generally need T4 and T3 together because the thyroid gland makes both of these hormones, and they are both required for optimal and normal thyroid status. Studies that have used T4 alone without T3 may have found "lack of effectiveness" not because the patients did not stand to benefit from thyroid hormone(s) but because the patients were given *inactive* T4 when they needed *active* T3, or a combination of T4 with T3. The three most common types of thyroid hormone replacement are described here:
      - Synthetic T4: L-thyroxine, Levothyroxine: L-thyroxine is synthetic T4; it is chemically the same as the hormone produced in the body. Because it is synthetic and not derived from animal tissue, it does not contain antigens that can provoke an immune response. Levothyroxine/T4 must be converted in the body to liothyronine/T3 in order to be active; therefore, T4 administration is more safe and "stable" than is the administration of T3. The standard allopathic medical approach is to use T4 *without T3*.[751,752]

---

[751] Escobar-Morreale HF, Botella-Carretero JI, Escobar del Rey F, Morreale de Escobar G. Treatment of hypothyroidism with combinations of levothyroxine plus liothyronine. *J Clin Endocrinol Metab.* 2005 Aug;90(8):4946-54

[752] Joffe RT, Brimacombe M, Levitt AJ, Stagnaro-Green A. Treatment of clinical hypothyroidism with thyroxine and triiodothyronine: a literature review and metaanalysis. *Psychosomatics.* 2007 Sep-Oct;48(5):379-84

- ▫ <u>Available dose forms (amount per tablet)</u>: 25,50,75,88,100,112,125,137,150,175,200,300 mcg.
- ▫ <u>Conversion equivalents of various forms of thyroid hormone</u>: levothyroxine 100 mcg = liothyronine 25 mcg = Liotrix 1 grain = thyroid (porcine) 1 grain.
- ▫ <u>Dose for adults</u>: 50-200 to a max of 300 mcg PO (by mouth) qd (daily) with a starting dose of 12.5-50 mcg PO qd; doses are smaller for children. Levothyroxine appears to be slightly more effective if taken at night rather than in the morning.[753]
- ▫ <u>Info</u>: Give on empty stomach between meals; specifically avoid soy products within 2 hours of thyroid hormone administration because constituents of soy bind thyroid hormone in the gastrointestinal tract.
- ▫ <u>Contraindications and cautions</u>: allergy, recent heart attack, adrenal insufficiency; caution with cardiovascular disease, cardiac arrhythmia, diabetes mellitus, and elderly patients.
- ▫ <u>Drug/botanical/nutrient interactions</u>: Lemon balm and L-carnitine impair thyroid hormone utilization and effect.
- ▫ <u>Adverse effects—generally not noted with proper dosing</u>: Unmasking of cardiac arrhythmias, angina if cardiovascular disease and arterial stenosis is present. Excessive dosing or overdose can cause palpitations, tachycardia, nervousness, tremor, weight loss, diaphoresis/sweating, diarrhea, abdominal cramps, anxiety
- ▫ <u>Safety/Monitoring</u>: *Pregnancy*: A, *Lactation*: Safe
- ▫ <u>Half-life</u>: 6-7 days
- ▪ <u>Synthetic T3—Liothyronine, Cytomel</u>: T3 is the active form of thyroid hormone and it is therefore rapidly utilized and thus has a shorter half-life than does T4. T3 is the preferred form of thyroid hormone administration for the treatment of the previously described peripheral/metabolic hypothyroidism, treatment of which must be accomplished via suppressing endogenous T4 production to reduce the amount of rT3 being produced by stress-induced physiologic/enzymatic adaptations.[754] Some but not all studies show clinical improvement in patients who use combination T4 and T3 rather than T4 alone.
  - ▫ <u>Available dose forms (amount per tablet)</u>: 5,25,50 mcg
  - ▫ <u>Conversion equivalents of various forms of thyroid hormone</u>: levothyroxine 100 mcg = liothyronine 25 mcg = Liotrix 1 grain = thyroid (porcine) 1 grain.
  - ▫ <u>Dose for adults</u>: 25-75 mcg PO qd; for severe hypothyroidism start with a low dose of 5-10 mcg PO qd.
  - ▫ <u>Info</u>: Give on empty stomach between meals; specifically avoid soy products within 2 hours of thyroid hormone administration because constituents of soy bind thyroid hormone in the gastrointestinal tract.
  - ▫ <u>Contraindications and cautions</u>: allergy, recent heart attack, adrenal insufficiency; caution with cardiovascular disease, cardiac arrhythmia, diabetes mellitus, and elderly patients.
  - ▫ <u>Adverse effects—generally not noted with proper dosing</u>: Unmasking of cardiac arrhythmias, angina if cardiovascular disease and arterial stenosis is present. Excessive dosing or overdose can cause palpitations, tachycardia, nervousness, tremor, weight loss, diaphoresis/sweating, diarrhea, abdominal cramps, anxiety

Contraindications to T3, liothyronine, Cytomel
<u>Absolute contraindications</u>:   • Anaphylaxis or severe hypersensitivity,   • Acute (current) myocardial infarction,   • Hyperthyroidism,   • Untreated adrenal insufficiency.
<u>Relative contraindications and cautions</u>:   • CAD, angina pectoris, or cardiac arrhythmia,   • Elderly patients—start with low dose and titrate as tolerated.
<u>Reference</u>: Epocrates.com August 2011

---

[753] "Levothyroxine taken at bedtime significantly improved thyroid hormone levels. Quality-of-life variables and plasma lipid levels showed no significant changes with bedtime vs morning intake. Clinicians should consider prescribing levothyroxine intake at bedtime." Bolk N, Visser TJ, Nijman J, Jongste IJ, Tijssen JG, Berghout A. Effects of evening vs morning levothyroxine intake: a randomized double-blind crossover trial. *Arch Intern Med.* 2010 Dec 13;170(22):1996-2003

[754] Friedman M, Miranda-Massari JR, Gonzalez MJ. Supraphysiological cyclic dosing of sustained release T3 in order to reset low basal body temperature. *P R Health Sci J.* 2006 Mar;25(1):23-9

- ▫ Safety/Monitoring: *Pregnancy*: A, *Lactation*: Safe
- ▫ Half-life: 1 day
- ▪ Synthetic T4 with synthetic T3—Liotrix, Thyrolar: This is a convenient yet more expensive way to obtain synthetic T4 along with synthetic T3 in an attempt to most closely mimic normal thyroid hormone production. It is dosed orally between meals in strengths of "1", "2", and "3". This product can be very difficult to obtain.
- ▪ Animal-derived glandular products with either T4 and T3, or T3 alone: Glandular products derived from the glands of cows and pigs contain T4 and T3 in their prescription forms such as Armour Thyroid and T3 in their nonprescription forms. Patients who show greater benefit with these products than they did with synthetic T4 alone are probably responding to the T3, but it is possible that other nutritive factors or hormones in the whole gland are providing benefit. My preference is to avoid the use of glandular products in patients with thyroid autoimmunity due to the possible exacerbation of the (auto)immune response, which can be monitored by measurement of blood levels of anti-TPO and anti-thyroglobulin antibodies.

> **Combination T4 and T3 (rather than T4 alone) provides a mood-elevating antidepressant effect**
>
> "Fourteen of 17 patients showed improvement. One patient saw no improvement and 2 dropped out due to side effects. The patients who benefited showed an average CGI improvement of 2.5 (SD: 0.52). The average dose used was 80 mcg (SD: 30.2, range: 25 mcg-150 mcg). The average length of time on T(3) was 24.2 months (SD: 19.4, range: 11.8-86.7). This case series shows that T(3) may be successfully employed as a long term treatment augmentation of major depression if over time dosage levels are increased beyond the traditional 50 mcg."
>
> Kelly TF, Lieberman DZ. Long term augmentation with T3 in refractory major depression. *J Affect Disord.* 2009 May

- o Selenium—200 mcg per day: Selenium, zinc, and iron are all necessary for the biochemical pathways necessary for the peripheral metabolism of thyroid hormones, specifically the conversion of T4 to T3; deficiency of these nutrients can induce a "metabolic hypothyroidism" or "nutritional hypothyroidism" due to impairment of thyroid hormone metabolism and utilization. Further, zinc and selenium support antioxidant defenses; whereas iron is an antioxidant a low doses and a potent pro-oxidant in when present in higher amounts. Several studies have shown that nutritional supplementation with selenium 200 micrograms (mcg) per day for adults lowers the levels of anti-thyroid antibodies within three months and to an even greater extent by the end of nine months.
- o Zinc—15-50 mg per day: Zinc is necessary for the proper metabolism of thyroid hormones. Many patients—especially the elderly—are deficient in zinc. Zinc supplementation is quite safe and the pill(s) should be taken with food in order to avoid stomach upset. Long-term high-dose zinc supplementation can cause deficiency of copper. I always recommend use of a high-potency multivitamin-multimineral supplement to patients as part of the foundational treatment plan—see my free article[755] on-line at http://InflammationMastery.com/spmd.html.
- o Iron—only for patients with iron deficiency documented by the lab test serum ferritin: Iron is necessary for the proper metabolism of thyroid hormones. Iron status is assessed with a lab test called serum ferritin, and the optimal range is 40-70 ng/mL for most people; for patients with restless leg syndrome their ferritin can be up to 100 ng/mL. Details about interpreting the serum ferritin test are provided in the chapter on clinical assessments and additional information is available at my website at http://InflammationMastery.com/hemochromatosis.html. Iron deficiency in adults can be a sign of gastrointestinal blood loss such as from a stomach ulcer or colon cancer and must therefore always be evaluated appropriately.
- o Food allergen avoidance, especially gluten: Among food allergy disorders associated with thyroid autoimmunity, allergy to the protein gluten found in grains such as wheat is clearly preeminent. A specific type of gluten intolerance—celiac disease—is associated with autoimmunity in general and thyroid autoimmunity in particular. Approximately 15% of patients with celiac disease have thyroid autoimmunity (i.e., Hashimoto's thyroiditis), and this is reversible in nearly all patients following the adoption of a gluten-free diet.

---

[755] Vasquez A. Revisiting the Five-Part Nutritional Wellness Protocol: The Supplemented Paleo-Mediterranean Diet. *Nutritional Perspectives* 2011 January

- *Coleus forskolii*: *Coleus forskolii* is a useful botanical medicine that is often stated to enhance thyroid function; but the research supporting this effect is weak at best. One recent study showed that the extract forskolin promoted weight loss and muscle gain in overweight and obese men, but these benefits were not attributed to improved thyroid function.
- 7-keto-DHEA, also called 7-oxo-DHEA: 7-keto-DHEA is a metabolite of the hormone DHEA (dehydroepiandrosterone) which is a weak androgen (i.e. similar to but less potent than testosterone); 7-keto-DHEA metabolite does not have hormonal effects per se. One small study showed that administration of 7-keto-DHEA resulted in an increase in T3 levels.

Date and Time Collected 02/04/10 11:41	Date Entered 02/04/10	Date and Time Reported 02/09/10 04:06ET	Physician Name	NPI	PI 190

Tests Ordered

Triiodothyronine (T3);Reverse T3;Triiodothyronine,Free,Serum

General Comments

PID: 8282293

TESTS	RESULT	FLAG	UNITS	REFERENCE INTERV
Triiodothyronine (T3)				
Triiodothyronine (T3)	57	Low	ng/dL	71-180
Reverse T3				
Reverse T3	312		pg/mL	90-350
Triiodothyronine,Free,Serum				
Triiodothyronine,Free,Serum	2.5		pg/mL	2.0-4.4

Case presentation: 38yo male under extreme psychological stress with a complaint of constantly cold extremities—testing performed in February 2010 by LabCorp: Review the labs and outline your treatment plan before reading the discussion below.

Step-by-step conversion from ng/dL to pg/mL—end result is multiply by 10 (i.e., 10x)

Original units	Convert ng to pg[756]	Convert dL to mL	Simplify the fraction
1 ng / 1 dL	1,000 pg/ 1 dL	1,000 pg/ 100 mL	10 pg/ 1 ml
57 ng/ 1 dL	57,000 pg / 1 dL	57,000 pg / 100 mL	570 pg / 1 mL

Discussion: In this case, because the T3 level is low, *prima facie* justification for administration of T3 is provided, assuming that the clinical picture is compatible and that no contraindications to treatment are present. To calculate the total T3/rT3 ratio, equilibrate the units (multiply total T3 in ng/dL x 10 to convert to pg/mL; 1 pg = 0.001 ng (1 ng = 1,000 pg); 1 dl = 100 ml). The total T3/rT3 ratio should be >10-14 (per McDaniel[757]), but in this patient's case 570/312 = 1.8. Remember, more T3 than rT3 is better; hence, the higher ratio is better. On-line calculators for this conversion have been developed[758] and surely more will be available in the future. This athletic and otherwise healthy 220-lb (100 kg) patient responded very well to T3 (liothyronine/Cytomel) with a starting dose of 150 mcg which was eventually tapered to 25 mcg and then to 12.5 mcg; in this patient's case, the initial high dose of T3 was well-tolerated because of the initially low level of T3, the elevated rT3 which appears to block T3 function, and the patient's overall excellent cardiovascular fitness. A reasonable dosage range for liothyronine/Cytomel supplementation is 12.5-50 mcg for most patients tapered to the constellation of patient tolerance, patient preference, heart rate, basal body temperature optimization to 98.6° F, suppression of TSH and T4, resolution of symptoms and objective markers, and clinician's impression and experience.

---

[756] Double-checked with http://www.unitconversion.org/weight/nanograms-to-picograms-conversion.html July 2011

[757] McDaniel AB. Thyroid Assessment: Controversies and Conundrums. Institute for Functional Medicine Fourteenth International Symposium. Tucson, AZ. May 23-26, 2007

[758] http://www.stopthethyroidmadness.com/rt3-ratio/ Accessed—but not necessarily endorsed—August 2011

```
FREE T3/REVERSE T3 RATIO
   FREE T3/REVERSE T3 RATIO                           0.93 L        1.05-1.91**
   FREE T3                           325                             230-420 pg/dL
   REVERSE T3                                          350 H         100-340*** pg/mL
```

**Ratio= Free T3 in pg/dL : reverse T3 in pg/mL. Ratio for reference range is calculated by dividing the lower and upper end of free T3 with the mean of reverse T3 (220 pg/mL).

***Observed reference range is reported for reverse T3 per client request.

This test was performed using a kit that has not been approved or cleared by the FDA. The analytical performance characteristics of this test have been determined by Quest Diagnostics Nichols Institute, San Juan Capistrano. This test should not be used for diagnosis without confirmation by other medically established means.

Presentation: A 42yo male with fatigue—testing performed by Quest Diagnostics in January 2010: Review the labs and outline your treatment plan before reading the discussion below. Note that the "optimal ratio" provided by the laboratory in this example was performed using free T3 rather than total T3 and without converting to equal units.

Step-by-step conversion from pg/dL to pg/mL—end result is divide by 100 (i.e., 0.01x): Provided for the sake of completeness even though the conversion is not necessary per the laboratory interpretation provided above.

Original units	Convert dL to mL	Simplify the fraction
1 pg / 1 dL	1 pg/ 100 mL	0.01 pg/ 1 mL
325 pg/ 1 dL	325 pg / 100 mL	3.25 pg / 1 mL

Discussion: Note that if the T3 had been tested without rT3 the results would have been reported as "normal" and that a "depressed" patient so assessed would have likely been given an "antidepressant" medication and a diagnosis of depression rather than the proper treatment with T3 and a diagnosis of functional hypothyroidism. Luckily for this patient, his clinician tested rT3 and upon finding it impressively elevated treated with patient with T3 to suppress rT3 production by temporarily suppressing T4 production. The ratio calculation is provided and interpreted by the laboratory; notice that the "ideal ratio" for **total** T3/rT3 (>10) differs from that of **free** T3/rT3 (>1.05) *and that per the ratio provided by the labotatory does not equilibriate the measurement units.* This method is acceptable but is not the preferred method for determining functional thyroid status. The preferred method is the one presented by McDaniel[759] at the Institute for Functional Medicine's 14th International Symposium in 2007 wherein he advocated using total T3 (not free T3) in comparison with rT3 interpreted by an optimal ratio of 10-14.

---

[759] McDaniel AB. Thyroid Assessment: Controversies and Conundrums. Institute for Functional Medicine Fourteenth International Symposium. Tucson, Az. May 23-26, 2007

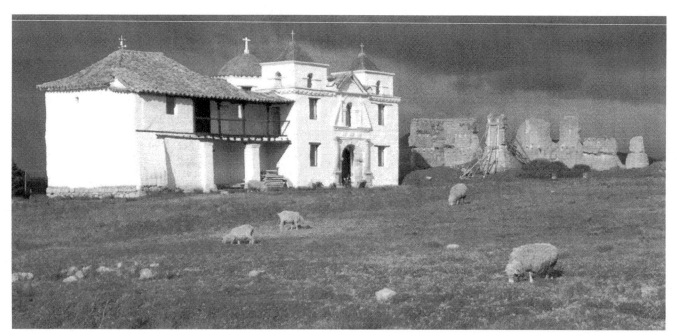

Grazing sheep near a 500-year-old church near Guasca, Colombia—2013 Dec. Photo by Dr Vasquez

Chapter 2:
Wellness Promotion
&
Re-Establishing the Foundation for Health

Introduction to Lifestyle Optimization, Wellness Promotion, and Disease Prevention

This section details the lifestyle modifications that support a wellness-promoting whole-health program.

Among the four major primary healthcare professions in the United States—chiropractic, osteopathy, naturopathy, and allopathy—the naturopathic profession stands preeminent in its emphasis upon wellness promotion and lifestyle optimization. This chapter reviews wellness promotion from the current author's perspective and experience—both personal and professional—which is consistent with but not officially representative of the naturopathic profession's concepts "re-establish the foundation of health" and "hierarchy of therapeutics."

This chapter originated many years ago as a handout for patients wherein it explained and described basic concepts that are foundational to health restoration, preservation, and optimization. Over the years that this handout has evolved into a chapter for my books, it has become more detailed and more relevant for clinicians treating patients. In essence, this chapter is a blueprint for the construction of a healthy lifestyle. While it may not cover every consideration, it covers the basics in sufficient detail so as to allow patients to change tracks from the downward descent of the disease-promoting lifestyle to the upward ascent of the health-promoting lifestyle.

Replacing the passive and disempowering drug-surgery paradigm with an active and empowering integrative/functional model of healthcare is one goal of this section.

This section can be thought of as a collection of essays. The review and consideration of a wide range of topics—which might otherwise appear random and nontopical to a reader accustomed to a more limited scope of discussion—is necessary due to the multifaceted nature of human experience and the widely ranging influences on health and disease outcomes.

<u>Topics</u>:

- **Re-establishing the Foundation for Health**
  - **Healthcare, Health, and Wellness**
  - **Daily living**
    - Lifestyle habits
    - Motivation: background and clinical applications
    - Exceptional living: the key to exceptional results
    - Recognize and affirm individual uniqueness
    - Individuation & conscious living: alternatives to common paradigms
    - Quality and quantity of sleep: concepts and clinical applications
    - Exercise, obesity, BMI, and proinflammatory activity of adipose tissue
  - **Diet is a powerful tool for the prevention and treatment of disease**
    - Make "whole foods" the foundation of the diet
    - Increase consumption of fruits and vegetables
    - Phytochemicals: food-derived anti-inflammatory nutrients
    - Eat the right amount of protein
    - Reducing consumption of sugars: exceptions for supercompensation
    - Avoiding artificial sweeteners, colors, and other additives, reducing caffeine
    - To the extent possible, eat "organic" foods
    - Recognize the importance of avoiding food allergens
    - Supplement your healthy diet with vitamins, minerals, and fatty acids
    - General guidelines for the safe use of nutritional supplements
  - **Advanced concepts in nutrition**
    - "Biochemical Individuality" and "Orthomolecular Medicine"
    - Nutrigenomics: Nutritional genomics
    - Putting it all together: *the supplemented Paleo-Mediterranean diet*
  - **Emotional, mental, and social health**
    - Stress management and authentic living
    - Stress always has a biochemical/physiologic component
    - The body functions as a whole
    - Healing past experiences
    - Autonomization, intradependence, emotional literacy, corrective experience
  - **Environmental health**
    - Environmental exposures and the importance of detoxification
    - Avoid unnecessary chemical medications and medical procedures
    - Intestinal health, bowel function, and introduction to dysbiosis
- **Natural holistic healthcare contrasted to standard medical treatment**
- **Opposite influences of health promotion vs. disease promotion**

Introduction to Wellness Promotion: Re-Establishing the Foundation for Health

> "The work of the naturopathic physician is to elicit healing by helping patients to create or recreate conditions for health to exist within them.
> **Health will occur where the conditions for health exist.**
> **Disease is the product of conditions which allow for it."** *Jared Zeff, N.D.*[1]

One of the most important concepts within the philosophy and practice of naturopathic medicine is that of "re-establishing the foundation for health." This means that instead of first looking to a specific treatment or "magic bullet" to solve a health problem, we first look at the environment in which the problem arose to determine if the patient's environment has initiated or perpetuated the problem. The term *environment* as used here means much more than the patient's immediate surroundings at home and work; it includes all modifiable factors that may have an effect on the patient's health, such as lifestyle, diet, exercise, supplementation, chronic and situational stress, medications with positive and negative effects, exposure to toxicants and microbes, nutritionally-modifiable genetic factors[2], emotions, feelings, and unconscious assumptions[3], and many other considerations. Although the genes that we and our patients have inherited cannot be changed, we can very often modulate the expression of those genes (e.g., via nutrigenomics, described later) by modifying the biochemical, microbial, toxicologic, and neurohormonal milieu that bathes our cells and thus our genes; this concept was expressed in a statement by the US Centers for Disease Control and Prevention in its "Gene-Environment Interaction Fact Sheet" available on-line.[4]

"Optimal health" does not and never will come in a pill or tonic—the human body and the interactions that we each have between our genes, outlooks, environments, and lifestyles are far too complex to ever be addressed wholly and completely by a simplistic paradigm or single treatment. Even a superficial observation of the complexity of human physiology and the complexity of our environments (including noise, toxins such as benzene and mercury, chemicals such as formaldehyde from building materials, work stress and multitasking, radiation exposure, microwaves, etc) shows that **our modern lifestyles subject the human body to many more "stressors" than ever before in the history of human existence.** Each of these stressors depletes our psychic and physiologic reserves, such that daily replenishment and protection are necessary.

> **Environment—lifestyle, diet, stresses, microbes, toxins—influences genetic expression and the manifestation of health or disease**
>
> "Virtually all human diseases result from the interaction of genetic susceptibility factors and modifiable environmental factors, broadly defined to include infectious, chemical, physical, nutritional, and behavioral factors. ...
>
> "Even so-called single-gene disorders actually develop from the interaction of both genetic and environmental factors. ...
>
> "We do not inherit a disease state per se. Instead, we inherit a set of a susceptibility factors to certain effects of environmental factors and therefore inherit a higher risk for certain diseases."
>
> Gene-Environment Interaction Fact Sheet by the Centers for Disease Control and Prevention, August 2000

Research in nutrition and physiology is revealing the mechanisms by which "simple" lifestyle practices and dietary interventions exert their powerful benefits. For example, whole foods such as fruits and vegetables contain over 8,000 phytochemicals with different physiologic effects[5], and simple practices such as meditation and massage can significantly alter hormone and neurotransmitter levels.[6,7] On the surface, a simple practice such as consumption of fruits and vegetables and a multivitamin/multimineral supplement may seem to be a way to

---

[1] Zeff JL. The process of healing: a unifying theory of naturopathic medicine. *Journal of Naturopathic Medicine* 1997; 7: 122-5
[2] Kaput J, Rodriguez LR. Nutritional genomics: the next frontier in the postgenomic era. *Physiol Genomics* 16: 166–177
http://physiolgenomics.physiology.org/cgi/content/full/16/2/166
[3] Miller A. *The truth will set you free: overcoming emotional blindness and finding your true adult self*. New York: Basic Books; 2001
[4] Gene-Environment Interaction Fact Sheet by the Centers for Disease Control and Prevention, August 2000 http://www.ashg.org/pdf/CDC%20Gene-Environment%20Interaction%20Fact%20Sheet.pdf
[5] "We propose that the additive and synergistic effects of phytochemicals in fruit and vegetables are responsible for their potent antioxidant and anticancer activities, and that the benefit of a diet rich in fruit and vegetables is attributed to the complex mixture of phytochemicals present in whole foods." Liu RH. Health benefits of fruit and vegetables are from additive and synergistic combinations of phytochemicals. *Am J Clin Nutr.* 2003 Sep;78(3 Suppl):517S-520S
[6] "The significant decrease of the catecholamine metabolite VMA (vanillic-mandelic acid) in meditators, that is associated with a reciprocal increase of 5-HIAA supports as a feedback necessity the "rest and fulfillment response" versus "fight and flight"." Bujatti M, Riederer P. Serotonin, noradrenaline, dopamine metabolites in transcendental meditation-technique. *J Neural Transm.* 1976;39(3):257-67
[7] "By the end of the study, the massage therapy group, as compared to the relaxation group, reported experiencing less pain, depression, anxiety and improved sleep. They also showed improved trunk and pain flexion performance, and their serotonin and dopamine levels were higher." Hernandez-Reif M, Field T, Krasnegor J, Theakston H. Lower back pain is reduced and range of motion increased after massage therapy. *Int J Neurosci* 2001;106(3-4):131-45

provide merely "good nutrition"; however the clinical effects can include antidepressant[8] and anti-inflammatory benefits[9] by enhancing the efficiency of biochemical reactions[10] and by reducing excess activity of NF-kappaB[11], respectively. The power of interventional nutrition utilizing high-doses and/or synergistic formulations of nutraceuticals and phytonutraceuticals becomes much more clinically apparent when patients first (re)establish a healthy foundation of diet and lifestyle practices upon which these treatments can be added; **I estimate that the effectiveness of treatments for complex illness such as inflammatory diseases and cancer is *at least* doubled when patients implement these lifestyle changes in addition to specific treatments rather than relying on specific treatments alone without a healthy supportive lifestyle.** In other words, "*foundation for health* + specific treatments" is much more effective than "*unhealthy lifestyle* + specific treatments." This explains, in part, the discrepancy between the relatively lackluster response seen in *single-intervention* clinical trials* compared to the better results that we attain clinically when using a holistic approach characterized by *multicomponent* treatment plans. The biochemical and "scientific" reasons for this positive/negative synergism will become more clear during the course of this chapter and textbook.

Single-intervention clinical trials (i.e., clinical trials that utilize only one treatment) are the "gold standard" in allopathic drug-based research because in that setting the goal is to quantify and qualify the nature of positive and negative responses to a single intervention, generally a drug. However, this approach loses much of its luster and relevance in clinical settings where neither patients nor their environments and treatment plans can be standardized due to the unique constitution, lifestyle, history, and other nuances of each patient. Single intervention clinical trials have a place in the researching of all treatments, including natural interventions. However, clinicians—especially recent graduates—must pry themselves away from this research tool when it comes to treating individual patients in clinical practice, where **single interventions are the antithesis of holistic treatment**.

Daily Living: Life occurs on a moment-to-moment and daily basis. Choices that we make in relationships, occupations, exercise, and diet have profound and powerful influence over the course of our lives—particularly our health and happiness. Despite the previous and current obfuscation of health information by allopathic groups[12,13,14,15,16] and the pharmaceutical industry[17,18], enough valid information and common sense is available to doctors and the public such that **ignorance is no longer a viable excuse for deferring responsibility for lifestyle-induced disease and misery.**[19] Eating too much sugar and fat while not eating enough fruits and vegetables is making a choice to have an increased probability of developing diabetes, cancer, heart disease, arthritis, and obesity. Exercising regularly, eating a healthy diet, and supplementing the diet with high-quality nutrients and botanicals is making the choice to greatly reduce one's risk of health problems[20,21] and to nurture one's life and one's body so that one can make the most of one's life experience and enjoy life, hobbies, life purpose(s), travel, creativity, community involvement, and time with friends and family.

When we were children, we looked to other people to provide for us and to "take care of us." **As adults, we have to assume responsibility for the course of our own lives, to make decisions based on long-term considerations rather than instant gratification and selective ignorance.** Of course, this does not mean that we have to abandon enjoyment; but it does mean that we can make decisions based on priorities, and if health is a

[8] Benton D, Haller J, Fordy J. Vitamin supplementation for 1 year improves mood. *Neuropsychobiology*. 1995;32(2):98-105

[9] Church TS, Earnest CP, Wood KA, Kampert JB. Reduction of C-reactive protein levels through use of a multivitamin. *Am J Med*. 2003;115(9):702-7

[10] Ames BN, Elson-Schwab I, Silver EA. High-dose vitamin therapy stimulates variant enzymes with decreased coenzyme binding affinity (increased K(m)): relevance to genetic disease and polymorphisms. *Am J Clin Nutr*. 2002 Apr;75(4):616-58 http://www.ajcn.org/cgi/content/full/75/4/616

[11] **Vasquez A**. Reducing pain and inflammation naturally - part 4: nutritional and botanical inhibition of NF-kappaB, the major intracellular amplifier of the inflammatory cascade. A practical clinical strategy exemplifying anti-inflammatory nutrigenomics. *Nutritional Perspectives*, July 2005:5-12

[12] Wolinsky H, Brune T. *The Serpent on the Staff: The Unhealthy Politics of the American Medical Association*. GP Putnam and Sons, New York, 1994

[13] Wilk CA. *Medicine, Monopolies, and Malice: How the Medical Establishment Tried to Destroy Chiropractic*. Garden City Park: Avery, 1996

[14] Carter JP. *Racketeering in Medicine: The Suppression of Alternatives*. Norfolk: Hampton Roads Pub; 1993

[15] National Alliance of Professional Psychology Providers. AMA Seeks To Control and Restrict Psychologist's Scope of Practice. http://www.nappp.org/scope.pdf 2006 Nov

[16] "In an effort to marshal the medical community's resources against the growing threat of expanding scope of practice for allied health professionals, the AMA has formed a national partnership to confront such initiatives nationwide... The committee will use $25,000..." Daly R, American Psychiatric Association. AMA Forms Coalition to Thwart Non-M.D. Practice Expansion. *Psychiatric News* 2006 March; 41: 17 http://pn.psychiatryonline.org/cgi/content/full/41/5/17-a?eaf Accessed November 25, 2006

[17] Angell M. *The Truth About the Drug Companies: How They Deceive Us and What to Do About it*. Random House; August 2004

[18] "It begins on the first day of medical school... It starts slowly and insidiously, like an addiction, and can end up influencing the very nature of medical decision-making and practice... Attempts to influence the judgment of doctors by commercial interests serving the medical industrial complex are nothing if not thorough." Editorial. Drug-company influence on medical education in USA. *Lancet*. 2000 Sep 2;356(9232):781

[19] "Error is not blindness, error is cowardice. Every acquisition, every step forward in knowledge is the result of courage, of severity towards oneself, of cleanliness with respect to oneself." Nietzsche FW. *Ecce Homo: How One Becomes What One Is*. [Translator: Hollingdale RJ] Penguin Books:1979,34

[20] Orme-Johnson DW, Herron RE. An innovative approach to reducing medical care utilization and expenditures. *Am J Manag Care*. 1997;3(1):135-44

[21] **Vasquez A**. Five-Part Nutritional Protocol that Produces Consistently Positive Results.*Nutr Wellness* 2005 Sept

priority then we should take steps to attain and maintain it. For people who have chosen to make their health a priority, sugar- and fat-laden food begins to lose its appeal, and exploring new health-building experiences such as healthy cooking, outdoor activities, and community involvement can become an empowering lifestyle that can be transformed into an art—one that is particularly amenable to building relationships and connections with other people. **The improved sense of well-being and improved physical and intellectual performance obtained from consumption of a health-promoting Paleo-Mediterranean diet (described later) supersedes any short-term**

Health living: lifestyle as living art
"What one should learn from artists: How can we make things beautiful, attractive, and desirable for us when they are not?—and I rather think that in themselves they never are! ... This we should learn from artists, while being wiser than they are in other matters. For with them this subtle power usually comes to an end where art ends and life begins; but we want to be the poets of our lives—first of all in the smallest, most everyday matters." Nietzsche FW. *Joyful Wisdom.* 1882. Essay #299.

gratification from the disease-promoting diet commonly referred to as the Standard American Diet (SAD). When people want to be healthy, exercising and spending enjoyable time outdoors becomes more fun than the inactivity and passivity of watching television. When we consider that the average American watches at least 3-4 hours of television per day then we should not be surprised that, with physical inactivity as such a major component of the day, Americans show progressively higher rates of obesity, cancer, heart disease, and diabetes. Such an inactive lifestyle also affects our children: on average, each American child watches more than 23 hours of television per week[22]—a national habit that unquestionably contributes to the high levels of obesity and (social) illiteracy demonstrated by America's youth. Adults who watch average amounts of television are exposed to—some might say "…indoctrinated by…") more than 30 hours of drug advertisements per year—far exceeding their exposure to other, potentially more authentic, health-promoting health information.[23] Not only does television siphon time and energy that could be used more productively, more socially, or more enjoyably, but at a cost of $50-100 per month ($600 to $1,200 per year) **cable television subtracts from the available resources (i.e., time, money, and attention) that could be directed toward health-promoting choices.** Cable television—because of its financial cost and time commitment—is only one of many examples of how everyday lifestyle choices can have an impact on long-term health/disease outcomes. **Clinicians should encourage patients to become mindful of their choices and the impact these choices have on long-term health and vitality.**

Lifestyle habits: Without the conscious decision that **health is a priority** and the realization that **optimal health has to be earned rather than taken for granted**, patients and doctors alike can fall into the belief that healthcare and health maintenance are *burdens* and *inconveniences* rather than opportunities for fulfillment and self-care. Taking an **empowered** and **pro-active** role in one's healthcare may include a coordinated program of diet changes (i.e., eating certain foods, avoiding other foods, modulating total intake), regular exercise, nutritional supplementation, stress reduction, and relationship improvement. Unhealthy habits such as eating junk foods, using tobacco, and watching too much television rob people of the time, energy, motivation, and financial resources that could otherwise be used to improve health and prevent unnecessary illness. As described later in this chapter, the choices that are made on a daily basis from this point forward are the most powerful predictors of future health and are generally more powerful than past habits or genetic inheritance. We can all greatly increase our probability of enjoying a future of high-energy health rather than painful illness by consistently choosing health-promoting options instead of foods, behaviors, and emotional states that promote illness.

---

[22] "American children view over 23 hours of television per week. * Teenagers view an average of 21 to 22 hours of television per week. * By the time today's children reach age 70, they will have spent 7 to 10 years of their lives watching television." American Academy of Pediatrics http://www.aapca1.org/aapca1/tv.html accessed September 30, 2003
[23] "…many ads may be targeted specifically at women and older viewers. Our findings suggest that Americans who watch average amounts of television may be exposed to more than 30 hours of direct-to-consumer drug advertisements each year, far surpassing their exposure to other forms of health communication." Brownfield ED, Bernhardt JM, Phan JL, Williams MV, Parker RM. Direct-to-consumer drug advertisements on network television: an exploration of quantity, frequency, and placement. *J Health Commun.* 2004 Nov-Dec;9(6):491-7

One hour of time per day and/or about $2 - $8 per day:

Active self-care lifestyle	*Distraction & inactive lifestyle*
1. Meditation 2. Yoga, stretching 3. Walking, jogging, biking, no-cost calisthenics 4. Martial arts, Tai Chi 5. Hot bath 6. Cooking new healthy meals 7. Herbal teas (especially green tea) provide anti-inflammatory, anticancer, and antioxidant benefits 8. Basic nutritional supplementation (less than $2 per day): 1) High-potency multivitamin and multimineral supplement, 2) Complete balanced, fatty acid supplementation, 3) 2,000 – 4,000 IU vitamin D per day for adults, 4) probiotics and/or symbiotic.	1. Cable television 2. 1 pack of cigarettes per day 3. Designer coffee such as Grande Café Latte
Benefits 1. Increased flexibility and joint mobility 2. Reduction in blood pressure 3. Reduced risk of cancer 4. Increased strength 5. Improved cognitive function 6. New and enjoyable meals 7. Relaxation 8. New life skills 9. Improved heart health 10. The opportunity to develop social skills and more friends and a better social support network 11. Reduced risk for Alzheimer's and Parkinson's diseases	**Results** 1. Cable television: Cost $2 - $4 per day = average $1,095 per year) 2. 1 pack of cigarettes per day ($3 per day = $1,095 per year) 3. Grande Café Latte ($4 per day = average $1,460 per year)
Cost: At $2 per day for meditation, stretching, calisthenics, (etc.) and basic supplementation, the total comes to $730 per year.	**Cost:** For cable television, cafe coffee, and cigarettes, the total comes to approximately $3,600 per year.

<u>Motivation</u>: We all have a combination of reasons, feelings, inclinations, and unconscious influences that support and perpetuate our health behaviors.[24,25,26] Getting in touch with those motivations can help us to better understand the healthy/functional (health-promoting) and unhealthy/dysfunctional (illness-promoting) aspects of our psyches. Uncovering and "upgrading" these motivations can help us and our patients to develop more authentic lives and improved health. Self-defeating behaviors, such as 1) a willingness to remain ignorant of factors which influence health, 2) a willingness to frequently consume disease-promoting processed convenience foods, and 3) submission to confinement within the boundaries of one's insurance coverage (which often confines one to drugs and surgery as the only treatment options), reflect—*at best*—the willingness to settle for mediocrity and—*at worst*—an unconscious movement in the direction of illness and early death—masochism and suicide by lifestyle. Conversely, an unencumbered drive toward health will create the greatest opportunity for wellness. Since **actions originate from beliefs and goals**, we can surmise much about undisclosed beliefs and goals in others and ourselves simply by observing outward behavior. Effectively changing actions (such as diet and lifestyle choices) therefore must include not only behavior modification but also careful examination and reconsideration of largely unconscious goals and beliefs that motivate and underlie those behaviors. **When a fully empowered motivation toward health is matched with accurate informational insight, we have the** *potential* **for health-promoting change**—*potential* **which only becomes** *manifest* **after the habitual application of appropriate** *action.* Patients and doctors alike can benefit from considering the factors that incline them *toward* or *away* from behaviors that promote health or disease.

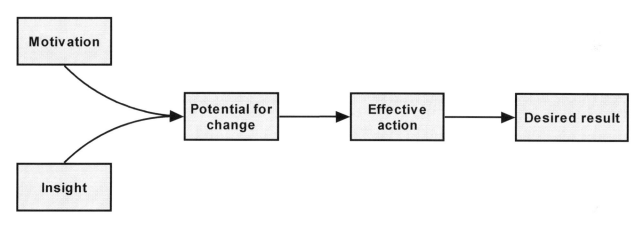

<u>Reasons and ways that I take good care of myself</u>:

_____

_____

_____

_____

_____

<u>Reasons and ways that I don't take good care of myself</u>:

_____

_____

_____

_____

_____

---

[24] Bradshaw J. *Healing the Shame that Binds You* [Audio Cassette (April 1990) Health Communications Audio; ISBN: 1558740430]
[25] Miller A. *The Drama of the Gifted Child: The Search for the True Self.* Basic Books; 1981
[26] Prochaska, JO, Norcross, JC, and DiClemente, CC (1994). *Changing for Good: A Revolutionary Six-Stage Program for Overcoming Bad Habits and Moving Your Life Positively Forward.* NY, William Morrow and Company; 1994

Motivation: moving from theory to practice: Many recently-graduated doctors start with the erroneous assumption that all patients actually want to become healthier, and furthermore, that all that the doctor has to do is "enlighten" them to the error of their ways and the patient will be dutifully compliant unto the attainment of his or her health-related goals. In reality, many people are surprisingly indifferent about their health. Many people do not care if they are 30 lbs overweight or have hypertension or will die early as a result of their lifestyle; they often have to be encouraged to begin to *consider* making positive changes.

Action determines outcome

"Knowing is not enough;
we must apply.
Willing is not enough;
we must do."

Johann Wolfgang von Goethe,
German novelist, poet, and scientist
(1749 - 1832)

At our 2004 Functional Medicine Symposium, Dr. James Prochaska[27] elucidated the different stages of patient preparedness, and we note that each of these five levels of thought and action produces specific results and requires different types of support from the doctor. I have summarized and modified Dr. Prochaska's lecture in the following table; for additional information and insights, obtain his lecture from the Institute for Functional Medicine (functionalmedicine.org) or obtain his book *Changing for Good*.[28]

Level of preparedness and readiness for change

Stage: representative statement	Doctor's interventions and social support
1. **Pre-contemplation**: "I am not seriously thinking about making a change to be healthier."	<ul><li>Outreach</li><li>Retainment</li></ul>
2. **Contemplation**: "I am thinking about making a change, but I am not ready for action."	<ul><li>Resolve resistance</li><li>Emphasize benefits</li><li>Address ambivalence</li></ul>
3. **Preparation**: "I am getting ready to make a change, but I am not taking effective action yet."	<ul><li>Ensure adequate preparation</li><li>Prevent relapse following initial action</li></ul>
4. **Action**: "I am beginning to make changes to become healthier."	<ul><li>Support (group support is best)</li><li>Encouragement</li><li>Reward system</li></ul>
5. **Maintenance**: "I take action every day and on a consistent basis to reach my goals."	<ul><li>Continued provision for continuation of health changes: facilities, supplements, social support, affirmation</li></ul>

Recognizing the different levels of patient preparedness and addressing individual patients with a customized approach not only for their *disease* but also for their *level of preparedness* for action can help doctors deliver more effective healthcare. Also, patients may have different levels of preparedness for different aspects of their treatment plans. He/she may be ready for **action** with regard to exercise, in **preparation** for dietary change, but in **precontemplation** for the use of supplements and botanicals.

---

[27] Prochaska JO. Changing for good: motivating diabetic patients. The Coming Storm: Reversing the Rising Pandemic of Diabetes and Metabolic Syndrome. The Eleventh International Symposium on Functional Medicine. May 13-15, 2004 in Vancouver, British Columbia, Canada. Pages 173-180
[28] Prochaska, JO, Norcross, JC, and DiClemente, CC (1994). *Changing for Good: A Revolutionary Six-Stage Program for Overcoming Bad Habits and Moving Your Life Positively Forward*. NY, William Morrow and Company; 1994

The secret to being exceptionally healthy: *One has to live in an exceptional (unique, personalized) way*. We cannot expect to achieve the goal of being vibrantly healthy or exceptionally happy if we live in the same way as everyone else, particularly when our fellow citizens are likely to be overweight, depressed, socially isolated[29], requiring multiple pharmaceutical medications[30], and experiencing a state of progressively declining health.[31] *Healthy lifestyle* not only includes the basics of adequate sleep, healthy whole-foods diet, supportive relationships, and regular exercise, but it also includes preventive medicine and pro-active healthcare.

> **Americans have poor health outcomes compared to citizens of other industrialized nations**
>
> "Basically, you die earlier and spend more time disabled if you're an American rather than a member of most other advanced countries."
>
> Christopher Murray MD PhD, Director of World Health Organization's Global Program on Evidence for Health Policy. Press release on June 4, 2000. http://www.who.int/inf-pr-2000/en/pr2000-life.html

Despite the fact that we in the United States (US) spend more on medical treatments than does any other country in the world, Americans have the worst health outcomes of all the major industrialized countries.[32,33,34] This is largely because *American medicine* is centered on a *disease-oriented model of medicine* which means that instead of having a healthcare system and social structure that proactively promotes health and prevents disease before it happens, our systems are *reactive—* treating disease *after* it occurs rather than emphasizing the prevention of disease *before* it occurs. The dominant allopathic model in the US is also reductionistic: focusing on the small problem (micromanagement) rather than the big picture (macromanagement).

> **Approximately 493 Americans are killed each day by hospital injuries and drug-prescribing errors**
>
> "Recent estimates suggest that each year more than 1 million patients are injured while in the hospital and approximately 180,000 die because of these injuries. Furthermore, drug-related morbidity and mortality are common and are estimated to cost more than $136 billion a year."
>
> Holland EG, Degruy FV. Drug-induced disorders. *Am Fam Physician.* 1997;56:1781-8, 1791-2

Clearly, the most effective method for avoiding expensive and potentially dangerous medical procedures and drug treatments is for us as a nation and as individuals to shift our thinking from a *disease treatment* model of healthcare to a more logical program of aggressive *disease prevention* and *wellness promotion* via the use of safe natural treatments rather than heroic interventions.[35,36] Of course, this means that our concept and view of health and healthcare will have to change. As noted by Shi[37], "**Redesigning the system of health care delivery in the United States may be the only viable option to improve the quality of health care.**" In the meantime, while we work for change on a national level, we are wise to change our personal habits and healthcare choices in favor of natural and preventive healthcare.

> **Medical drug (in)efficacy**
>
> "The vast majority of drugs —more than 90 percent— only work in 30 or 50 percent of the people."
>
> Allen Roses, M.D., worldwide vice-president of genetics at GlaxoSmithKline. Published Dec 8, 2003 http://commondreams.org/headlines03/1208-02.htm

Healthy lifestyle and biochemical individuality credo: Recognize and affirm that you are a unique individual with unique needs: For each of us, our "personality" extends far beyond and far deeper than our sense of humor and our choice of clothing; we are very unique on a physiologic and biochemical level as well. So-called *normal* and *apparently healthy* individuals vary greatly in their biochemical efficiency and nutritional needs. This is the concept of "biochemical individuality" which was first detailed in 1956 by the renowned scientist Roger J Williams from

---

[29] McPherson M, Smith-Lovin L, Brashears ME. Social Isolation in America: Changes in Core Discussion Networks over Two Decades. *American Sociological Review* 2006; 71: 353-75 http://www.asanet.org/galleries/default-file/June06ASRFeature.pdf

[30] "According to the latest available data, total health care costs reached $1.3 trillion in 2000. This represents a per capita health care expenditure of $4,637. The total prescription drug expenditure in 2000 was $121.8 billion, or approximately $430 per person." Presentation to the U.S. Senate Commerce Committee April 23, 2002 "Drug Pricing & Consumer Costs" Kathleen D. Jaeger, R.Ph., J.D. http://commerce.senate.gov/hearings/042302jaegar.pdf

[31] Zack MM, Moriarty DG, Stroup DF, Ford ES, Mokdad AH. Worsening trends in adult health-related quality of life and self-rated health-United States, 1993-2001. *Public Health Rep.* 2004 Sep-Oct;119(5):493-505 http://www.pubmedcentral.nih.gov/articlerender.fcgi?tool=pubmed&pubmedid=15313113

[32] "[America] also has the fewest hospital days per capita, the highest hospital expenditures per day, and substantially higher physician incomes than the other OECD countries. On the available outcome measures, the United States is generally in the bottom half, and its relative ranking has been declining since 1960." Anderson GF, Poullier JP. Health spending, access, and outcomes: trends in industrialized countries. *Health Aff* (Millwood) 1999 May-Jun;18(3):178-92 http://content.healthaffairs.org/cgi/reprint/18/3/178.pdf

[33] "However, on outcomes indicators such as life expectancy and infant mortality, the United States is frequently in the bottom quartile among the twenty-nine industrialized countries, and its relative ranking has been declining since 1960." Anderson GF. In search of value: an international comparison of cost, access, and outcomes. *Health Aff* 1997 Nov-Dec;16(6):163-71

[34] "Basically, you die earlier and spend more time disabled if you're an American rather than a member of most other advanced countries," says Christopher Murray, MD, PhD, Director of WHO's Global Program on Evidence for Health Policy. http://www.who.int/inf-pr-2000/en/pr2000-life.html

[35] "Systematic access to managed chiropractic care not only may prove to be clinically beneficial but also may reduce overall health care costs." Legorreta A, et al N. Comparative Analysis of Individuals With and Without Chiropractic Coverage. *Archives of Internal Medicine* 2004; 164: 1985-1992

[36] Orme-Johnson DW, Herron RE. An innovative approach to reducing medical care utilization and expenditures. *Am J Manag Care.* 1997;3(1):135-44

[37] Shi L. Health care spending, delivery, and outcome in developed countries: a cross-national comparison. *Am J Med Qual* 1997;12(2):83-93

the University of Texas. In his historic work _Biochemical Individuality: The Basis for the Genetotrophic Concept_, Dr. Williams[38] reviews research that conclusively proves that among _apparently healthy_ individuals, we can objectively determine great differences in physiology, organ efficiency, enzyme function, and nutritional needs. For example, variables that promote health include increased enzyme efficiency and efficient digestion and assimilation of nutrients, while internal factors that reduce health can include inadequate digestion, inefficient absorption, increased excretion of nutrients, impaired detoxification, poor enzyme function and "partial genetic blocks"—a term now understood to imply single nucleotide polymorphisms[39] and related enzyme defects, which result in **supradietary requirements for specific vitamins and minerals** for the prevention of disease and maintenance of health.[40] What this means for us as doctors and for our patients in practical terms is that in order for us to become as healthy as possible, we will almost certainly have to give attention to each person's unique biochemical abilities/disabilities in order to maximize the function of the various body systems, enzymes, and to optimize genetic expression.[41] This means that what works for one's neighbor, spouse, or best friend in terms of exercise, diet and nutrition may not work for one's unique physiology. We must all muster the courage to affirm that, in order to attain the goal of stable or progressively better health, we will each have to learn about how our unique bodies work—what conditions of health must be created. We will have to learn to make changes in lifestyle and daily routine which reflect and honor our bodies' ways of working. This may mean modifying work, sleep, and exercise schedules, avoiding some foods and eating others, and customizing nutrient intake to meet the body's needs as they are _in the present_—the health program that appears to have worked last year may not be appropriate at the present time. The process of learning how a person's body works requires time, patience, and the process of trial and error—from patient and doctor—but achieving the goal of improved health and increased energy are well worth the effort.

Individuation and the practice of conscious living: Our visions of reality are influenced by religious institutions, large corporations, advertising networks[42], corporate-owned mass media[43], and what Professors Stevens and Glatstein called "the medical-industrial complex."[44] Some of the paradigms that are advocated are both _unhistorical_ (having no historical precedent) and _antihistorical_ (contrary to the available historical precedent, which includes sustainability). Some of these companies and organizations offer us a view of reality and vision of our individual potentials that is fashioned in such a way as to promote the financial and political interests of the company or organization. Conversely, the

> **The importance of living consciously**
>
> "Consciousness is our basic tool for successful adaptation to reality. The more conscious we are in any situation, the more possibilities we tend to perceive, the more options we have, the more powerful we are — perhaps even the longer we will live.
>
> Living consciously means seeking to be aware of everything that bears on our actions, purposes, values, and goals — and behaving in accordance with that which we see and know."
>
> Branden N. _The Art of Living Consciously_.
> http://nathanielbranden.com Accessed Feb 2011

actualization of our true physical, emotional, intellectual, and spiritual potentials may require that we separate from or at least attain a conscious appreciation of the (pseudo)reality that we have been advised to follow.[45,46] Critiques of and reasonable alternatives to our current paradigms of school[47], work[48,49], and money[50] have been discussed elsewhere and are worthy of consideration. Becoming mindful of the paradigms and assumptions under which we live is the first step in true individuation, characterized by choosing (_creating_ the best option: freedom)

[38] Williams RJ. _Biochemical Individuality: The Basis for the Genetotrophic Concept_. Austin and London: University of Texas Press, 1956
[39] Ames BN. Cancer prevention and diet: help from single nucleotide polymorphisms. _Proc Natl Acad Sci U S A_. 1999 Oct 26;96(22):12216-8
[40] Ames BN, Elson-Schwab I, Silver EA. High-dose vitamin therapy stimulates variant enzymes with decreased coenzyme binding affinity (increased K(m)): relevance to genetic disease and polymorphisms. _Am J Clin Nutr_. 2002 Apr;75(4):616-58 http://www.ajcn.org/cgi/content/full/75/4/616
[41] "The combination of biochemical individuality and known functional utilities of allelic variants should converge to create a situation in which nutritional optima can be specified as part of comprehensive lifestyle prescriptions tailored to the needs of each person." Eckhardt RB. Genetic research and nutritional individuality. _J Nutr_ 2001;131(2):336S-9S
[42] "Patients' requests for medicines are a powerful driver of prescribing decisions. In most cases physicians prescribed requested medicines but were often ambivalent about the choice of treatment. If physicians prescribe requested drugs despite personal reservations, sales may increase but appropriateness of prescribing may suffer." Mintzes B, Barer ML, Kravitz RL, Kazanjian A, Bassett K, Lexchin J, Evans RG, Pan R, Marion SA. Influence of direct to consumer pharmaceutical advertising and patients' requests on prescribing decisions: two site cross sectional survey. _BMJ_. 2002 Feb 2; 324(7332): 278-9
[43] Manufacturing Consent: Noam Chomsky and the Media. Movie directed by Achbar M and Wintonick P. 1992. See also http://zeitgeistmovie.com/
Stevens CW, Glatstein E. Beware the Medical-Industrial Complex. _Oncologist_ 1996;1(4):IV-V http://theoncologist.alphamedpress.org/cgi/reprint/1/4/190-iv.pdf on July 4, 2004
[45] Breton D, Largent C. _The Paradigm Conspiracy_. Center City; Hazelden: 1996
[46] Pearce JC. _Exploring the Crack in the Cosmic Egg: Split Minds and Meta-Realities_. New York: Washington Square Press; 1974
[47] Gatto JT. _Dumbing us down: the hidden curriculum of compulsory education_. Gabriola Island, Canada; New Society Publishers: 2005
[48] "No one should ever work. In order to stop suffering, we have to stop working. That doesn't mean we have to stop doing things. It does mean creating a new way of life based on play..." Black B. The abolition of work and other essays. Port Townsend: Loompanics Unlimited; 1985, pages 17-33
[49] Jarow R. _Creating the Work You Love: Courage, Commitment and Career_; Inner Traditions Intl Ltd; 1995 [ISBN: 0892815426]
[50] Dominguez JR. _Transforming Your Relationship with Money_. Sounds True; Book and Cassette edition: 2001 Audio tape.

rather than deciding (*selecting* one of the offered options: the illusion of freedom). Various conscious thoughts and unconscious assumptions create our "working reality" which represents the way that we see things and the paradigm by which we *act in* and *interact with* the larger world. These layers come from our own families, schools, teachers, churches, companies, friends, parents, and ourselves—our previous interpretations and misinterpretations of ourselves and events; in sum, our responses to outer events combined with our internal experiences meld into our perception of ourselves (known as "the genesis of personal identity") and how we as individuals relate to our inner ourselves and [our perception of] the outer world. Becoming conscious of these realities and illusions allows us the opportunity to discard those views that are inaccurate, dysfunctional, and harmful and to accept a truer reality based on what we experience, feel, and know to be real—in the present, as adults. Once we are freed from *unreality*, we can live true to ourselves in a way that is authentically responsible to our own needs *and* the needs of our communities so that we can simultaneously sustain our obligations to society[51,52] while being free to be unique individuals.[53,54]

Examples of commonly accepted paradigms and their reasonable alternatives

Commonly advocated/accepted paradigms ↳ *Implication and effect*	*Alternate paradigm* ↳ *Implication and effect*
It is OK to be irresponsible in daily choices and then blame health problems on bad luck, bad genes, or both. ↳ Many people fail to take responsibility for their lives and thereby become victims of circumstances—negative circumstances that they themselves helped to create.	**Lifestyle, especially diet and nutrition, is the most powerful influence on health outcomes. Therefore, an educated patient is empowered to direct his/her health destiny.** ↳ Optimal health *per individual* is attained when people take responsibility for their lives, seek health information, and then incorporate this information into their daily routine in the form of healthy living: health-promoting lifestyle, eating, exercise, supplementation, relationships, and occupational and social activities, including socio-political involvement to protect the environment and resist the privatization of life and the spoliation of the environment in which we live and upon which our lives and health depend.[55,56]
In general, chemical medications are the answer to nearly all health problems. ↳ The belief in medications as the primary treatment of disease creates a patient population that is apathetic, disempowered, and dependent upon the medical-pharmaceutical industry, which grows richer and more powerful despite so-called 'earnest' attempts at cost containment.[57]	**Many acute and chronic problems can be more effectively managed in terms of prevention, safety, efficacy, and cost-effectiveness when phytonutritional interventions are either used as primary therapy or, when necessary, used in conjunction with medications.** ↳ A reduction in disease prevalence via health-promoting diet and lifestyle along with integrative treatments offers the best opportunity for benefit to patients, doctors, and third-party payers.[58]

---

[51] Bly R. The Sibling Society. Vintage Books USA; Reprint edition (June 1, 1997) ISBN: 0679781285 (Abridged audio edition (May 1, 1996)

[52] Bly R. Where have all the parents gone? A talk on the Sibling Society. New York: Sound Horizons, 1996 Highly recommended.

[53] Bradshaw J. Healing the Shame that Binds You [Audio Cassette (April 1990) Health Communications Audio; ISBN: 1558740430]

[54] Miller A. The truth will set you free: overcoming emotional blindness and finding your true adult self. New York: Basic Books; 2001

[55] "Your lack of interest in the past, your lack of involvement, your unwillingness to develop coherent strategies, your unwillingness to challenge authority - these have created a vacuum in decision-making, that has been filled by professional groups with close relationships with the chemical industries..." Samuel Epstein MD, 1993. Professor of Occupational and Environmental Medicine at the School of Public Health, University of Illinois Medical Center Chicago. http://www.converge.org.nz/pirm/pestican.htm

[56] Kristin S. Schafer, Margaret Reeves, Skip Spitzer, Susan E. Kegley. Chemical Trespass: Pesticides in Our Bodies and Corporate Accountability. Pesticide Action Network North America. May 2004 Available at http://www.panna.org/campaigns/docsTrespass/chemicalTrespass2004.dv.html on August 1, 2004

[57] "In this paper I offer four hypotheses to help explain why use of pharmaceuticals has continued to grow even as managed care and other cost containment efforts have flourished." Berndt ER. The U.S. pharmaceutical industry: why major growth in times of cost containment? *Health Aff* (Millwood). 2001 Mar-Apr;20(2):100-14

[58] "Hospital admission rates in the control group were 11.4 times higher than those in the MVAH group for cardiovascular disease, 3.3 times higher for cancer, and 6.7 times higher for mental health and substance abuse. ...MVAH patients older than age 45...had 88% fewer total patients days compared with control patients." Orme-Johnson DW, Herron RE. An innovative approach to reducing medical care utilization and expenditures. *Am J Manag Care*. 1997 Jan;3(1):135-44

Examples of commonly accepted paradigms and their reasonable alternatives—*continued*

Commonly accepted paradigms ↳ *Implication and effect*	Alternate paradigm ↳ *Implication and effect*
Work ethic: a belief that "hard work" has moral value and makes a person "better." ↳ Belief in the principle of "work ethic" encourages people to mindlessly engage in work for the sake of engaging in work without considering the implications of their actions or other alternatives that might produce a more beneficial outcome.[59]	**Work is the means rather than an end unto itself (except when the "work" is enjoyable, in which case it is no longer "work").** ↳ Occupations and professions can be designed for the enhancement of life (health, pleasure, relationships, the environment, care of the poor) rather than as an end to themselves at the expense of the individual, society, and the environment.
It is "normal" for adults to give 10.5-12 hours per day 5 days per week to work. ↳ In most corporate environments, employee's work at least 8.5 hours per day, with 1 additional hour spent in commuting[60] and another hour spent in preparation, transportation, and maintenance of work-related clothing, preparing work-related meals, maintaining the auto that is used for work-related tasks. With 10.5 hours given directly to work, 0.5-1 additional hours are needed for recuperation from work-related stress ("daily decompression"); thus the average amount of time given to work-related activities is much larger than commonly believed.[61] Because of the time and energies devoted to "work" the vast majority of people feel that they do not have sufficient time for themselves, their families and friends, their creativity, learning about the world, political involvement, and other more important aspects of life. "Not enough time" is the most common reason given by patients for not exercising.	**A paradigm of a 4-day workweek is just as valid and perhaps more valid than one that advocates a 5-day workweek. A paradigm of a 6-hour workday is at least as valid as one of an 8-10 hour workday.** ↳ Many people in our culture are chronically overworked, undernourished, tired and suffer from an insufficiency of time to simply be in community, to rest, to be creative. Living with such limitations and pressures should be expected to produce a population that is reactively hedonistic, impulsive, and prone to addiction. Behaviors that are addictive (e.g., drugs, alcohol) and destructive (e.g., over-eating, alcohol, sugar, fat) are simply frustrated and maladaptive coping strategies to combat the stress caused by a damaging, unnatural paradigm from which most people cannot escape.[62] Redesigning our societal structures and expectations in ways that conform to our natural humanity and biologic, nutritional, and emotional needs is more rational than forcing *en masse* all of humanity to contort and conform to an artificial posture and cadence of performance, productivity, "professionalism", and other unnatural expectations. Less time dedicated to work and all that it entails leaves more time for 1) healthy cooking, 2) relaxed, conscious, and enjoyable eating, 3) exercise, 4) creativity and hobbies, 5) keeping informed of and involved with political change, and 6) participation in social relationships.[63]

[59] "Conventional wisdom is the habitual, the unexamined life, absorbed into the culture and the fashion of the time, lost in the mad rush of accumulation, lulled to sleep by the easy lies of political hacks and newspaper scribblers, or by priests who wouldn't know a god if they met one." Nisker W. Crazy Wisdom. Berkeley; Ten Speed Press: 1990, page 7

[60] Monday, September 8, 2003 -- The average daily one-way commute to work in the United States takes just over 26 minutes, according to the Bureau of Transportation Statistics' Omnibus Household Survey. Omnibus Household Survey Shows Americans' Average Commuting Time is just over 26 Minutes. http://www.bts.gov/press_releases/2003/bts020_03/html/bts020_03.html on August 3, 2004

[61] Dominguez JR. Transforming Your Relationship with Money. Sounds True; Book and Cassette edition: 2001

[62] Breton D, Largent C. The Paradigm Conspiracy: Why Our Social Systems Violate Human Potential-And How We Can Change Them. Hazelden: 1998

[63] "Take back your time" is a major U.S./Canadian initiative to challenge the epidemic of overwork, over-scheduling and time famine that now threatens our health, our families and relationships, our communities and our environment. http://www.simpleliving.net/timeday/ on August 3, 2004

<u>Quality and quantity of sleep</u>: A sleep duration of less than 8 hours of deep solid sleep each night is physiologically insufficient for most of people; many people feel best with 9 hours of sleep, yet some people appear to function well on about 6 hours of sleep per night. Not only is it important to get a sufficient *quantity* of sleep, but we need to ensure that the *quality* of the sleep receives appropriate attention, as well. Sleep should be mostly continuous, not "broken" or interrupted. Some experts believe

The Importance of Sleep
Regulation of sleep-wake cycles and the regular satisfaction of sleep needs are important for preservation of immune function, intellectual performance, emotional stability, pain control, and the internal regulation of the body's inflammatory tendency.

that people should be able to recall their dreams at night, as this may be a sign of proper neurotransmitter status, especially with regard to serotonin, which is affected by pyridoxine[64] as well as other factors. Going to bed at a regular hour (not later than 10 or 11 at night) helps to synchronize the daily schedule with the body's inherent hormonal rhythms and "physiological clock" which expects one to be in deep sleep by midnight and to be waking at approximately 8 o'clock in the morning. Recent research has shown that **sleep deprivation causes a systemic inflammatory response manifested objectively by increases in high-sensitivity C-reactive protein (hsCRP)**.[65] Correspondingly, sleep apnea, a condition associated with repetitive sleep disturbances, is also associated with an elevation of CRP[66], and effective treatment of sleep apnea results in a normalization of CRP levels.[67] We could therefore conclude that **sleep deprivation creates a proinflammatory condition**. Furthermore, **sleep deprivation has been proven to impair intellectual functioning, emotional state, and immune function**, with abnormalities in immune status already evident the morning after sleep deprivation.[68] Wakefulness and exposure to light at night result in a suppression of melatonin production and may therefore contribute to cancer development since melatonin has anticancer actions that would be abrogated by its reduced endogenous production.[69,70] Limited evidence also suggests that melatonin production is altered in patients with the inflammatory conditions eczema[71] and psoriasis[72] and that this sleep-related hormone has anti-inflammatory/anti-autoimmune benefits that may be relevant for the suppression of diseases such as multiple sclerosis[73] and sarcoidosis.[74]

---

[64] " ...a significant difference in dream-salience scores (this is a composite score containing measures on vividness, bizarreness, emotionality, and color) between the 250-mg condition and placebo over the first three days of each treatment... An hypothesis is presented involving the role of B-6 in the conversion of tryptophan to serotonin." Ebben M, Lequerica A, Spielman A. Effects of pyridoxine on dreaming: a preliminary study. *Percept Mot Skills* 2002 Feb;94(1):135-40

[65] "CONCLUSIONS: Both acute total and short-term partial sleep deprivation resulted in elevated high-sensitivity CRP concentrations... We propose that sleep loss may be one of the ways that inflammatory processes are activated and contribute to the association of sleep complaints, short sleep duration, and cardiovascular morbidity observed in epidemiologic surveys." Meier-Ewert HK, Ridker PM, et al. Effect of sleep loss on C-reactive protein, an inflammatory marker of cardiovascular risk. *J Am Coll Cardiol.* 2004 Feb 18;43(4):678-83

[66] "OSA is associated with elevated levels of CRP, a marker of inflammation and of cardiovascular risk. The severity of OSA is proportional to the CRP level." Shamsuzzaman AS, Winnicki M, Lanfranchi P, et al. Elevated C-reactive protein in patients with obstructive sleep apnea. *Circulation.* 2002 May 28;105(21):2462-4

[67] "CONCLUSIONS: Levels of CRP and IL-6 and spontaneous production of IL-6 by monocytes are elevated in patients with OSAS but are decreased by nCPAP." Yokoe T, Minoguchi K, Matsuo H, Oda N, Minoguchi H, Yoshino G, Hirano T, Adachi M. Elevated levels of C-reactive protein and interleukin-6 in patients with obstructive sleep apnea syndrome are decreased by nasal continuous positive airway pressure. *Circulation.* 2003 Mar 4;107(8):1129-34 Available on-line at http://circ.ahajournals.org/cgi/reprint/107/8/1129.pdf on August 2, 2004

[68] "Taken together, SD induced a deterioration of both mood and ability to work, which was most prominent in the evening after SD, while the maximal alterations of the host defence system could be found twelve hours earlier, i.e., already in the morning following SD." Heiser P, et al. Alterations of host defense system after sleep deprivation are followed by impaired mood and psychosocial functioning. *World J Biol Psychiatry* 2001 Apr;2(2):89-94

[69] "Observational studies support an association between night work and cancer risk. We hypothesise that the potential primary culprit for this observed association is the lack of melatonin, a cancer-protective agent whose production is severely diminished in people exposed to light at night." Schernhammer ES, Schulmeister K. Melatonin and cancer risk: does light at night compromise physiologic cancer protection by lowering serum melatonin levels? *Br J Cancer.* 2004 Mar 8;90(5):941-3

[70] "This is the first biological evidence for a potential link between constant light exposure and increased human breast oncogenesis involving MLT suppression and stimulation of tumor LA metabolism." Blask DE, Dauchy RT, Sauer LA, Krause JA, Brainard GC. Growth and fatty acid metabolism of human breast cancer (MCF-7) xenografts in nude rats: impact of constant light-induced nocturnal melatonin suppression. *Breast Cancer Res Treat.* 2003 Jun;79(3):313-20

[71] "In 6 patients exhibiting low serum levels of melatonin, the circadian melatonin rhythm was found to be abolished. In 8 patients a diminished nocturnal melatonin increase was observed compared with the controls (n = 40)." Schwarz W, Birau N, Hornstein OP, Heubeck B, Schonberger A, Meyer C, Gottschalk J. Alterations of melatonin secretion in atopic eczema. *Acta Derm Venereol.* 1988;68(3):224-9

[72] "Our results show that psoriatic patients had lost the nocturnal peak and usual circadian rhythm of melatonin secretion." Mozzanica N, Tadini G, Radaelli A, et al. Plasma melatonin levels in psoriasis. *Acta Derm Venereol.* 1988;68(4):312-6

[73] "This hypothesis is supported by the observation that administration of melatonin (3 mg, orally) at 2:00 p.m., when the patient experienced severe blurring of vision, resulted within 15 minutes in a dramatic improvement in visual acuity and in normalization of the visual evoked potential latency after stimulation of the left eye." Sandyk R. Diurnal variations in vision and relations to circadian melatonin secretion in multiple sclerosis. *Int J Neurosci.* 1995 Nov;83(1-2):1-6

[74] Cagnoni ML, Lombardi A, Cerinic MC, Dedola GL, Pignone A. Melatonin for treatment of chronic refractory sarcoidosis. *Lancet.* 1995;346:1229-30

Helping patients improve quality and quantity of sleep

- Schedule sufficient time for sleep; generally this is 9 hours to allow time for "winding down" and "daily decompression" so that a full 8 hours of sleep can ensue.
- Reduce intake of stimulants such as caffeine, tobacco, and aspartame. Some patients will need to reduce intake only in the evening, while others will need to reduce intake even in the morning in order to have improved quality and quantity of sleep later at night.
- Exercise early in the day (morning or early afternoon) to promote restful sleep at night.
- Avoid aggressive or arousing physical activity in the evening to avoid increases in norepinephrine, epinephrine, and cortisol, which can discourage sleep.
- Dim lights at night to promote melatonin production. Beginning one to two hours before bedtime, turn off bright lights and use only dim lighting. Bright lights reduce melatonin secretion and stimulate neocortical activity and thereby inhibit sleep.
- Have an evening ritual/pattern that helps the psyche recognize that the time for sleep has arrived. Such practices can include relaxing warm tea, meditation, prayer, and daily reflection.
- For patients with a pattern of falling asleep and then waking approximately 4-6 hours later with feelings of hunger or anxiety (nocturnal hypoglycemia), they should eat a small meal or snack of complex carbohydrates, protein, and fat before going to bed. For example, the combination of nuts (or nut butter) with whole fruit such as apples provides protein, fat, and complex carbohydrate with a low glycemic index to provide sustenance throughout the night. Protein powders and other sources of "predigested" amino acids should generally be avoided late at night because an excess consumption of high protein foods can reduce tryptophan entry into the brain and thus reduce serotonin and melatonin synthesis. Most amino acid-derived neurotransmitters such as dopamine, glutamate, and norepinephrine are excitatory/stimulatory in nature.
- Vitamin and mineral supplementation is commonly beneficial, particularly with thiamine, methylcobalamin (weak evidence), and magnesium (particularly sleep disturbance associated with restless leg syndrome). Vitamins should be taken earlier in the day (with breakfast and lunch; not before bed); however calcium and magnesium can be taken before bed.
- Earplugs, window covers, and a quiet, snore-free environment are generally conducive to better sleep.
- For patients with difficulty falling asleep, consider 5-hydroxytryptophan consumed with simple carbohydrate (50-200 mg for adults, up to 2 mg/kg for children), melatonin (0.5-10 mg), valerian-hops tea or capsules 60-90 minutes before bedtime.

Exercise: Human existence has changed radically over the past few millennia, centuries, and decades, and one of the most profound changes has been in our relationship to physical activity. Paleologists and historical scientists agree that physical activity among humans is at its all-time historical low, and that levels of exertion that we now call "vigorous and frequent exercise" would have been *completely normal* in the daily lives of our ancestors, who engaged in at least four times more physical activity than their modern-day progeny.[75] At one time—a time in which vigorous physical activity was a normal part of daily life—probably no word existed for what modern people describe and often resist as "exercise."

Daily exercise is health-promoting and restorative

"The health rewards of exercise extend far beyond its benefits for specific diseases." Exercise reduces blood clotting, lowers blood pressure, lowers cholesterol, improves glucose tolerance and insulin sensitivity, enhances self-image, elevates mood, reduces stress, creates a feeling of well-being, reinforces other positive life-style changes, stimulates creative thinking, increases muscle mass, increases basal metabolic rate, promotes improved sleep, stimulates healthy intestinal function, promotes weight loss, and enhances appearance. "Furthermore, **the ability of exercise to restore function to organs, muscles, joints, and bones is not shared by drugs or surgery.**"

Harold Elrick, MD. Exercise is Medicine. *Physician and Sportsmedicine.* 1996 February: 24; 2

Our current mode of compulsory primary and secondary education (in America) prioritizes "being still" over physical exertion/expression for the vast majority of students' time. Thus having been separated from their inherent tendency to be physically active and emotionally expressive, many children grow into adults who have to be *retaught to inhabit their bodies* and to engage in physical activity on a daily basis. Basic science has proven that this is true: when animals are restrained, they show less activity when freed and no longer tied down. Conversely, when animals are rigorously exercised, they show higher levels of *spontaneous physical activity* when left to their own

---

Daily exercise is the body's physiological expectation

"Although modern technology has made physical exertion optional, it is still important to exercise as though our survival depended on it, and in a different way it still does. **We are genetically adapted to live an extremely physically active lifestyle.**"

O'Keefe JH Jr, Cordain L. Cardiovascular disease resulting from a diet and lifestyle at odds with our Paleolithic genome: how to become a 21st-century hunter-gatherer. *Mayo Clin Proc.* 2004 Jan;79(1):101-8

---

discretion. A probable sociological parallel is at work in human cultures where, under the guise of *work* and *entertainment*, people are corralled into lifestyles of physical inactivity in a wide range of apparently divergent activities. Watching television, driving a car, seeing a movie, doing computer/desk work at the office, attending a sports event or educational lecture, seeing the opera—all of these are simply different forms of **sitting**, of physical inactivity. Changing our social structure in a way that prioritizes *life* over *work*, such as moving toward a 4-day work week and/or a 6-hour work day, would allow people more time to live their lives, to pursue healthy diets and relationships, to be creative, and to engage in more physical activity; thus, "escape entertainment" such as fiction books and movies and processed "fast foods"—the latter of which are inherently unhealthy[76]—would become less necessary and less attractive.

Industrialized Westernized societies' disregard for connection with the body

"That I deemed it an imposition to have to make use of my perfectly adequate coordination, or resented—from unexamined principle—the use of time to fill a need, was an arbitrary assignment of values that [this other culture] did not share."

Liedloff J. *The Continuum Concept*. Cambridge, MA: Da Capo Press; 1977, page 15

---

[75] Eaton SB, Cordain L, Eaton SB. An evolutionary foundation for health promotion. *World Rev Nutr Diet* 2001; 90:5-12
[76] For an additional perspective see movie by Morgan Spurlock (director). Super Size Me. www.supersizeme.com released in 2004

Exploring the spectrum of physical activity from inactivity to athleticism

Inactivity	Minimally active	Active	Healthy	Athletic
• Bed-ridden • Chair-ridden • Minimal activity, such as walking to car or bathroom or to buy groceries • Activity in this category is equivalent to or barely above that which is necessary to sustain life	• Periodic performance of more activity than the minimal needed to sustain life, such as walking around the block after dinner, or taking a brief stroll at a park or at the beach	• Regular performance of low/moderate levels of activity at work or leisure, at least 30-60 minutes of physical activity per day	• 60-120 minutes of vigorous activity such as running, swimming, cycling, or other physical training 4-7 days per week	• More than 2 hours devoted to conditioning, strengthening, and skill-building 4-7 days per week

At least 30-45 minutes of exercise four days per week is the *absolute minimum*. Ideally, patients who have been sedentary and are over age 45 years would have a pre-exercise physical exam that might also include electrocardiography before embarking on a program of vigorous exercise. Patients who have been sedentary for many years can start slowly with their new exercise program, gradually increasing the duration and intensity. With the simple addition of regular exercise to their routine, patients will have significantly reduced risk for problems such as depression, chronic pain, cancer, coronary artery disease, stroke, hypertension, diabetes, arthritis, osteoporosis, dyslipidemia, obesity, chronic obstructive pulmonary disease, constipation, and other problems.[77] Furthermore, successful prevention and treatment of health problems with exercise and lifestyle modifications reduces dependency on pharmaceutical drugs, thereby further saving lives. O'Keefe and Cordain[78] report that **during the hunter-gatherer period, humans averaged 5-10 miles of daily running and walking**. Additionally, **other physical activities such as heavy lifting, digging, and climbing would have been considered "normal" aspects of daily life rather than "exercise"—an achievement for which modern/industrialized people seek recognition.** Thus, when sedentary patients achieve the first-step goal of walking around the block after dinner, we can commend them for making a significant stride forward in ultimately attaining better health, but we cannot stop there nor delude them into believing that this is adequate.

Common physical activities: a buffet of options from which to choose
☑ **"Boot camp"-style aerobics classes**: excellent variety and fast-pace maintains oxygen debt for the entire session (generally 60 minutes) even among reasonably well trained "healthy" people
☑ **Aerobic machines such as elliptical runners and stair-climbing machines**: easy on joints; accessible during inclement weather; easy to integrate with weight-lifting which is commonly available at the same facility
☑ **Baseball**: requires some skill in throwing and batting, but otherwise this is a very inactive sport
☑ **Football**: much of the game is spent in inactivity; most of the fitness comes from preparation for the game, not the game itself; high impact activity wherein injuries are expected
☑ **Hiking**: virtually free of expense; allows for conversation, exploration, and time in nature; mountains required
☑ **Indoor aerobics**: excellent for cardiovascular fitness and weight loss, requires and thus promotes coordination and timing
☑ **Indoor cycling**: excellent for cardiovascular fitness and weight loss, easy on the joints; accessible during inclement weather
☑ **Jogging and running**: easy, accessible, virtually free; allows for conversation and exploration; increases endorphin production and promotes a sense of well-being; detoxification via sweating
☑ **Kayaking and canoeing**: excellent combination of relaxation and exertion; develops upper body strength and balance
☑ **Martial arts**: requires more balance, coordination, timing, strategy, endurance; injuries are to be expected, as is enhanced sense of security and confidence
☑ **Outdoor cycling (mountain and trail)**: same as above; requires more balance and coordination
☑ **Outdoor cycling (road)**: same as above with added bonus of being outdoors; promotes independence from automobiles and petroleum products – thereby reducing pollution and sustaining the environment

---

[77] Harold Elrick, MD. Exercise is Medicine. *The Physician and Sportsmedicine* - Volume 24 - No. 2 - February 1996
[78] O'Keefe JH Jr, Cordain L. Cardiovascular disease resulting from a diet and lifestyle at odds with our Paleolithic genome: how to become a 21st-century hunter-gatherer. *Mayo Clin Proc*. 2004 Jan;79(1):101-8. Available on line at http://www.thepaleodiet.com/articles/Hunter-Gatherer%20Mayo.pdf on May 19, 2004

- ☑ **Rock-climbing (indoor and outdoor)**: requires upper body and grip strength; promotes agility, resourcefulness, courage, and trust; good for building stronger relationships assuming that your partner does not drop the rope or get distracted; carries some inherent risk
- ☑ **Skiing, snowboarding, cross-country skiing**: Require balance and coordination, costly equipment, and appropriate season and climate; risk of traumatic injury due to speed in skiing and snowboarding. Cross-country skiing is generally safe from trauma and provides excellent cardiovascular exertion, in addition to exposure to nature
- ☑ **Soccer**: excellent for lower-body conditioning, teamwork, and coordination, the rapid stops and turns can be hard on joints
- ☑ **Surfing**: paddling requires upper body endurance and strength; some leg strength is required but is not strongly developed during the riding portion of surfing, which is mostly technique and "style"; excellent proprioceptive training
- ☑ **Swimming**: requires access to a pool or suitable body of water; excellent for promoting fitness in a way that is generally easy on joints and muscles and is without impact; requires and thus promotes coordination and timing
- ☑ **Tennis and racket sports**: requires more balance, coordination, timing, strategy, endurance; the rapid stops, starts, and turns can be hard on joints; upper body exertion is asymmetric and can promote muscle imbalance
- ☑ **Volleyball**: good team activity; not highly exertional in terms of either aerobic fitness nor strength acquisition
- ☑ **Walking**: easy, accessible, virtually free; allows for conversation and exploration; allows for time outdoors
- ☑ **Weight lifting, bodybuilding, and powerlifting**: excellent for increasing lean body mass – one of the primary determinants of basal metabolic rate; promotes bone strengthening
- ☑ **Yoga, Calisthenics**: inexpensive, can be done alone or in groups; does not require much/any equipment, therefore costs are low and access is near universal

Obesity: Obesity is a major risk factor for cardiovascular disease, cancer, diabetes mellitus, depression, joint degeneration and pain. Obese people also commonly report difficulties with performing daily activities, and they also report higher rates of depression and social isolation than do people of normal weight. Adipose tissue is biologically active, promoting systemic inflammation and estrogen dominance, thereby promoting the development of inflammatory and malignant diseases such as psoriasis and cancers of the breast, prostate, and colon, respectively.

"Body Mass Index" is a clinically valuable measure of height-weight proportionality and therefore adiposity, since an excess of height-proportionate weight is more commonly due to excess adipose than to excess muscle. To calculate BMI simply chart height and weight in the table below. Numbers greater than 25 correlate with being "overweight" while numbers greater than 30 meet the criteria for "obesity." BMI determinations may not be reflective of disease risk for people who are pregnant, highly muscular, or for young children or the frail elderly.

Body mass index (BMI) interpretation

- ❑ Severely underweight: < 16.5
- ❑ Underweight: 16.5 - 18.4
- ❑ **Normal: 18.5 - 24.9**
- ❑ Overweight: 25 - 29.9

- ❑ Obese Class 1: 30 - 34.9
- ❑ Obese Class 2 (severe obesity): 35 - 39.9
- ❑ Obese Class 3 (morbid obesity): 40 - 47.9
- ❑ Obese Class 4 (supermorbid obesity): ≥ 48

WEIGHT in pounds

HEIGHT	100	110	120	130	140	150	160	170	180	190	200	210	220	230	240	250
5'0"	20	21	23	25	27	29	31	33	35	37	39	41	43	45	47	49
5'1"	19	21	23	25	26	28	30	32	34	36	38	40	42	43	45	47
5'2"	18	20	22	24	26	27	29	31	33	35	37	38	40	42	44	46
5'3"	18	19	21	23	25	27	28	30	32	34	35	37	39	41	43	44
5'4"	17	19	21	22	24	26	27	29	31	33	34	36	38	39	41	43
5'5"	17	18	20	22	23	25	27	28	30	32	33	35	37	38	40	42
5'6"	16	18	19	21	23	24	26	27	29	31	32	34	36	37	39	40
5'7"	16	17	19	20	22	23	25	27	28	30	31	33	34	36	38	39
5'8"	15	17	18	20	21	23	24	26	27	29	30	32	33	35	36	38
5'9"	15	16	18	19	21	22	24	25	27	28	30	31	32	34	35	37
5'10"	14	16	17	19	20	22	23	24	26	27	29	30	32	33	34	36
5'11"	14	15	17	18	20	21	22	24	25	26	27	28	30	32	33	35
6'0"	14	15	16	18	19	20	22	23	24	26	27	28	30	31	33	34
6'1"	13	15	16	17	18	20	21	22	24	25	26	28	29	30	32	33
6'2"	13	14	15	17	18	19	21	22	23	24	26	27	28	30	31	32
6'3"	12	14	15	16	17	19	20	21	22	24	25	26	27	29	30	31
6'4"	12	13	15	16	17	18	19	21	22	23	24	26	27	28	29	30

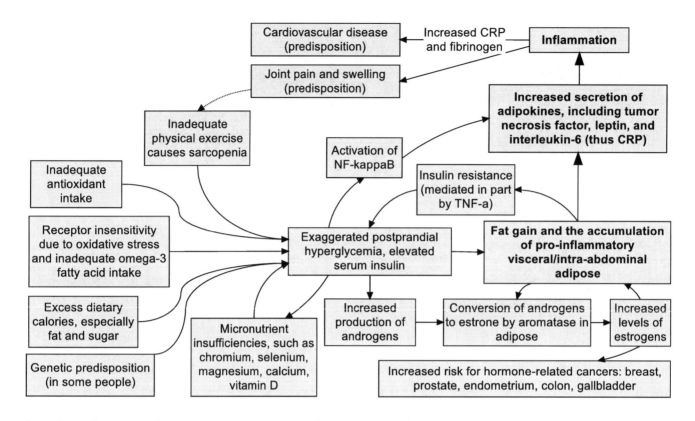

Overview of the proinflammatory and endocrinologic activity of adipose tissue: Adipose tissue is biologically active, promoting systemic inflammation and production of estrogens at the expense of androgens via the enzyme aromatase

The old view that fat (adipose) tissue was merely serving as an inert and inactive depot for lipid/energy storage is now replaced with the view that adipose tissue is biologically-active, influencing overall health via complex mechanisms that are biochemical-inflammatory-endocrinologic and not merely mechanical (i.e., excess weight, excess mass).[79] **Excess fat tissue—especially visceral/abdominal adipose—creates a systemic proinflammatory state** evidenced most readily by the elevations in hsCRP commonly seen in patients with obesity and the metabolic syndrome.[80] Adipokines are cytokines secreted by adipose tissue and include tumor necrosis factor-alpha, interleukin-6, and leptin—a cytokine derived from fat cells that promotes inflammation and immune activation; levels are higher in obese patients and decrease after weight loss. Obese patients also appear to have "leptin resistance" with regard to the suppression of appetite by leptin. **Adipose creates excess estrogens;** concomitant hyperglycemia increases androgen production[81], and these androgens are subsequently converted to estrogens by aromatase in the adipose tissue. For example, the adrenal gland makes androstenedione, which can be converted by aromatase in adipose tissue into estrone.[82] These proinflammatory and hormonal perturbations manifest clinically as an increased risk for breast, prostate, endometrial, colon and gallbladder cancers, and cardiovascular disease. This pattern of inflammation, reduced testosterone, and elevated estrogen is also a predisposition toward the development of autoimmune/inflammatory diseases.

---

[79] "The fat cell is a true endocrine cell that secretes a variety of factors, including metabolites such as lactate, fatty acids, prostaglandin derivatives and a variety of peptides, including cytokines (leptin, tumor necrosis factor, interleukin-1 and -6, adiponectin), angiotensinogen, complement D (adipsin), plasminogen activator inhibitor-1 and undoubtedly many others." Bray GA. The underlying basis for obesity: relationship to cancer. *J Nutr*. 2002 Nov;132(11 Suppl):3451S-3455S

[80] "Our results indicate a strong relationship between adipocytokines and inflammatory markers, and suggest that cytokines secreted by adipose tissue could play a role in increased inflammatory proteins secretion by the liver." Maachi M, Pieroni L, Bruckert E, Jardel C, Fellahi S, Hainque B, Capeau J, Bastard JP. Systemic low-grade inflammation is related to both circulating and adipose tissue TNFalpha, leptin and IL-6 levels in obese women. *Int J Obes Relat Metab Disord*. 2004;28:993-7

[81] Christensen L, Hagen C, Henriksen JE, Haug E. Elevated levels of sex hormones and sex hormone binding globulin in male patients with insulin dependent diabetes mellitus. Effect of improved blood glucose regulation. *Dan Med Bull*. 1997 Nov;44(5):547-50

[82] "The conversion of androstenedione secreted by the adrenal gland into estrone by aromatase in adipose tissue stroma provides an important source of estrogen for the postmenopausal woman. This estrogen may play an important role in the development of endometrial and breast cancer." Bray GA. The underlying basis for obesity: relationship to cancer. *J Nutr*. 2002 Nov;132(11 Suppl):3451S-3455S

The Daily Diet—Powerful Intervention for the Prevention and Treatment of Disease: "Whole foods" should form the foundation and majority of the diet. As doctors and patients, we should emphasize whole fruits, vegetables, nuts, seeds, berries, and lean sources of protein. "Whole foods" are foods that are found in nature, and they should be eaten as closely as possible to their natural state—preferably *unprocessed* and *raw*. Creating a diet based on whole, natural foods by emphasizing the consumption of fruits, vegetables, and lean meats and excluding high-fat factory meats, high-sugar foods like white potatoes, and milled grains like wheat and corn is essential for our efforts of promoting health by matching the human *diet* with the human *genome*.[83] Our genetic make-up was co-created over a period of more than 2.6 million years by interaction with the environment as it exists in its natural state. This environment mandated daily physical activity and a diet that was exclusively composed of 1) fresh fruits, 2) fresh vegetables (mostly uncooked), 3) raw nuts, seeds, berries, roots, and 4) generous portions of lean game meat that was rich in omega-3 fatty acids from free-living animals who were lean because they also ran, fasted, and dealt with limited food supplies. Humans have deviated from this original diet for the sake of ease, conformity, and short-term satisfaction at the expense of health and longevity. Peoples who consume traditional, natural diets have dramatically lower incidences *major* health problems such as cancer, cardiovascular disease, diabetes, obesity and also suffer much less from *milder* problems such as

> ### The Supplemented Paleo-Mediterranean Diet
> My conclusion after reading several hundred articles on epidemiology, nutritional biochemistry, and dietary intervention studies is that the Paleo-Mediterranean diet—particularly its pesco-vegetarian version—is the single most healthy dietary regimen for the broadest range of patients and for the prevention of the widest range of diseases including cancer, hypertension, diabetes, dermatitis, depression, obesity, arthritis and all inflammatory and autoimmune diseases. By definition, this is a diet that helps patients increase their intake of fruits and vegetables (fiber, antioxidants, phytonutrients), increases their intake of fish (for the anti-inflammatory omega-3 fats EPA and DHA) while reducing intake of the pro-cancer and pro-inflammatory omega-6 fats linoleic acid and arachidonic acid), and it is naturally low in sugars and cholesterol (for alleviating hyperglycemia and dyslipidemia). This dietary pattern helps patients avoid grains, particularly wheat (a common allergen), and it reduces the intake of the high-fermentation carbohydrates in breads, pasta, pastries, potatoes, and sucrose which promote overgrowth of bacteria and yeast in the intestines. Supplementing this pesco-vegetarian diet with vitamins, minerals, fatty acids such as fish oil and GLA (from borage oil), and protein from soy and whey makes this diet effective for both the treatment and prevention of many conditions; I have called this "the Supplemented Paleo-Mediterranean Diet."
>
> 1. Vasquez A. A Five-Part Nutritional Protocol that Produces Consistently Positive Results. *Nutritional Wellness* 2005 September
> 2. Vasquez A. Implementing the Five-Part Nutritional Wellness Protocol for the Treatment of Various Health Problems. *Nutritional Wellness* 2005 November
> 3. Vasquez A. Revisiting the Five-Part Nutritional Wellness Protocol: The Supplemented Paleo-Mediterranean Diet. *Nutritional Perspectives* 2011 January

acne, psoriasis, dental cavities, oral malocclusion, and chronic sinus congestion. Societies that are free of these disorders become overwhelmed with them *within only one or two generations* as soon as they adopt the American/Western style of eating. These facts were conclusively documented by Weston Price in his famous 1945 masterpiece *Nutrition and Physical Degeneration*[84] and have been reiterated recently in an excellent review by O'Keefe and Cordain in *Mayo Clinic Proceedings*.[85]

Most patients (and doctors) need to increase consumption of fruits and vegetables: Encourage consumption of collard greens, broccoli, kale, spinach, chard, lettuce, onions, red peppers, green beans, carrots, apples, oranges, nuts, blueberries and other fruits and vegetables. Patients can find or make a good low-carbohydrate dressing (such as lemon-garlic tahini[86]) to make these vegetables taste great. Fresh fruits and vegetables are best; but frozen fruits and vegetables are acceptable. Patients can buy a package of (organic) frozen vegetables; then when they are ready for a healthy-and-fast meal, simply thaw the vegetables or warm/steam them on the stovetop. In just a few minutes and with only minimal effort, by regularly eating vegetables, they will have significantly reduced their risk for heart disease, diabetes, cancer, hemorrhoids, constipation, and many other chronic health problems. Using frozen vegetables and eating vegetables only twice per day is not *optimal*—it is *minimal*. For many patients, consuming two servings of vegetables per day is a major lifestyle change. ***Ultimately, the goal is for fresh fruits and vegetables***

---

[83] O'Keefe JH Jr, Cordain L. Cardiovascular disease resulting from a diet and lifestyle at odds with our Paleolithic genome: how to become a 21st-century hunter-gatherer. *Mayo Clin Proc.* 2004 Jan;79(1):101-8

[84] Price WA. Nutrition and Physical Degeneration. Santa Monica; Price-Pottenger Nutrition Foundation: 1945

[85] O'Keefe JH Jr, Cordain L. Cardiovascular disease resulting from a diet and lifestyle at odds with our Paleolithic genome. *Mayo Clin Proc.* 2004;79:101-8

[86] Mollie Katzen. The New Moosewood Cookbook Ten Speed Press; page 103

to form a major portion of the diet, to be the main course rather than simply a side dish. A diet based on fruits and vegetables is a powerful nutritional strategy for reducing the risk for cancer, heart disease, and autoimmune and inflammatory disorders.[87]

Phytochemicals—important antioxidant and anti-inflammatory nutrients from fruits, vegetables, nuts, seeds, berries, and many herbs and spices: While we have all commonly thought of the benefits of fruits and vegetables as being derived from the vitamins, minerals, and fiber, we are learning from new research that many if not most of the health-promoting benefits of fruit and vegetable consumption comes from the unique plant-based chemicals—phytochemicals—contained therein. For example, while in the past we might have thought of the benefits of eating apples as being derived from the vitamin C content, we now know that vitamin C only provides 0.4% of the antioxidant action contained within a whole apple—obviously the other components of the apple, namely the phenolic compounds are responsible for most of an apple's antioxidant activity.[88] Recent research has shown that cranberries, apples, red grapes, and strawberries have the most antioxidant power of the fruits[89], while red peppers, broccoli, carrots, and spinach are the best antioxidant vegetables[90]; see the tables that follow. This is a very important concept to appreciate and remember: **the benefits derived from fruits and vegetables are _not_ derived principally from the vitamins and therefore can never be obtained from the use of multivitamin pills as a substitute for whole foods. Multivitamin and multimineral supplements are valuable and worthwhile _supplements_ to a whole-foods diet but should not be used as _substitutes_ for a whole-foods diet. Fruits and vegetables contain more than 8,000 phytochemicals, most of which have anti-inflammatory, anti-proliferative, and anti-cancer benefits[91]—the best and only way to benefit from these health-promoting chemicals is to change the diet in favor of relying principally on fruits and vegetables as the major component of the diet**, and the easiest way to do this is to eliminate carbohydrate-rich antioxidant-poor foods such as bread, pasta, rice, sweets, crackers, chips and "junk foods"—when people avoid unhealthy foods, they will trend toward using more healthy foods.

> **Proteins, fruits, vegetables—not grains**
>
> "Historical and archaeological evidence shows hunter-gatherers generally to be lean, fit, and largely free from signs and symptoms of chronic diseases. When hunter-gatherer societies transitioned to an agricultural grain-based diet, their general health deteriorated. ... When former hunter-gatherers adopt Western lifestyles, obesity, type-2 diabetes, atherosclerosis, and other diseases of civilization become commonplace."
>
> O'Keefe JH Jr, Cordain L. Cardiovascular disease resulting from a diet and lifestyle at odds with our Paleolithic genome. *Mayo Clin Proc.* 2004;79:101-8

Phenolic content and antioxidant capacity of common vegetables and fruits[92,93]

Vegetables		Fruits	
Phenolic content	*Antioxidant capacity*	*Phenolic content*	*Antioxidant capacity*
1. **Broccoli**	1. **Red pepper**	1. **Cranberry**	1. **Cranberry**
2. **Spinach**	2. **Broccoli**	2. **Apple**	2. **Apple**
3. **Yellow onion**	3. **Carrot**	3. **Red grape**	3. **Red grape**
4. **Red pepper**	4. **Spinach**	4. **Strawberry**	4. **Strawberry**
5. Carrot	5. Cabbage	5. Pineapple	5. Peach
6. Cabbage	6. Yellow onion	6. Banana	6. Lemon
7. Potato	7. Celery	7. Peach	7. Pear
8. Lettuce	8. Potato	8. Lemon	8. Banana
9. Celery	9. Lettuce	9. Orange	9. Orange
10. Cucumber	10. Cucumber	10. Pear	10. Grapefruit
		11. Grapefruit	11. Pineapple

---

[87] "...one of the most consistent research findings is that those who consume higher amounts of fruits and vegetables have lower rates of heart disease and stroke as well as cancer..." Seaman DR. The diet-induced proinflammatory state: a cause of chronic pain and other degenerative diseases? *J Manipulative Physiol Ther.* 2002;25(3):168-79

[88] "We propose that the additive and synergistic effects of phytochemicals in fruit and vegetables are responsible for their potent antioxidant and anticancer activities, and that the benefit of a diet rich in fruit and vegetables is attributed to the complex mixture of phytochemicals present in whole foods." Liu RH. Health benefits of fruit and vegetables are from additive and synergistic combinations of phytochemicals. *Am J Clin Nutr.* 2003 Sep;78(3 Suppl):517S-520S

[89] "Cranberry had the highest total antioxidant activity (177.0 +/- 4.3 micromol of vitamin C equiv/g of fruit), followed by apple, red grape, strawberry, peach, lemon, pear, banana, orange, grapefruit, and pineapple." Sun J, Chu YF, Wu X, Liu RH. Antioxidant and antiproliferative activities of common fruits. *J Agric Food Chem.* 2002 Dec 4;50(25):7449-54

[90] "Red pepper had the highest total antioxidant activity, followed by broccoli, carrot, spinach, cabbage, yellow onion, celery, potato, lettuce, and cucumber." Chu YF, Sun J, Wu X, Liu RH. Antioxidant and antiproliferative activities of common vegetables. *J Agric Food Chem.* 2002 Nov 6;50(23):6910-6

[91] Liu RH. Health benefits of fruit and vegetables are from additive and synergistic combinations of phytochemicals. *Am J Clin Nutr.* 2003 Sep;78(3 Suppl):517S-520S

[92] Chu YF, Sun J, Wu X, Liu RH. Antioxidant and antiproliferative activities of common vegetables. *J Agric Food Chem.* 2002;50:6910-6

[93] Sun J, Chu YF, Wu X, Liu RH. Antioxidant and antiproliferative activities of common fruits. *J Agric Food Chem.* 2002;50:7449-54

Different fruits and vegetables contain different types, quantities, and ratios of vitamins, minerals, and phytochemicals; therefore, *dietary diversity* **will therefore help patients obtain a broad spectrum of and maximum benefit from these different nutrients**. Taking appropriate action with the data that a fruit/vegetable-based diet has powerful health-promoting benefits means that we as doctors and patients have to change our lifestyles with regard to how we plan our meals, what we buy, what we prepare, and what we eat. Behavior modification is a tremendous challenge for people, especially those who lack sufficient motivation or insight. This text is providing the *insight*—the data, references, and concepts. But without *motivation*—from doctors to help their patients attain the highest levels of health, and from patients to change their lifestyles to become as healthy as possible—the research itself does little to promote health.

<u>Consuming the right amount of protein</u>: Dietary protein is eaten to provide the body with amino acids, which are the fundamental components that the body uses to create new tissues (such as skin, mucosal surfaces, hair, and nails), heal wounds (e.g., formation of collagen), fight off infections (e.g., formation of immunoglobulin proteins, antibodies), and to create specific hormones (such as insulin and thyroid hormones) and neurotransmitters, such as dopamine, serotonin, norepinephrine, and gamma-aminobutyric acid (GABA). Amino acid profiles in meats, eggs, and milk is similar to that of the human body and such dietary sources have been described as containing relatively more "complete protein" than most plant-based protein sources. For plant-based diets without concomitant use of animal proteins to provide sufficient quantity and quality of protein, foods must be combined with respect to one another's amino acid profiles.

For most people (without kidney or liver problems) the goal for daily protein intake should be 0.50-0.75 grams of protein per pound of lean body weight, depending on activity level and other health needs (see table).

Recommended <u>Grams of Protein</u> Per <u>Pound of Body Weight</u> Per Day[94]	
Infants and children ages 1-6 years[95]	0.68-0.45
RDA for sedentary adult and children ages 6-18 years[96]	0.4
Adult recreational exerciser	**0.5-0.75**
Adult competitive athlete	0.6-0.9
Adult building muscle mass	0.7-0.9
Dieting athlete	0.7-1.0
Growing teenage athlete	0.9-1.0
Pregnant women need additional protein	Add 15-30 grams/day[97]

Sufficient dietary protein is essential for patients with musculoskeletal injuries because tissue healing relies on the constant availability of amino acids and micronutrients[98], which should be supplied by a healthy, balanced, whole-foods diet that may be supplemented with specific vitamins, minerals, and phytonutrients. Low-protein diets suppress immune function, reduce muscle mass, and impair healing[99,100] whereas intakes of higher amounts of protein safely facilitate healing and the maintenance of muscle mass. Increased protein intake does not adversely affect bone health as long as dietary calcium intake is adequate.[101] According to the 1998 review by Lemon[102], "Those involved in strength training might need to consume as much as …1.7 g protein x kg(-1) x day(-1)…while those

---

[94] Slightly modified from Nancy Clark, MS, RD. Protein Power. *The Physician and Sportsmedicine* 1996, volume 24, number 4

[95] 1.5-1 g/kg/d (0.68-0.45 grams per pound of body weight. Younger people need proportionately more protein.) Brown ML (ed). <u>Present Knowledge in Nutrition. Sixth Edition</u>. Washington DC: International Life Sciences Institute Nutrition Foundation; 1990 page 68

[96] 0.83 g.kg-1.d-1 (equivalent to 0.37 grams per pound of body weight) Pellet PL. Protein requirements in humans. *Am J Clin Nutr* 1990 May;51:723-37

[97] Weinsier RL, Morgan SL (eds). <u>Fundamentals of Clinical Nutrition</u>. St. Louis: Mosby, 1993 page 50

[98] "Supplementation with protein and vitamins, specifically arginine and vitamins A, B, and C, provides optimum nutrient support of the healing wound." Meyer NA, Muller MJ, Herndon DN. Nutrient support of the healing wound. *New Horiz* 1994 May;2(2):202-14

[99] Castaneda C, Charnley JM, Evans WJ, Crim MC. Elderly women accommodate to a low-protein diet with losses of body cell mass, muscle function, and immune response. *Am J Clin Nutr* 1995 Jul;62(1):30-9 http://www.ajcn.org/cgi/reprint/62/1/30

[100] [No author listed]. Vegetarians and healing. *JAMA* 1995; 273: 910

[101] Heaney RP. Excess dietary protein may not adversely affect bone. *J Nutr* 1998 Jun;128(6):1054-7

[102] Lemon PW. Effects of exercise on dietary protein requirements. *Int J Sport Nutr 1998* Dec;8(4):426-47

undergoing endurance training might need about 1.2 to 1.6 g x kg(-1) x day(-1)**... ...there is no evidence that protein intakes in the range suggested will have adverse effects in healthy individuals.**"

For patients who are completely sedentary, multiply body weight in pounds by 0.4 and this will give the number of grams of protein that should be eaten each day.[103] For patients who are very active (frequent weight lifting, or competitive athlete), multiply body weight in pounds by 0.7-0.9 and this will give the number of grams of protein that should be eaten each day.

Again, compared with sedentary people, *sick people, injured people,* and *athletes* **need more protein** to maintain weight, fight infections, repair injuries, and build and maintain muscle. Not only can insufficient protein intake cause muscle weakness and loss of weight, but recent articles have also suggested that low-protein diets can cause suppression of the immune system[104] and impairment of healing after injury or surgery.[105]

For example, in most instances and according to the data presented in and reviewed for this section, a person weighing 120 pounds should aim for at least 60 grams of protein per day, or 90 grams of protein per day if he/she is more physically active, ill, or injured. A can of tuna has 30 grams of protein; one egg has 6 grams of protein. If she is going to eat eggs as a source of protein for a meal, she might have to eat as many as five eggs to reach a target of 30 grams of protein per meal. When eating meat, visualize the amount of meat in a can of tuna to estimate the amount of protein being eaten—for example, if the portion of meat at a given meal is about the size of a half can of tuna, then we can estimate that the serving contains 15-20 grams of high-quality protein. By knowing the "target intake" for the day, and by estimating the amount of protein eaten with each meal, patients will be able to modify their protein intake to ensure that they reach their protein intake goal.

Protein supplements—most common of which are based on concentrates of or isolated components of egg, soy, or cow's milk— can be used *in conjunction with a healthy diet*. Patients using a protein supplement should eat a healthy diet and then add protein supplements between regular meals. If they substitute a protein supplement for a regular meal, then they may not actually increase protein intake. Whole *real* foods should form the foundation for the diet—patients should not rely too heavily on *protein supplements* when patients can get better results *and improved overall health* with *whole foods*. Whey, casein, and lactalbumin are proteins from milk and dairy products, and may therefore be allergenic in people allergic to cow's milk. Soy protein is safe and a source of high-quality protein for adults[106], and research shows that consumption of soy protein can help reduce the risk of cancer and heart disease[107]; however, I do not recommend the use of large quantities of supplemental soy protein for pregnant women, or for children due to the potential for disrupting endocrine function. Patients may have to experiment with different products until they find one that is suitable in regard to taste, texture, digestibility, hypoallergenicity, nutritional effects, ease of preparation, and affordability.

Recall again that the goal is *improved health*, not simply *adequate protein intake*. If we focus solely on "grams of protein" then we might overlook adverse effects that are associated with certain protein sources. Cow's milk is a high quality protein, but it is commonly allergenic and can exacerbate joint pain in sensitive individuals.[108] Beef, liver, pork and other land animal meats are excellent sources of protein, but they are also generally rich sources of arachidonic acid[109] (if not grass-fed) and iron[110], both of which have been shown to exacerbate joint pain and inflammation. Fish is an excellent source of protein, but fish are often poisoned with mercury and other toxicants, which can be ingested by humans to produce negative health effects.[111,112]

---

[103] Pellet PL. Protein requirements in humans. *Am J Clin Nutr* 1990 May;51(5):723-37

[104] Castaneda C, Charnley JM, Evans WJ, Crim MC. Elderly women accommodate to a low-protein diet with losses of body cell mass, muscle function, and immune response. *Am J Clin Nutr* 1995 Jul;62(1):30-9

[105] Vegetarians and healing. *Journal of the American Medical Association* 1995; 273: 910

[106] "These results indicate that for healthy adults, the isolated soy protein is of high nutritional quality, comparable to that of animal protein sources, and that the methionine content is not limiting for adult protein maintenance." Young VR, Puig M, Queiroz E, Scrimshaw NS, Rand WM. Evaluation of the protein quality of an isolated soy protein in young men: relative nitrogen requirements and effect of methionine supplementation. *Am J Clin Nutr*. 1984 Jan;39(1):16-24

[107] Lissin LW, Cooke JP. Phytoestrogens and cardiovascular health. *J Am Coll Cardiol*. 2000 May;35(6):1403-10

[108] Golding DN. Is there an allergic synovitis? *J R Soc Med* 1990 May;83(5):312-4

[109] Adam O, Beringer C, Kless T, Lemmen C, Adam A, Wiseman M, Adam P, Klimmek R, Forth W. Anti-inflammatory effects of a low arachidonic acid diet and fish oil in patients with rheumatoid arthritis. *Rheumatol Int* 2003 Jan;23(1):27-36

[110] Dabbagh AJ, Trenam CW, Morris CJ, Blake DR. Iron in joint inflammation. *Ann Rheum Dis* 1993; 52:67-73

[111] "These fish often harbor high levels of methylmercury, a potent human neurotoxin." Evans EC. The FDA recommendations on fish intake during pregnancy. *J Obstet Gynecol Neonatal Nurs* 2002 Nov-Dec;31(6):715-20

[112] "Geometric mean mercury levels were almost 4-fold higher among women who ate 3 or more servings of fish in the past 30 days compared with women who ate no fish in that period.." Schober SE, Sinks TH, Jones RL, Bolger PM, McDowell M, Osterloh J, Garrett ES, Canady RA, Dillon CF, Sun Y, Joseph CB, Mahaffey KR. Blood mercury levels in US children and women of childbearing age, 1999-2000. *JAMA* 2003 Apr 2;289(13):1667-74

Eat complex carbohydrates to stabilize blood sugar, mood, and energy: Choose items with a "low glycemic index"[113] to stabilize blood sugar and—for many people—to lower triglycerides and cholesterol levels. Foods with a low Glycemic Index (GI < 55)[114] include yogurt, apple (36), whole orange (43), peach (28), legumes, lentils (28), and soybeans (18), cherries, dried apricots, nuts, most meats, and most vegetables. Healthy foods that have both a low *glycemic index* as well as a low *glycemic load* include: apples, carrots, chick peas, grapes, green peas, kidney beans, oranges, peaches, peanuts, pears, pinto beans, red lentils, and strawberries.[115]

Reduce or eliminate simple sugars from the diet (as necessary): Nearly everyone should minimize intake of table sugar (sucrose), fructose and high-fructose corn syrup, and all artificial sweeteners. Of important and recent note, high-fructose corn syrup has been shown to be contaminated by mercury due to the manufacturing process[116], and fructose has been shown to induce hypertension and the metabolic syndrome in humans.[117] Chronic overconsumption of refined carbohydrates promotes disease by 1) increasing urinary excretion of magnesium and calcium, 2) inducing oxidative stress, 3) promoting fat deposition and obesity, which then generally leads to insulin resistance and hyperinsulinemia with an increase in production of cholesterol, triglycerides, and proinflammatory adipokines[118], and 4) reducing function of leukocytes.[119] Among sweeteners, honey is the best choice since it is the only natural sweetener available with a wide range of health-promoting benefits including anti-inflammatory, antibacterial, antioxidant and anti-allergy effects.[120] Also consider the herb stevia as a non-caloric and nutritive sweetener. Occasional intake of sweets is likely to be of little consequence for people who are generally healthy and who are willing to sustain relatively short-term endothelial dysfunction[121], oxidative stress[122], increased LDL oxidation[123], and activation of NF-kappaB[124] as a result of their self-induced hyperglycemia. Postexertional hyperglycemia can be used to enhance athletic performance by sustaining and inducing glycogen storage following and during exercise (i.e., carbohydrate loading for glycogen "supercompensation"[125,126]). Similarly, consumption of "simple" carbohydrate without protein can be used to promote entry of tryptophan across the blood-brain barrier

---

[113] For more information on glycemic index, consult a nutrition book or website such as http://www.stanford.edu/~dep/gilists.htm last accessed August 16, 2003

[114] Janette Brand-Miller, Kaye Foster-Powell. Diets with a low glycemic index: from theory to practice. *Nutrition Today* 1999 March. Accessed on-line at: http://www.findarticles.com/cf_dls/m0841/2_34/54654508/p1/article.jhtml on August 16, 2003.

[115] Mendosa D. Glycemic Values of Common American Foods http://www.mendosa.com/common_foods.htm Accessed on August 4, 2004

[116] "Average daily consumption of high fructose corn syrup is about 50 grams per person in the United States. With respect to total mercury exposure, it may be necessary to account for this source of mercury in the diet of children and sensitive populations." Dufault R, LeBlanc B, Schnoll R, Cornett C, Schweitzer L, Wallinga D, Hightower J, Patrick L, Lukiw WJ. Mercury from chlor-alkali plants: measured concentrations in food product sugar. *Environ Health*. 2009 Jan 26;8:2. See also: "High fructose corn syrup has been shown to contain trace amounts of mercury as a result of some manufacturing processes, and its consumption can also lead to zinc loss." Dufault R, Schnoll R, Lukiw WJ, Leblanc B, Cornett C, Patrick L, Wallinga D, Gilbert SG, Crider R. Mercury exposure, nutritional deficiencies and metabolic disruptions may affect learning in children. *Behav Brain Funct*. 2009 Oct 27;5:44.

[117] News release from American Heart Association's 63rd High Blood Pressure Research Conference. High-sugar diet increases men's blood pressure; gout drug protective. Abstract P127. Sept. 23, 2009. http://americanheart.mediaroom.com/index.php?s=43&item=829 Accessed December 19, 2009

[118] "Because visceral and subcutaneous adipose tissues are the major sources of cytokines (adipokines), increased adipose tissue mass is associated with alteration in adipokine production (eg, overexpression of tumor necrosis factor-a, interleukin-6, plasminogen activator inhibitor-1, and underexpression of adiponectin in adipose tissue)." Aldahhi W, Hamdy O. Adipokines, inflammation, and the endothelium in diabetes. *Curr Diab Rep*. 2003 Aug;3(4):293-8

[119] Sanchez A, Reeser JL, Lau HS, Yahiku PY, Willard RE, McMillan PJ, Cho SY, Magie AR, Register UD. Role of sugars in human neutrophilic phagocytosis. *Am J Clin Nutr*. 1973 Nov;26(11):1180-4

[120] Al-Waili NS. Effects of daily consumption of honey solution on hematological indices and blood levels of minerals and enzymes in normal individuals. *J Med Food*. 2003 Summer;6(2):135-4

[121] "Modest hyperinsulinemia, mimicking fasting hyperinsulinemia of insulin-resistant states, abrogates endothelium-dependent vasodilation in large conduit arteries, probably by increasing oxidant stress. These data may provide a novel pathophysiological basis to the epidemiological link between hyperinsulinemia/insulin-resistance and atherosclerosis in humans." Arcaro G, Cretti A, Balzano S, Lechi A, Muggeo M, Bonora E, Bonadonna RC. Insulin causes endothelial dysfunction in humans: sites and mechanisms. *Circulation*. 2002 Feb 5;105(5):576-82

[122] "Hyperglycemia increased plasma MDA concentrations, but the activities of GSH-Px and SOD were significantly higher after a larger dose of glucose only. Plasma catecholamines were unchanged. These results indicate that the transient increase of plasma catecholamine and insulin concentrations did not induce oxidative damage, while glucose already in the low dose was an important triggering factor for oxidative stress." Koska J, Blazicek P, Marko M, Grna JD, Kvetnansky R, Vigas M. Insulin, catecholamines, glucose and antioxidant enzymes in oxidative damage during different loads in healthy humans. *Physiol Res*. 2000;49 Suppl 1:S95-100

[123] "In conclusion, insulin at physiological doses is associated with increased LDL peroxidation independent of the presence of hyperglycemia." Quinones-Galvan A, Sironi AM, Baldi S, Galetta F, Garbin U, Fratta-Pasini A, Cominacini L, Ferrannini E. Evidence that acute insulin administration enhances LDL cholesterol susceptibility to oxidation in healthy humans. *Arterioscler Thromb Vasc Biol*. 1999 Dec;19(12):2928-32

[124] "These data show that the intake of a mixed meal results in significant inflammatory changes characterized by a decrease in IkappaBalpha and an increase in NF-kappaB binding, plasma CRP, and the expression of IKKalpha, IKKbeta, and p47(phox) subunit." Aljada A, Mohanty P, Ghanim H, Abdo T, Tripathy D, Chaudhuri A, Dandona P. Increase in intranuclear nuclear factor kappaB and decrease in inhibitor kappaB in mononuclear cells after a mixed meal: evidence for a proinflammatory effect. *Am J Clin Nutr*. 2004 Apr;79(4):682-90

[125] "A significant glycogen sparing, as well as supercompensation within 24 h of recovery, was observed after [carbohydrate] supplementation." Brouns F, Saris WH, Beckers E, Adlercreutz H, van der Vusse GJ, Keizer HA, Kuipers H, Menheere P, Wagenmakers AJ, ten Hoor F. Metabolic changes induced by sustained exhaustive cycling and diet manipulation. *Int J Sports Med*. 1989 May;10 Suppl 1:S49-62

[126] "The accepted method of increasing muscle glycogen stores is by "glycogen loading," which classically involves depletion of muscle glycogen, usually by exercise, followed by consumption of a high-CHO diet for several days (e.g., 3, 39). ...increase muscle glycogen concentrations ([glycogen]) to between 150 and 200% of normal resting levels." Robinson TM, Sewell DA, Hultman E, Greenhaff PL. Role of submaximal exercise in promoting creatine and glycogen accumulation in human skeletal muscle. *J Appl Physiol*. 1999 Aug;87(2):598-604

and into the brain to promote serotonin synthesis.[127] In summary, *habitual overconsumption* of simple carbohydrates promotes disease by oxidative and proinflammatory mechanisms, while conversely *periodic consumption* of simple carbohydrates can be used to promote athletic performance and to increase intracerebral serotonin synthesis for the promotion of enhanced mood and cognitive performance and for the regulation of food intake.

Avoid artificial sweeteners, colors and other additives: Absolutely never use **aspartame**—this is a synthetic chemical that is easily converted to the toxin formaldehyde.[128] Aspartame causes cancer in animals and is strongly linked to brain tumors in humans.[129,130] **Sodium benzoate** is a food preservative that can cause asthma[131] and skin rashes[132] in sensitive individuals. **Tartrazine (yellow dye #5)** is a food/drug coloring agent that can cause asthma and skin rashes in sensitive individuals.[133] **Carrageenan** is a naturally-occurring carbohydrate extracted from red seaweed. Common sources of carrageenan are certain brands of "rice milk" and "soy milk." In addition to suppressing immune function[134], carrageenan causes intestinal ulcers and inflammatory bowel disease in animals[135] and some research indicates that carrageenan consumption is associated with an increased risk for cancer in humans.[136,137]

Consume sufficient daily water in the form of water and health-promoting teas and juices: Daily "water" intake should be approximately 30 ml/kg; thus, for a 150-lb (70-kg) person, fluid intake should be at least 2.1 liters, and for a person who weighs 220 lbs (100 kg) the daily intake should be approximately 3 liters. More fluids may be used during times of exercise, heat exposure, illness, or detoxification, while fluid restriction can be indicated in patients with heart failure, renal failure, anasarca (generalized edema), and hyponatremia.

Consider reducing or eliminating caffeine: This is especially important for people with reactive hypoglycemia, insomnia, anxiety, hypertension, low-back pain, and for women with fibrocystic breast disease. Caffeine ingestion also leads to the activation of brain noradrenergic receptors, which can cause inhibition of dopaminergic pathways.[138] For people who are in good health, 1-3 servings of caffeine per day are not harmful. Herbal teas and green tea appear to have significant health-promoting effects due to their phytonutrient components and antioxidant, anti-inflammatory, and anticancer properties.

To the extent possible, eat "organic" foods rather than industrially-produced foods: Organic foods (i.e., foods which are *naturally grown* rather than being treated with insect poisons, synthetic fertilizers, and chemicals to enhance shelf-life) tend to cost more than chemically-produced foods; but the increased phytonutrient content justifies the cost. Organic foods contain more nutrients than do chemically-produced foods.[139] More importantly, recent research has also indicated that organic foods are better able to prevent the genetic damage that can lead to cancer than are foods that have been grown in an environment of artificial fertilizers and pesticides.[140]

---

[127] "Our results suggest that high-carbohydrate meals have an influence on serotonin synthesis. We predict that carbohydrates with a high glycemic index would have a greater serotoninergic effect than carbohydrates with a low glycemic index." Lyons PM, Truswell AS. Serotonin precursor influenced by type of carbohydrate meal in healthy adults. *Am J Clin Nutr*. 1988 Mar;47(3):433-9

[128] Trocho C, Pardo R, Rafecas I, et al. Formaldehyde derived from dietary aspartame binds to tissue components in vivo. *Life Sci*. 1998;63(5):337-4949

[129] Compared to other environmental factors putatively linked to brain tumors, the artificial sweetener aspartame is a promising candidate to explain the recent increase in incidence and degree of malignancy of brain tumors. ...exceedingly high incidence of brain tumors in aspartame-fed rats compared to no brain tumors in concurrent controls..." Olney JW, Farber NB, Spitznagel E, Robins LN. Increasing brain tumor rates: is there a link to aspartame? *J Neuropathol Exp Neurol* 1996;55(11):1115-23

[130] Russell Blaylock MD. Excitotoxins. Health Press; December 1996 [ISBN: 0929173252] Pages 211-214

[131] "Adverse reactions to benzoate in this patient required avoidance of some drugs, some of those classically prescribed under the form of syrups in asthma." Petrus M, Bonaz S, Causse E, Rhabbour M, Moulie N, Netter JC, Bildstein G. [Asthma and intolerance to benzoates] [Article in French] *Arch Pediatr*. 1996;3(10):984-7

[132] Munoz FJ, et al. Perioral contact urticaria from sodium benzoate in a toothpaste. *Contact Dermatitis*. 1996 Jul;35(1):51

[133] "Tartrazine sensitivity is most frequently manifested by urticaria and asthma... Vasculitis, purpura and contact dermatitis infrequently occur as manifestations of tartrazine sensitivity." Dipalma JR. Tartrazine sensitivity. *Am Fam Physician*. 1990 Nov;42(5):1347-50

[134] "Impairment of complement activity and humoral responses to T-dependent antigens, depression of cell-mediated immunity, prolongation of graft survival and potentiation of tumour growth by carrageenans have been reported." Thomson AW, Fowler EF. Carrageenan: a review of its effects on the immune system. *Agents Actions*. 1981;11(3):265-73

[135] Watt J, Marcus R. Experimental ulcerative disease of the colon. *Methods Achiev Exp Pathol*. 1975;7:56-71

[136] Tobacman JK. Review of harmful gastrointestinal effects of carrageenan in animal experiments. *Environ Health Perspect*. 2001 Oct;109(10):983-94

[137] "However, the gum carrageenan which is comprised of linked, sulfated galactose residues has potent biological activity and undergoes acid hydrolysis to poligeenan, an acknowledged carcinogen." Tobacman JK, Wallace RB, Zimmerman MB. Consumption of carrageenan and other water-soluble polymers used as food additives and incidence of mammary carcinoma. *Med Hypotheses*. 2001 May;56(5):589-98

[138] "The results suggest that noradrenergic innervation of dopamine cells can directly inhibit the activity of dopamine cells." Paladini CA, Williams JT. Noradrenergic inhibition of midbrain dopamine neurons. *J Neurosci*. 2004 May 12;24(19):4568-75

[139] Smith B. Organic Foods versus Supermarket Foods: element levels. *Journal of Applied Nutrition* 1993; 45(1), p35-9

[140] "Against BaP, three species of OC vegetables showed 30-57% antimutagenecity, while GC ones did only 5-30%." Ren H, Endo H, Hayashi T. The superiority of organically cultivated vegetables to general ones regarding antimutagenic activities. *Mutat Res*. 2001 Sep 20;496(1-2):83-8

Recognize the importance of avoiding food allergens: Biomedical research has established that adverse food reactions, regardless of the underlying mechanisms or classification of allergy, intolerance, or sensitivity, can exacerbate a wide range of human illnesses, including thyroid disease[141], mental depression[142,143], asthma, rhinitis,[144] recurrent otitis media[145], migraine[146,147,148], attention deficit and hyperactivity disorders[149], epilepsy[150,151,152], gastrointestinal inflammation[153], hypertension[154], joint pain and inflammation[155,156,157,158,159,160,161,162] and a wide range of other health problems. Any program of health promotion and health maintenance must include consideration of food allergies, food intolerances, and food sensitivities. The elimination-and-challenge technique is the most cost-effective and it also teaches patients how to identify their own food allergies and intolerances, which may change for the better or worse over time; when the patient is empowered with this technique, he/she can take an active and on-going role in his/her own healthcare. Patients may be allergic to foods that are generally considered healthy, including whole organic foods. The more common food allergens—exemplified here by a list of offending foods identified in a study of patients with migraine[163]—are wheat (78%), orange (65%), eggs (45%), tea and coffee (40% each), chocolate and milk (37% each), beef (35%), and corn, cane sugar, and yeast (33% each).

Supplement the health-promoting whole-foods diet with specific vitamins, minerals, fatty acids, and probiotics: Despite the fact that America is one of the richest nations on earth, and that we produce more than enough food to feed ourselves and many other nations with a healthy diet, Americans tend to have poor dietary habits and inadequate levels of nutritional intake that do not meet the minimal standards, such as the Recommended Daily Allowance (RDA, now Daily Reference Intake (DRI)).[164] Many people are under the misperception that if they appear healthy or are even overweight then they could not possibly have nutritional deficiencies. The truths of this matter are that 1) gross/obvious nutritional deficiencies are common among "apparently healthy" individuals, 2) common situations like stress, poor diets, and use of medications predispose people to nutritional deficiencies, 3) hereditary/genetic disorders affect a large portion of the population and lead to an increased need for nutritional intake which can generally only be met with supplementation in addition to a healthy whole-foods diet. Taking a "one-a-day" multivitamin is insufficient for people who truly desire significant benefit from supplementation. These one-a-day preparations generally only provide the minimum daily allowance—this dose is not large enough to provide truly preventive medicine results; also, such one-a-day products tend to contain low-quality nutrients,

[141] Sategna-Guidetti C, Volta U, Ciacci C, Usai P, Carlino A, De Franceschi L, Camera A, Pelli A, Brossa C. Prevalence of thyroid disorders in untreated adult celiac disease patients and effect of gluten withdrawal: an Italian multicenter study. *Am J Gastroenterol.* 2001 Mar;96(3):751-7

[142] "The detection and treatment of psychological dysfunction related to food intolerance with particular reference to the problem of objective evaluation is discussed… Long-term follow-up revealed maintenance of marked improvements in psychological and physical functioning." Mills N. Depression and food intolerance: a single case study. *Hum Nutr Appl Nutr.* 1986 Apr;40(2):141-5

[143] "OBJECTIVE: To describe a patient with food intolerance probably contributing to depressive symptoms, intolerance to psychotropic medication and treatment resistance… RESULTS: The patient's course improved considerably with an elimination diet." Parker G, Watkins T. Treatment-resistant depression: when antidepressant drug intolerance may indicate food intolerance. *Aust N Z J Psychiatry.* 2002 Apr;36(2):263-5

[144] Speer F. The allergic child. *Am Fam Physician.* 1975 Feb;11(2):88-94

[145] Juntti H, Tikkanen S, Kokkonen J, Alho OP, Niinimaki A. Cow's milk allergy is associated with recurrent otitis media during childhood. *Acta Otolaryngol.* 1999;119(8):867-73

[146] "Foods which provoked migraine in 9 patients with severe migraine refractory to drug therapy were identified… These observations confirm that a food-allergic reaction is the cause of migraine in this group of patients." Monro J, Carini C, Brostoff J. Migraine is a food-allergic disease. *Lancet.* 1984 Sep 29;2(8405):719-21

[147] Egger J, Carter CM, Wilson J, et al. Is migraine food allergy? A double-blind controlled trial of oligoantigenic diet treatment. *Lancet.* 1983 Oct 15;2(8355):865-9

[148] Monro J, Brostoff J, Carini C, Zilkha K. Food allergy in migraine. Study of dietary exclusion and RAST. *Lancet.* 1980 Jul 5;2(8184):1-4

[149] Boris M, Mandel FS. Foods and additives are common causes of the attention deficit hyperactive disorder in children. *Ann Allergy.* 1994 May;72(5):462-8

[150] Egger J, Carter CM, Soothill JF, Wilson J. Oligoantigenic diet treatment of children with epilepsy and migraine. *J Pediatr.* 1989;114(1):51-8

[151] Pelliccia A, Lucarelli S, Frediani T, D'Ambrini G, Cerminara C, Barbato M, Vagnucci B, Cardi E. Partial cryptogenetic epilepsy and food allergy/intolerance. A causal or a chance relationship? Reflections on three clinical cases. *Minerva Pediatr.* 1999 May;51(5):153-7

[152] Frediani T, Lucarelli S, Pelliccia A, Vagnucci B, et al. Allergy and childhood epilepsy: a close relationship? *Acta Neurol Scand.* 2001;104(6):349-52

[153] Marr HY, Chen WC, Lin LH. Food protein-induced enterocolitis syndrome: report of one case. *Acta Paediatr Taiwan.* 2001;42(1):49-52

[154] Grant EC. Food allergies and migraine. *Lancet.* 1979 May 5;1(8123):966-9

[155] "Food allergy appeared to be responsible for the joint symptoms in three patients and in one it was possible to precipitate swelling of a knee due to synovitis with effusion by drinking milk a few hours beforehand, the synovial fluid having mildly inflammatory features and a relatively high eosinophil count." Golding DN. Is there an allergic synovitis? *J R Soc Med.* 1990 May;83(5):312-4

[156] Panush RS. Food induced ("allergic") arthritis: clinical and serologic studies. *J Rheumatol.* 1990 Mar;17(3):291-4

[157] Pacor ML, Lunardi C, Di Lorenzo G, Biasi D, Corrocher R. Food allergy and seronegative arthritis: report of two cases. *Clin Rheumatol.* 2001;20(4):279-81

[158] Schrander JJ, Marcelis C, de Vries MP, van Santen-Hoeufft HM. Does food intolerance play a role in juvenile chronic arthritis? *Br J Rheumatol.* 1997 Aug;36(8):905-8

[159] van de Laar MA, van der Korst JK. Food intolerance in rheumatoid arthritis. I. A double blind, controlled trial of the clinical effects of elimination of milk allergens and azo dyes. *Ann Rheum Dis.* 1992 Mar;51(3):298-302

[160] Haugen MA, Kjeldsen-Kragh J, Forre O. A pilot study of the effect of an elemental diet in the management of rheumatoid arthritis. *Clin Exp Rheumatol.* 1994;12(3):275-9

[161] van de Laar MA, Aalbers M, Bruins FG, et al. Food intolerance in rheumatoid arthritis. II. Clinical and histological aspects. *Ann Rheum Dis.* 1992;51(3):303-6

[162] Panush RS, Stroud RM, Webster EM. Food-induced (allergic) arthritis. Inflammatory arthritis exacerbated by milk. *Arthritis Rheum* 1986; 29(2): 220-6

[163] Grant EC. Food allergies and migraine. *Lancet.* 1979 May 5;1(8123):966-9

[164] "Most people do not consume an optimal amount of all vitamins by diet alone. Pending strong evidence of effectiveness from randomized trials, it appears prudent for all adults to take vitamin supplements." Fletcher RH, Fairfield KM. Vitamins for chronic disease prevention in adults: clinical applications. *JAMA* 2002 Jun 19;287(23):3127-9

such as ergocalciferol rather than cholecalciferol[165], cyanocobalamin rather than the hydroxyl-, methyl-, or adenosyl- forms[166], and DL-tocopherol or exclusively L-alpha-tocopherol rather than a mix of tocopherols with a high concentration (generally approximately 40%) of gamma tocopherol.[167]

For people still not convinced of the importance of a multi-vitamin/mineral supplement as part of the basic foundation of the health plan, please consider the following data from the medical research:

- Many people think that eating a "healthy diet" will supply them with the nutrients that they need and that they do not need to take a vitamin supplement. This may have been true 2000 years ago, but today's industrially produced "foods" are generally stripped of much of their nutritional value long before they leave the factory. Industrially-produced fruits and vegetables contain lower quantities of nutrients than does naturally raised "organic" produce. [168]

- The reason that people can be of normal weight or can even be overweight and obese and still have nutrient deficiencies is that the body lowers the metabolic rate when the intake of vitamins and minerals is low. This is referred to as the "physiologic adaptation to marginal malnutrition." Even though people may eat enough calories and protein, they can still suffer from growth retardation and behavioral problems as a result of micronutrient malnutrition, even though they *appear* nourished.[169]

- Most nutrition-oriented doctors will agree that magnesium is one of the most important nutrients, especially for helping prevent heart attack and stroke. **Magnesium deficiency is an epidemic in so-called "developed" nations, with 20-40% of different populations showing objective laboratory evidence of magnesium deficiency**.[170,171,172,173]

- Add to the above that every day we are confronted with more chronic emotional stress and toxic chemicals than has ever before existed on the planet, and it becomes easy to see that basic nutritional support and an organic whole foods diet is just the start of attaining improved health.

General Guidelines for the Safe Use of Nutritional Supplements: Supplementation with vitamins and minerals is generally safe, especially if the following guidelines are followed:

- <u>Vitamins and minerals should generally be taken with food in order to eliminate the possibility of nausea and to increase absorption</u>: Most vitamins and other supplements should be taken with food so that nausea is avoided.

- <u>Iron is potentially harmful</u>: Iron promotes the formation of reactive oxygen species ("free radicals") and is thus implicated in several diseases, such as infections, cancer, liver disease, diabetes, and cardiovascular disease. Iron supplements should not be consumed except by people who have been definitively diagnosed with iron deficiency by measurement of serum ferritin. Iron supplementation without documentation of iron deficiency by measurement of serum ferritin is inappropriate. [174]

- <u>Vitamin A is one of the only vitamins with the potential for serious toxicity even at low doses</u>: Attention should be given to vitamin A intake so that toxicity is avoided. Total intake of vitamin A must account for all sources—foods, fish oils, and vitamin supplements. Manifestations of vitamin A toxicity include: skin problems (dry skin, flaking skin, chapped or split lips, red skin rash, hair loss), joint pain, bone pain,

[165] "Vitamin D(2) potency is less than one third that of vitamin D(3). Physicians resorting to use of vitamin D(2) should be aware of its markedly lower potency and shorter duration of action relative to vitamin D(3)." Armas LA, Hollis BW, Heaney RP. Vitamin D2 is much less effective than vitamin D3 in humans. *J Clin Endocrinol Metab.* 2004 Nov;89(11):5387-91

[166] Freeman AG. Cyanocobalamin--a case for withdrawal: discussion paper. *J R Soc Med.* 1992 Nov;85(11):686–687
http://www.ncbi.nlm.nih.gov/pmc/articles/PMC1293728/pdf/jrsocmed00105-0046.pdf

[167] "gamma-tocopherol is the major form of vitamin E in many plant seeds and in the US diet, but has drawn little attention compared with alpha-tocopherol, the predominant form of vitamin E in tissues and the primary form in supplements. However, recent studies indicate that gamma-tocopherol may be important to human health and that it possesses unique features that distinguish it from alpha-tocopherol." Jiang Q, Christen S, Shigenaga MK, Ames BN. gamma-tocopherol, the major form of vitamin E in the US diet, deserves more attention. *Am J Clin Nutr.* 2001 Dec;74(6):714-22 http://www.ajcn.org/content/74/6/714.full.pdf

[168] Smith B. Organic Foods versus Supermarket Foods: element levels. *Journal of Applied Nutrition* 1993; 45(1), p35-9. I recently found that this article is also available on-line at http://journeytoforever.org/farm_library/bobsmith.html as of June 19, 2004

[169] Allen LH. The nutrition CRSP: what is marginal malnutrition, and does it affect human function? *Nutr Rev* 1993 Sep;51(9):255-67

[170] "The American diet is low in magnesium, and with modern water systems, very little is ingested in the drinking water." Innerarity S. Hypomagnesemia in acute and chronic illness. *Crit Care Nurs Q.* 2000 Aug;23(2):1-19

[171] "Altogether 43% of 113 trauma patients had low magnesium levels compared to 30% of noninjured cohorts." Frankel H, Haskell R, Lee SY, Miller D, Rotondo M, Schwab CW. Hypomagnesemia in trauma patients. *World J Surg.* 1999 Sep;23(9):966-9

[172] "There was a 20% overall prevalence of hypomagnesemia among this predominantly female, African American population." Fox CH, Ramsoomair D, Mahoney MC, Carter C, Young B, Graham R. An investigation of hypomagnesemia among ambulatory urban African Americans. *J Fam Pract.* 1999 Aug;48(8):636-9

[173] "Suboptimal levels were detected in 33.7 per cent of the population under study. These data clearly demonstrate that the Mg supply of the German population needs increased attention." Schimatschek HF, Rempis R. Prevalence of hypomagnesemia in an unselected German population of 16,000 individuals. *Magnes Res.* 2001 Dec;14(4):283-90

[174] Hollán S, Johansen KS. Adequate iron stores and the 'Nil nocere' principle.*Haematologia* (Budap). 1993;25(2):69-84

headaches, anorexia (loss of appetite), edema (water retention, weight gain, swollen ankles, difficulty breathing), fatigue, and/or liver damage. Whenever vitamin A is used in high doses, it must be used for a defined period of time in order to avoid the toxicity that will result from high-dose long-term vitamin A supplementation.

- o Adults: Women who are pregnant or might become pregnant and who are planning to carry the baby to full term delivery should not ingest more than 10,000 IU of vitamin A per day. Vitamin A toxicity is seen with chronic ingestion of therapeutic doses (for example: 25,000 IU per day for 6 years, or 100,000 IU per day for 2.5 years[175]). Most patients should not consume more than 25,000 IU of vitamin A per day for more than 2 months without express supervision by a healthcare provider. Vitamin A is present in some multivitamins, in animal liver and products such as fish liver oil, and in other supplements—read labels to ensure that the total daily intake is not greater than 25,000 IU per day.

- o Infants and Children: Different studies have used either daily or monthly schedules of vitamin A supplementation. In a study with extremely low-birth weight infants, 5,000 IU of vitamin A per day for 28 days was safely used.[176] In another study conducted in sick children, those aged less than 12 months received 100,000 IU on two consecutive days, while children between ages 12-60 months received a larger dose of 200,000 IU on two consecutive days.[177]

- Preexisting kidney problems (such as renal insufficiency) increase the risks associated with nutritional supplementation: Supplementation with vitamins and minerals does not cause kidney damage. However, if a patient already has kidney problems, then nutritional supplementation may become hazardous; this is particularly true with magnesium and potassium and perhaps also with vitamin C. Assessment of renal function with serum or urine tests is encouraged before beginning an aggressive plan of supplementation. Conditions which cause kidney damage include use of specific drugs (e.g., acetaminophen, aspirin, contrast and chemotherapy agents, cocaine), acute or chronic high blood pressure, diabetes mellitus and other diseases such as lupus (SLE), polycystic kidney disease, and scleroderma.

- Pre-existing medical conditions may make supplementation unsafe: A few rare medical conditions may cause nutritional supplementation to be unsafe, including severe liver disease, renal failure, electrolyte imbalances, hyperparathyroidism and other vitamin D hypersensitivity syndromes.

- Several drugs/medications may adversely interact with vitamin/mineral supplements and with botanical medicines: Vitamins/minerals may reduce the effectiveness of some prescription medications. For example, taking certain antibiotics such as ciprofloxacin or tetracycline with calcium reduces absorption of the drugs, therefore rendering the drugs much less effective. Taking botanical medicines with medications may make the drugs dangerously less effective (such as when St. John's Wort is combined with protease inhibitor drugs[178]) or may make the drug dangerously more effective (such when Kava is combined with the anti-anxiety drug alprazolam[179]). If vitamin D is used in doses greater than 1,000 IU/d in patients taking hydrochlorothiazide or other calcium-retaining drugs, serum calcium should be monitored at least monthly until safety (i.e., lack of hypercalcemia) has been established per patient.[180] Patients should not combine nutritional or botanical medicines with chemical/synthetic drugs without specific advice from a knowledgeable doctor. Do not increase vitamin K consumption from supplements or dietary improvements in patients taking coumadin/warfarin. A reasonable recommendation is that nutritional supplements be taken 2 hours away from pharmaceutical medications to avoid complications such as intraintestinal drug-nutrient binding.

---

[175] "The smallest continuous daily consumption leading to cirrhosis was 25,000 IU during 6 years, whereas higher daily doses (greater than or equal to 100,000 IU) taken during 2 1/2 years resulted in similar histological lesions. ... The data also indicate that prolonged and continuous consumption of doses in the low "therapeutic" range can result in life-threatening liver damage." Geubel AP, De Galocsy C, Alves N, Rahier J, Dive C. Liver damage caused by therapeutic vitamin A administration: estimate of dose-related toxicity in 41 cases. *Gastroenterology.* 1991 Jun;100(6):1701-9

[176] "Infants with birth weight < 1000 g were randomised at birth to receive oral vitamin A supplementation (5000 IU/day) or placebo for 28 days." Wardle SP, Hughes A, Chen S, Shaw NJ. Randomised controlled trial of oral vitamin A supplementation in preterm infants to prevent chronic lung disease. *Arch Dis Child Fetal Neonatal Ed* 2001 Jan;84:F9-F13

[177] "Children were assigned to oral doses of 200 000 IU vitamin A (half that dose if <12 months) or placebo on the day of admission, a second dose on the following day, and third and fourth doses at 4 and 8 months after discharge from the hospital, respectively." Villamor E, Mbise R, Spiegelman D, Hertzmark E, Fataki M, Peterson KE, Ndossi G, Fawzi WW. Vitamin A supplements ameliorate the adverse effect of HIV-1, malaria, and diarrheal infections on child growth. *Pediatrics.* 2002 Jan;109(1):E6

[178] Piscitelli SC, Burstein AH, Chaitt D, Alfaro RM, Falloon J. Indinavir concentrations and St John's wort. *Lancet.* 2000 Feb 12;355(9203):547-8

[179] Almeida JC, Grimsley EW. Coma from the health food store: interaction between kava and alprazolam. *Ann Intern Med.* 1996 Dec 1;125(11):940-1

[180] **Vasquez A** et al.. The clinical importance of vitamin D (cholecalciferol): a paradigm shift with implications for all healthcare providers. *Altern Ther Health Med.* 2004 Sep-Oct

Advanced concepts in nutrition—an introduction

Biochemical Individuality and Orthomolecular Medicine:

"Biochemical individuality" was the term coined by biochemist Dr. Roger Williams of the University of Texas[181] to describe the genetic and physiologic variations in human beings that produced different nutritional needs among individuals. Because we all have different genes, each of our bodies therefore creates different protein enzymes, and many of these enzymes—which are essential for proper cellular function—are adversely affected by defects in their construction (i.e., amino acid sequence) that reduce their efficiency. Dr. Linus Pauling[182] noted that single amino acid substitutions could produce dramatic alterations in protein function. Pauling discovered that sickle cell disease was caused by a single amino acid substitution in the hemoglobin molecule, and for this discovery he won the Nobel Prize in Chemistry in 1954.[183] With recognition of the importance of individual molecules in determining health or disease, Pauling coined the phrase "orthomolecular medicine" based on his thesis that many diseases could be effectively prevented and treated if we used the "right molecules" to correct abnormal

Orthomolecular precepts

- The functions of the body are dependent upon thousands of enzymes. Because of genetic defects that are common in the general population, some of these enzymes are commonly defective – even if only slightly – in large portions of the human population.
- Enzyme defects reduce the function and efficiency of important chemical reactions. Because enzymes are so important for normal function and the prevention of disease, defects in enzyme function can result in disruptions in physiology and the creation of what later manifests as "disease."
- Rather than treating these diseases with synthetic chemical drugs, it is commonly possible to prevent and treat disease with high-doses of vitamins, minerals, and other nutrients to compensate for or bypass metabolic dysfunctions, thus allowing for the promotion of optimal health by promoting optimal physiologic function.

Exemplary review: Ames BN, et al. High-dose vitamin therapy stimulates variant enzymes with decreased coenzyme binding affinity. _Am J Clin Nutr._ 2002 Apr

physiologic function. Pauling contrasted the clinical use of nutrients for the improvement of physiologic function (orthomolecular medicine) with the use of chemical drugs, which generally work by interfering with normal physiology (toximolecular medicine). Since nutrients are the fundamental elements of the human body from which all enzymes, chemicals, and cellular structures are formed, Pauling advocated that the use of customized nutrition and nutritional supplements could promote optimal health by optimizing cellular function and efficiency. More recently, Dr. Bruce Ames has thoroughly documented the science of the orthomolecular precepts[184] and has advocated optimal diets along with nutritional supplementation as a highly efficient and cost-effective method for preventing disease and optimizing health.[185,186] In sum, we see that 1) the foundational diet must be formed from whole foods such as fruits, nuts, seeds, vegetables, and lean meats, 2) processed and artificial foods should be avoided, and 3) the use of nutritional supplements is necessary to provide sufficiently high levels of nutrition to overcome defects in enzymatic activity.

Molecular rationale for high-dose nutrient supplementation

"As many as **one-third of mutations** in a gene result in the corresponding enzyme having an increased Michaelis constant, or Km, (decreased binding affinity) for a coenzyme, resulting in a lower rate of reaction. **About 50 human genetic dis-eases due to defective enzymes can be remedied or ameliorated by the administration of high doses of the vitamin component of the corresponding coenzyme**, which at least partially restores enzymatic activity." …
"**High doses of vitamins are used to treat many inheritable human diseases**. The molecular basis of disease arising from as many as one-third of the mutations in a gene is an increased Michaelis constant, or Km, (decreased binding affinity) of an enzyme for the vitamin-derived coenzyme or substrate, which in turn lowers the rate of the reaction."
Ames BN, Elson-Schwab I, Silver EA. _Am J Clin Nutr._ 2002 Apr ajcn.org/cgi/content/full/75/4/616

---

[181] "Every individual organism that has a distinctive genetic background has distinctive nutritional needs which must be met for optimal well-being. …[N]utrition applied with due concern for individual genetic variations…offers the solution to many baffling health problems." Williams RJ. Biochemical Individuality : The Basis for the Genetotrophic Concept. Austin and London: University of Texas Press, 1956. Page x

[182] "…the concentration of coenzyme [vitamins and minerals] needed to produce the amount of active enzyme required for optimum health may well be somewhat different for different individuals. …many individuals may require a considerably higher concentration of one or more coenzymes than other people do for optimum health…" Pauling L. On the Orthomolecular Environment of the Mind: Orthomolecular Theory. In: Williams RJ, Kalita DK. A Physician's Handbook on Orthomolecular Medicine. New Cannan; Keats Publishing: 1977. Page 76

[183] http://www.nobel.se/chemistry/laureates/1954/pauling-bio.html on April 4, 2004

[184] "About 50 human genetic dis-eases due to defective enzymes can be remedied or ameliorated by the administration of high doses of the vitamin component of the corresponding coenzyme, which at least partially restores enzymatic activity." Ames BN, Elson-Schwab I, Silver EA. High-dose vitamin therapy stimulates variant enzymes with decreased coenzyme binding affinity (increased K(m)): relevance to genetic disease and polymorphisms. _Am J Clin Nutr._ 2002 Apr;75(4):616-58

[185] "An optimum intake of micronutrients and metabolites, which varies with age and genetic constitution, would tune up metabolism and give a marked increase in health, particularly for the poor and elderly, at little cost." Ames BN. The metabolic tune-up: metabolic harmony and disease prevention. _J Nutr._ 2003 May;133(5 Suppl 1):1544S-8S

[186] "Optimizing micronutrient intake [through better diets, fortification of foods, or multivitamin-mineral pills] can have a major impact on public health at low cost." Ames BN. Cancer prevention and diet: help from single nucleotide polymorphisms. _Proc Natl Acad Sci U S A._ 1999 Oct 26;96(22):12216-8

Nutrigenomics—Nutritional Genomics:

"Genome" refers to all of the genetic material in an organism, and "genomics" is the field of study of this information. The field of nutritional genomics—nutrigenomics—refers to the clinical synthesis of 1) research on the human genome (e.g., the Human Genome Project[187]), and 2) the advancing science of clinical nutrition, including research on nutraceuticals (nutritional medicines) and phytomedicinals (botanical medicines). Nutrigenomics represents a major advance in our understanding of the underlying biochemical and physiologic mechanisms of the effects of nutrition.

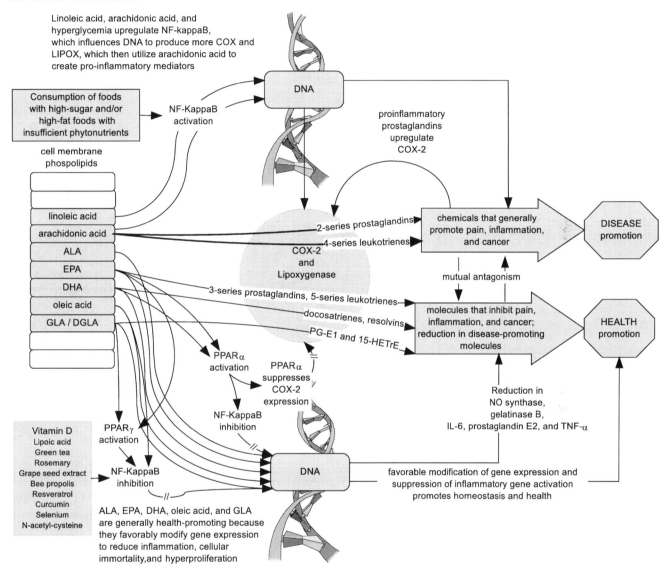

Nutrigenomics—a conceptual diagram: Nutrients influence gene transcription as well as post-translational metabolism.

Nutrition is far more than "fuel" for our biophysiologic machine; we know now that nutrition—the consumption of specific proteins, amino acids, vitamins, minerals, fatty acids, and phytochemicals—can alter genetic expression and can thus either promote health or disease at the very fundamental level of genetic expression. The commonly employed excuse that many patients use—"I just have bad genes"—now takes on a whole new meaning; it may be that these patients suffer from the expression of "bad genes" *because of the food that they eat.*

---

[187] "Begun formally in 1990, the U.S. Human Genome Project is a 13-year effort coordinated by the U.S. Department of Energy and the National Institutes of Health. The project originally was planned to last 15 years, but rapid technological advances have accelerated the expected completion date to 2003. Project goals are to identify all the approximate 30,000 genes in human DNA..." See the official Human Genome website at http://www.ornl.gov/sci/techresources/Human_Genome/home.shtml

The concept and phenomenon of nutrigenomics can be described by saying that each of us has the genes for health, as well as the genes for disease; what largely determines our level of health is how we treat our genes with environmental inputs, especially nutrition. We appear able, to a large extent, to "turn on" disease-promoting genes with poor nutrition and a pro-inflammatory lifestyle[188,189], while, to a lesser extent, we are able to activate or "turn on" health-promoting genes with a healthy diet[190] and with proper nutritional supplementation.[191] For additional details, see the literature cited in this section and the review article by Vasquez available on-line.[192]

Putting it all together with "the supplemented Paleo-Mediterranean diet": The health-promoting diet of choice for the majority of people is a diet based on abundant consumption of fruits, vegetables, seeds, nuts, omega-3 and monounsaturated fatty acids, and lean sources of protein such as lean meats, fatty cold-water fish, soy and whey proteins. This diet prohibits and obviates overconsumption of chemical preservatives, artificial sweeteners, and carbohydrate-dominant foods such as candies, pastries, breads, potatoes, grains, and other foods with a high glycemic load and high glycemic index. This "Paleo-Mediterranean Diet" is a combination of the "Paleolithic" or "Paleo diet" and the well-known "Mediterranean diet", both of which are well described in peer-reviewed journals and the lay press. The Mediterranean diet is characterized by increased proportions of legumes, nuts, seeds, whole grain products, fruits, vegetables (including potatoes), fish and lean meats, and monounsaturated and n-3 fatty acids.[193] Consumption of the Mediterranean diet is associated with improvements in insulin sensitivity and reductions in cardiovascular disease, diabetes, cancer, and all-cause mortality when contrasted to the effects of *ad libitum* eating, particularly in the standard American diet (SAD) eating pattern.[194] The Paleolithic diet detailed by collaborators Eaton[195], O'Keefe[196], and Cordain[197] is similar to the Mediterranean diet except for stronger emphasis on fruits and vegetables (preferably raw or minimally cooked), omega-3-rich lean meats, and reduced consumption of starchy foods such as potatoes and grains, the latter of which were not staples in the human diet until the last few thousand years. Emphasizing the olive oil and red wine of the Mediterranean diet and the absence of grains and potatoes per the Paleo diet appears to be the way to get the best of both dietary worlds; the remaining diet is characterized by fresh whole fruits, vegetables, nuts (especially almonds), seeds, berries, olive oil, lean meats rich in n-3 fatty acids, and red wine in moderation. In sum, this dietary plan along with the inclusion of garlic and dark chocolate (a rich source of cardioprotective, antioxidative, antihypertensive, and anti-inflammatory polyphenolic flavonoids[198,199]) is expected to reduce adverse cardiovascular events by more than 76%.[200] Biochemical justification for this type of diet is ample and is well supported by numerous long-term studies in humans wherein both Mediterranean and Paleolithic diets result in statistically significant and clinically meaningful reductions in disease-specific and all-cause mortality.[201,202,203,204] Diets rich in fruits and vegetables are sources of more than 8,000 phytochemicals, many of which have antioxidant, anti-inflammatory, and anti-cancer properties.[205] Oleic acid, squalene, and phenolics in olive oil and phenolics and resveratrol in red wine have antioxidant, anti-inflammatory,

[188] Rusyn I, Bradham CA, Cohn L, Schoonhoven R, Swenberg JA, Brenner DA, Thurman RG. Corn oil rapidly activates nuclear factor-kappaB in hepatic Kupffer cells by oxidant-dependent mechanisms. *Carcinogenesis*. 1999 Nov;20(11):2095-100 http://carcin.oxfordjournals.org/cgi/content/full/20/11/2095

[189] Aljada A, Mohanty P, Ghanim H, Abdo T, Tripathy D, Chaudhuri A, Dandona P. Increase in intranuclear nuclear factor kappaB and decrease in inhibitor kappaB in mononuclear cells after a mixed meal: evidence for a proinflammatory effect. *Am J Clin Nutr*. 2004 Apr;79(4):682-90

[190] OKeefe JH Jr,Cordain L.Cardiovascular disease resulting from a diet and lifestyle at odds with our Paleolithic genome.*Mayo Clin Proc*.2004;79:101-8

[191] Kaput J, Rodriguez LR. Nutritional genomics: the next frontier in the postgenomic era. *Physiol Genomics* 16: 166–177

[192] **Vasquez A**. Reducing pain and inflammation naturally - Part 4: Nutritional and Botanical Inhibition of NF-kappaB, the Major Intracellular Amplifier of the Inflammatory Cascade.A Clinical Strategy Exemplifying Anti-Inflammatory Nutrigenomics.*Nutr Perspec* 2005;Jul:5-12

[193] Curtis BM, O'Keefe JH Jr. Understanding the Mediterranean diet. Could this be the new "gold standard" for heart disease prevention? *Postgrad Med*. 2002 Aug;112(2):35-8, 41-5 http://www.postgradmed.com/issues/2002/08_02/curtis.htm

[194] Knoops KT, de Groot LC, Kromhout D, Perrin AE, Moreiras-Varela O, Menotti A, van Staveren WA. Mediterranean diet, lifestyle factors, and 10-year mortality in elderly European men and women: the HALE project. *JAMA*. 2004 Sep 22;292(12):1433-9

[195] Eaton SB, Shostak M, Konner M. *The Paleolithic Prescription: A program of diet & exercise and a design for living*, New York: Harper & Row, 1988

[196] O'Keefe JH Jr, Cordain L. Cardiovascular disease resulting from a diet and lifestyle at odds with our Paleolithic genome: how to become a 21st-century hunter-gatherer. *Mayo Clin Proc*. 2004 Jan;79(1):101-8

[197] Cordain L. *The Paleo Diet*. Indianapolis; John Wiley and Sons, 2002

[198] Schramm DD, Wang JF, Holt RR, Ensunsa JL, Gonsalves JL, Lazarus SA, Schmitz HH, German JB, Keen CL. Chocolate procyanidins decrease the leukotriene-prostacyclin ratio in humans and human aortic endothelial cells. *Am J Clin Nutr*. 2001;73(1):36-40

[199] Engler MB, Engler MM, Chen CY, et al. Flavonoid-rich dark chocolate improves endothelial function and increases plasma epicatechin concentrations in healthy adults. *J Am Coll Nutr*. 2004;23(3):197-204

[200] Franco OH, Bonneux L, de Laet C, Peeters A, Steyerberg EW, Mackenbach JP. The Polymeal: a more natural, safer, and probably tastier (than the Polypill) strategy to reduce cardiovascular disease by more than 75%. *BMJ*. 2004;329(7480):1447-50

[201] de Lorgeril et al. Mediterranean dietary pattern in a randomized trial: prolonged survival and possible reduced cancer rate. *Arch Intern Med*. 1998 Jun 8;158(11):1181-7

[202] Knoops KT, de Groot LC, Kromhout D, Perrin AE, Moreiras-Varela O, Menotti A, van Staveren WA. Mediterranean diet, lifestyle factors, and 10-year mortality in elderly European men and women: the HALE project. *JAMA*. 2004 Sep 22;292(12):1433-9

[203] Lindeberg S, Cordain L, and Eaton SB. Biological and clinical potential of a Paleolithic diet. *J Nutri Environ Med* 2003; 13:149-160

[204] O'Keefe JH Jr, Cordain L, et al. Optimal low-density lipoprotein is 50 to 70 mg/dl: lower is better and physiologically normal. *J Am Coll Cardiol*. 2004 Jun 2;43(11):2142-6

[205] Liu RH. Health benefits of fruit and vegetables are from additive and synergistic combinations of phytochemicals. *Am J Clin Nutr*. 2003;78(3 Sup):517S-520S

and anti-cancer properties and also protect against cardiovascular disease.[206] N-3 fatty acids have numerous health benefits via multiple mechanisms as described in the sections that follow. Increased intake of dietary fiber from fruits and vegetable favorably modifies gut flora, promotes xenobiotic elimination (via flora modification, laxation, and overall reductions in enterohepatic recirculation), and is associated with reductions in morbidity and mortality. Such a "Paleolithic diet" can also lead to urinary alkalinization (average urine pH of ≥ 7.5 according to Sebastian et al[207]) which increases renal *retention of minerals* for improved musculoskeletal health[208,209,210] and which increases *urinary elimination of many toxicants and xenobiotics* for a tremendous reduction in serum levels and thus adverse effects from chemical exposure or drug overdose.[211] Furthermore, therapeutic alkalinization was recently shown in an open trial with 82 patients to reduce symptoms and disability associated with low-back pain and to increase intracellular magnesium concentrations by 11%.[212] **Ample intake of amino acids via dietary proteins supports phase-2 detoxification** (amino acid and sulfate conjugation) for proper xenobiotic elimination[213,214], **provides amino acid precursors for neurotransmitter synthesis** and maintenance of mood, memory, and cognitive performance[215,216,217,218], **and prevents the immunosuppression and decrements in musculoskeletal status caused by low-protein diets.**[219] Described originally by the current author[220], the "supplemented Paleo-Mediterranean diet" provides patients the best of current knowledge in nutrition by relying on a foundational diet plan of fresh fruits, vegetables, nuts, seeds, berries, fish, and lean meats which is adorned with olive oil for its squalene, phenolic antioxidant/anti-inflammatory and monounsaturated fatty acid content. Inclusive of medical foods such as red wine, garlic, and dark chocolate which may synergize to effect at least a 76% reduction in cardiovascular disease[221], this diet also reduces the risk for cancer[222] and can be an integral component of a health-promoting lifestyle.[223] Competitive athletes are allowed increased carbohydrate consumption before and after training and competition to promote glycogen storage supercompensation.[224,225,226]

---

[206] Alarcon de la Lastra C, Barranco MD, Motilva V, Herrerias JM. Mediterranean diet and health: biological importance of olive oil. *Curr Pharm Des.* 2001;7:933-50

[207] Sebastian A, Frassetto LA, Sellmeyer DE, Merriam RL, Morris RC Jr. Estimation of the net acid load of the diet of ancestral preagricultural Homo sapiens and their hominid ancestors. *Am J Clin Nutr* 2002;76:1308-16

[208] Sebastian A, Harris ST, Ottaway JH, Todd KM, Morris RC Jr. Improved mineral balance and skeletal metabolism in postmenopausal women treated with potassium bicarbonate. *N Engl J Med.* 1994;330(25):1776-81

[209] Tucker KL, Hannan MT, Chen H, Cupples LA, Wilson PW, Kiel DP. Potassium, magnesium, and fruit and vegetable intakes are associated with greater bone mineral density in elderly men and women. *Am J Clin Nutr.* 1999;69(4):727-36

[210] Whiting SJ, Boyle JL, Thompson A, Mirwald RL, Faulkner RA. Dietary protein, phosphorus and potassium are beneficial to bone mineral density in adult men consuming adequate dietary calcium. *J Am Coll Nutr.* 2002;21(5):102-9

[211] Proudfoot AT, Krenzelok EP, Vale JA. Position Paper on urine alkalinization. *J Toxicol Clin Toxicol.* 2004;42(1):1-26

[212] "The results show that a disturbed acid-base balance may contribute to the symptoms of low back pain. The simple and safe addition of an alkaline multimineral preparate was able to reduce the pain symptoms in these patients with chronic low back pain." Vormann J,Worlitschek M,Goedecke T,Silver B. Supplementation with alkaline minerals reduces symptoms in patients with chronic low back pain. *J Trace Elem Med Biol.* 2001;15:179-83

[213] Liska DJ. The detoxification enzyme systems. *Altern Med Rev.* 1998;3:187-9

[214] Anderson KE, Kappas A. Dietary regulation of cytochrome P450. *Annu Rev Nutr.* 1991;11:141-67

[215] Rogers RD, Tunbridge EM, Bhagwagar Z, Drevets WC, Sahakian BJ, Carter CS. Tryptophan depletion alters the decision-making of healthy volunteers through altered processing of reward cues. *Neuropsychopharmacology.* 2003;28:153-62 Accessed at http://www.acnp.org/sciweb/journal/Npp062402336/default.htm on November 10, 2004

[216] Arnulf I, Quintin P, Alvarez JC, Vigil L, Touitou Y, Lebre AS, Bellenger A, Varoquaux O, Derenne JP, Allilaire JF, Benkelfat C, Leboyer M. Mid-morning tryptophan depletion delays REM sleep onset in healthy subjects. *Neuropsychopharmacology.* 2002;27(5):843-51 http://www.nature.com/npp/journal/v27/n5/pdf/1395948a.pdf

[217] Thomas JR,Lockwood PA,Singh A, Deuster PA.Tyrosine improves working memory in a multitasking environment.*Pharmacol Biochem Behav.*1999;64:495-500

[218] Markus CR, Olivier B, Panhuysen GE, Van Der Gugten J, Alles MS, Tuiten A, Westenberg HG, Fekkes D, Koppeschaar HF, de Haan EE. The bovine protein alpha-lactalbumin increases the plasma ratio of tryptophan to the other large neutral amino acids, and in vulnerable subjects raises brain serotonin activity, reduces cortisol concentration, and improves mood under stress. *Am J Clin Nutr.* 2000;71:1536-44

[219] Castaneda C, et al. Elderly women accommodate to a low-protein diet with losses of body cell mass, muscle function, and immune response. *Am J Clin Nutr.* 1995;62:30-9

[220] **Vasquez A.** Five-Part Nutritional Protocol that Produces Consistently Positive Results. *Nutritional Wellness* 2005 Sept

[221] Franco OH, Bonneux L, de Laet C, Peeters A, Steyerberg EW, Mackenbach JP. The Polymeal: a more natural, safer, and probably tastier (than the Polypill) strategy to reduce cardiovascular disease by more than 75%. *BMJ.* 2004;329(7480):1447-50

[222] "The combination of 4 low risk factors lowered the all-cause mortality rate to 0.35 (95% CI, 0.28-0.44). In total, lack of adherence to this low-risk pattern was associated with a population attributable risk of 60% of all deaths, 64% of deaths from coronary heart disease, 61% from cardiovascular diseases, and 60% from cancer." Knoops KT, de Groot LC, Kromhout D, et al. Mediterranean diet, lifestyle factors, and 10-year mortality in elderly European men and women: the HALE project. *JAMA.* 2004 Sep 22;292(12):1433-9

[223] Orme-Johnson DW, Herron RE. An innovative approach to reducing medical care utilization and expenditures. *Am J Manag Care.* 1997;3(1):135-44

[224] Cordain L, Friel J. The Paleo Diet for Athletes : A Nutritional Formula for Peak Athletic Performance: Rodale Books (September 23, 2005)

[225] "A significant glycogen sparing, as well as supercompensation within 24 h of recovery, was observed after [carbohydrate] supplementation." Brouns F, Saris WH, Beckers E, Adlercreutz H, et al. Metabolic changes induced by sustained exhaustive cycling and diet manipulation. *Int J Sports Med.* 1989 May;10 Suppl 1:S49-62

[226] "The accepted method of increasing muscle glycogen stores is by "glycogen loading," which classically involves depletion of muscle glycogen, usually by exercise, followed by consumption of a high-CHO diet for several days (e.g., 3, 39). ...increase muscle glycogen concentrations ([glycogen]) to between 150 and 200% of normal resting levels." Robinson et al. Role of submaximal exercise in promoting creatine and glycogen accumulation in human skeletal muscle. *J Appl Physiol.* 1999 Aug;87(2):598-604

Profile of the Supplemented Paleo-Mediterranean Diet[227]

Foods to consume: whole, natural, minimally processed foods include:	Foods to avoid: factory products, high-sugar foods, and chemicals

☺ **Lean sources of protein**
   • Fish (avoiding tuna which is commonly loaded with mercury)
   • Chicken and turkey
   • Lean cuts of free-range grass-fed meats: beef, buffalo, lamb are occasionally acceptable
   • Soy protein[228] and whey protein[229,230]
☺ **Fruits and fruit juices**
☺ **Vegetables and vegetable juices**
☺ **Nuts, seeds, berries**
☺ **Generous use of olive oil**: On sautéed vegetables and fresh salads
☺ **Daily vitamin/mineral supplementation**: With a high-potency broad-spectrum multivitamin and multimineral supplement[231]
☺ **Sun exposure or vitamin D3 supplementation**: To ensure provision of 2,000-5,000 IU of vitamin D3 per day for adults[232]
☺ **Balanced broad-spectrum fatty acid supplementation**: With ALA, GLA, EPA, and DHA[233]
☺ **Water, tea, home-made fruit/vegetable juices**: Commercial vegetable juices are commonly loaded with sodium chloride; choose appropriately. Fruit juices can be loaded with natural and superfluous sugars. Herbal teas can be selected based on the medicinal properties of the plant that is used.
	☒ **Avoid as much as possible fat-laden arachidonate-rich meats like beef, liver, pork, and lamb, as well as high-fat cream and other dairy products with emulsified, readily absorbed saturated fats and arachidonic acid**
	☒ **High-sugar pseudofoods**:
	   • Corn syrup
	   • Cola and soda
	   • Donuts, candy, etc...."junk food"
	☒ **Grains such as wheat, rye, barley**: These have only existed in the human diet for less than 10,000 years and are consistently associated with increased prevalence of degenerative diseases due to the allergic response they invoke and because of their high glycemic load and high glycemic index.
	☒ **Potatoes and rice**: High in sugar, low in phytonutrients
	☒ **Avoid allergens**: Determined per individual
	☒ **Chemicals to avoid**:
	   • Pesticides, Herbicides, Fungicides
	   • Carcinogenic sweeteners: aspartame[234]
	   • Artificial flavors
	   • Artificial colors: tartrazine
	   • Preservatives: benzoate
	   • Flavor enhancers: carrageenan and monosodium glutamate

[227] **Vasquez A**. Five-Part Nutritional Protocol that Produces Consistently Positive Results. *Nutritional Wellness* 2005 Sept. and Vasquez A. Revisiting the Five-Part Nutritional Wellness Protocol: The Supplemented Paleo-Mediterranean Diet. *Nutritional Perspectives* 2011 January. Both of these articles are included in this textbook and/or on-line at

[228] "These results indicate that for healthy adults, the isolated soy protein is of high nutritional quality, comparable to that of animal protein sources, and that the methionine content is not limiting for adult protein maintenance." Young VR, Puig M, Queiroz E, Scrimshaw NS, Rand WM. Evaluation of the protein quality of an isolated soy protein in young men: relative nitrogen requirements and effect of methionine supplementation. *Am J Clin Nutr*. 1984 Jan;39(1):16-24

[229] Bounous G. Whey protein concentrate (WPC) and glutathione modulation in cancer treatment. *Anticancer Res*. 2000 Nov-Dec;20(6C):4785-92

[230] Markus CR, Olivier B, Panhuysen GE, Van Der Gugten J, Alles MS, Tuiten A, Westenberg HG, Fekkes D, Koppeschaar HF, de Haan EE. The bovine protein alpha-lactalbumin increases the plasma ratio of tryptophan to the other large neutral amino acids, and in vulnerable subjects raises brain serotonin activity, reduces cortisol concentration, and improves mood under stress. *Am J Clin Nutr*. 2000 Jun;71(6):1536-44 http://www.ajcn.org/cgi/content/full/71/6/1536

[231] "Most people do not consume an optimal amount of all vitamins by diet alone. ...it appears prudent for all adults to take vitamin supplements." Fletcher RH, Fairfield KM. Vitamins for chronic disease prevention in adults: clinical applications. *JAMA*. 2002;287:3127-9

[232] **Vasquez A**, MansoG, CannellJ.The clinical importance of vitamin D (cholecalciferol).*Altern Ther Health Med*.2004Sep10:28-36 www.InflammationMastery.com

[233] **Vasquez A**. New Insights into Fatty Acid Supplementation and Its Effect on Eicosanoid Production and Genetic Expression. *Nutr Perspectives* 2005; Jan: 5-16

[234] "In the past two decades brain tumor rates have risen in several industrialized countries, including the United States... Compared to other environmental factors putatively linked to brain tumors, the artificial sweetener aspartame is a promising candidate to explain the recent increase in incidence and degree of malignancy of brain tumors." Olney JW, Farber NB, Spitznagel E, Robins LN. Increasing brain tumor rates: is there a link to aspartame? *J Neuropathol Exp Neurol* 1996 Nov;55(11):1115-23

Emotional, Mental, and Social Health

Stress management and authentic living: Mental, emotional, and physical "stress" describes any unpleasant living condition which can lead to negative effects on health, such as increased blood pressure, depression, apathy, increased muscle tension, and, according to some research, increased risk of serious health problems such as early death from cardiovascular disease and cancer. Many people find that their modern lives are characterized by excess amounts of multitasking, job responsibilities, family responsibilities, commuter traffic, financial pressures in combination with an insufficient amount of relaxation, sleep, community support, exercise, time in nature, healthy nutrition, and time to simply *be* rather than *do*. Stress comes in many different forms and includes malnutrition, trauma, insufficient exercise (epidemic), excess exercise (rare), sleep deprivation, emotional turmoil, and exposure to chemicals and radiation. When most people talk about "stress" they are referring to either chronic anxiety (such as with high-pressure work situations or dysfunctional interpersonal relationships) or the acute stress reaction that is typical of unpredictable rapid-onset events such as an injury, accident, or other physically threatening situation. **These "different types of stress" are not separate from each other; rather, they are interconnected:**

- Emotional stress causes nutritional depletion[235],
- Sleep deprivation alters immune response[236],
- Chemical exposure can disrupt endocrine function.[237]

Therefore, **any type of stress can cause other types of stress**. Avoiding stressful situations is, of course, an effective way to avoid being bothered or harmed by them. If work-related stress is the problem, then finding a new position or occupation is certainly an option worth considering and implementing. High-stress jobs are often high-paying jobs; but if in the process of making money, a person ruins her health and loses years from her life, then no one would ever say, "It was worth it." **Money, success, and freedom only have value for the person alive and healthy to enjoy them.**

Toxic relationships, whether at home or work, are relationships that cause more harm than good by re-injuring old emotional wounds and by creating new emotional injuries. We can all benefit from affirming our right to a happy and healthy life by minimizing/eliminating contact with people who cause emotional harm to us—this requires conscious effort.[238] Engel[239] provides a clear articulation and description of abusive relationships, along with checklists for their recognition and exercises for their remediation. Healthy relationships are difficult to create and maintain these days, and probably a few basic components contribute to this phenomenon. ❶ With the society-wide disintegration of the extended family, most people in our society have never even seen a healthy family unit and therefore have no model and no available mentors to help them recreate a lasting family structure. ❷ Due specifically to the structure of our educational systems and (pseudo)culture of entertainment, most people have very short attention spans and are accustomed to inattention, distraction, and externally derived entertainment and gratification. ❸ Modern schools and fragmented families both fail to teach conflict resolution and relationship skills. ❹ Poor nutritional status—very common in the general population—promotes impulsivity, irritability, depression, and mood instability.

"**Good relationships make you feel loved, wanted, and cared for**."

Malcolm LL. *Health Style*. Thorsons: 2001, p 133

---

[235] Ingenbleek Y, Bernstein L. The stressful condition as a nutritionally dependent adaptive dichotomy. *Nutrition* 1999 Apr;15(4):305-20

[236] Heiser P, e. Alterations of host defense system after sleep deprivation are followed by impaired mood and psychosocial functioning. *World J Biol Psychiatry* 2001 Apr;89-94

[237] "Evidence suggests that environmental exposure to some anthropogenic chemicals may result in disruption of endocrine systems in human and wildlife populations." http://www.epa.gov/endocrine on March 7, 2004

[238] Bryn C. Collins. *How to Recognize Emotional Unavailability and Make Healthier Relationship Choices*. [Mjf Books; ISBN: 1567313442] Recently reprinted as: Emotional Unavailability: Recognizing It, Understanding It, and Avoiding Its Trap [McGraw Hill - NTC (April 1998); ISBN: 0809229145]

[239] Engel B. *The Emotionally Abusive Relationship: How to Stop Being Abused and How to Stop Abusing*. Wiley Publishers: 2003

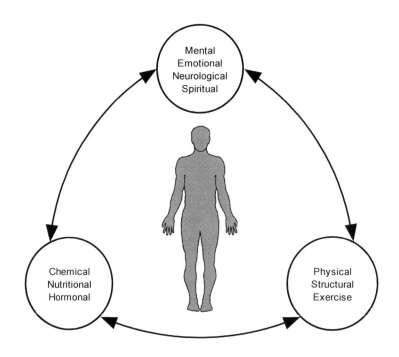

Stress affects the whole body.

Mental Emotional Neurological Spiritual

Chemical Nutritional Hormonal

Physical Structural Exercise

Therefore, a complete stress management program must address the whole body:

Physical Structural

Biochemical Hormonal Nutritional

Mental Emotional Spiritual

An important concept is that **stress is a "whole body" phenomenon**: affecting the mind, the brain, emotional state, the physical body (including musculoskeletal, immune, and cardiovascular systems), as well as the nutritional status of the individual. The adverse effects of stress can be reduced with an integrated combination of therapeutics that addresses each of the major body systems affected by stress, which are 1) mental/emotional, 2) physical, and 3) nutritional/biochemical.

Approaching stress management from a tripartite perspective

	Mental/emotional	Physical	Nutritional/biochemical
Therapeutic considerations	• Social support • Re-parenting • Conversational style[240] • Meditation, prayer • Healthy boundaries • Books, tapes, groups • Expressive writing[241] • Time to simply rest and relax	• Yoga • Massage • Exercise • Stretching • Swimming • Resting • Biking • Hiking • Affection	• Vitamins, including vitamin C[242] • Fish oil[243] • Hormones, cytokines, neurotransmitters, and eicosanoids • Tryptophan, pyridoxine • Botanical medicines such as *kava*[244], *Ashwaganda,* and *Eleutherococcus*

---

[240] Rick Brinkman ND and Rick Kirschner ND. *How to Deal With Difficult People* [Audio Cassette. Career Track, 1995]

[241] Smyth JM, Stone AA, Hurewitz A, Kaell A. Effects of writing about stressful experiences on symptom reduction in patients with asthma or rheumatoid arthritis: a randomized trial. *JAMA.* 1999 Apr 14;281(14):1304-9

[242] Brody S, Preut R, Schommer K, Schurmeyer TH. A randomized controlled trial of high dose ascorbic acid for reduction of blood pressure, cortisol, and subjective responses to psychological stress. *Psychopharmacology* (Berl). 2002 Jan;159(3):319-24

[243] Hamazaki T, Itomura M, Sawazaki S, Nagao Y. Anti-stress effects of DHA. *Biofactors.* 2000;13(1-4):41-5

[244] Cagnacci A, et al. Kava-Kava administration reduces anxiety in perimenopausal women. *Maturitas.* 2003 Feb 25;44(2):103-9

Sometimes a stressful situation can be modified into one that is less stressful or dysfunctional, so that the benefits are retained, yet the negative aspects are reduced. Of course, the best example of this is interpersonal relationships, which easily lend themselves to improvement with the application of conscious effort. Many audiotapes, books, and seminars are available for people interested in having improved interpersonal relationships. Selected resources are listed here:

- <u>Men and Women: Talking Together</u> by Deborah Tannen and Robert Bly [Sound Horizons, 1992. ISBN: 1879323095] A lively discussion of the different communication and relationship styles of men and women by two respected experts in their fields.
- <u>How to Deal with Difficult People</u> by Drs. Rick Brinkman and Rick Kirschner. [Audio Cassette. Career Track, 1995] An entertaining format with solutions to common workplace and situational difficulties. Authored and performed by two naturopathic physicians.
- <u>Men are From Mars, Women are From Venus</u> by John Gray. [Audio Cassette and Books]. Phenomenally popular concepts in understanding, accepting, and effectively integrating the differences between men and women.
- <u>The ManKind Project</u> (<u>www.mkp.org</u>). An international organization hosting events for men and women. The men's events, formats, and groups are authentic, clear, and healthy. The ManKind Project has an organization for women called The WomanWithin (<u>www.womanwithin.org</u>). No book or tape can substitute for the dynamics and personal attention that can be experienced by a conscious, empowered, and well-intended group.

When "the problem" cannot be avoided, and the interaction/relationship with the problem cannot be improved, a remaining option is to supplement the internal environment so that it is somewhat "strengthened" to deal with the stress of the bothersome event or situation. For example, when dealing with emotional stress, we can use counseling, support groups, or various relaxation techniques.[245] If we determine that the emotional stress has a biochemical component, then we can use specific botanical and nutritional supplementation to safely and naturally support and restore normal function. Moving deeper into the issue of "stress management" requires that we ask why a person is in a stressful situation to begin with. Of course, with *random acts of chaos* like car accidents, we cannot always ascribe the problem to the person, unless the accident resulted from their own negligence. But **when people are chronically stressed and unhappy about their jobs and/or relationships, then we need to employ more than stress reduction techniques**, and as clinicians we need to offer more than the latest adaptogen. **We have to ask why a person would subject himself/herself to such a situation, and what fears or limitations (self-imposed and/or externally applied) keep him/her from breaking free into a life that works**.[246,247,248,249,250,251]

---

[245] Martha Davis PhD, Matthew McKay MSW, Elizabeth Robbins Eshelman PhD. <u>The Relaxation & Stress Reduction Workbook 5th edition</u>. New Harbinger Publishers; 2000. [ISBN: 1572242140]

[246] Rick Jarow. *Creating the Work You Love: Courage, Commitment and Career*; Inner Traditions Intl Ltd; 1995 [ISBN: 0892815426]

[247] Breton D, Largent C. *The Paradigm Conspiracy: Why Our Social Systems Violate Human Potential-And How We Can Change Them*. Hazelden: 1998

[248] Dominguez JR. *Transforming Your Relationship with Money*. Sounds True; Book and Cassette edition: 2001 Audio tape.

[249] Miller A. *The truth will set you free: overcoming emotional blindness and finding your true adult self*. New York: Basic Books; 2001

[250] Bradshaw J. *Healing the Shame that Binds You* [Audio Cassette (April 1990) Health Communications Audio; ISBN: 1558740430]

[251] Miller A. *The Drama of the Gifted Child: The Search for the True Self*. Basic Books: 1981

Stress always has a biochemical/physiologic component: Regardless of its origins, stress always takes a toll on the body—*the whole body*. Well-documented effects of stress include:

1. Increased levels of cortisol—higher levels are associated with osteoporosis, memory loss, slow healing, and insulin resistance.
2. Reduced function of thyroid hormones[252] (i.e., induction of peripheral/metabolic hypothyroidism)
3. Reduced levels of testosterone (in men)
4. Increased intestinal permeability and "leaky gut"[253]
5. Increased excretion of minerals in the urine
6. Increased need for vitamins, minerals, and amino acids
7. Suppression of immune function and of natural killer cells that fight viral infections and tumors
8. Decreased production of sIgA—the main defense of the lungs, gastrointestinal tract, and genitourinary tract
9. Increased populations of harmful bacteria in the intestines and an associated increased rate of lung and upper respiratory tract infections
10. Increased incidence of food allergies[254]
11. Sleep disturbance

The body functions as a whole—not as independent, autonomous organ systems: Problems with one aspect of health create problems in other aspects of health. Treatment of disease and promotion of wellness must therefore improve overall health and functioning while simultaneously addressing the disease or presenting complaint.

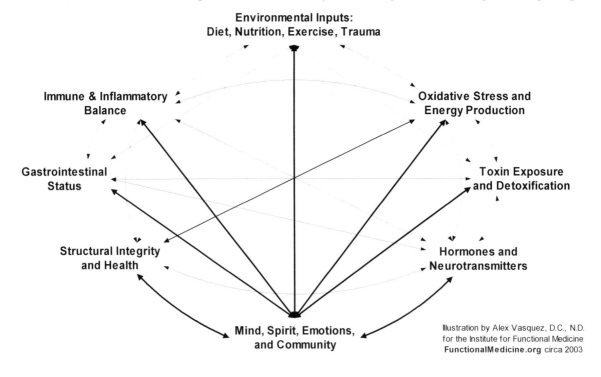

An earlier rendering of the Functional Medicine Matrix, circa 2003: The "Matrix" provides a graphic illustration of the interconnectedness and interdependency of physiologic factors and organ systems; this version was published in *Textbook of Functional Medicine* and published separately as Vasquez A. Web-like Interconnections of Physiological Factors. *Integrative Medicine* 2006, April, 32-37

---

[252] Ingenbleek Y, Bernstein L. The stressful condition as a nutritionally dependent adaptive dichotomy. *Nutrition* 1999 Apr;15(4):305-20
[253] Hart A, Kamm MA. Review article: mechanisms of initiation and perpetuation of gut inflammation by stress. *Aliment Pharmacol Ther* 2002;16(12):2017-28
[254] Anderzen I, Arnetz BB, Soderstrom T, Soderman E. Stress and sensitization in children: a controlled prospective psychophysiological study of children exposed to international relocation. *Journal of Psychosomatic Research* 1997; 43: 259-69

Autonomization, intradependence, emotional literacy, corrective experience:

> "None of us are completely developed people when we reach adulthood.
> We are each incomplete in our own way." *Merle Fossum*[255]

Consciousness-raising is a keystone gift that holistic physicians can impart to their patients and one which may be necessary for true healing to be manifested and maintained. Healthcare providers are quick to enlighten their patients to the details of diet, exercise, nutrition, medications, surgeries, and other *biomechanical* and *biochemical* aspects of health, but are routinely negligent when it comes to sharing with patients the emotional tools that may be necessary to repair or construct the "self" which is supposed to implement the treatment plan that the doctor has designed. Passivity and ignorance are not hindrances to the success of the *medical paradigm*, which requires that patients are "compliant" rather than self-directed; however, for *authentic, holistic healthcare* to be successful, it must empower the patient sufficiently such that he/she attains/regains appropriate *autonomy*—an "internal locus of control"—sufficient for lifelong internally-driven health maintenance. Health implications of autonomy (or its absence) are obvious and intuitive. Patients with an underdeveloped internal locus of control appear to experience greater degrees of social stress which can lead to hypercortisolemia and hippocampal atrophy.[256] A developed internal locus of control correlates strongly with the success of weight-loss programs, and for nonautonomous patients it is necessary to encourage the development of autonomous self-care behavior in addition to the provision of information about diet and exercise.[257]

Six fundamental components of self-esteem
1. Living consciously
2. Self-acceptance
3. Self-responsibility
4. Self-assertiveness
5. Living purposefully
6. Personal integrity
Branden N. *The Six Pillars of Self-Esteem*. Bantam: 1995

Completely formed internal identities are the natural result of the *continuum* of positive childhood experiences (inclusive of stability, "unconditional love", healthy parenting, and active, conscious intergenerational social contact) which are ideally merged into adolescent and adulthood experiences of success, acceptance, inclusion, independence, interdependence, and intradependence with the end result being a socially-conscious adult with an internal locus of control. Where the patient has experienced a relative absence of these natural and expected prerequisites, a truncated—wounded, reactive, shame-based, dissatisfied—self is likely to result. The failure to develop self-esteem and an internal locus of control largely explains why so many adult patients feign that they are incapable of action, "can't exercise", and "can't leave" their abusive jobs and relationships, and "can't resist" the dietary habits which daily contribute to their physical and psychoemotional decline. Thus, for more than a few patients, a therapeutic path must be explored which helps to re-create the foundation from which an autonomous adult and authentic self can grow—it is a *process* (not an event) of **emotional recovery**.[258] To this extent, interventional or therapeutic *autonomization* resembles a *recovery program* that can include various forms of conscious action, including goal-setting, positive reinforcement, developing emotional literacy[259] and emotional intelligence[260], and consciousness-raising experiences such as therapy and group work—all of which serve to intentionally (re)create and maintain the necessary climate for authentic selfhood. Therewith, the patient can accept challenges to further develop an *empowered self* by participating in exercises in which the ability to decide, choose, and act responsibly and appropriately are reinforced to eventually become second nature, replacing passivity, inaction, and ineffectiveness.[261]

"Empowerment" can only be authentic if it is built on the foundation of a developed self. While *emotional recovery* and *personal empowerment* are separate spheres of activity and attention, they are not mutually exclusive

---

[255] Fossum M. *Catching Fire: Men Coming Alive in Recovery*. New York; Harper/Hazelden: 1989, 4-7

[256] "Cumulative exposure to high levels of cortisol over the lifetime is known to be related to hippocampal atrophy... Self-esteem and internal locus of control were significantly correlated with hippocampal volume in both young and elderly subjects." Pruessner JC, Baldwin MW, Dedovic K, Renwick R, Mahani NK, Lord C, Meaney M, Lupien S. Self-esteem, locus of control, hippocampal volume, and cortisol regulation in young and old adulthood. *Neuroimage*. 2005 Dec;28(4):815-26

[257] "Their weight loss was significant and associated with an internal locus of control orientation (P < 0.05)... Participants with an internal orientation could be offered a standard weight reduction programme. Others, with a more external locus of control orientation, could be offered an adapted programme, which also focused on and encouraged the participants' internal orientation." Adolfsson B, Andersson I, Elofsson S, Rossner S, Unden AL. Locus of control and weight reduction. *Patient Educ Couns*. 2005 Jan;56(1):55-61

[258] Bradshaw J. *Healing the Shame that Binds You* [Audio Cassette (April 1990) Health Communications Audio; ISBN: 1558740430]

[259] Dayton T. *Trauma and Addiction: Ending the Cycle of Pain through Emotional Literacy*. Deerfield Beach; Health Communications, 2000

[260] Goleman D. *Emotional Intelligence*. New York; Bantam Books: 1995. Although the book as a whole was considered pioneering for its time, and the book continues to make a valuable contribution, a few of the concepts and author's personal stories are embarrassingly simplistic.

[261] Gatto JT. A Schooling Is Not An Education: interview by Barbara Dunlop. http://www.johntaylorgatto.com/bookstore/index.htm

and indeed are synergistic. However, emotional recovery—that process of recounting one's own history, delving into the depths of one's own psyche, and integrating what is found into a cohesive, functional and healthy whole—must occur before the program of personal development emphasizes empowerment. *Empowerment* cannot succeed without *recovery* because otherwise the so-called "empowerment" is likely to add to the defense mechanisms that protect against pain and thereby block the development of an authentic self. Stated concisely by Janov[262], "**Anything that builds a stronger defense system deepens the neurosis.**"

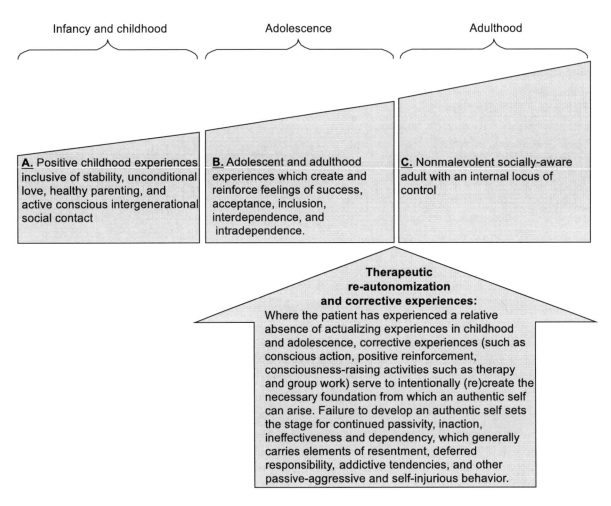

| Infancy and childhood | Adolescence | Adulthood |

A. Positive childhood experiences inclusive of stability, unconditional love, healthy parenting, and active conscious intergenerational social contact

B. Adolescent and adulthood experiences which create and reinforce feelings of success, acceptance, inclusion, interdependence, and intradependence.

C. Nonmalevolent socially-aware adult with an internal locus of control

Therapeutic re-autonomization and corrective experiences: Where the patient has experienced a relative absence of actualizing experiences in childhood and adolescence, corrective experiences (such as conscious action, positive reinforcement, consciousness-raising activities such as therapy and group work) serve to intentionally (re)create the necessary foundation from which an authentic self can arise. Failure to develop an authentic self sets the stage for continued passivity, inaction, ineffectiveness and dependency, which generally carries elements of resentment, deferred responsibility, addictive tendencies, and other passive-aggressive and self-injurious behavior.

Primary, secondary, and tertiary means for developing an autonomous, authentic self: Ideally, positive childhood experiences (A) merge into adolescent and adult experiences of confidence and maturity (B) for the development of a true adult (C). If A or B is lacking or insufficient, the result is an incomplete self often incapable of *effective* and *appropriate* action. Corrective experiences must then be pursued to re-establish the foundation from which an authentic self can arise.

Patients lacking an internal locus of control are much more likely to succumb to the tantalizing barrage of direct-to-consumer drug advertising[263] which infantilizes patients by 1) oversimplifying diseases, their causes, and treatments, 2) exonerating patients from responsibility and reinforcing the illusion of victimization and helplessness, and 3) encouraging a dependent, passively receptive role by telling patients that they have no proactive role other than to "ask your doctor if a prescription is right for you." Americans consume more prescription and OTC medications per capita than people in any other country.[264,265] With the combined and

[262] Janov A. *The Primal Scream*. New York; GP Putnam's Sons: 1970, page 20
[263] Aronson E. *The Social Animal*. San Fransisco; WH Freeman and company: 1972: 21-22, 53
[264] America the medicated. http://www.cbsnews.com/stories/2005/04/21/health/printable689997.shtml and http://www.msnbc.msn.com/id/7503122/ . See also http://usgovinfo.about.com/od/healthcare/a/usmedicated.htm Accessed September 17, 2005.
[265] Kivel P. *You Call This a Democracy*? Apex Press (August, 2004). ISBN: 1891843265 http://www.paulkivel.com/

synergistic effects of 1) the dissolution of first the extended family and now the nuclear family[266], 2) a society-wide famine of mentors, elders, and community[267,268,269], 3) a dearth of autonomous, genuine exploration from childhood to adulthood, and 4) primary and secondary "educational" institutions designed to squelch independence and autonomy in favor of the more efficient,

Integration promotes health
"The object of healing is…to move closer to wholeness." Kreinheder A. *Body and soul: the other side of illness*. Toronto, Canada; Inner City Books: 1991,38

predictable, and controllable conformity and "standardization"[270,271], **industrialized societies have raised generations of people who lack completely formed internal identities**. Lacking an internal locus of control and identity from which to think independently and critically, these "adults" are easy prey for slick and flashy drug advertisements that promise the illusion of perfect health in exchange for passivity, abdication, and lifelong medicalization. That the typical American watches four hours of television per day[272] is bad enough, what makes this worse is that "Americans who watch average amounts of television may be exposed to more than 30 hours of direct-to-consumer drug advertisements each year, far surpassing their exposure to other forms of health communication."[273] If we are to wean our suckling culture from undue dependence on the pharmaceutical industry, we have to address our patient population directly and transform them from *passive, nonautonomous, and ignorant about health and disease* to pro-active, autonomous, and well-informed about health and the means required to obtain and sustain it.

Insight into a patient's internal dynamic can provide the clinician with an understanding that explains the phenomena of *non-compliance* and *disease identification*. Rather than seeing non-compliance as "weakness of will", non-compliance as a form of "disobedience" may be a reflection of the patient's unconscious need to wrestle with and resolve parental introjects. For example, if a patient had a rejecting, nonaffirming parent, he/she may need to find another rejecting authority figure in order to continue playing the role of the child; by assuming this role and "setting the stage", the patient is unconsciously attempting to create a situation wherein the primary relationship can be healed.[274] Complicating this is *disease identification*—in which patients use their disease as a source of identity and secondary gain for martyrdom, social support, group participation, acceptance, admiration, purpose, excitement, and drama.

---

[266] Bly R. *Iron John*. Reading, Mass.: Addison Wesley, 1990
[267] Bly R. *The Sibling Society*. Vintage Books USA; Reprint edition (June 1, 1997) ISBN: 0679781285 (Abridged audio edition (May 1, 1996), ASIN: 0679451609)
[268] Bly R. *Where have all the parents gone? A talk on the Sibling Society*. New York: Sound Horizons, 1996 Highly recommended.
[269] Bly R, Hillman J, Meade M. Men and the Life of Desire. Oral Tradition Archives. ISBN: 1880155001. Audio Cassette
[270] Gatto JT. *Dumbing Us Down: the Hidden Curriculum of Compulsory Education*. Gabriola Island, Canada; New Society Publishers: 2005
[271] Gatto JT. *The Paradox of Extended Childhood*. [From a presentation in Cambridge, Mass. October 2000] http://www.johntaylorgatto.com/bookstore/index.htm
[272] "American children view over 23 hours of television per week. Teenagers view an average of 21 to 22 hours of television per week. By the time today's children reach age 70, they will have spent 7 to 10 years of their lives watching television." American Academy of Pediatrics http://www.aapca1.org/aapca1/tv.html See also TV-Turnoff Network. Facts and Figures About our TV Habit http://www.tvturnoff.org/factsheets.htm Accessed September 17, 2005
[273] Brownfield ED, et al. Direct-to-consumer drug advertisements on network television. *J Health Commun*. 2004 Nov-Dec;9(6):491-7
[274] Miller A. *The Drama of the Gifted Child: The Search for the True Self*. Basic Books: 1981, page 88

Helping patients create and maintain authentic selves

An absent or underdeveloped locus of control is the key problem that underlies many anxiety disorders, addictive behavioral traits such as overeating, overworking, codependency, as well as chronic ineffectiveness in the pursuit of one's goals. The solutions to this problem are logical, practical, and accessible to everyone; the major costs associated with each are open-mindedness, attentiveness, discipline and persistence. There is scant mention of this concept and its intervention in the biomedical literature; however, it is well described in the psychological literature, particularly that which focuses on various types of "recovery" such as that from addiction, co-dependence, and low self-esteem, the latter two of which are virtually synonymous with an insufficient internal locus of control.

There is no *single* path here. There are many paths. The goal is not to choose the right path; rather the goal is to travel several paths to the degree necessary, implement what has been learned, travel other paths, and return to the same path again to retrace one's steps in new ways. The process is similar to that of *ceremonial initiation*, the purpose of which is to formally mark the *beginning* of a process that is *ongoing* and *infinite*.[275] Each path and each process has its gifts, significance, and limitations. However, the ultimate goal of each must be a tangible and positive change in the ways which the patient feels and/or behaves in and interacts with the world on a day-to-day basis.

In no particular order (since the proper sequence will have to be customized to the situation and willingness of the patient), the following are some of the more commonly cited exercises, processes, and sources of additional information:

Apprenticeship and Mentoring: books, tapes, and lectures: Children and non-autonomous adults are pulled into authentic adulthood by mentors, elders, and true adults. The therapeutic encounters thus provided—whether interpersonal or vicarious in the form of lectures, books, or audiotapes— serve as sources of information from which new possibilities can be gleaned, and these therefore serve as infinitely valuable resources for expanding the narrow horizons that characterize an underdeveloped internal locus of control. In essence, books, tapes, and lectures allow the patient to become a student and to choose a vicarious mentor. *Advantages*: Books and tapes allow access to many of the best minds in psychology; books and tapes are inexpensive; allow patients to explore and benefit from many different perspectives; books and tapes are always available and are therefore amenable to various schedules of work and responsibility. *Disadvantages*: Books and tapes do not re-create the interpersonal bridge which is essential for authentic recovery; do not provide a direct and objective means of accountably, thus potentially allowing patients to delude themselves about the effectiveness (or lack thereof) of their recovery process. Examples of better-known books, tapes and recorded lectures on the *process* of emotional recovery:

- ***The Six Pillars of Self-Esteem*** by Nathaniel Branden PhD. This is a very accessible yet very structured work in which Dr Branden brilliantly elucidates key concepts in psychology relevant to self-efficacy and self-esteem; also available as an audiobook excellently narrated by Dr Branden.
- ***Healing the Shame that Binds You*** by John Bradshaw [Audio Cassette (April 1990) Health Communications Audio; ISBN: 1558740430] Available as book and cassette with identical titles and different content.
- ***A Little Book on the Human Shadow*** by Robert Bly. Certainly among the most concise, accessible, and complete books ever written on the processes involved in losing and recovering the self; also available as an audio presentation.
- ***The Drama of the Gifted Child*** by Alice Miller. This internationally acclaimed book is considered a true classic among therapists and patients alike. Available as book and a brilliantly performed audio cassette.
- ***You Can Heal Your Life*** by Louise Hay. Another standard for recovery; very "new age."
- ***Codependent No More: How to Stop Controlling Others and Start Caring for Yourself*** by Melody Beattie. Pioneering for its time.
- ***The Artist's Date Book*** by Julia Cameron. Each page has a new creative idea for creative expression and "creative recovery."
- ***The Psychology of Self-Esteem*** by Nathaniel Branden PhD. More advanced and perhaps less widely relevant than his "six pillars" work, this is also an excellent encapsulation of important concepts in personal psychology.

---

[275] Hillman J, Meade M, Some M. *Images of initiation*. Oral Tradition Archives; 1992

Therapy: *"Therapy is a conversation that matters."* Therapy in this context specifically means face-to-face, active interaction, either one-on-one or in a group setting, with the specific intention to give and/or provide support for personal growth. Whether 12-step groups such as Codependents Anonymous qualify as a form of therapy depends entirely upon the level of engagement of the participant; sitting in a room while *other people* do *their* work provides slow or no benefit for the passive observer. **Recovery is an *active* process, which is why it is antithetical to depression, which is a *passive* state of being.** Patients should go in knowing that this is a *process* and to not expect to be "fixed" after the first hour or even the first month. ***Advantages***: Therapists can provide crucial support and insight while the client wrestles with undecipherable and convoluted emotional and psychic data. Therapists can help the client set goals ("stretches" and "homework") by which the client reaches beyond his/her comfort zone to attain the next expansion in being and experience. Therapists must create a safe space or "container" in which ideas and feelings can be brought forth to intermingle and be consciously appreciated. ***Disadvantages***: Requires a flexible and disciplined schedule; costs money; bad therapists can do more harm than good if they misdirect their clients away from volatile and core issues and authentic expression.[276,277,278,279] Therapy can be disempowering if the patient continues to project his/her locus of control onto the therapist.

Some of the more commonly used tools of the psychotherapeutic trade include:
- **Active listening**
- **Insight, explanation of events**: their origins, reasons, and significance
- **Reminders** of previous conclusions and stories
- **Challenge old ideas and habits**: Therapy that generally or completely lacks confrontation and accountability is ineffective.
- **Encourage exploration and new modes of being and interacting**
- **Creating a safe container wherein the client can review the details, significance, and feelings associated with past events**
- **Modeling the expression of feeling**
- **Defining goals and helping the client focus on what is significant**
- **Correcting distortions of reality**
- **Asking patients to get in touch with and then express their feelings**
- **Support and encourage clients to take calculated risks for the sake of self-expansion**
- **Pointing out errors in logic**
- **Coaching patients in the proper and responsible use of emotional language**
- **Discouraging evasiveness; requiring accountability**[280]

Creativity: All types of self-expression reinforce and validate the patient's sense of self. Creative self-expression, such as writing about thoughts and feelings about significant experiences, can reduce symptomatology in patients with rheumatoid arthritis and asthma.[281]

Experiential: Corrective experiences can be obtained in therapy, with friends and family, in integration groups, and during "experiential" retreats. ***Advantages***: Experiential events orchestrated by therapists and various groups such as ManKind Project (mkp.org) and WomanWithin.org can rapidly facilitate personal growth while also providing an ongoing container and support system that encourages self-development rather than the ego-inflation that accompanies short-term events. ***Disadvantages***: "Adventures" like driving across the nation or climbing a mountain are unconscious and largely impotent attempts at self-initiation; authentic initiation has always been supervised by community elders. However, once a well-founded initiation has taken place, preferably with an on-going community that facilitates continued refinement and self-exploration, then "adventures" can be undertaken consciously to maintain and reinforce the experience of autonomy and competent selfhood. Eventually, transformative and sustentative experiences can be integrated and created in the daily life experience so that dramatic adventures become unnecessary for the continued renewal and "recharging" of the self.

276 Lee J. *Expressing Your Anger Appropriately* (Audio Cassette). Sounds True (June 1, 1990); ISBN: 1564550338
277 Bradshaw J. *Healing the Shame that Binds You* [Audio Cassette (April 1990) Health Communications Audio; ISBN: 1558740430]
278 Miller A. *The Drama of the Gifted Child: The Search for the True Self.* Basic Books; 1981
279 Miller A. *The truth will set you free: overcoming emotional blindness and finding your true adult self.* New York: Basic Books; 2001
280 Kottler JA. *The Compleat Therapist.* San Francisco; Jossey-Bass publishers; 1991, pages 134-174
281 Smyth JM, Stone AA, Hurewitz A, Kaell A. Effects of writing about stressful experiences on symptom reduction in patients with asthma or rheumatoid arthritis. *JAMA.* 1999 Apr 14;281(14):1304-9

Creating and Re-creating the Self:
An on-going process that involves various types of "therapy" such as healthy formal/informal interpersonal and group relationships, creative expression and exploration, the periodic infusion of new ideas from teachers and mentors, attendance in workshops and seminars (or other forms of on-going consciousness-raising), reflection, and the integration of transformative and sustentative significance into everyday life, in such a way that daily life itself becomes *therapeutic* and *affirmative*.

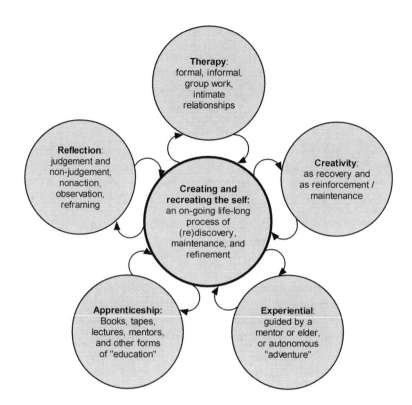

One possible sequence of events for effective, lasting, and authentic autonomization: The caterpillar does not blossom into a butterfly without spending time in its cocoon. The airborne seed descends into the earth for its nourishment before it sprouts and searches for the sun. Similarly, gratification of our ascentionist and impatient ego must be deferred for the sake of allowing the time and descent that provide "grounding" and developing of a solid foundation from which authentic growth can arise. The Western view of "personal development" idealizes a life course of constant ascension that is generally inconsistent with living in a real world fraught with imperfections; two of the major complications arising from such a perfectionistic paradigm are 1) that it causes people to feel anxious and ashamed when confronted with otherwise normal delays and failures, and 2) that it biases people into believing that improvement comes only from advancement rather than also from the return and short-term regression that are characteristic of most historically-proven societal traditions. With modification of the stepwise model proposed by Bradshaw[282], here I propose the following sequence:

1. *Short-term behavior modification*: For people whose behavior is acutely dysfunctional or harmful to themselves or others, they must stop the "acting out" that is the symptom of the underlying emotional injury or schism. Accepting abuse—at work or home—is a form of **acting out** that perpetuates old wounds and saps the strength required for recovery. Enacting addictive behavior is injurious to the psyche because self-injurious behavior reinforces the image of oneself as an object of contempt while also reinforcing the image of psychological dependency and emotional helplessness.

2. *Emotional recovery*: Complete healing is only possible when consciously pursued, and conscious healing can only be pursued after one has become conscious of the wounds, injuries, absences, dynamics, and events that lead to the current state. This process of recovery is referred to mythologically as the "descent" or the time of "eating ashes" that is a recurrent theme in various fairy tales ("Cinderella" literally means "ash girl") and cultural-religious histories (such as Jesus' *descent* into the tomb).[283] The biggest blockades to this process are 1) the ego, which prefers to ascend and to deny intrapersonal "negativity"[284], and 2) the challenge in finding elders and mentors in a society that constantly perpetuates and encourages immaturity, materialism, and superficiality.[285] In the words of famed psychologist Carl Jung, "One does not become enlightened by imagining figures of light, but by making the darkness *conscious*. The latter procedure, however, is disagreeable, and

[282] Bradshaw J. *Healing the Shame that Binds You* [Audio Cassette (April 1990) Health Communications Audio; ISBN: 1558740430]
[283] Bly R, Hillman J, Meade M. *Men and the Life of Desire*. Oral Tradition Archives. ISBN: 1880155001
[284] Robert Bly. *The Human Shadow*. Sound Horizons, New York 1991 [ISBN: 1879323001] and Bly R. *A Little Book on the Human Shadow* [ISBN: 0062548476]
[285] Bly R. *Where have all the parents gone? A talk on the Sibling Society*. New York: Sound Horizons, 1996

therefore unpopular." People often have tremendous resistances to the process of self-exploration and internal learning; as Jeffrey Kottler[286] wrote of his own experience in *The Compleat Therapist*, "…like most prospective consumers of therapy, I made up a bunch of excuses for why I could handle this on my own… I was smiling like an idiot…"

3. *Long-term behavior modification and integration*: Insight allows for an illumination of the internal mental-emotional landscape, and effective insight must then be manifested externally by changes/modifications in behavior, habits, and interaction in the world. **Externalized behaviors simultaneously reflect and reinforce thoughts and feelings.** According to Grieneeks[287], patients (and their healthcare providers) can "*think* their way into new ways of *acting*" and "*act* their way into new ways of *thinking*." Eventually, a consciously designed life can be created so that actions, interactions, thoughts, and feelings are melded together in such ways that everyday life itself becomes simultaneously *therapeutic*, *affirmative*, *sustentative*, and *empowering*. In this way, the person and his/her life are unified in such ways as to become self-perpetuating and self-sustaining cycles of ascents and descents, thought-feeling and action, reflection and courage, independence and interdependence—in sum: "a wheel rolling from its own center."[288] At this point the self is established, though it must be maintained and developed with the continuous application of consciousness, reflection, and action.

4. *Metapersonal involvement in community, religion, spirituality, and the world*: Many people are tempted to move from a state of woundedness, relative incompleteness and the feelings of shame and disempowerment to a state of illusory *perfection*, *enlightenment* and *omnipotence* without doing the requisite hard work that makes authentic personal growth possible. People with unhealed emotional wounds often seek to camouflage those deficiencies by becoming pious and projecting an image of completeness and of "having it all figured out" and "having it all together"; religion and the acquisition of power are often misused for this purpose. Many people are successful in wearing this mask for many years; but its crumbling—often manifested as the "midlife crisis"—heralds an opportunity for personal growth if not medicated with anti-depressants, vacations, affairs, gambling, or other distractions.[289] The temptation to bypass Stages 2 [emotional recovery] and 3 [integration] and leapfrog from Stage 1 [woundedness] to Stage 4 [spirituality] should be resisted because the religion or spirituality is then used as a shield *against authenticity* and as a tool for illusory control. Religion can be misused in this way by providing an "identity" and sense of redemption for people with incompletely formed identities and for those with incompletely reconciled shadows and unresolved childhood-parental introjects.[290,291,292] Nietzsche's[293] response to this problem was to encourage self-knowledge and self-reconciliation as prerequisites to religious devotion, hence his admonition, "By all means love your neighbor as yourself – but *first* be such that you love yourself." Historical and recent events remind us of how religion can be misused for misanthropic ends.[294] What is commonly referred to as "spiritual development"—a level of resolution, reconciliation, and autonomy that allows for compassionate interdependence with people, the planet and the larger "world"—is synergistic with and can be supported by religion; but the latter is not a substitute for the former.[295,296] Religion and other forms of metapersonal involvement (e.g., community participation and social generosity) are *important* and *necessary* extensions of self-development. In order for personal development to blossom from the germ of necessary narcissism into its flower of functional completeness, it must eventually manifest in the larger community and the world.

5. *Acceptance of mortality and death*: No individual person or any system of thought, whether scientific or religious, can feign completeness without accounting for the end of life and incorporating this account into its overarching paradigm. The

> "Once accepted, death is an integral component of every event, as the left hand to the right. The cultural death concept could only be instilled in a mind split from its own life flow."
>
> Pearce JC, *Exploring the Crack in the Cosmic Egg*. Washington Square Press; 1974, page 59

[286] Kottler JA. *The Compleat Therapist*. San Francisco; Jossey-Bass publishers; 1991, pages 2-3
[287] Keith Grieneeks PhD. "Psychological Assessment" taught in 1998 at Bastyr University.
[288] Friedrich Wilhelm Nietzsche, Walter Kaufmann (Translator). *Thus Spoke Zarathustra*. Penguin USA; 1978, page 27
[289] Robinson JC. *Death of a Hero, Birth of a Soul: Answering the Call of Midlife*. Council Oak Books, March 1997 ISBN: 1571780432
[290] Bradshaw J. *Healing the Shame that Binds You* [Audio Cassette (April 1990) Health Communications Audio; ISBN: 1558740430]
[291] Miller A. *The Drama of the Gifted Child: The Search for the True Self*. Basic Books; 1981
[292] Miller A. *The truth will set you free: overcoming emotional blindness and finding your true adult self*. New York: Basic Books; 2001
[293] Nietzsche N. *Thus spoke Zarathustra*. Read by Jon Cartwright and Alex Jennings and published by Naxos AudioBooks. I think this is among the more brilliant achievements in human history. http://naxosaudiobooks.com/nabusa/pages/432512.htm
[294] Bonhoeffer. (movie documentary by director/writer Martin Doblmeier) http://www.bonhoeffer.com/
[295] Lozoff B. *It's a Meaningful Life : It Just Takes Practice*. March 1, 2001. ISBN: 0140196242
[296] Bradshaw J. *Healing the Shame that Binds You* [Audio Cassette (April 1990) Health Communications Audio; ISBN: 1558740430]

event is too significant, and the fear and concerns it provokes are too weighty to not be addressed directly and held in consciousness on a periodic—if not frequent—basis. This topic is of practical importance, too, not only in our own lives and those of our friends and family, but also to the national healthcare system, which currently spends the bulk of its money and resources vainly attempting to preserve life in the last few years and months after which disease or age call unrelentingly for the end of life. Perhaps if we as individuals and as participants in the healthcare system could accept and deal with our own deaths, then we would not have to panic and participate in such superfluous expenditures of time, energy, emotion, and money when death seeks to arrive, either for our patients, our friends and family, or ourselves. Proximal to the panic and aversion that characterizes the West's relationship to death is the "subclinical" panic and aversion that infiltrate the lives, practices, and policies that we experience every day. Surely, many unconscious events and subconscious influences contribute to the "lives of quiet desperation"[297] and "universal anxiety"[298] that subtly yet powerfully afflict most

> "The event of death is not a tragedy—to rabbit, fox or man. But the *concept* of death *is* a tragedy, for man, and *indirectly* for poor fox, rabbit, bush, bird, just anything and everything in man's path."
>
> Pearce JC, *Exploring the Crack in the Cosmic Egg*. Washington Square Press; 1974, page 59

people; surely, lack of reconciliation with death is a major contributor. Especially in western cultures, death is commonly seen as some type of failure or shortcoming, either on behalf of the patient or his/her doctors, and the most common questions asked on the topic of death are *"how can this be avoided?"* before the event and *"who is to blame?"* after the event. Other cultures accept death as a natural part of life, and indeed, people are seen to have an obligation to die so that the next generations can have their turn in the cycle of life. Alternatives to western hysteria are founded on acceptance of death, and the prerequisites for the acceptance of death are 1) the dedication of sufficient time for its consideration (most people would rather watch a bad movie or attend spectator sports), 2) reframing the event in terms of its being a natural part of our lives, certainly nothing to be ashamed of (discussed below), 3) making necessary logistical preparations (e.g., writing of wills, providing for dependents, and other obvious technicalities), and 4) living as completely, consciously, compassionately, effectively, and authentically as possible so that remorse can be minimized, perhaps completely mitigated. Reframing the event of death begins with its description in general terms so that its enigma, from which its power over the hearts and minds of humanity is derived, can be deciphered and thus deflated. The main characteristics of death which precipitate its fear are 1) the unpredictability of its arrival, 2) the duration of the dying process, and 3) the quality of that process, for example whether it is painful or associated with or precipitated by severe illness or injury. The first characteristic of *timeliness*—the unpredictability of its arrival—stresses people because of their inadequate preparation and the feeling that they have only recently begun to live or have not quite yet begun to live their authentic lives. These concerns are allayed by preparation, both logistical and intrapersonal. Each of us has the responsibility to "become authentically whole" so that we do not inflict our incompleteness onto others, either directly through various forms of transference or deprivation or indirectly though the more subtle means of politics and cultural mores.[299,300] If a person can live with vitality, authenticity, compassion and effectiveness then little is left to want, and fears of death and its untimely arrival are diminished. The remaining variables are both controllable and uncontrollable; they are uncontrollable to the extent that we are all subject to chaos and accidents, whether in cars, planes, or bathtubs. *Duration* and *quality* are both controllable on an inpatient setting to the extent that palliative care and autonomous decision-making is made available.[301,302]

Life can only be authentically and completely experienced after one has created an authentic self and has thereafter accepted life *as it is*. Since death is part of life, the full engagement of life requires *acceptance of* and *reconciliation with* death. Acceptance of death does not necessarily entail that life becomes permeated with nihilistic resignation; on the contrary, it infuses daily events with significance and makes all experiences unique and worthy of appreciation.

[297] Throeau HD, (Thomas O, ed). *Walden and Civil Disobedience*. New York: WW Norton and Company; 1966, page 5

[298] Becker E. *The Denial of Death*. New York: Free Press; 1973, pages 11 and 21

[299] Miller A. *The Drama of the Gifted Child: The Search for the True Self*. Basic Books; 1981

[300] Robert Bly. *The Human Shadow*. Sound Horizons, New York 1991 [ISBN: 1879323001] and Bly R. *A Little Book on the Human Shadow* [ISBN: 0062548476

[301] Steinbrook R. Medical marijuana, physician-assisted suicide, and the Controlled Substances Act. *N Engl J Med*. 2004 Sep 30;351(14):1380-3

[302] "Failure to give an effective therapy to seriously ill patients, either adults or children, violates the core principles of both medicine and ethics... Therefore, in the patient's best interest, patients and parents/surrogates, have the right to request medical marijuana under certain circumstances and physicians have the duty to disclose medical marijuana as an option and prescribe it when appropriate." Clark PA. Medical marijuana: should minors have the same rights as adults? *Med Sci Monit*.2003;9:ET1-9

Growth, integration, and acceptance: Starting at the top, the progression of personal growth, emotional recovery, integration and daily practice is followed by the more advanced integration of one's chosen purpose, mission, and life work with one's chosen spiritual/religious practice, family and community involvement, and acceptance of and preparation for the end of life and the continuity of society and the environment.

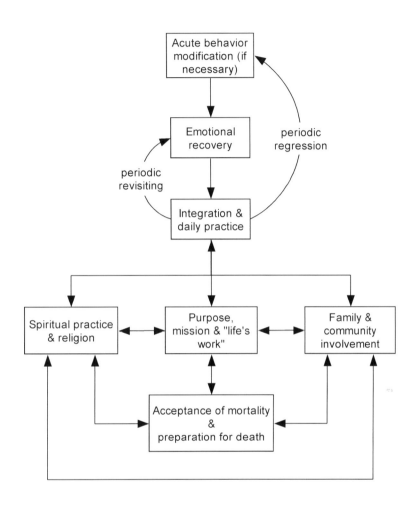

"They say there's no future for us.
            They're right,
                    which is fine with us."   *Rumi*[303]

[303] Rumi in Barks C (translator). *The Essential Rumi*. HarperSanFransisco: 1995, page 2

Environmental Health, Toxicity, and Detoxification

"Man's attitude toward nature is today critically important simply because we have now acquired a fateful power to alter and destroy nature. But man is a part of nature, and his war against nature is inevitably a war against himself." *Rachel Carson*[304]

Environmental exposures to chemicals and toxic substances: Studies using blood tests and tissue samples from Americans across the nation have consistently shown that all Americans have toxic chemical accumulation whether or not they work in chemical factories or are obviously exposed at home or work.[305,306] **The recent report from the CDC found toxic chemicals such as pesticides in all Americans, especially minorities, women, and children.**[307] Nearly all of these chemicals are known to contribute to health problems in humans—problems such as cancer, fatigue, poor memory, endocrinopathy, subfertility/infertility, Parkinson's disease, autoimmune diseases like lupus, and many other serious conditions. Therefore, ***detoxification programs are a necessity—not a luxury***.

Examples of toxicants commonly found in Americans

Environmental pollutant (population frequency)	Biologic effects as quoted from HSDB: Hazardous Substances Data Bank. National Library of Medicine, NIH[308] or other reference as noted
DDE (found in 99% of Americans): DDE is the main metabolite of DDT, a pesticide that was presumably banned in the US in 1972	• DDT is known to be immunosuppressive in animals. • A study published in 2004 showed that increasing levels of DDE in African-American male farmers in North Carolina correlated with a higher prevalence of antinuclear antibodies and up to 50% reductions in serum IgG.[309] • Other studies in humans have suggested an estrogenic or anti-androgenic effect.[310] • Virtually all US women have evidence of DDT/DDE accumulation. Women with higher levels of DDT and/or its metabolites show pregnancy and childbirth complications and have higher rates of infant mortality.[311]

[304] Rachel Carson. *Silent Spring*. Boston, Houghton Mifflin Company (2002). ISBN: 0395683297. See also Rachel Carson Dies of Cancer; 'Silent Spring' Author Was 56. New York Times 1956. http://www.rachelcarson.org/ on August 1, 2004

[305] "The average concentration of 2,3,7,8-tetrachlorodibenzo-p-dioxin in the adipose tissue of the US population was 5.38 pg/g, increasing from 1.98 pg/g in children under 14 years of age to 9.40 pg/g in adults over 45." Orban JE, Stanley JS, Schwemberger JG, Remmers JC. Dioxins and dibenzofurans in adipose tissue of the general US population and selected subpopulations. *Am J Public Health* 1994 Mar;84(3):439-45

[306] "Although the use of HCB as a fungicide has virtually been eliminated, detectable levels of HCB are still found in nearly all people in the USA." Robinson PE, Leczynski BA, Kutz FW, Remmers JC. An evaluation of hexachlorobenzene body-burden levels in the general population of the USA. *IARC Sci Publ* 1986;77:183-92

[307] "Many of the pesticides found in the test subjects have been linked to serious short- and long-term health effects including infertility, birth defects and childhood and adult cancers." http://www.panna.org/campaigns/docsTrespass/chemicalTrespass2004.dv.html July 25, 2004

[308] Primary source for this data is the Hazardous Substances Data Bank. National Library of Medicine, National Institutes of Health: http://toxnet.nlm.nih.gov/cgi-bin/sis/htmlgen?HSDB accessed on August 1, 2004

[309] Cooper GS, Martin SA, Longnecker MP, Sandler DP, Germolec DR. Associations between plasma DDE levels and immunologic measures in African-American farmers in North Carolina. *Environ Health Perspect*. 2004 Jul;112(10):1080-4

[310] Dalvie MA, Myers JE, Lou Thompson M, Dyer S, Robins TG, Omar S, Riebow J, Molekwa J, Kruger P, Millar R. The hormonal effects of long-term DDT exposure on malaria vector-control workers in Limpopo Province, South Africa. *Environ Res*. 2004 Sep;96(1):9-19

[311] "The findings strongly suggest that DDT use increases preterm births, which is a major contributor to infant mortality. If this association is causal, it should be included in any assessment of the costs and benefits of vector control with DDT." Longnecker MP, Klebanoff MA, Zhou H, Brock JW. Association between maternal serum concentration of the DDT metabolite DDE and preterm and small-for-gestational-age babies at birth. *Lancet*. 2001 Jul 14;358(9276):110-4

Examples of toxicants commonly found in Americans—*continued*

Environmental pollutant (population frequency)	*Biologic effects as quoted from HSDB*: Hazardous Substances Data Bank. *National Library of Medicine, NIH[312] or other reference*
2,5-dichlorophenol (88% nationally and up to 96% in select children populations): Dichlorophenols can occur in tap water as a result of standard chlorination treatment. General population may be exposed to 2,5-dichlorophenol through oral consumption or dermal contact with chlorinated tap water. 2,5-Dichlorophenol was identified in 96% of the urine samples of children residing in Arkansas near an herbicide plant at concentrations of 4-1,200 ppb. The sole manufacturer for herbicide use is Sandoz (Clariant Corporation).	• Human Toxicity Excerpts: 1. Burning pain in mouth and throat. White necrotic lesions in mouth, esophagus, and stomach. Abdominal pain, vomiting ... and bloody diarrhea. 2. Pallor, sweating, weakness, headache, dizziness, tinnitus. 3. Shock: Weak irregular pulse, hypotension, shallow respirations, cyanosis, pallor, and a profound fall in body temperature. 4. Possibly fleeting excitement and confusion, followed by unconsciousness. ... 5. Stentorous breathing, mucous rales, rhonchi, frothing at nose and mouth and other signs of pulmonary edema are sometimes seen. Characteristic odor of phenol on the breath. 6. Scanty, dark-colored ... urine ... moderately severe renal insufficiency may appear. 7. Methemoglobinemia, Heinz body hemolytic anemia and hyperbilirubinemia have been reported. ... 8. Death from respiratory, circulatory or cardiac failure. 9. If spilled on skin, pain is followed promptly by numbness. The skin becomes blanched, and a dry opaque eschar forms over the burn. When the eschar sloughs off, a brown stain remains.
Chlorpyrifos (found in 93% of Americans): Insecticide used on corn and cotton and for termite control. Conservative estimates hold that 80% of the chlorpyrifos in the US was produced directly or indirectly by Dow Chemical Corporation.[313] **This pesticide is routinely used in schools and is thus found in blood and tissue samples of nearly all American children.**	• Toxic if inhaled, in contact with skin, and if swallowed. • All the organophosphorus insecticides have a cumulative effect by progressive inhibition of cholinesterase. • The symptoms of chronic poisoning due to organophosphorus pesticides include headache, weakness, feeling of heaviness in head, decline of memory, quick onset of **fatigue**, **disturbed sleep**, loss of appetite, and loss of orientation. Other manifestations of accumulation include **tension, anxiety, restlessness, insomnia, headache, emotional instability, fatigue**… • Chlorpyrifos is a suspected endocrine disruptor.[314] • **Higher chlorpyrifos levels in children correlate with higher incidences attention problems, attention-deficit/hyperactivity disorder, and pervasive developmental disorder.[315]**

[312] Primary source for this data is the Hazardous Substances Data Bank, National Institutes of Health: http://toxnet.nlm.nih.gov/cgi-bin/sis/htmlgen?HSDB August 1, 2004
[313] Kristin S. Schafer, Margaret Reeves, Skip Spitzer, Susan E. Kegley. Chemical Trespass: Pesticides in Our Bodies and Corporate Accountability. Pesticide Action Network North America. May 2004 Available at http://www.panna.org/campaigns/docsTrespass/chemicalTrespass2004.dv.html on August 1, 2004
[314] http://www.panna.org/resources/documents/factsChlorpyrifos.dv.html accessed August 1, 2004
[315] "Highly exposed children (chlorpyrifos levels of >6.17 pg/g plasma) scored, on average, 6.5 points lower on the Bayley Psychomotor Development Index and 3.3 points lower on the Bayley Mental Development Index at 3 years of age compared with those with lower levels of exposure. Children exposed to higher, compared with lower, chlorpyrifos levels were also significantly more likely to experience Psychomotor Development Index and Mental Development Index delays, attention problems, attention-deficit/hyperactivity disorder problems, and pervasive developmental disorder problems at 3 years of age." Rauh VA, Garfinkel R, Perera FP, Andrews HF, Hoepner L, Barr DB, Whitehead R, Tang D, Whyatt RW. Impact of prenatal chlorpyrifos exposure on neurodevelopment in the first 3 years of life among inner-city children. *Pediatrics*. 2006 Dec;118(6):e1845-59

Examples of toxicants commonly found in Americans—*continued*

Environmental pollutant (population frequency)	*Biologic effects as quoted from HSDB*: Hazardous Substances Data Bank. National Library of Medicine, NIH[316] or other reference as noted
Mercury (8% of American women of reproductive age have mercury levels high enough to cause adverse health effects)	▪ Mercury is a well-known neurotoxin, immunotoxin, and nephrotoxin. Mercury toxicity is also a known cause of hypertension in humans. ▪ A recent study published in *JAMA—Journal of the American Medical Association*[317] noted that "Humans are exposed to methylmercury, a well-established neurotoxin, through fish consumption. The fetus is most sensitive to the adverse effects of exposure. … **approximately 8% of women had concentrations higher than the US EPA's recommended reference dose (5.8 microg/L),** below which exposures are considered to be without adverse effects." **The most obvious interpretation of this data published in *JAMA* is that 8% of American women have chronic mercury poisoning—poisoning in this case refers specifically to elevated blood levels of a known toxicant that consistently demonstrates adverse effects on human health.** Logical deduction holds that such a high prevalence of human poisoning should be unacceptable and should lead directly to legislative restrictions on corporate emissions to protect and salvage the health of the public.
2,4-dichlorophenol (found in 87% of Americans): Pesticide	▪ Human Toxicity Excerpts: same as for 2,5-dichlorophenol ▪ In males, significant increases in relative risk ratios for lung cancer, rectal cancer, and soft tissue sarcomas were reported; in females, there were increases in the relative risk of cervical cancer.

> **"The only thing necessary for the triumph of evil is for good men to do nothing."**
> **Edmond Burke (1729 – 1797)**
>
> "Your lack of interest in the past, your lack of involvement, your unwillingness to develop coherent strategies, your unwillingness to challenge authority - these have created a vacuum in decision-making, that has been filled by professional groups with close relationships with the chemical industries…" *Samuel Epstein, M.D.*[318]

Toxicity and detoxification—basics: The physiologic processes by which toxins—whether chemicals or metals—are referred to generally as "detoxification." Clinically, doctors can implement treatment interventions to promote and facilitate the removal of chemical and metal toxins; this, too, is generally referred to as detoxification or clinical/therapeutic detoxification programs. Detoxification programs are popular with patients and some doctors and are most often misused and misapplied.

The recent findings that mercury poisoning can result from once-weekly consumption of tuna[319] and that **the average American has 13 pesticides in his/her body**[320] should be seen as an indication of how dangerously toxic our environment has become, largely due to irresponsible corporate and government policies that value profitability over sustainability.

---

[316] Primary source for this data is the Hazardous Substances Data Bank, National Institutes of Health: http://toxnet.nlm.nih.gov/cgi-bin/sis/htmlgen?HSDB Accessed Aug 1, 2004
[317] Schober SE, Sinks TH, Jones RL, Bolger PM, McDowell M, Osterloh J, Garrett ES, Canady RA, Dillon CF, Sun Y, Joseph CB, Mahaffey KR. Blood mercury levels in US children and women of childbearing age, 1999-2000. *JAMA*. 2003 Apr 2;289(13):1667-74
[318] Samuel Epstein MD, 1993. Professor of Occupational and Environmental Medicine at the School of Public Health, University of Illinois Medical Center Chicago. http://www.converge.org.nz/pirm/pestican.htm accessed September 11, 2004
[319] "The neurobehavioral performance of subjects who consumed tuna fish regularly was significantly worse on color word reaction time, digit symbol reaction time and finger tapping speed (FT)." Carta P, Flore C, Alinovi R, Ibba A, Tocco MG, Aru G, Carta R, Girei E, Mutti A, Lucchini R, Randaccio FS. Sub-clinical neurobehavioral abnormalities associated with low level of mercury exposure through fish consumption. *Neurotoxicology*. 2003 Aug;24(4-5):617-23
[320] "A comprehensive survey of more than 1,300 Americans has found traces of weed- and bug-killers in the bodies of everyone tested, …. The survey, conducted by the U.S. Centers for Disease Control and Prevention, found that the body of the average American contained 13 of these chemicals." Martin Millelstaedt. 13 pesticides in body of average American. *The Globe and Mail*. Friday, May 21, 2004 - Page A17 Available on-line at http://www.theglobeandmail.com/servlet/ArticleNews/TPStory/LAC/20040521/HPEST21/TPEnvironment/ on August 6, 2004

Detoxification procedures: Though a detailed clinical explanation of detoxification procedures will not be included here, the general concepts for detoxification are as follows:

1. *Avoidance*: reduced exposure = reduced problem
   a. If there were less chemical pollution, then our environment would be less toxic and therefore we would not have such problems with environmental poisoning.
   b. Limit or eliminate exposure to paint fumes, car exhaust, new carpet, solvents, adhesives, artificial foods, synthetic chemical drugs, copier fumes, pesticides, herbicides, chemical fertilizers, etc.

2. *Depuration*: "The act or process of freeing from foreign or impure matter"[321]
   a. Exercise and sauna
   b. Bowel cleansing, fiber, probiotics, antibiotics, laxatives
   c. Liver and bile stimulators
   d. Cofactors for phase 1 oxidation and phase 2 conjugation
   e. Chelation for heavy metals
   f. Urine alkalinization

3. *Damage control*: managing the consequences of chemical and heavy metal toxicity
   a. Hormone replacement
   b. Antioxidant therapy
   c. Occupational and rehabilitative training
   d. Management of resultant diseases, particularly autoimmune diseases

4. *Political and social action*: Due in large part to corporate influence and government deregulation, environmental contamination with pesticides from American corporations has increased to such an extent over the past few decades that now all Americans show evidence of pesticide accumulation in their bodies. Failure to hold corporations to tight regulatory standards has jeopardized the future of humanity. Voter passivity combined with collusion between multinational corporations and government officials is the underlying problem. Political action is the solution. The past and recent history on this topic is clear and well documented for those who wish to access the facts.[322,323,324,325,326,327,328, 329,330]

---

[321] Webster's 1913 Dictionary

[322] Robert Van den Bosch. The pesticide conspiracy. Garden City, NY: Doubleday, 1978. ISBN: 0385133847

[323] "Monsanto Corporation is widely known for its production of the herbicide Roundup and genetically engineered Roundup-ready crops... altered to survive a dousing of the toxic herbicide. ...glyphosate, is known to cause eye soreness, headaches, diarrhea, and other flu-like symptoms, and has been linked to non-Hodgkin's lymphoma." Bush Names Former Monsanto Executive as EPA Deputy Administrator. Daily News Archive From March 29, 2001 http://www.beyondpesticides.org/NEWS/daily_news_archive/2001/03_29_01.htm accessed on August 1, 2004

[324] "They pointed to budgets cuts for research and enforcement, to steep declines in the number of cases filed against polluters, to efforts to relax portions of the Clean Air Act, to an acceleration of federal approvals for the spraying of restricted pesticides and more." Patricia Sullivan. Anne Gorsuch Burford, 62, Dies; Reagan EPA Director. *Washington Post*. Thursday, July 22, 2004; Page B06 http://www.washingtonpost.com/wp-dyn/articles/A3418-2004Jul21.html on August 2, 2004

[325] "In fact, amongst the crimes of Reagan and Bush which will go down in history are their emasculation of Federal regulatory apparatus... But in 1988, under the Bush administration, the EPA - illegally, in our view - revoked the Dellaney Law..." Samuel Epstein MD, 1993. Professor of Occupational and Environmental Medicine at the School of Public Health, University of Illinois Medical Center Chicago. http://www.converge.org.nz/pirm/pestican.htm accessed August 1, 2004

[326] "The Environmental Protection Agency will be free to approve pesticides without consulting wildlife agencies to determine if the chemical might harm plants and animals protected by the Endangered Species Act, according to new Bush administration rules.... It also is intended to head off future lawsuits, the officials said." Associated Press. Bush Eases Pesticide Laws http://www.cbsnews.com/stories/2004/07/29/tech/main633009.shtml accessed August 1, 2004

[327] "The new policy also could bolster pesticide makers' contention that federal labeling insulates them from suits alleging that their products cause illness or environmental damage, Olson says. 'It . . . could really be disastrous for public health.'" Bush Exempts Pesticide Companies from Lawsuits. Law on Pesticides Reinterpreted: Government Alters Policy in Effort to Protect Manufacturers. Peter Eisler. *USA TODAY*. October 6, 2003 http://www.organicconsumers.org/foodsafety/bushpesticides100703.cfm Accessed Aug 2004

[328] WASHINGTON (AP) — "The Environmental Protection Agency will be free to approve pesticides without consulting wildlife agencies to determine if the chemical might harm plants and animals protected by the Endangered Species Act, according to new Bush administration rules." Bush eases pesticide reviews for endangered species. http://www.usatoday.com/news/washington/2004-07-29-epa-pesticides_x.htm?csp=34 Accessed August 2004

[329] "It is simply intolerable that the EPA, instead of providing an example for open scientific discussion, has continuously violated key environmental legislation, stifling legitimate dissent. The failure of EPA to properly encourage and protect whistleblowing has undermined the ability of the EPA and state environmental agencies to enforce environmental laws." Letter to Carol Browner, Administrator U.S. Environmental Protection Agency from Stephen Kohn, Chair National Whistleblower Center Board of Directors dated March 23, 1999. Availble at http://www.whistleblowers.org/statements.htm on October 10, 2004

[330] "The Bush administration has imposed a gag order on the U.S. Environmental Protection Agency from publicly discussing perchlorate pollution, even as two new studies reveal high levels of the rocket-fuel component may be contaminating the nation's lettuce supply." Peter Waldman. Rocket Fuel Residues Found in Lettuce: Bush administration issues gag order on EPA discussions of possible rocket fuel tainted lettuce. *THE WALL STREET JOURNAL*. See http://www.organicconsumers.org/toxic/lettuce042903.cfm http://www.rhinoed.com/epa's_gag_order.htm http://www.peer.org/press/508.html http://yubanet.com/artman/publish/article_13637.shtml

Toxicant Exposure: solvents, pesticides, herbicides, plastics, fire-proofing, dioxins, exhaust, PCB, mercury, lead, cadmium, and thousands of others; the ultimate causes and therefore solutions are found primarily in addressing corporate environmental policies and influence on government regulations, societal structure/expectations regarding materialism/independence/convenience/passivity

Biological Persistence: lipolysis/redistribution; detoxification/reabsorption

Promote lipolysis with diet, exercise, sauna

lipophilic chemicals are deposited in cell membranes/adipose

metals circulate and are deposited in tissues where they impair function and thereby contribute to 'disease'

some heavy metals may alter detoxification

treatment

DMSA chelation

Phase One: activation / oxidation
Rapidly inducible by toxicant exposure and some drugs; the main clinical problems here are
1) **inhibition** by SNiPs, nutrient deficiencies, drugs, LPS, heavy metals
2) **relative excess activity**: rapid phase one in relation to slow conjugation: the body is not making a mistake here; it is simply responding to exposure; the solutions are to reduce exposure and support conjugation

Clinical Solutions:
1) nutritional supplementation and diet improvement,
2) reduce exposure to drugs and other 'inducers' including enterohepatic recirculation (check increased permeability and fecal b-glucuronidase)
3) clean the gut to restore mucosal integrity and reduce LPS and b-glucuronidase

hydration/urination, bile formation/expulsion, maintenance of conjugation, botanical adsorbents, daily defecation

failure

excretion in urine, excretion via bile flow and defecation

enterohepatic recirculation

insufficient oxidation

sufficient oxidation

sufficient oxidation

chemical toxicant accumulation: increased disease risk: autoimmunity, Parkinson's disease, cancer, multiple chemical sensitivity, adverse drug reactions

a few chemicals are excreted following Phase 1 (without Conjugation)

Phase Two: conjugation
Insufficiently induced by toxicant exposure; failure of conjugation following oxidation is highly problematic; the main clinical problems here are
1) **slow action**: phase 2 is commonly slower than phase 1; slow action can be caused by nutritional deficiencies, insufficient intake of vegetables/crucifers, and SNiPs, which are surprisingly common and are consistently associated with increased risk for disease;
2) **insufficient nutrient intake for conjugation**: recall that most conjugation factors are, of course, derived from foods: amino acids and sulphur

Clinical Solutions:
1) general nutritional supplementation and diet improvement,
2) reduce exposure to all endogenous and exogenous toxicants: drugs, chemicals, enterohepatic recirculation, hyperabsorption due to increased permeability and fecal b-glucuronidase
3) induce conjugation with cruciferous vegetables and specific botanicals
4) stimulate bile flow and bowel cleansing

insufficient conjugation

successful conjugation

hydration, healthy renal function (and alkalosis)

excretion in urine

Toxicant is solublized for excretion in bile or urine

failure of bile formation, blockage in bile flow, dehydration, dysbiosis causing deconjugation constipation promoting reabsorption, insufficient fiber

bile formation, bile expulsion, maintenance of conjugation, daily defecation

excretion via bile flow and defecation

enterohepatic recirculation

Overview of toxicant exposure and detoxification/depuration: Details are discussed in *Chapter 4*.[331]

[331] **Vasquez A**. *Integrative Rheumatology*. IBMRC: 2006, 2009. Updated as "*Inflammation Mastery*" starting in 2014.

Integrative/functional healthcare empowers patients with the ability to understand and effectively participate in the course of their life and health

Drug/surgery-based medicine	*Paradigm*	Holistic natural healthcare
• Doctor as "savior" and indifferent "objective" observer	*Role of the doctor*	• Doctor as "teacher" and active caring partner and co-participant in the process
• Helpless victim, disempowered, dependent	*Role of the patient*	• Active participant, empowered, responsible
• Illness is impossibly complex, and treating this with natural means is generally impossible • Treatment is simple: you have this disease, and you need to take one or more drugs for every problem • Diet and lifestyle modifications are generally viewed as secondary to drugs • The disease is more important than the patient	*Nature of illness*	• Multifactorial: involving many different aspects of lifestyle, diet, exercise, genetic inheritance, psychology, and environment • Many causes allows for many different treatment approaches and different ways of attaining health • Illness can be modified via selective dietary and lifestyle changes and a custom-tailored treatment plan • The patient is more important than the disease
• Disease-centered, drug-centered	*Viewpoint*	• Patient-centered, wellness-centered
• Drugs, including chemotherapy • Surgery • Radiation • Electroconvulsive treatment • Vaccinations	*Treatment and options*	• Diet and lifestyle improvement • Relationship/emotional work • Botanical and nutritional medicines • Physical medicine, chiropractic, exercise • Acupuncture • *Selective* rather than *first-line* use of pharmaceuticals and medical procedures
• Symptom suppression • Drug side-effects are a significant cause of death in the US • Only *treats disease*, does not *promote health*; cannot reach optimal health by only reactively treating established health problems • Enormous expense, often subsidized by private or public "insurance"	*Long-term outcome*	• Improved health • Potential for successful prevention, treatment or eradication of chronic disease • Potential to become optimally healthy • Proven cost-reduction
• Heightened risk, since drugs are foreign chemicals that have action in the body by interfering with the way that the body normally works • Every drug has side-effects, some of which can be life-threatening • Surgery causes irreparable changes to the body, often for the worse. • Radiation and chemotherapy can cause a secondary cancer to develop	*Risks*	• Reduced risk, since most of the botanical treatments and all of the nutritional medicines have been a major part of the human diet for centuries/millennia and have proven safety • Delayed onset of action: most treatments are not fast-acting enough to be of value in traumatic or acutely life-threatening situations • Patients must be willing to adopt healthier lifestyles
• Allows a doctor to see many patients within a short amount of time, thus increasing profitability • Since drugs do not cure problems, patients must return for lifelong prescription renewals • Therapeutic passivity: minimal action or effort required by patient and doctor • The doctor holds all the power, and the patient is completely dependent on the doctor for treatment	*Benefits*	• Improved short-term and long-term health • Empowerment • Understanding of body processes as well as healthcare directions and goals • Options

Health-promoting:

- Frequent exercise and physical activity
- Plenty of sleep
- Maintaining ideal body weight
- Avoiding exposure to chemicals, drugs, pollution, exhaust, tobacco smoke
- Daily consumption of fruits and vegetables
- Ideal protein intake for body size, physical activity, and health status
- Diet high in fiber and complex carbohydrates
- Use of health-promoting beverages such as green tea, fruit/vegetable juices, water, and light consumption of beer or red wine
- Increased intake of ALA, EPA, DHA, GLA, and oleic acid
- Multi-vitamin and multi-mineral supplementation
- Optimal vitamin D and iron status
- Beneficial gastrointestinal flora
- Natural and phytonutraceutical interventions to promote optimal health
- Pro-active healthcare
- Healthy and supportive relationships that foster responsibility, independence, interdependence, health and feelings of being wanted and cared for
- Work environments that promote collaboration and creativity and which appreciate personal time and allow for schedule flexibility

Disease-promoting:

- Physical inactivity and sedentary lifestyle
- Insufficient sleep
- Obesity
- Frequent exposure to chemicals, drugs, pollution, exhaust, tobacco smoke
- Daily consumption of processed and artificial foods
- Insufficient (common) or excessive (rare) protein
- Diet high in simple carbohydrates and sugars
- Use of disease-promoting beverages such as cola, artificially colored/flavored/sweetened drinks, and hard liquor
- Increased intake of linoleic acid (vegetable oils) and arachidonic acid (beef, liver, pork, lamb and most farm-raised land animals)
- Low intake of vitamins and minerals
- Excess iron and insufficient vitamin D
- Dysbiosis: intestinal overgrowth of yeast, parasites, and harmful bacteria
- Use of synthetic chemical drugs to suppress symptoms of poor health
- Reactive healthcare that only responds to problems after they have developed
- Dysfunctional relationships that enable and foster illness, dependency and isolation
- Work environments that promote isolation, pressure, perfectionism and which disapprove of creativity, personal time, and flexibility

Maximize factors that promote health ♦ Minimize factors that promote disease

Opposite influences of health promotion vs. disease promotion: Lifestyle concept: Improved clinical outcomes will be attained when doctors and patients attend to both **prescription of health-promoting activities** and **proscription of disease-promoting activities**. Indeed, attention needs to be given to the **ratio** of these disparate and opposing forces, which ultimately influence genetic expression and physiologic function of many organ systems.

Chapter 3:
Basic Concepts and Therapeutics in Musculoskeletal Care

Introduction
Nonpharmacologic management of musculoskeletal problem should be seen as the treatment of choice because of the collateral benefits, safety, and cost-effectiveness associated with manual, dietary, botanical, and physiologic/physiotherapeutic treatments. Note: In order for this book to be printed in a single volume (limit 630 pages) for the Bastyr University Rheumatology course, this chapter, which contains information which the Naturopathic Medicine students at Bastyr University have already covered in other courses, had to be shortened. Students wanting to review the information from this chapter can review the previous editions of *Integrative Rheaumatology* (2006, 2007) or the more complete version in *Integrative Orthopedics* (2012) or await the multivolume compete version of the new *Inflammation Mastery* series in 2014. In addition to reformatting this chapter by removing spacing, condensing sections, minimizing the font in the footnotes from 7 to 6 points and in the text from 10 to 9.5 points (for this chapter only), the following sections were removed: • Myofascial trigger points (MFTP): diagnosis and treatment • Musculoskeletal Manipulative Manual Medicine • Proprioceptive retraining/rehabilitation • Reasons to avoid the use of nonsteroidal anti-inflammatory drugs (NSAIDs) and COX-2 inhibitors (coxibs)

<u>Topics:</u>
- Comprehensive Musculoskeletal Care
  - Protect, prevent re-injury
  - Relative rest
  - Ice/heat, individualize treatment
  - Compression
  - Elevation, establish treatment program
  - Anti-inflammatory & analgesic treatments
  - Treat with physical/manual medicine
  - Uncover the underlying problem
  - Re-educate, rehabilitate, resourcefulness, return to active life, refer to specialist
  - Nutrition, diet, and supplements
- BENDSTEMS: A useful clinical acronym

<u>Introduction</u>: Whether dealing with a *recent and acutely painful injury* or an *exacerbation of a chronic injury or musculoskeletal disease*, all integrative clinicians are wise to have at their disposal a comprehensive protocol for the management of acute and subacute pain and exacerbations of joint inflammation. Incompetence in musculoskeletal medicine, which is common among allopathic physicians[1,2,3,4,5], forces doctors to overuse simplistic and dangerous treatments (i.e., pharmaceutical drugs) because they are unaware of better options.[6] Failure to understand how to arrive at an accurate diagnosis and subsequent failure to know how to manage musculoskeletal pain leaves doctors *and thus their patients* with no other option than the overuse of so-called anti-inflammatory drugs such as non-steroidal anti-inflammatory drugs (NSAIDs, such as

---

[1] Joy EA, Hala SV. Musculoskeletal Curricula in Medical Education: Filling In the Missing Pieces. *The Physician and Sportsmedicine*. 2004; 32: 42-45
[2] Freedman KB, Bernstein J. The adequacy of medical school education in musculoskeletal medicine. *J Bone Joint Surg Am*. 1998;80(10):1421-7
[3] Freedman KB, Bernstein J. Educational deficiencies in musculoskeletal medicine. *J Bone Joint Surg Am*. 2002;84-A(4):604-8
[4] Matzkin E, Smith ME, Freccero CD, Richardson AB. Adequacy of education in musculoskeletal medicine. *J Bone Joint Surg Am*. 2005 Feb;87-A(2):310-4
[5] Schmale GA. More evidence of educational inadequacies in musculoskeletal medicine. *Clin Orthop Relat Res*. 2005 Aug;(437):251-9
[6] Vasquez A. The Importance of Integrative Chiropractic Health Care in Treating Musculoskeletal Pain and Reducing the Nationwide Burden of Medical Expenses and Iatrogenic Injury and Death: Concise Review of Current Research and Implications for Clinical Practice and Healthcare Policy. *The Original Internist* 2005;12:159-182

aspirin), which kill at least 17,000 patients per year[7], and the cyclooxygenase-2 inhibiting drugs (COX-2 inhibitors, coxibs, such as Vioxx and Celebrex) which have killed tens of thousands of patients.[8,9,10,11] Previously, any medical treatment that was non-surgical was commonly described as "conservative" simply because it was *non-invasive/non-surgical*. However, many so-called "conservative" drug treatments are dangerously lethal and expensive, as the coxibs, with their lethality and high costs, have demonstrated. Further, "conservative" has become such a confusing term in modern politics that even people who identify themselves as such are often at a loss for an accurate definition of the term. Thus, I have replaced the previous "holistic conservative care" with the current "comprehensive acute care" to indicate the consideration and selective implementation of the treatments described in this chapter.

Throughout the other chapters this text, when the phrase "**comprehensive musculoskeletal care**" is included in the list of therapeutic considerations, readers should understand that this implies these treatments for musculoskeletal problems *in addition to reestablishing the foundation for health*, which was detailed in Chapter 2. While all of us are familiar with the components of basic care for injuries—"*rice*": r̲est, i̲ce, c̲ompression, e̲levation—I have expanded this list to include p̲rotect, prevent re-injury, r̲elative rest, i̲ce, individualize treatment, c̲ompression, e̲levation, establish treatment program, a̲nti-inflammatory and analgesic treatments, t̲reat with physical/manual medicine, u̲ncover the underlying problem, r̲e-educate, rehabilitation, retrain, resourcefulness, return to active life, and n̲utrition including diet and nutritional and botanical supplements. The mnemonic acronym spells "*price a turn*" which is cumbersome but perhaps easy to remember and therefore useful. The major point is to think outside of the "rice" box; as integrative clinicians, we have much more to offer our patients than rest, ice, compression, and elevation. Understanding the shorthand that is conveyed by *comprehensive musculoskeletal care* is important for grasping the important differences between our medicine and the myopic and pharmacocentric allopathic approach. Whereas the allopathic approach stops with minimal disease treatment and provides essentially nothing in terms of prevention or comprehensive patient management—let alone promotion of optimal health—the holistic and integrative approach is centered on the *patient* and seeks to help him/her attain optimal health while being treated for the musculoskeletal disorder. We can and must help our patients attain optimal health while effectively managing their acute and chronic musculoskeletal problems.[12,13,14] **Indeed, since for many patients their only interaction with the healthcare system is when they are injured, we must seize upon this opportunity to enroll patients in preventive and pro-active healthcare.**

Basic Treatment Concepts and Commonly Employed Therapeutics

The following pages summarize the basic therapeutics most commonly employed by integrative physicians in the treatment of acute and chronic musculoskeletal conditions. Knowledge of some of the clinical skills relied upon in orthopedics is necessary when treating rheumatic musculoskeletal problems because an acutely inflamed joint associated with a *chronic* and *systemic* disorder may need to be treated as if it were a *recent* and *focal* injury.

Orthopedics generally centers on the clinical management of 1) **acute injuries** (e.g., whiplash), 2) **chronic injuries** (tendonitis and myofasciitis/myofascitis), and 3) **congenital/developmental anomalies**, (odontoid hypoplasia and scoliosis). For most clinicians, management of congenital anomalies centers on accurate diagnosis and then either observation or appropriate referral. For the treatment of common acute and chronic injuries encountered in general practice, **comprehensive acute care** can include the facets described in the following section, modified for the clinical situation and individual patient. Although *rheumatology* is generally concerned with the treatment of *non-traumatic* disorders of an inflammatory or autoimmune nature, knowledge of orthopedics is necessary during the course of evaluating and treating patients with autoimmunity because differential diagnosis, qualification/quantification, and comanagement of joint disorders *within the same patient* are commonly necessary. For example, a patient with rheumatoid arthritis (chronic autoimmune disease) affecting the knees and hips may also develop carpal tunnel syndrome (orthopedic problem) and later present with neck pain and leg spasticity secondary to atlantoaxial instability (neuro-orthopedic emergency). Generally, different types and locations of injuries can be treated from a common framework of interventions that are then customized for the three following primary considerations:

[7] Singh G. Recent considerations in nonsteroidal anti-inflammatory drug gastropathy. *Am J Med.* 1998;105(1B):31S-38S
[8] "The results from VIGOR showed that the relative risk of developing a confirmed adjudicated thrombotic cardiovascular event (myocardial infarction, unstable angina, cardiac thrombus, resuscitated cardiac arrest, sudden or unexplained death, ischemic stroke, and transient ischemic attacks) with rofecoxib treatment compared with naproxen was 2.38." Mukherjee D, Nissen SE, Topol EJ. Risk of cardiovascular events associated with selective COX-2 inhibitors. *JAMA.* 2001 Aug 22-29;286(8):954-9
[9] Topol EJ. Failing the public health--rofecoxib, Merck, and the FDA. *N Engl J Med.* 2004 Oct 21;351(17):1707-9
[10] Ray WA, Griffin MR, Stein CM. Cardiovascular toxicity of valdecoxib. *N Engl J Med.* 2004;351(26):2767
[11] "Patients in the clinical trial taking 400 mg. of Celebrex twice daily had a 3.4 times greater risk of CV events compared to placebo. For patients in the trial taking 200 mg. of Celebrex twice daily, the risk was 2.5 times greater. The average duration of treatment in the trial was 33 months." FDA Statement on the Halting of a Clinical Trial of the cox-2 Inhibitor Celebrex. http://www.fda.gov/bbs/topics/news/2004/NEW01144.html Available on January 4, 2005
[12] Vasquez A. New Insights into Fatty Acid Supplementation and Its Effect on Eicosanoid Production and Genetic Expression. *Nutritional Perspectives* 2005; January: 5-16
[13] Vasquez A. Improving overall health while safely and effectively treating musculoskeletal pain. *Nutritional Perspectives* 2005; 28: 34-38, 40-42
[14] Vasquez A. The Importance of Integrative Chiropractic Health Care in Treating Musculoskeletal Pain and Reducing the Nationwide Burden of Medical Expenses and Iatrogenic Injury and Death: A Concise Review of Current Research and Implications for Clinical Practice and Healthcare Policy. *The Original Internist* 2005; 12(4): 159-182

1) <u>Location</u>: The specific location and associated functional considerations, e.g., lower extremity injuries may require crutches while upper extremity injuries may benefit from a brace or sling,

2) <u>Tissue</u>: The type of tissue that is injured—i.e., muscle, cartilage, tendons, or ligaments—may respond to a particular nutritional and rehabilitative protocol,

3) <u>Patient</u>: The specific goals, needs, comorbidities, medications, occupation, recreational activities, age, and other characteristics of the individual patient.

Protect & prevent re-injury:

- **Avoid motions and activities that cause significant pain, as pain indicates that damaged/inflamed tissues are being stressed.** The goals are 1) to allow healing of injured tissues, and 2) to promote maximal physical restoration and functional ability. An excess of rest promotes functional disability, muscle atrophy, and psychological dysfunction (e.g., iatrogenic neurosis, inaccurate perception of patient being permanently damaged or defective, loss of confidence, loss of social contact [especially for children, and adults for whom physical activity is important]). Returning to activities and work too quickly may not allow time for sufficient healing and may thus promote re-injury, temporary exacerbation, progression from mild to severe injury, and/or progression to repetitive strain injury.
- **Use bracing, taping, bandages, wrapping, canes, crutches, and walkers as needed.**[15,16]

Relative rest:

- **"Relative rest" simply means to take time away from the activities that either promote additional injury or that unnecessarily drain energies which could otherwise be used for healing and recuperation.** For some patients, this means avoiding certain exercises during a workout, while for other patients this may mean using a crutch or taking days off from work.
- "Bed rest" is generally to be avoided since it promotes muscle atrophy, intraarticular adhesions, loss of neuromuscular coordination, constipation, and patients' assumption of the sick role.[17]

Ice/heat:

- **First 48-72 hours after injury: Apply ice or cold pack for 10 minutes each 30-60 minutes for reduction in pain and inflammation.** The best protocol appears to be interrupted application of ice to maximize deep cooling of tissues while minimizing cold-induced damage to the skin.[18] Ice massage is more effective than stationary application of ice or an ice bag.[19] Intraarticular temperatures can be lowered with topical application of ice[20], and immersion into ice water appears to be the best method for reducing intraarticular temperature according to an animal study.[21] Greater skin thickness due to subcutaneous adipose increases the amount of time needed to achieve clinically significant cooling of deep tissues.[22] Avoid frostbite and cold injuries to skin and superficial nerves. Use caution in patients with decreased skin sensitivity, circulatory insufficiency, and/or suboptimal ability to follow directions and employ good judgment.
- **After 48-72 hours post-injury: Apply gentle heat as needed for the relief of pain and reduction in muscle spasm and to promote healing by increasing circulation.** Avoid heat injuries to skin. Use caution in patients with decreased skin sensitivity (e.g., diabetics and the elderly) or suboptimal ability to follow directions and employ good judgment.

Individualize treatment:

- **The cornerstone of effective holistic and integrative treatment is to design treatment plans that simultaneously 1) address "the problem" while also 2) improving the patient's overall health.** Often, serious and so-called "untreatable" diseases can be ameliorated or eradicated simply with general, non-specific, overall health improvement even when these conditions repeatedly fail to respond to specific "disease-targeting" medical treatments.

Compression:

- Snug bandages/wraps may help to reduce swelling and can provide support for injured tissues and weakened joints. Care must be utilized to avoid arterial, venous, or lymphatic obstruction.

[15] Van Hook FW, Demonbreun D, Weiss BD. Ambulatory devices for chronic gait disorders in the elderly. *Am Fam Physician*. 2003 Apr 15;67(8):1717-24 http://www.aafp.org/afp/20030415/1717.html
[16] Joyce BM, Kirby RL. Canes, crutches and walkers. *Am Fam Physician*. 1991 Feb;43(2):535-42
[17] "Glucose intolerance, anorexia, constipation, and pressure sores might develop. Central nervous system changes could affect balance and coordination and lead to increasing dependence on caregivers." Teasell R, Dittmer DK. Complications of immobilization and bed rest. Part 2: Other complications. *Can Fam Physician*. 1993 Jun;39:1440-2, 1445-6
[18] "The evidence from this systematic review suggests that melting iced water applied through a wet towel for repeated periods of 10 minutes is most effective." MacAuley DC. Ice therapy: how good is the evidence? *Int J Sports Med*. 2001 Jul;22(5):379-84
[19] Zemke JE, et al. Intramuscular temperature responses in the human leg to two forms of cryotherapy: ice massage and ice bag. *J Orthop Sports Phys Ther*. 1998 Apr;27(4):301-7
[20] Martin SS, Spindler KP, Tarter JW, Detwiler K, Petersen HA. Cryotherapy: an effective modality for decreasing intraarticular temperature after knee arthroscopy. *Am J Sports Med*. 2001 May-Jun;29:288-91
[21] Bocobo C, Fast A, Kingery W, Kaplan M. The effect of ice on intra-articular temperature in the knee of the dog. *Am J Phys Med Rehabil*. 1991 Aug;70(4):181-5
[22] Otte JW, Merrick MA, Ingersoll CD, Cordova ML. Subcutaneous adipose tissue thickness alters cooling time during cryotherapy. *Arch Phys Med Rehabil*. 2002 Nov;83(11):1501-5

<u>*Educate, establish treatment program, elevation*</u>:
- Educate patient about the injury.
- Educate patient about the need for appropriate follow-up office visits for reexamination, reassessment, and treatment.
- Estimate the amount of time during which most recovery will take place.
- Estimate the extent of return to previous status.
- Elevate the injured part to minimize swelling and edema.

<u>*Anti-inflammatory & analgesic treatments*</u>:
- <u>Anti-inflammation versus hemostasis</u>: Anti-inflammatory/analgesic medications that impair coagulation (e.g., aspirin) are contraindicated in patients with possible internal bleeding such as severe hematoma, hemarthrosis, spleen injury, intracranial hemorrhage (i.e., subdural hematoma following a whiplash injury) and in patients about to undergo surgery. Caution might also be used with nutritional/botanical supplements that have anti-coagulant effects, such as *Ginkgo biloba*[23] and garlic.[24]
- <u>Avoidance of pro-inflammatory foods</u>: **Arachidonic acid** (high in cow's milk, beef, liver, pork, and lamb) is the direct precursor to pro-inflammatory prostaglandins and leukotrienes[25] and pain-promoting isoprostanes.[26] **Saturated fats** promote inflammation by activating/enabling pro-inflammatory Toll-like receptors, which are otherwise "specific" for inducing pro-inflammatory responses to microorganisms.[27] Consumption of saturated fat in the form of **cream** creates marked oxidative stress and lipid peroxidation that lasts for at least 3 hours postprandially.[28] **Corn oil** rapidly activates NF-kappaB (in hepatic Kupffer cells) for a pro-inflammatory effect[29]; similarly, consumption of PUFA and linoleic acid promotes intracellular antioxidant depletion and may thus promote oxidation-mediated inflammation via activation of NF-kappaB. **Linoleic acid** causes intracellular oxidative stress and calcium influx and results in increased NF-kappaB-stimulated transcription of pro-inflammatory genes.[30] **High glycemic foods** cause oxidative stress[31,32] and inflammation via activation of NF-kappaB and other mechanisms—e.g., *white bread causes inflammation*[33] as **does a high-fat high-carbohydrate fast-food breakfast.**[34] **High glycemic foods** suppress immune function[35,36] and thus promote the development of infection/dysbiosis.[37] Delivery of a **high carbohydrate load** to the gastrointestinal lumen promotes bacterial overgrowth[38,39], which is inherently pro-inflammatory[40,41] and which appears to be myalgenic in humans[42] at least in part due to the ability of endotoxin to impair muscle function.[43] Overconsumption of high-carbohydrate low-phytonutrient **grains, potatoes, and manufactured foods** displaces phytonutrient-dense foods such as fruits,

[23] "A structured assessment of published case reports suggests a possible causal association between using ginkgo and bleeding events… Patients using ginkgo, particularly those with known bleeding risks, should be counseled about a possible increase in bleeding risk." Bent S, Goldberg H, Padula A, Avins AL. Spontaneous bleeding associated with ginkgo biloba: a case report and systematic review of the literature: a case report and systematic review of the literature. *J Gen Intern Med.* 2005 Jul;20(7):657-61 http://www.pubmedcentral.gov/picrender.fcgi?artid=1490168&blobtype=pdf

[24] "The authors report a case of spontaneous spinal epidural hematoma causing paraplegia secondary to a qualitative platelet disorder from excessive garlic ingestion." Rose KD, Croissant PD, Parliament CF, Levin MB. Spontaneous spinal epidural hematoma with associated platelet dysfunction from excessive garlic ingestion: a case report. *Neurosurgery.* 1990 May;26(5):880-2

[25] Vasquez A. Reducing Pain and Inflammation Naturally. Part 2: New Insights into Fatty Acid Supplementation and Its Effect on Eicosanoid Production and Genetic Expression. *Nutritional Perspectives* 2005; January: 5-16

[26] Evans AR, Junger H, Southall MD, Nicol GD, Sorkin LS, Broome JT, Bailey TW, Vasko MR. Isoprostanes, novel eicosanoids that produce nociception and sensitize rat sensory neurons. *J Pharmacol Exp Ther.* 2000 Jun;293(3):912-20

[27] Lee JY, Sohn KH, Rhee SH, Hwang D. Saturated fatty acids, but not unsaturated fatty acids, induce the expression of cyclooxygenase-2 mediated through Toll-like receptor 4. *J Biol Chem.* 2001 May 18;276(20):16683-9. Epub 2001 Mar 2 http://www.jbc.org/cgi/content/full/276/20/16683

[28] "CONCLUSIONS: Both fat and protein intakes stimulate ROS generation. The increase in ROS generation lasted 3 h after cream intake and 1 h after protein intake. Cream intake also caused a significant and prolonged increase in lipid peroxidation." Mohanty P, Ghanim H, Hamouda W, Aljada A, Garg R, Dandona P. Both lipid and protein intakes stimulate increased generation of reactive oxygen species by polymorphonuclear leukocytes and mononuclear cells. *Am J Clin Nutr.* 2002 Apr;75(4):767-72 http://www.ajcn.org/cgi/content/full/75/4/767

[29] Rusyn I, Bradham CA, Cohn L, Schoonhoven R, Swenberg JA, Brenner DA, Thurman RG. Corn oil rapidly activates nuclear factor-kappaB in hepatic Kupffer cells by oxidant-dependent mechanisms. *Carcinogenesis.* 1999 Nov;20(11):2095-100 http://carcin.oxfordjournals.org/cgi/content/full/20/11/2095

[30] "Exposing endothelial cells to 90 micromol linoleic acid/L for 6 h resulted in a significant increase in lipid hydroperoxides that coincided wih an increase in intracellular calcium concentrations." Hennig B, Toborek M, Joshi-Barve S, Barger SW, Barve S, Mattson MP, McClain CJ. Linoleic acid activates nuclear transcription factor-kappa B (NF-kappa B) and induces NF-kappa B-dependent transcription in cultured endothelial cells. *Am J Clin Nutr.* 1996 Mar;63(3):322-8 http://www.ajcn.org/cgi/reprint/63/3/322

[31] Mohanty P, Hamouda W, Garg R, Aljada A, Ghanim H, Dandona P. Glucose challenge stimulates reactive oxygen species (ROS) generation by leucocytes. *J Clin Endocrinol Metab.* 2000 Aug;85(8):2970-3 http://jcem.endojournals.org/cgi/content/full/85/8/2970 Glucose/carbohydrate and saturated fat consumption appear to be the two biggest offenders in the food-stimulated production of oxidative stress. The effect by protein is much less. "CONCLUSIONS: Both fat and protein intakes stimulate ROS generation. The increase in ROS generation lasted 3 h after cream intake and 1 h after protein intake. Cream intake also caused a significant and prolonged increase in lipid peroxidation." Mohanty P, Ghanim H, Hamouda W, Aljada A, Garg R, Dandona P. Both lipid and protein intakes stimulate increased generation of reactive oxygen species by polymorphonuclear leukocytes and mononuclear cells. *Am J Clin Nutr.* 2002 Apr;75(4):767-72 http://www.ajcn.org/cgi/content/full/75/4/767

[32] Koska J, Blazicek P, Marko M, Grna JD, Kvetnansky R, Vigas M. Insulin, catecholamines, glucose and antioxidant enzymes in oxidative damage during different loads in healthy humans. *Physiol Res.* 2000;49 Suppl 1:S95-100 http://www.biomed.cas.cz/physiolres/pdf/2000/49_S95.pdf

[33] "Conclusion - The present study shows that high GI carbohydrate, but not low GI carbohydrate, mediates an acute proinflammatory process as measured by NF-kappaB activity." Dickinson S, Hancock DP, Petocz P, Brand-Miller JC. High glycemic index carbohydrate mediates an acute proinflammatory process as measured by NF-kappaB activation. *Asia Pac J Clin Nutr.* 2005;14 Suppl:S120

[34] Aljada A, Mohanty P, Ghanim H, Abdo T, Tripathy D, Chaudhuri A, Dandona P. Increase in intranuclear nuclear factor kappaB and decrease in inhibitor kappaB in mononuclear cells after a mixed meal: evidence for a proinflammatory effect. *Am J Clin Nutr.* 2004 Apr;79(4):682-90 http://www.ajcn.org/cgi/content/full/79/4/682

[35] Sanchez A, Reeser JL, Lau HS, et al. Role of sugars in human neutrophilic phagocytosis. *Am J Clin Nutr.* 1973 Nov;26(11):1180-4

[36] "Postoperative infusion of carbohydrate solution leads to moderate fall in the serum concentration of inorganic phosphate. ... The hypophosphatemia was associated with significant reduction of neutrophil phagocytosis, intracellular killing, consumption of oxygen and generation of superoxide during phagocytosis." Rasmussen A, Segel E, Hessov I, Borregaard N. Reduced function of neutrophils during routine postoperative glucose infusion. *Acta Chir Scand.* 1988 Jul-Aug;154(7-8):429-33

[37] Vasquez A. Reducing Pain and Inflammation Naturally. Part 6: Nutritional and Botanical Treatments Against "Silent Infections" and Gastrointestinal Dysbiosis, Commonly Overlooked Causes of Neuromusculoskeletal Inflammation and Chronic Health Problems. *Nutritional Perspectives* 2006; January

[38] Ramakrishnan T, Stokes P. Beneficial effects of fasting and low carbohydrate diet in D-lactic acidosis associated with short-bowel syndrome. *JPEN J Parenter Enteral Nutr.* 1985 May-Jun;9(3):361-3

[39] Gottschall E. *Breaking the Vicious Cycle: Intestinal Health Through Diet.* Kirkton Press; Rev edition (August 1, 1994)

[40] Lin HC. Small intestinal bacterial overgrowth: a framework for understanding irritable bowel syndrome. *JAMA.* 2004 Aug 18;292(7):852-8

[41] Simmons SN, Wang J, Sartor RB, Bender D, Dalldorf FG, Schwab JH. Reactivation of arthritis induced by small bowel bacterial overgrowth in rats: role of cytokines, bacteria, and bacterial polymers. *Infect Immun.* 1995 Jun;63(6):2295-301

[42] Pimentel M, et al. A link between irritable bowel syndrome and fibromyalgia may be related to findings on lactulose breath testing. *Ann Rheum Dis.* 2004 Apr;63(4):450-2

[43] Bundgaard H, Kjeldsen K, Suarez Krabbe K, van Hall G, Simonsen L, Qvist J, Hansen CM, Moller K, Fonsmark L, Lav Madsen P, Klarlund Pedersen B. Endotoxemia stimulates skeletal muscle Na+-K+-ATPase and raises blood lactate under aerobic conditions in humans. *Am J Physiol Heart Circ Physiol.* 2003 Mar;284(3):H1028-34. Epub 2002 Nov 21 http://ajpheart.physiology.org/cgi/reprint/284/3/H1028

vegetables, nuts, seeds, and berries which contain more than 8,000 phytonutrients, many of which have antioxidant and thus anti-inflammatory actions.[44,45]

- Anti-inflammatory diet, the "supplemented Paleo-Mediterranean diet": The health-promoting diet of choice for the majority of people is a diet based on **abundant consumption of fruits, vegetables, seeds, nuts, berries, omega-3 and monounsaturated fatty acids, and lean sources of protein such as lean meats, fatty cold-water fish, soy and whey proteins.** This diet obviates overconsumption of chemical preservatives, artificial sweeteners, and carbohydrate-dominant foods such as candies, pastries, breads, potatoes, grains, and other foods with a high glycemic load and high glycemic index. This "Paleo-Mediterranean Diet" is a combination of the "Paleolithic" or "Paleo diet" and the well-known "Mediterranean diet", both of which are well described in peer-reviewed journals and the lay press, particularly by Eaton[46], O'Keefe[47], and Cordain.[48] See Chapter 2 and my other reviews[49,50] for details. This diet is the most nutrient-dense diet available, and its benefits are further enhanced by supplementation with vitamins, minerals, probiotics, and the health-promoting polyunsaturated fatty acids: ALA, GLA, EPA, DHA.

- Anti-inflammatory nutrients and botanicals: Nutritional and botanical therapeutics are prescribed *per patient* and *per condition*. Select botanicals and therapeutics are detailed later in this book. Doses listed are for adults and can be reduced when numerous interventions are simultaneously applied.
  - Fish oil, EPA with DHA: Three grams per day (3,000 mg/d) of combined EPA and DHA is a reasonable therapeutic dose[51] and is generally supplied in one tablespoon of liquid fish oil. Encapsulated fish oil supplements vary tremendously in their concentration of EPA and DHA and may require consumption of as few as five and as many as 21 capsules per day to achieve the same dosage and of EPA+DHA found in one tablespoon of liquid fish oil; encapsulated fish oil supplements also generally cost significantly more than do liquid fish oil supplements. The routine use of eicosapentaenoic acid (EPA) and docosahexaenoic acid (DHA) supplements is justified based on the following data:
    1. Most modern diets are profoundly deficient in omega-3 fatty acids.[52]
    2. Dietary/supplemental intake of omega-3 fatty acids is a necessary prerequisite to reducing the pro-inflammatory effects of omega-6 fatty acids.[53]
    3. Supplementation with EPA+DHA is safe and reduces all-cause mortality.[54]
    4. Supplementation with EPA+DHA consistently provides clinically significant benefits in the treatment of a wide range of inflammatory conditions.[55,56]
  - GLA, Gamma-linolenic acid: Approximately 500 mg per day is the common anti-inflammatory dose[57] although higher doses of 2.8 grams per day have been safely used in patients with rheumatoid arthritis.[58] Except in the rarest circumstances (perhaps including temporal lobe epilepsy[59]), **GLA (most concentrated in borage oil) should always be co-administered with EPA and DHA (from fish oil) in order to obtain maximal benefit and avoid the increased formation of arachidonic acid that occurs when GLA is administered alone and the reduction in GLA/DGLA that occurs when fish oil is**

---

[44] "We propose that the additive and synergistic effects of phytochemicals in fruit and vegetables are responsible for their potent antioxidant and anticancer activities, and that the benefit of a diet rich in fruit and vegetables is attributed to the complex mixture of phytochemicals present in whole foods." Liu RH. Health benefits of fruit and vegetables are from additive and synergistic combinations of phytochemicals. *Am J Clin Nutr*. 2003 Sep;78(3 Suppl):517S-520S

[45] Seaman DR. The diet-induced proinflammatory state: a cause of chronic pain and other degenerative diseases? *J Manipulative Physiol Ther*. 2002;25(3):168-79

[46] Eaton SB, Shostak M, Konner M. *The Paleolithic Prescription*, New York: Harper & Row, 1988

[47] O'Keefe JH Jr, Cordain L. Cardiovascular disease resulting from a diet and lifestyle at odds with our Paleolithic genome: how to become a 21st-century hunter-gatherer. *Mayo Clin Proc*. 2004 Jan;79:101-8

[48] Cordain L. *The Paleo Diet*. Indianapolis; John Wiley and Sons, 2002

[49] Vasquez A. A Five-Part Nutritional Protocol that Produces Consistently Positive Results. *Nutritional Wellness* 2005 September

[50] Vasquez A. Implementing the Five-Part Nutritional Wellness Protocol for the Treatment of Various Health Problems. *Nutritional Wellness* 2005 November

[51] "...clinical benefits of the n-3 fatty acids were not apparent until they were consumed for > or =12 wk. It appears that a minimum daily dose of 3 g eicosapentaenoic and docosahexaenoic acids is necessary to derive the expected benefits [in patients with rheumatoid arthritis]." Kremer JM. n-3 fatty acid supplements in rheumatoid arthritis. *Am J Clin Nutr*. 2000;71(1Suppl):349S-51S

[52] Simopoulos AP. Essential fatty acids in health and chronic disease. *Am J Clin Nutr*. 1999 Sep;70(3 Suppl):560S-569S

[53] Rubin D, Laposata M. Cellular interactions between n-6 and n-3 fatty acids: a mass analysis of fatty acid elongation/desaturation, distribution among complex lipids, and conversion to eicosanoids. *J Lipid Res*. 1992 Oct;33(10):1431-40.

[54] "The recent GISSI (Gruppo Italiano per lo Studio della Sopravvivenza nell'Infarto miocardico)-Prevention study of 11,324 patients showed a 45% decrease in risk of sudden cardiac death and a 20% reduction in all-cause mortality in the group taking 850 mg/d of omega-3 fatty acids. These fatty acids have potent anti-inflammatory effects and may also be antiatherogenic." O'Keefe JH Jr, Harris WS. From Inuit to implementation: omega-3 fatty acids come of age. *Mayo Clin Proc*. 2000 Jun;75(6):607-14

[55] "Many of the placebo-controlled trials of fish oil in chronic inflammatory diseases reveal significant benefit, including decreased disease activity and a lowered use of anti-inflammatory drugs." Simopoulos AP. Omega-3 fatty acids in inflammation and autoimmune diseases. *J Am Coll Nutr*. 2002 Dec;21(6):495-505

[56] Vasquez A. Reducing Pain and Inflammation Naturally. Part 2: New Insights into Fatty Acid Supplementation and Its Effect on Eicosanoid Production and Genetic Expression. *Nutritional Perspectives* 2005; January: 5-16

[57] "Forty patients with rheumatoid arthritis and upper gastrointestinal lesions due to non-steroidal anti-inflammatory drugs entered a prospective 6-month double-blind placebo controlled study of dietary supplementation with gamma-linolenic acid 540 mg/day..." Brzeski M, Madhok R, Capell HA. Evening primrose oil in patients with rheumatoid arthritis and side-effects of non-steroidal anti-inflammatory drugs. *Br J Rheumatol*. 1991 Oct;30(5):370-2

[58] Zurier RB, Rossetti RG, Jacobson EW, DeMarco DM, Liu NY, Temming JE, White BM, Laposata M. gamma-Linolenic acid treatment of rheumatoid arthritis. A randomized, placebo-controlled trial. *Arthritis Rheum*. 1996 Nov;39(11):1808-17

[59] "Three long-stay, hospitalised schizophrenics who had failed to respond adequately to conventional drug therapy were treated with gamma-linolenic acid and linoleic acid in the form of evening primrose oil. They became substantially worse and electroencephalographic features of temporal lobe epilepsy became apparent." Vaddadi KS. The use of gamma-linolenic acid and linoleic acid to differentiate between temporal lobe epilepsy and schizophrenia. *Prostaglandins Med*. 1981 Apr;6(4):375-9

administered alone. For more details on fatty acid metabolism, see the final chapter in this text on *Therapeutics* and the 2005 fatty acid review published by Vasquez available on-line.[60]

o *Uncaria guianensis* and *Uncaria tomentosa* ("cat's claw", "una de gato"): A double-blind placebo-controlled study using 100 mg daily of highly-concentrated freeze-dried aqueous extract of *Uncaria tomentosa* found significant pain relief (reduction by 36%) and minimal adverse effects after 4 weeks of treatment in 30 male patients with osteoarthritis of the knees, a benefit mediated via antioxidant activities and inhibition of NF-kappaB, TNFα, COX-2, and PGE-2 production.[61] Inhibition of NF-kappaB and iNOS are of primary importance in the treatment of inflammatory conditions.[62] A year-long study of patients with active rheumatoid arthritis (RA) treated with sulfasalazine or hydroxychloroquine showed "relative safety and modest benefit" of coadministration of *Uncaria tomentosa*.[63] Other studies with *Uncaria tomentosa* have shown enhancement of post-vaccination immunity[64] and enhancement of DNA repair in humans.[65] Traditional uses have included the use of the herb as a contraceptive and as treatment for gastrointestinal ulcers.

o Topical application of *Capsicum annuum, Capsicum frutescens* (Cayenne pepper, hot chili pepper): Controlled clinical trials have conclusively demonstrated capsaicin's ability to deplete sensory fibers of substance P to thus reduce pain. Capsaicin also blocks transport and de-novo synthesis of substance P. Topical capsaicin alleviates diabetic neuropathy[66], chronic low back pain[67], chronic neck pain[68], osteoarthritis[69], rheumatoid arthritis[70], notalgia paresthetica[71], reflex sympathetic dystrophy[72], and cluster headache (intranasal application).[73,74,75] Doctors should experiment on themselves with this treatment before administering to patients in order to gain understanding by experience.

o *Boswellia serrata*: *Boswellia* inhibits 5-lipoxygenase[76] with no apparent effect on cyclooxygenase[77] and has been shown effective in the treatment of osteoarthritis of the knees[78] as well as asthma[79] and ulcerative colitis.[80] When used as monotherapy, the target dose is approximately 150 mg of boswellic acids TID.

o *Zingiber officinale* (Ginger): Ginger is a well-known spice and food with a long history of use as an anti-inflammatory, anti-nausea, and gastroprotective agent[81], and components of ginger have been shown to reduce production of the leukotriene LTB4 by inhibiting 5-lipoxygenase and to reduce production of the prostaglandin PGE2 by inhibiting cyclooxygenase.[82,83] With its dual reduction in the formation of pro-inflammatory prostaglandins and leukotrienes, ginger has been shown to safely reduce nonspecific musculoskeletal pain[84,85] and to provide relief from osteoarthritis of the knees[86] and migraine

[60] Vasquez A. Reducing Pain and Inflammation Naturally. Part 2: New Insights into Fatty Acid Supplementation and Its Effect on Eicosanoid Production and Genetic Expression. *Nutritional Perspectives* 2005; January: 5-16

[61] Piscoya J, Rodriguez Z, Bustamante SA, Okuhama NN, Miller MJ, Sandoval M. Efficacy and safety of freeze-dried cat's claw in osteoarthritis of the knee: mechanisms of action of the species Uncaria guianensis. *Inflamm Res.* 2001 Sep;50(9):442-8

[62] Sandoval-Chacon M, Thompson JH, Zhang XJ, Liu X, Mannick EE, Sadowska-Krowicka H, Charbonnet RM, Clark DA, Miller MJ. Antiinflammatory actions of cat's claw: the role of NF-kappaB. *Aliment Pharmacol Ther.* 1998 Dec;12(12):1279-89

[63] "This small preliminary study demonstrates relative safety and modest benefit to the tender joint count of a highly purified extract from the pentacyclic chemotype of UT in patients with active RA taking sulfasalazine or hydroxychloroquine." Mur E, Hartig F, Eibl G, Schirmer M. Randomized double blind trial of an extract from the pentacyclic alkaloid-chemotype of uncaria tomentosa for the treatment of rheumatoid arthritis. *J Rheumatol.* 2002 Apr;29(4):678-81

[64] "...Uncaria tomentosa or Cat's Claw which is known to possess immune enhancing and antiinflammatory properties in animals. There were no toxic side effects observed as judged by medical examination, clinical chemistry and blood cell analysis. However, statistically significant immune enhancement for the individuals on C-Med-100 supplement was observed..." Lamm S, Sheng Y, Pero RW. Persistent response to pneumococcal vaccine in individuals supplemented with a novel water soluble extract of Uncaria tomentosa, C-Med-100. *Phytomedicine.* 2001;8(4):267-74

[65] Sheng Y, Li L, Holmgren K, Pero RW. DNA repair enhancement of aqueous extracts of Uncaria tomentosa in a human volunteer study. *Phytomedicine.* 2001 Jul;8(4):275-82

[66] "Study results suggest that topical capsaicin cream is safe and effective in treating painful diabetic neuropathy. "[No authors listed] Treatment of painful diabetic neuropathy with topical capsaicin. A multicenter, double-blind, vehicle-controlled study. The Capsaicin Study Group. *Arch Intern Med.* 1991 Nov;151(11):2225-9

[67] Keitel W, Frerick H, Kuhn U, Schmidt U, Kuhlmann M, Bredehorst A. Capsicum pain plaster in chronic non-specific low back pain. *Arzneimittelforschung.* 2001 Nov;51(11):896-903

[68] Mathias BJ, Dillingham TR, Zeigler DN, Chang AS, Belandres PV. Topical capsaicin for chronic neck pain. A pilot study. *Am J Phys Med Rehabil* 1995 Jan-Feb;74(1):39-44

[69] McCarthy GM, McCarty DJ. Effect of topical capsaicin in the therapy of painful osteoarthritis of the hands. *J Rheumatol.* 1992;19(4):604-7

[70] Deal CL, Schnitzer TJ, Lipstein E, Seibold JR, Stevens RM, Levy MD, Albert D, Renold F. Treatment of arthritis with topical capsaicin: a double-blind trial. *Clin Ther.* 1991 May-Jun;13(3):383-95

[71] Leibsohn E. Treatment of notalgia paresthetica with capsaicin. *Cutis* 1992 May;49(5):335-6

[72] "Capsaicin is effective for psoriasis, pruritus, and cluster headache; it is often helpful for the itching and pain of postmastectomy pain syndrome, oral mucositis, cutaneous allergy, loin pain/hematuria syndrome, neck pain, amputation stump pain, and skin tumor; and it may be beneficial for neural dysfunction (detrusor hyperreflexia, reflex sympathetic dystrophy, and rhinopathy)." Hautkappe M, Roizen MF, Toledano A, Roth S, Jeffries JA, Ostermeier AM. Review of the effectiveness of capsaicin for painful cutaneous disorders and neural dysfunction. *Clin J Pain* 1998 Jun;14(2):97-106

[73] "Capsaicin application to human nasal mucosa was found to induce painful sensation, sneezing, and nasal secretion. All of these factors exhibit desensitization upon repeated applications." Sicuteri F, Fusco BM, Marabini S, Campagnolo V, Maggi CA, Geppetti P, Fanciullacci M. Beneficial effect of capsaicin application to the nasal mucosa in cluster headache. *Clin J Pain.* 1989;5(1):49-53

[74] "The efficacy of repeated nasal applications of capsaicin in cluster headache is congruent with previous reports on the therapeutic effect of capsaicin in other pain syndromes (post-herpetic neuralgia, diabetic neuropathy, trigeminal neuralgia) and supports the use of the drug to produce a selective analgesia." Fusco BM, Marabini S, Maggi CA, Fiore G, Geppetti P. Preventative effect of repeated nasal applications of capsaicin in cluster headache. *Pain.* 1994 Dec;59(3):321-5

[75] "These results indicate that intranasal capsaicin may provide a new therapeutic option for the treatment of this disease." Marks DR, Rapoport A, Padla D, Weeks R, Rosum R, Sheftell F, Arrowsmith F. A double-blind placebo-controlled trial of intranasal capsaicin for cluster headache. *Cephalalgia.* 1993 Apr;13(2):114-6

[76] Wildfeuer A, Neu IS, Safayhi H, Metzger G, Wehrmann M, Vogel U, Ammon HP. Effects of boswellic acids extracted from a herbal medicine on the biosynthesis of leukotrienes and the course of experimental autoimmune encephalomyelitis. *Arzneimittelforschung* 1998 Jun;48(6):668-74

[77] Safayhi H, Mack T, Sabieraj J, Anazodo MI, Subramanian LR, Ammon HP. Boswellic acids: novel, specific, nonredox inhibitors of 5-lipoxygenase. *J Pharmacol Exp Ther* 1992 Jun;261(3):1143-6

[78] Kimmatkar N, Thawani V, Hingorani L, Khiyani R. Efficacy and tolerability of Boswellia serrata extract in treatment of osteoarthritis of knee--a randomized double blind placebo controlled trial. *Phytomedicine.* 2003 Jan;10(1):3-7

[79] Gupta I, Gupta V, Parihar A, Gupta S, Ludtke R, Safayhi H, Ammon HP. Effects of Boswellia serrata gum resin in patients with bronchial asthma: results of a double-blind, placebo-controlled, 6-week clinical study. *Eur J Med Res.* 1998 Nov 17;3(11):511-4

[80] Gupta I, Parihar A, Malhotra P, Singh GB, Ludtke R, Safayhi H, Ammon HP. Effects of Boswellia serrata gum resin in patients with ulcerative colitis. *Eur J Med Res.* 1997 Jan;2(1):37-43

[81] Langner E, Greifenberg S, Gruenwald J. Ginger: history and use. *Adv Ther* 1998 Jan-Feb;15(1):25-44

[82] Kiuchi F, Iwakami S, Shibuya M, Hanaoka F, Sankawa U. Inhibition of prostaglandin and leukotriene biosynthesis by gingerols and diarylheptanoids. *Chem Pharm Bull* (Tokyo) 1992 Feb;40(2):387-91

[83] Tjendraputra E, Tran VH, Liu-Brennan D, Roufogalis BD, Duke CC. Effect of ginger constituents and synthetic analogues on cyclooxygenase-2 enzyme in intact cells. *Bioorg Chem* 2001 Jun;29(3):156-63

[84] Srivastava KC, Mustafa T. Ginger (Zingiber officinale) in rheumatism and musculoskeletal disorders. *Med Hypotheses.* 1992 Dec;39(4):342-8

[85] Srivastava KC, Mustafa T. Ginger (Zingiber officinale) and rheumatic disorders. *Med Hypotheses.* 1989 May;29(1):25-8

[86] Altman RD, Marcussen KC. Effects of a ginger extract on knee pain in patients with osteoarthritis. *Arthritis Rheum.* 2001 Nov;44(11):2531-8

headaches.[87] Ginger can be consumed somewhat liberally as a supplement or as whole food, and it is safe for use in pregnancy up to one gram per day.[88]

- o *Harpagophytum procumbens* (Devil's claw): The safety and effectiveness of *Harpagophytum* has been established in patients with hip pain, low-back pain, and knee pain.[89,90,91] The mechanisms of action include weak anti-inflammatory effects and a stronger analgesic effect.[92,93] Research suggests that *Harpagophytum* is an effective analgesic for low back pain[94], including low back pain with radiculitis and radiculopathy.[95] The common dose is 60 mg harpagoside per day.[96]

- o Willow bark (*Salix* spp): In a double-blind placebo-controlled clinical trial in 210 patients with moderate/severe low-back pain (20% of patients had positive straight-leg raising test), willow bark extract showed a dose-dependent analgesic effect with benefits beginning in the first week of treatment.[97] In a head-to-head study of 228 patients comparing willow bark (standardized for 240 mg salicin) with Vioxx (rofecoxib), treatments were equally effective yet willow bark was safer and 40% less expensive.[98] Because willow bark's salicylates were the original source for the chemical manufacture of acetylsalicylic acid (aspirin), researchers and clinicians have erroneously mistaken willow bark to be synonymous with aspirin; this is certainly inaccurate and therefore clarification of willow's mechanism of action will be provided here. Aspirin has two primary effects via three primary mechanisms of action: 1) anticoagulant effects mediated by the acetylation and permanent inactivation of thromboxane-A synthase, which is the enzyme that makes the powerfully proaggregatory thromboxane-A2; 2) antiprostaglandin action via acetylation of both isoforms of cyclooxygenase (COX-1 inhibition 25-166x more than COX-2) with widespread inhibition of prostaglandin formation, and 3) antiprostaglandin formation via retroconversion of acetylsalicylate into salicylic acid which then inhibits cyclooxygenase-2 gene transcription.[99] Notice that the acetylation reactions are specific to aspirin and thus actions #1 and #2 are not seen with willow bark; whereas #3—inhibition of COX-2 transcription by salicylates—appears to be the major mechanism of action of willow bark extract. Proof of this principle is supported by the lack of adverse effects associated with willow bark in the research literature. If willow bark were pharmacodynamically synonymous with aspirin, then we would expect case reports of gastric ulceration, hemorrhage, and Reye's syndrome to permeate the research literature; this is not the case and therefore—**with the exception of possible allergic reactions in patients previously allergic/anaphylactic to aspirin and salicylates—extensive "warnings" on willow bark products[100] are unnecessary.[101]** Salicylates are widely present in fruits, vegetables, herbs and spices and are partly responsible for the anti-cancer, anti-inflammatory, and health-promoting benefits of fruit and vegetable consumption.[102,103] With willow bark products, the daily dose should not exceed 240 mg of salicin, and products should include other components of the whole plant. **Except for rare allergy in patients previously sensitized to aspirin or salicylates, no adverse effects are known**; to be on the medicolegal safe side, use is discouraged during pregnancy, before surgery, or when anti-coagulant medications are being used.

[87] Mustafa T, Srivastava KC. Ginger (Zingiber officinale) in migraine headache. *J Ethnopharmacol*. 1990 Jul;29(3):267-73

[88] "…oral ginger 1 g per day… No adverse effect of ginger on pregnancy outcome was detected." Vutyavanich T, Kraisarin T, Ruangsri R. Ginger for nausea and vomiting in pregnancy: randomized, double-masked, placebo-controlled trial. *Obstet Gynecol* 2001 Apr;97(4):577-82.

[89] Chrubasik S, Thanner J, Kunzel O, Conradt C, Black A, Pollak S. Comparison of outcome measures during treatment with the proprietary Harpagophytum extract doloteffin in patients with pain in the lower back, knee or hip. *Phytomedicine* 2002 Apr;9(3):181-94

[90] Chantre P, Cappelaere A, Leblan D, Guedon D, Vandermander J, Fournie B. Efficacy and tolerance of Harpagophytum procumbens versus diacerhein in treatment of osteoarthritis. *Phytomedicine* 2000 Jun;7(3):177-83

[91] Leblan D, Chantre P, Fournie B. Harpagophytum procumbens in the treatment of knee and hip osteoarthritis. Four-month results of a prospective, multicenter, double-blind trial versus diacerhein. *Joint Bone Spine* 2000;67(5):462-7

[92] Whitehouse LW, Znamirowska M, Paul CJ. Devil's Claw (Harpagophytum procumbens): no evidence for anti-inflammatory activity in the treatment of arthritic disease. *Can Med Assoc J* 1983 Aug 1;129(3):249-51

[93] Moussard C, Alber D, Toubin MM, Thevenon N, Henry JC. A drug used in traditional medicine, harpagophytum procumbens: no evidence for NSAID-like effect on whole blood eicosanoid production in human. *Prostaglandins Leukot Essent Fatty Acids* 1992 Aug;46(4):283-6

[94] Chrubasik S, Model A, Black A, Pollak S. A randomized double-blind pilot study comparing Doloteffin and Vioxx in the treatment of low back pain. *Rheumatology* (Oxford). 2003 Jan;42(1):141-8

[95] "The majority of responders' were patients who had suffered less than 42 days of pain, and subgroup analyses suggested that the effect was confined to patients with more severe and radiating pain accompanied by neurological deficit… There was no evidence for Harpagophytum-related side-effects, except possibly for mild and infrequent gastrointestinal symptoms." Chrubasik S, Junck H, Breitschwerdt H, Conradt C, Zappe H. Effectiveness of Harpagophytum extract WS 1531 in the treatment of exacerbation of low back pain: a randomized, placebo-controlled, double-blind study. *Eur J Anaesthesiol* 1999 Feb;16(2):118-29

[96] "They took an 8-week course of Doloteffin at a dose providing 60 mg harpagoside per day… Doloteffin is well worth considering for osteoarthritic knee and hip pain and nonspecific low back pain." Chrubasik S, Thanner J, Kunzel O, Conradt C, Black A, Pollak S. Comparison of outcome measures during treatment with the proprietary Harpagophytum extract doloteffin in patients with pain in the lower back, knee or hip. *Phytomedicine* 2002 Apr;9(3):181-94

[97] Chrubasik S, Eisenberg E, Balan E, Weinberger T, Luzzati R, Conradt C. Treatment of low-back pain exacerbations with willow bark extract: a randomized double-blind study. *Am J Med*. 2000;109:9-14

[98] Chrubasik S, Kunzel O, Model A, Conradt C, Black A. Treatment of low-back pain with a herbal or synthetic anti-rheumatic: a randomized controlled study. Willow bark extract for low-back pain. *Rheumatology* (Oxford). 2001;40:1388-93

[99] Hare LG, Woodside JV, Young IS. Dietary salicylates. *J Clin Pathol* 2003 Sep;56(9):649-50 http://jcp.bmj.com/cgi/content/full/56/9/649

[100] Clauson KA, Santamarina ML, Buettner CM, Cauffield JS. Evaluation of Presence of Aspirin-Related Warnings with Willow Bark (July/August). *Ann Pharmacother*. 2005 May 31; [Epub ahead of print]

[101] **Vasquez** A, Muanza DN. Evaluation of Presence of Aspirin-Related Warnings with Willow Bark: Comment on the Article by Clauson et al. *Ann Pharmacotherapy* 2005 Oct;39(10):1763

[102] Lawrence JR, Peter R, Baxter GJ, Robson J, Graham AB, Paterson JR. Urinary excretion of salicyluric and salicylic acids by non-vegetarians, vegetarians, and patients taking low dose aspirin. *J Clin Pathol*. 2003 Sep;56(9):651-3

[103] Paterson JR, Lawrence JR. Salicylic acid: a link between aspirin, diet and the prevention of colorectal cancer. *QJM*. 2001 Aug;94(8):445-8 http://qjmed.oxfordjournals.org/cgi/content/full/94/8/445

Treat with physical/manual medicine:

- Massage: Gentle massage provides comfort, increases circulation, reduces edema, and promotes healing. After the acute phase, deeper massage may help restore range of motion by breaking adhesions and reducing the feeling of vulnerability that may occur after injury. Research indicates that massage can reduce adolescent aggression[104], improve outcome in preterm infants[105], alleviate premenstrual syndrome[106], improve flexibility, reduce pain, increase serotonin and dopamine in patients with low back pain[107], and improve function and alleviate depression in patients with Parkinson's disease (Alexander technique).[108]
- Joint mobilization and manipulation as appropriate (after contraindications have been excluded) and to the level of patient comfort. Mechanisms of action are listed later in this section.
- Treatment of associated muscle spasm and myofascial trigger points (MFTP): Such treatment can increase range of motion and decrease pain. See notes on the diagnosis and treatment of MFTP in the following section in this chapter.
- Consider physiotherapy: As appropriate.

Uncover the underlying problem:

- In the case of most acute injuries, the underlying problem is often the injury itself. However, the physician must not be overly naïve and must conduct a thorough history and examination to assess for possible underlying pathologies that cause or contribute to the problem that "appears" to be injury related. Congenital anomalies, underlying pathology, previous injury, and psychoemotional disorders may have been present before the "injury."
  - o **In children and young adults, 5% of "sports-related" injuries are associated with preexisting infection, anomalies, or other conditions.**
  - o In adult women: "In three cases of carcinoma, the breast mass was not noticed until after the [auto accident] and was initially thought by the patient to have been caused by the trauma. **Indeed between 9% and 20% of women with breast cancer attribute their symptoms to previous trauma to the breast.**"[109]
- Look for leg length inequalities and biomechanical faults such as hyperpronation and pelvic torque.
- Assess and correct poor posture, poor ergonomics, lack of flexibility, muscle strength imbalances, and proprioceptive/coordination deficits.
- Patients may experience a reduction in pain—particularly low-back pain and osteoarthritis pain—when they eliminate coffee/caffeine, food allergens, and/or specific foods to which they are sensitive, most notably the *Solanaceae*/nightshade family—eggplant, tobacco, tomatoes, potatoes, and bell peppers. Foods in the *Solanaceae* family contain anti-acetylcholinesterases[110] that may effect increased synaptic transmission of afferent pain sensations, particularly via NMDA receptors.
- Correction of **diet-induced chronic metabolic acidosis** with the use of alkalinizing diets/supplements[111] can alleviate musculoskeletal pain[112], at least in part by raising/normalizing intracellular magnesium levels and by reducing intracellular calcium levels. Additional benefits of alkalinization include increased mineral retention, reduced bone resorption[113] and enhanced clearance of toxic xenobiotics[114], especially many pesticides and pharmacologic agents.

Re-educate, rehabilitate, resourcefulness, return to active life, reassure, referral:

- Educate patient on ways to avoid re-injury and to decrease likelihood of recurrence.

---

[104] Diego MA, Field T, Hernandez-Reif M, Shaw JA, Rothe EM, Castellanos D, Mesner L. Aggressive adolescents benefit from massage therapy. *Adolescence* 2002 Fall;37(147):597-607

[105] Mainous RO. Infant massage as a component of developmental care: past, present, and future. *Holist Nurs Pract* 2002 Oct;16(5):1-7

[106] Hernandez-Reif M, Martinez A, Field T, Quintero O, Hart S, Burman I. Premenstrual symptoms are relieved by massage therapy. *J Psychosom Obstet Gynaecol* 2000 Mar;21(1):9-15

[107] "RESULTS: By the end of the study, the massage therapy group, as compared to the relaxation group, reported experiencing less pain, depression, anxiety and improved sleep. They also showed improved trunk and pain flexion performance, and their serotonin and dopamine levels were higher." Hernandez-Reif M, Field T, Krasnegor J, Theakston H. Lower back pain is reduced and range of motion increased after massage therapy. *Int J Neurosci* 2001;106(3-4):131-45

[108] Stallibrass C, Sissons P, Chalmers C. Randomized controlled trial of the Alexander technique for idiopathic Parkinson's disease. *Clin Rehabil* 2002 Nov;16(7):695-708

[109] Seifert S. Medical Illness Simulating Trauma (MIST) syndrome: case reports and discussion of syndrome. *Fam Med* 1993 Apr;25(4):273-6

[110] Krasowski MD, McGehee DS, Moss J. Natural inhibitors of cholinesterases: implications for adverse drug reactions. *Can J Anaesth*. 1997 May;44(5 Pt 1):525-34 www.cja-jca.org/cgi/reprint/44/5/525.pdf

[111] For long-term out-patient treatment of patients who do not achieve alkalinization with diet alone, oral administration of potassium citrate and/or sodium bicarbonate can be implemented. See the following article for concepts: "Urine alkalinization is a treatment regimen that increases poison elimination by the administration of intravenous sodium bicarbonate to produce urine with a pH > or = 7.5." Proudfoot AT, Krenzelok EP, Vale JA. Position Paper on urine alkalinization. *J Toxicol Clin Toxicol*. 2004;42:1-26 http://www.eapcct.org/publicfile.php?folder=congress&file=PS_UrineAlkalinization.pdf Also see: Vormann J, Worlitschek M, Goedecke T, Silver B. Supplementation with alkaline minerals reduces symptoms in patients with chronic low back pain. *J Trace Elem Med Biol*. 2001;15(2-3):179-83 Also see: Maurer M, Riesen W, Muser J, Hulter HN, Krapf R. Neutralization of Western diet inhibits bone resorption independently of K intake and reduces cortisol secretion in humans. *Am J Physiol Renal Physiol*. 2003 Jan;284(1):F32-40. Epub 2002 Sep 24. http://ajprenal.physiology.org/cgi/content/full/284/1/F32

[112] "The results show that a disturbed acid-base balance may contribute to the symptoms of low back pain. The simple and safe addition of an alkaline multimineral preparate was able to reduce the pain symptoms in these patients with chronic low back pain." Vormann J, Worlitschek M, Goedecke T, Silver B. Supplementation with alkaline minerals reduces symptoms in patients with chronic low back pain. *J Trace Elem Med Biol*. 2001;15(2-3):179-83

[113] "In postmenopausal women, the oral administration of potassium bicarbonate at a dose sufficient to neutralize endogenous acid improves calcium and phosphorus balance, reduces bone resorption, and increases the rate of bone formation." Sebastian A, Harris ST, Ottaway JH, Todd KM, Morris RC Jr. Improved mineral balance and skeletal metabolism in postmenopausal women treated with potassium bicarbonate. *N Engl J Med*. 1994 Jun 23;330(25):1776-81 http://content.nejm.org/cgi/content/abstract/330/25/1776

[114] "Urine alkalinization is a treatment regimen that increases poison elimination by the administration of intravenous sodium bicarbonate to produce urine with a pH > or = 7.5." Proudfoot AT, Krenzelok EP, Vale JA. Position Paper on urine alkalinization. *J Toxicol Clin Toxicol*. 2004;42:1-26 http://www.eapcct.org/publicfile.php?folder=congress&file=PS_UrineAlkalinization.pdf

- Pre-rehabilitation assessment has three main goals: 1) identification of the type of injury, 2) quantification of the severity of the injury, and 3) determining the appropriate interventions.[115] Rehabilitative exercises **emphasizing strength, coordination, proprioception, range of motion, and functional utility** (appropriate per occupation and hobbies) should be employed.
- **Isometric exercises** can be used to maintain/increase muscle strength in patients for whom range-of-motion exercises are painful or contraindicated.
- **Work hardening** has been defined by the American Physical Therapy Association as "a highly structured goal-oriented, individualized treatment program designed to return a person to work. Work Hardening programs...use real or simulated work activities designed to restore physical, behavioral, and vocational functions."[116] Teperman[117] defined the specific goals of work hardening as:
  1. Improved lifting strength (loading and unloading) to/from different heights, including overhead,
  2. Improved carrying capacity (various objects, different distances, unilateral and bilateral),
  3. Improved functional tolerance (coordination and manipulation) at different levels,
  4. Improved cardiovascular endurance,
  5. Improved dexterity tasks (counting, weighing, sorting, packaging/unpacking)
  6. Improved biomechanics in any setting (work/leisure).
- **Work conditioning** has been defined as "a work-related, intensive, and goal-oriented treatment program specifically designed to restore an individual's systemic, neuromuscular (strength, endurance, flexibility, etc.) and cardiopulmonary function."[118] While overlaps exist between work hardening and work conditioning, and both are generally designed to "return the patient to work", work hardening is focused more on the performance of work-related tasks (task-oriented) while work conditioning tends to focus more on the cardiopulmonary and neuromuscular fitness of the patient (fitness-oriented).
- **Rehabilitation can become more than *restorative*; if the plan is comprehensive and it effects long-term improvements in overall health, then such a program can become *transformative.*** For example, while the oversimplified medical model as commonly practiced in HMO and PPO systems might describe a patient's problem as "low-back pain, refer for physiotherapy and begin Vioxx 25 mg b.i.d.", a more comprehensive assessment and treatment of the same patient's problem might be described as "low-back pain secondary to sedentary lifestyle, obesity, mild systemic inflammation, hypovitaminosis D, and proprioceptive deficits. Begin program of daily general exercise along with specific exercises for low-back region, low-carbohydrate diet to promote weight loss, balance training twice daily, begin supplementation with cholecalciferol 4,000 IU/d and fish oil 3 g/d." Notice that the typical allopathic plan *requires* and *thus ensures* patient passivity and does nothing to promote overall health, whereas the comprehensive natural/integrative plan is more in accord with current biomedical literature, requires active patient participation, offers the probability of improved overall health, and will reduce the severity and risk of present and future diseases, respectively.
- Patients should be supported in the tolerance of minor discomfort to avoid overuse of analgesics, to avoid an excessive reduction in activities, and to avoid playing the "sick role." While validating the patient's concerns, physicians should not encourage dysfunctional behavior or contribute to "iatrogenic neurosis."
- **Symptomatic treatment that provides no lasting benefit can foster therapeutic dependency and therapeutic passivity**. "Therapeutic dependency" describes the situation wherein the patient becomes dependent on treatment sessions for secondary gain of attention, physical contact, and time off from work (etc.) rather than focusing on the goal of getting as healthy as possible as quickly as possible. Therapeutic dependency is fostered by doctors who fail to educate patients to take an active role in their own care and by doctors who take on the role of "savior" rather than empowering patients to take effective action in improving their health. **Therapeutic passivity** is related to **therapeutic dependency** since patients who fail to take responsible action tend to become dependent on healthcare providers to "cure me", "fix me" and "rescue me."
- While detailed individual descriptions of therapeutic exercise and rehabilitative programs are not the subject of this book, we can readily appreciate the many options that are available to us for the rehabilitation of injuries:

---

[115] Geffen SJ. 3: Rehabilitation principles for treating chronic musculoskeletal injuries. *Med J Aust.* 2003 Mar 3;178(5):238-42

[116] American Physical Therapy Association, "Guidelines for Programs for Injured Workers" 1995. Quoted by Washington State Department of Labor and Industries. http://www.lni.wa.gov/Main/MostAskedQuestions/ClaimsIns/WorkHardFaq.asp. Accessed July 23, 2006

[117] Teperman LJ. Active functional restoration and work hardening program returns patient with 2½-year-old elbow fracture-dislocation to work after 6 months: a case report. *J Can Chiropr Assoc* 2002; 46(1): 22-30 http://www.jcca-online.org/client/cca/JCCA.nsf/objects/Active+functional+restoration+elbow+fracture-dislocation/$file/5-Teperman.pdf

[118] Howar JM. Keys to Effective Work Hardening and Limited Duty Programs. http://www.eh.doe.gov/feosh/contacts/LimitedDutyPrograms.pdf Accessed July 23, 2006. Ironically, even though the third page of this presentation clearly shows the use of spinal manipulation, chiropractic doctors are notably absent from the list of "Industrial Rehab Specialists" having been usurped even by Occupational Nurses.

- o **Therapeutic exercise**: Includes strength training, stretching, improving endurance, and functional training specific to the patient's occupational or athletic activities. These can be tailored to great detail to the patient's condition and goals.[119]
- o **Proprioceptive retraining/rehabilitation**: As discussed later in this chapter, restoration and optimization of proprioceptive function and balance control is especially important for the long-term functional improvement of patients with proprioceptive deficits, commonly seen in patients with chronic low-back pain[120], neck pain[121], knee arthritis[122], and ankle instability.[123]
- o **Weight optimization**: For the majority of patients living in our society where obesity is pandemic, weight reduction is important not only to improve overall health and to reduce mechanical stresses on joints, but perhaps even more importantly to reduce the production of proinflammatory chemicals made in adipose tissue (adipokines) which promote an overall internal climate of pain and inflammation. Some patients may need to gain muscle strength to promote healing and avoid re-injury; this can generally be achieved with resistance training and increased protein consumption.
- o **Eicosanoid modulation**: Historically, the balance of omega-3 to omega-6 fatty acids in the human diet has been approximately 1:1 or 1:2.[124] Since omega-3 fatty acids are generally *anti-inflammatory* while omega-6 fatty acids are generally proinflammatory (with the exception of GLA/DGLA), the former *quantitative* dietary balance translated to a *qualitative* balance with regard to the body's inherent inflammatory tendency. Modern diets today, however, provide a ratio of 1:30, with anti-inflammatory omega-3 fatty acids greatly outnumbered by the proinflammatory omega-6 fatty acids. Thus, human physiology has been altered by the widespread consumption of a ***pro-inflammatory diet***.[125] Correction of this problem at the level of dietary intake rather than by the use of anti-inflammatory medications is essential for the attainment of health and the long-term relief of pain and inflammation.[126,127]
- o **Alkalinization**: The American/Western style of eating results in subclinical diet-induced pathogenic chronic metabolic acidosis[128] which can be corrected with a Paleo-Mediterranean diet[129] or alkalinizing supplements[130] (including potassium citrate and sodium bicarbonate) for the alleviation of musculoskeletal pain in general and low-back pain in particular.[131]
- o **Analgesia**: Safe and effective natural means for achieving a timely reduction in pain include topical capsaicin, *Harpagophytum*, *Uncaria*, acupuncture, willow, and spinal manipulation.
- o **Anti-inflammatory botanicals and nutraceuticals**: Fish oil, GLA, vitamin E, *Boswellia*, willow bark, *Harpagophytum*, and *Zingiber* are just a few of the effective natural anti-inflammatory treatments available.
- o **Treatment of myofascial trigger points**: Since joint injuries and chronic pain—*especially in the neck, back and shoulder*—are commonly associated with trigger points[132], addressing this secondary and occult cause of pain is important to maximize pain relief and functional restoration.
- o **Manipulation, mobilization, and massage**: Joint manipulation has numerous physiologic and anatomic effects, most of which are relevant for the alleviation of pain and improvement of joint function. These mechanisms include:
  1. Releasing entrapped intraarticular menisci and synovial folds,
  2. Acutely reducing intradiscal pressure, thus promoting replacement of decentralized disc material,

[119] Basmajian JV (ed). *Therapeutic Exercise. Fourth Edition*. Baltimore: Williams and Wilkins. 1984

[120] Newcomer KL, Jacobson TD, Gabriel DA, Larson DR, Brey RH, An KN. Muscle activation patterns in subjects with and without low back pain. *Arch Phys Med Rehabil*. 2002;83(6):816-21

[121] McPartland JM, Brodeur RR, Hallgren RC. Chronic neck pain, standing balance, and suboccipital muscle atrophy--a pilot study. *J Manipulative Physiol Ther*. 1997 Jan;20(1):24-9

[122] Callaghan MJ, Selfe J, Bagley PJ, Oldham JA. The Effects of Patellar Taping on Knee Joint Proprioception. *J Athl Train*. 2002 Mar;37(1):19-24

[123] Olmsted LC, Carcia CR, Hertel J, Shultz SJ. Efficacy of the Star Excursion Balance Tests in Detecting Reach Deficits in Subjects With Chronic Ankle Instability. *J Athl Train*. 2002 Dec;37(4):501-506

[124] Simopoulos AP. Essential fatty acids in health and chronic disease. *Am J Clin Nutr*. 1999 Sep;70(3 Suppl):560S-569S

[125] Seaman DR. The diet-induced proinflammatory state: a cause of chronic pain and other degenerative diseases? *J Manipulative Physiol Ther*. 2002;25(3):168-79

[126] Vasquez A. A Five-Part Nutritional Protocol that Produces Consistently Positive Results. *Nutritional Wellness* 2005 September

[127] Vasquez A. Dietary, Nutritional and Botanical Interventions to Reduce Pain and Inflammation. *Naturopathy Digest* 2006, March *Nutritional Wellness* 2006, March

[128] "As a result, healthy adults consuming the standard US diet sustain a chronic, low-grade pathogenic metabolic acidosis that worsens with age as kidney function declines." Cordain L, Eaton SB, Sebastian A, Mann N, Lindeberg S, Watkins BA, O'Keefe JH, Brand-Miller J. Origins and evolution of the Western diet: health implications for the 21st century. *Am J Clin Nutr*. 2005 Feb;81(2):341-54 http://www.ajcn.org/cgi/content/full/81/2/341

[129] Cordain L. *The Paleo Diet: Lose Weight and Get Healthy by Eating the Food You Were Designed to Eat*. Indianapolis; John Wiley and Sons, 2002

[130] "An acidogenic Western diet results in mild metabolic acidosis in association with a state of cortisol excess, altered divalent ion metabolism, and increased bone resorptive indices." Maurer M, Riesen W, Muser J, Hulter HN, Krapf R. Neutralization of Western diet inhibits bone resorption independently of K intake and reduces cortisol secretion in humans. *Am J Physiol Renal Physiol*. 2003 Jan;284(1):F32-40. Epub 2002 Sep 24. http://ajprenal.physiology.org/cgi/content/full/284/1/F32

[131] "The results show that a disturbed acid-base balance may contribute to the symptoms of low back pain. The simple and safe addition of an alkaline multimineral preparate was able to reduce the pain symptoms in these patients with chronic low back pain." Vormann J, Worlitschek M, Goedecke T, Silver B. Supplementation with alkaline minerals reduces symptoms in patients with chronic low back pain. *J Trace Elem Med Biol*. 2001;15(2-3):179-83

[132] "The mean number of TrPs present on each neck pain patient was 4.3, of which 2.5 were latent and 1.8 were active TrPs. Control subjects also exhibited TrPs (mean: 2; SD: 0.8). All were latent TrPs." Fernandez-de-Las-Penas C, Alonso-Blanco C, Miangolarra JC. Myofascial trigger points in subjects presenting with mechanical neck pain: A blinded, controlled study. *Man Ther*. 2006 Jun 10

3. Stretching of deep periarticular muscles to break the cycle of chronic autonomous muscle contraction by lengthening the muscles and thereby releasing excessive actin-myosin binding,

4. Promoting restoration of proper kinesthesia and proprioception,

5. Promoting relaxation of paraspinal muscles by stretching facet joint capsules,

6. Promoting relaxation of paraspinal muscles via "postactivation depression", which is the temporary depletion of contractile neurotransmitters,

7. Temporarily elevating plasma beta-endorphin,

8. Temporarily enhancing phagocytic ability of neutrophils and monocytes,

9. Activating the diffuse descending pain inhibitory system located in the periaqueductal gray matter—this is an important aspect of nociceptive inhibition by intense sensory/mechanoreceptor stimulation, and

10. Improving neurotransmitter balance and reducing pain (soft-tissue manipulation).[133]

Additional details are provided in numerous published reviews and primary research[134,135,136,137,138,139,140] and by Leach[141], whose extensive description of the mechanisms of action of spinal manipulative therapy is unsurpassed. Given such a wide base of experimental and clinical support published in peer-reviewed journals and widely-available textbooks, denigrations directed toward spinal manipulation on the grounds that it is "unscientific" or "unsupported by research" are unfounded and are indicative of selective ignorance.[142]

o <u>Reassurance</u>: Education, explanation, reassurance, and support help to address the mental and emotional aspects of injury.

o **<u>Referral</u>: Patients with severe pain, serious conditions/complications, or documented noncompliance are excellent candidates for co-management or unidirectional referral.**

- Modify home and occupational workstations to minimize strain and stress on injured tissues. Educate patients to use tools, machines, props, and stepstools to work efficiently and to reduce unnecessary lifting and straining motions.

- Physical activities can be fully resumed when symptoms have decreased and when physical examination findings (e.g., reflexes, strength, range of motion, spinal segmental function, and trigger points) are within normal limits. Note that in many situations returning the patient to their previous duration, frequency, and intensity of activity may predispose to re-injury since the patient is re-entering the situation wherein the original injury occurred; therefore at least one of these lifestyle/occupational/recreational variables must change in order to reduce the likeliness of re-injury.

- Books, websites, and national/local support groups and organizations may be available for emotional, physical, psychological-emotional, and legal assistance.

Nutrition:

- <u>Protein</u>: In otherwise healthy patients with no liver, renal, or other metabolic disorders, ensure adequate intake of 0.5-0.9 gram of protein per pound of body weight.[143] Vegetarians may heal more slowly after injury than do omnivores; vegetarians and lacto-vegetarians undergoing cosmetic surgery reportedly have more complications and slower healing than do people eating a diet containing meat.[144] Additionally, low-protein diets have shown to reduce muscle mass and suppress immune function.[145] See the table below for protein intake recommendations:

[133] "RESULTS: By the end of the study, the massage therapy group, as compared to the relaxation group, reported experiencing less pain, depression, anxiety and improved sleep. They also showed improved trunk and pain flexion performance, and their serotonin and dopamine levels were higher." Hernandez-Reif M, Field T, Krasnegor J, Theakston H. Lower back pain is reduced and range of motion increased after massage therapy. *Int J Neurosci* 2001;106(3-4):131-45

[134] Maigne JY, Vautravers P. Mechanism of action of spinal manipulative therapy. *Joint Bone Spine*. 2003;70(5):336-41

[135] Brennan PC, Triano JJ, McGregor M, Kokjohn K, Hondras MA, Brennan DC. Enhanced neutrophil respiratory burst as a biological marker for manipulation forces: duration of the effect and association with substance P and tumor necrosis factor. *J Manipulative Physiol Ther*. 1992 Feb;15(2):83-9

[136] Brennan PC, Kokjohn K, Kaltinger CJ, Lohr GE, Glendening C, Hondras MA, McGregor M, Triano JJ. Enhanced phagocytic cell respiratory burst induced by spinal manipulation: potential role of substance P. *J Manipulative Physiol Ther*. 1991 Sep;14(7):399-408

[137] Heikkila H, Johansson M, Wenngren BI. Effects of acupuncture, cervical manipulation and NSAID therapy on dizziness and impaired head repositioning of suspected cervical origin: a pilot study. *Man Ther*. 2000 Aug;5(3):151-7

[138] Rogers RG. The effects of spinal manipulation on cervical kinesthesia in patients with chronic neck pain: a pilot study. *J Manipulative Physiol Ther*. 1997;20(2):80-5

[139] Bergman, Peterson, Lawrence. <u>Chiropractic Technique</u>. New York: Churchill Livingstone 1993. An updated edition is now availabe published by Mosby.

[140] Herzog WH. Mechanical and physiological responses to spinal manipulative treatments. *JNMS: J Neuromusculoskeltal System* 1995; 3: 1-9

[141] Leach RA. (ed) <u>The Chiropractic Theories: A Textbook of Scientific Research, Fourth Edition</u>. Baltimore: Lippincott, Williams & Wilkins, 2004

[142] Vasquez A. The Science of Chiropractic and Spinal Manipulation, Part 2. http://www.mercola.com/2005/mar/12/chiropractic_spine.htm

[143] Nancy Clark, MS, RD. The Power of Protein. *The Physician and Sportsmedicine* 1996, volume 24, number 4. http://www.physsportsmed.com/issues/1996/04_96/protein.htm

[144] Vegetarians and healing. *JAMA* 1995; 273: 910

[145] Castaneda C, Charnley JM, Evans WJ, Crim MC. Elderly women accommodate to a low-protein diet with losses of body cell mass, muscle function, and immune response. *Am J Clin Nutr* 1995 Jul;62(1):30-9

Recommended <u>Grams of Protein</u> Per <u>Pound of Body Weight</u> Per Day[146]	
Infants and children ages 1-6 years[147]	0.68-0.45
RDA for sedentary adult and children ages 6-18 years[148]	0.4
Adult recreational exerciser	**0.5-0.75**
Adult competitive athlete	0.6-0.9
Adult building muscle mass	0.7-0.9
Dieting athlete	0.7-1.0
Growing teenage athlete	0.9-1.0
Pregnant women need additional protein	Add 15-30 grams/day[149]

- Water: Adequate intake of water is important to flush out wastes, toxins, and to prevent constipation. Eight glasses per day is the classic recommendation; however increased fluid intake is appropriate during exercise, heat exposure, stress, and to promote clearance of nitrogenous wastes and xenobiotics. Fluid restriction may be appropriate for persons with adrenal insufficiency to avoid hyponatremia and those with cardiovascular failure, fluid overload, or edema.

- Vegetables, fruit, and fiber: Whole foods provide micronutrients, natural anti-inflammatory components, and immune modulators; the fiber/phytonutrient content provides positive effects on gut flora while maintaining proper waste elimination and reducing straining (e.g., reduced need for the Valsalva maneuver).

- Carbohydrates: Carbohydrate intake should be adequate to supply energy-expenditure needs and to support healing but should not be excessive such as to unfavorably increase body weight during times of decreased physical activity. Preferred sources of carbohydrates are fruits and vegetables.

- Identification and elimination of adverse food reactions: Adverse food reactions—regardless of the underlying mechanism(s) or classification of allergy, intolerance, or sensitivity—can precipitate joint pain and inflammation[150,151,152,153,154,155,156] and a wide range of other health problems.

- Supplementation with a high-potency broad-spectrum multivitamin and multimineral product: This will help correct common nutritional deficiencies and support optimal healing. Certain nutrients such as vitamin C, zinc, and copper are commonly considered "specific" for promoting optimal repair of connective tissue.

- Specific supplements/botanicals: Supplementation is tailored to the type of tissue that has been injured, such as calcium, magnesium, and vitamins D and K for bone fractures, glucosamine sulfate and niacinamide for cartilage injuries, and proteolytic enzymes for muscle strains.
  - Niacinamide: The niacinamide form of vitamin B3 was proven effective against osteoarthritis by Kaufman more than 50 years ago.[157] Furthermore, Kaufman's documentation of an "anti-aging" effect of vitamin supplementation in general and niacinamide therapy in particular[158] is consistent with recent experimental data demonstrating rapid reversion of aging phenotypes by niacinamide through modulation of histone acetylation.[159] A recent double-blind placebo-controlled repeat study found that niacinamide therapy improved joint mobility, reduced objective inflammation as assessed by ESR, reduced the impact of the arthritis on the activities of daily living, and allowed a reduction in analgesic/anti-inflammatory medication use.[160] While the mechanism of action is probably multifaceted, inhibition of joint-destroying nitric oxide appears to be an important benefit.[161] The standard dose of 500 mg given orally 6 times per day is more effective than 1,000 mg 3 times per day. Hepatic dysfunction is rare when daily doses are kept below 3,000 mg per day, yet Gaby[162] suggests measurement of liver

[146] Slightly modified from Nancy Clark, MS, RD. The Power of Protein. *The Physician and Sportsmedicine* 1996, volume 24, number 4

[147] 1.5-1 g/kg/d (0.68-0.45 grams per pound of body weight. Younger people need proportionately more protein.) Brown ML (ed). *Present Knowledge in Nutrition. Sixth Edition*. Washington DC: International Life Sciences Institute Nutrition Foundation; 1990 page 68

[148] 0.83 g.kg-1.d-1 (equivalent to 0.37 grams per pound of body weight) "By use of an age-specific scoring system and the mean amino acid composition and digestibility of the US diet, this allowance became 0.83 g.kg-1.d-1 of mixed US dietary protein--a value similar to the previous RDA but derived in a different manner." Pellet PL. Protein requirements in humans. *Am J Clin Nutr*. 1990 May;51(5):723-37

[149] Weinsier RL, Morgan SL (eds). *Fundamentals of Clinical Nutrition*. St. Louis: Mosby, 1993 page 50

[150] Golding DN. Is there an allergic synovitis? *J R Soc Med*. 1990 May;83(5):312-4

[151] Panush RS. Food induced ("allergic") arthritis: clinical and serologic studies. *J Rheumatol*. 1990 Mar;17(3):291-4

[152] Pacor ML, Lunardi C, Di Lorenzo G, Biasi D, Corrocher R. Food allergy and seronegative arthritis: report of two cases. *Clin Rheumatol*. 2001;20(4):279-81

[153] Schrander JJ, Marcelis C, de Vries MP, van Santen-Hoeufft HM. Does food intolerance play a role in juvenile chronic arthritis? *Br J Rheumatol*. 1997 Aug;36(8):905-8

[154] van de Laar MA, van der Korst JK. Food intolerance in rheumatoid arthritis. I. *Ann Rheum Dis*. 1992 Mar;51(3):298-302

[155] Haugen MA, Kjeldsen-Kragh J, Forre O. A pilot study of the effect of an elemental diet in the management of rheumatoid arthritis. *Clin Exp Rheumatol*. 1994 May-Jun;12(3):275-9

[156] van de Laar MA, Aalbers M, Bruins FG, van Dinther-Janssen AC, van der Korst JK, Meijer CJ. Food intolerance in rheumatoid arthritis. II. *Ann Rheum Dis*. 1992 Mar;51(3):303-6

[157] Kaufman W. Niacinamide therapy for joint mobility. Therapeutic reversal of a common clinical manifestation of the normal aging process. *Conn State Med J* 1953;17:584-591

[158] Kaufman W. The use of vitamin therapy to reverse certain concomitants of aging. *J Am Geriatr Soc* 1955;3:927-936

[159] Matuoka K, Chen KY, Takenawa T. Rapid reversion of aging phenotypes by nicotinamide through possible modulation of histone acetylation. *Cell Mol Life Sci*. 2001;58(14):2108-16

[160] Jonas WB, Rapoza CP, Blair WF. The effect of niacinamide on osteoarthritis: a pilot study. *Inflamm Res* 1996 Jul;45(7):330-4

[161] McCarty MF, Russell AL. Niacinamide therapy for osteoarthritis--does it inhibit nitric oxide synthase induction by interleukin 1 in chondrocytes? *Med Hypotheses*. 1999;53(4):350-60

[162] Gaby AR. Literature review and commentary: Niacinamide for osteoarthritis. *Townsend Letter for Doctors and Patients*. 2002; May; 32

enzymes after 3 months of treatment and yearly thereafter. Antirheumatic benefit is generally significant following 2-6 weeks of treatment, and patients may also notice an anxiolytic benefit, possibly mediated by the binding of niacinamide to GABA/benzodiazepine receptors.[163]

o Glucosamine sulfate and chondroitin sulfate: Glucosamine and chondroitin are the "building blocks" from which cartilage is built and oral supplementation is intended to enhance cartilage anabolism and to thus counteract the enhanced cartilage catabolism seen in destructive arthritic processes.[164] Clinical trials with glucosamine and chondroitin sulfates have shown consistently positive results in clinical trials involving patients with osteoarthritis of the hands, hips, knees, temporomandibular joint, and low-back.[165,166,167,168,169,170,171] For example, glucosamine sulfate was superior to placebo for pain reduction and preservation of joint space in a 3-year clinical trial in patients with knee osteoarthritis.[172] Arguments against the use of glucosamine due to inflated concern about inefficacy or exacerbation of diabetes[173] are without scientific merit[174,175] as evidenced by a 90-day trial of diabetic patients consuming 1500 mg of glucosamine hydrochloride with 1200 mg of chondroitin sulfate which showed no significant alterations in serum glucose or hemoglobin A1c[176] and by the previously cited 3-year study which found significant clinical benefit and no adverse effects on glucose homeostasis.[177] The adult dose of glucosamine sulfate is generally 1500-2000 mg per day in divided doses, and the dose of chondroitin sulfate is approximately 1000 mg daily; these treatments can be used singly, in combination, and with other treatments. Both treatments are safe for multiyear use, and rare adverse effects include allergy and nonpathologic gastrointestinal upset. Clinical benefit is generally significant following 4-6 weeks of treatment and is maintained for the duration of treatment. In contrast to coxib and other mislabeled "anti-inflammatory" drugs that consistently elevate the incidence of cardiovascular disease, death, and other adverse effects[178,179,180,181,182], supplementation with chondroitin sulfate appears to safely reduce the pain and disability associated with osteoarthritis while simultaneously reducing incidence of cardiovascular morbidity and mortality.[183,184] In a study with animals that spontaneously develop atherosclerosis[185], administration of chondroitin sulfate induced regression of existing atherosclerosis. In a six-year study with 120 patients with established cardiovascular disease, 60 chondroitin-treated patients suffered 6 coronary events and 4 deaths compared to 42 events and 14 deaths in a comparable group of 60 patients receiving "conventional" therapy; chondroitin-treated patients reported enhancement of well-being while no adverse clinical or laboratory effects were noted during the 6 years of treatment.[186]

o Pancreatic/proteolytic enzymes: Orally-administered pancreatic and proteolytic enzymes are absorbed from the gastrointestinal tract into the systemic circulation[187,188] to exert analgesic, anti-inflammatory,

[163] Mohler H, Polc P, Cumin R, Pieri L, Kettler R. Nicotinamide is a brain constituent with benzodiazepine-like actions. *Nature.* 1979; 278(5704): 563-5

[164] Vidal y Plana RR, Bizzarri D, Rovati AL. Articular cartilage pharmacology: I. In vitro studies on glucosamine and non steroidal antiinflammatory drugs. *Pharmacol Res Commun.* 1978 Jun;10(6):557-69

[165] "...patients taking GS had a significantly greater decrease in TMJ pain with function, effect of pain, and acetaminophen used between Day 90 and 120 compared with patients taking ibuprofen." Thie NM, Prasad NG, Major PW. Evaluation of glucosamine sulfate compared to ibuprofen for the treatment of temporomandibular joint osteoarthritis: a randomized double blind controlled 3 month clinical trial. *J Rheumatol.* 2001;28(6):1347-55

[166] Braham R, Dawson B, Goodman C. The effect of glucosamine supplementation on people experiencing regular knee pain. *Br J Sports Med.* 2003;37(1):45-9

[167] "...oral glucosamine therapy achieved a significantly greater improvement in articular pain score than ibuprofen, and the investigators rated treatment efficacy as 'good' in a significantly greater proportion of glucosamine than ibuprofen recipients. In comparison with piroxicam, glucosamine significantly improved arthritic symptoms after 12 weeks of therapy..." Matheson AJ, Perry CM. Glucosamine: a review of its use in the management of osteoarthritis. *Drugs Aging.* 2003; 20(14): 1041-60

[168] Uebelhart D, Malaise M, Marcolongo R, DeVathaire F, Piperno M, Mailleux E, Fioravanti A, Matoso L, Vignon E. Intermittent treatment of knee osteoarthritis with oral chondroitin sulfate: a one-year, randomized, double-blind, multicenter study versus placebo. *Osteoarthritis Cartilage.* 2004;12:269-76

[169] van Blitterswijk WJ, van de Nes JC, Wuisman PI. Glucosamine and chondroitin sulfate supplementation to treat symptomatic disc degeneration: biochemical rationale and case report. *BMC Complement Altern Med.* 2003;3(1):2

[170] Morreale P, et al. Comparison of the antiinflammatory efficacy of chondroitin sulfate and diclofenac sodium in patients with knee osteoarthritis. *J Rheumatol.* 1996;23(8):1385-91

[171] Mazieres B, et al. Chondroitin sulfate in osteoarthritis of the knee: a prospective, double blind, placebo controlled multicenter clinical study. *J Rheumatol.* 2001;28(1):173-81

[172] Reginster JY, Deroisy R, Rovati LC, Lee RL, Lejeune E, Bruyere O, Giacovelli G, Henrotin Y, Dacre JE, Gossett C. Long-term effects of glucosamine sulphate on osteoarthritis progression: a randomised, placebo-controlled clinical trial. *Lancet.* 2001;357(9252):251-6

[173] Adams ME. Hype about glucosamine. *Lancet.* 1999;354(9176):353-4

[174] Cumming A. Glucosamine in osteoarthritis. *Lancet.* 1999;354(9190):1640-1

[175] Rovati LC, Annefeld M, Giacovelli G, Schmid K, Setnikar I. *Glucosamine in osteoarthritis.* Lancet. 1999;354(9190):1640

[176] Scroggie DA, Albright A, Harris MD. The effect of glucosamine-chondroitin supplementation on glycosylated hemoglobin levels in patients with type 2 diabetes mellitus: a placebo-controlled, double-blinded, randomized clinical trial. *Arch Intern Med.* 2003;163(13):1587-9

[177] Reginster JY, et al. Long-term effects of glucosamine sulphate on osteoarthritis progression: a randomised, placebo-controlled clinical trial. *Lancet.* 2001;357(9252):251-6

[178] Topol EJ. Failing the public health--rofecoxib, Merck, and the FDA. *N Engl J Med.* 2004 Oct 21;351(17):1707-9

[179] Mukherjee D, Nissen SE, Topol EJ. Risk of cardiovascular events associated with selective cox-2 inhibitors. *JAMA* 2001; 286(8):954-9

[180] Ray WA, Griffin MR, Stein CM. Cardiovascular toxicity of valdecoxib. *N Engl J Med.* 2004;351(26):2767

[181] "Patients in the clinical trial taking 400 mg. of Celebrex twice daily had a 3.4 times greater risk of CV events compared to placebo. For patients in the trial taking 200 mg. of Celebrex twice daily, the risk was 2.5 times greater. The average duration of treatment in the trial was 33 months." FDA Statement on the Halting of a Clinical Trial of the cox-2 Inhibitor Celebrex. http://www.fda.gov/bbs/topics/news/2004/NEW01144.html Available on January 4, 2005

[182] "Preliminary information from the study showed some evidence of increased risk of cardiovascular events, when compared to placebo, to patients taking naproxen." FDA Statement on Naproxen. http://www.fda.gov/bbs/topics/news/2004/NEW01148.html Available on January 4, 2005

[183] Morrison LM. Treatment of coronary arteriosclerotic heart disease with chondroitin sulfate-A: preliminary report. *J Am Geriatr Soc.* 1968;16(7):779-85

[184] Morrison LM, Branwood AW, Ershoff BH, Murata K, Quilligan JJ Jr, Schjeide OA, Patek P, Bernick S, Freeman L, Dunn OJ, Rucker P. The prevention of coronary arteriosclerotic heart disease with chondroitin sulfate A: preliminary report. *Exp Med Surg.* 1969;27(3):278-89

[185] Morrison LM, Bajwa GS. Absence of naturally occurring coronary atherosclerosis in squirrel monkeys (Saimiri sciurea) treated with chondroitin sulfate A. *Experientia.* 1972 Dec 15;28(12):1410-1

[186] Morrison LM, Enrick N. Coronary heart disease: reduction of death rate by chondroitin sulfate A. *Angiology.* 1973 May;24(5):269-87

[187] Gotze H, Rothman SS. Enteropancreatic circulation of digestive enzymes as a conservative mechanism. *Nature* 1975; 257(5527): 607-609

[188] Liebow C, Rothman SS. Enteropancreatic Circulation of Digestive Enzymes. *Science* 1975; 189(4201): 472-474

anti-edematous benefits with therapeutic relevance for acute and chronic musculoskeletal disorders.[189,190,191,192]

- o <u>Vitamin C</u>: Doses of 1-2 grams per day have been suggested to reduce pain and the need for surgery in patients with low-back pain by improving disc integrity.[193] Vitamin C reduces production of isoprostanes, which promote inflammation and pain. Ascorbate is also necessary for the production of the anti-inflammatory prostaglandin E-1. Supplemental vitamin C may also reduce the severity and progression of osteoarthritis.[194]
- o <u>Vitamin E, with an emphasis on gamma-tocopherol</u>: The *gamma* form of vitamin E inhibits cyclooxygenase and thus has anti-inflammatory activity.[195] Clinical trials and case reports have suggested benefit of vitamin E supplementation in patients with rheumatoid arthritis[196,197], spondylosis and back pain[198], osteoarthritis[199,200,201], and autoimmune diseases including scleroderma, discoid lupus erythematosus, porphyria cutanea tarda, vasculitis, and polymyositis.[202,203,204]

Myofascial trigger points (MFTP)

<u>Description/pathophysiology</u>:

- Many patients suffer from chronic pain that originates from myofascial trigger points—localized areas within muscle tissue that produce chronic pain, promote muscle contraction and tightness, and which mediate autonomous autonomic responses. Physicians who take the time to locate and treat MFTP and educate patients about effective home care can often rapidly and permanently reduce their patients' pain in a safe and highly cost-effective manner.
- MFTP have been defined as "a highly localized and hyperirritable spot in a palpable taut band of skeletal muscle fibers"[205] characterized by the following:
  1. <u>Referred pain with compression</u>: Digital compression of the MFTP causes local pain and most often causes referred pain in a distribution similar or identical to the patient's presenting complaint. The distribution of pain may appear radicular and may thus be described as "pseudoradicular."
  2. <u>Twitch response</u>: When digital pressure is applied perpendicularly to the direction of muscle fibers at the location of the MFTP and the muscle is "plucked" or allowed to "snap" as if one were plucking a taut rubber band or the string of a guitar, the muscle being assessed undergoes a rapid contraction.
  3. <u>Muscle tightness</u>: The muscle involved is tighter than usual, and it is resistant to stretch.
  4. <u>Associated autonomic phenomena</u>: Regions of the body near a localized MFTP may display associated autonomic dysregulation such as vasoconstriction, sweating, pilomotor response, and the patient may experience nausea, dizziness, light-headedness[206] or atrial fibrillation.[207]
  5. <u>MFTP may be "active" or "latent"</u>: Active MFTP are those which cause spontaneous pain with joint motion or muscle contraction, whereas latent MFTP cause pain only when provoked by an examiner's deep palpation and physical compression.[208]

[189] Trickett P. Proteolytic enzymes in treatment of athletic injuries. *Appl Ther.* 1964;30:647-52
[190] Walker JA, Cerny FJ, Cotter JR, Burton HW. Attenuation of contraction-induced skeletal muscle injury by bromelain. *Med Sci Sports Exerc.* 1992 Jan;24(1):20-5
[191] Walker AF, et al. Bromelain reduces mild acute knee pain and improves well-being in a dose-dependent fashion in an open study of otherwise healthy adults. *Phytomedicine.* 2002; 9: 681-6
[192] Brien S, et al. Bromelain as a Treatment for Osteoarthritis: a Review of Clinical Studies. *Evidence-based Complementary and Alternative Medicine.* 2004;1(3)251–257
[193] Greenwood J. Optimum vitamin C intake as a factor in the preservation of disc integrity. *Med Ann Dist Columbia.* 1964 Jun;33:274-6
[194] "A 3-fold reduction in risk of OA progression was found for both the middle tertile and highest tertile of vitamin C intake. This related predominantly to a reduced risk of cartilage loss. Those with high vitamin C intake also had a reduced risk of developing knee pain." McAlindon TE, Jacques P, Zhang Y, Hannan MT, Aliabadi P, Weissman B, Rush D, Levy D, Felson DT. Do antioxidant micronutrients protect against the development and progression of knee osteoarthritis? *Arthritis Rheum.* 1996 Apr;39(4):648-56
[195] Jiang Q, Christen S, Shigenaga MK, Ames BN. gamma-tocopherol, the major form of vitamin E in the US diet, deserves more attention. *Am J Clin Nutr 2001 Dec;74(6):714-22*
[196] Helmy M, Shohayeb M, Helmy MH, el-Bassiouni EA. Antioxidants as adjuvant therapy in rheumatoid disease. A preliminary study. *Arzneimittelforschung.* 2001;51(4):293-8
[197] Edmonds SE, Winyard PG, Guo R, Kidd B, Merry P, Langrish-Smith A, Hansen C, Ramm S, Blake DR. Putative analgesic activity of repeated oral doses of vitamin E in the treatment of rheumatoid arthritis. Results of a prospective placebo controlled double blind trial. *Ann Rheum Dis.* 1997 Nov;56(11):649-55
[198] "Vitamin E administration at a dose of 100 mg daily for three weeks resulted in a significant increase in serum vitamin E level accompanied by complete relief of pain... The results therefore strongly indicate that vitamin E is effective in curing spondylosis and most probably due to its antioxidant activity." Mahmud Z, Ali SM. Role of vitamin A and E in spondylosis. *Bangladesh Med Res Counc Bull.* 1992 Apr;18(1):47-59
[199] "The results of this double-blind controlled clinical trial showed that vitamin E was superior to placebo with respect to the relief of pain (pain at rest, pain during movement, pressure-induced pain) and the necessity of additional analgetic treatment. Improvement of mobility was better in the group treated with vitamin E." Blankenhorn G. [Clinical effectiveness of Spondyvit (vitamin E) in activated arthroses. A multicenter placebo-controlled double-blind study] [Article in German] *Z Orthop Ihre Grenzgeb.* 1986 May-Jun;124(3):340-3
[200] This is a very interesting study because the clinical response to vitamin E was proportional to the increase in plasma levels of vitamin E, thus confirming the dose-response relationship that implies causality as well as indicating that the failure of such treatment in some patients may be due to malabsorption or unquenchable systemic oxidative stress rather than the inefficacy of vitamin E supplementation, per se. "There were no significant differences in the efficacy of the two drugs, although one patient of the V-group refused further treatment after 8 days because of inefficacy. V reduced or abolished the pain at rest in 77% (D in 85%), the pain on pressure in 67% (D in 50%), and the pain on movement in 62% (D in 63%). Both treatments appeared to be equally effective in reducing the circumference of the knee joints (p = 0.001) and the walking time (p less than 0.001) and in increasing the joint mobility (p less than 0.002)." Scherak O, Kolarz G, Schodl C, Blankenhorn G. [High dosage vitamin E therapy in patients with activated arthrosis] [Article in German] Z Rheumatol. 1990 Nov-Dec;49(6):369-73
[201] Machtey I, Ouaknine L. Tocopherol in Osteoarthritis: a controlled pilot study. *J Am Geriatr Soc.* 1978 Jul;26(7):328-30
[202] Killeen RN, Ayres S Jr, Mihan R. Polymyositis: response to vitamin E. *South Med J.* 1976 Oct;69(10):1372-4
[203] Ayres S Jr, Mihan R. Lupus erythematosus and vitamin E: an effective and nontoxic therapy. *Cutis.* 1979 Jan;23(1):49-52, 54
[204] Ayres S Jr, Mihan R. Is vitamin E involved in the autoimmune mechanism? *Cutis.* 1978 Mar;21(3):321-5
[205] Hong CZ, Simons DG. Pathophysiologic and electrophysiologic mechanisms of myofascial trigger points. *Arch Phys Med Rehabil.* 1998;79(7):863-72
[206] Hubbard DR, Berkoff GM. Myofascial trigger points show spontaneous needle EMG activity. *Spine.* 1993 Oct 1;18(13):1803-7
[207] Simons DG. Cardiology and myofascial trigger points: Janet G. Travell's contribution. *Tex Heart Inst J.* 2003;30(1):3-7
[208] Hubbard DR, Berkoff GM. Myofascial trigger points show spontaneous needle EMG activity. *Spine.* 1993 Oct 1;18(13):1803-7

6. <u>Normal muscle strength</u>: Muscle weakness and atrophy are not associated with MFTP unless the weakness or atrophy is secondary to pain.

- The initiation and perpetuation of MFTP is complex and commonly associated with previous injury or chronic static posturing (such as sitting in front of a computer for 8-14 hours per day) and also with emotional stress. Since **intrafusal fibers of muscle spindles receive direct sympathetic innervation**, and since adrenaline/epinephrine directly increases the contractile tone and tension of muscles, it is reasonable to conclude that attention to emotional stress and stress management techniques should be part of the comprehensive treatment plan for MFTP. A significant reduction in emotional tension and work-related repetitive strain injuries may follow a comprehensive and "body-based" approach to healthy living and appropriate career choices.[209]

- The pathogenesis and physiology-based treatment of MFTP follow this route are as follows:
  <u>Pathogenesis</u>[210]
  1. Excess calcium is released from the sarcoplasmic reticulum, leading to local muscle fiber contraction.
  2. Intense and chronic muscle contractions cause relative local ischemia.
  3. The reduction in local blood supply limits energy replacement and leads to the depletion of adenosine triphosphate (ATP).
  4. The muscle cell now has insufficient ATP for the active return of calcium from the contractile elements to the sarcoplasmic reticulum, thus maintaining the muscle fibers in a contracted state.
  <u>Physiology-based treatment</u>:
  5. Stretching the muscle fibers reduces the overlap between actin and myosin, which then leads to a reduction in energy demand of the cell and thus helps to "break the cycle" of **contraction** *leading to* **energy depletion** *leading to* **contraction** *leading to* **energy depletion…**
  6. Application of ice (or other benign, intense afferent stimuli such as capsaicin or spinal manipulation) floods the dorsal horn and thus blocks transmission of nociceptive stimuli via the hypothesized "gate control" mechanism of pain reception.
  7. Magnesium supplementation is appropriate for many patients with MFTP since many patients do not consume sufficient dietary magnesium and since magnesium inhibits calcium release from the sarcoplasmic reticulum[211] and thereby has a muscle relaxing effect. **Magnesium deficiency is an epidemic** in so-called "developed" nations, with 20-40% of different populations showing objective serologic/cytologic evidence of magnesium deficiency.[212,213,214,215]

<u>Clinical presentations</u>:
- The pain pattern from MFTP is varied and is dependent on the muscle(s) involved. Each muscle has a unique pattern of pain referral; e.g., a MFTP in the deltoid or supraspinatus may cause shoulder pain and arm pain that can mimic cervical radiculitis. MFTP in the sternocleidomastoid commonly causes "headache" and pain over the side of the face and TMJ; MFTP in the psoas can cause low back and leg pain. Patients may also subjectively notice numbness or tingling in addition to pain.[216] Differentiation of MFTP pain from radiculitis and radiculopathy should be pursued clinically and documented in the patient chart.

<u>Major differential diagnoses</u>:
- <u>Arthropathy and arthritis</u>: Passive joint provocation tests are negative with MFTP; no laboratory abnormalities (such as elevated CRP) are seen with MFTP.
- <u>Acute muscle injury, strain</u>: History of *recent* injury is often negative; history of *chronic* strain and *previous* injury are common with MFTP
- <u>Radiculitis</u>: The pain associated with MFTP is not dermatomal and is reproduced with local muscle compression, whereas the pain of radiculitis is dermatomal and reproduced with nerve tension tests.
- <u>Radiculopathy</u>: Radiculopathy is associated with muscle weakness, which is not a characteristic of MFTP.

---

[209] Jarrow R. *Creating the Work You Love: Courage, Commitment and Career*. Inner Traditions Intl Ltd; December 1995) [ISBN: 0892815426]
[210] Simons DG. Cardiology and myofascial trigger points: Janet G. Travell's contribution. *Tex Heart Inst J*. 2003;30(1):3-7
[211] "Mg2+ inhibits Ca2+ release from the sarcoplasmic reticulum." Mathew R, Altura BM. The role of magnesium in lung diseases: asthma, allergy and pulmonary hypertension. *Magnes Trace Elem*. 1991-92;10(2-4):220-8
[212] "The American diet is low in magnesium, and with modern water systems, very little is ingested in the drinking water." Innerarity S. Hypomagnesemia in acute and chronic illness. *Crit Care Nurs Q*. 2000 Aug;23(2):1-19
[213] "Altogether 43% of 113 trauma patients had low magnesium levels compared to 30% of noninjured cohorts." Frankel H, Haskell R, Lee SY, Miller D, Rotondo M, Schwab CW. Hypomagnesemia in trauma patients. *World J Surg*. 1999 Sep;23(9):966-9
[214] "There was a 20% overall prevalence of hypomagnesemia among this predominantly female, African American population." Fox CH, Ramsoomair D, Mahoney MC, Carter C, Young B, Graham R. An investigation of hypomagnesemia among ambulatory urban African Americans. *J Fam Pract*. 1999 Aug;48(8):636-9
[215] "Suboptimal levels were detected in 33.7 per cent of the population under study. These data clearly demonstrate that the Mg supply of the German population needs increased attention." Schimatschek HF, Rempis R. Prevalence of hypomagnesemia in an unselected German population of 16,000 individuals. *Magnes Res*. 2001 Dec;14(4):283-90
[216] Hubbard DR, Berkoff GM. Myofascial trigger points show spontaneous needle EMG activity. *Spine*. 1993 Oct 1;18(13):1803-7

Clinical assessments:
- _History/subjective_: Pain is always present (although it may be mild or latent).
- _Physical examination/objective_: The most reliable physical signs of MFTP are **1) spot tenderness within a taut band of muscle, 2) reproduction of pain and referred pain with palpation and provocation**, and 3) local twitch response with palpation and provocation.
- _Imaging & laboratory assessments_: Lab tests and imaging assessments are normal. Myofascial trigger points show spontaneous electromyographic activity.[217]

Establishing the diagnosis:
- Reasonable clinical exclusion of acute strain, radiculopathy and radiculitis combined with characteristic clinical findings mentioned above, including at least **1) spot tenderness within a taut band of muscle, 2) reproduction of pain and referred pain with palpation/provocation**.

Complications:
- Many patients with MFTP suffer from pain for years before being properly diagnosed. Many patients are prescribed hazardous and inappropriate medications to treat the pain and symptoms of MFTP, and surgical interventions are periodically used inappropriately in patents who have not been accurately diagnosed. For example when a patient with low back pain due to MFTP is found to have an incidental disc herniation, the patient may undergo surgery on the intervertebral disc only to have pain continue postoperatively until it is treated with simple techniques directed at the MFTP.[218]

Clinical management:
- Simple nutritional and physical treatments as described below.
- Patients should be advised that deep massage of the area is often necessary and that pain may be temporarily exacerbated.

Treatments:
- _Post-isometric stretching_: Lewit and Simons described this simple and highly effective treatment succinctly in a highly recommended article[219], "The post-isometric relaxation technique begins by placing the muscle in a stretched position. Then an isometric contraction is exerted against minimal resistance. Relaxation and then gentle stretch follow as the muscle releases." In a large study involving 244 patients, post-isometric stretching "produced **immediate pain relief in 94%, lasting pain relief in 63%**, as well as lasting relief of point tenderness in 23% of the sites treated. Patients who practiced autotherapy on a home program were more likely to realize lasting relief." Clinically the technique is simultaneously performed, explained, and taught by the clinician: 1) stretch the target muscle, 2) weakly contract the target muscle against resistance for 10 seconds, 3) stretch the target muscle to a greater length than before for at least 20 seconds, 4) repeat this procedure 2-3 times. Pretreatment heating or exercising of the target muscles along with post-treatment application of ice helps to increase treatment efficacy and minimize post-treatment soreness, respectively.
- _Cold and stretch_: The application of cold and the simultaneous stretching of the muscle is an effective treatment for MFTP.[220] Cold can be applied with ice. The previously popular "spray and stretch" technique that used a vapocoolant spray such as Fluori-Methane is unnecessary and is environmentally irresponsible.
- _Topical application_: Capsaicin helps to relieve neuromuscular pain, too, and may help break the cycle of pain and spasm by 1) providing afferent stimuli to block nociceptive stimuli, and 2) by depleting local tissues of substance P, which not only serves as a transmitter of pain sensations, but may also perpetuate muscle contraction and spasm. Another mechanism by which capsaicin can alleviate trigger points is by desensitizing the vanilloid receptor (VR-1) to ultimately decrease local neurotransmitter release.[221]
- _Dry needling or injection of local anesthetic or saline_: While local injection of anesthetic or saline may appear more complex and therefore more effective, dry needling (rapid insertion and withdrawal of a needle) directly into the MFTP is just as effective, safer, and is less complicated than using anesthetic or saline solution. Increased efficacy of this technique is associated with the elicitation of a local twitch response immediately upon insertion and withdrawal of the needle. The accuracy of the needle insertion directly into the "sensitive locus" of the MFTP is essential for the effectiveness of this approach. Common locations for MFTP correlate with commonly used

[217] Hubbard DR, Berkoff GM. Myofascial trigger points show spontaneous needle EMG activity. _Spine_. 1993 Oct 1;18(13):1803-7
[218] Rubin D. Myofascial trigger point syndromes: an approach to management. _Arch Phys Med Rehabil_. 1981 Mar;62(3):107-10
[219] Lewit K, Simons DG. Myofascial pain: relief by post-isometric relaxation. _Arch Phys Med Rehabil_. 1984 Aug;65(8):452-6
[220] Rubin D. Myofascial trigger point syndromes: an approach to management. _Arch Phys Med Rehabil_. 1981 Mar;62(3):107-10
[221] "Massage with capsaicin cream (0.075%, available over the counter) is useful for treating TrPs located in surgical scars,36 which are particularly refractory to treatment." McPartland JM. Travell trigger points--molecular and osteopathic perspectives. _J Am Osteopath Assoc_. 2004 Jun;104(6):244-9 http://www.jaoa.org/cgi/content/full/104/6/244

acupuncture points, and the technique of acupuncture is analogous to the dry needling technique except that dry needling is performed more quickly and with highly localized precision into the MFTP sensitive locus. [222]

- Adjunctive nutritional support: Supplementation with **magnesium** (600 mg per day or to bowel tolerance[223]) and **calcium** are often helpful, particularly when used with an **alkalinizing Paleo-Mediterranean diet** (as discussed in Chapter 2), which—at the very least—promotes renal retention of calcium and magnesium to thus facilitate mineral retention. Other treatments to reduce intracellular calcium levels (intracellular hypercalcinosis[224]) include supplementation with **physiologic doses of vitamin D3**[225] and **fish oil for EPA**[226] along with avoidance/reduction of factors which promote renal loss of calcium and magnesium such as caffeine, sugar, alcohol/ethanol, and psychoemotional stress.

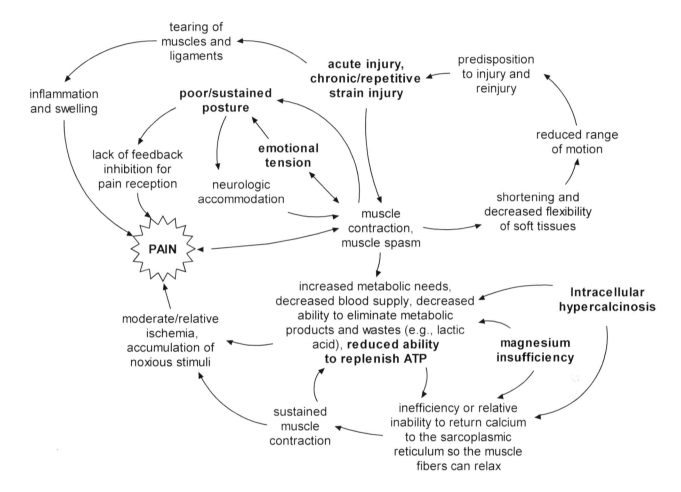

Hypothesized model for the initiation and promotion of myofascial trigger points with self-perpetuating cycles

[222] Hong CZ, Simons DG. Pathophysiologic and electrophysiologic mechanisms of myofascial trigger points. *Arch Phys Med Rehabil.* 1998 Jul;79(7):863-72

[223] "When the practitioner has been convinced to start Mg on the basis of his diagnosis or through insistence of the patient, the often recommended dose of 300 mg per day is insufficient. Experience of successful therapy indicates that no less than 600 mg per day is required." Liebscher DH, Liebscher DE. About the misdiagnosis of magnesium deficiency. *J Am Coll Nutr.* 2004 Dec;23(6):730S-1S http://www.coldcure.com/html/misdiagnosis-magnesium-deficiency.pdf

[224] See http://InflammationMastery.com/archives/intracellular-hypercalcinosis and www.naturopathydigest.com/archives/2006/sep/vasquez.php for additional discussion

[225] Vasquez A, Manso G, Cannell J. The clinical importance of vitamin D (cholecalciferol): a paradigm shift with implications for all healthcare providers. *Altern Ther Health Med.* 2004 Sep-Oct;10(5):28-36

[226] "This is a consequence of the ability of EPA to release Ca2+ from intracellular stores while inhibiting their refilling via capacitative Ca2+ influx that results in partial emptying of intracellular Ca2+ stores and thereby activation of protein kinase R." Palakurthi SS, Fluckiger R, Aktas H, Changolkar AK, Shahsafaei A, Harneit S, Kilic E, Halperin JA. Inhibition of translation initiation mediates the anticancer effect of the n-3 polyunsaturated fatty acid eicosapentaenoic acid. *Cancer Res.* 2000 Jun 1;60(11):2919-25

Another Clinically Useful Mnemonic Acronym: "B.e.n.d. S.t.e.m.s."

As an alternative to the "p.r.i.c.e. a. t.u.r.n." acronym as previously described and which is admittedly cumbersome, clinicians may use the following alternate, either additively or substitutionally. "B.end. s.t.e.m.s." is aesthetically more appealing, though it is less complete than *price a turn*. The goal, of course, is to have a useful memory key available when the clinician is formulating the treatment plan. Just as all doctors are familiar with the *s.o.a.p.* format for writing chart notes to ensure their inclusion of *subjective, objective, assessment*, and *plan* for each visit, when arriving to the "p" portion of the note, integrative clinicians can use *price a turn* and/or *bend stems* to help remember key components to integrative and holistic care.

B   **Botanical**: Numerous botanical medicines are available for a wide range of indications. Among the botanical medicines with the best research support for the treatment of musculoskeletal pain and inflammation are willow bark, *Boswellia*, *Harpagophytum*, *Uncaria*, ginger, and *Capsicum*.

E   **Ergonomics/posture and Exercise**: Patients can improve their ergonomics at home, at work, and (occasionally) in the car. Likewise, attention to posture—the "style" with which one holds one's body—is important in the prevention of repetitive strain injuries, particularly to the shoulders and neck region. Most patients are overweight, out of shape, weak, and neuromuscularly uncoordinated; problems correctible with exercise.

N   **Nutrition**: Nutritional supplements are extremely valuable in the treatment and prevention of a wide range of mild and serious health problems. Use of high-dose "supranutritional" levels of vitamins can be used to help patients overcome their enzyme and receptor defects to facilitate improved physiological function and improved overall health.[227]

D   **Diet**: In order to remain consistent with the time-proven wisdom of the *Hierarchy of Therapeutics* (discussed in Chapter 2) and to avoid becoming an aimless horde of drug-pushing symptom-suppressors, holistic integrative clinicians must always attend to the basics—the foundational influences which powerfully affect metabolism and thus overall health. Clearly, diet is one of those basics, along with emotions and lifestyle—exercise, work, stress management, outlook, and relationships.

S   **Stretching, strengthening, and stabilization**: Tight muscles can be stretched in the office, where the doctor is able to teach the patient proper methods and is able to refine the diagnosis and specificity of the stretch to ensure that targeted muscles are effectively addressed. Thereafter, the patient *must* continue these stretches at home—both physically and mentally. *Physical stretching* involves the therapeutic lengthening of muscles and fascia to maintain or restore ease of myofascial motion and to alleviate adhesions or restrictions that impair function. *Mental stretching* involves the patient's active use of reframing and discipline in order to attain a higher level of functioning and effectiveness in his/her relationships, lifestyle, work situation, mental outlook, habits and other phenomena in order to overcome the external or internal *adhesions* or *restrictions* that are impairing and preventing optimal function *of the patient as a whole*. Exercise and proprioceptive rehabilitation for spinal and peripheral joint stabilization are essential requirements for neuromusculoskeletal health.

T   **Trigger points**: Always remember to address the trigger point component (discussed previously in this chapter) when working with musculoskeletal pain. Seek and ye shall find; treat and the patient will improve. Think outside the region. A trigger point in the low-back or gluteal region may cause the patient to assume an antalgic posture that results in altered biomechanics and leads to a clinical presentation of shoulder or neck pain with chronic tension headaches; direct treatment of the painful shoulders or neck will provide improvement, but cure will not be effected until the cause—often distant from the region of complaint—is effectively addressed.[228]

E   **Educate and Ensure return**: Educate the patient about the condition, its cause and solutions. Educate about PAR-B— procedures, risks, alternatives, and benefits of treatment. Also, educate the patient *in writing* about the importance of follow-up visits and time limitations on treatments; failure to ensure that the patient was educated to return for follow-up visits is grounds for malpractice if the patient's condition changes or deteriorates due to complications associated with the presenting complaint at the last office visit.

M   **Manual medicine—mobilization, manipulation, massage**: Treat the problem effectively and directly with the skilled use of your hands. Practice produces proficiency.

S   **Spirituality (emotions, psychology)**: Perceptions create our emotional and mental realities, and from these subjective realities do we engage the world. Inaccurate perceptions skew and misshape one's interactions with the world. Creating more accurate perceptions—a process that requires intentionality and hard work—enhances *effectiveness* and ultimately *enjoyment* of one's life experience.

---

[227] Ames BN, Elson-Schwab I, Silver EA. High-dose vitamin therapy stimulates variant enzymes. *Am J Clin Nutr.* 2002 Apr;75(4):616-58 ajcn.org/cgi/content/full/75/4/616
[228] "This patient seemed to respond favorably to conservative care that included regions of spine not traditionally associated with headache pain." Stude DE, Sweere JJ. A holistic approach to severe headache symptoms in a patient unresponsive to regional manual therapy. *J Manipulative Physiol Ther.* 1996 Mar-Apr;19(3):202-7

Chapter 4:
Introduction to DrV's Functional Inflammology Protocol: The Seven Major Modifiable Factors in Systemic Inflammation, Allergy, and Autoimmunity

---

Major Modifiable Influences on Immune and Inflammatory Balance

This section reviews clinically-relevant information related to the pathogenesis and etiology of inflammatory/allergic/autoimmune conditions. Following extensive reviews of the research literature in conjunction with the author's own clinical experience with patients, the original version of this information was published in 2006 in the first edition of *Integrative Rheumatology*. This section is a distillation of thousands of research articles, abstracts, seminar notes, conversations with colleagues, one-on-one patient encounters and the author's own considerations and reflections.

Following my review and perusal of thousands of research articles in addition to the attentive application of my interest in these conditions throughout three doctoral programs, I have come to appreciate seven major modifiable factors that are chiefly relevant for the initial and long-term management of patients with inflammatory conditions and rheumatic diseases. These seven factors are:

1. Food: The pro-inflammatory effects of diet, including food allergies and intolerances,
2. Infections and dysbiosis: Chronic exposure to microbial effectors/effects,
3. Nutritional modulation of the immune system: Nutrigenomic modification of immunocytes phenotype,
4. Dysfunctional mitochondria: Especially the pro-inflammatory, pro-oxidant, and anti-apoptotic consequences of dysfunctional mitochondria,
5. Stress, sleep deprivation vs sleep sufficiency, spinal health, social and psychological considerations: Included in this section is a collection of important considerations which—in the first draft of this acronym—started with stress management, sleep hygiene, and pSychological and social factors. Later versions have included spinal health, surgery, specialized supplementation, and "stamp your passport"—sometimes we all just need to vacate for a while and implement some geographic cure for the sake of inspiration, life enhancement, exposure to new ideas and lifestyles, and the breaking of thought patterns.
6. Endocrine imbalances: Hormones can promote or retard the genesis and perpetuation of inflammation/allergy/autoimmunity; therapeutic correction with prescription or nonprescription interventions can have a profound anti-inflammatory benefit.
7. Xenobiotic immunotoxicity: Exposure to and accumulation of toxic chemicals and/or toxic metals can alter immune responses toward allergy and autoimmunity and away from immunosurveillance against infections and cancer.

Common diseases such as psoriasis and rheumatoid arthritis are greater public health concerns and are more commonly encountered in clinical practice than are the rare conditions; proportionate mention is made in the following section. Importantly, readers should appreciate that the information in various sections likely applies either conceptually or specifically to conditions described in other sections and that therefore the best way to understand inflammatory/allergic/autoimmune disorders in their totality is to appreciate the nuances of each and the common themes among all.

I am quite pleased to see that the original five variables that I defined in the first two editions of *Integrative Rheumatology* (2006, 2007) have stood the tests of time, science, and clinical practice: in fact, all have been strengthened in the intervening years.

Affirmation and consistency of common themes in an interconnected reality

"The fact that today I still stand by these ideas, **that in the intervening time they themselves have constantly become more strongly associated with one another, even to the point of growing into each other, intertwining, and becoming *one***, that has reinforced in me the joyful confidence that they may not have originally developed in me as single, random, or sporadic ideas, but up out of common roots, from some fundamental *will for knowledge* ruling from deep within, always speaking with greater clarity, always demanding greater clarity.

In fact, this is the only thing appropriate and proper for a philosopher. **We have no right to be isolated in any way: we are not permitted to make isolated mistakes or to run into isolated truths**. Our ideas, our values, our affirmations and denials, our if's and but's—these rather grow out of us from the same necessity which makes a tree bear its fruit—totally related and interlinked amongst each other: witnesses of one will, one health, one soil, one sun."

Nietzsche FW. *On the Genealogy of Morals*, 1887, Preface essay #2

Nutrition & FxMed for chronic immune-inflammatory disorders

Causes of Inflammation-Immune-Metabolic Imbalance:

1. Food, Lifestyle

2. Infection, Dysbiosis

3. Nutritional Immunomodulation

4. Dysfunctional mitochondria

5. Stress, Emotions, Psychology, Sociology, Lifestyle

6. Endocrine, Hormones

7. Xenobiotics, Toxins

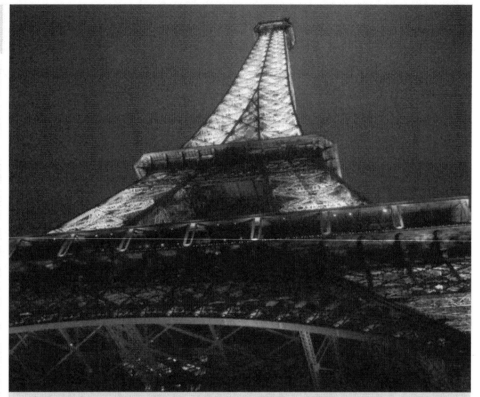

Notice that these 7 factors can be remembered by the acronym: **F.I.N.D. S.E.X.**

♥ First presented in Paris in 2012 ♥

The "Functional Immunology/Inflammology Protocol" and acronym: As the clinical protocol expanded from five components (diet, dysbiosis, xenobiotics, hormones, and stress) published in 2006 and 2007 to seven components (adding nutritional immunomodulation and mitochondrial dysfunction) in 2012, I realized that the time had come to attempt an acronym in order to facilitate student memorization and clinician application. I applied some priority to the sequence of the categories, and then experimented with a few acronyms. The rest, as is said, is history. This occurred just before a series of presentations in France (starting in Paris), Holland, and Belgium in March of 2012. The FINDSEX acronym is a registered trademark (e.g., ® and ™) in association with *Functional Immunology and Nutritional Immunomodulation*, *Inflammation Mastery*, and other books and videos.

❶ Food ❷ Infections ❸ Nutri-immunomod ❹ Dys mito ❺ Stress/Sleep/Socio/Surg/Sup ❻ Endo ❼ Xeno

❶ Food:
Diet and Basic Nutritional Supplementation

Major Concepts in this Section

"Food" is the first part of the protocol and the foundation of the overall plan, not simply for improving nutritional status, but for setting the stage for more profound improvements in immune balance, mitochondrial function, et al.

As it currently is, this first section on "Food" should be a bit elementary for naturopathic students, whose training in nutrition prior to the Rheumatology course should have already covered topics like TLR, AGE/RAGE, acid-base balance, fatty acid metabolism, allergies, probiotics, and hopefully topics like GP-120 and food-induced hypothalamic inflammation; such topics will be detailed in future editions of this book, namely the multivolume work that allows unlimited space.

Contents of this section:
1. Nutrigenomics
2. DrV's "Supplemented Paleo-Mediterranean Diet—previously published descriptions
3. DrV's perspectives on "food allergies", which must also be discussed in conjunction with the new information on nutritional immunomodulation

---

Pro-Inflammatory and Anti-Inflammatory Nutrigenomics

We must look beyond the nutritional properties of foods to appreciate that dietary patterns and the consumption of specific foods can influence genetic expression and either promote or retard the development of inflammation and related clinical disorders. The purpose of this section is to help clinicians attain a more profound understanding of the value of nutrition and its critical role as a foundational component in the treatment plan of patients with inflammatory disorders. The "correct" diet for the vast majority of patients with inflammatory disorders is the "supplemented Paleo-Mediterranean diet" which I have described in several other publications. The diet is modified for the specific exclusion of allergenic foods; it is implemented on a rotation basis, and it allows for periodic fasting and vegetarianism/veganism. The implementation of health-promoting dietary modifications is an *absolutely mandatory* component of the treatment plan, upon which other treatments depend for their success.

The study of how dietary components and nutritional supplements influence genetic expression is referred to as *nutrigenomics* or *nutritional genomics* and has been described as "the next frontier in the postgenomic era."[1] Various nutrients have been shown to modulate genetic expression and thus alter phenotypic manifestations of disease by upregulating or downregulating specific genes, interacting with nuclear receptors, altering hormone receptors, and modifying the influence of transcription factors, such as pro-inflammatory NF-kappaB (NFkB) and the anti-inflammatory peroxisome-proliferator activated receptors (PPARs).[2,3,4,5] **The previous view that nutrients only interact with human physiology at the metabolic/post-transcriptional level must be updated in light of current research showing that nutrients can, in fact, modify human physiology and phenotype at the genetic/pre-transcriptional level.**

---

[1] Kaput J, Rodriguez RL. Nutritional genomics: the next frontier in the postgenomic era. *Physiol Genomics*. 2004 Jan 15;16(2):166-77 http://physiolgenomics.physiology.org/cgi/content/full/16/2/166

[2] Vamecq J, Latruffe N. Medical significance of peroxisome proliferator-activated receptors. *Lancet*. 1999;354:141-8

[3] Ehrmann J Jr, Vavrusova N, Collan Y, Kolar Z. Peroxisome proliferator-activated receptors (PPARs) in health and disease. *Biomed Pap Med Fac Univ Palacky Olomouc Czech Repub*. 2002 Dec;146(2):11-4 http://publib.upol.cz/~obd/fulltext/Biomed/2002/2/11.pdf

[4] Kliewer SA, Xu HE, Lambert MH, Willson TM. Peroxisome proliferator-activated receptors: from genes to physiology. *Recent Prog Horm Res*. 2001;56:239-63

[5] Delerive P, Fruchart JC, Staels B. Peroxisome proliferator-activated receptors in inflammation control. *J Endocrinol*. 2001;169(3):453-9

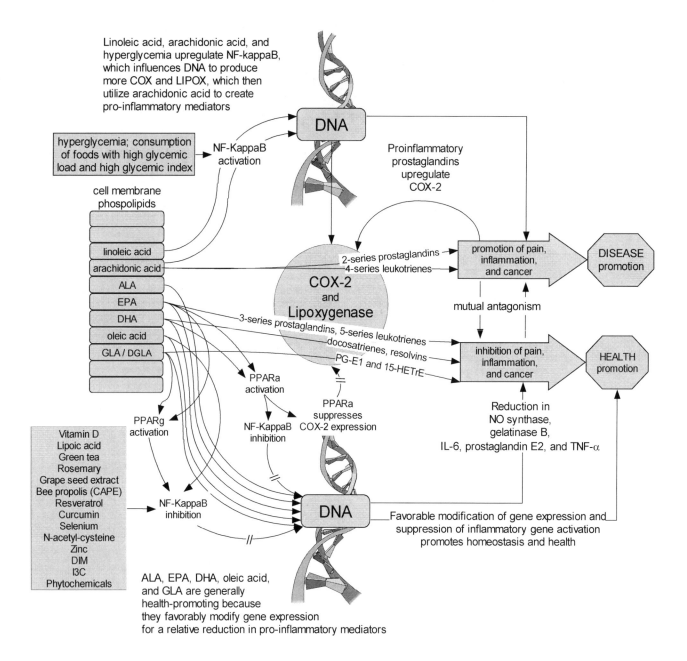

Schematic Representation of Simultaneous Nutrigenomic and Metabolic Effects of Nutrients[6]

Fatty acids and their *eicosanoid*, *leukotriene*, and *isoprostane* intermediates and end-products modulate genetic expression in several ways. In general, n-3 fatty acids decrease inflammation and promote health while n-6 fatty acids (except for GLA, which is generally health-promoting) increase inflammation, oxidative stress, and the manifestation of disease. Corn oil, probably as a result of its high n-6 LA (linoleic acid) content, rapidly activates NFkB and thus promotes tumor development, atherosclerosis, and elaboration of proinflammatory mediators such as TNFa.[7,8,9] Similarly n-6 arachidonic acid increases production of the free radical *superoxide* approximately 4-fold when added to isolated Kupffer cells *in vitro*. Prostaglandin-E2 is produced from arachidonic acid by cyclooxygenase and increases genetic expression of cyclooxygenase and IL-6; thus, an

[6] Vasquez A. New Insights into Fatty Acid Supplementation and Its Effect on Eicosanoid Production and Genetic Expression. *Nutritional Perspectives* 2005; Jan: 5-16
[7] Rusyn I, Bradham CA, Cohn L, Schoonhoven R, Swenberg JA, Brenner DA, Thurman RG. Corn oil rapidly activates nuclear factor-kappaB in hepatic Kupffer cells by oxidant-dependent mechanisms. *Carcinogenesis*. 1999 Nov;20(11):2095-100
[8] Rose DP, Hatala MA, Connolly JM, Rayburn J. Effect of diets containing different levels of linoleic acid on human breast cancer growth and lung metastasis in nude mice. *Cancer Res*. 1993 Oct 1;53(19):4686-90
[9] Dichtl W, Ares MP, Jonson AN, Jovinge S, Pachinger O, Giachelli CM, Hamsten A, Eriksson P, Nilsson J. Linoleic acid-stimulated vascular adhesion molecule-1 expression in endothelial cells depends on nuclear factor-kappaB activation. *Metabolism*. 2002 Mar;51(3):327-33

increase in PG-E2 leads to additive expression of cyclooxygenase, which further increases inflammation and elevates C-reactive protein.[10] Some of the unique health-promoting effects of GLA are nutrigenomically mediated via activation of PPAR-gamma, resultant inhibition of NFkB, and impairment of estrogen receptor function.[11,12] Supplementation with ALA leads to a dramatic reduction of prostaglandin formation in humans[13], and this effect is probably mediated by downregulation of proinflammatory gene transcription, as evidenced by reductions in CRP, IL-6, and serum amyloid A.[14] EPA appears to exert much of its anti-inflammatory benefit by suppressing NFkB activation and thus reducing elaboration of proinflammatory mediators.[15,16] EPA also indirectly modifies gene expression and cell growth by reducing intracellular calcium levels and thus activating protein kinase R which impairs eukaryotic initiation factor-2alpha and inhibits protein synthesis at the level of translation initiation, thereby mediating an anti-cancer benefit.[17] DHA is the precursor to docosatrienes and resolvins which downregulate gene expression for proinflammatory IL-1, inhibit of TNFa, and reduce neutrophil entry to sites of inflammation.[18] Oxidized EPA activates PPAR-alpha and thereby suppresses NFkB and the activation of proinflammatory genes.[19,20] Other nutrients that inhibit the activation of NFkB include vitamin D[21,22], lipoic acid[23], green tea[24], rosemary[25], grape seed extract[26], resveratrol[27,28], caffeic acid phenethyl ester (CAPE) from bee propolis[29], indole-3-carbinol[30], N-acetyl-L-cysteine[31], selenium[32], and

[10] Bagga D, Wang L, Farias-Eisner R, Glaspy JA, Reddy ST. Differential effects of prostaglandin derived from omega-6 and omega-3 polyunsaturated fatty acids on COX-2 expression and IL-6 secretion. *Proc Natl Acad Sci U S A.* 2003 Feb 18;100(4):1751-6. http://www.pnas.org/cgi/reprint/100/4/1751.pdf

[11] Menendez JA, Colomer R, Lupu R. Omega-6 polyunsaturated fatty acid gamma-linolenic acid (18:3n-6) is a selective estrogen-response modulator in human breast cancer cells: gamma-linolenic acid antagonizes estrogen receptor-dependent transcriptional activity, transcriptionally represses estrogen receptor expression and synergistically enhances tamoxifen and ICI 182,780 (Faslodex) efficacy in human breast cancer cells. *Int J Cancer.* 2004 May 10;109(6):949-54

[12] Jiang WG, Redfern A, Bryce RP, Mansel RE. Peroxisome proliferator activated receptor-gamma (PPAR-gamma) mediates the action of gamma linolenic acid in breast cancer cells. *Prostaglandins Leukot Essent Fatty Acids.* 2000 Feb;62(2):119-27

[13] Adam O, Wolfram G, Zollner N. Effect of alpha-linolenic acid in the human diet on linoleic acid metabolism and prostaglandin biosynthesis. *J Lipid Res.* 1986 Apr;27(4):421-6

[14] Rallidis LS, Paschos G, Liakos GK, Velissaridou AH, Anastasiadis G, Zampelas A. Dietary alpha-linolenic acid decreases C-reactive protein, serum amyloid A and interleukin-6 in dyslipidaemic patients. *Atherosclerosis.* 2003 Apr;167(2):237-42

[15] Zhao Y, Joshi-Barve S, Barve S, Chen LH. Eicosapentaenoic acid prevents LPS-induced TNF-alpha expression by preventing NF-kappaB activation. *J Am Coll Nutr.* 2004 Feb;23(1):71-8

[16] Mishra A, Chaudhary A, Sethi S. Oxidized omega-3 fatty acids inhibit NF-kappaB activation via a PPARalpha-dependent pathway. *Arterioscler Thromb Vasc Biol.* 2004 Sep;24(9):1621-7

[17] Palakurthi SS, Fluckiger R, Aktas H, Changolkar AK, Shahsafaei A, Harneit S, Kilic E, Halperin JA. Inhibition of translation initiation mediates the anti-cancer effect of the n-3 polyunsaturated fatty acid eicosapentaenoic acid. *Cancer Res.* 2000 Jun 1;60(11):2919-25

[18] "These results indicate that DHA is the precursor to potent protective mediators generated via enzymatic oxygenations to novel docosatrienes and 17S series resolvins that each regulate events of interest in inflammation and resolution." Hong S, Gronert K, Devchand PR, Moussignac RL, Serhan CN. Novel docosatrienes and 17S-resolvins generated from docosahexaenoic acid in murine brain, human blood, and glial cells. Autacoids in anti-inflammation. *J Biol Chem.* 2003 Apr 25;278(17):14677-87

[19] Mishra A, Chaudhary A, Sethi S. Oxidized omega-3 fatty acids inhibit NF-kappaB activation via a PPARalpha-dependent pathway. *Arterioscler Thromb Vasc Biol.* 2004 Sep;24(9):1621-7

[20] Delerive P, Fruchart JC, Staels B. Peroxisome proliferator-activated receptors in inflammation control. J Endocrinol. 2001;169(3):453-9

[21] "1Alpha,25-dihydroxyvitamin D3 (1,25-(OH)2-D3), the active metabolite of vitamin D, can inhibit NF-kappaB activity in human MRC-5 fibroblasts, targeting DNA binding of NF-kappaB but not translocation of its subunits p50 and p65." Harant H, Wolff B, Lindley IJ. 1Alpha,25-dihydroxyvitamin D3 decreases DNA binding of nuclear factor-kappaB in human fibroblasts. *FEBS Lett.* 1998 Oct 9;436(3):329-34

[22] "Thus, 1,25(OH)2D3 may negatively regulate IL-12 production by downregulation of NF-kB activation and binding to the p40-kB sequence." D'Ambrosio D, Cippitelli M, Cocciolo MG, Mazzeo D, Di Lucia P, Lang R, Sinigaglia F, Panina-Bordignon P. Inhibition of IL-12 production by 1,25-dihydroxyvitamin D3. Involvement of NF-kappaB downregulation in transcriptional repression of the p40 gene. *J Clin Invest.* 1998 Jan 1;101(1):252-62

[23] "ALA reduced the TNF-alpha-stimulated ICAM-1 expression in a dose-dependent manner, to levels observed in unstimulated cells. Alpha-lipoic acid also reduced NF-kappaB activity in these cells in a dose-dependent manner." Lee HA, Hughes DA. Alpha-lipoic acid modulates NF-kappaB activity in human monocytic cells by direct interaction with DNA. *Exp Gerontol.* 2002 Jan-Mar;37(2-3):401-10

[24] "In conclusion, EGCG is an effective inhibitor of IKK activity. This may explain, at least in part, some of the reported anti-inflammatory and anti-cancer effects of green tea." Yang F, Oz HS, Barve S, de Villiers WJ, McClain CJ, Varilek GW. The green tea polyphenol (-)-epigallocatechin-3-gallate blocks nuclear factor-kappa B activation by inhibiting I kappa B kinase activity in the intestinal epithelial cell line IEC-6. *Mol Pharmacol.* 2001 Sep;60(3):528-33

[25] "These results suggest that carnosol suppresses the NO production and iNOS gene expression by inhibiting NF-kappaB activation, and provide possible mechanisms for its anti-inflammatory and chemopreventive action." Lo AH, Liang YC, Lin-Shiau SY, Ho CT, Lin JK. Carnosol, an antioxidant in rosemary, suppresses inducible nitric oxide synthase through down-regulating nuclear factor-kappaB in mouse macrophages. *Carcinogenesis.* 2002 Jun;23(6):983-91

[26] "Constitutive and TNFalpha-induced NF-kappaB DNA binding activity was inhibited by GSE at doses > or =50 microg/ml and treatments for > or =12 h." Dhanalakshmi S, Agarwal R, Agarwal C. Inhibition of NF-kappaB pathway in grape seed extract-induced apoptotic death of human prostate carcinoma DU145 cells. *Int J Oncol.* 2003 Sep;23(3):721-7

[27] "Resveratrol's anticarcinogenic, anti-inflammatory, and growth-modulatory effects may thus be partially ascribed to the inhibition of activation of NF-kappaB and AP-1 and the associated kinases." Manna SK, Mukhopadhyay A, Aggarwal BB. Resveratrol suppresses TNF-induced activation of nuclear transcription factors NF-kappa B, activator protein-1, and apoptosis: potential role of reactive oxygen intermediates and lipid peroxidation. *J Immunol.* 2000 Jun 15;164(12):6509-19

[28] "Both resveratrol and quercetin inhibited NF-kappaB-, AP-1- and CREB-dependent transcription to a greater extent than the glucocorticosteroid, dexamethasone." Donnelly LE, Newton R, Kennedy GE, Fenwick PS, Leung RH, Ito K, Russell RE, Barnes PJ. Anti-inflammatory Effects of Resveratrol in Lung Epithelial Cells: Molecular Mechanisms. *Am J Physiol Lung Cell Mol Physiol.* 2004 Jun 4 [Epub ahead of print]

[29] "Caffeic acid phenethyl ester (CAPE) is an anti-inflammatory component of propolis (honeybee resin). CAPE is reportedly a specific inhibitor of nuclear factor-kappaB (NF-kappaB)." Fitzpatrick LR, Wang J, Le T. Caffeic acid phenethyl ester, an inhibitor of nuclear factor-kappaB, attenuates bacterial peptidoglycan polysaccharide-induced colitis in rats. *J Pharmacol Exp Ther.* 2001 Dec;299(3):915-20

[30] Takada Y, Andreeff M, Aggarwal BB. Indole-3-carbinol suppresses NF-{kappa}B and I{kappa}B{alpha} kinase activation causing inhibition of expression of NF-{kappa}B-regulated antiapoptotic and metastatic gene products and enhancement of apoptosis in myeloid and leukemia cells. Blood. 2005 Apr 5; [Epub ahead of print]

[31] Paterson RL, Galley HF, Webster NR. The effect of N-acetylcysteine on nuclear factor-kappa B activation, interleukin-6, interleukin-8, and intercellular adhesion molecule-1 expression in patients with sepsis. Crit Care Med. 2003 Nov;31(11):2574-8

[32] Faure P, Ramon O, Favier A, Halimi S. Selenium supplementation decreases nuclear factor-kappa B activity in peripheral blood mononuclear cells from type 2 diabetic patients. *Eur J Clin Invest.* 2004;34(7):475-81

zinc.[33] **Therefore, we see that fatty acids and nutrients directly affect gene expression by complex and multiple mechanisms, as graphically illustrated in the accompanying diagram, and the synergism and potency of these anti-inflammatory nutraceuticals supports the rationale for the use of nutrition and select botanicals for the safe and effective treatment of inflammatory disorders.**

A Five-Part Nutritional Wellness Protocol That Produces Consistently Positive Results: Brief Review of Scientific Rationale

This article was originally published in *Nutritional Wellness*
http://www.nutritionalwellness.com/archives/2005/sep/09_vasquez.php

When I am lecturing here in the U.S., as well as in Europe, doctors often ask if I will share the details of my protocols with them. Thus, in 2004, I published a 486-page textbook for doctors that includes several protocols and important concepts for the promotion of wellness and treatment of musculoskeletal disorders.[34] In this article, I will share with you what I consider a basic protocol for wellness promotion. I've implemented this protocol as part of the treatment plan for a wide range of clinical problems. In my next column, I will provide several case reports of patients from my office to exemplify the effectiveness of this program and show how it can be the foundation upon which additional treatments can be added as necessary.

Nutrients are required in the proper amounts, forms, and approximate ratios for essential physiologic function; if nutrients are lacking, the body cannot function normally, let alone optimally. Impaired function results in subjective and objective manifestations of what is commonly labeled as "disease." Thus, a powerful and effective alternative to treating diseases with drugs is to re-establish normal/optimal physiologic function by replenishing the body with essential nutrients.

Of course, many diseases are multifactorial and therefore require multicomponent treatment plans, and some diseases actually require the use of drugs. However, while only a relatively small portion of patients actually need drugs for their problems, I am sure we all agree that everyone needs a foundational nutrition plan, as outlined and substantiated below.

1. <u>Health-promoting diet</u>: Following an extensive review of the research literature, I developed what I call the "supplemented Paleo-Mediterranean diet," which I have described in greater detail elsewhere.[35] In essence, this diet plan combines the best of the Mediterranean diet with the best of the Paleolithic diet, the latter of which has been detailed most recently by Dr. Loren Cordain in his book, The Paleo Diet, and his numerous scientific articles.[36] This diet places emphasis on fruits, vegetables, nuts, seeds, and berries that meet the body's needs for fiber, carbohydrates, and most importantly, the 8,000+ phytonutrients that have additive and synergistic health benefits.[37] Preferred protein sources are lean meats such as fish and poultry. In contrast to Cordain's Paleo diet, I also advocate soy and whey for their high-quality protein and anticancer, cardioprotective, and mood-enhancing benefits. Rice and potatoes are discouraged due to their relatively high glycemic indexes and high glycemic loads, and their lack of fiber and phytonutrients (compared to other fruits and vegetables). Generally speaking, grains such as wheat and rye are discouraged due to the high glycemic loads/indexes of most breads and pastries, as well as the allergenicity of gluten, a protein that appears to help trigger disorders such as migraine, celiac disease, psoriasis, epilepsy, and autoimmunity. Sources of simple sugars such as high-fructose corn syrup (e.g., cola, soda) and processed foods (e.g., "TV dinners" and other manufactured snacks and convenience foods) are strictly forbidden. Chemical preservatives, colorants, sweeteners and carrageenan are likewise prohibited. In summary, this diet plan provides plenty of variety, as most dishes comprised of poultry, fish, soy, fruits, vegetables, nuts, berries, and seeds are allowed. The diet also provides plenty of fiber, phytonutrients, carbohydrates, potassium, and protein, while simultaneously being low in fat, sodium,

[33] Uzzo RG, Leavis P, Hatch W, Gabai VL, Dulin N, Zvartau N, Kolenko VM. Zinc inhibits nuclear factor-kappa B activation and sensitizes prostate cancer cells to cytotoxic agents. *Clin Cancer Res.* 2002;8(11):3579-83

[34] **Vasquez A**. *Integrative Orthopedics: The Art of Creating Wellness While Managing Acute and Chronic Musculoskeletal Disorders.* 2004, 2007

[35] **Vasquez A**. The Importance of Integrative Chiropractic Health Care in Treating Musculoskeletal Pain and Reducing the Nationwide Burden of Medical Expenses and Iatrogenic Injury and Death: Concise Review of Current Research and Implications for Clinical Practice and Healthcare Policy. *The Original Internist* 2005; 12(4): 159-182

[36] Cordain L. *The Paleo Diet*. (John Wiley and Sons, 2002). Also: Cordain L. Cereal grains: humanity's double edged sword. *World Rev Nutr Diet* 1999;84:19-73 Access to most of Dr Cordain's articles is available at http://thepaleodiet.com/

[37] Liu RH. Health benefits of fruit and vegetables are from additive and synergistic combinations of phytochemicals. *Am J Clin Nutr* 2003;78(3 Suppl):517S-520S

arachidonic acid, and "simple sugars." The diet must be customized with regard to total protein and calorie intake, as determined by the size, status, and activity level of the patient, and individual food allergens should be avoided. Regular consumption of this diet has shown the ability to reduce hypertension, alleviate diabetes, ameliorate migraine headaches, and result in improvement of overall health and a lessening of the severity of many common "diseases." This diet is supplemented with vitamins, minerals, and fatty acids as described below.

2. Multivitamin and multimineral supplementation: Vitamin and mineral supplementation finally received endorsement from "mainstream" medicine when researchers from Harvard Medical School published a review article in *Journal of the American Medical Association* that concluded, "Most people do not consume an optimal amount of all vitamins by diet alone. ...It appears prudent for all adults to take vitamin supplements."[38] Long-term nutritional insufficiencies experienced by "most people" promote the development of "long-latency deficiency diseases" such as cancer, neuroemotional deterioration, and cardiovascular disease.[39] Impressively, the benefits of multivitamin/multimineral supplementation have been demonstrated in numerous clinical trials. Multivitamin/multimineral supplementation has been shown to improve nutritional status and reduce the risk for chronic diseases[40]. improve mood[41], potentiate antidepressant drug treatment[42], alleviate migraine headaches (when used with diet improvement and fatty acids[43]), improve immune function and infectious disease outcomes in the elderly[44] (especially diabetics[45]), reduce morbidity and mortality in patients with HIV infection[46,47] alleviate premenstrual syndrome[48,49] and bipolar disorder[50], reduce violence and antisocial behavior in children[51] and incarcerated young adults (when used with essential fatty acids[52]), and improve scores of intelligence in children.[53] Vitamin supplementation has anti-inflammatory benefits, as evidenced by significant reduction in C-reactive protein, (CRP) in a double-blind, placebo-controlled trial.[54] The ability to safely and affordably deliver these benefits makes multimineral-multivitamin supplementation and essential component of any and all health-promoting and disease-prevention strategies. Vitamin A can result in liver damage with chronic consumption of 25,000 IU or more, and intake should generally not exceed 10,000 IU per day in women of childbearing age. Iron should not be supplemented except in patients diagnosed with iron deficiency by a blood test (serum ferritin). Additional vitamin D should be used, as described in the next section.

3. Physiologic doses of vitamin D3: The prevalence of vitamin D deficiency varies from 40 percent (general population) to almost 100 percent (patients with musculoskeletal pain) in the American population. I described the many benefits of vitamin D3 supplementation in the previous issue of *Nutritional Wellness* and in the major monograph published last year.[55] In summary, vitamin D deficiency causes or contributes to depression, hypertension, seizures, migraine, polycystic ovary syndrome, inflammation,

[38] Fletcher RH, Fairfield KM. Vitamins for chronic disease prevention in adults: clinical applications. *JAMA* 2002;287:3127-9

[39] Heaney RP. Long-latency deficiency disease: insights from calcium and vitamin D. *Am J Clin Nutr* 2003;78:912-9

[40] McKay DL, Perrone G, Rasmussen H, Dallal G, Hartman W, Cao G, Prior RL, Roubenoff R, Blumberg JB. The effects of a multivitamin/mineral supplement on micronutrient status, antioxidant capacity and cytokine production in healthy older adults consuming a fortified diet. *J Am Coll Nutr* 2000;19(5):613-21

[41] Benton D, Haller J, Fordy J. Vitamin supplementation for 1 year improves mood. *Neuropsychobiology* 1995;32(2):98-105

[42] Coppen A, Bailey J. Enhancement of the antidepressant action of fluoxetine by folic acid: a randomised, placebo controlled trial. *J Affect Disord* 2000;60:121-30

[43] Wagner W, Nootbaar-Wagner U. Prophylactic treatment of migraine with gamma-linolenic and alpha-linolenic acids. *Cephalalgia* 1997;17:127-30

[44] Langkamp-Henken B, Bender BS, Gardner EM, Herrlinger-Garcia KA, Kelley MJ, Murasko DM, Schaller JP, Stechmiller JK, Thomas DJ, Wood SM. Nutritional formula enhanced immune function and reduced days of symptoms of upper respiratory tract infection in seniors. *J Am Geriatr Soc* 2004;52:3-12

[45] Barringer TA, Kirk JK, Santaniello AC, Foley KL, Michielutte R. Effect of a multivitamin and mineral supplement on infection and quality of life. A randomized, double-blind, placebo-controlled trial. *Ann Intern Med* 2003;138:365-71

[46] Fawzi WW, Msamanga GI, et al. A randomized trial of multivitamin supplements and HIV disease progression and mortality. *N Engl J Med* 2004;351:23-32

[47] Burbano X, Miguez-Burbano MJ, McCollister K, Zhang G, Rodriguez A, Ruiz P, Lecusay R, Shor-Posner G. Impact of a selenium chemoprevention clinical trial on hospital admissions of HIV-infected participants. *HIV Clin Trials* 2002;3:483-91

[48] Abraham GE. Nutritional factors in the etiology of the premenstrual tension syndromes. *J Reprod Med* 1983;28(7):446-64

[49] Stewart A. Clinical and biochemical effects of nutritional supplementation on the premenstrual syndrome. *J Reprod Med* 1987;32:435-41

[50] Kaplan BJ, Simpson JS, Ferre RC, Gorman CP, McMullen DM, Crawford SG. Effective mood stabilization with a chelated mineral supplement: an open-label trial in bipolar disorder. *J Clin Psychiatry* 2001;62:936-44

[51] Kaplan BJ, Crawford SG, Gardner B, Farrelly G. Treatment of mood lability and explosive rage with minerals and vitamins: two case studies in children. *J Child Adolesc Psychopharmacol* 2002;12(3):205-19

[52] Gesch CB, Hammond SM, Hampson SE, Eves A, Crowder MJ. Influence of supplementary vitamins, minerals and essential fatty acids on the antisocial behaviour of young adult prisoners. Randomised, placebo-controlled trial. *Br J Psychiatry* 2002;181:22-8

[53] Benton D. Micro-nutrient supplementation and the intelligence of children. *Neurosci Biobehav Rev* 2001;25:297-309

[54] Church TS, Earnest CP, Wood KA, Kampert JB. Reduction of C-reactive protein levels through use of a multivitamin. *Am J Med* 2003;115:702-7

[55] **Vasquez A**, Manso G, Cannell J. The clinical importance of vitamin D (cholecalciferol): a paradigm shift with implications for all healthcare providers. *Alternative Therapies in Health and Medicine* 2004;10:28-37

autoimmunity, and musculoskeletal pain such as low-back pain. Clinical trials using vitamin D supplementation have proven the cause-and-effect relationship between vitamin D deficiency and these conditions by showing that each of these could be cured or alleviated with vitamin D supplementation. In our review of the literature, we concluded that daily vitamin D doses should be 1,000 IU for infants, 2,000 IU for children, and 4,000 IU for adults. Cautions and contraindications include the use of thiazide diuretics (e.g., hydrochlorothiazide) or any other medications that can promote hypercalcemia, as well as granulomatous diseases such as sarcoidosis, tuberculosis, and certain types of cancer, especially lymphoma. Effectiveness is monitored by measuring serum 25-OH-vitamin D, and safety is monitored by measuring serum calcium.

4. <u>Balanced and complete fatty acid supplementation</u>: A detailed survey of the literature shows there are at least five health-promoting fatty acids commonly found in the human diet.[56] These are alpha-linolenic acid (ALA; omega-3, from flaxseed oil), eicosapentaenoic acid (EPA; omega-3, from fish oil), docosahexaenoic acid (DHA; omega-3, from fish oil and algae), gamma-linolenic acid (GLA; omega-6, most concentrated in borage oil), and oleic acid (omega-9, from olive oil, also flaxseed and borage oils). Each of these fatty acids has health benefits that cannot be fully attained from supplementing a different fatty acid. The benefits of GLA (borage oil) are not attained by consumption of EPA and DHA (fish oil); in fact, consumption of fish oil can actually promote a deficiency of GLA.[57] Likewise, consumption of GLA alone can reduce EPA levels while increasing levels of proinflammatory arachidonic acid; both of these problems are avoided with co-administration of fish oil any time borage oil is used. Using ALA (flaxseed oil) alone only slightly increases EPA but generally leads to no improvement in DHA status and can lead to a reduction of oleic acid; thus, fish oil, olive oil (and borage oil) should be supplemented when flaxseed oil is used.[58] Obviously, the goal here is a balanced intake of all of the health-promoting fatty acids; using only one or two sources of fatty acids is not balanced and results in suboptimal improvement, at best. In clinical practice, I routinely use combination fatty acid therapy comprised of ALA, EPA, DHA, and GLA for essentially all patients. The product also contains a modest amount of oleic acid, and I encourage use of olive oil for salads and cooking. This approach results in complete and balanced fatty acid intake, and the clinical benefits are impressive.

5. <u>Probiotics/gut flora modification</u>: Proper levels of good bacteria promote intestinal health, proper immune function, and support overall health. Excess bacteria or yeast, or the presence of harmful bacteria, yeast, or "parasites" such as amoebas and protozoas, can cause "leaky gut," systemic inflammation, and a wide range of clinical problems. Intestinal flora can become imbalanced by poor diets, excess stress, immunosuppressive drugs, antibiotics, or exposure to contaminated food or water, all of which are common among American patients. Thus, as a rule, I reinstate the good bacteria by the use of probiotics (good bacteria and yeast), prebiotics (fiber, arabinogalactan, and inulin), and the use of fermented foods such as kefir (in patients not allergic to milk). Harmful yeast, bacteria, and other "parasites" can be eradicated with the combination of dietary change, drugs, and/or herbal extracts. For example, oregano oil in an emulsified, time-released form has proven safe and effective for the elimination of various parasites encountered in clinical practice.[59] Likewise, the herb *Artemisia annua* (sweet wormwood) commonly is used to eradicate specific bacteria and has been used for thousands of years in Asia for the treatment and prevention of infectious diseases, including malaria.[60]

<u>Conclusion</u>: In this brief review, I have outlined and scientifically substantiated a fundamental protocol that can serve as effective therapy for patients with a wide range of "diseases." Customizing the Paleo-Mediterranean diet to avoid food allergens, using vitamin-mineral supplements along with physiologic doses of vitamin D and broad-spectrum balanced fatty acid supplementation, and ensuring gastrointestinal health

---

[56] **Vasquez A**. Reducing Pain and Inflammation Naturally. Part 2: New Insights into Fatty Acid Supplementation and Its Effect on Eicosanoid Production and Genetic Expression. *Nutritional Perspectives* 2005; January: 5-16

[57] Cleland LG, Gibson RA, Neumann M, French JK. The effect of dietary fish oil supplement upon the content of dihomo-gammalinolenic acid in human plasma phospholipids. *Prostaglandins Leukot Essent Fatty Acids* 1990 May;40(1):9-12

[58] Jantti J, Nikkari T, Solakivi T, Vapaatalo H, Isomaki H. Evening primrose oil in rheumatoid arthritis: changes in serum lipids and fatty acids. *Ann Rheum Dis* 1989;48(2):124-7

[59] Force M, Sparks WS, Ronzio RA. Inhibition of enteric parasites by emulsified oil of oregano in vivo. *Phytother Res* 2000;14:213-4

[60] Schuster BG. Demonstrating the validity of natural products as anti-infective drugs. *J Altern Complement Med* 2001;7 Suppl 1:S73-82

with the skillful use of probiotics, prebiotics, and antimicrobial treatments provides an excellent health-promoting and disease-eliminating foundation and lifestyle for many patients. Often, this simple protocol is all that is needed for the effective treatment of a wide range of clinical problems. For other patients with more complex illnesses, of course, additional interventions and laboratory assessments can be used to customize the treatment plan. However, we must always remember that the attainment and preservation of health requires that we meet the body's basic nutritional needs. This five-step protocol begins the process of meeting those needs. In my next article, I'll give you some examples from my clinical practice and additional references to show how safe and effective this protocol can be.

Implementing the Five-Part Nutritional Wellness Protocol for the Treatment of Various Health Problems

This article was originally published in *Nutritional Wellness*
http://www.nutritionalwellness.com/archives/2005/nov/11_vasquez.php

In my last article in *Nutritional Wellness* I described a 5-part nutritional protocol that can be used in the vast majority of patients without adverse effects and with major benefits. For many patients, the basic protocol consisting of 1) the Paleo-Mediterranean diet, 2) multivitamin/multimineral supplementation, 3) additional vitamin D3, 4) combination fatty acid therapy with an optimal balance of ALA, GLA, EPA, DHA, and oleic acid, and 5) probiotics (including the identification and eradication of harmful yeast, bacteria, and other "parasites") is all the treatment that they need. For patients who need additional treatment, this foundational plan still serves as the core of the biochemical aspect of their intervention. Of course, in some cases, we have to use other lifestyle modifications (such as exercise), additional supplements (such as policosanol or antimicrobial herbs), manual treatments (including spinal manipulation) and occasionally select medications (such has hormone modulators) to obtain our goal of maximum improvement.

The following examples show how the 5-part protocol serves to benefit patients with a wide range of conditions. For the sake of saving space, I will use only highly specific citations to the research literature, since I have provided the other references in the previous issue of *Nutritional Wellness* and elsewhere.[61]

- A Man with High Cholesterol: This patient is a 41-year-old slightly overweight man with very high cholesterol. His total cholesterol was 290 (normal < 200), LDL cholesterol was 212 (normal <130), and his triglycerides were 148 (optimal <100). I am quite certain that nearly every medical doctor would have put this man on cholesterol-lowering statin drugs for life. *Treatment*: In contrast, I advised a low-carb Paleo-Mediterranean diet because such diets have been shown to reduce cardiovascular mortality more powerfully that "statin" cholesterol-lowing drugs in older patients.[62] Likewise, fatty acid supplementation is more effective than statin drugs for reducing cardiac and all-cause mortality.[63] We added probiotics, because supplementation with *Lactobacillus* and *Bifidobacterium* has been shown to lower cholesterol levels in humans with high cholesterol.[64] Finally, I also prescribed 20 mg of policosanol for its well-known ability to favorably modify cholesterol levels.[65] *Results*: Within *one month* the patient had lost weight, felt better, and his total cholesterol had dropped to normal at 196 (from 290!), LDL was reduced to 141, and triglycerides were reduced to 80. Basically, this treatment plan was "the protocol + policosanol." Drug treatment of this patient would have been more expensive, more risky, and would not have resulted in global health improvements.

- A Child with Intractable Seizures: This is a 4-year-old nonverbal boy with 3-5 seizures per day despite being on two anti-seizure medications and having previously had several other "last resort" medical and surgical procedures. He also had a history of food allergies. *Treatment*: Obviously, there was no room for error in this case. We implemented a moderately low-carb hypoallergenic diet since both carbohydrate

---

[61] **Vasquez A.** Integrative Orthopedics. www.InflammationMastery.com and Chiropractic and Naturopathic Medicine for the Promotion of Optimal Health and Alleviation of Pain and Inflammation. http://InflammationMastery.com/monograph05

[62] Knoops KT, et al. Mediterranean diet, lifestyle factors, and 10-year mortality in elderly European men and women: the HALE project. *JAMA*. 2004 Sep 22;292(12):1433-9

[63] Studer M, et al. Effect of different antilipidemic agents and diets on mortality: a systematic review. *Arch Intern Med*. 2005;165:725-30

[64] Xiao JZ, et al. Effects of milk products fermented by Bifidobacterium longum on blood lipids in rats and healthy adult male volunteers. *J Dairy Sci*. 2003;86:2452-61

[65] Cholesterol-lowering action of policosanol compares well to that of pravastatin and lovastatin. *Cardiovasc J S Afr*. 2003;14(3):161

restriction[66] and allergy avoidance[67] can reduce the frequency and severity of seizures. Since many "anti-seizure" medications actually cause seizures by causing vitamin D deficiency[68], I added 800 IU per day of emulsified vitamin D3 for its antiseizure benefit.[69] We used 1 tsp per day of a combination fatty acid supplement that provides balanced amounts of ALA, GLA, EPA, and DHA, since fatty acids appear to have potential antiseizure benefits.[70] Vitamin B-6 (250 mg of P5P) and magnesium (bowel tolerance) were also added to reduce brain hyperexcitability.[71] Stool testing showed an absence of *Bifidobacteria* and *Lactobacillus*; probiotics were added for their anti-allergy benefits.[72] **Results**: Within about 2 months seizure frequency reduced from 3-5 per day to one seizure every other day: *an 87% reduction in seizure frequency*. Patient was able to discontinue one of the anti-seizure medications. His parents also noted several global improvements: the boy started making eye contact with people, he was learning again, and intellectually he was "making gains every day." His parents considered this an "amazing difference." Going from 30 seizures per week to 4 seizures per week while reducing medication use by 50% is a major achievement. Notice that we simply used the basic wellness protocol with some additional B6 and magnesium. It is highly unlikely that B6 and magnesium alone would have produced such a favorable response.

- A Young Woman with Full-Body Psoriasis Unresponsive to Drug Treatment: This is a 17-year-old woman with head-to-toe psoriasis since childhood. She wears long pants and long-sleeved shirts year-round, and the psoriasis is a major interference to her social life. Medications have ceased to help. **Treatment**: The Paleo-Mediterranean diet was implemented with an emphasis on food allergy identification.[1] We used a multivitamin-mineral supplement with 200 mcg selenium to compensate for the nutritional insufficiencies and selenium deficiency that are common in patients with psoriasis; likewise 10 mg of folic acid was added to address the relative vitamin deficiencies and elevated homocysteine that are common in these patients.[73] Combination fatty acid therapy with EPA and DHA from fish oil and GLA from borage oil was used for the anti-inflammatory and skin-healing benefits.[74] Vitamin E (1200 IU of mixed tocopherols) and lipoic acid (1,000 mg per day) were added for their anti-inflammatory benefits and to combat the oxidative stress that is characteristic of psoriasis.[75] Of course, probiotics were used to modify gut flora, which is commonly deranged in patients with psoriasis.[76] **Results**: Within a few weeks, this patient's "lifelong psoriasis" was essentially gone. Food allergy identification and avoidance played a major role in the success of this case. When I saw the patient again 9 months later for her second visit, she had no visible evidence of psoriasis. Her "medically untreatable" condition was essentially cured by the use of my basic protocol, with the addition of a few extra nutrients.

- A Man with Fatigue and Recurrent Numbness in Hands and Feet. This 40-year-old man had seen numerous neurologists and had spent tens of thousands of dollars on MRIs, CT scans, lumbar punctures, and other diagnostic procedures. No diagnosis had been found, and no effective treatment had been rendered by medical specialists. **Assessments**: We performed a modest battery of lab tests which revealed elevations of fibrinogen and C-reactive protein (CRP), two markers of acute inflammation. Assessment of intestinal permeability with the lactulose-mannitol assay showed major intestinal damage ("leaky gut"). Follow-up parasite testing on different occasions showed dysbiosis caused by *Proteus*, *Enterobacter*, *Klebsiella*, *Citrobacter*, and *Pseudomonas aeruginosa*—of course, these are gram-negative bacteria that can induce immune dysfunction and autoimmunity, as described elsewhere.[1] Specifically, *Pseudomonas aeruginosa* has been linked to the development of nervous system autoimmunity, such as multiple sclerosis.[77] **Treatment**: We implemented a plan of diet modification, vitamins, minerals, fatty acids, and probiotics. The dysbiosis was further addressed with specific antimicrobial herbs (including caprylic acid and emulsified oregano

[66] Freeman JM, et al. The efficacy of the ketogenic diet-1998: a prospective evaluation of intervention in 150 children. *Pediatrics*. 1998;102:1358-63

[67] Egger J, Carter CM, Soothill JF, Wilson J. Oligoantigenic diet treatment of children with epilepsy and migraine. *J Pediatr*. 1989;114:51-8

[68] Ali FE, Al-Bustan MA, Al-Busairi WA, Al-Mulla FA. Loss of seizure control due to anticonvulsant-induced hypocalcemia. *Ann Pharmacother*. 2004;38:1002-5

[69] Christiansen C, Rodbro P, Sjo O. "Anticonvulsant action" of vitamin D in epileptic patients? A controlled pilot study. *Br Med J*. 1974 May 4;2(913):258-9

[70] Yuen AW, et al. Omega-3 fatty acid supplementation in patients with chronic epilepsy: A randomized trial. *Epilepsy Behav*. 2005 Sep;7(2):253-8

[71] Mousain-Bosc M, et al. Magnesium VitB6 intake reduces central nervous system hyperexcitability in children. *J Am Coll Nutr*. 2004;23(5):545S-548S

[72] Majamaa H, Isolauri E. Probiotics: a novel approach in the management of food allergy. *J Allergy Clin Immunol*. 1997 Feb;99(2):179-85

[73] Vanizor Kural B, et al. Plasma homocysteine and its relationships with atherothrombotic markers in psoriatic patients. *Clin Chim Acta*. 2003 Jun;332(1-2):23-3

[74] **Vasquez A**. Reducing Pain and Inflammation Naturally. Part 2: New Insights into Fatty Acid Supplementation and Its Effect on Eicosanoid Production and Genetic Expression. *Nutritional Perspectives* 2005; January: 5-16

[75] Kokcam I, Naziroglu M. Antioxidants and lipid peroxidation status in the blood of patients with psoriasis. *Clin Chim Acta*. 1999 Nov;289(1-2):23-31

[76] Waldman A, et al. Incidence of Candida in psoriasis--a study on the fungal flora of psoriatic patients. *Mycoses*. 2001 May;44(3-4):77-81

[77] Hughes LE, et al. Antibody responses to Acinetobacter spp. and Pseudomonas aeruginosa in multiple sclerosis: prospects for diagnosis using the myelin-acinetobacter-neurofilament antibody index. *Clin Diagn Lab Immunol*. 2001;8(6):1181-8

oil[78]) and drugs (such as tetracycline, Bactrim, and augmentin). The antibiotic drugs proved to be ineffective based on repeat stool testing. ***Results***: Within one month we witnessed impressive improvements, both subjectively and objectively. Subjectively, the patient reported that the numbness and tingling almost completely resolved. Fatigue was reduced, and energy was improved. Objectively, the patient's elevated CRP plummeted from abnormally high at 11 down to completely normal at 1. Eighteen months later, the patient's CRP had dropped to less than 1 and fatigue and numbness were no longer problematic. Notice that this treatment plan was basically "the protocol" with additional attention to eradicating the dysbiosis we found with specialized stool testing.

- A 50-year-old Man with Rheumatoid Arthritis. This patient presented with a 3-year history of rheumatoid arthritis that had been treated unsuccessfully with drugs (methotrexate and intravenous Remicade). The first time I tested his hsCRP level, it was astronomically high at 124 (normal is <3). Because of the severe inflammation and other risk factors for sudden cardiac death, I referred this patient to an osteopathic internist for immune-suppressing drugs; the patient refused, stating that he was no longer willing to rely on immune-suppressing chemical medications. His treatment was entirely up to me. ***Assessments and Treatments***: We implemented the Paleo-Mediterranean diet and a program of vitamins, minerals, optimal combination fatty acid therapy (providing ALA, GLA, EPA, DHA, and oleic acid), and 4000 IU of vitamin D in emulsified form to overcome defects in absorption that are seen in older patients and those with gastrointestinal problems.[79] Hormone testing showed abnormally low DHEA, low testosterone, and slightly elevated estrogen; these problems were corrected with DHEA supplementation and the use of a hormone-modulating drug (Arimidex) that lowers estrogen and raises testosterone. Specialized stool testing showed absence of *Lactobacillus* and *Bifidobacteria* and intestinal overgrowth of *Citrobacter* and *Enterobacter* which was corrected with probiotics and antimicrobial treatments including undecylenic acid and emulsified oregano oil. Importantly, I also decided to inhibit NF-kappaB (the primary transcription factor that upregulates the pro-inflammatory response[80]) by using a combination botanical formula that contains curcumin, piperine, lipoic acid, green tea extract, propolis, rosemary, resveratrol, ginger, and phytolens (an antioxidant extract from lentils that may inhibit autoimmunity[81])—all of these herbs and nutrients have been shown to inhibit NF-kappaB and to thus downregulate inflammatory responses.[82] ***Results***: Within 6 weeks, this patient had happily lost 10 lbs of excess weight and was able to work without pain for the first time in years. Follow-up testing showed that his previously astronomical hsCRP had dropped from 124 to 7—a drop of 114 points in less than one month: better than had ever been achieved even with the use of intravenous immune-suppressing drugs! This patient continues to make significant progress. Obviously this case was complex, and we needed to do more than the basic protocol. Nonetheless, the basic protocol still served as the foundation for the treatment plan. Note that vitamin D has significant anti-inflammatory benefits and can cause major reductions in inflammation measured by CRP.[83] The correction of the hormonal abnormalities and the dysbiosis, and downregulating NF-kappaB with several botanical extracts were also critical components of this successful treatment plan.

Summary and Conclusions: These examples show how the nutritional wellness protocol that I described in the September issue of *Nutritional Wellness* can be used as the foundational treatment for a wide range of health problems. In many cases, implementation of the basic protocol is all that is needed. In more complex situations, we use the basic protocol and then add more specific treatments to address dysbiosis and hormonal problems, and we can add additional nutrients as needed. However, there will never be a substitute for a healthy diet, sufficiencies of vitamin D and all five of the health-promoting fatty acids (i.e., ALA, GLA, EPA, DHA, and oleic acid), and normalization of gastrointestinal flora. Without these basics, survival and the appearance of

---

[78] Force M, Sparks WS, Ronzio RA. Inhibition of enteric parasites by emulsified oil of oregano in vivo. *Phytother Res*. 2000 May;14(3):213-4
[79] **Vasquez A**. Subphysiologic Doses of Vitamin D are Subtherapeutic: Comment on the Study by The Record Trial Group. *TheLancet.com* Accessed June 16, 2005
[80] Tak PP, Firestein GS. NF-kappaB: a key role in inflammatory diseases. *J Clin Invest*. 2001 Jan;107(1):7-11
[81] Sandoval M, et al. Peroxynitrite-induced apoptosis in epithelial (T84) and macrophage (RAW 264.7) cell lines: effect of legume-derived polyphenols (phytolens). *Nitric Oxide*. 1997;1(6):476-83
[82] **Vasquez A**. Reducing pain and inflammation naturally - Part 4: Nutritional and Botanical Inhibition of NF-kappaB, the Major Intracellular Amplifier of the Inflammatory Cascade. A Practical Clinical Strategy Exemplifying Anti-Inflammatory Nutrigenomics. *Nutritional Perspectives* 2005;July: 5-12
[83] Timms PM, et al. Circulating MMP9, vitamin D and variation in the TIMP-1 response with VDR genotype. *QJM*. 2002 Dec;95(12):787-96

health are possible, but true health and recovery from "untreatable" illnesses is not possible. In order to attain optimal health, we have to create the conditions that allow for health to be attained, and we start this process by supplying the body with the nutrients that it needs to function optimally. In the words of naturopathic physician Jared Zeff from the *Journal of Naturopathic Medicine*, "*The work of the naturopathic physician is to elicit healing by helping patients to create or recreate the conditions for health to exist within them. Health will occur where the conditions for health exist. Disease is the product of the conditions which allow for it.*"[84]

Common Oversights and Shortcomings in the Study and Implementation of Nutritional Supplementation

This article was originally published in *Naturopathy Digest*
http://www.naturopathydigest.com/archives/2007/jun/vasquez.php

Introduction: An impressive discrepancy often exists between the low efficacy of nutritional interventions reported in the research literature and the higher efficacy achieved in the clinical practices of clinicians trained in the use of interventional nutrition (i.e., naturopathic physicians). This discrepancy is dangerous for at least two reasons. First, it results in an undervaluation of the efficacy of nutritional supplementation, which ultimately leaves otherwise treatable patients untreated. Second, such untreated and undertreated patients are often then forced to use dangerous and expensive pharmaceutical drugs and surgical interventions to treat conditions that could have otherwise been easily and safely treated with nutritional supplementation and diet modification. Consequently, the burden of suffering, disease, and healthcare expense in the US is higher than it would be if nutritionally-trained clinicians were more fully integrated into the healthcare system.

Obstacles to Efficacy in the Use of Nutritional Supplementation: Below are listed some of the most common causes for the underachievement of nutritional supplementation in practice and in published research. While this list is not all-inclusive, it will serve as a review for clinicians and an introduction for chiropractic/naturopathic students. In both practice and research, the problems listed below often overlap and function synergistically to reduce the efficacy of nutritional supplementation.

1. Inadequate dosing (quantity): Many clinical trials published in major journals and many doctors in clinical practice have used inadequate doses of vitamins (and other natural therapeutics) and have thus failed to achieve the results that would have easily been obtained had they implemented their protocol with the proper physiologic or supraphysiologic dose of intervention. The best example in my experience centers on vitamin D, where so many of the studies are performed with doses of 400-800 IU per day only to conclude that vitamin supplementation is ineffective for the condition being treated. The problem here is that the researchers failed to appreciate that the physiologic requirement for vitamin D3 in adults is approximately 3,000-5,000 IU per day[85] and that therefore their supplemental dose of 400-800 IU is only 10-20% of what is required. Subphysiologic doses are generally subtherapeutic. In this regard, I have had to correct journals such as *The Lancet*[86], *JAMA*[87], and *British Medical Journal*[88] from misleading their readers (many of whom are major policymakers) from concluding that nutritional supplementation is impotent; rather, their researchers and editors were not sufficiently educated in the design and review of studies using nutritional interventions. These journals should hire chiropractic and naturopathic physicians so that they have staff trained in natural treatments and who can thus provide an educated review of studies on these topics.[89]

2. Inadequate dosing (duration): Often the effects of long-term nutritional deficiency are not fully reversible and/or may require a treatment period of months or years to achieve maximal clinical response. For example, full replacement of fatty acids in human brain phospholipids is an ongoing process that occurs over a period of several years; thus studies using fatty acid supplements for a period of weeks or 2-3

---

[84] Zeff JL. The process of healing: a unifying theory of naturopathic medicine. *Journal of Naturopathic Medicine* 1997; 7: 122-5

[85] Heaney RP, Davies KM, Chen TC, Holick MF, Barger-Lux MJ. Human serum 25-hydroxycholecalciferol response to extended oral dosing with cholecalciferol. *Am J Clin Nutr*. 2003 Jan;77(1):204-10 http://www.ajcn.org/cgi/content/full/77/1/204

[86] **Vasquez A**. Subphysiologic Doses of Vitamin D are Subtherapeutic: Comment on the Study by The Record Trial Group. *The Lancet* 2005 Published on-line May 6

[87] Muanza DN, **Vasquez A**, Cannell J, Grant WB. Isoflavones and Postmenopausal Women. [letter] *JAMA* 2004; 292: 2337

[88] **Vasquez A**, Cannell J. Calcium and vitamin D in preventing fractures: data are not sufficient to show inefficacy. [letter] *BMJ: British Medical Journal* 2005;331:108-9

[89] **Vasquez A**. Allopathic Usurpation of Natural Medicine. *Naturopathy Digest* 2006 Feb naturopathydigest.com/archives/2006/feb/vasquez.php

months generally underestimate the enhanced effectiveness that can be obtained with administration over many months or several years of treatment. Relatedly, recovery from vitamin D deficiency takes several weeks of high-dose supplementation in order to achieve tissue saturation and subsequent cellular replenishment; studies of short duration are destined to underestimate the results that could have been achieved with supplementation carried out over several months.[90]

3. <u>Failure to use proper forms of nutrients (quality)</u>: Nutrients are often available in different forms, not the least of which are "active" versus "inactive" and "natural" versus "unnatural." Most vitamin supplements, particularly high-potency B vitamins, are manufactured synthetically and are not from "natural sources" despite the marketing hype promulgated by companies that, for example, mix their synthetic vitamins with a vegetable powder and then call their vitamin supplements "natural." The simple fact is that production of high-potency supplements from purely natural sources would be prohibitively wasteful, inefficient, and expensive. Thus, while it is not necessary for vitamins to be "natural" in order to be useful, it is necessary that the vitamins are useable and preferably not "unnatural." The best example of the use of unnatural supplements is the use of synthetic DL-tocopherol in the so-called "vitamin E" studies; DL-tocopherol is by definition 50% comprised of the L-isomer of tocopherol which is not only unusable by the human body but is actually harmful in that it interferes with normal metabolism and can exacerbate hypertension and cause symptomatic complications (e.g., headaches). Further, tocopherols exist within the body in relationship with the individual forms of the vitamin, such that supplementation with one form (e.g., alpha-tocopherol) can result in a relative deficiency of another form (e.g., gamma-tocopherol). One final example of the failure to use proper forms of nutrients is in the use of pyridoxine HCl as a form of vitamin B6; while this practice itself is not harmful, clinicians need to remember that pyridoxine HCl is ineffective until converted to the more active forms of the vitamin including pyridoxal-5-phosphate. Since this conversion requires co-nutrients such as magnesium and zinc, we can easily see that the reputed failure of B6 supplementation when administered in the form of pyridoxine HCl might actually be due to untreated insufficiencies of required co-nutrients, as discussed in the following section.

4. <u>Failure to ensure adequacy of co-nutrients</u>: Vitamins, minerals, amino acids, and fatty acids work together in an intricately choreographed and delicately orchestrated dance that culminates in the successful completion of interconnected physiologic functions. If any of the performers in this event are missing (i.e., nutritional deficiency) or if successive interconversions are impaired due to lack of enzyme function, then the show cannot go on, or—if it does go on—impaired metabolism and defective function will result. So, if we take a patient with "vitamin B6 deficiency" and give him vitamin B6 in the absence of other co-nutrients needed for the proper activation and metabolic utilization of vitamin B6, we cannot honestly expect the "nutritional supplementation" to work in this case; rather, we might see a marginal benefit or perhaps even a negative outcome as an imbalanced system is pushed into a different state of imbalance despite supplementation with the "correct" vitamin. In the case of vitamin B6, necessary co-nutrients include zinc, magnesium, and riboflavin; deficiency of any of these will result in a relative "failure" of B6 supplementation even if a patient has a B6-responsive condition. Notably, overt magnesium deficiency is alarmingly common among patients and citizens in industrialized nations[91,92,93], and this epidemic of magnesium deficiency is due not only to insufficient intake but also to excessive excretion caused by consumption of high-glycemic foods, caffeine, and a diet that promotes chronic metabolic acidosis with resultant urinary acidification.

5. <u>Failure to achieve urinary alkalinization</u>: Western/American-style diets typified by overconsumption of grains, dairy, sugar, and salt result in a state of subclinical chronic metabolic acidosis which results in

[90] **Vasquez A**, Manso G, Cannell J. The clinical importance of vitamin D (cholecalciferol): a paradigm shift with implications for all healthcare providers. *Altern Ther Health Med.* 2004 Sep-Oct;10(5):28-36

[91] "Altogether 43% of 113 trauma patients had low magnesium levels compared to 30% of noninjured cohorts." Frankel H, Haskell R, Lee SY, Miller D, Rotondo M, Schwab CW. Hypomagnesemia in trauma patients. *World J Surg.* 1999 Sep;23(9):966-9

[92] "There was a 20% overall prevalence of hypomagnesemia among this predominantly female, African American population." Fox CH, Ramsoomair D, Mahoney MC, Carter C, Young B, Graham R. An investigation of hypomagnesemia among ambulatory urban African Americans. *J Fam Pract.* 1999 Aug;48(8):636-9

[93] "Suboptimal levels were detected in 33.7 per cent of the population under study. These data clearly demonstrate that the Mg supply of the German population needs increased attention." Schimatschek HF, Rempis R. Prevalence of hypomagnesemia in an unselected German population of 16,000 individuals. *Magnes Res.* 2001 Dec;14(4):283-90

urinary acidification, relative hypercortisolemia, and consequent hyperexcretion of minerals such as calcium and magnesium.[94] [95] Thus, the common conundrum of magnesium replenishment requires not only magnesium supplementation but also dietary interventions to change the internal climate to one that is conducive to bodily retention and cellular uptake of magnesium.[96]

6. <u>Use of mislabeled supplements</u>: Even in the professional arena of nutritional supplement manufacturers, some companies habitually underdose their products either in an attempt to spend less in the manufacture of their products or as a consequence of poor quality control. If a product is labeled to contain 1,000 IU of vitamin D but only contains 836 IU of the nutrient, then obviously full clinical efficacy will not be achieved; this was a problem in a recent clinical trial involving vitamin D.[97] The problem for clinicians is in trusting the companies that supply nutritional supplements; some companies do "in house" testing which lacks independent review, while other companies use questionable "independent testing" which is not infrequently performed by a laboratory that is a wholly owned subsidiary of the parent nutritional company. Manufacturing regulations that are sweeping through the industry will cleanse the nutritional supplement world of poorly made products, and these same regulations will sweep some unprepared companies right out the door when they are unable to meet the regulatory requirements.

7. <u>Failure to ensure/assess bioavailability and optimal serum/cellular levels</u>: Clinical trials with nutritional therapies need to monitor serum or cellular levels to ensure absorption, product bioavailability, and the attainment of optimal serum levels. This is particularly relevant in the treatment of chronic disorders such as the autoimmune diseases, wherein so many of these patients have gastrointestinal dysbiosis and often have concomitant nutrient malabsorption.[98] Simply dosing these patients with supplements is not always efficacious; often the gut must be cleared of dysbiosis so that the mucosal lining can be repaired and optimal nutrient absorption can be reestablished.

8. <u>Coadministration of food with nutritional supplements (sometimes right, sometimes wrong)</u>: Food can help or hinder the absorption of nutritional supplements. Phytate and tannins in grains and teas, respectively, are notorious for inhibiting mineral absorption. Some supplements, like coenzyme Q10, should be administered with fatty food to enhance absorption. Other supplements, like amino acids, should be administered away from protein-rich foods and are often better administered with simple carbohydrate to enhance cellular uptake; this is especially true with tryptophan.

9. <u>Correction of gross dietary imbalances enhances supplement effectiveness</u>: If the diet is grossly imbalanced, then nutritional supplementation is less likely to be effective. The best example of this is in the use of fatty acid supplements, particularly in the treatment of inflammatory disorders. If the diet is laden with dairy, beef, and other sources of arachidonate, then fatty acid supplementation with EPA, DHA, and GLA is much less likely to be effective, or much higher doses of the supplements will need to be used in order to help restore fatty acid balance. Generally speaking, the diet needs to be optimized to enhance the efficacy of nutritional supplementation.

<u>Conclusion</u>: In this brief review, I have listed and discussed some of the most common impediments to the success of nutritional supplementation. I hope that naturopathic students, clinicians, and researchers will find these points helpful in their design of clinical treatment protocols.

[94] Cordain L, Eaton SB, Sebastian A, Mann N, Lindeberg S, Watkins BA, O'Keefe JH, Brand-Miller J. Origins and evolution of the Western diet: health implications for the 21st century. *Am J Clin Nutr.* 2005 Feb;81(2):341-54

[95] Maurer M, Riesen W, Muser J, Hulter HN, Krapf R. Neutralization of Western diet inhibits bone resorption independently of K intake and reduces cortisol secretion in humans. *Am J Physiol Renal Physiol.* 2003 Jan;284(1):F32-40

[96] Vormann J, Worlitschek M, Goedecke T, Silver B. Supplementation with alkaline minerals reduces symptoms in patients with chronic low back pain. *J Trace Elem Med Biol.* 2001;15(2-3):179-83

[97] Heaney RP, Davies KM, Chen TC, Holick MF, Barger-Lux MJ. Human serum 25-hydroxycholecalciferol response to extended oral dosing with cholecalciferol. *Am J Clin Nutr.* 2003 Jan;77(1):204-10 http://www.ajcn.org/cgi/content/full/77/1/204

[98] **Vasquez A**. Reducing Pain and Inflammation Naturally. Part 6: Nutritional and Botanical Treatments Against "Silent Infections" and Gastrointestinal Dysbiosis, Commonly Overlooked Causes of Neuromusculoskeletal Inflammation and Chronic Health Problems. *Nutritional Perspectives* 2006; January

Revisiting the Five-Part Nutritional Wellness Protocol: The Supplemented Paleo-Mediterranean Diet

This article was originally published in the January 2011 issue of the American Chiropractic Association's Council on Nutrition's journal *Nutritional Perspectives*

Abstract: This article reviews the five-part nutritional protocol that incorporates a health-promoting nutrient-dense diet and essential supplementation with vitamins/minerals, specific fatty acids, probiotics, and physiologic doses of vitamin D3. This foundational nutritional protocol has proven benefits for disease treatment, disease prevention, and health maintenance and restoration. Additional treatments such as botanical medicines, additional nutritional supplements, and pharmaceutical drugs can be used atop this foundational protocol to further optimize clinical effectiveness. The rationale for this five-part protocol is presented, and consideration is given to adding iodine-iodide as the sixth component of the protocol.

<u>Introduction</u>: In 2004 and 2005 I first published a "five-part nutrition protocol"[99,100] that provides the foundational treatment plan for a wide range of health disorders. This protocol served and continues to serve as the foundation upon which other treatments are commonly added, and without which those other treatments are likely to fail, or attain suboptimal results at best.[101] Now as then, I will share with you what I consider a basic foundational protocol for wellness promotion and disease treatment. I have used this protocol in my own self-care for many years and have used it in the treatment of a wide range of health-disease conditions in clinical practice.

This nutritional protocol is validated by biochemistry, physiology, experimental research, peer-reviewed human trials, and the clinical application of common sense. It is the most nutrient-dense diet available, satisfying nutritional needs and thereby optimizing metabolic processes while promoting satiety and weight loss/optimization. Nutrients are required in the proper amounts, forms, and approximate ratios for critical and innumerable physiologic functions; if nutrients are lacking, the body cannot function *normally*, let alone *optimally*. Impaired function results in subjective and objective manifestations of what is eventually labeled as "disease." Thus, a powerful and effective alternative to treating diseases with drugs is to re-establish normal/optimal physiologic function by replenishing the body with essential nutrients, reestablishing hormonal balance ("orthoendocrinology"), promoting detoxification of environmental toxins, and by reestablishing the optimal microbial milieu, especially the eradication of (multifocal) dysbiosis; this multifaceted approach can be applied to several diseases, especially those of the inflammatory and autoimmune varieties.[102]

Of course, most diseases are multifactorial and therefore require multicomponent treatment plans, and some diseases actually require the use of drugs in conjunction with assertive interventional nutrition. However, while only a smaller portion of patients actually need drugs for the long-term management their problems, all clinicians should agree that everyone needs a foundational nutrition plan because nutrients—not drugs—are universally required for life and health. This five-part nutrition protocol is briefly outlined below; a much more detailed substantiation of the underlying science and clinical application of this protocol was recently published in a review of more than 650 pages and approximately 3,500 citations.[103]

1. <u>Health-promoting Paleo-Mediterranean diet</u>: Following an extensive review of the research literature, I developed what I call the "supplemented Paleo-Mediterranean diet." In essence, this diet plan combines the best of the Mediterranean diet with the best of the Paleolithic diet, the latter of which has been best distilled by Dr. Loren Cordain in his book "The Paleo Diet"[104] and his numerous scientific articles.[105,106,107]

[99] **Vasquez A**. *Integrative Orthopedics: The Art of Creating Wellness While Managing Acute and Chronic Musculoskeletal Disorders*. 2004, 2007

[100] Vasquez A.Five-Part Nutritional Protocol that Produces Consistently Positive Results.*NutrWellness*2005Sep nutritionalwellness.com/archives/2005/sep/09_vasquez.php

[101] **Vasquez A.** Common Oversights and Shortcomings in the Study and Implementation of Nutritional Supplementation. *Naturopathy Digest* 2007 June. http://www.naturopathydigest.com/archives/2007/jun/vasquez.php

[102] **Vasquez A**. Integrative Rheumatology. IBMRC: 2006, 2009

[103] **Vasquez A**. Chiropractic and Naturopathic Mastery of Common Clinical Disorders. IBMRC: 2009

[104] Cordain L. *The Paleo Diet*. John Wiley and Sons, 2002

[105] O'Keefe JH Jr, Cordain L. Cardiovascular disease resulting from a diet and lifestyle at odds with our Paleolithic genome: how to become a 21st-century hunter-gatherer. *Mayo Clin Proc*. 2004 Jan;79(1):101-8

[106] Cordain L. Cereal grains: humanity's double edged sword. *World Rev Nutr Diet* 1999;84:19-73

[107] Cordain L, Eaton SB, Sebastian A, Mann N, Lindeberg S, Watkins BA, O'Keefe JH, Brand-Miller J. Origins and evolution of the Western diet: health implications for the 21st century. *Am J Clin Nutr*. 2005 Feb;81(2):341-54

The Paleolithic diet is superior to the Mediterranean diet in nutrient density for promoting satiety, weight loss, and improvements/normalization in overall metabolic function.[108,109] This diet places emphasis on fruits, vegetables, nuts, seeds, and berries that meet the body's needs for fiber, carbohydrates, and most importantly, the 8,000+ phytonutrients that have additive and synergistic health effects[110]—including immunomodulating, antioxidant, anti-inflammatory, and anti-cancer benefits. High-quality protein sources such as fish, poultry, eggs, and grass-fed meats are emphasized. Slightly modifying Cordain's paleo diet, I also advocate soy and whey protein isolates for their high-quality protein and their anticancer, cardioprotective, and mood-enhancing (due to the high tryptophan content) benefits. Potatoes and other starchy vegetables, wheat and other grains including rice are discouraged due to their high glycemic indexes and high glycemic loads, and their relative insufficiency of fiber and phytonutrients compared to fruits and vegetables. Grains such as wheat, barley, and rye are discouraged due to the high glycemic loads/indexes of most breads, pastries, and other grain-derived products, as well as due to the immunogenicity of constituents such as gluten, a protein composite (consisting of a prolamin and a glutelin) that can contribute to disorders such as migraine, epilepsy, eczema, arthritis, celiac disease, psoriasis and other types of autoimmunity. Sources of simple sugars and foreign chemicals such as colas/sodas (which contain artificial colors, flavors, and high-fructose corn syrup, which contains mercury[111] and which can cause the hypertensive-diabetic metabolic syndrome[112]) and processed foods (e.g., "TV dinners" and other manufactured snacks and convenience foods) are strictly forbidden. Chemical preservatives, colorants, sweeteners, flavor-enhancers such as monosodium glutamate and carrageenan are likewise avoided. In summary, this diet plan provides plenty of variety, as most dishes comprised of poultry, fish, lean meats, soy, eggs, fruits, vegetables, nuts, berries, and seeds are allowed. The diet provides an abundance of fiber, phytonutrients, carbohydrates, potassium, and protein, while simultaneously being low in fat, sodium, arachidonic acid, and "simple sugars." The diet must be customized with regard to total protein and calorie intake, as determined by the size, status, and activity level of the patient; individual per-patient food allergens should be avoided. Regular consumption of this diet has shown the ability to reduce hypertension, alleviate diabetes, ameliorate migraine headaches, and result in improvement of overall health and a lessening of the severity of many common "diseases", particularly those with an autoimmune or inflammatory component. This Paleo-Mediterranean diet is supplemented with vitamins, minerals, fatty acids, and probiotics—making it the "supplemented Paleo-Mediterranean diet" as described below.

2. <u>Multivitamin and multimineral supplementation</u>: Vitamin and mineral supplementation has been advocated for decades by the chiropractic/naturopathic professions while being scorned by so-called "mainstream medicine." Vitamin and mineral supplementation finally received bipartisan endorsement when researchers from Harvard Medical School published a review article in *Journal of the American Medical Association* that concluded, "Most people do not consume an optimal amount of all vitamins by diet alone. ...it appears prudent for all adults to take vitamin supplements."[113] Long-term nutritional insufficiencies experienced by "most people" promote the development of "long-latency deficiency diseases"[114] such as cancer, neuroemotional deterioration, and cardiovascular disease. Impressively, the

---

[108] "A high micronutrient density diet mitigates the unpleasant aspects of the experience of hunger even though it is lower in calories. Hunger is one of the major impediments to successful weight loss. Our findings suggest that it is not simply the caloric content, but more importantly, the micronutrient density of a diet that influences the experience of hunger. It appears that a high nutrient density diet, after an initial phase of adjustment during which a person experiences "toxic hunger" due to withdrawal from pro-inflammatory foods, can result in a sustainable eating pattern that leads to weight loss and improved health." Fuhrman J, Sarter B, Glaser D, Acocella S. Changing perceptions of hunger on a high nutrient density diet. *Nutr J*. 2010 Nov 7;9:51 http://www.nutritionj.com/content/9/1/51

[109] "The Paleolithic group were as satiated as the Mediterranean group but consumed less energy per day (5.8 MJ/day vs. 7.6 MJ/day, Paleolithic vs. Mediterranean, p=0.04). Consequently, the quotients of mean change in satiety during meal and mean consumed energy from food and drink were higher in the Paleolithic group (p=0.03). Also, there was a strong trend for greater Satiety Quotient for energy in the Paleolithic group (p=0.057). Leptin decreased by 31% in the Paleolithic group and by 18% in the Mediterranean group with a trend for greater relative decrease of leptin in the Paleolithic group." Jonsson T, Granfeldt Y, Erlanson-Albertsson C, Ahren B, Lindeberg S. A Paleolithic diet is more satiating per calorie than a Mediterranean-like diet in individuals with ischemic heart disease. *Nutr Metab* (Lond). 2010 Nov 30;7(1):85.

[110] Liu RH. Health benefits of fruit and vegetables are from additive and synergistic combinations of phytochemicals. *Am J Clin Nutr* 2003;78(3 Suppl):517S-520S

[111] "With daily per capita consumption of HFCS in the US averaging about 50 grams and daily mercury intakes from HFCS ranging up to 28 μg, this potential source of mercury may exceed other major sources of mercury especially in high-end consumers of beverages sweetened with HFCS." Dufault R, LeBlanc B, Schnoll R, Cornett C, Schweitzer L, Wallinga D, Hightower J, Patrick L, Lukiw WJ. Mercury from chlor-alkali plants: measured concentrations in food product sugar. *Environ Health*. 2009 Jan 26;8:2 http://www.ehjournal.net/content/8/1/2

[112] **Vasquez A**. Integrative Medicine and Functional Medicine for Chronic Hypertension: An Evidence-based Patient-Centered Monograph for Advanced Clinicians. IBMRC; 2011. See also: Reungjui S, Roncal CA, Mu W, Srinivas TR, Sirivongs D, Johnson RJ, Nakagawa T. Thiazide diuretics exacerbate fructose-induced metabolic syndrome. *J Am Soc Nephrol*. 2007 Oct;18(10):2724-31 http://jasn.asnjournals.org/content/18/10/2724.full.pdf

[113] Fletcher RH, Fairfield KM. Vitamins for chronic disease prevention in adults: clinical applications. *JAMA* 2002;287:3127-9

[114] Heaney RP. Long-latency deficiency disease: insights from calcium and vitamin D. *Am J Clin Nutr* 2003;78:912-9

benefits of multivitamin/multimineral supplementation have been demonstrated in numerous clinical trials. Multivitamin/multimineral supplementation has been shown to improve nutritional status and reduce the risk for chronic diseases[115], improve mood[116], potentiate antidepressant drug treatment[117], alleviate migraine headaches (when used with diet improvement and fatty acids[118]), improve immune function and infectious disease outcomes in the elderly[119] (especially diabetics[120]), reduce morbidity and mortality in patients with HIV infection[121,122], alleviate premenstrual syndrome[123,124] and bipolar disorder[125], reduce violence and antisocial behavior in children[126] and incarcerated young adults (when used with essential fatty acids[127]), and improve scores of intelligence in children.[128] Multivitamin and multimineral supplementation provides anti-inflammatory benefits, as evidenced by significant reduction in C-reactive protein (CRP) in a double-blind, placebo-controlled trial.[129] The ability to safely and affordably deliver these benefits makes multimineral-multivitamin supplementation an essential component of any and all health-promoting and disease-prevention strategies. A few cautions need to be observed; for example, vitamin A can (rarely) result in liver damage with chronic consumption of 25,000 IU or more, and intake should generally not exceed 10,000 IU per day in women of childbearing age. Also, iron should not be supplemented except in patients diagnosed with iron deficiency by a blood test (serum ferritin).

3. Physiologic doses of vitamin D3: The prevalence of vitamin D deficiency varies from 40-80 percent (general population) to almost 100 percent (patients with musculoskeletal pain) among Americans and Europeans. Vasquez, Manso, and Cannell described the many benefits of vitamin D3 supplementation in an assertive review published in 2004.[130] Our publication showed that vitamin D deficiency causes or contributes to depression, hypertension, seizures, migraine, polycystic ovary syndrome, inflammation, autoimmunity, and musculoskeletal pain, particularly low-back pain. Clinical trials using vitamin D supplementation have proven the cause-and-effect relationship between vitamin D deficiency and most of these conditions by showing that each could be cured or alleviated with vitamin D supplementation. In our review of the literature, we concluded that daily vitamin D doses should be 1,000 IU for infants, 2,000 IU for children, and 4,000 IU for adults, although some adults respond better to higher doses of 10,000 IU per day. Cautions and contraindications include the use of thiazide diuretics (e.g., hydrochlorothiazide) or any other medications that promote hypercalcemia, as well as granulomatous diseases such as sarcoidosis, tuberculosis, and certain types of cancer, especially lymphoma. Effectiveness is monitored by measuring serum 25-OH-vitamin D, and safety is monitored by measuring serum calcium. Dosing should be tailored for the attainment of optimal serum levels of 25-hydroxy-vitamin D3, generally 50-100 ng/ml (125-250 nmol/l) as illustrated.

[115] McKay DL, Perrone G, Rasmussen H, Dallal G, Hartman W, Cao G, Prior RL, Roubenoff R, Blumberg JB. The effects of a multivitamin/mineral supplement on micronutrient status, antioxidant capacity and cytokine production in healthy older adults consuming a fortified diet. *J Am Coll Nutr* 2000;19(5):613-21

[116] Benton D, Haller J, Fordy J. Vitamin supplementation for 1 year improves mood. *Neuropsychobiology* 1995;32(2):98-105

[117] Coppen A, Bailey J. Enhancement of the antidepressant action of fluoxetine by folic acid: a randomised, placebo controlled trial. *J Affect Disord* 2000;60:121-30

[118] Wagner W, Nootbaar-Wagner U. Prophylactic treatment of migraine with gamma-linolenic and alpha-linolenic acids. *Cephalalgia* 1997;17:127-30

[119] Langkamp-Henken B, Bender BS, Gardner EM, Herrlinger-Garcia KA, Kelley MJ, Murasko DM, Schaller JP, Stechmiller JK, Thomas DJ, Wood SM. Nutritional formula enhanced immune function and reduced days of symptoms of upper respiratory tract infection in seniors. *J Am Geriatr Soc* 2004;52:3-12

[120] Barringer TA, Kirk JK, Santaniello AC, Foley KL, Michielutte R. Effect of a multivitamin and mineral supplement on infection and quality of life. A randomized, double-blind, placebo-controlled trial. *Ann Intern Med* 2003;138:365-71

[121] Fawzi WW, Msamanga GI, et al. A randomized trial of multivitamin supplements and HIV disease progression and mortality. *N Engl J Med* 2004;351:23-32

[122] Burbano X, Miguez-Burbano MJ, McCollister K, Zhang G, Rodriguez A, Ruiz P, Lecusay R, Shor-Posner G. Impact of a selenium chemoprevention clinical trial on hospital admissions of HIV-infected participants. *HIV Clin Trials* 2002;3:483-91

[123] Abraham GE. Nutritional factors in the etiology of the premenstrual tension syndromes. *J Reprod Med* 1983;28(7):446-64

[124] Stewart A. Clinical and biochemical effects of nutritional supplementation on the premenstrual syndrome. *J Reprod Med* 1987;32:435-41

[125] Kaplan BJ, Simpson JS, Ferre RC, Gorman CP, McMullen DM, Crawford SG. Effective mood stabilization with a chelated mineral supplement: an open-label trial in bipolar disorder. *J Clin Psychiatry* 2001;62:936-44

[126] Kaplan BJ, Crawford SG, Gardner B, Farrelly G. Treatment of mood lability and explosive rage with minerals and vitamins: two case studies in children. *J Child Adolesc Psychopharmacol* 2002;12(3):205-19

[127] Gesch CB, Hammond SM, Hampson SE, Eves A, Crowder MJ. Influence of supplementary vitamins, minerals and essential fatty acids on the antisocial behaviour of young adult prisoners. Randomised, placebo-controlled trial. *Br J Psychiatry* 2002;181:22-8

[128] Benton D. Micro-nutrient supplementation and the intelligence of children. *Neurosci Biobehav Rev* 2001;25:297-309

[129] Church TS, Earnest CP, Wood KA, Kampert JB. Reduction of C-reactive protein levels through use of a multivitamin. *Am J Med* 2003;115:702-7

[130] **Vasquez A**, Manso G, Cannell J. The clinical importance of vitamin D (cholecalciferol): a paradigm shift with implications for all healthcare providers. *Alternative Therapies in Health and Medicine* 2004;10:28-37

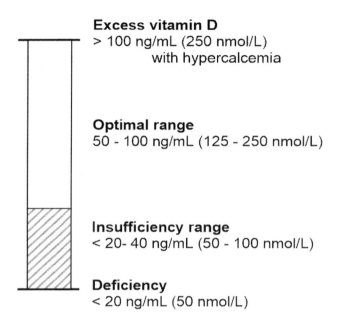

Excess vitamin D
> 100 ng/mL (250 nmol/L)
with hypercalcemia

Optimal range
50 - 100 ng/mL (125 - 250 nmol/L)

Insufficiency range
< 20- 40 ng/mL (50 - 100 nmol/L)

Deficiency
< 20 ng/mL (50 nmol/L)

Interpretation of serum 25(OH) vitamin D levels.
Modified from Vasquez et al, *Alternative Therapies in Health and Medicine* 2004 and Vasquez A. *Musculoskeletal Pain: Expanded Clinical Strategies* (Institute for Functional Medicine) 2008.

4. <u>Balanced and complete fatty acid supplementation</u>: A detailed survey of the literature shows that five fatty acids have major health-promoting disease-preventing benefits and should therefore be incorporated into the daily diet and/or regularly consumed as dietary supplements.[131] These are alpha-linolenic acid (ALA; omega-3, from flaxseed oil), eicosapentaenoic acid (EPA; omega-3, from fish oil), docosahexaenoic acid (DHA; omega-3, from fish oil and algae), gamma-linolenic acid (GLA; omega-6, most concentrated in borage oil but also present in evening primrose oil, hemp seed oil, black currant seed oil), and oleic acid (omega-9, most concentrated in olive oil, which contains in addition to oleic acid many anti-inflammatory, antioxidant, and anticancer phytonutrients). Supplementing with one fatty acid can exacerbate an insufficiency of other fatty acids; hence the importance of balanced combination supplementation. Each of these fatty acids has health benefits that cannot be fully attained from supplementing a different fatty acid; hence, again, the importance of balanced combination supplementation. The benefits of GLA are not attained by consumption of EPA and DHA; in fact, consumption of fish oil can actually promote a deficiency of GLA.[132] Likewise, consumption of GLA alone can reduce EPA levels while increasing levels of proinflammatory arachidonic acid; both of these problems are avoided with co-administration of EPA any time GLA is used because EPA inhibits delta-5-desaturase, which converts dihomo-GLA into arachidonic acid. Using ALA alone only slightly increases EPA but generally leads to no improvement in DHA status and can lead to a reduction of oleic acid; thus, DHA and oleic acid should be supplemented when flaxseed oil is used.[133] Obviously, the goal here is physiologically-optimal (i.e., "balanced") intake of all of the health-promoting fatty acids; using only one or two sources of fatty acids is not balanced and results in suboptimal improvement. In clinical practice, I routinely use combination fatty acid therapy comprised of ALA, EPA, DHA, and GLA for essentially all patients; when one appreciates that the average daily Paleolithic intake of n-3 fatty acids was 7 grams per day contrasted to the average daily American

---

[131] **Vasquez A**. New Insights into Fatty Acid Biochemistry and the Influence of Diet. *Nutritional Perspectives* 2004; October: 5, 7-10, 12, 14
[132] Cleland LG, Gibson RA, Neumann M, French JK. The effect of dietary fish oil supplement upon the content of dihomo-gammalinolenic acid in human plasma phospholipids. *Prostaglandins Leukot Essent Fatty Acids* 1990 May;40(1):9-12
[133] Jantti J, Nikkari T, Solakivi T, Vapaatalo H, Isomaki H. Evening primrose oil in rheumatoid arthritis: changes in serum lipids and fatty acids. *Ann Rheum Dis* 1989;48(2):124-7

intake of 1 gram per day, we can see that—by using combination fatty acid therapy emphasizing n-3 fatty acids—we are simply meeting physiologic expectations via supplementation, rather than performing an act of recklessness or heroism. The product I use also contains a modest amount of oleic acid that occurs naturally in flax and borage seed oils, and I encourage use of olive oil for salads and cooking. This approach results in complete and balanced fatty acid intake, and the clinical benefits are impressive. Benefits are to be expected in the treatment of premenstrual syndrome, diabetic neuropathy, respiratory distress syndrome, Crohn's disease, lupus, rheumatoid arthritis, cardiovascular disease, hypertension, psoriasis, eczema, migraine headaches, bipolar disorder, borderline personality disorder, mental depression, schizophrenia, osteoporosis, polycystic ovary syndrome, multiple sclerosis, and musculoskeletal pain. The discovery in September 2010 that the G protein-coupled receptor 120 (GPR120) functions as an n-3 fatty acid receptor that, when stimulated with EPA or DHA, exerts broad anti-inflammatory effects (in cell experiments) and enhances systemic insulin sensitivity (in animal study) confirms a new mechanism of action of fatty acid supplementation and shows that we as clinician-researchers are still learning the details of the beneficial effects of commonly used treatments.[134]

5. Probiotics /gut flora modification: Proper levels of good bacteria promote intestinal health, support proper immune function, and encourage overall health. Excess bacteria or yeast, or the presence of harmful bacteria, yeast, or "parasites" such as amoebas and protozoas, can cause "leaky gut," systemic inflammation, and a wide range of clinical problems, especially autoimmunity. Intestinal flora can become imbalanced by poor diets, excess stress, immunosuppressive drugs, and antibiotics, and all of these factors are common among American patients. Thus, as a rule, I reinstate the good bacteria by the use of probiotics (good bacteria and yeast), prebiotics (fiber, arabinogalactan, and inulin), and the use of fermented foods such as kefir and yogurt for patients not allergic to milk. Harmful yeast, bacteria, and other "parasites" can be eradicated with the combination of dietary change, antimicrobial drugs, and/or herbal extracts. For example, oregano oil in an emulsified, time-released form has proven safe and effective for the elimination of various parasites encountered in clinical practice.[135] Likewise, the herb *Artemisia annua* (sweet wormwood) commonly is used to eradicate specific bacteria and has been used for thousands of years in Asia for the treatment and prevention of infectious diseases, including drug-resistant malaria.[136] Restoring microbial balance by providing probiotics, restoring immune function (immunorestoration) and eliminating sources of dysbiosis, especially in the gastrointestinal tract, genitourinary tract, and oropharynx, is a very important component in the treatment plan of autoimmunity and systemic inflammation.[137]

Should combinations of iodine and iodide be the sixth component of the Protocol?**: Both iodine and iodide have biological activity in humans. An increasing number of clinicians are using combination iodine-iodide products to provide approximately 12 mg/d; this is consistent with the average daily intake of iodine-iodide in countries such as Japan with a high intake of seafood, including fish, shellfish, and seaweed. Collectively, iodine and iodide provide antioxidant, antimicrobial, mucolytic, immunosupportive, antiestrogen, and anticancer benefits that extend far beyond the mere incorporation of iodine into thyroid hormones.[5] Benefits of iodine/iodide in the treatment of asthma[138,139] and systemic fungal infections[140,141] have been documented, and many clinicians use combination iodine/iodide supplementation for the treatment of estrogen-driven conditions such as fibrocystic breast disease.[142] While additional research is needed and already underway to

[134] Oh da Y, Talukdar S, Bae EJ, Imamura T, Morinaga H, Fan W, Li P, Lu WJ, Watkins SM, Olefsky JM. GPR120 is an omega-3 fatty acid receptor mediating potent anti-inflammatory and insulin-sensitizing effects. Cell. 2010 Sep 3;142(5):687-98 http://www.cell.com/abstract/S0092-8674%2810%2900888-3?switch=standard

[135] Force M, Sparks WS, Ronzio RA. Inhibition of enteric parasites by emulsified oil of oregano in vivo. *Phytother Res* 2000;14:213-4

[136] Schuster BG. Demonstrating the validity of natural products as anti-infective drugs. *J Altern Complement Med* 2001;7 Suppl 1:S73-82

[137] **Vasquez A**. Integrative Rheumatology. IBMRC: 2006, 2009.

[138] Tuft L. Iodides in bronchial asthma. *J Allergy Clin Immunol.* 1981 Jun;67(6):497

[139] Falliers CJ, McCann WP, Chai H, Ellis EF, Yazdi N. Controlled study of iodotherapy for childhood asthma. *J Allergy.* 1966 Sep;38(3):183-92

[140] Tripathy S, Vijayashree J, Mishra M, Jena DK, Behera B, Mohapatra A. Rhinofacial zygomycosis successfully treated with oral saturated solution of potassium iodide: a case report. *J Eur Acad Dermatol Venereol.* 2007 Jan;21(1):117-9

[141] Bonifaz A, Saúl A, Paredes-Solis V, Fierro L, Rosales A, Palacios C, Araiza J. Sporotrichosis in childhood: clinical and therapeutic experience in 25 patients. *Pediatr Dermatol.* 2007 Jul-Aug;24(4):369-72

[142] Ghent WR, Eskin BA, Low DA, Hill LP. Iodine replacement in fibrocystic disease of the breast. *Can J Surg.* 1993 Oct;36(5):453-60

further establish the role of iodine-iodide as a routine component of clinical care, clinicians should begin incorporating this nutrient into their protocols based on the above-mentioned physiologic roles and clinical benefits.**

*** See update and addendum following this reprint*

<u>Summary and Conclusions</u>: In this brief review, I have described and substantiated a fundamental protocol that can serve as effective therapy for patients with a wide range of diseases and health disorders. Customizing the Paleo-Mediterranean diet to avoid patient-specific food allergens, using vitamin-mineral supplements along with physiologic doses of vitamin D and broad-spectrum balanced fatty acid supplementation, and ensuring "immunomicrobial" health with the skillful use of probiotics, prebiotics, immunorestoration, and antimicrobial treatments provides an excellent health-promoting and disease-eliminating foundation and lifestyle for many patients. Often, this simple protocol is all that is needed for the effective treatment of a wide range of clinical problems, even those that have been "medical failures" for many years. For other patients with more complex illnesses, of course, additional interventions and laboratory assessments can be used to optimize and further customize the treatment plan. Clinicians should avoid seeking "silver bullet" treatments that ignore overall metabolism, immune function, and inflammatory balance, and we must always remember that the attainment and preservation of health requires that we first meet the body's basic nutritional and physiologic needs. This five-step protocol begins the process of meeting those needs. With it, health can be restored and the need for disease-specific treatment is obviated or reduced; without it, fundamental physiologic needs are not met, and health cannot be obtained and maintained. Addressing core physiologic needs empowers doctors to deliver the most effective healthcare possible, and it allows patients to benefit from such treatment.

**Update and addendum to information on iodine and iodide:

- <u>Authoritative enthusiasm for high-dose iodine-iodide</u>: Several authoritative articles/authors stated that an advisable level of intake for iodine-iodide for the prevention and treatment of various conditions is approximately 12 mg/d. Because of these well-referenced and apparently authoritative publications, many clinicians and nutrition professionals began using higher doses iodine-iodide with patients and clients, quite often with benefit and nearly always with the absence of serious adverse effects. Several popular nutritional supplements used by clinicians and nutritionists contain both iodi<u>n</u>e (the <u>n</u>atural, diatomic form) and iodi<u>d</u>e (the <u>d</u>ivided/ionic form most commonly consumed in <u>d</u>ietary supplements, such as potassium iodi<u>d</u>e); both forms of this volatile metal have biologic properties in humans. Benefits of iodine-iodide supplementation focus mostly on the mucolytic, antimicrobial, and anti-estrogen effects.
  - <u>Dr Jonathan V Wright</u> (<u>*Nutrition and Healing* 2002 Nov and 2005 May</u>): In *Nutrition and Healing* (2002 Nov), well-respected nutrition expert, pioneer, and clinician Jonathan V. Wright MD advocated high-dose iodine-iodide for a wide range of conditions, particularly those related to inflammation, excess estrogen, and microbial infections. In another issue of *Nutrition and Healing* (2005 May) Dr Wright wrote "12.5 milligrams (that's 12,500 micrograms) is the optimal daily amount of iodine, not only for your thyroid but for the rest of your body, too." In that same article, Dr Wright stated, "The Japanese have traditionally consumed more iodine, mostly from seaweed, than any other population. The average daily intake of iodine in Japan [is] 13.8 milligrams…", and throughout the article Dr Wright advocates that 12.5 mg/d is "the optimal daily dose" of combined iodine-iodine.
  - <u>Extrathyroidal benefits of iodine</u> (<u>*Journal of American Physicians and Surgeons* 2006 Winter</u>): Independently and in a peer-reviewed publication, Donald Miller MD (Professor of Surgery, Division of Cardiothoracic Surgery, University of Washington School of Medicine) supported the daily intake of 12.5 mg/d in *Journal of American Physicians and Surgeons* and even supported higher doses with the statement "More than 4,000 patients in this project [Iodine Project] take iodine in daily doses ranging from 12.5 to 50 mg, and those with diabetes can take up to 100 mg /day." Miller also noted that dermatologists "treat inflammatory dermatoses, like nodular vasculitis and pyoderma gangrenosum, with SSKI (supersaturated potassium iodide), beginning with an iodine

dose of 900 mg/day, followed by weekly increases of up to 6 g/day as tolerated. Fungal eruptions, like sporotrichosis, are treated initially in gram amounts with great effect."

- o Iodine deficiency and therapeutic considerations (*Alternative Medicine Review* 2008 Jun): In 2008, Patrick wrote "Estimates of the average daily Japanese iodine consumption vary from 5,280 mcg to 13,800 mcg..." and this again supported and reinforced enthusiasm for doses of approximately 12 mg/d of iodine-iodine. However, in this article, Patrick did not advocate any specific daily dosage, citing 3-6 mg/d as beneficial and without adverse effect.

- Review, reanalysis, and caution: Soon after these enthusiastic publications, Alan Gaby MD published in several magazines, presented in post-graduate educational events, and discussed in his book *Nutritional Medicine* a review and reanalysis of the original data and concluded that the estimated average daily intake of iodine-iodine in Japan had been *overestimated* by a mathematical error (mistakenly interchanging wet and dry weights of seaweed and thus overestimating the daily Japanese intake of iodine-iodine). Per Gaby (*Nutritional Medicine*, page 175), the true intake of iodine-iodide in Japan averages 330-500 mcg/d, which is 25-fold lower than the estimate of 13.8 mg/d, upon which rested much of the rationale for implementing high-dose iodine-iodide supplementation empirically and routinely.

- Benefits, perspectives, and additional research: Many clinicians including the current author have used high-dose iodine-iodide ranging from approximately 12-48 mg/d for variable periods of time without personally experiencing or clinically observing apparent adverse effects; that statement does not imply endorsement of routine universal high-dose iodine-iodide supplementation. Some degree of caution is advised in consideration of the risks of inducing thyroid dysfunction (hyperthyroidism, hypothyroidism), intestinal hemorrhage[143], and anaphylaxis-like reactions.[144] Topical and systemic antimicrobial benefits of iodine-iodide are well known and well documented; oral high-dose iodine-iodide has been used to treat drug-resistant fungal infections (cited below). When applied for sufficient concentrations and durations, both diatomic iodine and ionic iodide possess potent broad-spectrum antimicrobial properties; essentially no "drug resistance" against iodine-iodide exists for bacteria, fungi, viruses, and protozoans. Iodine also has documented molecular and clinical anti-estrogen effects, thus providing scientific explanation for its ability to treat and prevent estrogen-related disorders ranging from fibrocystic breast disease to cancer. Indeed, iodine treatment of breast cancer cells has been shown to increase the mRNA levels of several genes involved in estrogen metabolism and "detoxification" such as cytochrome p450-1A1 while also decreasing the levels of estrogen responsive genes such as TFF1 and WISP2; also noted following iodine treatment is upregulation of gene expression for the enzyme glutathione peroxidase, an important selenium-dependent component of antioxidant defense mechanisms.[145]

  - o Ultra-high dose iodide for sporotrichosis in childhood (*Pediatric Dermatology* 2007 Jul-Aug): Nineteen pediatric patients with proven sporotrichosis were successfully treated with potassium iodide per the following quoted protocol: "All patients were initially treated with potassium iodide (KI), and only those who were unresponsive or who developed side effects were given itraconazole. The dose of KI used was 1–3 g/day, starting at 1 g/day and increasing until the dose of 3 g/day was reached. ... Treatments were sustained until remission was reached, which ranged from 3 to 6 months."[146] Per the review by Miller[147] cited previously, KI 1g (1,000 mg) contains 770 mg of iodide. **Thus, the pediatric patients in this case series were treated with 770-2,310 mg/d of iodide for successful antimycotic treatment.** Two patients from the original group of 23 patients experienced nausea and vomiting from the KI and were switched to itraconazole; two other patients were lost to follow-up. The authors note that, "Side effects occur in 5% to 10% of patients,

---

[143] Kinoshita et al. Severe duodenal hemorrhage induced by Lugol's solution administered for thyroid crisis treatment. *Intern Med.* 2010;49(8):759-61
[144] Indraccolo et al. Anaphylactic-like reaction to Lugol solution during colposcopy. *South Med J* 2009 Jan;102(1):96-7
[145] "Quantitative RT-PCR confirmed the array data demonstrating that iodine/iodide treatment increased the mRNA levels of several genes involved in estrogen metabolism (CYP1A1, CYP1B1, and AKR1C1) while decreasing the levels of the estrogen responsive genes TFF1 and WISP2." Stoddard FR 2nd, et al. Iodine alters gene expression in the MCF7 breast cancer cell line: evidence for an anti-estrogen effect of iodine. *Int J Med Sci.* 2008 Jul 8;5(4):189-96
[146] Bonifaz A, et al. Sporotrichosis in childhood: clinical and therapeutic experience in 25 patients. *Pediatr Dermatol.* 2007 Jul-Aug;24(4):369-72
[147] Said of KI, "The standard dose was 1g, which contains 770 mg of iodine." Miller DW. Extrathyroidal benefits of iodine. *J Am Physicians Surgeons* 2006;Winter,106-10

mainly presenting as gastrointestinal symptoms as well as headache and rhinorrhea to a lesser extent."

- o Ultra-high dose iodide for rhinofacial zygomycosis—case report (*Journal of European Academy of Dermatology and Venereology* 2007 Jan): A 19-year-old male "was put on oral SSKI at an initial dose of 0.5 mL three times daily. This was gradually increased by 0.1 mL/dose/day until a dose of 5 mL three times daily was reached."[148] Generic formulation of "saturated solution of potassium iodide" (SSKI) contains 1000 mg of KI per mL of solution, which provides roughly 750 mg iodide; thus, SSKI dosed at 5 mL thrice daily = 15 mL/d = **11,250 mg/d (slightly more than 11 grams per day) of iodide for this adult patient with rhinofacial zygomycosis**. Treatment was continued for at least 12 months without report of adverse effect.

- o Modest dose iodine replacement in fibrocystic disease of the breast (*Canadian Journal of Surgery* 1993 Oct): Ghent and colleagues[149] sought to determine the response of patients with fibrocystic breast disease to "iodine replacement therapy" and reviewed three clinical studies of different design containing 233, 145 (later up to 1365), and 23 subjects; overall, subjective alleviation of pain and objective alleviation of breast fibrosis was seen in approximately 70% of patients. Consistent with other reports and impressions, the authors noted that, "**Molecular iodine is nonthyrotropic** and was the most beneficial." **The dose of molecular iodine averaged 0.08 mg/kg body weight, which for an average 140-lb (63-kg) patient equates to approximately 5 mg/d.**

- o Modest dose iodine in patients with cyclic mastalgia (*Breast Journal* 2004 Jul-Aug): Kessler[150] reports a randomized, double-blind, placebo-controlled, multicenter clinical trial was conducted with 111 otherwise healthy euthyroid women with a history of breast pain and fibrosis; subjects received molecular iodine for 6 months. Physicians assessed breast pain, tenderness, and nodularity each cycle; patients assessed breast pain and tenderness with the Lewin breast pain scale at 3-month intervals and with a VAS at each cycle. All iodine-treated subjects improved compared to no improvement seen in the placebo group. "Reductions in all three physician assessments were observed in patients after 5 months of therapy in the 3.0 mg/day (7/28; 25%) and 6.0 mg/day (15/27; 18.5%) treatment groups, but not the 1.5 mg/day or placebo group. **Patients recorded statistically significant decreases in pain by month 3 in the 3.0 and 6.0 mg/day treatment groups**, but not the 1.5 mg/day or placebo group; more than 50% of the 6.0 mg/day treatment group recorded a clinically significant reduction in overall pain. All doses were associated with an acceptable safety profile. No dose-related increase in any adverse event was observed." Notably, the failure of the 1.5 mg/day dose implies that this dose is inadequate and thereby justifies higher routine dosing.

- Clinical implementation and the author's perspective: Iodide has a stronger effect on thyroid function and provides tissue-penetrating antimicrobial benefits from oral administration. Molecular iodine has anti-estrogen effects that correlate with the clinical alleviation of cyclic breast pain and fibrocystic breast disease; other anti-estrogen benefits such as an anti-cancer benefit are reasonably anticipated from supplemental iodine. Products with combined iodine and iodide are available and reasonable for clinical use, and a daily dose range of 3-6 mg does not appear unreasonable and has been shown to be beneficial in human studies. Iodine and iodide are impressively well tolerated. Nicely summarized in a personal email from Michael Gonzalez DSc PhD in November 2012, an overview of iodine-iodine's clinical applications may be stated as follows:

   "Different tissues of the body respond to different forms of iodine. The Iodide form is believed to be particularly useful for the thyroid. But the supplement of choice for the breast is "iodine" not "iodide." Lugol's formula is Iodine 5% + Potassium iodide (KI) 10% in distilled water. Because different tissues concentrate different forms of iodine, using a supplement that contains both iodine and iodide is preferable to using a supplement that contains only one form. With different tissues responding to different forms of iodine, it would make common sense that a greater therapeutic

[148] Tripathy S, et al. Rhinofacial zygomycosis successfully treated with oral saturated solution of potassium iodide: a case report. *J Eur Acad Dermatol Venereol.* 2007;21(1):117-9

[149] Ghent et al. Iodine replacement in fibrocystic disease of the breast. *Can J Surg.* 1993 Oct;36(5):453-60

[150] Kessler JH. The effect of supraphysiologic levels of iodine on patients with cyclic mastalgia. *Breast J.* 2004 Jul-Aug;10(4):328-36

benefit from iodine will be achieved by using a combination of iodide and iodine. ... The most frequent adverse reactions to potassium iodide are stomach upset, diarrhea, nausea, vomiting, stomach pain, salivary gland swelling/tenderness, acne and skin rash."

Antioxidant support in general and supplementation with selenium in particular are recommended always, and particularly when iodine-iodide doses greater than 1-3 mg/d are used. Selenium 200 mcg/d has been shown in several studies to have an ameliorating effect on thyroid autoimmunity and a supportive effect on peripheral thyroid hormone metabolism. Although iodi*ne* is generally considered *n*onthyrotropic, periodic assessment of thyroid function and for thyroid autoimmunity is reasonable for patients taking long-term high-dose treatment. Clinicians should take advantage of iodine-iodide's safe and effective mucolytic, antimicrobial, and anti-estrogen benefits.

Distinguishing iodiNe from iodiDe

IodiNe
- **Natural** elemental form—diatomic.
- **Nonthyrotropic**—no immediate adverse effects on thyroid function.
- **Nuclear**—affects gene expression, for example by promoting estrogen detoxification and reducing estrogen responsiveness.
- **Nixes microbes**, antimicrobial—very broad spectrum; povidone iodine is one of the most widely used topical antimicrobials in the history of microbiology and medicine.

IodiDe
- **Divided**—ionic, nondiatomic.
- **Dietary** form, such as in iodized salt which typically contains potassium iodate, potassium iodide, sodium iodate, or sodium iodide.
- **Dissolves mucus**—mucolytic benefits advantageous in the treatment of asthma, bronchitis and respiratory tract infections. Potassium iodide is thought to act as an expectorant by increasing respiratory tract secretions and thereby decreasing the viscosity of mucus; iodide levels increase in respiratory secretions within approximately 15 minutes after oral administration.
- **Directly thyrotropic**—necessary for thyroid hormone production; high doses can cause thyroid dysfunction, which may be problematic (exacerbation of thyroid autoimmunity, hypothyroidism, or hyperthyroidism) or therapeutic (inhibition of thyroid hormone production during hyperthyroidism).
- **Deals death to microbes**, antimicrobial—very broad spectrum, used in the form of potassium iodide (KI, SSKI) for the treatment of microbial infections such as zygomycosis and sporotrichosis.

Food Allergy and Adverse Food Reactions: A few considerations and perspectives

"**Adverse food reactions**" is a broad and general category that includes food allergy, food sensitivity, and food intolerance. The term "food" here means anything that is ingested other than drugs and medications and includes food, drink, food additives, preservatives, and food dyes. Many studies in the medical literature underestimate the high prevalence and clinical importance of food allergies because of inconsistent terminology, imperfect laboratory assessments[151], and the assumption that an "apparently healthy" person would only be allergic/sensitive to one or two foods—this is an erroneous assumption considering that many patients with food allergy/sensitivity/intolerance must avoid several (common range 3-10) commonly eaten foods to obtain clinical response and maximal improvement.[152,153] Clinical practice differs from basic research in that we as clinicians must often do what is effective while having neither the need nor the luxury for determining the molecular and physiologic basis for the effectiveness of each treatment in each patient. Clinical research has scientifically proven that adverse food reactions, regardless of the underlying mechanism(s) or classification of allergy, intolerance, or sensitivity, can exacerbate a wide range of human illnesses, including

---

[151] Bindslev-Jensen C, Skov PS, Madsen F, Poulsen LK. Food allergy and food intolerance--what is the difference? *Ann Allergy.* 1994 Apr;72(4):317-20
[152] Grant EC. Food allergies and migraine. *Lancet.* 1979 May 5;1(8123):966-9
[153] Speer F. Multiple food allergy. *Ann Allergy.* 1975 Feb;34(2):71-6

thyroid disease[154], mental depression[155,156], asthma, rhinitis,[157] recurrent otitis media[158], migraine[159,160,161], attention deficit and hyperactivity disorders[162], epilepsy[163,164,165], gastrointestinal inflammation[166], hypertension[167], joint pain[168,169,170,171,172,173,174,] and other health problems.

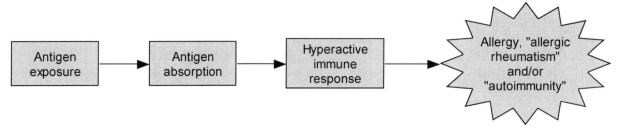

The common view of allergic phenomena it is incomplete and therefore inaccurate because it fails to include the prerequisite immune dysfunction and complex physiologic interconnections

"**Food allergy**" generally refers to adverse food reactions that are specifically immunoglobulin-mediated. Classically, food allergy is seen with immediate-onset allergy mediated via IgE antibodies which initiate mast cell degranulation and histamine release. The classic symptoms of immediate-onset allergies are skin rash, abdominal pain, angioedema, and bronchoconstriction. However, many doctors recognize the possibility of IgG-mediated allergies and suggest that these might be responsible for the delayed-onset or "hidden" food allergies which are clinically significant but more subtle and difficult to diagnose than the classic IgE-mediated allergies. The binding of antigens with immunoglobulins forms immune complexes that can deposit in parenchymal and synovial tissues where a localized immune response causes inflammation and organ dysfunction. "**Food sensitivity**" refers to immune-mediated adverse food reactions that are not antibody-mediated but are mediated by some other aspect of the immune/inflammatory system. An example of this is the increased production of specific prostaglandins in food-induced irritable bowel syndrome.[175] "**Food intolerance**" refers to adverse food reactions which are associated with poor nutritional status and/or impaired hepatic detoxification and which are *not* immune-mediated. Classic and well-known examples of this category of adverse food reaction include MSG sensitivity (associated with deficiency of vitamin B-6 and subsequent defects in hepatic transamination), tyramine intolerance that can result in hypertension and headaches, and histamine intolerance that can result in bronchoconstriction.[176] From a practical clinical standpoint, the following facts are self-evident for any doctor working in the field of nutrition:

1. Some people have adverse food reactions from the foods that they eat.

[154] Sategna-Guidetti C, Volta U, Ciacci C, Usai P, Carlino A, De Franceschi L, Camera A, Pelli A, Brossa C. Prevalence of thyroid disorders in untreated adult celiac disease patients and effect of gluten withdrawal: an Italian multicenter study. *Am J Gastroenterol*. 2001 Mar;96(3):751-7

[155] Mills N. Depression and food intolerance: a single case study. *Hum Nutr Appl Nutr*. 1986 Apr;40(2):141-5

[156] Parker G, Watkins T. Treatment-resistant depression: when antidepressant drug intolerance may indicate food intolerance. *Aust N Z J Psychiatry*. 2002 Apr;36(2):263-5

[157] Speer F. The allergic child. *Am Fam Physician*. 1975 Feb;11(2):88-94

[158] Juntti H, Tikkanen S, Kokkonen J, et al. Cow's milk allergy is associated with recurrent otitis media during childhood. *Acta Otolaryngol*. 1999;119(8):867-73

[159] Monro J, Carini C, Brostoff J. Migraine is a food-allergic disease. *Lancet*. 1984 Sep 29;2(8405):719-21

[160] Egger J, Carter CM, Wilson J,et al. Is migraine food allergy? A double-blind controlled trial of oligoantigenic diet treatment. *Lancet*. 1983 Oct 15;2(8355):865-9

[161] Monro J, Brostoff J, Carini C, Zilkha K. Food allergy in migraine. Study of dietary exclusion and RAST. *Lancet*. 1980 Jul 5;2(8184):1-4

[162] Boris M, Mandel FS. Foods and additives are common causes of the attention deficit hyperactive disorder in children. *Ann Allergy*. 1994 May;72(5):462-8

[163] Egger J, Carter CM, Soothill JF, Wilson J. Oligoantigenic diet treatment of children with epilepsy and migraine. *J Pediatr*. 1989;114(1):51-8

[164] Pelliccia A, Lucarelli S, Frediani T, D'Ambrini G, Cerminara C, Barbato M, Vagnucci B, Cardi E. Partial cryptogenetic epilepsy and food allergy/intolerance. A causal or a chance relationship? Reflections on three clinical cases. *Minerva Pediatr*. 1999 May;51(5):153-7

[165] Frediani T, Lucarelli S, Pelliccia A, et al. Allergy and childhood epilepsy: a close relationship? *Acta Neurol Scand*. 2001 Dec;104(6):349-52

[166] Marr HY, Chen WC, Lin LH. Food protein-induced enterocolitis syndrome: report of one case. *Acta Paediatr Taiwan*. 2001;42(1):49-52

[167] Grant EC. Food allergies and migraine. *Lancet*. 1979 May 5;1(8123):966-9

[168] Golding DN. Is there an allergic synovitis? *J R Soc Med*. 1990 May;83(5):312-4

[169] Panush RS. Food induced ("allergic") arthritis: clinical and serologic studies. *J Rheumatol*. 1990 Mar;17(3):291-4

[170] Pacor ML, Lunardi C, Di Lorenzo G, Biasi D, Corrocher R. Food allergy and seronegative arthritis: report of two cases. *Clin Rheumatol*. 2001;20(4):279-81

[171] Schrander JJ, Marcelis C, de Vries MP, van Santen-Hoeufft HM. Does food intolerance play a role in juvenile chronic arthritis? *Br J Rheumatol*. 1997;36(8):905-8

[172] van de Laar MA, van der Korst JK. Food intolerance in rheumatoid arthritis. I. A double blind, controlled trial of the clinical effects of elimination of milk allergens and azo dyes. *Ann Rheum Dis*. 1992 Mar;51(3):298-302

[173] Haugen MA, Kjeldsen-Kragh J, Forre O. A pilot study of the effect of an elemental diet in the management of rheumatoid arthritis. *Clin Exp Rheumatol*. 1994 May-Jun;12(3):275-9

[174] van de Laar MA, Aalbers M, Bruins FG, van Dinther-Janssen AC, van der Korst JK, Meijer CJ. Food intolerance in rheumatoid arthritis. II. Clinical and histological aspects. *Ann Rheum Dis*. 1992 Mar;51(3):303-6

[175] "Food intolerance associated with prostaglandin production is an important factor in the pathogenesis of IBS." Jones VA, McLaughlan P, Shorthouse M, Workman E, Hunter JO. Food intolerance: a major factor in the pathogenesis of irritable bowel syndrome. *Lancet*. 1982 Nov 20;2(8308):1115-7

[176] Wantke F, Hemmer W, Haglmuller T, Gotz M, Jarisch R. Histamine in wine. Bronchoconstriction after a double-blind placebo-controlled red wine provocation test. *Int Arch Allergy Immunol*. 1996 Aug;110(4):397-400

2. Food-induced reactions may be either immediate-onset (i.e., within minutes) or delayed-onset (within days) of eating the triggering food.

3. The same patient might have immediate-onset reactions to food X with symptoms A and B and simultaneously have a delayed-onset reaction to food Y with symptom C.

4. Food X might cause symptoms D and E in one patient and symptoms F and G in another patient.

5. By avoiding allergens and/or improving immune function, many "diseases" go away with out direct treatment and the patient experiences an improved state of health.

6. Failure to identify and avoid problematic foods combined with failure to correct the underlying immune dysfunction often makes the "disease" recalcitrant to remediation even with "generally effective" treatment. This has been demonstrated in migraine, hypertension[177], and drug-resistant mental depression.[178]

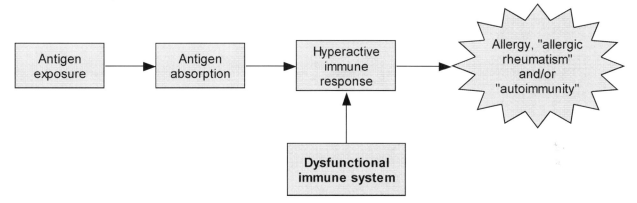

Potential roles of "food allergy" in the induction and perpetuation of autoimmunity and inflammation

Food allergy both *results from* and *contributes to* immune dysfunction and a systemic proinflammatory state. Food allergy contributes to "autoimmunity" and musculoskeletal inflammation via several mechanisms, including but not limited to the following:

1. Stimulation of cytokine release: As will be discussed later, the term "superantigen" classically refers to microbial—viral, bacterial, or fungal—antigens which have the ability to induce production of excessive levels of cytokines and other inflammatory effectors[179], and superantigens appear to be involved in the pathogenesis of inflammatory musculoskeletal disorders such as rheumatoid arthritis.[180,181] **In this section I propose that since food allergens appear capable of inducing cytokine production, they should in certain circumstances be considered "dietary superantigens"** since they invoke cytokine release similarly as do microbial superantigens. An important distinction here, however, is that microbial superantigens generally stimulate cytokine release as an inherent property in *all* patients, whereas **the production of cytokines by dietary (super)antigens is dependent on previous sensitization**; thus cytokine production by allergens is patient-dependent and not an inherent property of the allergen itself. **Mononuclear cells from egg-allergic patients produce much**

[177] "When an average of ten common foods were avoided there was a dramatic fall in the number of headaches per month, 85% of patients becoming headache-free. The 25% of patients with hypertension became normotensive." Grant EC. Food allergies and migraine. *Lancet.* 1979 May 5;1(8123):966-9

[178] "The prevalence of food intolerance as a contributing factor to depressive disorders requires clarification. Clinicians should be aware of the possible syndrome and that it may be worsened by psychotropic medication." Parker G, Watkins T. Treatment-resistant depression: when antidepressant drug intolerance may indicate food intolerance. *Aust N Z J Psychiatry.* 2002 Apr;36(2):263-5

[179] "The basis of autoimmune disorders due to superantigen is due to greater stimulation of T-lymphocytes and elaborate cytokine production." Hemalatha V, Srikanth P, Mallika M. Superantigens - Concepts, clinical disease and therapy. *Indian J Med Microbiol* 2004;22:204-211

[180] "They also suggest that the etiology of RA may involve initial activation of V beta 14+ T cells by a V beta 14-specific superantigen with subsequent recruitment of a few activated autoreactive v beta 14+ T cell clones to the joints while the majority of other V beta 14+ T cells disappear." Paliard X, West SG, Lafferty JA, Clements JR, Kappler JW, Marrack P, Kotzin BL. Evidence for the effects of a superantigen in rheumatoid arthritis. *Science.* 1991 Jul 19;253(5017):325-9

[181] "Given that binding sites for superantigens have been mapped to the CDR4s of TCR beta chains, the synovial localization of T cells bearing V beta s with significant CDR4 homology indicates that V beta-specific T-cell activation by superantigen may play a role in RA." Howell MD, Diveley JP, Lundeen KA, Esty A, Winters ST, Carlo DJ, Brostoff SW. Limited T-cell receptor beta-chain heterogeneity among interleukin 2 receptor-positive synovial T cells suggests a role for superantigen in rheumatoid arthritis. *Proc Natl Acad Sci* U S A. 1991 Dec 1;88(23):10921-5

more proinflammatory cytokine (interferon) than do those from nonallergic patients.[182] Similarly, in children with autism, who commonly demonstrate immune dysfunction and neuroautoimmunity[183], exposure to food allergens greatly increases cytokine release compared to controls.[184] Food allergy, NFkB activation, cytokine release, and increased intestinal permeability form a self-perpetuating vicious cycle because consumption of dietary allergens causes damage to the intestinal mucosa and stimulates NFkB activation and cytokine release which then increases intestinal permeability, thus allowing for increased absorption of dietary and microbial immunogens for the perpetuation and exacerbation of allergy and immune dysfunction.[185] Generally speaking, cytokines are proinflammatory and would be expected to contribute to autoimmune disease induction via mechanisms such as bystander activation and increased autoantigen processing regardless of their original stimuli.

2. Immune complex formation and deposition: **Dietary antigen-antibody immune complexes are formed following the consumption of allergenic foods by patients with allergy to those foods**[186,187] and these anti-food and anti-IgE immune complexes contribute to allergic symptomatology by a mechanism that has been described as "chronic serum sickness."[188] These immune complexes are then deposited in the joints to localize the resultant proinflammatory response. In the study by Carini et al[189], the authors found that **patients with food-induced joint pain and inflammation had anti-IgE IgG antibodies which formed large immune complexes that were detectable in synovial fluid and which probably contributed to the arthritis**. Anti-IgE IgG antibodies are commonly elevated in patients with allergic/inflammatory diseases such as eczema[190], asthma[191], and Crohn's disease[192] and thus tissue damage in these conditions appears mediated at least in part by anti-immunoglobulin immune complexes (i.e., anti-IgE IgG complexed with IgE) rather than the classic antigen-antibody immune complexes. In this way, food allergies cause joint pain and inflammation by the deposition of immune complexes into the synovium and joint cartilage.[193] Conversely, the consumption of a relatively hypoallergenic diet reduces intake of food antigens and helps reduce IgE levels. This explains, in part, the success of hypoallergenic diets in the treatment of immune-complex-mediated diseases such as mixed cryoglobulinemia[194,195], hypersensitivity vasculitis[196], and leukocystoclastic vasculitis with arthritis.[197] In patients with rheumatoid arthritis, the symptomatic and clinical

---

[182] "The levels of IFN-gamma production of only IL-2-stimulated or both ovalbumin-stimulated and IL-2-stimulated peripheral blood mononuclear cells from egg-sensitive patients with atopic dermatitis was significantly higher than that of healthy children and that of egg-sensitive patients with immediate allergic symptoms." Shinbara M, Kondo N, Agata H, Fukutomi O, Kuwabara N, Kobayashi Y, Miura M, Orii T. Interferon-gamma and interleukin-4 production of ovalbumin-stimulated lymphocytes in egg-sensitive children. *Ann Allergy Asthma Immunol*. 1996;77(1):60-6

[183] "Autistic children, but not normal children, had antibodies to caudate nucleus (49% positive sera), cerebral cortex (18% positive sera) and cerebellum (9% positive sera)." Singh VK, Rivas WH. Prevalence of serum antibodies to caudate nucleus in autistic children. *Neurosci Lett*. 2004 Jan 23;355(1-2):53-6

[184] Jyonouchi H, Sun S, Itokazu N. Innate immunity associated with inflammatory responses and cytokine production against common dietary proteins in patients with autism spectrum disorder. *Neuropsychobiology*. 2002;46(2):76-84

[185] Ma TY, Iwamoto GK, Hoa NT, Akotia V, Pedram A, Boivin MA, Said HM. TNF-alpha-induced increase in intestinal epithelial tight junction permeability requires NF-kappa B activation. Am *J Physiol Gastrointest Liver Physiol*. 2004 Mar;286(3):G367-76 http://ajpgi.physiology.org/cgi/content/full/286/3/G367

[186] "Antigen entry and the formation of immune complexes occur in atopic subjects after food ingestion. ...Food allergic subjects showed, after food challenge, the presence of IgE and IgG immune complexes, which correlates with the subsequent occurrence of symptoms." Carini C, Brostoff J. Evidence for circulating IgE complexes in food allergy. *Ric Clin Lab*. 1987 Oct-Dec;17(4):309-22

[187] "Following challenge, immune complexes containing IgE, IgG, and antigen are detectable in the circulation. Their appearance correlates with the production of symptoms." Carini C, Brostoff J, Wraith DG. IgE complexes in food allergy. *Ann Allergy*. 1987 Aug;59(2):110-7

[188] Marinkovich V. "Immunology and Food Allergy" in "Applying Functional Medicine in Clinical Practice" hosted by the Institute for Functional Medicine. Seattle, Washington: March 2005

[189] "In three food-allergic patients IgG anti-IgE was detectable in a complexed form in the serum samples examined before and after food challenge. The finding of IgG anti-IgE autoantibody in a group of patients with allergic arthralgia is quite exciting." Carini C, Fratazzi C, Aiuti F. Immune complexes in food-induced arthralgia. *Ann Allergy*. 1987 Dec;59(6):422-8

[190] "An IgG type of antibody directed against IgE has been studied in serum from healthy and allergic individuals. ... Significantly raised levels of anti-IgE autoantibody were found in patients suffering from atopic disorders in comparison to the controls." Carini C, Fratazzi C, Barbato M. IgG autoantibody to IgE in atopic patients. *Ann Allergy*. 1988 Jan;60(1):48-52

[191] "Significantly enhanced levels of IgE/anti-IgE IC were detected in children with asthma." Ritter C, Battig M, Kraemer R, Stadler BM. IgE hidden in immune complexes with anti-IgE autoantibodies in children with asthma. *J Allergy Clin Immunol*. 1991 Nov;88(5):793-801

[192] "In CD sera no food-specific IgE could be detected, but levels of immune complexes of IgE and IgG anti-IgE autoantibodies were statistically significantly increased compared to healthy controls." Huber A, Genser D, Spitzauer S, Scheiner O, Jensen-Jarolim E. IgE/anti-IgE immune complexes in sera from patients with Crohn's disease do not contain food-specific IgE. *Int Arch Allergy Immunol*. 1998 Jan;115(1):67-72

[193] Inman RD. Antigens, the gastrointestinal tract, and arthritis. *Rheum Dis Clin North Am*. 1991 May;17(2):309-21

[194] "CONCLUSION: These data show that an LAC diet decreases the amount of circulating immune complexes in MC and can modify certain signs and symptoms of the disease." Ferri C, Pietrogrande M, Cecchetti R, et al. Low-antigen-content diet in the treatment of patients with mixed cryoglobulinemia. *Am J Med*. 1989 Nov:519-24

[195] Pietrogrande M, Cefalo A, Nicora F, Marchesini D. Dietetic treatment of essential mixed cryoglobulinemia. *Ric Clin Lab*. 1986 Apr-Jun;16(2):413-6

[196] "In three cases the vasculitis relapsed following the introduction of food additives; in one case with the addition of potatoes and green vegetables (i.e., beans and green peas) and in the last case with the addition of eggs to the diet." Lunardi C, Bambara LM, Biasi D, Zagni P, Caramaschi P, Pacor ML. Elimination diet in the treatment of selected patients with hypersensitivity vasculitis. *Clin Exp Rheumatol*. 1992 Mar-Apr;10(2):131-5

[197] "Described in this report are two children with severe vasculitis caused by specific foods." Businco L, Falconieri P, Bellioni-Businco B, Bahna SL. Severe food-induced vasculitis in two children. *Pediatr Allergy Immunol*. 2002 Feb;13(1):68-71

improvement induced by hypoallergenic diets correlates with reductions in antibodies to food antigens.[198]

3. <u>Damage to the intestinal mucosa with resultant increased absorption of dietary and microbial antigens</u>: Consumption of food allergens increases intestinal permeability[199] and thus amplifies the absorption of intestinal contents—dietary and microbial antigens. Patients with food allergy have "leaky gut" that is exacerbated by consumption of allergenic foods; thus lactulose-mannitol assays can be used to assist the diagnosis of food allergy.[200,201] By increasing intestinal permeability, consumption of dietary antigens serves to exacerbate the adverse effects of gastrointestinal dysbiosis by increasing antigen and (anti)metabolite absorption. Since both dietary allergens and bacterial endotoxin stimulate production of cytokines[202], **concomitant exposure to both allergens and intra-intestinal endotoxin leads to an additive increase in proinflammatory cytokine production.[203] Thus, consumption of allergenic foods in the presence of gastrointestinal dysbiosis would be expected to lead to more severe and more diverse adverse physiologic and clinical consequences than would be experienced following exposure to either allergens or dysbiosis alone.**

4. <u>Dietary haptenization</u>: **Dietary antigens can complex with human tissues to form *neoantigens* that are immunostimulatory.** The best example of this appears to be the induction of autoimmunity by wheat-derived gliadin which haptenizes with intestinal tissue transglutaminase and other extracellular matrix proteins and results in the allergic-autoimmune disease celiac disease.[204,205] **The finding that gliadin proteins haptenize with collagen and can induce the formation of anti-collagen antibodies in humans[206] makes clear the pathomechanism by which "wheat allergy" can directly precipitate systemic musculoskeletal autoimmunity.** Once initiated and perpetuated by dietary gliadin from wheat, additional autoimmunity ensues (perhaps mediated directly by epitope spreading and/or indirectly by deposition of immune complexes) which is directed against various tissues, most notably the thyroid gland[207], brain[208], and musculoskeletal system.[209] Given the association between lupus and celiac disease[210,211,212], we may speculate that allergy becomes systemic autoimmunity in certain circumstances and in susceptible patients.

---

[198] Hafstrom I, Ringertz B, Spangberg A, von Zweigbergk L, Brannemark S, Nylander I, Ronnelid J, Laasonen L, Klareskog L. A vegan diet free of gluten improves the signs and symptoms of rheumatoid arthritis: the effects on arthritis correlate with a reduction in antibodies to food antigens. *Rheumatology* (Oxford). 2001 Oct;40(10):1175-9 http://rheumatology.oxfordjournals.org/cgi/content/full/40/10/1175

[199] "When compared to the control group, the 11 patients of the allergic group presented a normal mannitol urinary excretion (16.5 +/- 13.4%, p = NS, Student's t-test) and an increase in the lactulose excretion (1.36 +/- 0.92%, p < 0.001). Moreover, the allergic group showed a lactulose/mannitol ratio that was significantly different (0.105 +/- 0.071, p < 0.001)." Laudat A, et al. The intestinal permeability test applied to the diagnosis of food allergy in paediatrics. *West Indian Med J.* 1994 Sep;43(3):87-8

[200] "After ingestion of food allergens by the patients, mean mannitol recovery fell to 11.57% and mean recovery of lactulose rose to 1.04%, both values being significantly different from those obtained in the fasting patients." Andre C, Andre F, Colin L, Cavagna S. Measurement of intestinal permeability to mannitol and lactulose as a means of diagnosing food allergy and evaluating therapeutic effectiveness of disodium cromoglycate. *Ann Allergy.* 1987 Nov;59(5 Pt 2):127-30

[201] "A provocation IPT with food induced significant L/M ratio changes only in the group in which the food was proved to be responsible for the exacerbation of skin lesions." Dupont C, Barau E, Molkhou P, Raynaud F, Barbet JP, Dehennin L. Food-induced alterations of intestinal permeability in children with cow's milk-sensitive enteropathy and atopic dermatitis. *J Pediatr Gastroenterol Nutr.* 1989 May;8(4):459-65

[202] Jyonouchi H, Sun S, Itokazu N. Innate immunity associated with inflammatory responses and cytokine production against common dietary proteins in patients with autism spectrum disorder. *Neuropsychobiology.* 2002;46(2):76-84

[203] "Thus, endotoxin and allergen acting together could play a role in up-regulating the response of the human asthmatic airway to adenosine. However, our data suggest that the interaction would be additive rather than synergistic." Karmouty Quintana H, Mazzoni L, Fozard JR. Effects of endotoxin and allergen alone and in combination on the sensitivity of the rat airways to adenosine. *Auton Autacoid Pharmacol.* 2005 Oct;25(4):167-70

[204] "Our findings firstly demonstrated that gliadin was directly bound to tTG in duodenal mucosa of coeliacs and controls, and the ability of circulating tTG-autoantibodies to recognize and immunoprecipitate the tTG-gliadin complexes." Ciccocioppo R, Di Sabatino A, Ara C, Biagi F, Perilli M, Amicosante G, Cifone MG, Corazza GR. Gliadin and tissue transglutaminase complexes in normal and coeliac duodenal mucosa. *Clin Exp Immunol.* 2003 Dec;134(3):516-24

[205] "Thus, modification of gluten peptides by tTG, especially deamidation of certain glutamine residues, can enhance their binding to HLA-DQ2 or -DQ8 and potentiate T cell stimulation. Furthermore, tTG-catalyzed cross-linking and consequent haptenization of gluten with extracellular matrix proteins allows for storage and extended availability of gluten in the mucosa." Dieterich W, Esslinger B, Schuppan D. Pathomechanisms in celiac disease. *Int Arch Allergy Immunol.* 2003 Oct;132(2):98-108

[206] "Gliadins alpha1-alpha11, gamma1- gamma6, omega1-omega3, and omega5 were substrates for tTG. tTG catalyzed the crosslinking of gliadin peptides with interstitial collagens type I, III and VI. Coeliac patients showed increased antibody titers against the collagens I, III, V and VI." Dieterich W, Esslinger B, Trapp D, Hahn E, Huff T, Seilmeier W, Wieser H, Schuppan D. Crosslinking to tissue transglutaminase and collagen favours gliadin toxicity in coeliac disease. *Gut.* 2005 Sep 27

[207] "Elevated titres of antithyroid antibodies observed in children with coeliac disease (41.1%) in comparison to control group (3.56%) indicate the need for performing the screening tests for antithyroid antibodies in children with CD." Kowalska E, Wasowska-Krolikowska K, Toporowska-Kowalska E. Estimation of antithyroid antibodies occurrence in children with coeliac disease. *Med Sci Monit.* 2000 Jul-Aug;6(4):719-2 http://www.medscimonit.com/pub/vol_6/no_4/1240.pdf

[208] Kieslich M, Errazuriz G, Posselt HG, Moeller-Hartmann W, Zanella F, Boehles H. Brain white-matter lesions in celiac disease: a prospective study of 75 diet-treated patients. *Pediatrics.* 2001 Aug;108(2):E21 http://pediatrics.aappublications.org/cgi/content/full/108/2/e21

[209] "JIA children have an increased prevalence of autoimmune thyroiditis, subclinical hypothyroidism and coeliac disease." Stagi S, Giani T, Simonini G, Falcini F. Thyroid function, autoimmune thyroiditis and coeliac disease in juvenile idiopathic arthritis. *Rheumatology* (Oxford). 2005 Apr;44(4):517-2

[210] Zitouni M, Daoud W, Kallel M, Makni S. Systemic lupus erythematosus with celiac disease: a report of five cases. *Joint Bone Spine.* 2004 Jul;71(4):344-6

[211] Komatireddy GR, Marshall JB, Aqel R, Spollen LE, Sharp GC. Association of systemic lupus erythematosus and gluten enteropathy. *South Med J.* 1995 Jun;88:673-6

[212] Rustgi AK, Peppercorn MA. Gluten-sensitive enteropathy and systemic lupus erythematosus. *Arch Intern Med.* 1988 Jul;148(7):1583-4

- Review and proposal: Hapten exposure might predispose to atopic disease—the hapten-atopy hypothesis (*Trends Immunol* 2009 Feb[213] and SkinAndAllergyNews.com 2010 Oct[214]): Dr McFadden and his colleagues propose that **orally-consumed chemicals—commonly consumed as processed foods—bind to and alter endogenous proteins to result in hapten-protein neoantigens that stimulate immunologic disease, particularly allergic conditions** such as atopic dermatitis (eczema), asthma and seasonal respiratory allergies. Per an interview with Jancin, McFadden explained that "Haptens are low-molecular-weight organic chemicals that aren't allergenic on their own but can bind to a peptide or protein, thereby altering its configuration and rendering it foreign and allergenic. Examples of haptens include antibiotics and some other drugs, as well as chemicals present in toiletries, processed foods, powdered milk, preservatives used in vaccines, and metal jewelry. … **Various brands of powdered milk contain a mean of 12 haptens each**. … Also, epidemiologic studies show that certain maternal occupations predispose to the birth of atopic children. Among these occupations are hairdresser, beautician, cleaner, electroplater, bar staff, dental assistant, confectionary maker, and book binder. What these diverse occupations have in common is increased environmental exposure to haptens."

5. Dietary molecular mimicry: Just as microbes produce structures similar to human molecules which then incite a cross-reacting immune response—**molecular mimicry** (discussed elsewhere in this chapter in the section on dysbiosis)—certain dietary antigens appear capable of inducing cross reactions. For example, Vojdani et al[215] recently demonstrated **cross-reactivity between anti-gliadin antibodies and anti-cerebellar antibodies in an experimental model that may partly explain the anti-brain autoimmunity seen in autism.** Further expanding this concept of dietary molecular mimicry is the finding that "the virulence factor of C albicans-hyphal wall protein 1 (HWP1)-contains amino acid sequences that are identical or highly homologous to known coeliac disease-related alpha-gliadin and gamma-gliadin T-cell epitopes."[216] This raises three interrelated possibilities: 1) that gastrointestinal overgrowth of *Candida albicans* and the resultant elaboration of HWP1 and immunostimulation may result in sensitivity to gluten, particularly as HWP1 and gliadin are both substrates for transglutaminase, 2) that consumption of wheat gluten may trigger sensitivity to *Candida albicans*, and 3) that wheat gluten and *Candida albicans* must both be present for the development of celiac disease and the ensuant autoimmunity. Additional details on the ability of *C. albicans* to contribute to autoimmunity are discussed in the section on dysbiosis.

6. Enhanced processing of autoantigens: Food-allergic patients may produce autoimmunity-stimulating autoantigens following exposure to foods to which they are sensitized. This has been demonstrated in autistic children, **exposure of lymphocytes from autistic patients to dietary antigens (gliadin and casein peptides) stimulates production of autoantigens that presumably incite and perpetuate autoimmunity**.[217] Thus, at least in autistic patients, we have evidence that food allergy can segue into autoimmunity. This phenomenon is probably not restricted only to autistic patients, as suggested by the association between celiac disease and the systemic autoimmune disease lupus.[218,219,220]

7. Diet-derived xenobiotic immunotoxicity: Foods commonly contain trace amounts of xenobiotics such as pesticides, fungicides, fumigants, fertilizers, preservatives, military propellants such as

---

[213] McFadden JP, White JM, Basketter DA, Kimber I. Does hapten exposure predispose to atopic disease? The hapten-atopy hypothesis. *Trends Immunol.* 2009 Feb;30(2):67-74

[214] Article by Bruce Jancin of the Skin & Allergy News Digital Network; interview with Dr. John P. McFadden. Expert Analysis from the Annual Congress of the European Academy of Dermatology and Venereology: Exploring the Hapten Hypothesis of Atopic Disease. http://www.skinandallergynews.com/news/medical-dermatology/single-article/eadv-exploring-the-hapten-hypothesis-of-atopic-disease/e7df2851ed.html Posted 10/26/10 and accessed May 31, 2011.

[215] "This cross-reaction was further confirmed by DOT-immunoblot and inhibition studies. We conclude that a subgroup of patients with autism produce antibodies against Purkinje cells and gliadin peptides, which may be responsible for some of the neurological symptoms in autism." Vojdani A, O'Bryan T, Green JA, Mccandless J, Woeller KN, Vojdani E, Nourian AA, Cooper EL. Immune response to dietary proteins, gliadin and cerebellar peptides in children with autism. *Nutr Neurosci.* 2004 Jun;7:151-61

[216] "Subsequently, C albicans might function as an adjuvant that stimulates antibody formation against HWP1 and gluten, and formation of autoreactive antibodies against tissue transglutaminase and endomysium." Nieuwenhuizen WF, Pieters RH, Knippels LM, Jansen MC, Koppelman SJ. Is Candida albicans a trigger in the onset of coeliac disease? *Lancet.* 2003;361(9375):2152-4

[217] Vojdani A, Pangborn JB, Vojdani E, Cooper EL. Infections, toxic chemicals and dietary peptides binding to lymphocyte receptors and tissue enzymes are major instigators of autoimmunity in autism. *Int J Immunopathol Pharmacol.* 2003 Sep-Dec;16(3):189-99

[218] Zitouni M, Daoud W, Kallel M, Makni S. Systemic lupus erythematosus with celiac disease: a report of five cases. *Joint Bone Spine.* 2004 Jul;71(4):344-6

[219] Komatireddy GR, Marshall JB, Aqel R, Spollen LE, Sharp GC. Association of systemic lupus erythematosus and gluten enteropathy. *South Med J.* 1995 Jun;88:673-6

[220] Rustgi AK, Peppercorn MA. Gluten-sensitive enteropathy and systemic lupus erythematosus. *Arch Intern Med.* 1988 Jul;148(7):1583-4

perchlorate[221], and toxic metals such as mercury. Some of these xenobiotics have been insufficiently studied in humans, while others such as mercury are well-known immunotoxins capable of inducing immune dysfunction which may contribute to autoimmunity. **Mercury poisoning/accumulation can occur in humans as a result of consumption of contaminated foods—especially seafood such as shark, swordfish, king mackerel, tilefish, and albacore ("white") tuna**[222], and the immunologic effects of organic and/or inorganic mercury include immunosuppression, immunostimulation, formation of antinucleolar antibodies targeting fibrillarin, and formation and deposition of immune-complexes, resulting in a syndrome called "mercury-induced autoimmunity" which can be induced by exposure of susceptible animals to mercury.[223] Mercury/"silver" amalgam dental fillings rank highly among the most significant source of mercury exposure in humans, and **implantation of mercury-silver dental amalgams in susceptible animals causes chronic stimulation of the immune system with induction of systemic autoimmunity.**[224] Besides being **a neurotoxin with no safe exposure limit**[225], **mercury is known to modify/antigenize endogenous proteins to promote autoimmunity**[226], and **mercury may also promote autoimmunity by contributing to a pro-inflammatory environment that awakens quiescent autoreactive immunocytes via bystander activation**[227] (detailed later). For example, administration of mercury to "susceptible" mice induces autoimmunity via modification of the nucleolar protein *fibrillarin*[228]; noteworthy in this regard is the fact that antifibrillarin antibodies are characteristic of the autoimmune disease **scleroderma**.[229] Mercury toxicity is commonly encountered in clinical practice (diagnosis and treatment are discussed later), and a recent study published in *JAMA* showed that 8% of American women of childbearing age have sufficient levels of mercury in their bodies to produce neurologic damage in their children.[230] **The mercury-based preservative thimerosol is a type-IV (delayed hypersensitivity) sensitizing agent**[231], and **recent research implicates mercury as an important contributor to the clinical manifestations of autism**[232,233] **and eczema.**[234] Preliminary clinical evidence shows that removal of mercury amalgams, particularly along

[221] "The Bush administration has imposed a gag order on the U.S. Environmental Protection Agency from publicly discussing perchlorate pollution, even as two new studies reveal high levels of the rocket-fuel component may be contaminating the nation's lettuce supply." Peter Waldman. Rocket Fuel Residues Found in Lettuce: Bush administration issues gag order on EPA discussions of possible rocket fuel tainted lettuce. *THE WALL STREET JOURNAL*. See http://www.organicconsumers.org/toxic/lettuce042903.cfm http://www.rhinoed.com/epa's_gag_order.htm http://www.peer.org/press/508.html http://yubanet.com/artman/publish/article_13637.shtml

[222] See http://www.cfsan.fda.gov/~dms/admehg3.html for the white-washed version; see http://www.ewg.org/issues/mercury/20040319/index.php for a more accurate and complete perspective.

[223] Havarinasab S, Hultman P. Organic mercury compounds and autoimmunity. *Autoimmun Rev.* 2005;4(5):270-5 www.generationrescue.org/pdf/havarinasab.pdf Accessed December 27, 2005

[224] "We hypothesize that under appropriate conditions of genetic susceptibility and adequate body burden, heavy metal exposure from dental amalgam may contribute to immunological aberrations, which could lead to overt autoimmunity." Hultman P, Johansson U, Turley SJ, Lindh U, Enestrom S, Pollard KM. Adverse immunological effects and autoimmunity induced by dental amalgam and alloy in mice. *FASEB J.* 1994 Nov;8(14):1183-90 http://www.fasebj.org/cgi/reprint/8/14/1183

[225] University of Calgary Faculty of Medicine. How Mercury Causes Brain Neuron Degeneration http://commons.ucalgary.ca/mercury/

[226] Havarinasab S, Hultman P. Organic mercury compounds and autoimmunity. *Autoimmun Rev.* 2005 Jun;4(5):270-5

[227] "It is therefore theoretically possible that compounds present in vaccines such as thiomersal or aluminium hydroxyde can trigger autoimmune reactions through bystander effects." Fournie GJ, Mas M, Cautain B, Savignac M, Subra JF, Pelletier L, Saoudi A, Lagrange D, Calise M, Druet P. Induction of autoimmunity through bystander effects. Lessons from immunological disorders induced by heavy metals. *J Autoimmun.* 2001 May;16(3):319-26

[228] Nielsen JB, Hultman P. Mercury-induced autoimmunity in mice. *Environ Health Perspect.* 2002 Oct;110 Suppl 5:877-81 http://ehp.niehs.nih.gov/docs/2002/suppl-5/877-88 1nielsen/abstract.html

[229] "Since anti-fibrillarin antibodies are specific markers of scleroderma, the present animal model may be valuable for studies of the immunological aberrations which are likely to induce this autoimmune response." Hultman P, Enestrom S, Pollard KM, Tan EM. Anti-fibrillarin autoantibodies in mercury-treated mice. *Clin Exp Immunol.* 1989 Dec;78(3):470-7

[230] "However, approximately 8% of women had concentrations higher than the US Environmental Protection Agency's recommended reference dose (5.8 microg/L), below which exposures are considered to be without adverse effects. Women who are pregnant or who intend to become pregnant should follow federal and state advisories on consumption of fish." Schober SE, Sinks TH, Jones RL, Bolger PM, McDowell M, Osterloh J, Garrett ES, Canady RA, Dillon CF, Sun Y, Joseph CB, Mahaffey KR. Blood mercury levels in US children and women of childbearing age, 1999-2000. *JAMA.* 2003 Apr 2;289(13):1667-74

[231] "Thimerosal is an important preservative in vaccines and ophthalmologic preparations. The substance is known to be a type IV sensitizing agent. High sensitization rates were observed in contact-allergic patients and in health care workers who had been exposed to thimerosal-preserved vaccines." Westphal GA, Schnuch A, Schulz TG, Reich K, Aberer W, Brasch J, Koch P, Wessbecher R, Szliska C, Bauer A, Hallier E. Homozygous gene deletions of the glutathione S-transferases M1 and T1 are associated with thimerosal sensitization. *Int Arch Occup Environ Health.* 2000 Aug;73(6):384-8

[232] Vojdani A, Pangborn JB, Vojdani E, Cooper EL. Infections, toxic chemicals and dietary peptides binding to lymphocyte receptors and tissue enzymes are major instigators of autoimmunity in autism. *Int J Immunopathol Pharmacol.* 2003 Sep-Dec;16(3):189-99

[233] Geier DA, Geier MR. A comparative evaluation of the effects of MMR immunization and mercury doses from thimerosal-containing childhood vaccines on the population prevalence of autism. *Med Sci Monit.* 2004 Mar;10(3):PI33-9. Epub 2004 Mar 1. http://www.medscimonit.com/pub/vol_10/no_3/3986.pdf

[234] Weidinger S, Kramer U, Dunemann L, Mohrenschlager M, Ring J, Behrendt H. Body burden of mercury is associated with acute atopic eczema and total IgE in children from southern Germany. *J Allergy Clin Immunol.* 2004 Aug;114(2):457-9

with implementation of antioxidant therapy and/or mercury chelation, benefits the biochemical status and/or clinical course of autoimmune disease.[235,236]

8. <u>Diet-derived dysbiosis</u>: Induction and exacerbation of dysbiosis following chronic consumption of allergenic foods has been reported to occur in humans. Raw vegetables and salad greens are thoroughly contaminated with bacteria and occasionally other microbes. Food can be contaminated with pathogenic microbes via improper preparation, storage, or handling by chefs with contagious diseases and poor hygiene. An inflammatory "reactive" arthritis can result from consumption of food that is contaminated by microorganisms, most commonly *Salmonella*[237,238,239] and *Campylobacter* species.[240] Long-term autoimmune/inflammatory complications of gastrointestinal infections/colonization sourced from food include Reiter's syndrome, Guillain-Barre syndrome (peripheral nerve autoimmunity), uveitis, sacroiliitis, and ankylosing spondylitis.

9. <u>Diet-derived immunodysregulation</u>: Certain foods contain constituents that cause immune dysfunction and the induction or exacerbation of autoimmunity. L-Canavanine sulfate is a non-protein amino acid found in alfalfa sprouts which triggers a condition similar to systemic lupus erythematosus in monkeys[241,242] and which may exacerbate SLE in humans.

10. <u>Dietary xenobiotics</u>: Artificial sweeteners, thickeners, flavor enhancers, emulsifiers, and plasticizers can be found in foods, particularly those which are manufactured and processed. Some of these chemicals have the potential to alter immune mechanisms in favor of autoimmunity. These dietary xenobiotics may be particularly relevant for initiating and promoting Crohn's disease.[243]

11. <u>Immunogenicity induced by cooking—the Maillard reaction (non-enzymatic glycosylation)</u>: Heated exposure of lysine, arginine, and tryptophan to reducing sugars such as fructose and lactose results in the non-enzymatic binding (glycosylation) of the sugar with the amino acid. If the amino acid is a component of a protein, then the structure and antigenicity of the protein is altered as it is now a glycoprotein, which may either serve as a neoantigen or may increase the allergenicity of a protein that was previously hypoallergenic, as seen with the roasting of peanuts.[244,245] Glycoproteins formed from the baking and browning of foods are also called ***glycotoxins*** and are capable of exacerbating

[235] Prochazkova J, Sterzl I, Kucerova H, Bartova J, Stejskal VD. The beneficial effect of amalgam replacement on health in patients with autoimmunity. *Neuro Endocrinol Lett*. 2004 Jun;25(3):211-8. See also: "The MELISA Test is reproducible, sensitive, specific, and reliable for detecting metal sensitivity in metal-sensitive patients." Valentine-Thon E, Schiwara HW. Validity of MELISA for metal sensitivity testing. *Neuro Endocrinol Lett*. 2003 Feb-Apr;24(1-2):57-64. See also: "The hypothesis that metal exposure from dental amalgam can cause ill health in a susceptible part of the exposed population was supported." Lindh U, Hudecek R, Danersund A, Eriksson S, Lindvall A. Removal of dental amalgam and other metal alloys supported by antioxidant therapy alleviates symptoms and improves quality of life in patients with amalgam-associated ill health. *Neuro Endocrinol Lett*. 2002 Oct-Dec;23(5-6):459-82 http://www.nel.edu/23_56/NEL235602A12_Lindh.htm and http://www.nel.edu/pdf_w/23_56/NEL235602A12_Lindh_wr.pdf

[236] "This study documents objective biochemical changes following the removal of these fillings along with other dental materials, utilizing a new health care model of multidisciplinary planning and treatment." Huggins HA, Levy TE. Cerebrospinal fluid protein changes in multiple sclerosis after dental amalgam removal. *Altern Med Rev*. 1998 Aug;3(4):295-300 http://www.thorne.com/altmedrev/.fulltext/3/4/295.pdf

[237] "We describe the case of a patient who became ill with Salmonella Blockley food poisoning while working in Cyprus in August 1994. As his diarrhoea resolved he began to suffer from lower limb joint pains which were diagnosed as acute salmonella reactive arthritis." Wilson IG, Whitehead E. Long-term post-Salmonella reactive arthritis due to Salmonella Blockley. *Jpn J Infect Dis*. 2004 Oct;57(5):210-1

[238] "Reactive joint symptoms after food-borne Salmonella infection may be more frequent than previously thought. The duration of diarrhea is strongly correlated with the occurrence of joint symptoms." Locht H, Molbak K, Krogfelt KA. High frequency of reactive joint symptoms after an outbreak of Salmonella enteritidis. *J Rheumatol*. 2002 Apr;29(4):767-71

[239] Leirisalo-Repo M, Helenius P, Hannu T, Lehtinen A, Kreula J, Taavitsainen M, Koskimies S. Long-term prognosis of reactive salmonella arthritis. *Ann Rheum Dis*. 1997 Sep;56(9):516-20 http://ard.bmjjournals.com/cgi/content/full/56/9/516

[240] "Campylobacter jejuni is the most commonly reported bacterial cause of foodborne infection in the United States. Adding to the human and economic costs are chronic sequelae associated with C. jejuni infection--Guillain-Barre syndrome and reactive arthritis." Altekruse SF, Stern NJ, Fields PI, Swerdlow DL. Campylobacter jejuni--an emerging foodborne pathogen. *Emerg Infect Dis*. 1999 Jan-Feb;5(1):28-35

[241] "L-Canavanine sulfate, a constituent of alfalfa sprouts, was incorporated into the diet and reactivated the syndrome in monkeys in which an SLE-like syndrome had previously been induced by the ingestion of alfalfa seeds or sprouts." Malinow MR, Bardana EJ Jr, Pirofsky B, Craig S, McLaughlin P. Systemic lupus erythematosus-like syndrome in monkeys fed alfalfa sprouts: role of a nonprotein amino acid. *Science*. 1982 Apr 23;216(4544):415-7

[242] "Occurrence of autoimmune hemolytic anemia and exacerbation of SLE have been linked to ingestion of alfalfa tablets containing L-canavanine." Alcocer-Varela J, Iglesias A, Llorente L, Alarcon-Segovia D. Effects of L-canavanine on T cells may explain the induction of systemic lupus erythematosus by alfalfa. *Arthritis Rheum*. 1985 Jan;28(1):52-7

[243] "Various food additives, especially emulsifiants, thickeners, surface-finishing agents and contaminants like plasticizers share structural domains with mycobacterial lipids. It is therefore hypothesized, that these compounds are able to stimulate by molecular mimicry the CD1 system in the gastrointestinal mucosa and to trigger the pro-inflammatory cytokine cascade." Traunmuller F. Etiology of Crohn's disease: Do certain food additives cause intestinal inflammation by molecular mimicry of mycobacterial lipids? *Med Hypotheses*. 2005;65(5):859-64

[244] "Roasted peanuts exhibited a higher level of IgE binding, which was correlated with a higher level of AGE adducts. We concluded that there is an association between AGE adducts and increased IgE binding (i.e., allergenicity) of roasted peanuts." Chung SY, Champagne ET. Association of end-product adducts with increased IgE binding of roasted peanuts. *J Agric Food Chem*. 2001 Aug;49(8):3911-6

[245] "The data presented here indicate that thermal processing may play an important role in enhancing the allergenic properties of peanuts and that the protein modifications made by the Maillard reaction contribute to this effect." Maleki SJ, Chung SY, Champagne ET, Raufman JP.The effects of roasting on the allergenic properties of peanut proteins. *J Allergy Clin Immunol*. 2000 Oct;106(4):763-8

inflammation in patients with diabetes.[246] Similar to the formation of **glycotoxins** is the formation of **acrylamide**, a possible carcinogen, in fried and baked foods.

Common allergy treatments advocated by the pharmaceutical industry create an overly simplistic and inaccurate view of the allergic process which obfuscates the identification and correction of the underlying processes, only two of which are antigen exposure and histamine release. Nutritionally oriented doctors, too, often emphasize the identification and elimination of allergen exposure as the sole means of addressing allergic diathesis with the presumption that allergen avoidance cures the allergy. These simplistic models and the incomplete treatments based upon them fail to address the underlying cause of the allergic phenomenon: immune dysfunction. Allergic manifestations always require at least two factors: 1) exposure of the antigen to the immune system (antigen absorption) and 2) a dysfunctional immune system that "overreacts" to the otherwise benign antigen. Allergy treatment that fails to address the underlying immune dysfunction is incomplete. Allergy treatment that addresses the underlying immune dysfunction has the opportunity to correct the *total problem*, rather than merely reducing the manifestations of the problem. Therefore, treatment of the allergic diathesis must always address issues of antigen exposure, antigen absorption, ***and the dysfunctional immune system*** that results in the hyperactive immune response that we call "allergy." Elimination of either antigen exposure or antigen absorption eliminates allergic manifestations, but does not necessarily correct the underlying immune defect(s). Complete correction of the underlying immune defect obviates the need for the identification and avoidance of the allergen. In clinical practice, a combination of both approaches—allergen avoidance and immune modulation—is the most effective approach, affording relatively high effectiveness in symptom reduction even with only modest compliance.

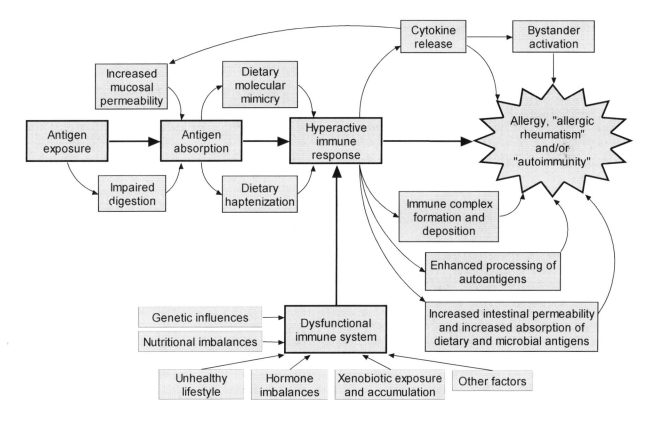

Approaching a More Comprehensive Understanding of "Food Allergy" and Its Contribution to Immune Dysfunction and Musculoskeletal Inflammation

---

[246] "A study now reveals that the consumption of foods rich in browned and oxidized products (so-called glycotoxins) induces a chronic inflammatory state in diabetic individuals." Monnier VM, Obrenovich ME. Wake up and smell the maillard reaction. *Sci Aging Knowledge Environ.* 2002 Dec 18;2002(50):pe21

Orthomolecular Immunomodulation: The Author's Approach to Alleviating Allergy

My clinical approach to improving immune function in patients with allergy begins with supplementation of vitamin E, CoQ-10, vitamin B-12, vitamin C, bioflavonoids, honey, and fish oil. Thereafter, I look at hormones, particularly DHEA, estrogen (quantitative and qualitative), testosterone, and cortisol. I also look at diet and bowel health with respect to putrefaction and intestinal permeability. Although rarely powerful when used in isolation, these treatments when used in combinations tailored to the individual patient often result in an impressive reduction in allergic manifestations even when allergen avoidance is either not pursued or not feasible. The process of alleviating allergic disorders is, however, arduous and time-consuming unless the doctor uses a group of protocols such as those described herein which address the most common contributing factors to allergic problems. Here I extend my previous three-step process[247] into a four-tiered approach, with the fourth step including selected pharmaceutical drugs.

Step 1: From initial patient assessment to the first phase of treatment

In a patient with presumed "allergy" who is in otherwise good health, following a basic health assessment and exclusion of significant disease, I begin by correcting problems that are common to patients with allergy. Minor improvements in allergy symptoms as a result of a low-cost low-risk interventions can be multiplied with a specified group of interventions; we aim for a modest improvement with several treatments rather than a "silver bullet" miracle cure with a single intervention. For example, 10% improvement in symptoms may be insignificant in itself; however a 10% improvement from six interventions results in a 60% improvement and enhances patient confidence long enough for other interventions and assessments to be implemented, if necessary. The goal with the first step of treatment is to correct the most common and most likely problems, namely fatty acid imbalances, micronutrient deficiencies, phytonutrient insufficiencies, and dysbiosis.

> **CoQ-10 for allergy treatment**
>
> The mechanisms involved with this benefit are likely mediated primarily via improved mitochondrial function which ultimately manifests as reduced inflammation, oxidant stress, and enhanced Treg formation, as well as direct inhibition of NFkB by CoQ-10.

- Avoidance of suspected food allergens: The most common allergens are wheat, cow's milk, and eggs; however any patient can be allergic to any food. It is not uncommon for patients to have to avoid up to 10 foods before attaining maximal improvement, and up to 85% of migraine patients can be cured of their headaches by the use of allergy avoidance alone.[248] Food allergy avoidance for 1 month helps achieve symptomatic relief and allows the gut to heal and the immune system to recalibrate. The diet should emphasize consumption of lean meats, fruits, vegetables, nuts, seeds, and berries to ensure a systemic anti-inflammatory effect and increased consumption of anti-inflammatory phytonutrients, especially flavonoids. High-glycemic foods are avoided as are "food additives" such as tartrazine, which is known to exacerbate allergic asthma. Some foods like tuna, certain cheeses and wines are high in histamine; frequent consumption of these foods by an allergic individual is analogous to adding fuel to a fire that the patient is simultaneously trying to extinguish. Recall that in breast-feeding infants, the mother will have to consume a hypoallergenic diet to prevent passage of allergens[249] and allergen-antibody immune complexes[250] in breast milk.

- Rotation diet: While select foods should be completely avoided, the remaining foods that are consumed should be rotated in and out of the diet with a periodicity of 3-5 days. Patients should avoid "dietary monotony"[251] by consuming a variety of foods. By rotating different foods in and out of the diet, patients are more likely to consume a nutritious diet and are less likely to develop or perpetuate food allergies.

---

[247] Vasquez A. Improving neuromusculoskeletal health by optimizing immune function and reducing allergic reactions: a review of 16 treatments and a 3-step clinical approach. *Nutritional Perspectives* 2005; October: 27-35, 40

[248] Grant EC. Food allergies and migraine. *Lancet*. 1979 May 5;1(8123):966-9

[249] "In all, clinical disappearance of symptoms was observed after removal of milk from the mother's diet and/or elimination from the child's diet of any cow's-milk-based hypoallergenic formula." Barau E, Dupont C. Allergy to cow's milk proteins in mother's milk or in hydrolyzed cow's milk infant formulas as assessed by intestinal permeability measurements. *Allergy*. 1994 Apr;49(4):295-8

[250] The finding of egg-allergen immune complex in breast milk inplies 1) egg protein escapes complete digestion/degradation in the gastrointestinal tract, 2) egg protein is absorbed intact through the mucosa, 3) egg protein escapes filtration by the liver, 4) egg protein stimulates formation IgA immune complexes, and 5) egg-IgA immune complexes are secreted in milk which would then expose the infant to both allergen and immune complex, possibly resulting in clinical disease. Hirose J, Ito S, Hirata N, Kido S, Kitabatake N, Narita H. Occurrence of the major food allergen, ovomucoid, in human breast milk as an immune complex. *Biosci Biotechnol Biochem*. 2001 Jun;65(6):1438-40 http://www.jstage.jst.go.jp/article/bbb/65/6/1438/_pdf

[251] Pelchat ML, Schaefer S. Dietary monotony and food cravings in young and elderly adults. *Physiol Behav*. 2000 Jan;68(3):353-9

- <u>CoQ-10</u>: CoQ-10 levels are low in approximately 40% of patients with allergies, according to a small study conducted by Folkers and Pfeiffer.[252] Asthmatics also have lower levels of CoQ-10 compared to healthy people.[253] In my experience, clinical improvement is commonly seen in allergic patients after supplementation with CoQ-10. I generally prescribe 100-300mg/day of CoQ-10 for adults.

- <u>Probiotics</u>: Supplementation with probiotics (beneficial strains of bacteria and yeast) appears to improve intestinal barrier function, promote microecological balance in the gastrointestinal tract, modulate immune function, and thus reduce manifestations of allergic disease.[254,255,256]

- <u>Vitamin E</u>: Vitamin E has been shown to reduce IgE levels in humans and to reduce the manifestations of allergy-related disease.[257] I commonly prescribe 800-2,000 IU per day of mixed tocopherols with approximately 40% gamma tocopherol for patients with allergy.

- <u>Vitamin C</u>: A recent clinical trial showed that 2 grams per day of ascorbic acid reduced blood histamine levels by 38%.[258] Cathcart hypothesized that high doses of vitamin C (i.e., bowel tolerance) may impair the adsorption of IgE with allergens and thus retard the allergic cascade from being initiated.[259] Either of these two mechanisms, perhaps in addition to other mechanisms, may explain the anti-allergy effects of ascorbic acid.[260]

> **Nutritional immunomodulation for the treatment of "allergies"**
>
> Very importantly, the new treatment approach of "nutritional immunomodulation" as described in this textbook is a very important advance in the treatment of allergic conditions; this approach stimulates phenotypic switching in favor of regulatory T-cells (Treg) and thereby supports natural, endogenous anti-inflammatory anti-allergy anti-autoimmune benefits.

- <u>Bioflavonoids</u>: Bioflavonoids stabilize mast cell membranes and thus reduce the liberation of histamine. Additionally, quercetin and catechin inhibit the action of histidine decarboxylase, which converts histidine into histamine. Many fruits, vegetables, and herbal teas are excellent sources of flavonoids, which can also be consumed in the form of tablets and capsules.

- <u>Vitamin B-12</u>: Vitamin B-12 has been shown to reduce physiologic manifestations of allergy in ovalbumin-sensitized mice.[261] Since vitamin B-12 is safe, non-toxic, and bioavailable when administered orally in large doses to humans, I commonly prescribe 2,500-5,000 mcg per day for allergic patients for a one-month trial. Although the benefit of vitamin B-12 in patients with sulfite-sensitive asthma is biochemically mediated rather than immunologically mediated[262], this research adds tangential support to the use of high-dose vitamin B-12 in selected patients with allergy (particularly asthma), at least for a short-term clinical trial. Hydroxocobalamin and methylcobalamin are preferred over cyanocobalamin due to the content of cyanide in the latter.[263]

---

[252] Ye CQ, Folkers K, Tamagawa H, Pfeiffer C. A modified determination of coenzyme Q10 in human blood and CoQ10 blood levels in diverse patients with allergies. *Biofactors*. 1988 Dec;1(4):303-6

[253] Gazdik F, Gvozdjakova A, Nadvornikova R, Repicka L, Jahnova E, Kucharska J, Pijak MR, Gazdikova K. Decreased levels of coenzyme Q(10) in patients with bronchial asthma. *Allergy*. 2002 Sep;57(9):811-4

[254] Majamaa H, Isolauri E. Probiotics: a novel approach in the management of food allergy. *J Allergy Clin Immunol* 1997 Feb;99(2):179-85

[255] von der Weid T, Ibnou-Zekri N, Pfeifer A. Novel probiotics for the management of allergic inflammation. *Dig Liver Dis*. 2002 Sep;34 Suppl 2:S25-8

[256] "The administration of probiotics, strains of bacteria from the healthy human gut microbiota, have been shown to stimulate antiinflammatory, tolerogenic immune responses, the lack of which has been implied in the development of atopic disorders. Thus probiotics may prove beneficial in the prevention and alleviation of allergic disease." Rautava S, Isolauri E. The development of gut immune responses and gut microbiota: effects of probiotics in prevention and treatment of allergic disease. *Curr Issues Intest Microbiol*. 2002 Mar;3(1):15-22

[257] Tsoureli-Nikita E, Hercogova J, Lotti T, Menchini G. Evaluation of dietary intake of vitamin E in the treatment of atopic dermatitis: a study of the clinical course and evaluation of the immunoglobulin E serum levels. *Int J Dermatol*. 2002 Mar;41(3):146-50

[258] "Chemotaxis was inversely correlated to blood histamine (r = -0.32, p = 0.045), and, compared to baseline and withdrawal values, histamine levels were depressed 38% following VC supplementation. ... These data indicate that VC may indirectly enhance chemotaxis by detoxifying histamine in vivo." Johnston CS, Martin LJ, Cai X. Antihistamine effect of supplemental ascorbic acid and neutrophil chemotaxis. *J Am Coll Nutr*. 1992 Apr;11(2):172-6

[259] "Allergic and sensitivity reactions are frequently ameliorated and sometimes completely blocked by massive doses of ascorbate. I now hypothesize that one mechanism in blocking of allergic symptoms is the reducing of the disulfide bonds between the chains in antibody molecules making their bonding antigen impossible." Cathcart RF 3rd. The vitamin C treatment of allergy and the normally unprimed state of antibodies. *Med Hypotheses*. 1986 Nov;21(3):307-21

[260] Bucca C, Rolla G, Oliva A, Farina JC. Effect of vitamin C on histamine bronchial responsiveness of patients with allergic rhinitis. *Ann Allergy*. 1990 Oct;65(4):311-4

[261] "We infer that Cbl administration significantly reduced the IL-2 concentration, and secondarily the IL-4, IgE and histamine concentrations." Funada U, Wada M, Kawata T, Tanaka N, Tadokoro T, Maekawa A. Effect of cobalamin on the allergic response in mice. *Biosci Biotechnol Biochem* 2000 Oct;64(10):2053-8

[262] Anibarro B, Caballero T, Garcia-Ara C, Diaz-Pena JM, Ojeda JA. Asthma with sulfite intolerance in children: a blocking study with cyanocobalamin. *J Allergy Clin Immunol*. 1992 Jul;90(1):103-9

[263] Freeman AG. Cyanocobalamin--a case for withdrawal: discussion paper. *J R Soc Med*. 1992 Nov;85(11):686-7

<u>Step 2: Additional interventions for moderate or unresponsive allergies</u>: For patients who do not respond sufficiently to the first phase of treatment, the following interventions can be considered.

- <u>Pancreatic and proteolytic enzymes</u>: Pancreatic enzymes have been shown to alleviate symptoms of food allergy in a controlled clinical trial.[264] Administration of enzyme preparations can alleviate intestinal and extra-intestinal manifestations of food allergy.[265] Proteolytic enzymes are safe and effective for the relief of musculoskeletal pain, as reviewed later in this text and elsewhere.[266] When taken with food, pancreatic/proteolytic enzymes facilitate hydrolysis of proteins, fats, and carbohydrates and are then absorbed into the systemic circulation for an anti-inflammatory effect. Although individual enzymes may be used in isolation, enzyme therapy is generally delivered in the form of polyenzyme preparations containing pancreatin, bromelain, papain, amylase, lipase, trypsin and alpha-chymotrypsin.

- <u>NFkB inhibitors</u>: The clinical significance of NFkB and its phytonutritional modulation is detailed later in this book and elsewhere.[267] Nutrients that can be used to downregulate inflammatory responses are vitamin D, curcumin (requires piperine for absorption), lipoic acid, green tea, rosemary, grape seed extract, propolis, resveratrol, selenium, zinc, and N-acetyl-cysteine.

- <u>Eradication of harmful intestinal yeast, bacteria, and other "parasites"</u>: I have seen several patients become cured of their "allergies" once we eradicated the dysbiotic bacteria, yeast, amoebas, or other microorganisms from their gastrointestinal tract. Intestinal colonization with harmful bacteria/yeast/protozoa/amebas can cause mucosal injury and result in macromolecular absorption and thus promotes immune sensitization to dietary antigens; in these situations, correction of dysbiosis via eradication of harmful microorganisms can lead to an impressive reduction in food-associated allergic phenomena. Although many indirect mechanisms will be discussed later, the most direct means by which dysbiosis may contribute to "allergy" is via endogenous formation of histamine via bacterial histidine decarboxylase. Galland and Lee[268] reported that eradication of *Giardia lamblia* in patients with chronic digestive complaints lessened the severity of food intolerance/allergy in 54% of patients. The supremely important topic of gastrointestinal dysbiosis is detailed later in this chapter.

<u>Step 3: Treatment for severe allergies</u>: For some patients with severe allergies, we start with selected treatments from Step 2 or Step 3 on the first visit *in addition to* the treatments included in Step 1. Implementation is customized based on history, examination, laboratory findings, and the doctor's experience and good judgment.

- <u>Calcium and magnesium butyrate</u>: Butyrate is a short-chain fatty acid which can be obtained from 1) a limited number of foods, namely butter, 2) intestinal fermentation of carbohydrates by probiotic bacteria, and 3) use of nutritional supplements. It is increasingly well-established that probiotic bacteria have immune-normalizing and "anti-allergy" effects, and this benefit is probably mediated at least in part by probiotic production of butyrate. The mechanisms of the anti-allergy effect of butyrate are manifold, and as a fatty acid butyrate activates peroxisome-proliferator activated receptor-alpha (PPAR-alpha) and thereby results in an immunomodulatory action and a suppressive effect on NFkB.[269,270] Butyrate is also a primary fuel for enterocytes and may improve enterocyte metabolism for the normalization of intestinal permeability. In the treatment of patients with inflammatory bowel disease, 4 grams per day of orally administered butyrate salts safely improves

---

[264] Raithel M, Weidenhiller M, Schwab D, Winterkamp S, Hahn EG. Pancreatic enzymes: a new group of antiallergic drugs? *Inflamm Res*. 2002 Apr;51 Suppl 1:S13-4
[265] Gaby AR. Pancreatic enzymes block food allergy reactions. *Townsend Letter for Doctors and Patients* 2002; Nov. http://www.townsendletter.com/Nov_2002/gabyliteraturereview1102.htm
[266] Vasquez A. Reducing pain and inflammation naturally - Part 3: Improving overall health while safely and effectively treating musculoskeletal pain. *Nutritional Perspectives* 2005; 28: 34-38, 40-42
[267] Vasquez A. Reducing pain and inflammation naturally - part 4: nutritional and botanical inhibition of NF-kappaB, the major intracellular amplifier of the inflammatory cascade. A practical clinical strategy exemplifying anti-inflammatory nutrigenomics. *Nutritional Perspectives*, July 2005:5-12.
[268] Galland L, Lee M. Abstract #170 High frequency of giardiasis in patients with chronic digestive complaints. *Am J Gastroenterol* 1989;84:1181
[269] Zapolska-Downar D, Siennicka A, Kaczmarczyk M, Kolodziej B, Naruszewicz M. Butyrate inhibits cytokine-induced VCAM-1 and ICAM-1 expression in cultured endothelial cells: the role of NF-kappaB and PPARalpha. *J Nutr Biochem*. 2004 Apr;15(4):220-8
[270] Luhrs H, Gerke T, Muller JG, Melcher R, Schauber J, Boxberge F, Scheppach W, Menzel T. Butyrate inhibits NF-kappaB activation in lamina propria macrophages of patients with ulcerative colitis. *Scand J Gastroenterol*. 2002 Apr;37(4):458-66

the action of mesalamine[271] as does topical application of butyrate in distal ulcerative colitis.[272] As a normal dietary component and product of the gastrointestinal tract, supplemental calcium and magnesium salts of butyrate are safe and effective for human consumption at doses of 1,000 – 4,500 mg butyrate per day for the alleviation of allergic diseases.[273,274]

- Purified chondroitin sulfate and glucosamine sulfate: Doctors and patients everywhere should already know that chondroitin sulfate and glucosamine sulfate are safe and effective for the treatment of osteoarthritis. Furthermore, purified chondroitin sulfate is cardioprotective and that it helps to reduce the vessel occlusion characteristic of atherosclerosis.[275] Additionally, new experimental evidence shows that chondroitin sulfate and glucosamine sulfate can inhibit allergic reactions.[276] With this in mind, it is reasonable to speculate that many arthritic patients who respond to glucosamine and chondroitin may actually be responding to the anti-allergy benefits of chondroitin and glucosamine *rather than* or *in addition to* the "cartilage building" properties of these supplements. Furthermore, there is evidence that purified chondroitin sulfate can act as a "decoy" and reduce adhesion of harmful bacteria; the role of harmful gastrointestinal bacteria in the genesis and perpetuation of joint pain and inflammation will be discussed in the next article in this series. For now, it will suffice to say that occult gastrointestinal infections (i.e., gastrointestinal dysbiosis) are a major contributor to the systemic pain and inflammation seen in conditions such as rheumatoid arthritis and ankylosing spondylitis.

- Hormones: DHEA, progesterone, testosterone, and cortisol tend to be lower in allergic/autoimmune individuals than in healthy controls. I use either serum testing and/or 24-hour urine samples before prescribing hormones, though I will empirically use progesterone in a woman or a 3-month trial of DHEA in a man with allergies if I find sufficient indications and no contraindications. Treatment is customized per patient. I discuss the hormonal contributions to autoimmunity later in this chapter under the heading of "orthoendocrinology." Much of what applies to "allergy" also applies to "autoimmunity" and visa versa; they are both manifestations of immune dysfunction.[277]

Step 4: Drug treatments: We must acknowledge a place for drug therapy in patients with recalcitrant or severe allergies.
- Prednisone: For patients with allergies that are inconsolable, prednisone becomes a reasonable consideration. The lowest effective dose should be used for the shortest possible period of time. Discontinuation of treatment that has lasted longer than 4 days must be gradual in order to avoid adrenal insufficiency. Topical rather than systemic therapy should be used when appropriate.
- Sodium cromoglycate: Cromoglycate is a mast cell stabilizer which can be applied nasally for allergic rhinitis (Nasalcrom) or taken orally (Gastrocrom) by patients with food allergy to inhibit the local response to type-1 allergies.[278] The drug is poorly absorbed; therefore its anti-allergy effect is mediated at the gastrointestinal mucosa even though the benefits are systemic. Although not officially "approved" in the US for the treatment of food allergy, numerous studies support its use for this purpose.[279] Cromoglycate has been shown to reduce allergy-induced migraine[280] and eczema[281] and prevent the formation of immune complexes following the consumption of allergenic foods. In

---

[271] Vernia P, Monteleone G, Grandinetti G, Villotti G, Di Giulio E, Frieri G, Marcheggiano A, Pallone F, Caprilli R, Torsoli A. Combined oral sodium butyrate and mesalazine treatment compared to oral mesalazine alone in ulcerative colitis: randomized, double-blind, placebo-controlled pilot study. *Dig Dis Sci.* 2000 May;45:976-81

[272] Vernia P, Annese V, Bresci G, d'Albasio G, D'Inca R, Giaccari S, Ingrosso M, Mansi C, Riegler G, Valpiani D, Caprilli R; Gruppo Italiano per lo Studio del Colon and del Retto. Topical butyrate improves efficacy of 5-ASA in refractory distal ulcerative colitis: results of a multicentre trial. *Eur J Clin Invest.* 2003 Mar;33(3):244-8

[273] Neesby TE. Method for desensitizing the gastrointestinal tract from food allergies. United States Patent 4,721,716. January 26, 1988

[274] Neesby TE. Method for desensitizing the gastrointestinal tract from food allergies. United States Patent 4,735,967. April 5, 1988

[275] Morrison LM, Enrick N. Coronary heart disease: reduction of death rate by chondroitin sulfate A. *Angiology.* 1973 May;24(5):269-87

[276] Theoharides TC, Bielory L. Mast cells and mast cell mediators as targets of dietary supplements. *Ann Allergy Asthma Immunol.* 2004 Aug;93(2 Suppl 1):S24-34

[277] Vasquez A. In *Textbook of Functional Medicine.*

[278] http://www.drugs.com/MMX/Cromolyn_Sodium.html Accessed November 24, 2005

[279] "Both the clinician's and patient's preferences and the clinician's evaluation of the specific response to challenge showed a significant benefit from SCG." Dannaeus A, Foucard T, Johansson SG. The effect of orally administered sodium cromoglycate on symptoms of food allergy. *Clin Allergy.* 1977 Mar;7(2):109-15

[280] "Immune complexes were not produced in those patients who were protected by sodium cromoglycate. These observations confirm that a food-allergic reaction is the cause of migraine in this group of patients." Monro J, Carini C, Brostoff J. Migraine is a food-allergic disease. *Lancet.* 1984 Sep 29;2(8405):719-21

[281] "The same atopic patients pretreated with oral sodium cromoglycate had less antigen entry, diminished immune-complex formation, and no atopic symptoms." Paganelli R, Levinsky RJ, Brostoff J, Wraith DG. Immune complexes containing food proteins in normal and atopic subjects after oral challenge and effect of sodium cromoglycate on antigen absorption. *Lancet.* 1979 Jun 16;1(8129):1270-2

addition to preventing the allergic phenomena related directly to the consumption of allergenic foods, an additional mechanism of action of sodium cromoglycate is probably that it reduces the allergy-induced increase in intestinal permeability[282] and thereby prohibits absorption of bacterial and other microbial antigens and metabolites; stated differently, some of the manifestations attributed to "food allergy" are probably not mediated by the response to food allergens directly but result from the adverse immunologic and metabolic responses toward gut-derived microbial antigens and metabolites which are absorbed in increased amounts following the consumption of allergenic foods which increase intestinal permeability and absorption of "foreign" and "toxic" intraluminal contents which would have otherwise been excluded. Common doses for children are 100 mg 30 minutes before food (up to 400 mg per day) and 100-200 mg qid for adults 30 minutes before meals. Capsules or ampules should be mixed in plain water before consumption.

- Leukotriene antagonists: Montelukast (Singulair®, Merck) is an orally active leukotriene receptor antagonist that blocks leukotriene D4 from the cysteinyl leukotriene CysLT-1 receptor and thereby reduces vasodilation, eosinophilic inflammation, and vascular hyperpermeability. Montelukast is used in the medical treatment of asthma, rhinitis, and eczema.

Objective means for the identification of allergens: skin-prick testing, serum IgE and IgG assays, double-blind placebo-controlled food challenges, and the elimination and challenge technique

- Skin prick testing: IgE-dependent immediate-onset allergies as assessed with a skin-prick test are indicative of immediate-onset allergy to the particular allergen, and provide the identity of the allergen, quantification of the severity of the allergic response, *and evidence of underlying immune dysfunction*. Skin-prick testing does not assess for delayed-onset allergies, thus leaving at least one class of adverse food reactions literally unassessed.

- Allergen-specific serum levels of IgE and IgG: Elevated serum levels of IgE and IgG, which are identified as specific for certain foods, also provide the identity of the allergen *and evidence of underlying immune dysfunction*. These "objective" tools are part of the clinician's repertoire for identifying food allergens, while keeping in mind that both skin-prick testing and serum testing are prone to both false positives and false negatives. Serum IgE testing does not assess IgG-mediated allergies, nor does it assess for sensitivity (immune but not immunoglobulin-mediated responses) or intolerance, which tends to be biochemical rather than immunologic. IgG assays and the subclasses of IgG-4 assays have not gained acceptance for their sensitivity or specificity, even though clinicians order them and patients pay for them.

- Double-blind placebo-controlled food challenge: Another commonly mentioned objective means for identifying food allergens is the "double-blind placebo-controlled food challenge" (DBPCFC) wherein food is administered a double-blind fashion with placebo control generally via either capsules or nasogastric tube. Unfortunately, DBPCFC is commonly considered the gold standard for the identification of particular allergens and the establishment of an allergic diathesis. This is unfortunate because the hospital admission and associated costs are expensive, cumbersome and therefore inaccessible for most patients. Some patients will have a false-negative response when challenged with isolated foods because of the lack of "accessory antigens", "accomplice antigens", or "bystander antigens."[283] Some patients will have adverse food reactions only when foods are eaten either with *high frequency* or in *specific combinations* or when *gastrointestinal problems* (e.g., dysbiosis or increased intestinal permeability) are present at the same time as the food challenge. For example, while the patient may tolerate eggs alone and wheat alone without the manifestation of allergic symptoms, the additive insult of the combination of both eggs and wheat may cause sufficient intestinal damage and/or immune activation that clinical manifestations become apparent. With single food challenges

---

[282] "It is suggested that a local IgE-mediated mechanism acts as a "trigger" for the entry of antigen and the formation of immune complexes by altering the permeability of the gut mucosa. The resulting delayed onset symptoms could be viewed as a form of serum sickness with few or many target organs affected." Carini C, Brostoff J, Wraith DG. IgE complexes in food allergy. *Ann Allergy*. 1987 Aug;59(2):110-7

[283] "The mechanisms of enhanced permeability to specific and bystander antigens have been delineated as well as the molecular events involved in the sequential phases of allergic reactions." Heyman M. Gut barrier dysfunction in food allergy. *Eur J Gastroenterol Hepatol*. 2005 Dec;17(12):1279-1285

given with **DBPCFC**, "real life" situations are not reproduced, and false negative results may erroneously suggest that either the patient has no allergies or that a particular food is not offensive.

- Elimination and challenge: The "**elimination and challenge**" technique (more accurately described as "avoidance and challenge") requires that the patient first clear the diet of all possible offending foods, either by **fasting** or by **consuming a simple diet of unlikely-to-be-allergenic foods**, such as the classic triad of rice, lamb, and pears or a relatively hypoallergenic hydrolyzed formula such as Vivonex. After 7-14 days of elimination (i.e., avoidance) *and the clearing of symptoms thought to be allergy-mediated*, an offending food is reintroduced by intense consumption (i.e., eaten with every meal) for a period of up to two days. Every two to four days, a new food is added back into the diet, and a correlation is searched for between consumption of a given food and the exacerbation of symptoms. If the symptoms do not abate or disappear with the fasting/elimination phase, then confirming the nature of the disorder as allergic is more difficult and determining the identity of the allergen is additionally unlikely. However, in some cases, clinical signs and symptoms that are indeed allergy-mediated will fail to regress significantly during the brief washout period. This is because the underlying tissue damage is too great to be healed in such a short time. A good example is the thyroid disease induced by gluten-containing grains in people with the severe gluten allergy called celiac disease; simply avoiding gluten for 1-2 weeks does not restore endocrine function because the body needs more time to reacquire homeostasis and to heal injured tissues. A common scenario is one in which symptoms remit during fasting/elimination and then return *gradually* rather than *immediately* when the offending food is eaten. In these situations, the most likely explanations are either 1) a threshold of time was necessary for physiologic abnormalities (e.g., immune complex deposition, increased intestinal permeability, dysbiosis, accumulative immune stimulation) to culminate in the reproduction of symptoms, or 2) synergistic factors may have to be combined in order to produce the symptoms of allergy, such as the induction of IgE-mediated increased intestinal permeability by food R which then leads to the increased absorption of food S, to which the peripheral immune system then responds with an IgG-mediated reaction with resultant clinical manifestations. In the latter case, food R or food S *when eaten alone or on a rotation basis* may be insufficient to produce allergic manifestations, but the combination of R+S, which would not be identified with skin-prick testing, serum tests, or one-at-a-time DBPCFC, may produce allergic manifestations. Since, in real life, foods are eaten in combination when they cause allergic disease (e.g. a headache or joint pain after eating a hamburger with wheat/gluten, cheese/milk, mayonnaise/egg, and pickle/tartrazine/yeast), a reasonable conclusion is that foods will have to be avoided in specific combinations to attain maximal improvement in allergic symptoms since complex foods probably work synergistically to produce allergic manifestations in affected people. Creating chronological distance between the consumption of allergenic foods explains the success of the **rotation diets** in alleviating allergic manifestations, but it does little to address the underlying immune dysfunction other than to reduce the total allergenic load to which the immune system is exposed. **Intestinal dysbiosis** can also increase intestinal permeability and result in increased absorption of food antigens and depletion of detoxification co-factors, which can mimic or perpetuate immune-mediated food allergies. Correction of this problem can begin to normalize immune function and eliminate symptoms attributed to the consumption of specific foods.

Objective Assessments for Adverse Food Reactions—A Quick Clinical Guide

	Advantages	Disadvantages
Skin-prick testing	<ul><li>Proves presence of allergic diathesis.</li><li>Identifies allergen that is being responded to by IgE-mediated reaction.</li><li>Can be used for both food and inhalant allergies.</li></ul>	<ul><li>Numerically impossible to test for all probable allergens due to method of testing, which can be quite painful</li><li>Allergen preparations may not contain full spectrum of immunogenic epitopes that are present in "real food" thus patient may not respond to offensive food, resulting in clinically relevant false negative results.</li><li>Subcutaneous injection is not the natural or physiologic route of allergen exposure.</li><li>Does not assess for IgG or other delayed-onset allergies, thus resulting in clinically relevant false negative results.</li><li>Does not assess for reactions that are mediated by immune complexes, thus resulting in clinically relevant false negative results.</li><li>Procedure is moderately expensive.</li><li>Does not assess for intolerances or biochemical perturbations, thus resulting in clinically relevant false negative results.</li></ul>
Serum IgE assay	<ul><li>Identifies allergen that is being responded to by IgE-mediated reaction.</li><li>Can be used for both food and inhalant allergies.</li><li>Procedure is relatively painless and provides "objective evidence" of food allergies.</li></ul>	<ul><li>Numerically impossible to test for all probable allergens due to method of testing.</li><li>Allergen preparations may not contain full spectrum of immunogenic epitopes that are present in "real food" thus patient may not respond to offensive food, resulting in clinically relevant false negative results.</li><li>Does not assess for IgG or other delayed-onset allergies, thus resulting in clinically relevant false negative results.</li><li>Does not assess for reactions that are mediated by IgG, IgM, or IgA immune complexes, thus resulting in clinically relevant false-negative results.</li><li>Does not assess for intolerances or biochemical perturbations, thus resulting in clinically relevant false negative results.</li></ul>
Serum IgG4 assay	<ul><li>Identifies allergen that is being responded to by IgG-mediated reaction.</li><li>Mostly used in an attempt to identify delayed-onset food allergies.</li><li>Procedure is relatively painless.</li><li>Procedure provides "objective evidence" of food allergies.</li></ul>	<ul><li>Numerically impossible to test for all probable allergens due to method of testing.</li><li>Allergen preparations may not contain full spectrum of immunogenic epitopes that are present in "real food" thus patient may not respond to offensive food, resulting in clinically relevant false negative results.</li><li>Does not assess for IgE or other immediate-onset allergies, thus resulting in clinically relevant false negative results.</li><li>Does not assess for reactions that are mediated by immune complexes, thus resulting in clinically relevant false negative results.</li><li>Procedure is moderately expensive.</li><li>Does not assess for intolerances or biochemical perturbations, thus resulting in clinically relevant false negative results.</li><li>The clinical relevance of IgG4 antibodies to food is controversial.[284]</li></ul>

---

[284] "...it seems unlikely that increased IgG4 antibody levels against egg white is a cause of egg hypersensitivity, and one should pay much attention to IgG1 antibodies ...it is possible that increased IgG4 may reduce the effect of complement-fixing antibodies like IgG1 and/or interfere the action of IgE antibodies." Nakagawa T. Egg white-specific IgE and IgG subclass antibodies and their associations with clinical egg hypersensitivity. *N Engl Reg Allergy Proc.* 1988 Jan-Feb;9(1):67-73

Objective Assessments for Adverse Food Reactions—A Quick Clinical Guide *continued*

	Advantages	Disadvantages
Double-blind placebo-controlled food challenges	<ul><li>Allows for control of interfering factors.</li><li>Removes psychological cues and triggers that can be mistakenly interpreted as adverse food reactions.</li><li>Procedure provides "objective evidence" of food allergies.</li></ul>	<ul><li>Setting and experiment are artificial and not representative of the real environment in which the patient lives and is exposed to allergen(s).</li><li>Testing of single antigens alone is not reflective of real life wherein antigens are consumed in combination.</li><li>Numerically impossible to test for all probable allergens due to method of testing.</li><li>Allergen preparations may not contain full spectrum of immunogenic epitopes that are present in "real food" thus patient may not respond to offensive food, resulting in clinically relevant false negative results.</li><li>Procedure is time-consuming and cumbersome and requires the preparation of both food challenge and placebo, which are administered either by capsules or by nasogastric tube.</li><li>Due to small quantity of allergen and limited time of observation, does not assess for reactions that are quantity-dependent, delayed-onset, or mediated by immune complexes, thus resulting in clinically relevant false negative results.</li><li>Procedure is moderately expensive.</li><li>Does not assess for intolerances or biochemical perturbations, thus resulting in clinically relevant false negative results.</li></ul>
Elimination and challenge	<ul><li>Represents "real life" situations with psychological influences, daily stress, and combinations of foods.</li><li>No financial cost.</li><li>Easy to implement for motivated patients.</li><li>Trains patients to be active in their healthcare and to learn how to diagnose and treat themselves—the true goals of wellness promotion.</li></ul>	<ul><li>Compliance is a challenge for unmotivated or undisciplined patients.</li><li>Identification of offending allergen may take time and repeated cycles of elimination and challenge before the allergen is conclusively identified.</li></ul>

❷ Infections:
Dysbiosis and Persistent Microbial Colonization

Major Concepts in this Section
This section reviews in detail the mechanisms by which dysbiosis—also described as multifocal polydysbiosis, subclinical infections, microbial colonizations—contributes to immune dysfunction that results in systemic inflammation generally and rheumatic diseases specifically. Understanding this section and taking appropriate clinical action is of the highest importance in the successful treatment of inflammatory/rheumatic disorders. Readers of this section must attain 1) an appreciation of the mechanisms by which microbes and their molecular effects contribute to pro-inflammatory immune dysfunction, and 2) an appreciation that exclusive therapeutic focus on the eradication of microbe is fraught with inefficacy if it fails to address the intrinsic patient-specific imbalances that allowed that individual patient to be susceptible to microbe-induced inflammation and immune imbalance. "Dysbiosis" is not simply about the effects of microbes in inflammatory disease, the detection and eradication of those microbes. Although this section focuses on microbes and their effects, detection, and treatment, the complete treatment of dysbiosis needs to contain three major components: ❶ microbe-specific treatment, ❷ restoration of immune function and other means by which to make the human host less hospitable to re-colonization, ❸ promotion of immune and inflammatory tolerance.

Multifocal Dysbiosis: A Major Promoter of Chronic Inflammation and "Autoimmunity"

Microbes contribute to noninfectious human diseases—including chronic inflammation and autoimmunity—by mechanisms which are *numerous, complex, direct* and *indirect*. For the purposes of this discussion, I will use a broad definition of dysbiosis that implies "a relationship of non-acute host-microorganism interaction that adversely affects the human host"; the subtype of dysbiosis can be distinguished based on location: gastrointestinal, orodental, sinorespiratory, genitourinary, dermal, or environmental. Patients may have more than one dysbiotic loci at a time with microbes from more than one kingdom. One of the best clinical examples of autoimmunity/inflammation perpetuated by multifocal dysbiosis is Behcet's syndrome, characterized by subclinical pulmonary infection (sinorespiratory dysbiosis) with *Chlamydia pneumonia*[285], cutaneous colonization (dermal dysbiosis) with *Staphylococcus aureus*[286], and orodental dysbiosis with *Streptococcus sanguis*.[287] Combine with multifocal dysbiosis a few pro-rheumatic genetic traits (especially HLA-B27) and subclinical proinflammatory nutritional imbalances[288], and it becomes easy to see why rheumatic diseases are generally still considered "idiopathic" when reviewed from a reductionistic medical paradigm that fails to appreciate the interconnected and "holistic" web of influences that synergize to produce systemic inflammation. For the majority of patients in outpatient clinical practice, the location of their dysbiosis is the gut, which is easily assessed with specialized stool testing and parasitology examinations, and which is easily treated with oral botanical antimicrobials and dietary modification. In my own clinical practice, I consider stool testing extremely valuable and estimate that 80% of parasitology examinations return with at least one clinically-relevant abnormality. **Testing for and treating dysbiosis is absolutely essential in patients with chronic fatigue, fibromyalgia, autoimmunity, and any type of "inflammatory arthritis."**[289,290]

---

[285] "These finding provide serological evidence of chronic C. pneumoniae infection in association with Behcet's disease." Ayaslioglu E, Duzgun N, Erkek E, Inal A. Evidence of chronic Chlamydia pneumoniae infection in patients with Behcet's disease. *Scand J Infect Dis*. 2004;36(6-7):428-30

[286] "Staphylococcus aureus (41/70, 58.6%, p = 0.008) and Prevotella spp (17/70, 24.3%, p = 0.002) were significantly more common in pustules from BS patients..." Hatemi G, Bahar H, Uysal S, Mat C, Gogus F, Masatlioglu S, Altas K, Yazici H. The pustular skin lesions in Behcet's syndrome are not sterile. *Ann Rheum Dis*. 2004 Nov;63(11):1450-2

[287] "These data indicate that the BD patients are infected with IgA protease-producing S. sanguis strains, which cause an increase of IgA titer against these organisms and IgA protease antigen." Yokota K, Oguma K. IgA protease produced by Streptococcus sanguis and antibody production against IgA protease in patients with Behcet's disease. *Microbiol Immunol*. 1997;41(12):925-31

[288] Seaman DR. The diet-induced proinflammatory state: a cause of chronic pain and other degenerative diseases? *J Manipulative Physiol Ther*. 2002 Mar-Apr;25:168-79

[289] Vasquez A. Reducing Pain and Inflammation Naturally. Part 6: Nutritional and Botanical Treatments Against "Silent Infections" and Gastrointestinal Dysbiosis, Commonly Overlooked Causes of Neuromusculoskeletal Inflammation and Chronic Health Problems. Nutritional Perspectives 2006; January

[290] Vasquez A. Multifocal Dysbiosis: Pathophysiology, Relevance for Inflammatory and Autoimmune Diseases, and Treatment with Nutritional and Botanical Interventions. *Naturopathy Digest* 2006 June http://www.naturopathydigest.com/archives/2006/jun/vasquez.php

Readers should appreciate that the "total dysbiotic load" (TDL) or "total microbial load" (TML) from all sources—skin, gastrointestinal tract, genitourinary tract, sinorespiratory tract, orodental cavity, environment, and any subclinical parenchymal/tissue foci—contributes to the total inflammatory load (TIL) and total xenobiotic load (TXL) which the immune system must process and which the hepatobiliary system must detoxify, respectively.

At least 70% of patients with chronic arthritis are carriers of "silent infections", according to a 1992 article published in the peer-reviewed medical journal *Annals of the Rheumatic Diseases*.[291] A 2001 article in this same journal which focused exclusively on five bacteria showed that **56% of patients with idiopathic inflammatory arthritis had gastrointestinal or genitourinary dysbiosis**.[292] Indeed, published research strongly and consistently indicates that bacteria, yeast/fungi, amebas, protozoa, and other "parasites" (rarely including helminths/worms) are underappreciated causes of neuromusculoskeletal inflammation. This section will explain the mechanisms by which **silent infections**, **noninfectious microbial colonization**, and **dysbiosis** can cause and perpetuate numerous health problems, and I will also discuss basic assessment and treatment measures that can be used clinically to help patients with microbe-induced musculoskeletal inflammation.

A problem that plagues many healthcare providers of all professions is that most doctors are still under the spell of the "Pasteurian paradigm of infectious disease", namely that pathogenic microorganisms cause *disease* by causing "*infection*." Relatedly, Koch's Postulates first published in 1884 held that "the organism must be found in all animals suffering from the disease, but not in healthy animals" and "the cultured organism should cause disease when introduced into a healthy animal."[293] Such contributions by Pasteur, Koch, and other researchers were essential in providing a preliminary understanding of the role of microorganisms in the genesis of human disease; however, we must appreciate that these simplistic, linear, and rather primitive models do not suffice for explaining all microbe-induced disorders. The major problems with the paradigms proposed by Pasteur and Koch are that both of these models fail to appreciate 1) adverse microbe-host

> **Dysbiosis definitions and descriptions**
>
> **Dysbiosis**: A relationship of non-acute non-infectious host-microorganism interaction that adversely affects the human host.
>
> **Dysbiosis subtypes** (based on location):
> 1. Orodental
> 2. Sinorespiratory
> 3. Gastrointestinal
> 4. Parenchymal, tissue
> 5. Genitourinary
> 6. Cutaneous
> 7. Environmental
>
> **Multifocal dysbiosis**: A clinical condition characterized by a patient's having more than one foci/location of dysbiosis; generally the adverse physiologic and clinical consequences are additive and synergistic.

interactions which may not *result in* nor *result from* a true "infection" (thus refuting the Pasteurian paradigm), and 2) the importance of the patient's biochemical individuality and genetic uniqueness which influence the clinical manifestations of dysbiosis-induced disease such that a) not all patients exposed to a pathogenic microbe will express the stereotypic disease, and b) some patients exposed to microorganisms that are generally considered benign commensals will produce a dramatic inflammatory response which results in clinical disease (thus refuting Koch's postulates). Supported amply by the research reviewed herein, **healthcare providers have an obligation to move beyond these simplistic "pathogenic" "infection-based" models of microorganism-induced disease to apprehend the more common "functional" disorders that can result from exposure to microbes.** Readers will note that these new concepts and ideas are amply supported by the references to the biomedical research that are included in the footnotes.[294,295]

---

[291] "At the time of initial evaluation, 57 (69%) of the patients with oligoarthritis and 4/20 (20%) of the control subjects were carriers of clinically silent infections." Weyand CM, Goronzy JJ. Clinically silent infections in patients with oligoarthritis: results of a prospective study. *Ann Rheum Dis*. 1992 Feb;51(2):253-8

[292] Fendler C, Laitko S, Sorensen H, Gripenberg-Lerche C, Groh A, Uksila J, Granfors K, Braun J, Sieper J. Frequency of triggering bacteria in patients with reactive arthritis and undifferentiated oligoarthritis and the relative importance of the tests used for diagnosis. *Ann Rheum Dis*. 2001 Apr;60(4):337-43 http://ard.bmjjournals.com/cgi/content/full/60/4/337

[293] Koch's Postulates. http://encyclopedia.thefreedictionary.com/Koch%27s+postulates Accessed October 4, 2005

[294] Noah PW. The role of microorganisms in psoriasis. *Semin Dermatol*. 1990 Dec;9(4):269-76

[295] Samarkos M, Vaiopoulos G. The role of infections in the pathogenesis of autoimmune diseases. *Curr Drug Targets Inflamm Allergy*. 2005 Feb;4(1):99-10 http://www.bentham.org/cdtia/sample/cdtia4-1/0016L.pdf

One of the common rhetorical positions espoused by undertrained skeptics is, "If infections caused autoimmunity, then antibiotics would cure autoimmune disease." This rhetoric is biophysiologically illogical for several reasons:

Mechanisms of autoimmunity-induction by microorganisms

"Infectious agents can cause autoimmune disease by different mechanisms, which fall into two categories: *antigen specific* in which pathogen products or elements have a central role e.g. **superantigens** or epitope **(molecular) mimicry**, and *antigen non-specific* in which the pathogen provides the appropriate inflammatory setting for **bystander activation**."

Samarkos, Vaiopoulos. The role of infections in the pathogenesis of autoimmune diseases. *Curr Drug Targets Inflamm Allergy.* 2005 Feb

1. First, autoimmunity may be incited by microbes and then persist in the absence of those same microbes; when a hammer breaks a window, removing the hammer does not repair the window. Autoimmunity—whether induced by xenobiotics or microorganisms—may have a tendency to persist due to the immune sensitization toward autoantigens that have been haptenized, exposed, or otherwise immunogenized, and due to the secondary endocrinologic changes and xenobiotic accumulation that have been induced by the disease process and which perpetuate the dysregulated proinflammatory state. The autoimmune "reactive arthritis" that follows microbial infection responds only partially to early antibiotic treatment[296], thus indicating that microbe-induced musculoskeletal inflammation—once induced—may persist despite [supposedly] effective antimicrobial treatment. **Pro-inflammatory antigens can persist in synovial immunocytes for years following a bacterial infection that results in chronic inflammatory arthritis.**[297] Conversely, the observation that antimicrobial intervention, particularly with more powerful treatments, can significantly reduce (not eliminate) the development of "autoimmune" phenomena in patients following bacterial infection[298] appears to indicate that 1) microorganisms, particularly bacteria, contribute directly to the genesis of specific inflammatory/autoimmune disorders, and that 2) antimicrobial treatment of autoimmune disorders is warranted.

2. Second, all clinicians are aware that no antimicrobial treatment eradicates *all* microbes from *all* surfaces; for example, an orally administered broad-spectrum antibiotic is not appropriate for eradicating a fungal infection located in the sinuses. **Microbial drug resistance is an increasingly large problem in outpatient and hospital-based medicine**[299] where antimicrobial drug therapies are the mainstay treatment of bacterial infections and no consideration is given to effective botanical antimicrobials (reviewed later) and to strengthening host defenses (described throughout this text and particularly in sections on diet and immunonutrition).

3. Third, the administration of antimicrobial therapeutics of a limited scope for a limited time may allow the dysbiosis to return when the antimicrobials are discontinued. The autoimmune condition problem may continue or recur despite even "appropriate" antimicrobial treatment if the duration of antimicrobial treatment is too brief.

4. Fourth, even when the microbe is eradicated, its antigens may persist. **Microbial antigens can persist within the human body for years following clearance of the primary infection.**[300,301,302]

5. Fifth, the microbe-autoimmunity model of autoimmune disease induction does not state that microbes are the *sole cause* of autoimmunity. What I have documented here with an abundance of research is

---

[296] Laasila K, Laasonen L, Leirisalo-Repo M. Antibiotic treatment and long term prognosis of reactive arthritis. *Ann Rheum Dis.* 2003 Jul;62(7):655-8 http://ard.bmjjournals.com/cgi/content/full/62/7/655

[297] "Extensive bacterial cultures of the synovial fluid were negative... We conclude that in patients with reactive arthritis after yersinia infection, microbial antigens can be found in synovial-fluid cells from the affected joints." Granfors K, Jalkanen S, von Essen R, Lahesmaa-Rantala R, Isomaki O, Pekkola-Heino K, Merilahti-Palo R, Saario R, Isomaki H, Toivanen A. Yersinia antigens in synovial-fluid cells from patients with reactive arthritis. *N Engl J Med.* 1989 Jan 26;320(4):216-2

[298] Yli-Kerttula T, Luukkainen R, Yli-Kerttula U, Mottonen T, Hakola M, Korpela M, Sanila M, Uksila J, Toivanen A. Effect of a three month course of ciprofloxacin on the late prognosis of reactive arthritis. *Ann Rheum Dis.* 2003 Sep;62(9):880-4 http://ard.bmjjournals.com/cgi/content/full/62/9/880

[299] Sharma R, Sharma CL, Kapoor B. Antibacterial resistance: Current problems and possible solutions. *Indian J Med Sci* [serial online] 2005 [cited 2005 Dec 27];59:120-129. Available from: http://www.indianjmedsci.org/article.asp?issn=0019-5359;year=2005;volume=59;issue=3;spage=120;epage=129;aulast=Sharma

[300] Inman RD. Antigens, the gastrointestinal tract, and arthritis. *Rheum Dis Clin North Am.* 1991 May;17(2):309-21

[301] "These samples were studied by immunochemical techniques for the presence of Yersinia antigens at the beginning of infection and up to 4 years thereafter... This study has, for the first time, directly demonstrated that bacterial antigens persist for a long time in patients who develop ReA after Y. enterocolitica O:3 infection." Granfors K, Merilahti-Palo R, Luukkainen R, Mottonen T, Lahesmaa R, Probst P, Marker-Hermann E, Toivanen P. Persistence of Yersinia antigens in peripheral blood cells from patients with Yersinia enterocolitica O:3 infection with or without reactive arthritis. *Arthritis Rheum.* 1998 May;41(5):855-62

[302] "Extensive bacterial cultures of the synovial fluid were negative... We conclude that in patients with reactive arthritis after yersinia infection, microbial antigens can be found in synovial-fluid cells from the affected joints." Granfors K, Jalkanen S, von Essen R, Lahesmaa-Rantala R, Isomaki O, Pekkola-Heino K, Merilahti-Palo R, Saario R, Isomaki H, Toivanen A. Yersinia antigens in synovial-fluid cells from patients with reactive arthritis. *N Engl J Med.* 1989 Jan 26;320(4):216-2

that **microbes are a major contributor to autoimmunity** and that **dysbiosis works in concert with hormonal abnormalities, xenobiotic immunotoxicity, food intolerances, and a proinflammatory lifestyle which synergize to create proinflammatory immune dysfunction that happens to destroy body tissues in a phenomenon that gets labeled "autoimmunity."**

Despite the ability of autoimmunity/inflammation to persist despite the eradication of causative microorganisms, clinicians (and patients) will be pleased to learn that effective oligomicrobial eradication can result in dramatic clinical improvements in patients with autoimmunity. This observation is not merely anecdote from practicing clinicians; **published research and relatively large clinical trials are increasingly documenting that comprehensive antimicrobial treatments do indeed** *promote regression* **and** *initiate cure* **in a growing list of previously "untreatable" autoimmune diseases.**

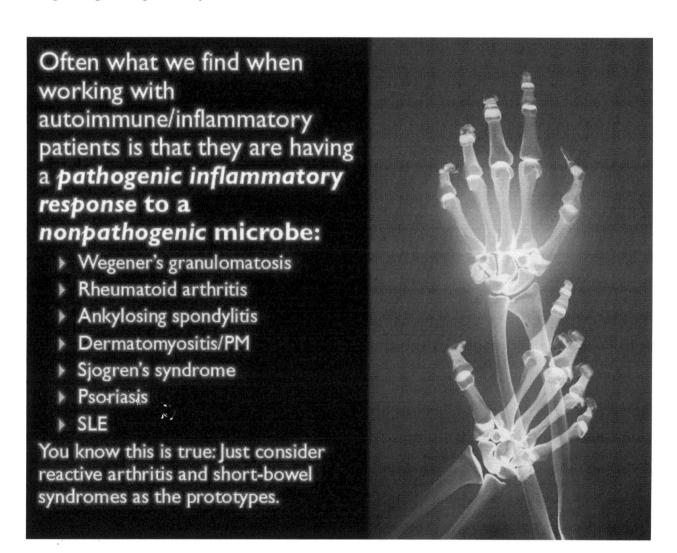

Often what we find when working with autoimmune/inflammatory patients is that they are having a *pathogenic inflammatory response* to a *nonpathogenic microbe*:

▸ Wegener's granulomatosis
▸ Rheumatoid arthritis
▸ Ankylosing spondylitis
▸ Dermatomyositis/PM
▸ Sjogren's syndrome
▸ Psoriasis
▸ SLE

You know this is true: Just consider reactive arthritis and short-bowel syndromes as the prototypes.

Dysbiotic inflammation—beyond the microbe: Often what we find when working with autoimmune/inflammatory patients is that they are having a pathogenic inflammatory response to a nonpathogenic microbe. Remember, we are not looking for classic "infection" here; we are looking to determine which underlying disruptions may be exacerbating inflammation and the patient's symptomatology. We have to look beyond the disease-associated characteristics of the microbe to see the patient's individualized response to the microbe. Dysbiosis in one patient may present with dermatitis, while [what appears to be] the same microbial imbalance in another patient can present as peripheral neuropathy or inflammatory arthritis.

Mechanisms of Autoimmune Disease Induction by Microorganisms

I have identified at least seventeen mechanisms by which microorganisms can cause immune dysfunction that promotes musculoskeletal inflammation. Each of the following exemplifies a mechanism by which microbes can cause "disease" without causing an "infection." Mechanisms by which microorganisms can contribute to musculoskeletal inflammation without causing "infection" include but are not limited to the following:

1. <u>Molecular mimicry</u>: Several microbes have peptides and other structures that resemble or "mimic" the peptides and cell structures found in human tissues. Thus, when the immune system fights against the microbe, the antibodies and T-cells can "cross-react" with the tissues of the human host. In this way, the immune system begins attacking the human body, which is otherwise an innocent bystander—the victim of "friendly fire."[303] As reviewed by Ringrose[304], evidence clearly indicates that specific microbial proteins have amino acid homology with human proteins and/or that homologous bacterial peptides appear to stimulate (auto)immunity toward similar neighboring human peptides. Therefore the two underlying bases for autoimmune induction by molecular mimicry—namely 1) homology between human and microbial amino acid sequences, and 2) stimulation of immunity against human peptides—do indeed occur *in vivo*. **Molecular mimicry is strongly implicated in the pathogenesis of reactive arthritis and ankylosing spondylitis.**[305,306]

   - <u>Psoriasis and molecular mimicry—Ex vivo experimental study using human T-cells (*Clin Exp Immunol* 1999 Sep[307])</u>: The authors of this paper introduce their topic by noting that psoriasis is an inflammatory disease mediated largely by T-cells in the skin and that psoriasis has a strong association with infections by group-A beta-hemolytic streptococci bacteria, also known as *Streptococcus pyogenes*. The authors cite their previous work which showed that patients with active psoriasis have Th1-like cells that respond to a 20 amino acid (AA) sequence shared between a protein made by streptococcal bacteria (M protein) that has the same AA sequence as the human protein found in the skin named keratin, specifically kerakin 17. ("Keratin" is a group of fibrous structural proteins forming the key structural material of the outer layer of human skin; keratin is also the key structural component of hair and nails. Keratin 17 is not expressed in normal skin except for hair follicles, sweat/sebaceous glands, and basal cells in the scalp; however, keratin 17 is expressed in suprabasal keratinocytes in lesional psoriatic skin, thus making its presence in skin a unique feature of psoriasis lesions. Increased production of keratin 17 can be induced by the pro-inflammatory cytokines gamma-interferon, which plays a key role as a mediator of psoriatic inflammation, and IL-6, which is abundant in psoriatic lesions. Langerhans cells are the dentritic cells of the epidermis; as such, they function as antigen-presenting cells (APC). Given that keratin within skin cells exists as an intracellular structural (cytoskeletal) protein, its ability to be exposed to the immune system is required for it to function as an autoantigen, a target of self-induced immunologic attack. The authors of this paper note that "cytoplasmic processes of Langerhans cells can extend into the cytoplasm of adjacent keratinocytes with frequent absence of intervening plasma membranes at the apices of these processes"; thus these epidermal APCs can uptake and present antigen via MHC class 1 and class 2 molecules to CD8 and CD4 T-cells, respectively.)

Molecular mimicry in psoriatic skin and bacterial proteins
These amino acid sequences are found in human keratin and M-protein from the bacteria *Streptococcus pyogenes*.
1.   ALEEAN,
2.   LRR-LD,
3.   AKLEA,
4.   AKLEAE.
Gudmundsdottir et al. Is an epitope on keratin 17 a major target for autoreactive T lymphocytes in psoriasis? *Clin Exp Immunol.* 1999 Sep

---

[303] Wucherpfennig KW. Mechanisms for the induction of autoimmunity by infectious agents. *J Clin Invest.* 2001 Oct;108(8):1097-104 http://www.jci.org/cgi/reprint/108/8/1097

[304] Ringrose JH. HLA-B27 associated spondyloarthropathy, an autoimmune disease based on crossreactivity between bacteria and HLA-B27? *Ann Rheum Dis.* 1999 Oct;58(10):598-610 http://ard.bmjjournals.com/cgi/content/full/58/10/598

[305] "HLA-B27 and proteins from enteric bacteria are structurally related, in a manner that may affect T cell response to enteric pathogens." Inman RD, Scofield RH. Etiopathogenesis of ankylosing spondylitis and reactive arthritis. *Curr Opin Rheumatol.* 1994 Jul;6(4):360-70

[306] "With respect to bacterial infection, recent findings in bacterial antigenicity, host response through interactions of antigen-presenting cells, T cells, and cytokines are providing new understanding of host-pathogen interactions and the pathogenesis of arthritis." Kim TH, Uhm WS, Inman RD. Pathogenesis of ankylosing spondylitis and reactive arthritis. *Curr Opin Rheumatol.* 2005 Jul;17(4):400-5

[307] Gudmundsdottir AS, Sigmundsdottir H, Sigurgeirsson B, Good MF, Valdimarsson H, Jonsdottir I. Is an epitope on keratin 17 a major target for autoreactive T lymphocytes in psoriasis? *Clin Exp Immunol.* 1999 Sep;117(3):580-6

These same Th1-like cells are deleted following treatment with ultraviolet B (UVB) radiation that induces clinical remission; the fact that the disappeaerance of these cells correlates with clinical improvement following treatment implies that these cells may have a direct causative role in the skin inflammation of psoriasis. In the ex vivo experiment, the authors took T-cells from the blood of 17 psoriatic patients and 17 healthy controls and then challenged these T-cells with keratin peptides and M-peptides to monitor for increased production of gamma-interferon [IFNg]), which implies specificity for the corresponding amino acid sequences. Results of the investigation showed that the most frequent and strongest responses were observed to a peptide from keratin 17 that shares a specific AA sequence with M-protein. Specifically, the overlapping AA sequence is A-L-E-E-A-N. In fact, T-cell responses to the ALEEAN sequence were stronger than to the corresponding M-peptide containing the ALEEAN sequence; this implies that sensitized T-cells preferentially attack keratin rather than the bacterial peptide. The ALEEAN sequence present in keratin 17 is also found in keratin subtype 14, which is overexpressed in psoriatic skin; thus, for T-cells already primed to respond to ALEEAN following exposure to *Streptococcus pyogenes*, the dual exposure to ALEEAN in keratins 14 and 17—both of which are uniquely present in psoriatic skin—may promote localized attack by T-cells against keratinocytes, ie, immune cross-reactivity via molecular mimicry. UVB treatment abolished T-cell responses to keratin and M protein, while responses to other bacterial antigens (streptokinase [SK] and streptodornase [SD]) were not affected. The authors conclude, "These findings are consistent with the notion that AA sequences which keratin has in common with M-protein may be a major target for autoreactive T cells in psoriasis." Per Table 2 of their article, 13 of 17 psoriatic patients demonstrated a T-cell response to peptide 146-K17 (from human keratins subtypes 14 and 17) contrasted to only 4 of 17 healthy controls; interestingly, three patients and eight controls showed no responses to either keratin or M protein. This lack of perfect concordance indicates that molecular mimickry and the resulting immune cross-reaction does not account for the entirety of the pathogenesis of psoriasis, or that ❶ the research methods employed in the study were imperfect resulting in a few false negatives and/or false positives, or ❷ seasonal variation in streptococcal infections caused varying intensities of immune responsiveness, ❸ seasonal vitamin D fluctuations caused varying intensities of immune responsiveness, ❹ that a variable unaccounted for (eg, sun exposure, medication use, etc) influenced these results, or that ❺ other nonstreptococal infections/microbes—as very well documented by Noah and collecgues[308]—and dysbiotic microbial relationships may have been causative in some cases of psoriasis. Readers and clinicians should note that the ALEEAN sequence is not the only sequence shared between human keratin and staphylococcal M-protein; other homologous sequences include LRR-LD, AKLEA, and AKLEAE.

Peptide identification and source	*Peptide amino acid (AA) sequence*
Peptide 146-M from *Streptococcus pyogenes*	**AKKQVEKALEEANSKLAALE**
Peptide 146-M49 from *Streptococcus pyogenes*	AKKKVEADLAEANSKLQALE
Peptide 146-K17* from human keratin subtypes 14 and 17	**SYLDKVRALEEANADLEVK**
Peptide 146-K9 from human keratin	SYLDKVQALEEANNDLENKI

Data from Figure 1 and Table 1 of Gudmundsdottir et al. *Clin Exp Immunol*. 1999 Sep;117(3):580-6
* Based on the frequency of IFN-g-producing T-cells of patients and controls after stimulation with M- and keratin peptides sharing the ALEEAN sequence, peptide 146-K17 is the only peptide which elicited significantly stronger responses in psoriatic patients than in healthy controls

---

308 Rosenberg EW, Noah PW, Skinner RB Jr. Microorganisms and psoriasis. *J Natl Med Assoc*. 1994 Apr;86(4):305-10

- Psoriasis and molecular mimicry—Psoriasis is an autoimmune disease caused in whole or in part by molecular mimicry. (*Trends Immunol* 2009 Oct[309]): The authors of this paper note that T cells in psoriatic lesions are oligoclonal and that these T-cells recognize amino acid sequences (determinants) common to streptococcal M-protein and human skin keratin; they propose that CD8(+) T cells in psoriatic epidermis respond mainly to such determinants. Further, they note that streptococcal peptidoglycan may act as an adjuvant for this immune response and that, likewise, a streptococcal superantigen may promote an inflammatory/cytokine mileau that advances skin-homing of tonsillar T cells. They conclude their abstract/summary by stating that if the above bases are correct, then "tonsillectomy should be associated with fewer T cells that recognize keratin and streptococcal determinants." These conclusions are conceptually consistent with previously published literature, in particular the work of Noah and colleagues[310], which has also emphasized the microbial link to psoriasis and has noted the documented benefit of tonsillectomy. I included citation to this article for the additional reason that it is one of the first articles to boldly state *in its title* that molecular mimicry is a defining pathoetiologic aspect of psoriasis, thus emphasizing the role of this mechanism in the condition previously acquiesced by the medical profession to the realms of esotericity and idiopathicity in order to justifty perpetual pharmaceuticalization of these patients.[311]

2. Superantigens: Many viral, bacterial, and fungal microbes produce superantigens—molecules which are capable of causing widespread, nonspecific, and unregulated proinflammatory immune activation. One of the hallmarks of superantigens is their ability to induce polyclonal T- and B-lymphocyte activation and the production of excessive levels of cytokines and other inflammatory effectors.[312] Solanki et al[313] described superantigens as "microbial or viral toxins" which behave as "immunostimulatory molecules" and "extremely potent polyclonal T-cell mitogens" which "bind major histocompatibility complex (MHC) class-II molecules without any prior processing and stimulate large number of T cells (up to 20% of all T cells)" due to "their **unique ability to cross-link MHC class II [found on antigen-presenting cells] and the T-cell receptor (TCR),** forming a trimolecular complex."; these authors concisely note that superantigens "activate antigen-presenting dendritic cells by producing increased expression of HLA-DR antigen and co-stimulatory molecules (CD54, CD83 and CD86) and the production of tumor necrosis factor TNF-alpha [as well as TNF-beta, IL-2, and gamma-interferon]." Obviously, when the body is in such a state of unregulated hyper-inflammation, inevitably some of this inflammation will affect the structures of the musculoskeletal system, especially since articular tissues are predisposed to immune attack, if for no other reasons than their proclivity to retain antigens and immune complexes[314,315] to which an exaggerated inflammatory response is promoted by superantigen stimulation. Several research groups have found evidence of superantigen involvement in the pathogenesis of rheumatoid

> **Important concepts about superantigens**
>
> Bacteria and other microorganisms (microbes) can each produce several—not just one—superantigens. The implications are that 1) one single microbe can promote inflammation and immune dysfunction via elaboration of several different superantigens, and that 2) researchers have to test for several superantigens per microbe per patient per disease in order to fully appreciate the role of a microbe's superantigen repertoire in association with a particular disease. Further adding to the complexity of these associations is the fact that other molecules—beside and beyond the classic/known/prototypic superantigens—can also contribute to pro-inflammatory immune dysfunction; bacterial DNA is known to be immunostimulatory.

---

[309] Valdimarsson H, Thorleifsdottir RH, Sigurdardottir SL, Gudjonsson JE, Johnston A. Psoriasis--as an autoimmune disease caused by molecular mimicry. *Trends Immunol*. 2009 Oct;30(10):494-501

[310] Rosenberg EW, Noah PW, Skinner RB Jr. Microorganisms and psoriasis. *J Natl Med Assoc*. 1994 Apr;86(4):305-10

[311] Vasquez A. Twilight of the Idiopathic Era and the Dawn of New Possibilities in Health and Healthcare. *Naturopathy Digest* 2006 Mar

[312] "The basis of autoimmune disorders due to superantigen is due to greater stimulation of T-lymphocytes and elaborate cytokine production." Hemalatha V, Srikanth P, Mallika M. Superantigens - Concepts, clinical disease and therapy. *Indian J Med Microbiol* 2004;22:204-211

[313] Solanki LS, Srivastava N, Singh S. Superantigens: a brief review with special emphasis on dermatologic diseases. *Dermatology Online Journal* 2008 Feb 28;14(2):3 http://dermatology.cdlib.org/142/reviews/superantigens/singh.html

[314] Inman RD. Antigens, the gastrointestinal tract, and arthritis. *Rheum Dis Clin North Am*. 1991 May;17(2):309-21

[315] "Other factors, like the specific properties of synovial vessels and the adhesion molecules responsible for synovium-specific homing, will contribute to the guiding of the monocytes from the mucosal areas into the joints." Wuorela M, Tohka S, Granfors K, Jalkanen S. Monocytes that have ingested Yersinia enterocolitica serotype O:3 acquire enhanced capacity to bind to nonstimulated vascular endothelial cells via P-selectin. *Infect Immun*. 1999 Feb;67(2):726-32 iai.asm.org/cgi/content/full/67/2/726

arthritis.[316,317] Superantigens can be categorized as ❶ **endogenous superantigens**—these are encoded by viruses such as Epstein-Barr virus, ❷ **exogenous superantigens**—these are elaborated by bacteria and include staphylococcal enterotoxins and streptococcal pyrogenic exotoxins, and ❸ **B-cell superantigens**—these predominantly stimulate B-cells to produce antibodies/immunoglobulins; an example of a B-cell superantigen is staphylococcal proteins A and Fv. Very noteworthy is the fact that superantigens, which are directly immunologically active at very low concentrations, are resistant to degradation by protein-digesting enzymes (proteases) and that they are absorbed intact directly through the skin and mucosal surfaces; therefore, a direct positive relationship is likely to exist between microbial production and physiologic effects of superantigens.

- Skin disorders and superantigens—Superantigens in dermatologic diseases. (*Dermatology Online Journal* 2008 Feb[318]): In this excellent review of molecular biology and clinical disorders, the authors note that microbial superantigens are associated with many important clinical disease that affect the skin, including staphylococcal toxic shock syndrome, staphylococcal scalded skin syndrome, guttate psoriasis, psoriasis vulgaris (chronic plaque psoriasis), Kawasaki syndrome, atopic dermatitis, cutaneous T-cell lymphoma, and acute juvenile pityriasis rubra pilaris. The authors state, "Evidence shows that T-cells in psoriasis are triggered by conventional antigens and superantigens. It is suggested that although **the process is initiated by bacterial superantigens, molecular mimicry between the bacterial antigens and keratin 17 leads to activation of autoreactive T-cells and persistence of disease**." The authors note that all streptococci secrete SPEC, a superantigen known to stimulate marked expansion of T-cells which display a particular marker "Vβ2"; these Vβ2 T-cells are found in increased quantities in acute skin lesions of patients with guttate psoriasis.

- Psoriasis and superantigens—High prevalence of *Staphylococcus aureus* cultivation and superantigen production in patients with psoriasis. (*Eur J Dermatol* 2009 May-Jun[319]): This excellent research—conducted in by assessing the skin and nasal cavities (nostrils, nares) of 50 psoriatics and 50 healthy controls—demonstrates the following associations between psoriasis and active colonization with the bacteria *Staphylococcus aureus*:

  ❶ Psoriatic skin lesions have more *Staphylococcus aureus* than does nearby unaffected skin: In patients with psoriasis, skin lesions are more likely to culture *Staphylococcus aureus* (64%) than is the unaffected non-lesional skin (14%).

  ❷ Psoriatic patients are more likely to harbor *Staphylococcus aureus* in their nares/nostrils than are healthy people: "*Staphylococcus aureus* was cultivated from the nares in 25 (50%) of 50 patients with psoriasis and in 17 (34%) of 50 healthy controls."

  ❸ The *Staphylococcus aureus* found at the site of psoriatic lesions is more likely to be a strain of bacteria that produces distinct toxins: "In psoriasis patients, 31 (96.8%) out of the 32 strains isolated from the lesional skin and 3 (42.3%) out of the 7 strains isolated from the non-lesional skin were toxigenic (p = 0.01)." This means that psoriasis is quantitatively (more bacteria) and qualitatively (more toxin-producing bacteria) linked with *Staphylococcus aureus*. A very important contribution of this study is the finding that *Staphylococcus aureus* produces numerous—not only one—superantigens capable of inducing a significant part of the pathophysiology of psoriasis; these superantigens can be described as "non-classical

[316] "They also suggest that the etiology of RA may involve initial activation of V beta 14+ T cells by a V beta 14-specific superantigen with subsequent recruitment of a few activated autoreactive v beta 14+ T cell clones to the joints while the majority of other V beta 14+ T cells disappear." Paliard X, West SG, Lafferty JA, Clements JR, Kappler JW, Marrack P, Kotzin BL. Evidence for the effects of a superantigen in rheumatoid arthritis. *Science.* 1991 Jul 19;253(5017):325-9

[317] "Given that binding sites for superantigens have been mapped to the CDR4s of TCR beta chains, the synovial localization of T cells bearing V beta s with significant CDR4 homology indicates that V beta-specific T-cell activation by superantigen may play a role in RA." Howell MD, Diveley JP, Lundeen KA, Esty A, Winters ST, Carlo DJ, Brostoff SW. Limited T-cell receptor beta-chain heterogeneity among interleukin 2 receptor-positive synovial T cells suggests a role for superantigen in rheumatoid arthritis. *Proc Natl Acad Sci* U S A. 1991 Dec 1;88(23):10921-5

[318] Solanki LS, Srivastava N, Singh S. Superantigens: a brief review with special emphasis on dermatologic diseases. *Dermatology Online Journal* 2008 Feb 28;14(2):3 http://dermatology.cdlib.org/142/reviews/superantigens/singh.html

[319] Balci DD, Duran N, Ozer B, Gunesacar R, Onlen Y, Yenin JZ. High prevalence of Staphylococcus aureus cultivation and superantigen production in patients with psoriasis. *Eur J Dermatol.* 2009 May-Jun;19(3):238-42 http://www.john-libbey-eurotext.fr/e-docs/00/04/49/59/vers_alt/VersionPDF.pdf

superantigens" such as methicillin resistance gene (*mecA*), *etb*, *eta* and *see* as well as "classical superantigens such as *sea*, *seb*, *sec*, *sed* and *tst*.

❹ The *Staphylococcus aureus* found in the nares/nostrils of psoriatic patients is more likely to be a strain of bacteria that produces distinct toxins: "Isolated strains from the nares were toxigenic in 96% (24/25) for patients with psoriasis and in 41.2% (7/17) for healthy controls, respectively (p = 0.006)." A strong correlation of approximately 70% was found between the *Staphylococcus aureus* in the nares and on the skin of patients with psoriasis; this means that cross-contamination from skin to nares and from nares to skin is very likely.

❺ Psoriatic patients with lesions that culture positive for *Staphylococcus aureus* have worse disease activity than psoriatic patients with negative cultures: "Patients with cultivation-positive in lesional skin had a significantly higher PASI score than patients who were cultivation-negative in lesional skin (8.28 +/- 3.97 vs. 5.89 +/- 2.98, p = 0.031)." More *Staphylococcus aureus* in psoriasis lesions could be cause (i.e., the *Staphylococcus aureus* are directly contributing to the psoriatic lesions) or effect (i.e., the psoriatic lesions are more likely to become colonized with *Staphylococcus aureus*). However, given the established molecular role of superantigens in two primary hallmarks of psoriasis—inflammation and cytokine-induced cellular hyperproliferation—the most logical interpretation is that the association between *Staphylococcus aureus* and psoriasis is causal rather than casual.

The authors conclude by stating, "Our results confirm that *S. aureus* colonization and its toxigenic-strains are associated with psoriasis. According to our findings, non-classical superantigens such as methicillin resistance gene (*mecA*), *see* and *etb* may also be associated with psoriasis."

3. Enhanced production/processing of autoantigens: When the immune system perceives the presence of microbial molecules, mechanisms are enhanced which facilitate the processing and presentation of preexistent antigens to the immune system, which then targets these antigens for destruction. Of course, this is beneficial when fighting a true infection; but recent evidence shows that chronic silent infections can facilitate the processing and presentation of the body's own antigens (autoantigens) which are then attacked. Clinically, we see the immune system attacking the body, and we call this an "autoimmune disease" even though the original cause of the problem may have been an occult infection or exposure to specific microbial molecules. Ringrose et al[320] showed that infecting HLA-B27-positive human cells with *Salmonella typhimurium* and *Shigella flexneri* caused these cells to express autoantigens, namely human histone H3, human ribosomal protein S17 (two separate amino acid sequences) and the heavy chain of HLA-B27. A similar phenomenon has been demonstrated in autistic children wherein patients exposed to bacterial antigens (streptokinase), toxic chemicals (Thimerosal, ethyl-mercury), and dietary antigens (gliadin and casein peptides) produce autoantigens that appear capable of inciting and perpetuating autoimmunity.[321] **Therefore, we have experimental evidence with human cells *in vitro* which demonstrates that *enhanced processing of autoantigens* occurs following exposure to bacterial antigens, dietary allergens, and xenobiotics**.

- Psoriasis and microbially-evoked autoantigens—Ex vivo experimental study using human T-cells (see especially *Clin Exp Immunol* 1999 Sep[322]): Amino acid sequences in skin keratin subtypes 14 and 17 have homology with peptides from the bacterium *Streptococcus pyogenes*, thereby providing clear evidence of molecular mimicry between an infectious agent and chronic human disease, as reviewed in a previous section. Evidence has shown that psoriatic patients have T-cells which specifically target keratin 17 thereby indicating that keratin 17 serves as an autoantigen in psoriasis; Johnston et al[323] wrote, "…psoriatic individuals have CD8(+) T cells that recognize keratin self-antigens." As noted earlier in this chapter, increased production of keratin

[320] Ringrose JH, Muijsers AO, Pannekoek Y, Yard BA, Boog CJ, van Alphen L, Dankert J, Feltkamp TE. Influence of infection of cells with bacteria associated with reactive arthritis on the peptide repertoire presented by HLA-B27. *J Med Microbiol*. 2001 Apr;50(4):385-9 http://jmm.sgmjournals.org/cgi/reprint/50/4/385
[321] Vojdani A, Pangborn JB, Vojdani E, Cooper EL. Infections, toxic chemicals and dietary peptides binding to lymphocyte receptors and tissue enzymes are major instigators of autoimmunity in autism. *Int J Immunopathol Pharmacol*. 2003 Sep-Dec;16(3):189-99
[322] Gudmundsdottir AS, Sigmundsdottir H, Sigurgeirsson B, Good MF, Valdimarsson H, Jonsdottir I. Is an epitope on keratin 17 a major target for autoreactive T lymphocytes in psoriasis? *Clin Exp Immunol*. 1999 Sep;117(3):580-6
[323] Johnston A, Gudjonsson JE, Sigmundsdottir H, Love TJ, Valdimarsson H. Peripheral blood T cell responses to keratin peptides that share sequences with streptococcal M proteins are largely restricted to skin-homing CD8(+) T cells. *Clin Exp Immunol*. 2004 Oct;138(1):83-93 http://www.ncbi.nlm.nih.gov/pmc/articles/PMC1809187/pdf/cei0138-0083.pdf

17 can be induced by the pro-inflammatory cytokines gamma-interferon, which plays a key role as a mediator of psoriatic inflammation, and IL-6, which is abundant in psoriatic lesions. Factors that can increase IFN-g and/or IL-6 production are numerous and include such phenomena as infection, injury, obesity, and consumption of a pro-inflammatory diet; increased production of IFN-g and IL-6 is characteristic of nearly any immune response and is certainly not specific to psoriasis or any other rheumatic condition. As noted previously, the ALEEAN sequence present in keratin 17 is also found in keratin subtype 14, which is overexpressed in psoriatic skin; thus, for T-cells already primed to respond to ALEEAN following exposure to *Streptococcus pyogenes*, the dual exposure to ALEEAN in keratins 14 and 17—both of which are uniquely present in psoriatic skin—may promote localized attack by T-cells against keratinocytes, ie, immune cross-reactivity via molecular mimicry. In sum, the totality of data supports the following:

❶ Exposure to microbes induces IFNg and/or IL-6: IFN-g and IL-6 production is increased during overt or occult infection/colonization/dysbiosis, such as with *Streptococcus pyogenes* and other pathogenic microorganisms.

❷ Increased production of IFN-g and IL-6 increases production of keratin-17: Increased production of IFN-g and IL-6 increases production of keratin-17.

❸ Keratin-17 is an autoantigen in psoriatic skin: Keratin-17 is a clinically-important autoantigen in psoriasis based on its location, molecular homology with proteins made by *Streptococcus pyogenes* which is a known trigger in psoriasis, and the identification of T-cells which are specifically responsive to keratin-17

❹ Therefore, <u>microbial exposure</u> → <u>IFN-g and IL-6</u> → <u>increased keratin-17</u> = *increased autoantigen production induced by proinflammatory cytokines induced by microbial exposure.*

❺ Furthermore, increased production of autoantigen keratin-17 by IFN-g and IL-6 is probably not microbe-dependent. Of note, obesity in general and visceral adipose tissue in particular are causally associated with increased production of these inflammatory cytokines. If non-microbial induction of IFN-g and IL-6 can stimulate increased production of autoantigen keratin-17, then we would expect conditions such as obesity/hyperadiposity to be associated with more severe psoriasis; indeed this appears to be the case, as recently shown in studies showing that obese young women are at increased risk for severe psoriasis[324] and that weight loss treatments can improve psoriasis.[325]

4. Bystander activation: Evidence suggests that we all have immunocytes capable of attacking our body tissues, and thus we all have the potential to develop autoimmune disease. Normally, these autoreactive cells are kept anergic, dormant, quiescent, and otherwise inactive through various mechanisms that regulate the immune system; in this way, such autoreactive cells can be considered "bystanders" because they are not really doing anything and are basically "standing by." Bystander activation occurs when these cells are awakened by the cascade of inflammatory processes that occur as a result of superantigen exposure, molecular mimicry, immune complex deposition, or xenobiotic immunotoxicity. Bystander activation appears to contribute to the development of certain

---

[324] "Multivariate analysis demonstrated an association between excess increase in body mass index and psoriasis in females only. Being overweight in adole-scence was the main factor behind this observation." Bryld LE, Sørensen TI, Andersen KK, Jemec GB, Baker JL. High body mass index in adolescent girls precedes psoriasis hospitalization. *Acta Derm Venereol.* 2010 Sep;90(5):488-93

[325] "There are two recent reports of chronic severe psoriasis improving with weight loss after Roux-en-Y gastric bypass surgery. We have observed two patients with body mass indices greater than 50 kg/m(2) who had marked improvement in their psoriasis after gastric bypass surgery." Hossler EW, Maroon MS, Mowad CM. Gastric bypass surgery improves psoriasis. *J Am Acad Dermatol.* 2010 Jul 21. [Epub ahead of print]

autoimmune conditions, such as **drug-induced lupus**[326], and it may be a contributing pathogenic mechanism in **heavy/toxic metal-induced autoimmunity**.[327]

> ▪ <u>Psoriasis and bystander activation</u>—Keratinocytes are immunologically active cells that present bacterial-derived superantigens to T lymphocytes. (*J Dermatol Sci* 1993 Oct[328]): Most doctors and researchers have believed that epidermal keratinocytes were relatively passive components of the outer layers of the skin where these cells form a mechanical barrier against injury and infection; likewise, their role in skin diseases was considered passive, with keratinocytes acting as passive targets and "**innocent bystanders**." However, newer research mandates that we reclassify keratinocytes from passive barrier cells to "fully fledged members of the immune system (i.e. immunocytes)" based on the findings that keratinocytes produce important cytokines, adhesion molecules, and mononuclear cell chemotactic factors. Activated keratinocytes "can initiate and perpetuate the inflammatory and immunological reactions in the skin which contribute to the pathobiology of psoriasis." Specifically, cytokine-activated keratinocytes can present bacterial superantigens to T-cells, resulting in activation and proliferation of these effectors of psoriasis.

> ▪ <u>Thyroid autoimmunity induced by hepatitis C virus via bystander activation</u>—Binding of hepatitis C virus E2 protein to thyroid cells may cause thyroid autoimmunty via bystander activation (*J Autoimmun* 2008 Dec[329]): Hepatitis C virus (HCV) infection is well-known to be causally associated with thyroid autoimmunity (eg, Hashimoto's thyroiditis) but the molecular mechanism by which this association manifests has not been previously elucidated. In this study, researchers Akeno, Blackard, and Tomer showed that thyroid cells express a surface receptor called CD81, which is a binding site for the HCV protein E2. When HCV E2 binds to CD81, the proinflammatory cytokine IL-8 is produced. These authors concluded, "In summary, we have shown that CD81 is expressed in thyroid cells and can bind HCV envelope protein E2 leading to IL-8 production. These data suggest that local effects of HCV proteins can induce thyroiditis by bystander activation mechanisms." Although their conclusion might be premature insofar as their data showed deductive probability rather than objective certainty, it may be considered pragmatically sufficient.

5. <u>Haptenization and the formation of neoantigens/neoautoantigens</u>: **A nonantigenic microbial molecule may bind to a nonantigenic human molecule and result in the formation of a new hybridized or "haptenized" molecule—neoantigen—which stimulates immunologic attack**. Haptenization may be the underlying mechanism by which viruses induce autoimmunity[330] and appears to be a primary mechanism by which *Staphylococcus aureus* contributes to autoimmune vasculitis in **Wegener's granulomatosis**, namely by producing an antigenic acid phosphatase enzyme which binds with human endothelial cells by a charge interaction—the resultant **hybrid/hapten/neoantigen** formed by the antigen-endothelium complex becomes the target of immune attack, thus creating the phenomenon of "autoimmunity" and the clinical consequences of vasculitis.[331] Similarly, Hwp1 (Hyphal wall protein-1) of *Candida albicans* is a substrate for the tissue transglutaminase enzyme and cross-links with proteins in the mammalian mucosa[332]; the resultant

---

[326] "Several mechanisms for induction of autoimmunity will be discussed, including bystander activation of autoreactive lymphocytes due to drug-specific immunity or to non-specific activation of lymphocytes, direct cytotoxicity with release of autoantigens and disruption of central T-cell tolerance." Rubin RL. Drug-induced lupus. *Toxicology*. 2005 Apr 15;209(2):135-47

[327] "It is therefore theoretically possible that compounds present in vaccines such as thiomersal or aluminium hydroxyde can trigger autoimmune reactions through bystander effects." Fournie GJ, Mas M, Cautain B, Savignac M, Subra JF, Pelletier L, Saoudi A, Lagrange D, Calise M, Druet P. Induction of autoimmunity through bystander effects. Lessons from immunological disorders induced by heavy metals. *J Autoimmun*. 2001 May;16(3):319-26

[328] Nickoloff BJ, Mitra RS, Green J, Shimizu Y, Thompson C, Turka LA. Activated keratinocytes present bacterial-derived superantigens to T lymphocytes: relevance to psoriasis. *J Dermatol Sci*. 1993 Oct;6(2):127-33

[329] Akeno N, Blackard JT, Tomer Y. HCV E2 protein binds directly to thyroid cells and induces IL-8 production: a new mechanism for HCV induced thyroid autoimmunity. *J Autoimmun*. 2008 Dec;31(4):339-44 http://www.ncbi.nlm.nih.gov/pmc/articles/PMC2641008/pdf/nihms84111.pdf

[330] Van Ghelue M, Moens U, Bendiksen S, Rekvig OP. Autoimmunity to nucleosomes related to viral infection: a focus on hapten-carrier complex formation. *J Autoimmun*. 2003;20(2):171-82

[331] Brons RH, Bakker HI, Van Wijk RT, et al. Staphylococcal acid phosphatase binds to endothelial cells via charge interaction; a pathogenic role in Wegener's granulomatosis? *Clin Exp Immunol*. 2000 Mar;119(3):566-73 http://www.blackwell-synergy.com/doi/abs/10.1046/j.1365-2249.2000.01172.x

[332] "By serving as a microbial substrate for epithelial cell transglutaminase, Hwp1 (Hyphal wall protein 1) of Candida albicans participates in cross-links with proteins on the mammalian mucosa." Staab JF, Bahn YS, Tai CH, Cook PF, Sundstrom P. Expression of transglutaminase substrate activity on Candida albicans germ tubes through a coiled, disulfide-bonded N-terminal domain of Hwp1 requires C-terminal glycosylphosphatidylinositol modification. *J Biol Chem*. 2004 Sep 24;279(39):40737-47 http://www.jbc.org/cgi/content/full/279/39/40737

neoantigen that results from this microbe-human haptenization would be a prime candidate to incite autoimmunity, as has been demonstrated by the transglutaminase-mediated haptenization of gliadin with human collagen *in vivo*.[333,334] In fact, since both Hwp1 and gliadin are substrates for tissue transglutaminase, *Candida albicans* may be synergistic with gluten/gliadin in the production of the systemic inflammatory/autoimmune/allergic condition known as **celiac disease**[335]; this may exemplify the interrelated nature of dysbiosis, food allergy, and autoimmunity. Lastly, since many toxic metals, xenobiotics, and drugs appear to trigger autoimmunity via haptenization[336,337,338], the adverse effects of these toxicants will be enhanced by microbe-induced alterations in xenobiotic detoxification and/or the proinflammatory effects of peptidoglycans, exotoxins, endotoxins, lipoteichoic acid, and other antigens and superantigens. In a recent animal study, exposure to bacterial endotoxin exacerbated metal-induced autoimmunity.[339] Endotoxin from gram-negative bacteria impairs detoxification by inhibiting the first cytochrome-p450-mediated step of detoxification[340]; this inhibition of detoxification increases the risk for drug toxicity and chemical accumulation. Bacteria can also adversely affect detoxification by elaborating beta-glucuronidase in the lumen of the intestine which cleaves bile-secreted toxins from their water-soluble conjugation moieties, resulting in increased "enterohepatic recycling"[341] or "enterohepatic recirculation"[342] as discussed below; increased re-exposure to previously detoxified endogenous and exogenous toxins can result in an upregulation of Phase 1 (cytochrome-p450-mediated biotransformation) leading to the formation of reactive intermediates and a condition commonly described by clinicians as "imbalanced detoxification" or "pathological detoxification."

- Wegener's granulomatosis and bacterial enzyme haptenization—Staphylococcal enzyme acid phosphatase binds to (i.e., haptenizes) endothelial cells via charge interaction in Wegener's vasculitis (*Clin Exp Immunol* 2000 Mar[343]): Wegener's granulomatosis is an autoimmune vasculitic condition with a high mortality; the majority of untreated patients die an average of 5 months following diagnosis, and 2-year survival without treatment is 10%. Histologically, the condition demonstrates focal accumulations of inflammation and immune cell activity (ie, granulomas); however, the main clinical concern is the vasculitis in general and in particular the vasculitis affecting the kidneys and which commonly leads to kidney failure, a leading cause of death in affected patients. This excellent study by Brons and coworkers shows that the bacteria

[333] "Our findings firstly demonstrated that gliadin was directly bound to tTG in duodenal mucosa of coeliacs and controls, and the ability of circulating tTG-autoantibodies to recognize and immunoprecipitate the tTG-gliadin complexes." Ciccocioppo R, Di Sabatino A, Ara C, Biagi F, Perilli M, Amicosante G, Cifone MG, Corazza GR. Gliadin and tissue transglutaminase complexes in normal and coeliac duodenal mucosa. *Clin Exp Immunol*. 2003 Dec;134(3):516-24

[334] "Thus, modification of gluten peptides by tTG, especially deamidation of certain glutamine residues, can enhance their binding to HLA-DQ2 or -DQ8 and potentiate T cell stimulation. Furthermore, tTG-catalyzed cross-linking and consequent haptenization of gluten with extracellular matrix proteins allows for storage and extended availability of gluten in the mucosa." Dieterich W, Esslinger B, Schuppan D. Pathomechanisms in celiac disease. *Int Arch Allergy Immunol*. 2003 Oct;132(2):98-108

[335] "Subsequently, C albicans might function as an adjuvant that stimulates antibody formation against HWP1 and gluten, and formation of autoreactive antibodies against tissue transglutaminase and endomysium." Nieuwenhuizen WF, Pieters RH, Knippels LM, Jansen MC, Koppelman SJ. Is Candida albicans a trigger in the onset of coeliac disease? *Lancet*. 2003;361(9375):2152-4

[336] Rao T, Richardson B. Environmentally induced autoimmune diseases: potential mechanisms. *Environ Health Perspect*. 1999 Oct;107 Suppl 5:737-42 http://ehp.niehs.nih.gov/members/1999/suppl-5/737-742rao/rao-full.html

[337] "Here, Peter Griem and colleagues focus on several aspects of neoantigen formation by xenobiotics: metabolism of xenobiotics into reactive, haptenic metabolites; polymorphisms of metabolizing enzymes; induction of costimulatory signals; and sensitization of T cells." Griem P, Wulferink M, Sachs B, Gonzalez JB, Gleichmann E.Allergic and autoimmune reactions to xenobiotics: how do they arise? *Immunol Today*. 1998 Mar;19(3):133-4

[338] "It appears that the patients' antibodies recognize epitopes consisting of shared structural features of the protein carriers (100 kDa, 76 kDa, 59 kDa, 57 kDa and 54 kDa), not the TFA hapten alone." Kenna JG, Satoh H, Christ DD, Pohl LR. Metabolic basis for a drug hypersensitivity: antibodies in sera from patients with halothane hepatitis recognize liver neoantigens that contain the trifluoroacetyl group derived from halothane. *J Pharmacol Exp Ther*. 1988 Jun;245(3):1103-9 As an extension of this work, also see: "These investigations have further revealed that the antibodies are directed against distinct polypeptide fractions (100 kDa, 76 kDa, 59 kDa, 57 kDa, 54 kDa) that have been covalently modified by the reactive trifluoroacetyl halide metabolite of halothane." Satoh H, Martin BM, Schulick AH, Christ DD, Kenna JG, Pohl LR. Human anti-endoplasmic reticulum antibodies in sera of patients with halothane-induced hepatitis are directed against a trifluoroacetylated carboxylesterase. *Proc Natl Acad Sci U S A*. 1989 Jan;86(1):322-6 http://www.pnas.org/cgi/reprint/86/1/322

[339] Abedi-Valugerdi M, Nilsson C, Zargari A, Gharibdoost F, DePierre JW, Hassan M. Bacterial lipopolysaccharide both renders resistant mice susceptible to mercury-induced autoimmunity and exacerbates such autoimmunity in susceptible mice. *Clin Exp Immunol*. 2005 Aug;141(2):238-47

[340] Shedlofsky SI, Israel BC, McClain CJ, Hill DB, Blouin RA. Endotoxin administration to humans inhibits hepatic cytochrome P450-mediated drug metabolism. *J Clin Invest*. 1994 Dec;94(6):2209-14

[341] "Enterohepatic recycling occurs by biliary excretion and intestinal reabsorption of a solute, sometimes with hepatic conjugation and intestinal deconjugation. ... Of particular importance is the potential amplifying effect of enterohepatic variability in defining differences in the bioavailability, apparent volume of distribution and clearance of a given compound." Roberts MS, Magnusson BM, Burczynski FJ, Weiss M. Enterohepatic circulation: physiological, pharmacokinetic and clinical implications. *Clin Pharmacokinet*. 2002;41(10):751-90

[342] Liska DJ. The detoxification enzyme systems. *Altern Med Rev*. 1998 Jun;3(3):187-98

[343] Brons RH, Bakker HI, Van Wijk RT, et al. Staphylococcal acid phosphatase binds to endothelial cells via charge interaction; a pathogenic role in Wegener's granulomatosis? *Clin Exp Immunol*. 2000 Mar;119(3):566-73

Staphyloccus areus produces an enzyme—acid phosphatase—which binds to endothelial cells, the cells that form the inner linings of arteries and all blood vessels. This positively-charged enzyme has also been shown to bind to the renal basement membrane, a target of immune attack in inflammatory/autoimmune renal diseases described as as crescentic glomerulonephritis, a type of immune-mediated renal disease seen in several autoimmune conditions such as Goodpasture syndrome, IgA nephropathy, and systemic lupus erythematosus. Because the staphylococcal acid phosphatase is a foreign non-self protein, the human immune system forms antibodies against it; these antibodies are measurable in the blood of patients with Wegener's vasculitis. Thus, when the staphylococcal acid phosphatase binds to endothelial cells, the antibodies directed against the the acid phosphatase induce a vigorous immune response and inflammatory reaction on the surface of the vessel wall—this is the hallmark of vasculitis. The authors conclude that "Since antibodies directed against staphylococcal acid phosphatase are present in patients with WG and these antibodies recognize endothelial cell-bound staphylococcal acid phosphatase, we suggest that the results published in this study support the hypothesis that staphylococcal acid phosphatase may play a role in the initiation of vasculitis and glomerulonephritis in patients with WG by acting as a planted antigen." For this discussion, "planted antigen" and "hapten" are synonymous and interchangeable.

6. Peptidoglycans, teichoic acid, and exotoxins from gram-positive bacteria: Peptidoglycan (PG), a major cell-wall component of Gram-positive bacteria. Peptidoglycans from gram-positive bacteria such as group-A streptococci can cause malaise, fever, dermatosis, tenosynovitis, cryoglobulinemia (an immune complex disease), and arthritis.[344] Experimental arthritis can be induced in animals by exposing them to group-B streptococci isolated from the nasopharynx of human patients with rheumatoid arthritis.[345] *Staphylococcus aureus* is a gram-positive bacterium, certain strains of which produce the toxic shock syndrome toxin-1 (TSST-1) that causes scalded skin syndrome, toxic shock syndrome, and food poisoning; other strains of *Staphylococcus aureus* that do not produce TSST-1 are also capable of causing toxic shock syndrome from colonization of bone, vagina, wounds, or rectum.[346] Experimental evidence has shown that peptidoglycan-polysaccharide complexes from "good" and "normal" bacteria such as Bifidobacteria and *Lactobacillus casei* can also induce an inflammatory arthritis; this speaks against the "more is better" approach to probiotic supplementation and also demonstrates how **bacterial overgrowth of the small bowel (detailed later) can induce joint pain and inflammation even in the absence of so-called "pathogens."**[347,348]

- Psoriasis and peptidoglycans—Peptidoglycan appears to be a major causative factor for psoriasis (*Trends Immunol* 2006 Dec[349]): Peptidoglycan is a major cell-wall component of Gram-positive bacteria and has been detected within antigen-presenting cells of patients with psoriasis. Furthermore, the skin of patients with psoriasis shows Th1 cells that are specifically responsive to streptococcal and/or staphylococcal peptidoglycans; this indicates that peptidoglycan is probably an important T-cell stimulator which contributes to psoriasis. Additionally, patients with psoriasis appear to be genetically predisposed to disorders associated with peptidoglycans because their immune cells are altered in such a way as to allow for enhanced T-cell response to the bacterial antigens such as peptidoglycans. The authors conclude, "These observations suggest that peptidoglycan is a major aetiological factor for psoriasis and emphasize the importance of peptidoglycan in bacterial-infection-induced inflammatory disease."

---

[344] "A characteristic intermittent neutrophilic dermatosis, associated with polyarthritis, tenosynovitis, malaise, fever, and cryoglobulinemia, occurs in 20% of patients who undergo ileojejunal bypass surgery for the treatment of morbid obesity... Peptidoglycans from numerous intestinal bacteria…are suggested as causative of the toxic and immunologic features of this syndrome." Ely PH. The bowel bypass syndrome: a response to bacterial peptidoglycans. *J Am Acad Dermatol*. 1980 Jun;2(6):473-87

[345] "The origin of rheumatoid arthritis (RA) is in our opinion a bacterial infection." Svartz N. The origin of rheumatoid arthritis. *Rheumatology*. 1975;6:322-8

[346] Shandera WX, Moran A. "Infectious diseases: viral and rickettsial." In Tierney LM, McPhee SJ Papadakis MA (eds). Current Medical Diagnosis and Treatment. 44th edition. New York: Lange; 2005, page 1356-8

[347] Simelyte E, Rimpilainen M, Lehtonen L, Zhang X, Toivanen P. Bacterial cell wall-induced arthritis: chemical composition and tissue distribution of four Lactobacillus strains. *Infect Immun*. 2000 Jun;68(6):3535-40 http://iai.asm.org/cgi/reprint/68/6/3535

[348] Toivanen P. Normal intestinal microbiota in the aetiopathogenesis of rheumatoid arthritis. *Ann Rheum Dis*. 2003 Sep;62(9):807-11 http://ard.bmjjournals.com/cgi/reprint/62/9/807

[349] Baker BS, Powles A, Fry L. Peptidoglycan: a major aetiological factor for psoriasis? *Trends Immunol*. 2006 Dec;27(12):545-51

- Psoriasis and peptidoglycans—Patients with cutaneous and arthritic psoriasis have elevated IgA antibodies against streptococcal peptidoglycan-polysaccharide. (*Clin Exp Rheumatol* 1997 Jul-Aug[350]): Patients with psoriasis and psoriatic arthritis have elevated IgA levels specific to streptococcal peptidoglycan-polysaccharide (PG-PS); antibody levels do no vary with disease severity. Very remarkably, the authors concluded by stating, "**The results suggest chronic mucosal stimulation of lymphocytes by long-lived streptococcal antigens in patients with psoriasis**..." Readers should appreciate that the evidence linking psoriasis with mucosal infections with the streptococcal bacteria is consistent and very strong. The mucosal surfaces of the nose, sinuses, and throat are the most common locations for chronic streptococcal bacteria colonization/dysbiosis.

- Psoriasis and peptidoglycans and teichoic acid—Contribution of *Staphylococcus aureus* cell wall products teichoic acid and peptidoglycan to immunoglobulin (IgE, IgA, IgG) synthesis and CD23 expression in patients with atopic dermatitis (*Immunology* 1992 Jan[351]): Patients with the inflammatory pruritic skin condition atopic dermatitis (eczema) have increased skin and nasal colonization with the bacteria *Staphylococcus aureus* and that the immune response induced by living or dead *Staphylococcus aureus* differs in eczema patients from that seen in normal healthy patients; in patients with eczema, exposure to fragments of *Staphylococcus aureus* actually causes immunosuppression (reductions in IgA and IgG) rather than the expected immune upregulation that should occur following exposure to a pathogenic microbe. Furthermore, in patients with eczema, exposure to *Staphylococcus aureus* cell wall fragments causes increased production of IgE and histamine, two pathophysiologic factors inextricably associated with the skin inflammation and discomfort/itchiness of eczema. The finding that bacterial cell wall fragments can lead to reduced production of IgA and IgG implies that mucous membrane and/or skin colonization with *Staphylococcus aureus* (and perhaps *Bordetella pertussis*, *Haemophilus influenzae* and Gram-negative bacteria which produce lipopolysaccharide [LPS]) can promote local and systemic immune suppression which favors (poly)microbial colonization and persistence while also contributing to skin inflammation and irritation via enhanced production of IgE and histamine. Readers should appreciate that psoriatic patients also have increased nasal and skin colonization with *Staphylococcus aureus* and that psoriasis—like eczema—is a chronic inflammatory skin disorder; thus, *Staphylococcus aureus* probably acts via similar molecular mechanisms to produce these two disorders, which differ from each other yet at the same time can be seen as variants on the theme of microorganism-triggered "patterns of inflammation."

- Rheumatoid arthritis and peptidoglycans: Normal intestinal bacteria appear to contribute to rheumatoid arthritis and other inflammatory [joint] diseases (*Ann Rheum Dis* 2003 Sep[352]): In this article Professor Toivanen reviews 61 published articles to advance the model of inflammatory disease induction by bacteria, particularly what might generally be considered normal intestinal bacteria. Professor Toivanen notes several interesting items of fact: ❶ bacteria that are genetically identical per PCR testing can have subtle differences in their peptidoglycan structure, and these minute differences in peptidoglycan structure [perhaps due to epigenetic factors] can effect profound differences in pathophysiologic responses, ie, either promoting or suppressing inflammatory responses by the immune system, ❷ bacterial peptidoglycan can stimulate the production of the autoantibody **rheumatoid factor**, which for many decades was considered the primary serologic diagnostic marker for rheumatoid arthritis (80% positivity), and which is present in other autoimmune disorders such as Sjogren's syndrome (70% positivity), and which contributes directly to joint and tissue injury and inflammation via direct deposition, particularly

[350] Rantakokko K, Rimpiläinen M, Uksila J, Jansèn C, Luukkainen R, Toivanen P. Antibodies to streptococcal cell wall in psoriatic arthritis and cutaneous psoriasis. *Clin Exp Rheumatol*. 1997 Jul-Aug;15(4):399-404
[351] Neuber K, König K. Effects of Staphylococcus aureus cell wall products (teichoic acid, peptidoglycan) and enterotoxin B on immunoglobulin (IgE, IgA, IgG) synthesis and CD23 expression in patients with atopic dermatitis. *Immunology*. 1992 January; 75(1): 23–28 http://www.ncbi.nlm.nih.gov/pmc/articles/PMC1384797/
[352] Toivanen P. Normal intestinal microbiota in the aetiopathogenesis of rheumatoid arthritis. *Ann Rheum Dis*. 2003 Sep;62(9):807-11 http://www.ncbi.nlm.nih.gov/pmc/articles/PMC1754679/?tool=pubmed

in the form of immune complexes, and ❸ peptidoglycans induce inflammatory reponses following binding with Toll-like receptor 2 (TLR-2). Three successive sentences are particularly worthy of quotation:

> "The ability of bacterial cell walls to induce chronic, erosive arthritis was first described in the rat by using *Streptococcus pyogenes*. Self perpetuating arthritis, closely resembling human rheumatoid arthritis by histological criteria, develops in susceptible rat strains after a single intraperitoneal injection of the bacterial cell wall. In addition to *Streptococcus pyogenes*, several bacterial species representing Lactobacillus, Bifidobacterium, Eubacterium, Collinsella, and Clostridium have been observed to have a similar ability."

The important observation that, in experiemental models with genetically susceptible animals, chronic inflammatory arthritis can be induced by a one-time exposure to commonly encountered bacteria provides clear objective proof that bacteria and—importantly—their nonviable cell wall fragments can induce chronic inflammatory disease. Readers should note the evidence showing that *Streptococcus pyogenes* can contribute to inflammatory *arthritis* in certain models, while contributing to inflammatory *dermatitis* in others.

- Skin disorders and peptidoglycans—Beta-blocking drugs and bacterial peptidoglycan promote Th1-mediated inflammatory reponses in skin (*Brain Behav Immun* 2008 Jan[353]): The authors of this paper note that many inflammatory diseases such as psoriasis, atopic dermatitis, lichen planus, and vitiligo have also been associated with emotional stress and local alterations of the sympathetic (adrenergic) nervous system. Using a unique experimental model, the authors show that peptidoglycan from Gram-positive bacteria—but not lipopolysacharide from Gram-negative bacteria—promoted a local Th1-type proinflammatory response. Based on the responses elicited by adrenergic receptor (AR)-blocking drugs, the authors conclude that the Th1 polarization is mediated by inhibition of both beta1- and beta2-AR. The local pro-inflammatory response includes enhanced local expression of IFN-gamma, IL-12 and IL-23 as well as of IFN-beta and CXCR3 ligands. The local inflammatory response resulted in an increase of antigen-positive plasmacytoid dendritic cells (pDCs) in the draining lymph node. In sum, these results suggest that "altered sympathetic nervous activity together with selected pattern recognition receptors activation might serve as initiation and/or persistence factors for numerous Th1-sustained inflammatory skin diseases." Psoriasis is a known Th1-sustained inflammatory skin disease; more recent research has demonstrated a strong Th-17 component as well.

7. Endotoxins (lipopolysaccharide) from gram-negative bacteria: Many different species of gram-negative bacteria produce endotoxin, also known as bacterial lipopolysaccharide (LPS). Even in the absence of viable bacteria, the exposure of humans to endotoxin, say for example by intravenous administration for the purpose of experimentation, produces a wide range of adverse physiologic consequences, including 1) triggering an acute proinflammatory response resembling febrile illness or sepsis, 2) increasing intestinal permeability, causing "leaky gut"[354], 3) inhibiting hepatic detoxification[355], 4) disrupting the blood-brain barrier and promoting neurodegeneration via neuroinflammation.[356,357,358] The pathophysiologic effects of endotoxin/LPS are often *similar to* and *synergistic with* those of superantigens to effect altered tissue function and widespread inflammation. **LPS and antigens from gram-negative bacteria (in the absence of viable bacteria) exacerbate**

[353] Manni M, Maestroni GJ. Sympathetic nervous modulation of the skin innate and adaptive immune response to peptidoglycan but not lipopolysaccharide: involvement of beta-adrenoceptors and relevance in inflammatory diseases. *Brain Behav Immun*. 2008 Jan;22(1):80-8

[354] "After endotoxin administration systemic absorption and excretion of lactulose increased almost two-fold... These data suggest that a brief exposure to circulating endotoxin increases the permeability of the normal gut." O'Dwyer ST, Michie HR, Ziegler TR, Revhaug A, Smith RJ, Wilmore DW. A single dose of endotoxin increases intestinal permeability in healthy humans. *Arch Surg*. 1988 Dec;123(12):1459-64

[355] Shedlofsky SI, Israel BC, Tosheva R, Blouin RA. Endotoxin depresses hepatic cytochrome P450-mediated drug metabolism in women. *Br J Clin Pharmacol*. 1997 Jun;43(6):627-32

[356] "Following administration of lipopolysaccharide (LPS) to immunized mice, antibodies gain access to the brain. They bind preferentially to hippocampal neurons and cause neuronal death with resulting cognitive dysfunction and altered hippocampal metabolism..." Kowal C, DeGiorgio LA, Nakaoka T, Hetherington H, Huerta PT, Diamond B, Volpe BT. Cognition and immunity; antibody impairs memory. *Immunity*. 2004 Aug;21(2):179-88 http://www.immunity.com/content/article/abstract?uid=PIIS1074761304001980

[357] Fassbender K, et al . The LPS receptor (CD14) links innate immunity with Alzheimer's disease. *FASEB J*. 2004 Jan;18(1):203-5. fasebj.org/cgi/reprint/03-0364fjev1

[358] Laflamme N, Rivest S. Toll-like receptor 4: the missing link of the cerebral innate immune response triggered by circulating gram-negative bacterial cell wall components. *FASEB J*. 2001 Jan;15(1):155-163 http://www.fasebj.org/cgi/reprint/15/1/155.pdf

arthritis in experimental models[359] and trigger inflammatory arthropathy (reactive arthritis) in humans.[360]

- Psoriasis and lipopolysaccharide from Gram-negative bacteria—Proposed explanation for the exacerbation of psoriasis in AIDS with a discussion of substance P and gram-negative bacteria (*Autoimmunity* 2004 Feb[361]): The author of this paper proposes that the well-known induction or exacerbation of psoriasis by HIV infection may be due to a variety of factors, including ❶ increased colonization of skin by *Staphylococcus aureus*, ❷ increased release of substance P by immunocytes rather than neurons, and ❸ increased infections/colonization with Gram-negative bacteria which elaborate endotoxin/lipopolysaccharide, which is potently pro-inflammatory. Also proposed is the model of a vicious cycle wherein psoriatic lesions produce substance P, which then promotes HIV replication and exacerbation of HIV-related disease, which then leads to exacerbations of psoriasis, which leads to more substance P elaboration and HIV replication. Other researchers have noted that psoriatic lesions show increased nerve growth and increased elaboration from nerves of substance P, which is a pro-inflammatory neuropeptide.[362]

- Psoriasis and endotoxin/LPS from Gram-negative bacteria—Improvement of psoriasis with cholestyramine (*Arch Dermatol* 1982 Mar[363]): In this letter to the editor, the authors report the rapid improvement of psoriasis after the oral administration of cholestyramine resin in five patients with psoriasis. The rationale for this intervention is to reduce the patient's total inflammatory load by reducing the amount of bacterial endotoxin/LPS absorbed from the gastrointestinal tract. Five patients were treated with orally administered cholestyramine 4 grams 4 times daily and topical chlorhexidine soap.

- Psoriasis—Endotoxin/lipopolysaccharide (LPS) from intestinal Gram-negative bacteria and the effect of binding with orally administered bile acids (*Pathophysiology* 2003 Dec[364]): This is an impressively large and impressively innovative stuty. The authors tested the hypothesis that an insufficiency in bile acid production by the liver results in increased bacterial endotoxin absorption from the intestines and that this endotoxin contributes to the immune dysfunction and systemic inflammation of psoriasis. The authors note that, under normal conditions, bile acids secreted from the hepatobiliary system act as detergents by degrading intestinal endotoxins and thereby protecting the host from their pathophysiologic sequelae. Bile acids thereby participate in "physico-chemical defense" by splitting endotoxin/lipopolysaccharide into nontoxic fragments and thus preventing the consequent release of inflammatory cytokines. In this clinical trial, total of 800 psoriasis patients participated in the study and 551 were treated with oral bile acid (dehydrocholic acid) supplementation for 1-8 weeks. Treatment efficacy was evaluated clinically and by use of the standard Psoriasis Area Severity Index (PASI) score. The authors note remarkable improvement; "During this treatment, 434 patients (78.8%) became asymptomatic. Of 249 psoriatics receiving the conventional therapy, only 62 (24.9%) showed clinical recovery during the same period of time (P<0.05)." Patients with more acute and short-term psoriais showed very high rates of improvement; 95% of these patients had resolution of their psoriasis. After two years of treatment, 319 of 551 (57.9%) psoriasis patients treated with bile acids were asymptomatic, compared to only 15 of 249 (6.0%) patients receiving the standard drug treatment. As for the subset of patients with acute psoriasis, at the end of two years, 147 of

---

[359] "The results showed that administration of LPS was followed by reactivation of AIA in a dose-related fashion." Yoshino S, Yamaki K, Taneda S, Yanagisawa R, Takano H. Reactivation of antigen-induced arthritis in mice by oral administration of lipopolysaccharide. *Scand J Immunol.* 2005 Aug;62(2):117-22

[360] "Extensive bacterial cultures of the synovial fluid were negative... We conclude that in patients with reactive arthritis after yersinia infection, microbial antigens can be found in synovial-fluid cells from the affected joints." Granfors K, Jalkanen S, von Essen R, Lahesmaa-Rantala R, Isomaki O, Pekkola-Heino K, Merilahti-Palo R, Saario R, Isomaki H, Toivanen A. Yersinia antigens in synovial-fluid cells from patients with reactive arthritis. *N Engl J Med.* 1989 Jan 26;320(4):216-2

[361] Namazi MR. Paradoxical exacerbation of psoriasis in AIDS: proposed explanations including the potential roles of substance P and gram-negative bacteria. *Autoimmunity.* 2004 Feb;37(1):67-71

[362] "Indeed, we have noted marked proliferation of nerve fibers in transplanted psoriatic plaques compared with the few nerves in transplanted normal human skin. By double label immunofluorescence staining, we have further demonstrated that in these terminal cutaneous nerves there is a marked upregulation of neuropeptides, such as substance P and calcitonin gene-related protein." Raychaudhuri SP, Raychaudhuri SK. Role of NGF and neurogenic inflammation in the pathogenesis of psoriasis. *Prog Brain Res.* 2004;146:433-7

[363] Skinner RB, Rosenberg EW, Belew PW, Marley WM. Improvement of psoriasis with cholestyramine. [letter] *Arch Dermatol.* 1982 Mar;118(3):144

[364] Gyurcsovics K, Bertók L. Pathophysiology of psoriasis: coping endotoxins with bile acid therapy. *Pathophysiology.* 2003 Dec;10(1):57-61

184 (79.9%) of psoriatic patients treated with bile acids were asymptomatic; only 10 of 139 (7.2%) acute psoriasis patients receiving standard drug treatment were cured. The authors summarize, "To conclude, the results obtained suggest that psoriasis can be treated with success by oral bile acid supplementation presumably affecting the microflora and endotoxins released and their uptake in the gut." These findings are consistent with the facts that ❶ psoriasis manifests most obviously as dermal hyperproliferation induced by cytokines and that ❷ endotoxin/LPS is one of the most powerful inducers of cytokine release.

- Psoriasis: 6 of 11 (54%) patients were shown to have endotoxinemia—measurable blood levels of bacterial lipopolysaccharide/endotoxin from Gram-negative bacteria (*Archives of Dermatology* 1982 Mar[365]): The authors introduce their letter by stating, "Our interest in the possibility of endotoxemia in psoriasis followed recent demonstrations of alterations in levels of alternative complement pathway components and of circulating IgA immune complexes in psoriasis. Endotoxin and immune IgA complexes each activate the alternative complement pathway." These authors report finding **circulating blood levels of endotoxin/lipopolysaccharide in 6 of 11 (54%) of their tested psoriatic patients**. Research laboratory methods are described.

- Psoriasis—Use of cholestyramine to bind intestinal endotoxin, and nutrient treatment of severe psoriasis in alcoholics (*J Drugs Dermatol* 2010 Apr[366]): Alcoholism increases the risk of initiation/exacerbation of psoriasis by as much as 800%, with the effect being strongest in men. Of course, alcoholism causes other health problems, too; notable for this discussion are ❶ increased intestinal permeability leading to bacterial endotoxin absorption, and ❷ vitamin and mineral deficiencies commonly causing elevated homocysteine levels and hypomagnesemia, respectively. The two patients in this 2-case report and brief review were treated with magnesium 600 mg, folic acid 5 mg, pyridoxine 100 mg, and cobalamin 1 mg in addition to routine topical and oral medications for psoriasis, acute infections (one patient was treated with Bactrim for MRSA); one patient was treated with cholestyramine 4 grams 4 times per day for 5 days repeated for 3 courses. In the discussion section of the article, the authors review that alcoholism causes increased intestinal permeability and resultant increased absorption of endotoxin with immunogenic/inflammatory consequences. Additionally, cholestyramine while being appropriate for alcoholics to bind endotoxin might exacerbate magnesium deficiency via reduced intestinal absorption (ie, binding) and by increased urinary excretion, the latter according to an animal study. As has been noted elsewhere, the authors of this report note that both psoriatics and alcoholics tend to have higher levels of homocysteine; less widely appreciated is the fact that homocysteine primes neutrophils for inflammatory responses, tissue homing, and induction of increased oxidative stress and tissue damage, some of which is relevant and somewhat specific for the pathogenesis of psoriasis. A separate publication cited by these authors noted that homocysteine levels correlated positively and folate levels correlated negatively with the severity and extent of psoriasis. Homocysteine causes intracellular depletion of magnesium; this problem is ameliorated by supplementation with magnesium, folate, pyridoxine, and cobalamin. Not mentioned in this report is the possibility that hypomagnesemia contributes to psoriasis via enhancement/derepression of neurogenic inflammation, and that folate and other coenzymes are necessary for the epigenetic modifications (most obviously, DNA methylation) that might favorably influence the psoriatic and proinflammatory phenotype.

8. Immunostimulation by bacterial DNA: **Bacterial DNA stimulates a proinflammatory response that is comparable to that induced by endotoxin/LPS.** Exposure to single-stranded *bacterial* DNA induces formation of antibodies against single-stranded *mammalian* DNA. These findings may be particularly relevant to patients with systemic lupus erythematosus—a disorder for which the pathogenic hallmark is the formation of anti-DNA antibodies—since these patients have an impaired ability to clear bacterial DNA from the serum and therefore experienced prolonged pro-inflammatory

[365] Belew PW, Rosenberg EW, Skinner RB Jr, Marley WM. Endotoxemia in psoriasis. *Arch Dermatol.* [Letter] 1982 Mar;118(3):142-3
[366] Aronson PJ, Malick F. Towards rational treatment of severe psoriasis in alcoholics: report of two cases. *J Drugs Dermatol.* 2010 Apr;9(4):405-8

stimulation when exposed to bacterial DNA.[367] Chronic exposure to immunostimulating antigens is a recognized means for the induction of autoimmunity in animal models.

- Psoriasis and immunostimulation via bacterial DNA—Enhanced activation of blood mononuclear cells in patients with psoriasis vulgaris mediated by streptococcal antigen with bacterial DNA (*J Invest Dermatol* 2009 Nov[368]): The authors note that streptococcal infection has an intimate relationship with psoriasis even though the specific role of streptococcal DNA has not been previously clarified. Therefore, these researchers investigated the effect of streptococcal DNA on lymphocyte proliferation and activation as well as cytokine secretion in psoriasis. As has been previously reported by other researchers, the authors of this paper also found that peripheral blood mononuclear cells (PBMCs) from psoriatic patients had higher proliferative responses upon stimulation by streptococcal antigens (SA) when compared with those from healthy individuals. Pretreatment of the streptococcal antigens with an enzyme that degrades DNA (DNase-1) reduced the amount of immune stimulation elicited following exposure of immune cells to streptococcal antigens, thus implicating streptococcal DNA as having an important role in the induction of the pro-inflammatory response elicited by streptococcal antigens in psoriatic immune cells. The authors conclude, "This study demonstrates the integral function of SA, particularly streptococcal DNA, in the pathogenesis of psoriasis."

9. Activation of Toll-like receptors (TLR) and NF-kappaB (NFkB): Microbial products such as peptidoglycans and endotoxins (as well as others) promote inflammation and arthritogenesis by activating receptors and nuclear transcription factors with the resultant non-specific upregulation of proinflammatory genetic expression. Nuclear transcription factor kappaB (NFkB) is considered one of the most important nuclear transcription factors for stimulating genetic expression of proinflammatory genes, and NFkB is activated by microbes and their structures including viruses and endotoxins.[369] Similar to NFkB are the Toll-like receptors (TLRs), which promote an inflammatory response by NFKB-dependent and NFKB-independent pathways following exposure to microbial structures including but not limited to peptidoglycans and lipopolysaccharides.[370] About a dozen different TLRs have been identified, and these play an important role in the joint destruction seen in the classic example of dysbiotic arthropathy—rheumatoid arthritis.[371] From a nutritional perspective, we see that **Toll-like receptor activity is stimulated by saturated fatty acids and inhibited by polyunsaturated fatty acids, especially the omega-3 fatty acid docosahexaenoic acid.**[372] Likewise, NFkB activity can be modulated by numerous nutrients as I have reviewed later in this text and elsewhere.[373] Of course, nutritional, botanical, or pharmacologic modulation of inflammation should not supersede investigation and correction of the underlying cause(s) of inflammation.

- Psoriasis and bacterial activation of TLRs and NFkB—Toll-like receptors in skin (*Adv Dermatol* 2008[374]): The author cites research showing that keratinocytes in **psoriatic lesions have increased levels of TLRs 1, 2, 4, 5 and 9 compared with normal skin**; this suggests the probability of enhanced responsiveness to microbial immunogens. Whether this upregulated expression of TLRs is a nonspecific response to inflammation or a specific response to the presence of microorganisms is not clear; however what is very obvious is that the presence of microbe-sensing TLRs with the presence of additional bacteria on the skin of psoriatic paitents certainly

[367] "The immunostimulatory activities of bacterial DNA are varied and encompass the mitogenicity of B cells and the induction of cytokines including IFN-α/β, IFN-γ, tumor necrosis factor alpha, interleukin 6 (IL-6), and IL-12 (17, 21, 23). Together, these activities resemble those of endotoxin..." Pisetsky DS. Antibody responses to DNA in normal immunity and aberrant immunity. *Clin Diagn Lab Immunol.* 1998 Jan;5(1):1-6 http://cvi.asm.org/cgi/reprint/5/1/1
[368] Cai YH, Lu ZY, Shi RF, Xue F, Chen XY, Pan M, Yuan WR, Xu H, Li WP, Zheng J. Enhanced proliferation and activation of peripheral blood mononuclear cells in patients with psoriasis vulgaris mediated by streptococcal antigen with bacterial DNA. *J Invest Dermatol.* 2009 Nov;129:2653-60
[369] Tak PP, Firestein GS. NF-kappaB: a key role in inflammatory diseases. *J Clin Invest.* 2001;107(1):7-11 http://www.jci.org/cgi/content/full/107/1/7
[370] Armant MA, Fenton MJ. Toll-like receptors: a family of pattern-recognition receptors in mammals. Genome Biol. 2002 Jul 29;3(8):REVIEWS3011. Epub 2002 Jul 29 http://genomebiology.com/2002/3/8/REVIEWS/3011
[371] Ospelt C, Kyburz D, Pierer M, Seibl R, Kurowska M, Distler O, Neidhart M, Muller-Ladner U, Pap T, Gay RE, Gay S. Toll-like receptors in rheumatoid arthritis joint destruction mediated by two distinct pathways. *Ann Rheum Dis.* 2004 Nov;63 Suppl 2:ii90-ii91 http://ard.bmjjournals.com/cgi/content/full/63/suppl_2/ii90
[372] Lee JY, Sohn KH, Rhee SH, Hwang D. Saturated fatty acids, but not unsaturated fatty acids, induce the _expression of cyclooxygenase-2 mediated through Toll-like receptor 4. J Biol Chem. 2001 May 18;276(20):16683-9. Epub 2001 Mar 2 http://www.jbc.org/cgi/content/full/276/20/16683
[373] Vasquez A. Reducing pain and inflammation naturally - part 4: nutritional and botanical inhibition of NF-kappaB, the major intracellular amplifier of the inflammatory cascade. A practical clinical strategy exemplifying anti-inflammatory nutrigenomics. *Nutritional Perspectives*, July 2005:5-12.
[374] Miller LS. Toll-like receptors in skin. *Adv Dermatol.* 2008;24:71-87

provides a well-set stage for dermatologic inflammation. "Thus," the author notes, "TLR activation may also play a role in the pathophysiology of psoriasis by exacerbating the disease process." Also noted is the very important observation that **the antimicrobial peptide cathelicidin (LL-37), which is found at high levels in psoriatic skin, can convert non-stimulatory self-DNA into a potent activator of TLR-9** on dendritic cells (plasmacytoid DCs) resulting in production of IFN-alpha, leading to the conclusion that "This may be one important mechanism of how **TLRs can promote autoimmunity in psoriasis.**" Per review by Lamphier et al[375], TLR-9 is expressed intracellularly and is activated in response to DNA, in particular DNA containing unmethylated CpG motifs that are more prevalent in microbial than mammalian DNA; however, under certain conditions, TLR-9 can recognize self-DNA and this may promote immune responses against DNA such as noted in the autoimmune disease systemic lupus erythematosis (SLE) particularly as TLR-9 binds rather indiscriminately to a broad range of DNAs. Notice the implications and four-step stream of probable events: ❶ microbe-induced skin inflammation and tissue injury → ❷ upregulation of TLRs (esp. TLR-9) and antimicrobial peptides (esp. cathelicidin) → ❸ cathelicidin-induced conversion of nonoffensive self-DNA into an autoinflammatory immunogen, which then potently activates the already upregulated TLR-9 = ❹ thereby, microbial inflammation results in autoimmunity/autoinflammation (to self-DNA). **A well-known function of TLRs is, via their transmembrane domain and a cytoplasmic tail domain that is homologous to the interleukin-1 receptor, the initiation of various intracellular signaling cascades, including activation of nuclear factor-kB (NFkB), which is a key transcription factor that promotes transcription of genes coding for pro-inflammatory molecules** such as cytokines, chemokines, co-stimulatory molecules (needed for immune responsiveness), and adhesion molecules (needed for the homing of immunocytes to inflamed/damaged tissue).

10. <u>Immune complex formation and deposition</u>: Chronic infection generally results in the increased production of immune complexes, which are polymeric antigen-antibody combinations. Antigen-antibody combinations are formed almost anytime the humoral immune system is fighting against a virus, bacteria, yeast, or food allergen. Although essential for the destruction and clearance of pathogenic antigens, immune complexes pose a problem for the body due to 1) the difficulty in clearing them from the systemic circulation, and 2) their proclivity for deposition in the skin and joints.[376] Indeed, **immune complexes are significant contributors to most "autoimmune" diseases; immune complex deposition is responsible for triggering joint inflammation in rheumatoid arthritis[377] and for the facial rash and many of the other clinical manifestations which characterize systemic lupus erythematosus (SLE, lupus).** Immune complex deposition directly contributes to the renal disease and vasculitis common in patients with autoimmune disease. Patients with autoimmune disease commonly have circulating IgM and IgA antibodies against bacteria from the gastrointestinal and genitourinary tracts[378] clearly indicating an active immune response against these bacteria and suggesting breaches in mucosal integrity. Since IgA-containing immune complexes are cleared from the serum by hepatocytes and are secreted intact into the bile[379,380,381], hepatobiliary phytostimulation

---

[375] Lamphier MS, Sirois CM, Verma A, Golenbock DT, Latz E. TLR9 and the recognition of self and non-self nucleic acids. *Ann N Y Acad Sci.* 2006 Oct;1082:31-43

[376] Inman RD. Antigens, the gastrointestinal tract, and arthritis. *Rheum Dis Clin North Am.* 1991 May;17(2):309-21

[377] Abramson SB. Mediators of inflammation, tissue destruction, and repair: cellular constituents." In Klippel JH. <u>Primer on the rheumatic diseases. 11th edition</u>. Atlanta: Arthritis Foundation; 1997, page 39

[378] "IgM and IgA anti-Proteus antibodies were significantly higher in patients with RF-positive RA compared with all other patient groups." Newkirk MM, Goldbach-Mansky R, Senior BW, Klippel J, Schumacher HR Jr, El-Gabalawy HS. Elevated levels of IgM and IgA antibodies to Proteus mirabilis and IgM antibodies to Escherichia coli are associated with early rheumatoid factor (RF)-positive rheumatoid arthritis. *Rheumatology* (Oxford). 2005 Aug 9; [Epub ahead of print]

[379] "Clearance of IgA immune complexes was delayed after bile duct ligation." Harmatz PR, Kleinman RE, Bunnell BW, McClenathan DT, Walker WA, Bloch KJ. The effect of bile duct obstruction on the clearance of circulating IgA immune complexes. *Hepatology.* 1984 Jan-Feb;4(1):96-100

[380] Lemaitre-Coelho I, Jackson GD, Vaerman JP. High levels of secretory IgA and free secretory component in the serum of rats with bile duct obstruction. *J Exp Med.* 1978 Mar 1;147(3):934-9 http://www.jem.org/cgi/reprint/147/3/934

[381] "CONCLUSIONS: Biliary obstruction secondary to both calculus or malignancy of the hepatobiliary system causes suppression of bile IgA secretion and elevated serum level of secretory IgA. Bile secretory IgA secretion recovers with endoscopic drainage of the obstructed system." Sung JJ, Leung JC, Tsui CP, Chung SS, Lai KN. Biliary IgA secretion in obstructive jaundice: the effects of endoscopic drainage. *Gastrointest Endosc* 1995 Nov;42:439-44

may thereby produce an anti-rheumatic benefit; however, this hypothesis requires serologic and outcomes-based validation in a clinical trial.[382]

- Psoriasis and immune complexes—Circulating IgA immune complexes in patients with psoriasis (*J Invest Dermatol* 1983 Jun[383]): Using a sensitive and specific Raji cell radioimmunoassay, authors of this study analyzed the sera of 35 patients with psoriatic arthritis for IgA-containing circulating immune complexes (IgA-CIC). Additionally, measurements for circulating immune complexes (CIC) containing IgG or IgM were performed using the 125I-Clq binding assay and the Raji IgG radio-immunoassay. Results showed that, "**Twenty-eight of thirty five (80%) patients with PsA were found to have IgA-containing circulating immune complexes.** In contrast, only 13 of 35 (37%) had IgG-containing circulating immune complexes detected using the Raji IgG assay and 10 of 33 (33%) had IgG- or IgM-containing immune complexes detected using the 125I-Clq binding assay." Frequency, level, or subclass of immune complexes did not correlate with different types or severities of cutaneous psoriasis. However, **the level of IgA-CIC did significantly correlate with the severity of psoriatic arthritis**—higher levels of IgA-CIC corresponded with more severe psoriatic arthritis. The authors concluded, "The finding of IgA-containing circulating immune complexes in 80% of patients with psoriatic arthritis as well as the significantly higher levels of these complexes in the patients with more severe arthritis suggests that IgA-containing circulating immune complexes may play a role in the pathogenesis of psoriatic arthritis." Generally speaking, because IgA is the subclass of antibody/immunoglobulin that is used to defend mucosal surfaces such as the mouth, throat, respiratory tract, and the gastrointestinal and genitourinary tracts, elevations of IgA and IgA-CIC naturally incline physicians to strongly consider microbial colonization of one or more mucosal surfaces. Additionally, since IgA-CIC are cleared by the liver for excretion into the bile and therefore into the intestines, additional attention (phytotherapeutic and physiologic) to ensuring optimal hepatobiliary and intestinal functions is likely to be of clinical benefit.[384]

- Psoriasis and immune complexes—IgA-containing immune complexes in patients with psoriatic arthritis (*Clin Exp Rheumatol* 1984 Jul-Sep-5[385]): In this study, blood samples from 21 patients with psoriasis were examined for the presence of IgA-CIC using the Raji IgA radioimmunoassay. Further, the Raji IgG radioimmunoassay and 125I-Clq binding assay were used to detect IgG-CIC and IgM-CIC. Results from the patients with psoriatic arthritis were contrasted against results from 25 patients with various nonpsoriatic hyperkeratotic skin disorders. Patients were given systemic therapy with etretinate (20 patients) or 13-cis-retinoic acid (1 patient)[Note 386]; blood from of 15 patients treated with etretinate were studied before, during, and after therapy. Whereas fourteen of 21 (67%) patients with psoriasis had evidence of IgA-CIC during the course of their disease, only 1 of 25 patients (4%) with other hyperkeratotic skin disorders showed this finding. Among the psoriatic patients, only 2 of 19 (11%) had evidence of IgG-CIC using the Raji IgG assay, and only 1 of 19 (5%) had evidence of IgG-CIC or IgM-CIC using the 125I-Clq binding assay. As was found in their previous study[387], these authors again showed a positive correlation between the extent of *psoriatic* disease and the level of IgA-CIC. Among 15 patients followed during therapy, results showed that levels of IgA-CIC did not change in response to positive response to treatment. Thus, given the correlation of IgA-CIC with the severity of psoriatic arthritis, the lack of correlation of IgA-CIC with improvement, and the lack of correlation of IgG-CIC and IgM-CIC with psoriasis, the authors concluded that, "...IgA-containing CIC are not

[382] Vasquez A. Do the Benefits of Botanical and Physiotherapeutic Hepatobiliary Stimulation Result From Enhanced Excretion of IgA Immune Complexes? *Naturopathy Digest* 2006; January: http://www.naturopathydigest.com/archives/2006/jan/vasquez_immune.php

[383] Hall RP, Peck GL, Lawley TJ. Circulating IgA immune complexes in patients with psoriasis. *J Invest Dermatol*. 1983 Jun;80(6):465-8

[384] Vasquez A. Do the Benefits of Botanical and Physiotherapeutic Hepatobiliary Stimulation Result From Enhanced Excretion of IgA Immune Complexes? http://www.naturopathydigest.com/archives/2006/jan/vasquez_immune.php

[385] Hall RP, Gerber LH, Lawley TJ. IgA-containing immune complexes in patients with psoriatic arthritis. *Clin Exp Rheumatol*. 1984 Jul-Sep;2(3):221-5

[386] Of note, etretinate is an aromatic retinoid which was approved for severe psoriasis in 1986 and removed from the Canadian market in 1996 and the United States market in 1998 due to the high risk of birth defects; it has been somewhat replaced by acitretin, a safer metabolite of etretinate. 13-cis-retinoic acid is more commonly known as isotretinoin and is available by prescription; like other synthetic variants of vitamin A, it is highly teratogenic (ie, isotretinoin causes severe birth defects.).

[387] Hall RP, Gerber LH, Lawley TJ. IgA-containing immune complexes in patients with psoriatic arthritis. *Clin Exp Rheumatol*. 1984 Jul-Sep;2(3):221-5

directly related to the cutaneous manifestations of psoriasis, but may be important in the modification of immune or inflammatory responses in these patients." Another more likely explanation in the opinion of the current author (Dr Vasquez) is that IgA-CIC contribute to and represent the underlying pathophysiology of psoriasis (ie, mucosal colonization with antigentic microbes and/or exposure to dietary antigens) which exists in proportion to the severity of the illness (ie, serving as a reflection of both antigenic stimulation and abnormally increased mucosal permeability) and which persists despite clearance of skin lesions (ie, the most superficial manifestation of the illness).

11. <u>Antimetabolites</u>: Yeast and bacteria can produce certain molecules which *jam up, monkey wrench*, or otherwise interfere with normal human cellular metabolism. The best example is **D-lactic acid**, which impairs human metabolic pathways that are designed to work with the "human" form of this metabolite—the levo isomer—L-lactic acid. Commonly resulting in headache, fatigue, depression, and sometimes death, D-lactic acidosis is extensively well documented in the medical research literature and commonly occurs in association with bacterial overgrowth of the intestine, particularly following intestinal bypass surgery.[388] Other antimetabolites produced from (intestinal) microbes which are associated with human disease and dysfunction include **ammonia, tryptamine, tyramine, octopamine, mercaptes, aldehydes, alcohol (ethanol), tartaric acid, indolepropionic acid, indoleacetic acid, skatole, indole, putrescine, and cadaverine**. Many of these metabolites are seen in higher amounts in patients with migraine, depression, weakness, confusion, schizophrenia, agitation, hepatic encephalopathy, chronic arthritis and rheumatoid arthritis. **Gut-derived neurotoxins** from bacteria and yeast may contribute to autistic symptomatology[389,390], and case reports have consistently demonstrated that excess absorption of bacterial metabolites can alter behavior in humans and result in acute neurocognitive decline and behavioral abnormalities in children.[391] **Hydrogen sulfide**, produced by intestinal bacteria such as *Citrobacter freundii*[392], is a mitochondrial poison[393] and is strongly associated with disease activity in ulcerative colitis.[394] Degradation of tryptophan by bacterial tryptophanase predisposes to a "functional tryptophan deficiency" and may result in insufficiency of serotonin which would contribute to hyperalgesia, depression, impaired adrenal responsiveness[395] ("hypoadrenalism"), and insomnia; **indole** and **skatole**, which are gut-derived bacterial degradation products of tryptophan, produce an inflammatory arthritis that is identical to rheumatoid arthritis in animal models.[396,397]

- Chronic fatigue syndrome: Increased D-lactic acid intestinal bacteria in patients with chronic fatigue syndrome (*In Vivo* 2009 Jul-Aug[398]): These researchers begin by noting that the symptoms of cognitive dysfunction and neurological impairment which are commonly seen in patients with chronic fatigue syndrome (CFS) are also classic presenting complaints in patients with D-lactic

---

[388] "D-Lactic acidosis is a potentially fatal clinical condition seen in patients with a short small intestine and an intact colon. Excessive production of D-lactate by abnormal bowel flora overwhelms normal metabolism of D-lactate and leads to an accumulation of this enantiomer in the blood." Vella A, Farrugia G. D-lactic acidosis: pathologic consequence of saprophytism. *Mayo Clin Proc*. 1998 May;73(5):451-6

[389] Sandler RH, Finegold SM, Bolte ER, et al. Short-term benefit from oral vancomycin treatment of regressive-onset autism. *J Child Neurol*. 2000 Jul;15(7):429-35

[390] Shaw W, Kassen E, Chaves E. Increased urinary excretion of analogs of Krebs cycle metabolites and arabinose in two brothers with autistic features. *Clin Chem*. 1995;41(8 Pt 1):1094-104

[391] "The neurological features consisted of a depressed conscious state, confusion, aggressive behaviour, slurred speech and ataxia. The organic acid profile of urine demonstrated increased amounts of lactic, 3-hydroxypropionic, 3-hydroxyisobutyric, 2-hydroxyisocaproic, phenyllactic, 4-hydroxyphenylacetic and 4-hydroxyphenyllactic acids. Of the lactic acid 99% was D-lactic acid." Haan E, Brown G, Bankier A, et al. Severe illness caused by the products of bacterial metabolism in a child with a short gut. *Eur J Pediatr*. 1985 May;144(1):63-5

[392] Lennette EH (editor in chief). Manual of Clinical Microbiology. Fourth Edition. Washington DC; American Society for Microbiology: 1985, page 269. See also http://web.indstate.edu/thcme/micro/GI/general/sld038.htm Accessed 10/27/2005

[393] "Treatment of H2S poisoning may benefit from interventions aimed at minimizing ROS-induced damage and reducing mitochondrial damage." Eghbal MA, Pennefather PS, O'Brien PJ. H2S cytotoxicity mechanism involves reactive oxygen species formation and mitochondrial depolarisation. *Toxicology*. 2004 Oct 15;203(1-3):69-76

[394] "CONCLUSIONS: Metabolic effects of sodium hydrogen sulfide on butyrate oxidation along the length of the colon closely mirror metabolic abnormalities observed in active ulcerative colitis, and the increased production of sulfide in ulcerative colitis suggests that the action of mercaptides may be involved in the genesis of ulcerative colitis." Roediger WE, Duncan A, Kapaniris O, Millard S. Reducing sulfur compounds of the colon impair colonocyte nutrition: implications for ulcerative colitis. *Gastroenterology*. 1993 Mar;104(3):802-9

[395] "This hypothesis is supported by the findings in chronic MS patients of a significantly diminished adrenal cortisol reactivity to insulin-induced hypoglycemia which is considered a stress response mediated through the 5-HT system. Consequently, since patients with MS exhibit an abnormal response to stress it follows that increased tryptophan availability through dietary supplementation would diminish their vulnerability to psychological stress." Sandyk R. Tryptophan availability and the susceptibility to stress in multiple sclerosis: a hypothesis. *Int J Neurosci*. 1996 Jul;86(1-2):47-53

[396] Nakoneczna I, Forbes JC, Rogers KS. The arthritogenic effect of indole, skatole and other tryptophan metabolites in rabbits. *Am J Pathol*. 1969 Dec;57(3):523-38

[397] Rogers KS, Forbes JC, Nakoneczna I. Arthritogenic properties of lipophilic, aryl molecules. *Proc Soc Exp Biol Med*. 1969 Jun;131(2):670-2

[398] Sheedy JR, Wettenhall RE, Scanlon D, Gooley PR, Lewis DP, McGregor N, Stapleton DI, Butt HL, DE Meirleir KL. Increased d-lactic Acid intestinal bacteria in patients with chronic fatigue syndrome. *In Vivo*. 2009 Jul-Aug;23(4):621-8

acidosis, which is always caused by bacterial overgrowth of the small bowel and/or (more rarely) by the patient's inability to metabolize/detoxify products of bacterial metabolism produced in the small and/or large bowel. The authors report finding a **significant increase of Gram-positive facultative anaerobic faecal microorganisms** in 108 CFS patients as compared to 177 control subjects. Specifically, they found that, "The viable count of D-lactic acid producing *Enterococcus* and *Streptococcus* spp. in the faecal samples from the CFS group (3.5 x 10(7) cfu/L and 9.8 x 10(7) cfu/L respectively) were significantly higher than those for the control group (5.0 x 10(6) cfu/L and 8.9 x 10(4) cfu/L respectively). **Readers should note that this is approximately a 10-fold increase in *Enterococcus* and a 1,000-fold increase in *Streptococcus* in the CFS group compared with the control group. These Gram-positive bacteria produced not only more lactic acid in general but specifically they produced more of the dextro isomer D-lactic acid** than the Gram negative *Escherichia coli*. The authors correctly conclude that these findings "might explain not only neurocognitive dysfunction in CFS patients but also mitochondrial dysfunction, these findings may have important clinical implications." As a note of personal experience, the current author (Dr Vasquez) had one event of severe headache and dyscognition following consumption of a symbiotic supplement during his 6-year bout with a CFS-related syndrome; from this experience, I furthered my understanding of dysbiosis and would continue to do so for the following 10 years. Of further note, based on my personal and clinical experiences as well as review of the biomedical literature, I proposed in 2008 in my monograph *Musculoskeletal Pain: Expanded Clinical Strategies* published by the Institute for Functional Medicine that D-lactic acidosis was one of the pathophysiologic mechanisms by which microbial overgrowth of the intestines causes fibromyalgia; I was therefore gratified to see this article—published in 2009, a full 18 months after I had proposed this mechanism—verifying my proposed mechanism.

- Short bowel syndrome and D-lactic acidosis: Case report (*Arch Dis Child* 1980 Oct[399]): The three-sentence abstract of this case report reads, "Metabolic acidosis in a 3-year-old child with short bowel syndrome led to the discovery of massive D-lactic aciduria. After normalisation of the intestinal bacterial flora, D-lactate disappeared together with the acidosis. Dysbacteriosis with excessive production of D-lactate by intestinal bacteria (unidentified) and subsequent absorption explains this unusual cause of metabolic acidosis." Note the use of the term "dysbacteriosis" which is more commonly abbreviated to "dysbiosis", with the latter term being more accurate in terms of its nonspecificity since the disease-producing microbes may be from several different kingdoms. The young boy in this case report underwent bowel resection secondary to multiple congenital malformations and complications from infection, ie, mesenteric thrombosis tertiary to dehydration secondary to infectious diarrhea. After several episodes of neurocognitive dysfunction including weakness and dyspnea, the child was eventually diagnosed with multiple nutritional deficiencies, malabsorption, and lactic acidosis secondary to intestinal overgrowth of Gram-positive D-lactate-producing bacteria and an insufficiency of Gram-negative bacteria. The child was treated only with probiotic supplementation—no antibiotics were given—and D-lactate levels fell quickly within 4 days and were virtually undetectable by day 11. Thus, probiotic therapy alone may be sufficient treatment for some cases of D-lactic acidosis, particularly when an "insufficiency dysbiosis" of Gram-negative bacteria and a relative or absolute "overgrowth dysbiosis" of Gram-positive bacteria is identified or suspected.

12. Autointoxication, auto-brewery syndrome, hepatic encephalopathy: The term "autointoxication" fell out of favor among American allopaths in the 1940s despite the recognition and objective documentation that systemically absorbed microbial metabolites/toxins from the colon could adversely affect systemic health, particularly neurocognitive function.[400] "Hepatic encephalopathy" seems to be one of the currently acceptable terms for this phenomenon, and it is probable that the

---

[399] Schoorel EP, Giesberts MA, Blom W, van Gelderen HH. D-Lactic acidosis in a boy with short bowel syndrome. *Arch Dis Child*. 1980 Oct;55(10):810-2
[400] Person JR, Bernhard JD. Autointoxication revisited. *J Am Acad Dermatol*. 1986;15(3):559-63

condition exists among some outpatients to a milder degree than that which is classically seen in patients with fulminant liver failure. Recognition that excess or abnormal microbes in the gut could cause neuropsychiatric symptoms contributed to the rationale for the use of colonic irrigation in clinical practice which was fully endorsed by the American Medical Association in a position paper published in 1932.[401] Concurrently, an article published in the *New England Journal of Medicine*[402] in this same year documented the clinical benefits of colonic irrigation in patients with mental disease; the treatment was deemed effective against most cases of dementia, depression, neurosis and many cases of irritability, headaches, and hypertension. Enemas and colonics, which promote hepatobiliary detoxification[403,404] and cleanse the bowel of harmful microbes, were valued by clinicians as a cure or adjunctive treatment for numerous systemic diseases.[405] Although the term "autointoxication" is eschewed as "unscientific", all medical professionals recognize that gastrointestinal dysbiosis—particularly generalized overgrowth of yeast and bacteria—can cause clinical conditions characterized by inflammatory vasculitis, dermatitis, arthritis as well as neurological symptoms ranging from confusion and disorientation to somnolence and death. Of a less dramatic but much more frequent note, bacterial overgrowth of the small bowel is also a cause of gastroesophageal reflux disease (GERD) because products of bacterial fermentation relax the lower esophageal sphincter[406] and retard intestinal transit[407]; ameliorating the intestinal bacterial overgrowth by simply "starving" the bacteria of carbohydrate by implementation of a **low-carbohydrate diet** alleviates GERD symptoms and substantiates the cause-and-effect relationship.[408,409]

One of the liver's chief functions is that of "detoxifying" envionronmentally ingested and endogenously produced metabolites and toxins, including those of microbial origin produced de novo within the gastrointestinal tract. The metabolic activity of the microbial population within the intestinal lumen is quantitatively enormous, physiologically important, and clinically significant; an estimated ten trillion microorganisms reside within the intestinal lumen of each human. Being very small of course creates very large surface-to-volume ratios for microorganisms; if we take as given that an average bacterium of spherical shape has surface area of approximately 12 micrometers squared, then multiplying this surface area by 10 trillion in order to give some appreciation of the mass of lipopolysaccharide and peptidoglycan mass yields a surface area of 120 trillion micrometers squared or 120 billion meters squared, equal to approximately 29,652,645 acres or 12,000,000 hectares. Given that the total surface of the bacterial community is constantly being shed and replaced by individual microbes throughout each unit of time and also per death of each microbe, then the "functional surface area" of the microbial population is massive beyond comprehension, leaving an inquantifiable quantity of debris to be either physically excluded or immunologially processed. In addition to this "physical debris", microbes secrete even more metabolic molecules, some of which are intentionally and directly toxic and all of which have to be processed/detoxified/eliminated if and when they are absorbed systemically. As stated previously in this chapter, readers should appreciate that the "total dysbiotic load" (TDL) from all sources—skin, gastrointestinal tract, genitourinary tract, sinorespiratory tract, orodental cavity, environment, and any subclinical parenchymal foci—

[401] Bastedo WA. Colon irrigations: their administration therapeutic applications and dangers. *Journal of the American Medical Association* 1932;98:734-6

[402] Marshall HK, Thomson CR. Colon irrigation in the treatment of mental disease. N Engl J Med 1932; 207 (Sept 8): 454-7

[403] Garbat, AL, Jacobi, HG: Secretion of Bile in Response to Rectal Installations. *Arch Intern Med* 1929; 44: 455-462

[404] "Caffeine enemas cause dilation of bile ducts, which facilitates excretion of toxic cancer breakdown products by the liver and dialysis of toxic products from blood across the colonic wall. The therapy must be used as an integrated whole." Gerson M. The cure of advanced cancer by diet therapy: a summary of 30 years of clinical experimentation. *Physiol Chem Phys.* 1978;10(5):449-64

[405] Snyder RG. The value of colonic irrigations in countering auto-intoxication of intestinal origin. *Medical Clinics of North America* 1939; May:781-788

[406] "In summary, we have shown that colonic fermentation, through the production of SCFAs, exerts a controlled feedback on LES motor function." Piche T, Zerbib F, Varannes SB, Cherbut C, Anini Y, Roze C, le Quellec A, Galmiche JP. Modulation by colonic fermentation of LES function in humans. *Am J Physiol Gastrointest Liver Physiol.* 2000 Apr;278(4):G578-84 http://ajpgi.physiology.org/cgi/content/full/278/4/G578

[407] "Altered gastrointestinal motility and sensation, changed activity of the central nervous system, and increased sympathetic drive and immune activation may be understood as consequences of the host response to SIBO." Lin HC. Small intestinal bacterial overgrowth: a framework for understanding irritable bowel syndrome. *JAMA.* 2004 Aug 18;292(7):852-8

[408] "These data suggest that a very low-carbohydrate diet in obese individuals with GERD significantly reduces distal esophageal acid exposure and improves symptoms." Austin GL, Thiny MT, Westman EC, Yancy WS Jr, Shaheen NJ. A very low-carbohydrate diet improves gastroesophageal reflux and its symptoms. *Dig Dis Sci.* 2006 Aug;51(8):1307-12

[409] "The 5 individuals described in these case reports experienced resolution of GERD symptoms after self-initiation of a low-carbohydrate diet." Yancy WS Jr, Provenzale D, Westman EC. Improvement of gastroesophageal reflux disease after initiation of a low-carbohydrate diet: five brief case reports. *Altern Ther Health Med.* 2001 Nov-Dec;7(6):120, 116-9

contributes to the total inflammatory load (TIL) and total xenobiotic load (TXL) which the immune system must process and which the hepatobiliary system must detoxify.

In a review article[410] published in 2010 which applies specifically to the gastrointestinal subtype of dysbiosis, the authors start their paper by stating, "Detoxification of gut-derived toxins and microbial products from gut-derived microbes is a major role of the liver. While the full repertoire of gut-derived microbial products that reach the liver in health and disease is yet to be explored, the levels of bacterial lipopolysaccharide (LPS), a component of Gram-negative bacteria, is increased in the portal and/or systemic circulation in several types of chronic liver diseases." The total metablilic and toxic load from the microbes in the gut can be of such a volume that the body's ability to detoxify/metabolize these toxins is overwhelmed.

- Autointoxication, auto-brewery syndrome: A child with ethanol intoxication secondary to bacterial/fungal overgrowth of the intestines (*J Pediatr Gastroenterol Nutr* 2001 Aug[411]): In this case report and review of the literature, the authors begin their article by noting that, "The term **auto-brewery syndrome** has been used to describe patients who become repeatedly inebriated after ingestion of food of high carbohydrate nature in the presence of abnormal yeast proliferation, particularly of *Candida* species." The case report centers on a 13-year-old girl who had bowel recection for important reasons when a neonate and who later had "recurrent episodes of bizarre behavior, somnolence, disorientation, and a fruity odor of her breath and was suspected to be abusing alcohol." **The young girl was diagnosed with alcohol intoxication when ethanol blood levels were repeatedly elevated in the range of 250 mg/dL to 350 mg/dL**; she persistently denied any intake of alcoholic beverages. Readers should note that in most states in the United States, a blood alcohol concentration (BAC) of or greater than 100 mg/dL is the legal definition of intoxication and drunkenness.[412] The young girl's father—a physician—began testing the girl's breath alcohol level at home and noticed a strong correlation between her elevated ethanol levels and the intake of carbohydrate-rich meals or fructose-containing drinks, such as fruit juices. The girl was treated empirically for bacterial overgrowth of the intestines with courses of the anti-bacterial drugs Bactrim, Flagyl, and Augmentin and attained zero benefit. The girl was then submitted for underwent upper gastrointestinal endoscopy study to obtain aspirates for microbial analysis; the aspirate grew abundant *Candida glabrata* and *Sacchromyces cerevisiae*. **Sensitivity-directed treatment with fluconazole resolved all symptoms and prevented recurrence of the elevated ethanol levels**. The combination of bacterial with fungal overgrowth was likely synergistic; bacterial LPS blocked Cyp450 detoxificiation and thereby heightened sensitivity to the fungally-produced ethanol.

The molecular evidence
Immune complexes in intestinal bypass arthritis contain IgG, IgM, and IgA antibodies directed against bacterial antigens from *E. coli*, *Bacteroides*, *Lactobacilli*, and Group D (gamma) streptococcus.
Ross CB, Scott HW, Pincus T. Jejunoileal bypass arthritis. *Baillieres Clin Rheumatol*. 1989 Aug

13. Dysbiotic arthropathy, dysbiotic dermatitis, dysbiotic vasculitis (etc): .....; current terms for this condition include "bowel-associated dermatosis-arthritis syndrome"[413], "intestinal arthritis-dermatitis syndrome"[414], and "bypass disease"[415]—all of which are largely mediated by the gut-derived absorption of antigens, mucosal and systemic antibody formation, and antigen-antibody binding in the circulation and tissues followed by systemic deposition of immune complexes in skin, joints, kidneys, and vascular endothelium.

[410] Szabo G, Bala S, Petrasek J, Gattu A. Gut-liver axis and sensing microbes. *Dig Dis*. 2010;28(6):737-44

[411] Dahshan A, Donovan K. Auto-brewery syndrome in a child with short gut syndrome: case report and review of the literature. *J Pediatr Gastroenterol Nutr*. 2001 Aug;33(2):214-5

[412] Cohen JS. (Plantz SH, Talavera F, Anker A, editors). Alcohol Intoxication. http://www.emedicinehealth.com/alcohol_intoxication/page2_em.htm June 9, 2011

[413] Jorizzo JL, Apisarnthanarax P, Subrt P, et al. Bowel-bypass syndrome without bowel bypass. Bowel-associated dermatosis-arthritis syndrome. *Arch Intern Med*. 1983 Mar;143(3):457-61

[414] Stein HB, Schlappner OL, Boyko W, Gourlay RH, Reeve CE. The intestinal bypass: arthritis-dermatitis syndrome. *Arthritis Rheum*. 1981 May;24(5):684-90

[415] Utsinger PD. Systemic immune complex disease following intestinal bypass surgery: bypass disease. *J Am Acad Dermatol*. 1980 Jun;2(6):488-95

- <u>Authoritative review: Jejunoileal bypass arthritis</u> (*Baillieres Clin Rheumatol 1989 Aug*[416]): In this 17-page review chapter, authors Ross, Scott, and Pincus discuss the allopathic medicosurgical use of jejunoileal bypass, a surgical procedure wherein the jejunum is connected to the terminal ileum, thereby bypassing the absorptive surface of the jejunum, causing a surgically-induced malabsorption and diarrhea-induced nausea and anorexia which results in weight loss for the "treatment" of obesity. The procedure was used on more than 100,000 patients between the years 1954-1983 when it was discarded due to the high rates of clinically important post-operative complications, noted in up to 58% of patients. Interestingly, studying the rheumatologic complications of jejunoileal bypass contributed to scientific knowledge about the relationship of microbial dysbiosis and inflammatory diseases, particularly skin inflammation and joint inflammation; the authors write, "However, important advances in the understanding of inflammatory joing disease emerged from studies of the prominent rheumatological compliation of intestinal bypass known as the **arthritis-dermatitis syndrome**. Furthermore, the symptoms of "**bypass arthritis**" have been recognized in individuals who have not undergone intestinal bypass, but who had perturbations of intestinal anatomy secondary to postoperative, inflammatory or diverticular conditions." The pathophysiology of bypass arthritis-dermatitis syndrome is straightforward

Intestinal arthritis-dermatitis syndrome: rheumatic-inflammatory complications of gastrointestinal dysbiosis-induced systemic inflammation and immune complex deposition
1. **Arthritis***,‡—Most commonly of the peripheral joints but may also include the spine and sacroiliac joints; may be destructive or nondestructive, with or without RF and serologic evidence of immune complex mediation such as hypocomplimentemia.
2. **Dermatitis***,‡—"The most common non-articular inflammatory findings in patients with intestinal bypass arthritis involve the skin, reported in as many as 77% of patients." Rashes may be urticarial, maculopapular, papulovesicular or vesiculopustular affecting any part of the face, trunk or extremities.
3. Myalgia,
4. Myositis, polymyositis‡,
5. Pleuritis‡,
6. Pericarditis‡,
7. Raynaud's phenomenon‡,
8. Vasculitis, leukocytoclastic angiitis*,‡,
9. Oral ulceration‡,
10. Tenosynovitis,
11. Paresthesias, peripheral neuropathy*,
12. Carpal tunnel syndrome,

* Note that these are common clinical manifestations of underlying immune complex pathophysiology.
‡ Note that many of these clinical manifestations of bypass-induced intestinal dysbiosis are clinical manifestations of—and indeed components of the diagnostic criteria for—prototypic autoimmune diseases such as systemic lupus erythematosus.

Ross et al. Jejunoileal bypass arthritis. *Baillieres Clin Rheumatol.* 1989 Aug

and linear and easy to understand: ❶ altered intestinal structure and function leads to bacterial overgrowth and compromise of the intestinal mucosa, ❷ bacterial overgrowth and compromise of the intestinal mucosa leads to increased absorption of bacteria and bacterial antigens, perhaps as well as food antigens, ❸ increased absorption of bacteria and bacterial antigens leads to antibody formation, ❹ combination of bacterial antigens with antibodies leads to immune complex formation, ❺ immune complexes have a biologic proclivity for deposition in the joints, vessels, kidneys, skin, alveoli, and serosal surfaces, ❻ deposition of immune complex in any tissue results in a localized immune response with resultant inflammation regardless of the primary origin of the antigens from the overgrowth/overcolonization of bacteria. Per the authors, "The pathogenesis of intestinal bypass arthritis involves bacterial overgrowth and mucosal alterations in the defunctionalized segment of small intestine, ie, the 'blind loop'. ... "The blunted villi allow increased absorption of bacteria and bacterial products, leading to dissemination of high molecular weight immune complexes containing bacterial products." These "immune complexes of enteric antigens" are then deposited in the joints, skin, vessels, kidneys, and pulmonary alveoli to produce arthritis, dermatitis, vasculitis, nephritis, and pneumonitis, respectively.

---

[416] Ross CB, Scott HW, Pincus T. Jejunoileal bypass arthritis. *Baillieres Clin Rheumatol.* 1989 Aug;3(2):339-55

New-onset inflammatory joint symptoms are noted in 6-52% of patients following jejunoileal bypass. Most commonly the inflammatory arthritis is seen in females, and the presentation "mimics early rheumatoid arthriritis" with involvement of the hands, wrists, and knees and less commonly the spine and sacroiliac joints. Morning stiffness—a finding classic for inflammatory joint disease—is common. The arthritis is generally nondestructive; however, some post-bypass patients will develop periarticular erosions and sclerosis—findings common to rheumatoid arthritis. Tests for antinuclear antibodies (ANA), rheumatoid factor (RF), and serum complement are generally normal, but some patients will develop cryoglobulinemia due to immune

> **Dysbiosis-induced immune complex formation and deposition accounts for the primary underlying pathophysiology of bypass arthritis and arthritis-dermatitis syndrome**
>
> "The pathogenesis of intestinal bypass arthritis involves bacterial overgrowth and mucosal alterations in the defunctionalized segment of small intestine, ie, the 'blind loop'. ... "The blunted villi allow increased absorption of bacteria and bacterial products, leading to dissemination of high molecular weight immune complexes containing bacterial products." These "immune complexes of enteric antigens" are then deposited in the joints, skin, vessels, kidneys, and pulmonary alveoli to produce <u>arthritis</u>, <u>dermatitis</u>, <u>vasculitis</u>, <u>nephritis</u>, and <u>pneumonitis</u>, respectively.
>
> Ross et al. Jejunoileal bypass arthritis. *Baillieres Clin Rheumatol*. 1989 Aug

complex formation and others positive for HLA-B27 will develop spondylitis. "Therefore", the authors note in 1989, "the diagnosis of intestinal bypass arthritis remains primarily clinical." Very interestingly, one patient developed "classic rheumatoid arthritis with erosions and rheumatoid factors following jejunoileal bypass. ... ...the patient experienced complete remission of muculoskeletal disease soon after revision [surgical reversal] of the bypass..." The vast majority (up to 77%) of patients with bypass-induced dysbiotic arthritis develop skin inflammation alongside; "The most common non-articular inflammatory findings in patients with intestinal bypass arthritis involve the skin, reported in as many as 77% of patients. ... Typical rashes may be uricarial, maculopapular, papulovesicular or vesiculopustular... Any part of the face, trunk or extremities may be involved."

Beside and beyond the merely symptomatic treatments such as NSAIDs—which notoriously increase intestinal permeability and may therefore contribute to the pathophysiology of intestinal dysbiosis—ultimate treatments for bypass dermatitis-arthitis syndrome are either antimicrobial therapy to eradicate the intestinal bacterial overgrowth or surgical restoration of the original intestinal anatomy. Impressively, surgical restoration of normal anatomy can completely resolve the condition within 48 hours, thereby proving the cause-and-effect relationship. **Broad-spectrum antimicrobial drugs are use empirically: tetracycline, metronidazole, trimethoprim/sulphamethoxazole, and clindamycin.** Oral corticosteroids may be used to help control the inflammation; adverse effects including exacerbation of diabetes and hypertension, as well as promotion of additional bacterial overgrowth due to intestinal immunosuppression are well-known. Importantly, "bowel bypass disease without bowel bypass" can occur secondary to any condition that promotes bacterial overgrowth of the intestines and the resultant immune complex formation; the term used to describe this phenomenon is "bowel-associated dermatitis and arthritis."

- <u>Pro-inflammatory effect of *Lactobacillus rhamnosus Lcr35* (*PLoS One* 2011 Apr[417])</u>: This experimental study shows that some intestinal bacteria—in this case, a specific strain of *Lactobacillus* identified as *Lactobacillus rhamnosus Lcr35*—can incite a proinflammatory effect. The possibility exists that the physiologic consequences of an individual bacteria might be different *in vivo* when intermixed with the effects of other microbes; however, the most reasonable

---

[417] Evrard B, Coudeyras S, Dosgilbert A, Charbonnel N, Alamé J, Tridon A, Forestier C. Dose-Dependent Immunomodulation of Human Dendritic Cells by the Probiotic Lactobacillus rhamnosus Lcr35. *PLoS One*. 2011 Apr 18;6(4):e18735

interpretation of this data is that *Lactobacillus rhamnosus* promotes inflammation and should therefore be avoided in patients already experiencing excessive inflammation. The authors introduce their paper appropriately by stating, "Some [probiotic] strains modulate the cytokine production of dendritic cells (DCs) in vitro and induce a regulatory response, while others induce conversely a pro-inflammatory response." Results of this experiement showed that, by use of DNA microarray and qRT-PCR analysis, the probiotic induced a large-scale change in gene expression (nearly 1,700 modulated genes, with 3-fold changes), but only with high doses (multiplicity of infection [MOI] of 100x [range 0.01 to 100]). Flow cytometry analysis showed an upregulated expression of CD86, CD83, HLA-DR and TLR4 and reduced expression of DC-SIGN, MR and CD14. Cytokine measurements showed strong dose-dependent increases in pro-Th1/Th17 cytokine levels (TNFα, IL-1β, IL-12p70, IL-12p40 and IL-23) contrasted with only a slight increase in antiinflammatory IL-10. The authors concluded therefore that, "The probiotic *L. rhamnosus* Lcr35 [leads to], at high doses, to the semi-maturation of the [dendritic] cells and to a strong pro-inflammatory effect." This article is noteworthy for showing the molecular evidence of dose-dependent inflammation induction by a bacterium generally considered to be among a group of benefical bacteria; many people consider "*Lactobacillus*" as a group to be exclusively beneficial while this evidence demonstrates pro-inflammatory effects. Bacterial overgrowth of the small bowel (aka, small intestine bacterial overgrowth [SIBO]) commonly includes a mix of Gram-negatives with Gram-positives, anaerobes with aerobes, and so-called "beneficial" bacteria along with pathogens and potential pathogens.

14. <u>Damage to the intestinal mucosa</u>: One of the indirect ways by which gastrointestinal microbes can cause non-infectious disease is by damaging the intestinal mucosa, a situation which results in "leaky gut." The increased absorption of molecular debris from the gut—"antigen overload" from otherwise benign yeast, bacteria, and foods—results in systemic inflammation[418] and immune activation[419], which contribute to enhanced autoantigen processing and bystander activation as discussed above. Exacerbations and relapse of the autoimmune diseases ulcerative colitis and Crohn's disease are preceded by increases in intestinal permeability; this is direct evidence of "leaky gut" preceding clinical disease.[420] Evidence of "leaky gut" is seen in several systemic inflammatory disorders, including asthma[421], eczema[422], psoriasis[423], Behcet's disease[424], seronegative spondyloarthritis[425] and ankylosing spondylitis[426] and nearly all of the so-called "idiopathic" juvenile arthropathies such as enteropathic spondyloarthropathy and oligoarticular juvenile idiopathic arthritis.[427] A "leaky gut" type of intestinal disease (protein-losing enteropathy) has also been documented in some patients with lupus.[428]

- <u>Psoriasis and intestinal permeability</u>—<u>!ntestinal permeability in patients with psoriasis (*J Dermatol Sci* 1991 Jul[429])</u>: In this study of 15 psoriatic patients and 15 healthy volunteers, intestinal permeability was evaluated using the 51Cr-labeled EDTA absorption test. 24-h urine excretion

[418] Campbell DI, Elia M, Lunn PG. Growth faltering in rural Gambian infants is associated with impaired small intestinal barrier function, leading to endotoxemia and systemic inflammation. *J Nutr*. 2003 May;133(5):1332-8

[419] "Altered gastrointestinal motility and sensation, changed activity of the central nervous system, and increased sympathetic drive and immune activation may be understood as consequences of the host response to SIBO." Lin HC. Small intestinal bacterial overgrowth: a framework for understanding irritable bowel syndrome. *JAMA*. 2004 Aug 18;292(7):852-8

[420] Wyatt J, Vogelsang H, Hubl W, Waldhoer T, Lochs H. Intestinal permeability and the prediction of relapse in Crohn's disease. *Lancet*. 1993 Jun 5;341(8858):1437-9

[421] Hijazi Z, Molla AM, Al-Habashi H, Muawad WM, Molla AM, Sharma PN. Intestinal permeability is increased in bronchial asthma. *Arch Dis Child*. 2004 Mar;89(3):227-9

[422] Ukabam SO, Mann RJ, Cooper BT. Small intestinal permeability to sugars in patients with atopic eczema. *Br J Dermatol*. 1984 Jun;110(6):649-52

[423] "The 24-h urine excretion of 51Cr-EDTA from psoriatic patients was 2.46 +/- 0.81%. These results differed significantly from controls (1.95 +/- 0.36%; P less than 0.05)." Humbert P, Bidet A, Treffel P, Drobacheff C, Agache P. Intestinal permeability in patients with psoriasis. *J Dermatol Sci*. 1991 Jul;2(4):324-6

[424] Fresko I, Hamuryudan V, Demir M, Hizli N, Sayman H, Melikoglu M, Tunc R, Yurdakul S, Yazici H. Intestinal permeability in Behcet's syndrome. *Ann Rheum Dis*. 2001 Jan;60(1):65-6

[425] Di Leo V, D'Inca R, Bettini MB, Podswiadek M, Punzi L, Mastropaolo G, Sturniolo GC. Effect of Helicobacter pylori and eradication therapy on gastrointestinal permeability. Implications for patients with seronegative spondyloarthritis. *J Rheumatol*. 2005 Feb;32(2):295-300

[426] "Patients with AS have altered small intestinal, but not gastric, permeability. NSAID use cannot explain all the abnormality. Bowel permeability abnormalities, possibly genetically determined, may antedate development of bowel or joint symptoms." Vaile JH, Meddings JB, Yacyshyn BR, Russell AS, Maksymowych WP. Bowel permeability and CD45RO expression on circulating CD20+ B cells in patients with ankylosing spondylitis and their relatives. *J Rheumatol*. 1999 Jan;26(1):128-35

[427] Picco P, Gattorno M, Marchese N, Vignola S, Sormani MP, Barabino A, Buoncompagni A. Increased gut permeability in juvenile chronic arthritides. A multivariate analysis of the diagnostic parameters. *Clin Exp Rheumatol*. 2000 Nov-Dec;18(6):773-8

[428] "Fourteen cases of primary lupus-associated protein-losing enteropathy have now been reported in the English-language literature." Perednia DA, Curosh NA. Lupus-associated protein-losing enteropathy. *Arch Intern Med*. 1990 Sep;150(9):1806-10

[429] Humbert P, Bidet A, Treffel P, Drobacheff C, Agache P. Intestinal permeability in patients with psoriasis. *J Dermatol Sci*. 1991 Jul;2(4):324-6

of 51Cr-EDTA from psoriatic patients was 2.46% which was significantly higher than the results from controls at 1.95% and therefore indicated increased intestinal permeability among patients with psoriasis. Clinical implications of these results include 1) that psoriasis not merely a skin condition and that it affects other vital structures, in this instance, the gastrointestinal tract, and 2) that enhanced intestinal absorption of food antigens and microbial metabolites and immunogenic debris is ensured among psoriatic patients and would be expected to contribute to systemic inflammation and immunologic sensitization. This study was published in 1991 and used urinary measurement of orally administered 51Cr-EDTA to determine intestinal permeability; in modern outpatient practice, we use the lactulose-mannitol assay as a more sensitive and reliable indicator of mucosal permeability status.

- <u>Skin diseases and intestinal permeability</u>—Small intestinal permeability in dermatological disease (*Quarterly Journal of Medicine* 1985 Sep[430]): The authors of this study assessed small intestinal permeability using the cellobiose/mannitol differential sugar absorption test (using urinary excretion of absorbed cellobiose and mannitol to determine intestinal permeability). Test subjects included 62 patients with atopic eczema, 29 with psoriasis, and 18 with dermatitis herpetiformis. Results of testing were *generally* unremarkable among *most* psoriatics and eczema patients when compared to the control population. However, some patients showed distinct abnormalities. Among the 62 patients with eczema, 7 (11%) had abnormal cellobiose/mannitol absorption as measured by urinary excretion; 6 of these patients underwent jejunal biopsy, and one patient was found to have celiac disease. Among the 29 patients with psoriasis, 7 (24%) had abnormal cellobiose/mannitol recovery. Among the 18 patients with dermatitis herpetiformis, 11 (61%) had abnormal cellobiose/mannitol recovery; this is not surprising give the intimate causative association between celiac disease and dermatitis herpetiformis. Thus, reasonable interpretations of this data are that ❶ a clinically significant number of patients with eczema, psoriasis, and dermatitis herpetiforms have abnormal intestinal permeability, ❷ that these "skin conditions" and apperant "dermatological diseases" are systemic disorders which commonly occur with gastrointestinal components, and ❸ given the important role of intestinal mucosa integrity as a barometer of health and as a determinant of systemic inflammation and immune responses, attention to gastrointestinal (dys)function in these patients is worthy of additional investigation by researchers and attention by clinicians. This study was published in 1985 and used urinary measurement of orally administered cellobiose and mannitol to determine intestinal permeability; in modern outpatient practice, we use the lactulose and mannitol assay as a more sensitive and reliable indicator of mucosal permeability status.

---

[430] Hamilton I, Fairris GM, Rothwell J, Cunliffe WJ, Dixon MF, Axon AT. Small intestinal permeability in dermatological disease. *Q J Med.* 1985 Sep;56(221):559-67

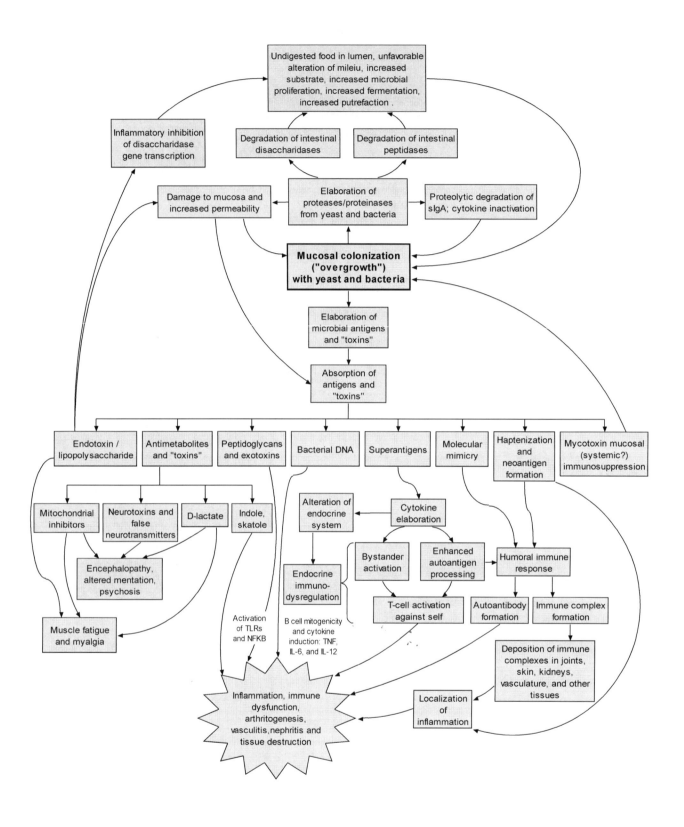

Schematic Representation of the Interconnected Physiologic Pathways Involved in Dysbiosis-Induced musculoskeletal Inflammation and "Autoimmunity"

15. <u>Insufficiency dysbiosis—an absolute or relative lack of benefical bacteria</u>: Clinicians performing stool tests on a regular basis—current author included—common find that patients simultaneously have—in addition to other problems—"too many bad bacteria and not enough good bacteria", as is commonly explained to patients. Benefical bacteria in general but particularly those in the gastrointestinal tract exert many positive benefits for the host which might be summarized as follows: ❶ maintaining the health and permeability integrity of the mucosa, ❷ providing fuel—butyrate—for enterocytes and specifically colonocytes, ❸ maintaining a slightly acidic pH due to elaboration of metabolic acids, ❹ blocking colonization by harmful yeasts and bacteria via several mechanisms such as by *directly* producing antimicrobial factors and *indirectly* inducing enhanced secretion of secretory IgA from mucosal plasma cells, ❺ metabolism/processing of phytonutrients for absorption and enhanced physiologic function, ❻ co-feeding other probiotic bacteria, for example, bifidobacteria convert carbohydrate substrate to lactate and acetate which are then further metabolized by *Lactobaccilus* into butyrate; in this way, probiotic bacteria "support each other" and are dependent/interdependent, ❼

> ## Probiotic mutualism via cross-feeding ultimately affects human gene expression, enterocyte health, and intestinal permeability
>
> Oral supplementation with synbiotics provides inulin and fructooligosaccharides to *Bifidobacterium* and *Lactobacillus* which partially metabolize carbohydrate substrates to acetate and lactate which then serve as substrate for butyrogenic microbes such as *Roseburia intestinalis* and *Anaerostipes caccae* for the production of butyrate, which provides anti-inflammatory nutrigenomic benefits via suppression of NF-kappaB, serves as a major fuel source for enterocytes especially colonocytes, and improves epithelial barrier integrity by modulating the expression of certain tight junction proteins such as cingulin, intercellular ZO (zonula occludens) proteins, and occludin. In this way, one can see how food intake influences/supports microbial mutualism for production of a metabolite that affects the tissue physiology and cellular molecular biology of the human host.
>
> Bosscher et al. Food-based strategies to modulate the composition of the intestinal microbiota and their associated health effects. *J Physiol Pharmacol.* 2009 Dec

maintaining a favorable biochemical and immunologic milieu for other benefical bacteria, ❽ promoting elaboration of anti-inflammatory cytokines and suppression of pro-inflammatory cytokines, specifically inducing tolerogenic DCs producing lowered amounts of pro-inflammatory IFN-gamma and elevated amounts of anti-inflammatory IL-10, ❾ helping to ameliorate allergy in general and food allergy in particular by the above mechanisms, and ❿ promoting maturation of undifferentiated/naïve T-cells into regulatory T-cells (Treg) for the suppression/modulation of pro-inflammatory Th17-cells which are some of the primary pathologic effectors of autoimmune-mediated tissue damage, particularly in multiple sclerosis. Induction of Foxp3+ Treg from mature Th2-type memory T-cells by use of combination treatment including retinoic acid (an active form of vitamin A) has been performed experimentally[431], probably occurs in vivo in humans, and is reviewed elsewhere in this book. Several of these aforementioned mechanisms are well-known and/or self-evident; however, induction of Treg by probiotics is a relatively new concept and is of supreme clinical importance and will be given additional detail here:

- <u>Probiotic induction of Treg and DCreg: Generation of regulatory dendritic cells and CD4+Foxp3+ T cells by probiotics administration suppresses immune disorders (*Proc Natl Acad Sci USA* 2010 Feb[432])</u>: In this study, the authors used a probiotic mixture which was found to achieve several very important goals: ❶ up-regulate CD4(+)Foxp3(+) regulatory T cells (Tregs) from the CD4(+)CD25(-) population, ❷ induced both T-cell and B-cell hyporesponsiveness, ❸ down-regulated T helper (Th) 1, Th2, and Th17 cytokines without apoptosis induction—the significance here is that the goal is to regulate and modulate the immune system, not induce death in key

---

[431] Kim BS, Kim IK, Park YJ, Kim YS, Kim YJ, Chang WS, Lee YS, Kweon MN, Chung Y, Kang CY. Conversion of Th2 memory cells into Foxp3+ regulatory T cells suppressing Th2-mediated allergic asthma. *Proc Natl Acad Sci USA.* 2010 May 11;107(19):8742-7

[432] Kwon HK, Lee CG, So JS, Chae CS, Hwang JS, Sahoo A, Nam JH, Rhee JH, Hwang KC, Im SH. Generation of regulatory dendritic cells and CD4+Foxp3+ T cells by probiotics administration suppresses immune disorders. *Proc Natl Acad Sci USA.* 2010 Feb 2;107(5):2159-64

elements, and ❹ increased the suppressor activity of naturally occurring CD4(+)CD25(+) Tregs. The authors note that conversion of T-cells into Foxp3(+) Tregs is directly mediated by regulatory dendritic cells (DCreg) that express high levels of IL-10, TGF-beta, COX-2, and indoleamine 2,3-dioxygenase (IDO)—an enzyme involved in tryptophan degradation and the expression of which is very important for the formation of DCregs and therefore Tregs—and they also note that therapeutic benefits in animal models of experimental inflammatory bowel disease, atopic dermatitis, and rheumatoid arthritis is associated with and likely directly due to the enrichment of CD4(+)Foxp3(+) Tregs in the inflamed regions, following their maturation/promotion in the environement of the GALT—gut-associated lymphoid tissue.

- Probiotic induction of anti-inflammatory IL-10: Oral probiotic administration induces interleukin-10 production and prevents spontaneous autoimmune diabetes in the NOD mouse (_Diabetologia_ 2005 Aug[433]): Researchers used the probiotic supplement VSL#3 on diabetes-prone mice (the non-obese diabetic [NOD] mouse develops a spontaneous form of autoimmune diabetes similar to the human disease). Results showed that probiotic administration prevented diabetes development in NOD mice and that the mice treated with the probiotic "showed reduced insulitis and a decreased rate of beta cell destruction. Prevention was associated with an increased production of IL-10 from Peyer's patches and the spleen and with increased IL-10 expression in the pancreas, where IL-10-positive islet-infiltrating mononuclear cells were detected." This is a very interesting experiment showing that marrow-derrived immunocytes are re-programmed in gut-associated lymphoid tissue (GALT) and subsequently redistribute to the periphery to effect cellular immunomodulation and thereby prevent autoimmune-mediated tissue injury.

- Probiotic induction via IL-10 of Treg: Alleviation of experimental autoimmune encephalomyelitis by probiotics (_PLoS One_ 2010 Feb[434]): Experimental autoimmune encephalomyelitis (EAE) is the experimental animal model of the human disease multiple sclerosis (MS), a chronic inflammatory autoimmune disease of the central nervous system (CNS). The authors note that, "One potential therapeutic strategy for MS is to induce regulatory cells that mediate immunological tolerance." Probiotics, including lactobacilli, have been shown to have immunomodulatory activity. Accordingly, they tested various _Lactobacillus_ strains for suppression of EAE; tested strains included _L. paracasei DSM 13434, L. plantarum DSM 15312_ and _DSM 15313_, each of which reduced inflammation in CNS and autoreactive T cell responses. The research showed that "_**L. paracasei** and **L. plantarum DSM 15312** induced_ **CD4(+)CD25(+)Foxp3(+) regulatory T cells (Tregs)** in mesenteric lymph nodes (MLNs) and enhanced production of serum TGF-beta1, while _**L. plantarum DSM 15313** increased serum IL-27 levels._" Work by other researchers has shown that IL-27 suppresses Th17 activity while apparently promoting Th1 activity. Very interestingly and of high clinical importance is the finding that "each monostrain probiotic failed to be therapeutic in diseased mice, while a mixture of the three lactobacilli strains suppressed the progression and reversed the clinical and histological signs of EAE." As would be expected in a classic scenario, _Lactobacillus_-induced suppressive activity "correlated with attenuation of pro-inflammatory Th1 and Th17 cytokines followed by IL-10 induction in MLNs, spleen and blood." In a separate experiment, the researchers showed **that IL-10-producing CD4(+)CD25(+) Tregs played the main role in the anti-inflammatory effects induced by probiotic administration**.

[433] Calcinaro F, Dionisi S, Marinaro M, Candeloro P, Bonato V, Marzotti S, Corneli RB, Ferretti E, Gulino A, Grasso F, De Simone C, Di Mario U, Falorni A, Boirivant M, Dotta F. Oral probiotic administration induces interleukin-10 production and prevents spontaneous autoimmune diabetes in the non-obese diabetic mouse. _Diabetologia._ 2005 Aug;48(8):1565-75
[434] Lavasani S, Dzhambazov B, Nouri M, Fåk F, Buske S, Molin G, Thorlacius H, Alenfall J, Jeppsson B, Weström B. A novel probiotic mixture exerts a therapeutic effect on experimental autoimmune encephalomyelitis mediated by IL-10 producing regulatory T cells. _PLoS One._ 2010 Feb 2;5(2):e9009

16. <u>Inhibition of detoxification</u>: **All clinicians must appreciate that bioaccumulation of toxic chemicals can cause autoimmunity.**[435,436,437] Examples of this include the increased autoimmunity seen in humans exposed to pesticides[438,439], the scleroderma-like disease that results from exposure to vinyl chloride[440], the association of mercury and pesticide exposure with lupus[441], and the well-recognized connection between drug and chemical exposure and various autoimmune syndromes such as drug-induced lupus.[442] Indeed, more than 40 pharmaceutical drugs are known to cause drug-induced lupus, and bystander activation appears to be one of the primary mechanisms involved.[443] Thus having established the general premise that *chemical exposure can cause autoimmune disease*, it seems logical and probable that

> **Immune alteration associated with exposure to toxic chemicals**
>
> "Autoimmunity due to chemical exposure was evidenced by elevation of TA1 phenotype frequencies and presence of rheumatoid factor, immune complexes, ANA, and antimyelin basic protein antibodies. **We conclude that chemical exposure may induce immune abnormalities including immune suppression and autoimmunity.**"
>
> Vojdani et al. Immune alteration associated with exposure to toxic chemicals. *Toxicol Ind Health*. 1992 Sep-Oct

anything which would inhibit the body's ability to detoxify these chemicals would likewise increase the risk for autoimmunity. Stated differently, factors that inhibit detoxification and which therefore increase the body-burden of immunotoxic xenobiotics would serve to indirectly contribute to immunodysfunction and the resultant autoimmunity. Indeed, **patients with lupus and systemic sclerosis show defects in detoxification**[444], **and different detoxification defects have been documented in patients with ankylosing spondylitis.**[445] Surmounting detoxification defects and xenobiotic exposure by the use of comprehensive detoxification programs (discussed later) is clinically beneficial.[446,447,448,449] Dysbiotic bacterial overgrowth of the gastrointestinal tract directly impairs detoxification via the following four mechanisms:

[435] "Autoimmunity due to chemical exposure was evidenced by elevation of TA1 phenotype frequencies and presence of rheumatoid factor, immune complexes, ANA, and anti myelin basic protein antibodies. We conclude that chemical exposure may induce immune abnormalities including immune suppression and autoimmunity." Vojdani A, Ghoneum M, Brautbar N. Immune alteration associated with exposure to toxic chemicals. *Toxicol Ind Health* 1992;8:239-253

[436] Crinnion WJ. Results of a decade of naturopathic treatment for environmental illnesses. *J Naturopathic Med* 1994;17:21-27

[437] Crinnion WJ. Environmental medicine, part one: the human burden of environmental toxins and their common health effects. *Altern Med Rev*. 2000 Feb;5(1):52-63 http://www.thorne.com/altmedrev/.fulltext/5/1/52.pdf See also: Crinnion WJ. Environmental medicine, part 2 - health effects of and protection from ubiquitous airborne solvent exposure. *Altern Med Rev*. 2000 Apr;5(2):133-43 http://www.thorne.com/altmedrev/.fulltext/5/2/133.pdf

[438] "IgG levels decreased with increasing p,p'-DDE levels, with a statistically significant decrease of approximately 50% in the highest two categories of exposure. Sixteen (12%) were positive for antinuclear antibodies... These analyses provide evidence that p,p'-DDE modulates immune responses in humans." Cooper GS, Martin SA, Longnecker MP, Sandler DP, Germolec DR. Associations between plasma DDE levels and immunologic measures in African-American farmers in North Carolina. *Environ Health Perspect*. 2004 Jul;112(10):1080-4

[439] "Twelve individuals who were exposed to chlorpyrifos were studied 1-4.5 y following exposure to determine changes in the peripheral immune system. The subjects were found to have a high rate of atopy and antibiotic sensitivities, elevated CD26 cells (p < .01), and a higher rate of autoimmunity, compared with two control groups." Thrasher JO, Madison R, Broughton A. Immunologic abnormalities in humans exposed to chlorpyrifos: preliminary observations. *Arch Environ Health* 1993;48:89-93

[440] "Vinyl chloride (VC) monomer can induce a scleroderma-like syndrome in a proportion of workers exposed to it during production of polyvinyl chloride." Black CM, Welsh KI, Walker AE, Bernstein RM, Catoggio LJ, McGregor AR, Jones JK. Genetic susceptibility to scleroderma-like syndrome induced by vinyl chloride. *Lancet*. 1983 Jan 1;1(8314-5):53-5

[441] "...reported occupational exposure to mercury (OR 3.6), mixing pesticides for agricultural work (OR 7.4), and among dental workers (OR 7.1, 95% CI 2.2, 23.4). ...these associations were fairly strong and statistically significant..." Cooper GS, Parks CG, Treadwell EL, St Clair EW, Gilkeson GS, Dooley MA. Occupational risk factors for the development of systemic lupus erythematosus. *J Rheumatol*. 2004 Oct;31(10):1928-33

[442] Hess EV. Environmental chemicals and autoimmune disease: cause and effect. *Toxicology*. 2002 Dec 27;181-182:65-70

[443] "Drug-induced lupus has been reported as a side-effect of long-term therapy with over 40 medications... Several mechanisms for induction of autoimmunity will be discussed, including bystander activation of autoreactive lymphocytes due to drug-specific immunity or to non-specific activation of lymphocytes, direct cytotoxicity with release of autoantigens ..." Rubin RL. Drug-induced lupus. *Toxicology*. 2005;209(2):135-47

[444] "The observed increased frequencies of the CYP1A1 mutant Val-allele and the slow acetylator phenotype in idiopathic autoimmune disease support our concept that in slow acetylators non-acetylated xenobiotics may accumulate and are subsequently metabolized by other enzymes into reactive intermediates. Thus, enhanced formation of reactive metabolites could alter self-proteins..." von Schmiedeberg S, Fritsche E, Ronnau AC, Specker C, Golka K, Richter-Hintz D, Schuppe HC, Lehmann P, Ruzicka T, Esser C, Abel J, Gleichmann E. Polymorphisms of the xenobiotic-metabolizing enzymes CYP1A1 and NAT-2 in systemic sclerosis and lupus erythematosus. *Adv Exp Med Biol*. 1999;455:147-52

[445] "Homozygosity for poor metabolizer alleles was found to be associated with AS... Significant within-family association of CYP2D6*4 alleles and AS was demonstrated. Weak linkage was also demonstrated between CYP2D6 and AS. We postulate that altered metabolism of a natural toxin or antigen by the CYP2D6 gene may increase susceptibility to AS." Brown MA, Edwards S, Hoyle E, Campbell S, Laval S, Daly AK, Pile KD, Calin A, Ebringer A, Weeks DE, Wordsworth BP. Polymorphisms of the CYP2D6 gene increase susceptibility to ankylosing spondylitis. *Hum Mol Genet*. 2000 Jul 1;9(11):1563-6 http://hmg.oxfordjournals.org/cgi/content/full/9/11/1563

[446] Crinnion WJ. Results of a decade of naturopathic treatment for environmental illnesses. *J Naturopathic Med* 1994;17:21-27

[447] Crinnion WJ. Environmental medicine, part one: the human burden of environmental toxins and their common health effects. *Altern Med Rev*. 2000 Feb;5(1):52-63 http://www.thorne.com/altmedrev/.fulltext/5/1/52.pdf See also: Crinnion WJ. Environmental medicine, part 2 - health effects of and protection from ubiquitous airborne solvent exposure. *Altern Med Rev*. 2000 Apr;5(2):133-43 http://www.thorne.com/altmedrev/.fulltext/5/2/133.pdf

[448] Krop J. Chemical sensitivity after intoxication at work with solvents: response to sauna therapy. *J Altern Complement Med*. 1998 Spring;4(1):77-86

[449] "Retesting following the detoxification program showed significantly improved scores on: three memory tests, block design, trails B, and embedded figures. Thus, there was significant reversibility of impairment after the detoxification interval." Kilburn KH, Warsaw RH, Shields MG. Neurobehavioral dysfunction in firemen exposed to polychlorinated biphenyls (PCBs): possible improvement after detoxification. *Arch Environ Health*. 1989 Nov-Dec;44(6):345-50

❶ cP450/phase-1 inhibition: Bacterial lipopolysaccharide (endotoxin) has been shown to significantly impair Phase 1 of chemical detoxification.[450] Obviously when major cytochrome p450 pathways are inhibited by endotoxin, then detoxification/biotransformation of xenobiotics and drugs is greatly impaired.[451]

❷ Deconjugation and enterohepatic recirculation: Several species of bacteria produce deconjugating enzymes (such as beta-glucuronidase) that cleave previously "detoxified" toxins from their water-soluble moieties thus allowing the toxin to be reabsorbed in a mechanism termed "enterohepatic recycling"[452] or "enterohepatic recirculation."[453]

❸ Increased intestinal permeability: Damage to the intestinal mucosa increases absorption of intraluminal contents and thus increase the toxic load placed on the detoxification mechanisms, which are mostly located in the liver; eventually these pathways become depleted, rendering the host susceptible to the consequences of nutritional depletion and impaired detoxification.[454]

❹ Constipation: Bacterial overgrowth can lead to excess production of methane which causes constipation[455] and thus increases the "toxic load" in the colon which then increases the load on the liver via the portal circulation. Likewise, hydrogen sulfide also promotes constipation; however, often, constipation leads to laxation/diarrhea once a sufficient amount of microbial toxins/debris/metabolites have accumulated.

Taken together, these enterometabolic mechanisms are consistent with the observance of increased risk for xenobiotic-associated diseases such as breast cancer[456,457] and Parkinson's disease[458,459] in patients with chronic constipation. With regard to Phase-1 acetylation, Evans[460] noted in a review published in 1984 that slow acetylation has been strongly noted in patients with Gilbert's disease and also bladder cancer, whereas the rapid acetylator phenotype is associated with diabetes mellitus. We would expect that patients with endotoxin-producing bacterial overgrowth of the small intestine would be more susceptible to the chemical accumulation that leads to multiple chemical sensitivity syndrome (MCS) and the xenobiotic-induced immune dysfunction that may result. In my own clinical practice, I have seen many patients with **multiple chemical sensitivity** respond very favorably to the eradication of their intestinal bacterial overgrowth, and I consider this treatment essential for all patients with autoimmune disease.

- Psoriasis—Genetic variants in drug metabolizing enzymes as risk factors for psoriasis (*Journal of Investigative Dermatology* 2003 May[461]): Foreign chemicals (xenobiotics) and drugs such as antimalarials and beta-blockers can trigger the onset or exacerbation of psoriasis; other exposures such as lithium, ACE inhibitors, nonsteroidal anti-inflammatory drugs, terbinacne, cigarette smoking, and heavy consumption of alcohol are also associated with the onset and exacerbation of psoriasis. Abnormalities in detoxification processes, such as different metabolic efficiencies caused by variant alleles of xenobiotic metabolizing enzymes, often leads to the accumulation of

[450] Shedlofsky SI, Israel BC, McClain CJ, Hill DB, Blouin RA. Endotoxin administration to humans inhibits hepatic cytochrome P450-mediated drug metabolism. *J Clin Invest*. 1994 Dec;94(6):2209-14 http://www.pubmedcentral.nih.gov.proxy.hsc.unt.edu/articlerender.fcgi?tool=pubmed&pubmedid=7989576

[451] "CONCLUSIONS: These data show that endotoxin-induced inflammation decreases hepatic cytochrome P450-mediated metabolism of selected probe drugs in women as it does in men." Shedlofsky SI, Israel BC, Tosheva R, Blouin RA. Endotoxin depresses hepatic cytochrome P450-mediated drug metabolism in women. *Br J Clin Pharmacol*. 1997 Jun;43(6):627-32

[452] "Enterohepatic recycling occurs by biliary excretion and intestinal reabsorption of a solute, sometimes with hepatic conjugation and intestinal deconjugation. ... Of particular importance is the potential amplifying effect of enterohepatic variability in defining differences in the bioavailability, apparent volume of distribution and clearance of a given compound." Roberts MS, Magnusson BM, Burczynski FJ, Weiss M. Enterohepatic circulation: physiological, pharmacokinetic and clinical implications. *Clin Pharmacokinet*. 2002;41(10):751-90

[453] Liska DJ. The detoxification enzyme systems. *Altern Med Rev*. 1998 Jun;3(3):187-98

[454] Lunn PG, Northrop-Clewes CA, Downes RM. Intestinal permeability, mucosal injury, and growth faltering in Gambian infants. *Lancet*. 1991 Oct 12;338(8772):907-1

[455] Lin HC. Small intestinal bacterial overgrowth: a framework for understanding irritable bowel syndrome. *JAMA*. 2004 Aug 18;292(7):852-8

[456] "These observations are consistent with an hypothesized association between constipation and increased risk of breast cancer." Micozzi MS, Carter CL, Albanes D, Taylor PR, Licitra LM. Bowel function and breast cancer in US women. *Am J Public Health*. 1989 Jan;79(1):73-5

[457] Petrakis NL, King EB. Cytological abnormalities in nipple aspirates of breast fluid from women with severe constipation. *Lancet*. 1981 Nov 28;2(8257):1203-4

[458] "...lower frequency bowel movements predict the future risk of PD. ...They also hypothesize that some yet undefined toxins break through the mucosal barrier of the intestine and are incorporated into the axon terminal of the vagus nerve and transported in a retrograde manner to the vagus nucleus." Ueki A, Otsuka M. Life style risks of Parkinson's disease: association between decreased water intake and constipation. *J Neurol*. 2004 Oct;251 Suppl 7:vII18-23

[459] "CONCLUSIONS: Findings indicate that infrequent bowel movements are associated with an elevated risk of future PD." Abbott RD, Petrovitch H, White LR, Masaki KH, Tanner CM, Curb JD, Grandinetti A, Blanchette PL, Popper JS, Ross GW. Frequency of bowel movements and the future risk of Parkinson's disease. *Neurology*. 2001 Aug 14;57(3):456-62

[460] Evans DA. Survey of the human acetylator polymorphism in spontaneous disorders. *J Med Genet*. 1984 Aug;21(4):243-53

[461] Richter-Hintz D, Their R, Steinwachs S, Kronenberg S, Fritsche E, Sachs B, Wulferink M, Tonn T, Esser C. Allelic variants of drug metabolizing enzymes as risk factors in psoriasis. *Journal of Investigative Dermatology*. 2003 May;120(5):765-70 http://www.nature.com/jid/journal/v120/n5/pdf/5601800a.pdf

xenobiotics and/or their reactive metabolites. Accumulation of xenobiotics and/or their metabolites in tissues can result in the formation of neoantigens (ie, haptens) and/or the exposure of cryptic peptides (eg, autoantigens); these neoantigens and exposed autoantigens can then initiate and stimulate an aggressive T-cell response, resulting in tissue inflammation and injury. In this study, the authors analyzed xenobiotic-metabolizing enzymes in 327 Caucasian psoriasis patients and 235 control persons. Gene variants were tested for four phase I (oxidation) enzymes and three phase II (conjugation) enzymes. CYP1A1 alleles *2A and *2C were found more often in healthy controls, suggesting a protective role for these gene variants. The authors note that no significant difference between patients and controls could be found for the phase I alleles 1B1*1, 1B1*3, 2E1*1A, and 2E1*5B nor for the phase II enzymes GSTT1 or NQOR when considered in isolation. However, an increased risk for psoriasis was associated with genetic variations in GSTM1 and with heterozygosity for CYP2C19 alleles *1A and *2A. The combination of CYP1A1*1A (reduced enzyme activity) with CYP2C19*1A increased the odds ratio (OR) in favor of psoriasis by 3.3 (OR=3.3) while the combination of CYP1A1*1A with GSTM1 increased the OR to 4.84. CYP1A1*2C encodes for an enzyme of greater detoxification activity and reduces the risk for developing psoriasis (OR=0.44). The authors conclude, "This is the first large-scale study on these enzymes and the results obtained support the concept that **different activities of metabolizing enzymes can contribute to disease etiology and progression**." This article supports the concept that genetic/inheritable abnormalities in detoxification abilities can increase the risk for developing psoriasis; if the increased risk is indeed due to the defective detoxification and not due to the gene products themselves per se, then any condition—importantly for this discussion the influence of bacteria—that alters detoxification could also increase the risk for psoriasis. The best singular example of this reality is the inhibition of CYP enzymes by bacterial endotoxin/lipopolysaccharide.

- Psoriasis—Evidence of impaired Phase-1 acetylation in psoriatics and psoriatics with psoriatic siblings (*Dermatologica* 1989[462]): Researchers conducting this study assessed acetylation ability using sulfamethazine as a probe in 64 psoriatic patients and in. Among the 157 normal

---

Impaired detoxification and illness

Clinically, three patterns of impaired detoxification are important and are particularly worthy of our understanding and appreciation:

1. Slow CYP activation: If "Phase-1" is slow, then toxins cannot be cleared from the system, and they accumulate. This leads to adverse effects from the toxins or the medications to which the patient is exposed. Patients with slow CYP activation are prone to adverse medication responses and environmental sensitivity because they are unable to normally clear drugs and chemicals from their system.

2. Fast CYP activation: If "Phase-1" is too fast, then toxins are converted into "reactive intermediates" which can bind to DNA or other cellular structures, resulting in genetic mutations or neoantigenization/haptenization. Patients with too-fast CYP activation may have more beneficial or adverse effects from medication if taking a medication that requires activation by the liver for function, or they may have less beneficial or adverse effects from medication if taking a medication that is inactivated by CYP oxidation.

3. Slow Phase-2 conjugation: Conjugation is the second phase of detoxification following Phase-1 oxidation. If Phase-2 is too slow in relation to Phase-1, we call this "imbalanced detoxification" or "pathological detoxification" because the reactive intermediates produced from Phase-1 oxidation cannot be cleared from the body yet are capable of binding to DNA and other vitally crucial cellular structures. Patients with slow Phase-2 conjugation are prone to adverse medication responses and environmental sensitivity because they are unable to normally clear drugs and chemicals from their system.

Variations in the rate and therefore quality and quantity of detoxification can be induced by genetic variations or by factors in the environment such as chemical exposures, gastrointestinal dysbiosis, nutrient status, and the consumption of specific foods. Each component of detoxification has several different subcomponents and therefore complex combinations of "too fast" and "too slow" can and do occur.

---

[462] Jiménez-Nieto LC, Ladero JM, Fernández-Gundín MJ, Robledo A. Acetylator phenotype in psoriasis. *Dermatologica*. 1989;178(3):136-7

control subjects, 90 (57.3%) were slow acetylators. Among the 64 psoriatic patients, 40 (62.5%) were slow acetylators. Among the 27 psoriatic patients who had a sibling with psoriasis, 22 (81%) were slow acetylators (p less than 0.05). The authors concluded, "**Slow acetylator phenotype may be a genetic risk factor for the development of psoriasis.**" These results show that psoriatic patients have impaired detoxification ability when compared to normal healthy people, and that psoriatic patients with a sporiatic sibling—the familiality of the disorder suggests common genotrophic factors (e.g., inefficient acetylation alleles) or environmental factors (e.g., susceptibility to intestinal overgrowth of Gram-negative bacteria) which adversely affect detoxification ability—have a greater probability of developing psoriasis. Interestingly, the slow acetylator phenotype noted above to be associated with psoriasis is also, per a 1984 review by Evans[463], associated with diabetes mellitus; clinical-epidemiologic research has consistently linked psoriasis and diabetes mellitus.

17. <u>Impairment of mucosal and systemic defenses</u>: Microbial colonization of mucosal surfaces can result in impaired local immunity by causing loss of protective secretory IgA or by causing direct tissue damage that results in increased absorption of microbial, dietary, or environmental antigens. Several microorganisms such as *Entamoeba histolytica*[464], *Streptococcus sanguis*[465], and *Candida albicans*[466] externalize a protein-digesting enzyme (proteinase) that "digests" defensive immunoglobulins, including secretory IgA and humoral immunoglobulins. The proteinases produced by *Candida* are capable of lysing not only sIgA but also keratin and collagen[467], obviously providing for a breach of protection from other infections and antigens. In this way, mucosal microbial colonization with yeast/bacteria that secrete proteases/proteinases can "open the door" to previously excluded microbes or antigens to promote the resultant "infection" or "allergy", respectively. Furthermore, because IgA is destroyed by the protease, the infection is allowed to fester, resulting in on-going immune stimulation and its consequences such as bystander activation. This may explain why women with chronic vaginal candidiasis, which always implies chronic yeast overgrowth of the intestine[468], have nearly double the incidence of allergic rhinitis compared to patients without chronic yeast overgrowth.[469] Further supporting the link between yeast and allergy is another recent study showing that allergy/atopy is more common in patients with chronic yeast infections.[470] *Candida* produces an immunotoxin called "gliotoxin", which suppresses human immune function.[471] The combination of mucosal damage, destruction of sIgA, immunosuppression, and microbial overgrowth synergize to sensitize the systemic immune system toward allergic and proinflammatory disease.[472] Lastly, bacterial proteases work synergistically with biofilm formation to nullify immunologic attack (via immunosuppression and cytokine inactivation) and are important for the establishment of chronic mucosal colonization.[473] Impairment of mucosal defenses and—o a lesser extent systemic defenses as been sufficiently reviewed in this paragraph such that additional disease-specific discussions are unnecessary.

[463] Evans DA. Survey of the human acetylator polymorphism in spontaneous disorders. *J Med Genet*. 1984 Aug;21(4):243-53

[464] Kelsall BL, Ravdin JI. Degradation of human IgA by Entamoeba histolytica. *J Infect Dis*. 1993 Nov;168(5):1319-22

[465] "These data indicate that the BD patients are infected with IgA protease-producing S. sanguis strains, which cause an increase of IgA titer against these organisms and IgA protease antigen." Yokota K, Oguma K. IgA protease produced by Streptococcus sanguis and antibody production against IgA protease in patients with Behcet's disease. *Microbiol Immunol*. 1997;41(12):925-31

[466] Kaminishi H, Miyaguchi H, Tamaki T, et al. Degradation of humoral host defense by Candida albicans proteinase. *Infect Immun*. 1995 Mar;63(3):984-8

[467] "The enzymes produced by these yeasts are all carboxyl proteinases capable of degrading secretory IgA, the major immunoglobulin of mucous membranes. Some have keratino- or collagenolytic activity." Douglas LJ. Candida proteinases and candidosis. *Crit Rev Biotechnol*. 1988;8(2):121-9

[468] "The results showed that if C albicans was cultured from the vagina, it was always found in the stool... The gut-reservoir concept may well apply to other forms of candidiasis." Miles MR, Olsen L, Rogers A. Recurrent vaginal candidiasis. Importance of an intestinal reservoir. *JAMA*. 1977 Oct 24;238(17):1836-7

[469] Moraes PS. Recurrent vaginal candidiasis and allergic rhinitis: a common association. *Ann Allergy Asthma Immunol*. 1998 Aug;81(2):165-9

[470] Neves NA, Carvalho LP, De Oliveira MA, et al. Association between atopy and recurrent vaginal candidiasis. *Clin Exp Immunol*. 2005 Oct;142(1):167-71

[471] "This study suggests a previously unrecognized potential virulence factor of C. albicans that could contribute to persistence of yeast colonization or recurrence of symptomatic infection through diminished host resistance." Shah DT, Jackman S, Engle J, Larsen B. Effect of gliotoxin on human polymorphonuclear neutrophils. *Infect Dis Obstet Gynecol* 1998;6(4):168-75

[472] "Studies performed in humans show that selective IgA deficiency, preterm delivery, intestinal helminth infection and type of feeding during the neonatal period may influence antigen uptake by the intestinal epithelium. These conditions...may cause increased absorption of intraluminal antigens and result in the triggering of allergic type responses." Reinhardt MC. Macromolecular absorption of food antigens in health and disease. *Ann Allergy*. 1984 Dec;53(6 Pt 2):597-601

[473] "The two proteases, alkaline protease and elastase, inhibit the function of the cells of the immune system (phagocytes, NK cells, T cells), inactivate several cytokines (IL-1, IL-2, IFN-r, TNF), cleave immunoglobulins and inactivate complement. Inhibition of the local immune response by bacterial proteases provides an environment for the colonization and establishment of chronic infection." Kharazmi A. Mechanisms involved in the evasion of the host defence by Pseudomonas aeruginosa. *Immunol Lett*. 1991 Oct;30(2):201-5

18. <u>Impairment of mucosal digestion by microbial proteases and inflammation</u>: Similar to the degradation of human IgA by microbial proteases/proteinases is the degradation of mucosal digestive enzymes such as the disaccharidases (sucrase, maltase, lactase, and isomaltase) and dipeptidases. First, impaired digestion of carbohydrates skews the intestinal milieu toward one favorable to bacterial/yeast overgrowth by increasing the levels of carbohydrate substrate upon which microbes feed. Impaired peptide breakdown promotes immune sensitization, protein malnutrition, and putrefaction. Second, inflammation resultant from intestinal dysbiosis further impairs carbohydrate digestion via downregulation of sucrase-isomaltase gene expression by inflammatory cytokines.[474] Third, destruction of microvilli exacerbates loss of mucosal enzymes and leads to additional malabsorption, maldigestion, and increased macromolecular absorption, such as seen in patients with intestinal giardiasis.[475] Impairment/reduction of disaccharidases and dipeptidases is also seen in patients with inflammatory bowel disease.[476]

19. <u>Inflammation-induced endocrine dysfunction</u>: Although research in this area is less conclusive, the pattern of emerging research indicates that the multifaceted phenomenon of inflammation, particularly the elaboration of cytokines, alters endocrine function, and these inflammation-induced endocrine alterations further promote additional musculoskeletal inflammation. Endocrine changes induced by chronic inflammation include increased production of proinflammatory **prolactin**, reduced production of anti-inflammatory and immunoregulatory **cortisol** and **androgens**. The effects of altered endocrine function is discussed in the following section detailing orthoendocrinology. The link between dysbiosis and inflammation-induced changes in endocrine status has only recently begun to be documented, and some of these conclusions are logical though somewhat speculative. However, the nature of holistic healthcare requires us to consider *all* potentially significant contributions and interconnections, and thus microbe-endocrine links are briefly outlined here based on *highly suggestive*—yet not *wholly conclusive*—data. What is very clear is that autoimmune patients have alterations in hypothalamic-pituitary-adrenal/gonadal function. What is not yet clear is whether or not these are primary initiators of disease or secondary results of the disease process. Here I propose that both of these statements are true, namely that 1) endocrine dysfunction predisposes to the immune dysfunction that results in autoimmunity, and that 2) systemic inflammation further exacerbates endocrine dysfunction. Further, I speculate and add that 3) in some patients, chronic dysbiosis and subclinical inflammation and bacterial endotoxinemia/exotoxinemia can initiate the endocrine dysfunction and pro-inflammatory state that can eventually cross a diagnostic threshold to become overt clinical autoimmunity. Research support is provided here:

    - <u>Altered hypothalamic responsiveness and circadian rhythm</u>: The region of the basal hypothalamus is not protected by the blood-brain barrier and is sensitive and vulnerable to substances in the blood.[477] Because of this, hypothalamic and thus pituitary responses can be tuned to and/or altered by circulating prostaglandins, cytokines, and bacterial endotoxins and exotoxins. Patients with rheumatoid arthritis show hypothalamic/endocrine disturbances including blunted responsiveness to ACTH, abnormal circadian rhythm of prolactin and cortisol, and abnormalities in growth hormone secretion.[478] Furthermore, arginine vasopressin (AVP) is secreted from the hypothalamus in response to stress, is inherently pro-inflammatory, and is capable of augmenting prolactin secretion to further increase inflammation.[479]

---

[474] Ziambaras T, Rubin DC, Perlmutter DH. Regulation of sucrase-isomaltase gene expression in human intestinal epithelial cells by inflammatory cytokines. *J Biol Chem.* 1996 Jan 12;271(2):1237-42 http://www.jbc.org/cgi/content/full/271/2/1237

[475] Buret AG. Immunopathology of giardiasis. *Mem Inst Oswaldo Cruz.* 2005 Mar;100 Suppl 1:185-90 http://www.scielo.br/pdf/mioc/v100s1/v100ns1a31.pdf

[476] "A significant reduction of the specific activity of disaccharidases (lactase, sucrase and trehalase) in jejunal mucosal homogenate occurred in patients with inflammatory bowel disease. ... Several dipeptidases such as glycyl-leucine, leucyl-glycine, glycyl-glycine and valyl-proline hydrolase activities were lower in patients with inflammatory bowel disease than in controls." Arvanitakis C. Abnormalities of jejunal mucosal enzymes in ulcerative colitis and Crohn's disease. *Digestion.* 1979;19(4):259-66

[477] Waxman SG. <u>Clinical Neuroanatomy 25th Edition</u>. McGraw Hill Medical, New York, 2003, p 160

[478] Anisman H, Baines MG, Berczi I, Bernstein CN, Blennerhassett MG, Gorczynski RM, Greenberg AH, Kisil FT, Mathison RD, Nagy E, Nance DM, Perdue MH, Pomerantz DK, Sabbadini ER, Stanisz A, Warrington RJ. Neuroimmune mechanisms in health and disease: 2. Disease. *CMAJ.* 1996 Oct 15;155(8):1075-82 http://www.pubmedcentral.nih.gov/articlerender.fcgi?tool=pubmed&pubmedid=8873636

[479] Chikanza IC, Grossman AS. Hypothalamic-pituitary-mediated immunomodulation: arginine vasopressin is a neuroendocrine immune mediator. *Br J Rheumatol.* 1998 Feb;37(2):131-6 http://rheumatology.oxfordjournals.org/cgi/reprint/37/2/131

- Irritable bowel syndrome as a clinical model of intestinal bacterial overgrowth dysbiosis: Dysregulation of the hypothalamic-pituitary-adrenal (HPA) axis in irritable bowel syndrome (*Journal of Neurogastroenterology and Motility* 2009 Feb[480]): In order to utilize irritable bowel syndrome (IBS) as a model of dysbiosis (subtype: microbial overgrowth within the intestines) and to thereby describe the hypothalamic and neuro-endocrine alterations as exemplifications of dysbiosis-induced alterations in neuro-endocrine function, a brief review to (re)acquaint readers with the fundamental cause of IBS will be provided (part 1) which will be followed by a brief overview of the neuro-endocrine abnormalities caused by dysbiosis in this condition (part 2). ❶ IBS was erroneously assumed to be enigmatic and esoteric by clinicians well-versed in the idiopathic ideology of allopathic/pharmaocococentric medicine; meanwhile, the fact seemed quite obvious to the rest of us that so-called IBS was simply a manifestation of small intestine bacterial overgrowth (SIBO). Thankfully, the correct viewpoint—after years of clinical validation in integrative practices—has finally received widespread publication, although not necessarily widespread acceptance by scientific nihilists and therapeutic obstructionists. The masterful review by Lin[481] "Small intestinal bacterial overgrowth: a framework for understanding irritable bowel syndrome" published in *JAMA-Journal of the American Medicial Assoiation* in 2004 should have laid to rest the search for the major direct cause of IBS, particularly since follow-up studies using orally-administered nonabsorbable antibiotics[482,483,484,485] have shown consistent benefit despite the limited scope of the pharmacologic intervention, failure to perform microbial identification and sensitivity testing, and the general failure to use probiotic therapy and dietary improvements which are required to (re)establish eubiosis. Thus, having established IBS to be a manifestation of intestinal dysbiosis generally and SIBO—or more accurately SIMO for "small intestinal microbial overgrowth" since the microbes may be yeast/fungi, amoebas or protozoas rather than exclusively bacteria—specifically, let us now look at the hypothalamic abnormalities seen in patients with "SIMO-induced IBS" (redundancy noted). ❷ Chang et al[486] in 2009 found evidence HPA axis dysregulation in women with IBS without psychiatric comorbidity as evidenced by SIMO-IBS patients' significantly lower basal secretion of adrenocorticotrophic hormone (ACTH) with slightly elevated and asynchronic secretion of cortisol contrasted with the findings in the control group. FitzGerald et al[487] showed that "women with IBS display blunted ACTH and cortisol responses to the LP (lumbar puncture used as a psychological stressor) along with a profile of affective responsiveness suggestive of chronic psychosocial stress, although no CRF (corticotrophin-releasing hormone in cerebrospinal fluid) differences between groups are observed." Whether these hypothalamic-pituitary dysfunctions are a contributing cause to or a result of SIMO-IBS could only be established by clinical trials with a 5-part protocol (ie, 1. assessment of normal subjects, 2. intentional induction of SIMO-IBS, 3. reassessment, 4. successful treatment, 5. reassessment) which would be logistically cumbersome and ethically untenable.
- Increased production of prolactin: Prolactin is a highly proinflammatory hormone produced by the anterior pituitary gland as well as by peripheral lymphocytes. As a model of infection-induced inflammation, **sepsis is generally associated with increased prolactin production in humans.**[488] Prolactin levels increase due to chronic psychoemotional stress. **The classic exemplification of**

[480] Chang L, Sundaresh S, Elliott J, Anton PA, Baldi P, Licudine A, Mayer M, Vuong T, Hirano M, Naliboff BD, Ameen VZ, Mayer EA. Dysregulation of the hypothalamic-pituitary-adrenal (HPA) axis in irritable bowel syndrome. *Neurogastroenterol Motil.* 2009 Feb;21(2):149-59

[481] Lin HC. Small intestinal bacterial overgrowth: a framework for understanding irritable bowel syndrome. *JAMA.* 2004 Aug 18;292(7):852-8

[482] Esposito I, de Leone A, Di Gregorio G, Giaquinto S, de Magistris L, Ferrieri A, Riegler G. Breath test for differential diagnosis between small intestinal bacterial overgrowth and irritable bowel disease: an observation on non-absorbable antibiotics. *World J Gastroenterol.* 2007 Dec 7;13(45):6016-21

[483] Peralta S, Cottone C, Doveri T, Almasio PL, Craxi A. Small intestine bacterial overgrowth and irritable bowel syndrome-related symptoms: experience with Rifaximin. *World J Gastroenterol.* 2009 Jun 7;15(21):2628-31

[484] Majewski M, McCallum RW. Results of small intestinal bacterial overgrowth testing in irritable bowel syndrome patients: clinical profiles and effects of antibiotic trial. *Adv Med Sci.* 2007;52:139-42

[485] Cuoco L, Salvagnini M. Small intestine bacterial overgrowth in irritable bowel syndrome: a retrospective study with rifaximin. *Minerva Gastroenterol Dietol.* 2006 Mar;52(1):89-95

[486] Chang L, Sundaresh S, Elliott J, Anton PA, Baldi P, Licudine A, Mayer M, Vuong T, Hirano M, Naliboff BD, Ameen VZ, Mayer EA. Dysregulation of the hypothalamic-pituitary-adrenal (HPA) axis in irritable bowel syndrome. *Neurogastroenterol Motil.* 2009 Feb;21(2):149-59

[487] FitzGerald LZ, Kehoe P, Sinha K. Hypothalamic--pituitary-- adrenal axis dysregulation in women with irritable bowel syndrome in response to acute physical stress. *West J Nurs Res.* 2009 Nov;31(7):818-36

[488] "Prolactin levels are regularly elevated in sepsis although to variable degrees." Dennhardt R, Gramm HJ, Meinhold K, Voigt K. Patterns of endocrine secretion during sepsis. *Prog Clin Biol Res.* 1989;308:751-6

dysbiosis-induced musculoskeletal inflammation—reactive arthritis—is frequently associated with hyperprolactinemia.[489]

- ▪ Infection-induced arthritis: Elevated prolactin in reactive arthritis (*J Rheumatol* 1994 Jul[490]): Without any question whatsoever, reactive arthritis—formerly called Reiter's syndrome—is one of the prototypes of inflammatory arthritis and "autoimmunity" triggered by microorganisms, whether as an acute infection such as a urinary tract infection or gastroenteritis or as a chronic subclinical infection. This classic association—that between the microbe and the induction of arthritis and systemic inflammation—is discussed in all textbooks of pathology and all thorough textbooks of microbiology; it is therefore a matter of "medical fact." Therefore, the identification of hormonal abnormalies in patients with this prototypic microbe-induced autoimmune/inflammatory syndrome would be supportive of either/both of the following: ❶ microbial infection or colonization can result in hormone imbalances, such as elevated prolactin, and/or ❷ hormone imbalances such as elevated prolactin function synergistically with microbial colonization to result in systemic inflammation and dysbiotic rheumatism. In this study, the authors measured serum prolactin (PRL) in patients with reactive arthritis and groups of other patients. Results showed that elevated PRL levels > 20 ng/ml were found in 9 of 25 (36%) patients with reactive arthritis but almost none of the other patients. Furthermore, a direct positive correlation between serum prolactin levels and the clinical intensity of conjunctivitis, urethritis, dysentery, and uveitis was noted.

- • Reduced production of cortisol: Cortisol is an immunoregulatory hormone which tends to suppress excess immune activity, and relative reductions in cortisol production are commonly seen in patients with autoimmunity and allergic disorders.[491,492] **Cortisol production is reduced by chronic psychoemotional stress**[493], and the stress of chronic inflammation due to dysbiosis and the resultant disease, pain, disability, and disfigurement may impair normal endocrine function.

  - ▪ Allergies, autoimmunity, and fatigue-related syndromes—Mild adrenocortical deficiency and the work of Jefferies (*Med Hypotheses* 1994 Mar[494]): In his textbook *Safe Uses of Cortisol* and peer-reviewed articles, Jefferies has been the strongest proponent of the idea that patients with chronic allergies, autoimmune disorders, and chronic fatigue syndrome have mild adrenocortical deficiency resulting in low physiologic reserve and immune abnormalities that would be better treated with physiologic doses of bioidentical cortisol rather than high doses of synthetic cortisol mimetics. Dr Jefferies approach—using physiologic amounts of cortisol at doses less than 20 mg per day—does not cause adrenal suppression or adverse effects which are commonly seen when synthetic cortisol mimetics such as prednisone are used. Allergies and autoimmune disorders are commonly treated with synthetic cortisol mimetics as part of standard medical practice; this can be viewed as appreciation for the role of cortisol in immunomodulation. Relatedly, a clinical trial by

---

[489] "Hyperprolactinemia (PRL > 20 ng/ml) was found in 9 of 25 (36%) patients with RS." Jara LJ, Silveira LH, Cuellar ML, Pineda CJ, Scopelitis E, Espinoza LR. Hyperprolactinemia in Reiter's syndrome. *J Rheumatol*. 1994 Jul;21(7):1292-7

[490] Jara et al. Hyperprolactinemia in Reiter's syndrome. *J Rheumatol*. 1994 Jul;21(7):1292-7

[491] "Yet evidence that patients with rheumatoid arthritis improved with small, physiologic dosages of cortisol or cortisone acetate was reported over 25 years ago, and that patients with chronic allergic disorders or unexplained chronic fatigue also improved with administration of such small dosages was reported over 15 years ago..." Jefferies WM. Mild adrenocortical deficiency, chronic allergies, autoimmune disorders and the chronic fatigue syndrome: a continuation of the cortisone story. *Med Hypotheses*. 1994 Mar;42(3):183-9 http://www.thebuteykocentre.com/Irish_%20Buteykocenter_files/further_studies/med_hyp2.pdf and http://members.westnet.com.au/pkolb/med_hyp2.pdf

[492] "The etiology of rheumatoid arthritis ...explained by a combination of three factors: (i) a relatively mild deficiency of cortisol, ..., (ii) a deficiency of DHEA, ...and (iii) infection by organisms such as mycoplasma,..." Jefferies WM. The etiology of rheumatoid arthritis. *Med Hypotheses*. 1998 Aug;51(2):111-4

[493] "Prolonged psychological stress is associated with a transient suppression of the HPA axis, manifested by low morning cortisol and reduced cortisol response to ACTH. The reduction of cortisol response is sufficient to cause false diagnosis of HPA insufficiency." Zarkovic M, Stefanova E, Ciric J, Penezic Z, Kostic V, Sumarac-Dumanovic M, Macut D, Ivovic MS, Gligorovic PV. Prolonged psychological stress suppresses cortisol secretion. *Clin Endocrinol* (Oxf). 2003 Dec;59(6):811-6

[494] Jefferies WM. Mild adrenocortical deficiency, chronic allergies, autoimmune disorders and the chronic fatigue syndrome: a continuation of the cortisone story. *Med Hypotheses*. 1994 Mar;42(3):183-9

Cleare et al[495] among patients with chronic fatigue syndrome (CFS) showed that low-dose cortisol in amounts of 5-10 mg per day provided significant benefit.

- **Reduced production and bioavailability of androgens—testosterone and/or dehydroepiandrosterone (DHEA)**: High-intensity stress associated with military training leads to 60-80% reductions in androgens[496]; the chronic stress and pain associated with musculoskeletal inflammation may contribute to a similar profile on a subacute and chronic basis. Hyperprolactinemia further complicates this problem by simulating hepatic production of sex hormone binding globulin (SHBG) which adsorbs androgens and reduces their bioavailability. Indeed, the clinical manifestations of hypogonadism—including probably inflammatory/rheumatic complications—can be seen despite adequate production of androgens when elevated prolactin stimulates increased SHBG production and results in reduced bioavailability of androgens.[497]

  - **Inflammatory bowel disease and dysbiosis—Patients with chronic inflammatory bowel disease have low levels of DHEA (*Clin Exp Rheumatol* 1998 Sep-Oct[498])**: Readers should note that both of the major forms of inflammatory bowel disease (IBD)—Crohn disease (CD) and ulcerative colitis (UC)—are very closely associated with gastrointestinal dysbiosis; in fact, a very strong case can be made that IBD is one of the prototypic manifestations of gastrointestinal dysbiosis.[499] In this study, DHEA-sulfate (DHEA-s) levels were measured in blood from 112 patients with IBD (66 with CD and 46 with UC), and the levels were compared with those in 80 healthy controls. DHEA-s concentrations were measured in tissue samples from 40 patients (28 patients with IBD and 12 with other bowel disorders) who had undergone intestinal surgery. Results of these analyses showed that average blood DHEA-s were markedly lower in the two IBD groups (1350 nmol/l in UC and 1850 nmol/l in CD vs. 3300 nmol/l in controls); readers should note that the DHEA-s levels in the IBD patients were rougly half—50%—of normal. Andus et al[500] showed that DHEA 200mg/d provided important benefits for patients with treatment-resistant CD and UC.

  - **HIV/AIDS—Testosterone deficiency is common in men and women infected with HIV (*Clin Infect Dis* 2001 Sep[501])**: The authors note, "Androgen deficiency is a common endocrine abnormality among men and women with human immunodeficiency virus (HIV) infection. … The most useful laboratory indicator is the serum bioavailable (free) **testosterone** concentration." Clinical benefits of the correction of hypoadrogenism—specifically serum free testosterone and/or serum total testosterone—include improvements in lean body mass, energy, quality of life, and mood-depression scores.

In conclusion, **this survey of the literature has supported the concept that dysbiosis can contribute to systemic pain, inflammation, and immune activation by numerous mechanisms, and that many of these "silent infections" are self-perpetuating by inducing alterations in local milieu and systemic immunity**. Clinical experience has demonstrated again and again that eradicating dysbiosis helps normalize immune function, alleviate autoimmunity and allergy, reduce inflammation, improve detoxification, and to help "cure" people of their previously "incurable" multiple chemical sensitivity, environmental illness, and autoimmunity.

---

[495] Cleare AJ, Heap E, Malhi GS, Wessely S, O'Keane V, Miell J. Low-dose hydrocortisone in chronic fatigue syndrome: a randomised crossover trial. *Lancet*. 1999 Feb 6;353(9151):455-8

[496] "Plasma levels of testosterone, free testosterone, dehydroepiandrosterone, 17 alpha-hydroxyprogesterone, and androstenedione decreased by 60-80% during the course." Opstad PK. Androgenic hormones during prolonged physical stress, sleep, and energy deficiency. *J Clin Endocrinol Metab*. 1992 May;74(5):1176-83

[497] "The pitfalls of measuring only total serum testosterone are illustrated by a 52 year old man whose hyperprolactinaemia was associated with normal total serum testosterone but a raised sex-hormone-binding globulin, giving a low free testosterone. Prolactin suppression with bromocriptine normalized sex-hormone-binding globulin and free testosterone…" Hardy KJ, Seckl JR. Endocrine assessment of impotence--pitfalls of measuring serum testosterone without sex-hormone-binding globulin. *Postgrad Med J*. 1994 Nov;70(829):836-7

[498] de la Torre B, Hedman M, Befrits R. Blood and tissue dehydroepiandrosterone sulphate levels and their relationship to chronic inflammatory bowel disease. *Clin Exp Rheumatol*. 1998 Sep-Oct;16(5):579-82

[499] Tamboli CP, Neut C, Desreumaux P, Colombel JF. Dysbiosis in inflammatory bowel disease. *Gut*. 2004 Jan;53(1):1-4

[500] Andus T, Klebl F, Rogler G, Bregenzer N, Schölmerich J, Straub RH. Patients with refractory Crohn's disease or ulcerative colitis respond to dehydroepiandrosterone: a pilot study. *Aliment Pharmacol Ther*. 2003 Feb;17(3):409-14

[501] Mylonakis E, Koutkia P, Grinspoon S. Diagnosis and treatment of androgen deficiency in human immunodeficiency virus-infected men and women. *Clin Infect Dis*. 2001 Sep 15;33(6):857-64

The Seven Main Loci of Dysbiosis

For a microorganism to induce a systemic proinflammatory immunodysregulatory response in a human, the microbe or its metabolic products must be exposed to a susceptible host. Non-infectious microbial overgrowth can occur inside the body (gastrointestinal, sinus, respiratory tract and lungs, genitourinary, or orodental), on the surface of the body (dermal), or outside of the body (environmental). The adverse physiologic and clinical effects can be similar regardless of the location of the microorganism. The term "dysbiosis" is classically applied to harmful, non-infectious relationships between the human host and yeast, bacteria, protozoans, amoebas, or other "parasites" located specifically in the gastrointestinal tract, and "dysbiosis" is now an accepted term in the medical literature.[502] However, we must also appreciate that harmful, noninfectious microbe-host interactions can also occur when microbes are localized in the sinuses, oral cavity, genitourinary tract, skin, and in the external environment. I prefer to use a broad definition of dysbiosis that implies "a relationship of non-infectious host-microorganism interaction that adversely affects the human host" and then to specify the subtype based on the location: gastrointestinal, oral, sinus, genitourinary, dermatologic, or environmental. Gastrointestinal dysbiosis is clearly the prototype for understanding other types of dysbiosis; this is because it seems to be the most common form of dysbiosis, perhaps due to the large numbers and types of microbes in the gut and the extensive surface area of the gastrointestinal tract. Clinicians must appreciate the anatomical interconnections that can segue one type of loci of dysbiosis into another. Orodental dysbiosis may result in gastrointestinal dysbiosis if the microbes can survive in the gastrointestinal tract. Sinus dysbiosis could likewise drain into the lungs and gastrointestinal tract. In women, close relationships between gastrointestinal dysbiosis and vaginal dysbiosis are well documented.[503] Bacterial and fungal superantigens from the surrounding environment can contribute to a proinflammatory response in the lungs and on the skin and which becomes systemic, leading to autoimmunity.[504,505]

Correlation of Dysbiosis with Autoimmune and Rheumatic Diseases

Disease & dysbiosis	Gastro-intestinal	Orodental	Sino-respiratory	Genito-urinary	Tissue	Cutaneous	Environ-mental
SLE	+		+				
RA	✓	✓	✓	✓	+ osteomyel		
ReA	✓		✓	✓	✓ pneumonia		
Psor	✓	✓	✓	✓		✓	✓
PM-DM	+	+	+				
Spond-AS	✓			✓			
Sclerod	+						
Weg	+	✓	✓				
Vasc	✓				✓ viral hep		
Sarc			✓				
Behc		✓	✓			✓	
Neuro	✓			✓			✓

✓ = Positive research and clinical evidence in humans; + = Weak research in humans, substantive research in animal models, biologic plausibility; N = Negative findings; No correlation; SLE = lupus; RA = rheumatoid arthritis; ReA = reactive arthritis; Psor = Psoriasis or psoriatic arthritis; PM-DM = polymyositis/dermatomyositis; PMR = polymyalgia rheumatica; Sjo = Sjogren's syndrome; Spond-AS = spondyloarthropathy and ankylosing spondylitis; Sclerod = scleroderma; Weg = Wegener's granulomatosis; Vasc = vasculitis; Sarc = sarcoidosis; Behc = Behcet's syndrome; Neuro = neurologic autoimmunity, which is not detailed in this text.

[502] Tamboli CP, Neut C, Desreumaux P, Colombel JF. Dysbiosis in inflammatory bowel disease. *Gut*. 2004 Jan;53(1):1-4
[503] "The results showed that if C albicans was cultured from the vagina, it was always found in the stool... The gut-reservoir concept may well apply to other forms of candidiasis." Miles MR, Olsen L, Rogers A. Recurrent vaginal candidiasis. Importance of an intestinal reservoir. *JAMA*. 1977 Oct 24;238(17):1836-7
[504] Campbell AW, Thrasher JD, Madison RA, Vojdani A, Gray MR, Johnson A. Neural autoantibodies and neurophysiologic abnormalities in patients exposed to molds in water-damaged buildings. *Arch Environ Health*. 2003 Aug;58(8):464-74
[505] Gray MR, Thrasher JD, Crago R, Madison RA, Arnold L, Campbell AW, Vojdani A. Mixed mold mycotoxicosis: immunological changes in humans following exposure in water-damaged buildings. *Arch Environ Health*. 2003 Jul;58(7):410-20

Gastrointestinal Dysbiosis*: Overview of the Prototype of All Forms of Dysbiosis*

We all have bacteria and occasionally small quantities of yeast in our intestines, and this is normal and generally healthy. However, problems arise when these yeast/bacteria become imbalanced or when *harmful* yeast, bacteria, parasites take up residence within the gut. Particularly in the European research literature, this condition has been more widely researched and described as "dysbacteriosis" or "dysbacterosis."[506] These latter terms are somewhat unfortunate because they imply that the problem has a *bacterial* origin, which is partially (and therefore significantly) misleading since dysbiosis commonly involves bacteria *and yeast* (including but not limited to *Candida albicans*) and commonly other harmful non-bacterial microbes such as *Giardia lamblia, Blastocystis hominis, Endolimax nana, Entamoeba histolytica* and a cast of other malcontents that adversely affect the overall health of their human host.[507] "Candidiasis" and yeast-related problems have been described in the research literature and general press.[508] Dysbiosis is probably a major aspect of the phenomenon that was previously referred to in the medical literature as "autointoxication" and which was effectively treated with dietary modifications, nutritional supplementation, and colonic irrigation.[509] **Given that endotoxin/lipopolysaccharide is one of the major activators of nuclear factor kappa-B (NFkB)[510], and that NFkB activation is a major rate-limiting step in the production of proinflammatory cytokines and in the induction of proinflammatory enzymes such as cyclooxygenase, lipoxygenase, and inducible nitric oxide synthase,[511] then the link between dysbiosis and systemic inflammation becomes clear: gastrointestinal bacterial overgrowth leads to excess production and absorption of endotoxin, which then initiates immune dysfunction and a systemic proinflammatory response.** Intestinal overgrowth of gram-negative bacteria is, in this author's opinion, highly problematic since endotoxin/lipopolysaccharide, of which there are varying degrees of toxicity, can cause intestinal inflammation, leaky gut, inhibition of hepatic detoxification, hyperalgesia[512], brain dysfunction[513] and immune dysfunction by acting as superantigens.[514] **Indeed, many of the systemic manifestations associated with dysbiosis are clearly not mediated by the infecting organism but are mediated by the host response to microbial toxins and to the systemic dysfunction induced by increased intestinal permeability and subsequent alterations in hepatic and immune function. Thus, the sequelae of dysbiosis are mediated by alterations in human physiology rather than being directly caused by the microbe.** Current research has linked several microbes with human autoimmune/inflammatory diseases, for example *Entamoeba histolytica* has been linked with Henoch Schonlein purpura[515], *Klebsiella pneumoniae* with ankylosing spondylitis[516], *Proteus mirabilis* with rheumatoid arthritis[517,518] and ankylosing spondylitis[519], *Pseudomonas aeruginosa* with multiple sclerosis[520], and *Helicobacter pylori* with reactive arthritis.[521]

---

[506] Lizko NN. Problems of microbial ecology in man space mission. *Acta Astronaut.* 1991;23:163-9

[507] Galland L. Intestinal protozoan infection is a common unsuspected cause of chronic illness. *J Advancement Med.* 1989;2: 539-552

[508] Crook W. The Yeast Connection. Professional Books. Jackson. Tennessee. 1983

[509] "The writer has observed numerous cases suffering from such conditions as chronic arthritis, hypertension, coronary disease, chronic abdominal distention, constipation, and colitis, in which the element of constipation, auto-intoxication and possible colon infection seemed to play a prominent part, which responded very satisfactorily to colonic irrigations after failure to improve following the usual forms of medical treatment." Snyder RG. The value of colonic irrigations in countering auto-intoxication of intestinal origin. *Medl Clin North America* 1939; May: 781-788

[510] D'Acquisto F, May MJ, Ghosh S. Inhibition of Nuclear Factor Kappa B (NF-B). *Mol Interv.* 2002 Feb;2(1):22-35 molinterv.aspetjournals.org/cgi/content/full/2/1/22

[511] Tak PP, Firestein GS. NF-kappaB: a key role in inflammatory diseases. *J Clin Invest.* 2001 Jan;107(1):7-1 http://www.jci.org/cgi/content/full/107/1/7

[512] "We have recently shown that 'illness'-inducing agents, such as intraperitoneally administered lipopolysaccharide (LPS; bacterial endotoxin), can produce prolonged hyperalgesia." Watkins et al. Illness-induced hyperalgesia is mediated by spinal neuropeptides and excitatory amino acids. *Brain Res.* 1994 Nov 21;664(1-2):17-24

[513] "The immunogen E. coli lipopolysaccharide (LPS, endotoxin) has been widely used to stimulate immune/inflammatory responses both systemically and in the CNS... LPS appears to release glutamate, which then acts at non-NMDA receptors to remove the voltage-sensitive Mg2+ block of NMDA receptors, thus permitting NMDA receptors to be activated..." Wang YS, White TD. The bacterial endotoxin lipopolysaccharide causes rapid inappropriate excitation in rat cortex. *J Neurochem.* 1999 Feb;72(2):652-60

[514] "Superantigens are potent activators of CD4+ T cells, causing rapid and massive proliferation of cells and cytokine production... Superantigens have also been implicated in acute diseases such as food poisoning and TSS, and in chronic diseases such as psoriasis and rheumatoid arthritis." Torres BA, Kominsky S, Perrin GQ, Hobeika AC, Johnson HM. Superantigens: the good, the bad, and the ugly. *Exp Biol Med* (Maywood). 2001 Mar;226(3):164-76

[515] Demircin G, Oner A, Erdogan O, Bulbul M, Memis L. Henoch Schonlein purpura and amebiasis. *Acta Paediatr Jpn.* 1998 Oct; 40(5): 489-91

[516] Ahmadi K, Wilson C, Tiwana H, Binder A, Ebringer A. Antibodies to Klebsiella pneumoniae lipopolysaccharide in patients with ankylosing spondylitis. *Br J Rheumatol.* 1998 Dec;37(12):1330-3

[517] Ebringer A, Rashid T, Wilson C. Rheumatoid arthritis: proposal for the use of anti-microbial therapy in early cases. *Scand J Rheumatol* 2003;32(1):2-11

[518] Rashid T, Darlington G, Kjeldsen-Kragh J, Forre O, Collado A, Ebringer A. Proteus IgG antibodies and C-reactive protein in English, Norwegian and Spanish patients with rheumatoid arthritis. *Clin Rheumatol* 1999;18(3):190-5

[519] Wilson C, Rashid T, Tiwana H, Beyan H, Hughes L, Bansal S, Ebringer A, Binder A. Cytotoxicity responses to Peptide antigens in rheumatoid arthritis and ankylosing spondylitis. *J Rheumatol* 2003 May;30(5):972-8

[520] Hughes LE, Bonell S, Natt RS, Wilson C, Tiwana H, Ebringer A, Cunningham P, Chamoun V, Thompson EJ, Croker J, Vowles J. Antibody responses to Acinetobacter spp. and Pseudomonas aeruginosa in multiple sclerosis: prospects for diagnosis using the myelin-acinetobacter-neurofilament antibody index. *Clin Diagn Lab Immunol.* 2001 Nov;8(6):1181-8

[521] "Our findings suggest that HP may be included in the list of possible arthritis triggering microbes." Melby KK, Kvien TK, Glennas A. Helicobacter pylori--a trigger of reactive arthritis? *Infection.* 1999;27:252-5

Gastrointestinal Dysbiosis: Subtypes and Categorization

Building upon a previous four-subtype categorization proposed by Galland[522], here I describe six different types of gastrointestinal dysbiosis:

1. <u>Insufficiency dysbiosis</u>: This results when there is an insufficient quantity of the "good bacteria." Absence of "good bacteria" such as *Bifidobacteria* and *Lactobacillus* leaves the gastrointestinal tract vulnerable to colonization with pathogens and is associated with increased risk for bacterial overgrowth and other intestinal diseases. Furthermore, **beneficial bacteria in the intestines helps to normalize systemic immune response and promote proper digestion, elimination and nutrient absorption**. Numerous scientific studies have documented the powerful benefits of supplementing with good bacteria (probiotics), supporting their growth with fermentable carbohydrates such as inulin and fructooligosaccharides (prebiotics), and by co-administering probiotics with prebiotics (synbiotics).

2. <u>Bacterial overgrowth</u>: This is a quantitative excess of yeast and bacteria in the gut. Bacterial overgrowth of the small bowel is a well-established medical problem that is particularly common in patients who are diabetic, elderly, immunosuppressed (such as with corticosteroids/prednisone[523,524]), naturally hypochlorhydric or iatrogenically hypochlorhydric due to "antacid" drugs.[525] This commonly results in gas, bloating, malabsorption, constipation and/or diarrhea, "irritable bowel syndrome", as well as myalgias and systemic immune activation.[526] **Animal studies have proven that it is possible to reactivate peripheral arthritis by inducing bacterial overgrowth of the small bowel; endotoxins and other microbial products stimulate a systemic proinflammatory state which re-activates inflammation of joints and periarticular structures**.[527] Bacterial overgrowth of the small intestine is seen in 84% of patients with irritable bowel syndrome[528] and in **100% of patients with fibromyalgia**.[529] Researchers recently demonstrated that endotoxins can lead to impairment of muscle function and a lowered lactate threshold[530], thereby explaining the link between intestinal dysbiosis and chronic musculoskeletal pain that is not responsive to drugs or manual therapies. Drs. Over and Bucknall[531] describe a patient with **systemic sclerosis** who achieved **long-term remission** of her disease following **antibiotic treatment for intestinal bacterial overgrowth**. Bacterial overgrowth generally leads to pathologically synergistic clinical effects mediated by fermentation, putrefaction, constipation, increased enterohepatic recycling, bile acid deconjugation, malabsorption (particularly fat-soluble nutrients and vitamin B-12), nutritional deficiencies, sugar cravings, increased intestinal permeability, immune complex formation, and induction of a systemic proinflammatory response with immune complexes that is particularly prone to manifest as vasculitis and arthritis.[532,533,534]

---

[522] Attributed to Galland L. "Fire in the belly: update on gut fermentation." Presented to Great Lakes Association of Clinical Medicine, circa 1996. Also, personal email from Leo Galland dated October 28, 2005: "I have used the concept of 4 types of dysbiosis (putrefaction, fermentation, depletion and immune activation forms) in several presentations and in one written document."

[523] "A 63-year-old man with systemic lupus erythematosus and selective IgA deficiency developed intractable diarrhoea the day after treatment with prednisone, 50 mg daily, was started. The diarrhoea was considered to be caused by bacterial overgrowth and was later successfully treated with doxycycline." Denison H, Wallerstedt S. Bacterial overgrowth after high-dose corticosteroid treatment. *Scand J Gastroenterol*. 1989 Jun;24(5):561-4

[524] "These bacteria also translocated to the mesenteric lymph nodes in mice injected with cyclophosphamide or prednisone." Berg RD, Wommack E, Deitch EA. Immunosuppression and intestinal bacterial overgrowth synergistically promote bacterial translocation. *Arch Surg*. 1988 Nov;123(11):1359-64

[525] Saltzman JR, Russell RM. Nutritional consequences of intestinal bacterial overgrowth. *Compr Ther*. 1994;20(9):523-30

[526] Lin HC. Small intestinal bacterial overgrowth: a framework for understanding irritable bowel syndrome. *JAMA*. 2004 Aug 18;292(7):852-8

[527] Lichtman SN, Wang J, Sartor RB, Zhang C, Bender D, Dalldorf FG, Schwab JH. Reactivation of arthritis induced by small bowel bacterial overgrowth in rats: role of cytokines, bacteria, and bacterial polymers. *Infect Immun*. 1995 Jun;63(6):2295-301

[528] Lin HC. Small intestinal bacterial overgrowth: a framework for understanding irritable bowel syndrome. *JAMA*. 2004 Aug 18;292(7):852-8

[529] Pimentel M, et al. A link between irritable bowel syndrome and fibromyalgia may be related to findings on lactulose breath testing. *Ann Rheum Dis*. 2004 Apr;63(4):450-2

[530] Bundgaard H, Kjeldsen K, Suarez Krabbe K, et al. Endotoxemia stimulates skeletal muscle Na+-K+-ATPase and raises blood lactate under aerobic conditions in humans. *Am J Physiol Heart Circ Physiol*. 2003 Mar;284(3):H1028-34. http://ajpheart.physiology.org/cgi/reprint/284/3/H1028

[531] Over KE, Bucknall RC. Regression of skin changes in a patient with systemic sclerosis following treatment for bacterial overgrowth with ciprofloxacin. *Br J Rheumatol*. 1998 Jun;37(6):696

[532] Lin HC. Small intestinal bacterial overgrowth: a framework for understanding irritable bowel syndrome. *JAMA*. 2004 Aug 18;292(7):852-8

[533] Zaidel O, Lin HC. Uninvited guests: the impact of small intestinal bacterial overgrowth on nutrition. *Practical Gastroenterology* 2003; 27(7):27-34 http://www.healthsystem.virginia.edu/internet/digestive-health/zaidelarticle.pdf

[534] "The initial skin changes were frankly vasculitic with "target' lesions, whilst older lesions showed a psoriasiform scale and a tendency to central clearing. The illness was associated with raised levels of IgM and IgG containing circulating immune complexes and deposition of IgM and IgG in the dermis." Fairris GM, Ashworth J, Cotterill JA. A dermatosis associated with bacterial overgrowth in jejunal diverticula. *Br J Dermatol*. 1985 Jun;112(6):709-13

3. <u>Immunosuppressive dysbiosis</u>: Some microbes, particularly yeast, produce toxins that suppress immune function. The immunosuppressive mycotoxin produced by *Candia albicans* is called gliotoxin[535], and it is produced at the site of yeast overgrowth, thus suppressing local—and possibly, systemic—immune function.[536] Since secretory IgA is the first line of defense against allergens and infections in the gastrointestinal tract, its destruction by microbes such as *Candida albicans* and *Entamoeba histolytica* retards this immune barrier, and this can be considered a form of local immunosuppression.

4. <u>Hypersensitivity/allergic dysbiosis</u>: **Some people have an exaggerated immune response to otherwise "normal" yeast and bacteria. In this situation, we have to eradicate their "normal" yeast or bacteria in order to alleviate their hypersensitivity reaction.** The best example of this is the **severe intestinal inflammation that some patients develop in response to intestinal colonization with *Candida albicans*,** which is generally considered "nonpathogenic" in small amounts. In susceptible patients, *Candida* can induce a severe local inflammatory reaction, such as colitis, that only remits with antifungal treatment.[537] **Gastrointestinal overgrowth of *Candida albicans* and *C. glabrata* caused near-fatal hypersensitivity alveolitis that remitted with eradication of gastrointestinal candidiasis.**[538] Some women become "allergic" to their own vaginal *Candida albicans*[539]; undoubtedly there are also men who are likewise allergic to their own intestinal yeast. In patients with lupus, gastrointestinal bacteria are abnormal (decreased colonization resistance[540]), and it is possible that gastrointestinal bacteria in these patients may translocate into the systemic circulation to induce formation of antibodies that cross-react with double-stranded DNA to produce the clinical manifestations of the disease.[541,542] With regard to dermal dysbiosis, **most (57%) of patients with atopic dermatitis show evidence of IgE-mediated histamine release (i.e., "allergy") to exotoxins secreted from *Staphylococcus aureus*,** which commonly colonizes eczematous skin[543]; in other words: most eczema patients are allergic to their own dermal bacteria and can thus be said to have *hypersensitivity dermal dysbiosis*.

5. <u>Inflammatory dysbiosis and reactive arthritis</u>: People with specific genotypes and HLA markers are susceptible to a proinflammatory "autoimmune" syndrome that occurs following exposure to specific microbial molecules that are structurally similar to human body tissues—a phenomenon previously described as molecular mimicry. The best-known example of systemic musculoskeletal inflammation caused by microbial exposure is "reactive arthritis" such as Reiter's syndrome, which is classically seen in patients with the genotype HLA-B27 following urogenital exposure to *Chlamydia trachomatis*.

6. <u>Amoebas, cysts, protozoas, and other parasites</u>: In this case when we use the term "parasites'" we are not talking about worms/helminths, *per se*, although these are occasionally found with parasitology examinations. Certain microorganisms are not consistent with optimal health and should be eliminated even though the microbe is not classically identified as a "pathogen." Interestingly, 97% of patients severely infected with the gastrointestinal "parasite" *Entamoeba histolytica* develop self-destructive ANCA[544], suggesting the possibility that this microbe can induce or sustain autoimmunity.

---

[535] "Candida albicans is known to produce gliotoxin, which has several prominent biological effects, including immunosuppression." Shah DT, Jackman S, Engle J, Larsen B. Effect of gliotoxin on human polymorphonuclear neutrophils. *Infect Dis Obstet Gynecol*. 1998;6(4):168-75

[536] "Based on the recent finding that C. albicans is able to produce an immunosuppressive mycotoxin, gliotoxin, we analyzed vaginal samples of 3 women severely symptomatic for vaginal candidiasis and found that they contained significant levels of gliotoxin." Shah DT, Glover DD, Larsen B. In situ mycotoxin production by Candida albicans in women with vaginitis. *Gynecol Obstet Invest*. 1995;39(1):67-9

[537] Doby T. Monilial esophagitis and colitis. *J Maine Med Assoc*. 1971 May;62(5):109-14

[538] "We conclude that the disease was induced by C.a.-antigen reaching the lungs from the intestinal tract via the bloodstream." Schreiber J, Struben C, Rosahl W, Amthor M. Hypersensitivity alveolitis induced by endogenous candida species. *Eur J Med Res*. 2000 Mar 27;5(3):126

[539] Ramirez De Knott HM, McCormick TS, Do SO, Goodman W, Ghannoum MA, Cooper KD, Nedorost ST. Cutaneous hypersensitivity to Candida albicans in idiopathic vulvodynia. *Contact Dermatitis*. 2005 Oct;53(4):214-8

[540] Colonization Resistance (CR)...tended to be lower in active SLE patients than in healthy individuals. This could indicate that in SLE more and different bacteria translocate across the gut wall due to a lower CR. Some of these may serve as polyclonal B cell activators or as antigens cross-reacting with DNA." Apperloo-Renkema HZ, Bootsma H, Mulder BI, Kallenberg CG, van der Waaij D. Host-microflora interaction in systemic lupus erythematosus (SLE): colonization resistance of the indigenous bacteria of the intestinal tract. *Epidemiol Infect*. 1994;112(2):367-73

[541] "The lower IgG antibacterial antibody titres in active SLE might possibly result from sequestration of these IgG antibodies in immune complexes, indicating a possible role for antibacterial antibodies in exacerbations of SLE." Apperloo-Renkema HZ, Bootsma H, Mulder BI, Kallenberg CG, van der Waaij D. Host-microflora interaction in systemic lupus erythematosus (SLE): circulating antibodies to the indigenous bacteria of the intestinal tract. *Epidemiol Infect*. 1995 Feb;114(1):133-41

[542] Pisetsky DS. Antibody responses to DNA in normal immunity and aberrant immunity. *Clin Diagn Lab Immunol* 1998;5:1-6 http://cdli.asm.org/cgi/content/full/5/1/1?view=long&pmid=9455870

[543] "These data indicate that a subset of patients with AD mount an IgE response to SEs that can be grown from their skin." Leung DY, Harbeck R, Bina P, Reiser RF, Yang E, Norris DA, Hanifin JM, Sampson HA. Presence of IgE antibodies to staphylococcal exotoxins on the skin of patients with atopic dermatitis. Evidence for a new group of allergens. *J Clin Invest*. 1993 Sep;92(3):1374-80 http://www.pubmedcentral.gov/articlerender.fcgi?tool=pubmed&pubmedid=7690780

[544] George J, Levy Y, Kallenberg CG, Shoenfeld Y. Infections and Wegener's granulomatosis--a cause and effect relationship? *QJM*. 1997 May;90(5):367-73 http://qjmed.oxfordjournals.org/cgi/reprint/90/5/367

Gastrointestinal Dysbiosis: Assessments

- **History**: Clinicians should suspect gastrointestinal dysbiosis in their patients with gas, bloating, alternating constipation/diarrhea, irritable bowel syndrome, fibromyalgia, chronic fatigue syndrome, multiple chemical sensitivity, severe allergies, and autoimmunity, especially Crohn's disease, ulcerative colitis, rheumatoid arthritis, and ankylosing spondylitis. Frequent gas and bloating indicates excess gastrointestinal fermentation by yeast and/or overgrowth of aerobic bacteria. Abdominal pain, chronic constipation, and/or diarrhea are clear indications for stool testing; however, clinicians must remember that **many very heavily colonized patients will have no gastrointestinal symptoms**. Thus, **assessment and treatment for gastrointestinal dysbiosis is *not un*necessary simply because the patient lacks gastrointestinal symptoms.**

- **Breath testing**: Bacterial overgrowth of the small bowel can be objectively documented with measurement of a **post-carbohydrate hydrogen/methane breath test**, but I consider a history of postprandial gas and bloating to be sufficiently diagnostic.

- **Lactulose-mannitol assay for "leaky gut"**: The intestinal wall should function as a tightly regulated barrier that accomplishes two tasks: 1) **efficient absorption** of nutrients, and 2) **selective exclusion** of antigens, foreign debris, microbes and microbial antigens, and indigestible food residues. Compromise of the intestinal barrier results in impairments in nutrient absorption and/or toxin exclusion. Impaired nutrient absorption predisposes to and commonly results in micro- or macro-nutrient deficiencies. Impaired exclusion results in increased absorption of microbes, antigens, waste products, and debris into the systemic circulation. This phenomenon of altered intestinal permeability is referred to in the lay public and increasingly in the medical literature as "leaky gut" or "leaky gut syndrome."[545,546] In many patients this injury is occult, and **they have no gastrointestinal symptoms at all**; other patients may have a spectrum of signs and symptoms including diarrhea, constipation, abdominal pain, fatigue, general malaise, dyscognition, and an increase in the number and severity of food allergies, food sensitivities, and food intolerances. The **lactulose and mannitol assay** evaluates paracellular (pathologic) and transcellular (physiologic) absorption, respectively; and an increased lactulose:mannitol ratio is a non-specific finding that indicates gastrointestinal damage, generally due to 1) enterotoxin consumption such as with alcohol or NSAIDs, 2) malnutrition, 3) food allergy including celiac disease, 4) inflammatory bowel disease, and/or 5) dysbiosis—excess/harmful yeast, bacteria, or parasites. **Recall that "leaky gut" is only a symptom or manifestation of another, larger problem.**

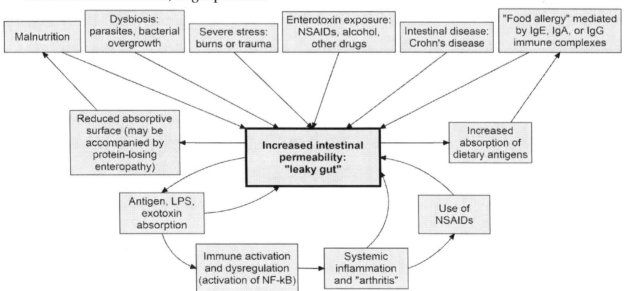

Appreciating some of the factors involved with disregulated intestinal permeability: Note vicious cycles.

---

[545] Hollander D. Intestinal permeability, leaky gut, and intestinal disorders. *Curr Gastroenterol Rep.* 1999 Oct;1(5):410-6

[546] Keshavarzian A, Holmes EW, Patel M, Iber F, Fields JZ, Pethkar S. Leaky gut in alcoholic cirrhosis. *Am J Gastroenterol.* 1999 Jan;94(1):200-7

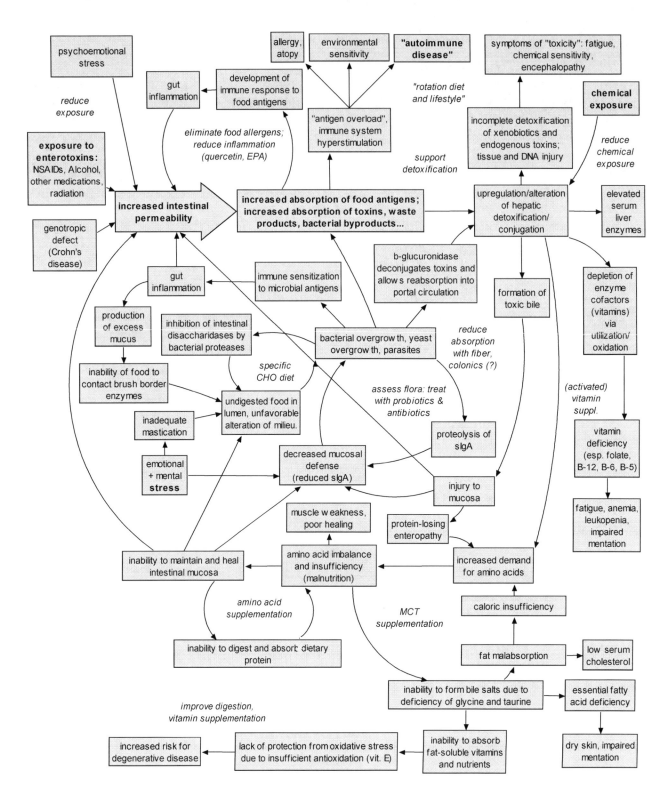

Gastrointestinal Dysbiosis, "Leaky Gut" and Impaired Detoxification: A Sampe Model of Interconnected Scenarios and Some Clinical Remediation: Therapeutic considerations are italicized.[547]

- **Comprehensive stool analysis and comprehensive parasitology**: The single best test for the assessment of gastrointestinal dysbiosis is a comprehensive stool analysis and comprehensive parasitology examination performed by a specialty laboratory that provides bacterial culture, yeast culture, microscopic exam, and measurement of sIgA to assess mucosal immune response, along with markers of inflammation

---

[547] Originally published in Vasquez A. *Integrative Orthopedics*, 2004

such as lactoferrin, calprotectin, and/or lysozyme. Comprehensive parasitology examinations (x3) to assess for bacteria, yeast, and parasites should be followed by culture and sensitivity to fine-tune the identification of the microbes and to guide treatment. These tests should be performed by a specialty laboratory rather than a regular medical or hospital laboratory. Additional markers can help put microbiological findings into the proper context; for example, in a patient with no "pathogens" other than normal *Candida albicans*, the finding of an exaggerated inflammatory response suggests a hypersensitivity/allergic dysbiosis that should be eradicated. **Stool testing must be performed by a specialty laboratory** because the quality of testing provided by most standard "medical labs" and hospitals is completely inadequate. Initial samples should be collected on three separate occasions by the patient and each sample should be analyzed separately by the laboratory. Important qualitative and quantitative markers include the following:

- o Beneficial bacteria (" probiotics"): Microbiological testing should quantify and identify various beneficial bacteria, which should be present at "+4" levels on a 0-4 scale.
- o Harmful and potentially harmful bacteria, protozoans, amebas, etc.: Questionable or harmful microbes should be eradicated even if they are not identified as true pathogens in the paleo-classic Pasteurian/Kochian sense.[548]
- o Yeast and mycology: At least two tests must be performed for a complete assessment: 1) yeast culture, and 2) microscopic examination for yeast elements. (See Chapter 1 for additional discussion.)
- o Microbial sensitivity testing: An important component to parasitology testing is the determination of which anti-microbial agents (natural and synthetic) the microbe is sensitive to. This helps to guide and enhance the effectiveness of anti-microbial therapy.
- o Secretory IgA: SIgA levels are elevated in patients who are having an immune response to either food or microbial antigens.[549] Thus, in a patient with minimal dysbiosis, say for example with *Candida albicans*, an elevated sIgA can indicate that the patient is having a hypersensitivity reaction to an otherwise benign microbe—in this case, eradication of the microbe is warranted and may result in a positive clinical response. Low sIgA suggests either primary or secondary immune defect such as selective sIgA deficiency[550] or malnutrition, stress, prednisone/corticosteroids, or possibly mycotoxicosis (immunosuppression due to fungal immunotoxins).
- o Short-chain fatty acids: These are produced by intestinal bacteria. Quantitative excess indicates bacterial overgrowth of the intestines, while insufficiency indicates a lack of probiotics or an insufficiency of dietary substrate, i.e., soluble fiber. Abnormal patterns of individual short-chain fatty acids indicate qualitative/quantitative abnormalities in gastrointestinal microflora, particularly anaerobic bacteria that cannot be identified with routine bacterial cultures.
- o Beta-glucuronidase: This is an enzyme produced by several different intestinal bacteria. High levels of beta-glucuronidase in the intestinal lumen serve to nullify the benefits of detoxification (specifically glucuronidation) by cleaving the toxicant from its glucuronide conjugate. This can result in re-absorption of the toxicant through the intestinal mucosa which then re-exposes the patient to the toxin that was previously detoxified ("enterohepatic recirculation" or "enterohepatic recycling"[551]). This is an exemplary aspect of "auto-intoxication" that results in chronic fatigue and upregulation of Phase 1 detoxification systems (chapter 4 of *Integrative Rheumatology*).
- o Lactoferrin: The iron-binding glycoprotein lactoferrin is an inflammatory marker that helps distinguish functional disorders (i.e., IBS) from more serious diseases (i.e., IBD).

---

[548] Vasquez A. Reducing Pain and Inflammation Naturally. Part 6: Nutritional and Botanical Treatments Against "Silent Infections" and Gastrointestinal Dysbiosis, Commonly Overlooked Causes of Neuromusculoskeletal Inflammation and Chronic Health Problems. *Nutr Perspect* 2006; Jan

[549] Quig DW, Higley M. Noninvasive assessment of intestinal inflammation: inflammatory bowel disease vs. irritable bowel syndrome. *Townsend Letter for Doctors and Patients* 2006;Jan:74-5

[550] "Selective IgA deficiency is the most common form of immunodeficiency. Certain select populations, including allergic individuals, patients with autoimmune and gastrointestinal tract disease and patients with recurrent upper respiratory tract illnesses, have an increased incidence of this disorder." Burks AW Jr, Steele RW. Selective IgA deficiency. *Ann Allergy*. 1986;57:3-13

[551] Parker RJ, Hirom PC, Millburn P.Enterohepatic recycling of phenolphthalein, morphine, lysergic acid diethylamide (LSD) and diphenylacetic acid in the rat. Hydrolysis of glucuronic acid conjugates in the gut lumen. *Xenobiotica*. 1980 Sep;10(9):689-70

- o __Lysozyme__: Elevated in proportion to intestinal inflammation in dysbiosis and IBD.
- o __Other markers__: Other markers of digestion, inflammation, and absorption are reported with the more comprehensive panels performed on stool samples. These tests are not always necessary, but such additional information is always helpful when working with complex patients. These markers are relatively self-explanatory and/or are described on the results of the test by the laboratory.

Orodental Dysbiosis

- • __Introduction__: The human oral cavity is heavily populated by microbes, and these microbes and their products such as endotoxin can enter the bloodstream to induce a proinflammatory response via "metastatic infection" and "__metastatic inflammation__", respectively.[552] The systemic inflammatory response triggered by mild oral/dental "infections" is now believed to exacerbate conditions associated with inflammation, such as cardiovascular disease and diabetes mellitus.[553] __Patients with rheumatoid arthritis have heightened antibody levels against common oral bacteria. IgG levels against__ *Porphyromonas gingivalis*, *Prevotella melaninogenica*, *Bacteroides forsythus*, __and__ *Prevotella intermedia* __were found to be significantly higher in RA patients when compared with those of controls.__[554] In the first human clinical trial to test the hypothesis that treatment of orodental dysbiosis would provide subjective and objective clinical benefits for patients with RA, Al-Katma et al[555] showed that __periodontal treatment consisting of scaling/root planing and oral hygiene instruction reduced symptom scores and ESR levels in patients with RA.__
- • __Assessments__: Obviously, any major microbial infestations of the mouth, such as gingivitis or thrush, need to be treated regardless of the presence or absence of systemic inflammatory disease. __Culture of mouth, throat, dentures for yeast and bacteria can be performed__ (see Noah[556]). Palpation/provocation of the gums and teeth should not cause pain; the presence of pain suggests underlying inflammation, which in turn indicates underlying infection. If flossing causes bleeding and pain, this is indicative of unhealthy gums due to an overgrowth of bacteria below the gum line. Mild gum regression and the development of deep dental pockets is an indication for intervention with fastidious oral hygiene and professional dental care. Patients with systemic disease including chronic unwellness may have asymptomatic infections of the mandible that can only be detected with non-standard imaging techniques such as computer-enhanced mandibular ultrasound (Cavitat).[557]
- • __Specific treatment considerations__: A professional cleaning by a dentist or oral hygienist is a reasonable start. Thereafter, twice-daily brushing, flossing, and the use of an antiseptic mouthwash and a plaque-removing solution should be employed. Toothbrushes should be periodically disinfected and replaced. Electric toothbrushes are more efficient than manual toothbrushes, and three-dimensional and ultrasound toothbrushes can cleanse below the gum line. Avoiding sucrose and refined carbohydrates is essential. Sugar-free chewing gums help to reduce bacterial loads at least in part by stimulating saliva production, and chewing gums with xylitol significantly reduce bacterial colonization of the oral cavity.[558,559] Immunonutrition as described later should be used to improve overall systemic defenses; particular

[552] Li X, Kolltveit KM, Tronstad L, Olsen I. Systemic diseases caused by oral infection. *Clin Microbiol Rev.* 2000 Oct;13(4):547-58 http://cmr.asm.org/cgi/content/full/13/4/547

[553] Amar S, Han X. The impact of periodontal infection on systemic diseases. *Med Sci Monit.* 2003 Dec;9(12):RA291-9 http://www.medscimonit.com/pub/vol_9/no_12/3776.pdf

[554] Ogrendik M, Kokino S, Ozdemir F, et al. Serum antibodies to oral anaerobic bacteria in patients with rheumatoid arthritis. *MedGenMed.* 2005 Jun 16;7(2):2

[555] "There was a statistically significant difference in DAS28 (4.3 +/- 1.6 vs. 5.1 +/- 1.2) and erythrocyte sedimentation rate (31.4 +/- 24.3 vs. 42.7 +/- 22) between the treatment and the control groups." Al-Katma MK, Bissada NF, Bordeaux JM, Sue J, Askari AD. Control of periodontal infection reduces the severity of active rheumatoid arthritis. *J Clin Rheumatol.* 2007 Jun;13(3):134-7

[556] Noah PW. The role of microorganisms in psoriasis. *Semin Dermatol.* 1990 Dec;9(4):269-76

[557] "Through-transmission alveolar ultrasonography (TAU) is a novel imaging modality in dental medicine. A brief introduction to through-transmission ultrasonography (TTU) is followed by a description of the first commercially available TAU device, the Cavitat CAV 4000 (Cavitat Medical Technologies, Inc., Alba, TX)." Imbeau J. Introduction to through-transmission alveolar ultrasonography (TAU) in dental medicine. *Cranio.* 2005 Apr;23(2):100-12. Cavitat Medical Technologies appears to have been involved in some litigation and regulatory issues and may have closed per internet information and http://www.fda.gov/ohrms/dockets/dailys/01/aug01/080801/cp0001.pdf surveyed 2014 Jan.

[558] "Chewing 100% xylitol gum caused significant reductions on salivary MS scores (p < 0.025) which was little different from the 55% xylitol group. The results suggest that the use of xylitol chewing gum can reduce the levels of MS in plaque and saliva." Thaweboon S, Thaweboon B, Soo-Ampon S. The effect of xylitol chewing gum on mutans streptococci in saliva and dental plaque. *Southeast Asian J Trop Med Public Health.* 2004 Dec;35(4):1024-7

[559] "Especially xylitol-containing chewing gum may significantly reduce the growth of mutans streptococci and dental plaque which may be associated with dental caries." Makinen KK, Isotupa KP, Makinen PL, Soderling E, Song KB, Nam SH, Jeong SH. Six-month polyol chewing-gum programme in kindergarten-age children: a feasibility study focusing on mutans streptococci and dental plaque. *Int Dent J.* 2005 Apr;55(2):81-8

attention should be given to glutamine, bovine colostrum and IgG, and thymus extract. In an animal study of experimental dental disease, administration of thymus extract was shown to normalize immune function and reduce orodental dysbiosis.[560]

Sinorespiratory Dysbiosis

- _Introduction_: **Sinorespiratory dysbiosis refers to adverse health consequences resultant from noninfectious colonization of the respiratory tract.** Patients with acute and chronic rhinosinusitis commonly display a rich mixture of bacteria and fungi in their sinuses. Regarding bacteria, both anaerobic and aerobic bacteria are seen, as are gram-positives such as *Staphylococcus aureus*, *Streptococcus* sp, Peptococcus/Peptostreptococcus, and gram-negative (endotoxin-producing) species including *Klebsiella pneumoniae*, *Proteus mirabilis*, *Bacteroides*, *Haemophilus parainfluenzae*, and *Haemophilus influenzae*.[561,562] Regarding fungi, **almost all patients with chronic sinus congestion have occult fungal sinus infections**, as shown in a landmark article wherein the authors concluded, *"Fungal cultures of nasal secretions were positive in 202 (96%) of 210 consecutive chronic rhinosinusitis patients."*[563] **Reactive arthritis** and **cutaneous vasculitis** have been reported in an HLA-B27-negative patient with *Chlamydia pneumoniae* pneumonia.[564] Perhaps the best current exemplification of the link between sinus infections and chronic inflammatory disease is seen in patients with **Wegener's granulomatosis**, who have a high incidence of sinus colonization with *Staphylococcus aureus*. In these patients, *Staphylococcus aureus* produces a superantigen as well as an antigenic acid phosphatase which induces autoimmune vasculitis, nephritis, the production of antineutrophil anticytoplasmic antibody (ANCA), and the formation of immune complexes. **Antimicrobial treatment to eradicate *Staphylococcus aureus* results in clinical remission of the "autoimmune" disease[565], thus proving the microbe-autoimmune link.** Increased nasal colonization with *Staphylococcus aureus* has also been documented in other inflammatory/autoimmune diseases, including **systemic lupus erythematosus[566]** and **psoriasis.**[567]

- _Assessments_: Several studies documenting fungal and bacterial colonization of the sinuses have used diagnostic/surgical techniques that are not routinely available to clinicians working in outpatient settings. **Nasal swab and culture, throat culture for bacteria and yeasts should be performed** (see Noah[568]). Accessing the sinuses is generally not feasible on a clinical/nonsurgical basis. Response to antimicrobial treatment implies cure of the occult infection. In severe cases, MRI or CT can be used to assess for occult infectious sinusitis.

- _Specific treatment considerations_: Systemic antibiotics are commonly used by allopaths when treating sinus infections. Nasal lavage with saline is highly efficacious for relieving sinus congestion.[569] The basic solution is approximately one cup of warm water with one-half teaspoon of salt (sodium chloride) and one-half teaspoon baking soda (sodium bicarbonate). Distilled, bottled, or otherwise filtered and purified water may be preferred to avoid the microbial contaminants that are found in municipal tap water. To this can be added antimicrobial botanicals such as berberine, hyperforin (highly effective against *Staphylococcus*

---

[560] Manti F, Kornman K, Goldschneider I. Effects of an immunomodulating agent on peripheral blood lymphocytes and subgingival microflora in ligature-induced periodontitis. *Infect Immun*. 1984 Jul;45(1):172-9 http://www.pubmedcentral.gov/articlerender.fcgi?tool=pubmed&pubmedid=6234232

[561] "Aspirates of 72 chronically inflamed maxillary sinuses were processed for aerobic and anaerobic bacteria. Bacterial growth was present in 66 of the 72 specimens (92%).... The predominant anaerobic organisms were anaerobic cocci and Bacteroides sp, and the predominant aerobes or facultatives were Streptococcus sp and Staphylococcus aureus." Brook I. Bacteriology of chronic maxillary sinusitis in adults. *Ann Otol Rhinol Laryngol*. 1989 Jun;98(6):426-8

[562] "The most frequently isolated bacteria were Streptococcus viridans, Klebsiella pneumoniae, Proteus mirabilis, and Hemophilus parainfluenzae." Jiang RS, Hsu CY, Leu JF. Bacteriology of ethmoid sinus in chronic sinusitis. *Am J Rhinol*. 1997 Mar-Apr;11(2):133-7

[563] Ponikau JU, Sherris DA, Kern EB, Homburger HA, Frigas E, Gaffey TA, Roberts GD. The diagnosis and incidence of allergic fungal sinusitis. *Mayo Clin Proc*. 1999 Sep;74(9):877-84 http://www.aspergillus.man.ac.uk/secure/laboratory_protocols/Ponikau.pdf

[564] "Here we present the case history of a patient with C. pneumoniae community acquired pneumonia (CAP) who subsequently developed a ReA and a cutaneous vasculitis." Cascina A, Marone Bianco A, Mangiarotti P, Montecucco CM, Meloni F. Cutaneous vasculitis and reactive arthritis following respiratory infection due to Chlamydia pneumoniae: report of a case. *Clin Exp Rheumatol*. 2002 Nov-Dec;20(6):845-7

[565] Popa et al. Staphylococcus aureus and Wegener's granulomatosis. *Arthritis Res*. 2002;4(2):77-9 http://arthritis-research.com/content/4/2/077

[566] Medline abstract from Polish research: "In 9 from 14 patients with (64.3%) a.b. very massive growth of Staphylococcus aureus in culture from vestibulae of the nose swab was, in other cultures very massive growth of physiological flora was seen. ...clinical significance of asymptomatic bacteriuria and pathogenic bacteria colonisation of nostrils as a precedence to symptomatic infections needs further investigations." Koseda-Dragan M, Hebanowski M, Galinski J, Krzywinska E, Bakowska A. [Asymptomatic bacteriuria in women diagnosed with systemic lupus erythematosus (SLE)] *Pol Arch Med Wewn*. 1998 Oct;100(4):321-30.

[567] "The nasal carriage rate of Staphylococcus aureus in psoriatics was higher ...." Singh G, Rao DJ. Bacteriology of psoriatic plaques. *Dermatologica*. 1978;157(1):21-7

[568] Noah PW. The role of microorganisms in psoriasis. *Semin Dermatol*. 1990 Dec;9(4):269-76

[569] "Endonasal irrigations with salt solutions are effective in the treatment of chronic sinusitis..." Bachmann G, Hommel G, Michel O. Effect of irrigation of the nose with isotonic salt solution on adult patients with chronic paranasal sinus disease. *Eur Arch Otorhinolaryngol*. 2000 Dec;257(10):537-41

aureus[570]), artemisinin, and others (discussed later) as well as diluted iodine[571] and powdered Nystatin (sugar-free only.) Irrigation with a bulb syringe (such as used to clear an infant's nostrils) or Neti lota pot (aka: Neti pot, or Jala neti pot) can be performed by the patient while leaning over the sink. In the author's experience, 10-15 drops of povidone iodine 10% solution can be added to one cup of nasal lavage; higher amounts of iodine cause a burning sensation. Irrigating while kneeling with the head on the floor is the most effective technique for irrigating the maxillary sinuses and frontal recess; however most techniques are inefficient for accessing the sphenoid and frontal sinuses.[572] Nasal sprays and nebulizers with saline and/or antimicrobial herbs and medications can also be utilized.[573] However, clinicians and patients must remember that the creation of microbial imbalance is possible in the sinuses just as it is in the gastrointestinal tract; thus, the use of an antibacterial agent may result in fungal overgrowth or proliferation of resistant microbes. Patients with sinus dysbiosis can integrate antimicrobial sinus lavage into their daily hygiene routine, e.g., as at the same time they brush their teeth in the

> **DrV's favorite way of explaining dysbiosis: Often what we find when working with autoimmune/inflammatory patients is that they are having a pathogenic inflammatory response to nonpathogenic microbes**
>
> - "Saint Louis University researchers have analyzed the microbiomes of people with chronic rhinosinusitis and healthy volunteers and found evidence that **some chronic sinus issues may be the result of inflammation triggered by an immune response to otherwise harmless microorganisms in the sinus membranes**.
> - "Further study findings suggested that bacteria and fungi are not causing an infection in the sinuses, but rather, that the **immune system was responding to commensals, microorganisms that, themselves, do not harm the human body**.
> - "When the immune system reacts in a hyper-responsive way, unnecessarily fighting off a harmless microorganism, it can initiate an immune response like inflammation. The body can then get locked into a cycle where inflammation generates more inflammation, causing a chronic condition.
> - "Patients with CRS are hyper-responsive to normal microbiota," said Aurora. "Our take-home message is that the problem doesn't lie in the microbiota. The inflammatory response and the resulting damage from the prolonged inflammation are caused by the body's own immune response to harmless microbiota."
>
> With Sinus Study, Harmless Members of Microbiome Spark Immune Reaction. sciencedaily.com/releases/2013/12/131219134455.htm Dec. 19, 2013. Original source: With Sinus Study, SLU Researchers Find that Harmless Members of Microbiome Spark Immune Reaction: Investigators Add Immune System Dimension to Discussion of Microbiota and Disease. www.slu.edu/x89847.xml

morning and evening. Perhaps we will find that many cases of recalcitrant gastrointestinal dysbiosis have recurred because of the gastrointestinal "seeding" of dysbiotic microbes from the sinorespiratory tract.

Tissue Dysbiosis

- **Introduction**: Infections and microbial colonization of internal organs is generally incompatible with life and unlikely to be a silent/asymptomatic locus of inflammatory stimuli due to the appropriate febrile response that typically characterizes such infections. However, exceptions to these rules do exist, and infections of parenchymal tissue—especially of liver or bone—have been reported as initiators/mimickers of systemic rheumatic/inflammatory disease. **Viral hepatitis may present with polyarthropathy while the hepatitis is asymptomatic and serum levels of**

> **"Blood Microbiota Dysbiosis" is Associated with the Onset of Cardiovascular Events in a Large Population**
>
> "The main finding of the study is that a **dysbiosis in blood microbiota**, defined by a decrease in blood bacterial DNA content and an increase in the proportion of Proteobacteria phylum within blood microbiota, predicts long-term cardiovascular prognosis."
>
> Amar J, et al. *PLoS ONE* 2013:8(1); e54461

---

[570] Schempp CM, Pelz K, Wittmer A, Schopf E, Simon JC. Antibacterial activity of hyperforin from St John's wort, against multiresistant Staphylococcus aureus and gram-positive bacteria. *Lancet*. 1999 Jun 19;353(9170):2129

[571] "Gargling with povidone-iodine before oral intubation reduces the transport of bacteria into the trachea." Ogata J, Minami K, Miyamoto H, Horishita T, Ogawa M, Sata T, Taniguchi H. Gargling with povidone-iodine reduces the transport of bacteria during oral intubation. *Can J Anaesth*. 2004 Nov;51(9):932-6 http://www.cja-jca.org/cgi/content/full/51/9/932 See also: "...a technique with facial, nasal vestibule and nasal cavity disinfection with a povidone-iodine solution followed by a cleansing of the nasal cavity (N = 87 patients and 166 samples)." Rombaux P, Collet S, Hamoir M, Eloy P, Bertrand B, Jamart F, Gigi J. The role of nasal cavity disinfection in the bacteriology of chronic sinusitis. *Rhinology*. 2005 Jun;43(2):125-9

[572] "...nasal douching while kneeling with the head on the floor. ...Nasal douches are more effective in distributing irrigation solution to the maxillary sinus and frontal recess. This should be the method of choice for irrigating these areas." Wormald PJ, Cain T, Oates L, Hawke L, Wong I. A comparative study of three methods of nasal irrigation. *Laryngoscope*. 2004 Dec;114(12):2224-7

[573] "Therapy with a 4-week course of large-particle nebulized aerosol therapy improves symptomatology and objective parameters of rhinosinusitis in patients refractory to surgical and medical therapies. Addition of tobramycin appears of minimal benefit." Desrosiers MY, Salas-Prato M. Treatment of chronic rhinosinusitis refractory to other treatments with topical antibiotic therapy delivered by means of a large-particle nebulizer: results of a controlled trial. *Otolaryngol Head Neck Surg*. 2001 Sep;125(3):265-9

liver enzymes are within normal limits; in these cases, the underlying dysbiosis/infection is identified with the use of specific serologic testing.[574] **Polyarteritis nodosa** is an autoimmune/inflammatory vasculitic syndrome strongly associated with hepatitis B infection, and 90% of patients with the immune complex vasculitis cryoglobulinemia have hepatitis C.[575] Robertson and Hickling[576] describe the case of a young girl who was **tentatively diagnosed with juvenile rheumatoid arthritis before being more accurately diagnosed with "recurrent multifocal osteomyelitis."** Dysbiosis (characterized by the acute nature of the microbial colonization) can segue into a true "infection." An advantage to the term *dysbiosis* in this situation is that it encourages clinicians to search for inflammation-generating microbial foci that may exist despite the absence of organ failure or classic/standard characteristics associated with parenchymal infection.

- *Assessments*: Given the increasing prevalence of viral hepatitis and its protean manifestations, specific serologic testing for viral hepatitis is warranted in patients with constitutional symptoms and inflammatory/idiopathic arthralgia. Likewise, occult osteomyelitis—particularly of the mandible—is increasingly appreciated, particularly as newer imaging techniques are facilitating detection. Bone scans can detect clinically occult bone infections.

- *Specific treatment considerations*: Treatment is determined by the underlying identity, nature, and location of the infection(s). Laboratory assessments are reviewed in Chapter 1.

> **"Tissue bacteria" DNA levels in blood predict diabetes (9 years, ~3,300 subjects)**
>
> - "RESULTS: We analysed 3,280 participants without diabetes or obesity at baseline. **The 16S rDNA concentration was higher in those destined to have diabetes**. No difference was observed regarding obesity. However, the 16S rDNA concentration was higher in those who had abdominal adiposity at the end of follow-up. The adjusted OR for incident diabetes and for abdominal adiposity were 1.35 and 1.18, respectively. Moreover, pyrosequencing analyses showed that participants destined to have diabetes and the controls shared a core blood microbiota, mostly composed of the Proteobacteria phylum (85-90%).
> - "CONCLUSIONS/INTERPRETATION: 16S rDNA was shown to be an independent marker of the risk of diabetes. These findings are **evidence for the concept that tissue bacteria are involved in the onset of diabetes in humans.**"
>
> Amar et al. Involvement of tissue bacteria in the onset of diabetes in humans. *Diabetologia*. 2011 Dec

---

Genitourinary dysbiosis

- *Introduction*: All doctors know that genitourinary infection with *Chlamydia trachomatis* can produce inflammatory arthropathy—"**reactive arthritis**"—and result in the condition previously known as Reiter's syndrome.[577] Often fatal, **toxic shock syndrome results from the absorption of toxins and superantigens from *Staphylococcus aureus* directly through the genitourinary mucosa. In a study of 234 patients with inflammatory arthritis, 44% of patients had a silent genitourinary infection, mostly due to *Chlamydia*, *Mycoplasma*, or *Ureaplasma*.**[578] Men with chronic prostatitis have elevated endotoxin levels in their expressed prostatic secretions[579], and plasma endotoxin levels are elevated in all types of chronic urinary tract infections[580], thus clearly

> **Reactive arthritis: urogenital swab culture to detect arthritogenic infection**
>
> "Urogenital swab culture is a sensitive diagnostic method to identify the triggering infection in reactive arthritis."
>
> Erlacher et al. *Br J Rheumatol*. 1995 Sep

---

[574] "HCV arthritis should be considered in the differential diagnosis of seronegative arthritis of undetermined etiology even in the setting of normal liver chemistries." Akhtar AJ, Funnye AS. Hepatitis C virus associated arthritis in absence of clinical, biochemical and histological evidence of liver disease--responding to interferon therapy. *Med Sci Monit*. 2005 Jul;11(7):CS37-9 http://www.medscimonit.com/pub/vol_11/no_7/6300.pdf

[575] Tierney ML. McPhee SJ, Papadakis MA (eds). Current Medical Diagnosis and Treatment 2006. 45th edition. New York; Lange Medical Books: 2006, pages 844-850

[576] Robertson LP, Hickling P. Chronic recurrent multifocal osteomyelitis is a differential diagnosis of juvenile idiopathic arthritis. *Ann Rheum Dis*. 2001 Sep;60(9):828-31 http://ard.bmjjournals.com/cgi/reprint/60/9/828

[577] Kobayashi S, Kida I. Reactive arthritis: recent advances and clinical manifestations. *Intern Med*. 2005 May;44(5):408-12 http://www.jstage.jst.go.jp/article/internalmedicine/44/5/408/_pdf

[578] "Urogenital swab cultures showed a microbial infection in 44% of the patients with oligoarthritis (15% Chlamydia, 14% Mycoplasma, 28% Ureaplasma), whereas in the control group only 26% had a positive result (4% Chlamydia, 7% Mycoplasma, 21% Ureaplasma)." Erlacher L, et al. Reactive arthritis: urogenital swab culture is the only useful diagnostic method for the detection of the arthritogenic infection in extra-articularly asymptomatic patients with undifferentiated oligoarthritis. *Br J Rheumatol*. 1995 Sep;34(9):838-42 http://rheumatology.oxfordjournals.org/cgi/content/abstract/34/9/838

[579] Dai YP, Sun XZ, Zheng KL. Endotoxins in the prostatic secretions of chronic prostatitis patients. *Asian J Androl*. 2005 Mar;7:45-7 blackwell-synergy.com/toc/ajan/7/1

[580] "RESULTS: The mean plasma endotoxin concentrations in patients with sterile pyuria, chronic complicated cystitis, acute uncomplicated pyelonephritis or acute exacerbation of chronic complicated pyelonephritis, chronic complicated pyelonephritis, and acute bacterial prostatitis or epididymitis were significantly higher than those

demonstrating the *systemic* inflammatory nature of these *localized* infections. **Microbial contamination of the genitourinary tract can cause a systemic pro-inflammatory arthritogenic response in susceptible individuals.**[581]

- *Assessments*: Basic assessment begins with a serum chemistry/metabolic panel to assess basic renal function, CBC to screen for any signs of classic infection, and urinalysis to assess for WBC, mucus, leukocyte esterase, bacteria and other basic markers. Serum tests for STDs can be performed. Urethral/vaginal swab for culture and DNA polymerase chain reaction is generally sufficient for the detection of the majority of urogenital infections. **Culture and sensitivity testing should be performed for all organisms from clean-catch urine specimens; assessment of sexual partners is advised** (see excellent review by Noah[582]). Women should undergo complete pelvic examinations, and men should undergo assessment of expressed prostatic secretions. Similar to the protocol evaluation of men with elevated PSA, a clinical trial of antibiotics/antimicrobials may reduce systemic inflammation and thereby implicate a dysbiotic stimulus to the inflammation.

- *Specific treatment considerations*: Asymptomatic genitourinary colonization with immunodysregulatory and arthritogentic dysbiotic microbes is impressively common; sufficiently common to warrant routine/empiric treaetment. In women, particular attention must be given to correcting gastrointestinal dysbiosis due to the close anatomical proximity and therefore microbiologic communication between the anus (and therefore gastrointestinal tract) and vagina.[583] Sexual partners should be tested; barrier methods (e.g., condoms) and postponment of oral-genital contact should be discussed to reduce transmission/cross-contamination during treatment. Orally administered products including Uva Ursi[584], buchu[585] and cranberry[586], ciprofloxacin, metronidazole, are commonly used for genitourinary infections/colonizations.

  - Reactive arthritis induced by bacterial vaginosis (*Int J Prev Med* 2013 Jul[587]): Paraphrased from the abstract with additional information from the complete text and additional sources: The authors report a 42-year-old woman with **reactive arthritis induced by bacterial vaginosis who presented with oligoarthritis, arthralgia, and enthesitis** — the classic musculoskeletal manifestations of reactive arthritis and findings consistenet (as perceived by some clinicians) with seronegative rheumatoid arthritis. She had zero history of diarrhea or dysuria or vaginal secretion, or sexually transmitted infections (STIs). Laboratory tests were normal except for a high erythrocyte sedimentation rate (ESR). Her pelvic examination revealed homogeneous white grey and malodorous vaginal discharge on the vaginal wall and Pap smear and Gram-stained smear of vaginal swab was consistent with bacterial vaginosis. "On physical examination, she had difficulty walking due to heel pain, a fever (38.8 degrees Celsius = 101.84 degrees Fahrenheit), swelling of her right ankle and right metatarsophalangeal joints." She responded to **metronidazole therapy [dose and duration not specified in article; however, treatment for bacterial vaginosis per *Epocrates*[588] "metronidazole 500 mg PO q12h x7 days; Info: may also consider 250 mg PO q8h x7 days in pregnant pts"]** and her six-month follow up hasn't shown recurrence of arthritis. As reactive arthritis (ReA) is a paradigm of a rheumatic disease in which the initiating infectious cause is known, so early use of antimicrobial drugs may prevent the development of musculoskeletal symptoms which are triggered by infections.

in healthy individuals and in patients with acute uncomplicated cystitis." Goto T, Makinose S, Ohi Y. Plasma endotoxin concentrations in patients with urinary tract infections. *Int J Urol.* 1995 Sep;2(4):238-42

[581] "Urogenital swab cultures showed a microbial infection in 44% of the patients with oligoarthritis (15% Chlamydia, 14% Mycoplasma, 28% Ureaplasma), whereas in the control group only 26% had a positive result (4% Chlamydia, 7% Mycoplasma, 21% Ureaplasma)." Erlacher et al. Reactive arthritis: urogenital swab culture is the only useful diagnostic method for the detection of the arthritogenic infection in extra-articularly asymptomatic patients with undifferentiated oligoarthritis. *Br J Rheumatol.* 1995 Sep;34(9):838-42 http://rheumatology.oxfordjournals.org/cgi/content/abstract/34/9/838

[582] Noah PW. The role of microorganisms in psoriasis. *Semin Dermatol.* 1990 Dec;9(4):269-76

[583] "The results showed that if C albicans was cultured from the vagina, it was always found in the stool... The gut-reservoir concept may well apply to other forms of candidiasis." Miles MR, Olsen L, Rogers A. Recurrent vaginal candidiasis. Importance of an intestinal reservoir. *JAMA.* 1977 Oct 24;238(17):1836-7

[584] Yarnell E. Botanical medicines for the urinary tract. *World J Urol.* 2002 Nov;20(5):285-93

[585] "Buchu preparations are now used as a diuretic and for a wide range of conditions including stomach aches, rheumatism, bladder and kidney infections and coughs and colds." Simpson D. Buchu--South Africa's amazing herbal remedy. *Scott Med J* 1998 Dec;43(6):189-91

[586] Lynch DM. Cranberry for prevention of urinary tract infections. *Am Fam Physician.* 2004 Dec 1;70(11):2175-7 http://www.aafp.org/afp/20041201/2175.pdf

[587] Aminzadeh Z, Fadaeian A. Reactive arthritis induced by bacterial vaginosis: prevention with an effective treatment. *Int J Prev Med.* 2013 Jul;4(7):841-4

[588] https://online.epocrates.com/noFrame/showPage.do?method=drugs&MonographId=256&ActiveSectionId=10   2014 Jan

Cutaneous Dysbiosis, Dermal Dysbiosis

- *Introduction*: Microorganisms from dermal infections such as acne can incite systemic inflammation either by dermal absorption of bacterial[589] and fungal[590] (super)antigens and by serving as loci for metastatic infections which produce septic arthritis.[591] **Patients with the autoimmune vasculitic syndrome known as Behcet's disease are more likely to develop arthritis if their skin lesions are infected, thus implicating absorption of an inflammatory immunogen.**[592] Most (57%) of patients with atopic dermatitis show evidence of IgE-mediated histamine release (i.e., "allergy") to exotoxins secreted from *Staphylococcus aureus*, which commonly colonizes eczematous skin[593]; in other words: most eczema patients are allergic to their own dermal bacteria and can thus be said to have *hypersensitivity dermal dysbiosis*.

- *Assessments*: Routine physical examination of the skin and scalp is generally sufficient to screen for obvious infections and any lesions that may be presumed to be colonized. Dermal scrapings and swabs are taken for bacterial, viral, and fungal cultures and microscopic examination. Skin/nail culture, Giemsa staining, culture of lesioned skin on blood agar, MacConkey agar, Sabouraud plates can be performed; see the review by Noah[594] for additional details. For many patients, especially those with atopic dermatitis, treatment can be empiric, per the protocol that follows, and clinically effective antimicrobial and immunorestorative treatment confirms the diagnosis of dysbiosis retrospectively; in other words, a successful clinical intervention—*therapeutic trial*—can provide diagnostic data—*diagnostic trial*.

- *Specific treatment considerations*: Topical and/or systemic antimicrobial treatment along with immunonutrition (detailed later) may be necessary for complete treatment of patients with inflammation perpetuated by dermal dysbiosis. Topical *Mahonia/Berberis aquifolium* is effective for dermal psoriasis[595] via its combined anti-inflammatory and antimicrobial benefits. Other botanical antimicrobials available in topical creams, gels, and soaps include grape seed extract, artemesinin from *Artemisia annua*, and tea tree oil. A complete outline of therapeutic interventions is as follows:

  1. Orally administered antimicrobial drugs to reduce total microbial load (TML), especially targeting *Staphylococcus aureus*: For example, cephalexin 50 mg/kg per day (maximum of 2 g/day), divided into 3 daily doses, for 2 weeks.[596]

  2. Intranasal antimicrobial treatment: Topical 5% povidone iodine is the fastest, most broadly antimicrobial, and least expensive; mupirocin ointment has been used in several studies.[597] Patients and their household members are instructed to apply intranasal treatment twice daily for five consecutive days of each month.

  3. Diluted bleach bath to reduce the total microbial load (TML) on the skin: Detailed in the accompanying textbox and in the following summaries:

     o Efficacy and safety of sodium hypochlorite (bleach) baths in patients with moderate to severe atopic dermatitis in Malaysia (*J Dermatol* 2013 Sep[598]): *Staphylococcus aureus* on skin and in nares contributes to disease pathogenesis in atopic dermatitis (AD). Patients between 2 and 30 years old with moderate to severe AD were enrolled in a prospective, randomized, placebo-controlled study. Patients soaked in diluted bleach (treatment) or distilled water baths (placebo) for 10 min, twice a week for 2 months. Patients in the treatment group showed

---

[589] Delyle LG, Vittecoq O, Bourdel A, Duparc F, Michot C, Le Loet X. Chronic destructive oligoarthritis associated with Propionibacterium acnes in a female patient with acne vulgaris: septic-reactive arthritis? *Arthritis Rheum*. 2000 Dec;43(12):2843-7

[590] Hemalatha V, Srikanth P, Mallika M. Superantigens - Concepts, clinical disease and therapy. *Indian J Med Microbiol* 2004;22:204-211

[591] Schaeverbeke T, Lequen L, de Barbeyrac B, Labbe L, Bebear CM, Morrier Y, Bannwarth B, Bebear C, Dehais J. Propionibacterium acnes isolated from synovial tissue and fluid in a patient with oligoarthritis associated with acne and pustulosis. *Arthritis Rheum*. 1998 Oct;41(10):1889-93

[592] Diri E, Mat C, Hamuryudan V, Yurdakul S, Hizli N, Yazici H. Papulopustular skin lesions are seen more frequently in patients with Behcet's syndrome who have arthritis: a controlled and masked study. *Ann Rheum Dis*. 2001 Nov;60(11):1074-6

[593] "These data indicate that a subset of patients with AD mount an IgE response to SEs that can be grown from their skin." Leung DY, Harbeck R, Bina P, Reiser RF, Yang E, Norris DA, Hanifin JM, Sampson HA. Presence of IgE antibodies to staphylococcal exotoxins on the skin of patients with atopic dermatitis. Evidence for a new group of allergens. *J Clin Invest*. 1993 Sep;92(3):1374-80 http://www.pubmedcentral.gov/articlerender.fcgi?tool=pubmed&pubmedid=7690780

[594] Noah PW. The role of microorganisms in psoriasis. *Semin Dermatol*. 1990 Dec;9(4):269-76

[595] "Taken together, these clinical studies conducted by several investigators in several countries indicate that Mahonia aquifolium is a safe and effective treatment of patients with mild to moderate psoriasis." Gulliver WP, Donsky HJ. A report on three recent clinical trials using Mahonia aquifolium 10% topical cream and a review of the worldwide clinical experience with Mahonia aquifolium for the treatment of plaque psoriasis. *Am J Ther*. 2005 Sep-Oct;12(5):398-406

[596] Huang JT et al. Treatment of Staphylococcus aureus colonization in atopic dermatitis decreases disease severity. *Pediatrics*. 2009 May;123(5):e808-14

[597] Huang JT et al. Treatment of Staphylococcus aureus colonization in atopic dermatitis decreases disease severity. *Pediatrics*. 2009 May;123(5):e808-14

[598] Wong SM, et al R. Efficacy and safety of sodium hypochlorite (bleach) baths in patients with moderate to severe atopic dermatitis in Malaysia. *J Dermatol*. 2013 Sep 20

significant reductions in Eczema Area and Severity Index (EASI) scores. **A 41.9% reduction in S. aureus density from baseline was seen at 1 month further reducing to 53.3% at 2 months**. Equal numbers of patients in both groups experienced mild side-effects. This study demonstrates that **diluted bleach baths clinically improved AD in as little as 1 month**. No patient withdrew from the treatment arm because of intolerance to the baths.

- o Treatment of Staphylococcus aureus colonization in atopic dermatitis decreases disease severity (*Pediatrics* 2009 May[599]): "METHODS: A randomized, investigator-blinded, placebo-controlled study was conducted with 31 patients, 6 months to 17 years of age, with moderate to severe atopic dermatitis and clinical signs of secondary bacterial infections. All patients received **orally administered cephalexin for 14 days** and were assigned randomly to receive **intranasal mupirocin ointment** treatment and **sodium hypochlorite (bleach) baths** (treatment arm) or intranasal petrolatum ointment treatment and plain water baths (placebo arm) for 3 months. The primary outcome measure was the Eczema Area and Severity Index score. RESULTS: The prevalence of community-acquired methicillin-resistant S aureus in our study (7.4% of our S aureus-positive skin cultures and 4% of our S aureus-positive nasal cultures) was much lower than that in the general population with cultures at Children's Memorial Hospital (75%-85%). **Patients in the group that received both the dilute bleach baths and intranasal mupirocin treatment showed significantly greater mean reductions from baseline in Eczema Area and Severity Index scores**, compared with the placebo group, at the 1-month and 3-month visits. The mean Eczema Area and Severity Index scores for the head and neck did not decrease for patients in the treatment group, whereas scores for other body sites (submerged in the dilute bleach baths) decreased at 1 and 3 months, in comparison with placebo-treated patients.

4. Nutritional immunorestoration: Patient-appropriate doses of vitamin A (not beta-cartene), zinc, vitamin D3, glutamine, arginine, etc.

5. Environmental decontamination: For example, bed sheets, towels, clothing, and furniture should all be cleaned thoroughly, preferably with an antimicrobial agent (as appropriate) such as bleach, alcohol, or povidone iodine. Clothes, bedding, and the environments in the car, home, and work should be disinfected and/or routinely washed; see section on *environmental dysbiosis*.

"Bleach bath" treatment for dermal dysbiosis
• Fill the bathtub with lukewarm water: approximately 40 gallons of water,
• Stir in one-quarter to one-half cup of common bleach (sodium hypochlorite 5-6% solution) solution to the bath water; the goal is to make a modified Dakin's solution with a final concentration of about 0.005%,
• Have patients soak in the chlorinated water for 5 to 10 minutes,
• Rinse thoroughly and pat (not rub) dry; use skin creams and emollients/moisturizers (if any) as usual,
• Perform bleach baths 2–3 times a week or as prescribed by the physician.
• Do not apply nondiluted bleach to skin; diluted bleach solution is generally well tolerated (same hypochlorite concentration as swimming pool water) but may likewise cause dryness and irritation, especially at skin lesions; avoid use or use extra caution in patients with contact allergy to chlorine.

Krakowski AC, et al. Management of atopic dermatitis in the pediatric population. *Pediatrics*. 2008 Oct

---

[599] Huang JT, Abrams M, Tlougan B, Rademaker A, Paller AS. Treatment of Staphylococcus aureus colonization in atopic dermatitis decreases disease severity. *Pediatrics*. 2009 May;123(5):e808-14

Environmental dysbiosis

- *Introduction*: Patients may develop inflammation/autoimmunity from exposures to microbial toxins from their home, work, or recreational environments. Many microorganisms, particularly yeasts/molds, defend themselves via elaboration of toxins to fend off other microbes that might otherwise invade their territory. Environmental and occupational researchers appreciate that **yeast/mold commonly elaborate immunomodulating bioaerosols, while gram-negative bacteria exude endotoxin, which is a common contaminant of "house dust."**[600] We may reasonably speculate that a susceptible person might have a systemic inflammatory response from the inhalation of bioaerosols and/or endotoxin in the air of their home and/or work environments. **Airborne immunogens include fungi, bacteria, actinomycetes, endotoxin, ß(1,3)-glucans, peptidoglycans, microbial volatile organic compounds (MVOC), and mycotoxins.**[601] "Toxic mold syndrome" and more recently "mixed mold mycotoxicosis"[602] describes patients with systemic health problems resultant from exposure to fungal bioaeresols, classically associated with mold-contaminated buildings following water damage. Such individuals develop systemic autoimmunity that resembles **multiple sclerosis** and **chronic inflammatory polyneuropathy** mediated in part by antibodies against endogenous neuronal structures.[603] Additional evidence proves that **mold exposure can lead to proinflammatory immune activation and resultant multisystem (especially neurologic) autoimmunity.**[604] This is yet another example of how microorganisms can cause human disease without causing "infection." Obviously, patients with inflammatory lung disorders such as asthma, idiopathic pulmonary fibrosis, and especially **acute pulmonary hemorrhage in infants**[605] are candidates for environmental evaluation and intervention. Patients with **Crohn's disease** are well-known to have exquisite sensitivity to the yeast *Saccharomyces cerevisiae*, and a few doctors have reported improvement in Crohn's patients following environmental disinfection. Of related interest is the finding that intraperitoneal exposure of autoimmune-prone mice to fungal components stimulates **autoimmune arthritis resembling rheumatoid arthritis**.[606]

- *Assessments*: Location-specific exacerbation of symptoms is an important historical indicator. Home, work, and recreational environments can be surveyed for microbial contamination, particularly mold. Pier-and-beam homes should be inspected for mold and water in the crawlspace; likewise, attics should be inspected for occult leaks and mold. Mold plates, Petri dishes, and filter cartridges can be used to identify airborne microbes. *Fusarium*, *Trichoderma*, and *Stachybotrys* produce mycotoxins.[607] Thorough cleaning/sanitization of wigs, shoes, furniture, whirlpool/pool water should be implemented; again, see the review by Noah.[608]

- *Specific treatment considerations*: Walls, windows, utility closets, bathrooms, and under-sink cabinets should be assessed for mold and thoroughly cleaned. High-efficiency air filters can be used in the HVAC system; stand-alone air purifiers and dehumidifiers can be used. Bedding, sheets, blankets, pillows, carpets, furniture and drapes should be inspected for contamination and thoroughly cleaned. Eucalyptus

---

[600] Douwes J, Thorne P, Pearce N, Heederik D. Bioaerosol health effects and exposure assessment: progress and prospects. *Ann Occup Hyg*. 2003 Apr;47(3):187-200 http://annhyg.oxfordjournals.org/cgi/content/full/47/3/187

[601] Douwes J, Thorne P, Pearce N, Heederik D. Bioaerosol health effects and exposure assessment: progress and prospects. *Ann Occup Hyg*. 2003 Apr;47(3):187-200

[602] Gray MR, Thrasher JD, Crago R, Madison RA, Arnold L, Campbell AW, Vojdani A. Mixed mold mycotoxicosis: immunological changes in humans following exposure in water-damaged buildings. *Arch Environ Health*. 2003 Jul;58(7):410-20

[603] "The authors concluded that exposure to molds in water-damaged buildings increased the risk for development of neural autoantibodies, peripheral neuropathy, and neurophysiologic abnormalities in exposed individuals." Campbell AW, Thrasher JD, Madison RA, Vojdani A, Gray MR, Johnson A. Neural autoantibodies and neurophysiologic abnormalities in patients exposed to molds in water-damaged buildings. *Arch Environ Health*. 2003 Aug;58(8):464-74

[604] "Abnormally high levels of ANA, ASM, and CNS myelin (immunoglobulins [Ig]G, IgM, IgA) and PNS myelin (IgG, IgM, IgA)... showing an increased risk for autoimmunity. ...exposure to mixed molds and their associated mycotoxins in water-damaged buildings leads to multiple health problems involving the CNS and the immune system... Mold exposure also initiates inflammatory processes." Gray MR, Thrasher JD, Crago R, Madison RA, Arnold L, Campbell AW, Vojdani A. Mixed mold mycotoxicosis: immunological changes in humans following exposure in water-damaged buildings. *Arch Environ Health*. 2003 Jul;58(7):410-20

[605] "Mean colony counts for all fungi averaged 29227 colony-forming units (CFU)/m3 in homes of patients and 707 CFU/m3 in homes of controls... Conclusion Infants with pulmonary hemorrhage and hemosiderosis were more likely than controls to live in homes with toxigenic S atra and other fungi in the indoor air." Etzel RA, Montana E, Sorenson WG, et al. Acute pulmonary hemorrhage in infants associated with exposure to Stachybotrys atra and other fungi. *Arch Pediatr Adolesc Med*. 1998 Aug;152(8):757-62

[606] Yoshitomi H, Sakaguchi N, Kobayashi K, et al. A role for fungal {beta}-glucans and their receptor Dectin-1 in the induction of autoimmune arthritis in genetically susceptible mice. *J Exp Med*. 2005 Mar 21;201(6):949-60 http://www.jem.org/cgi/content/full/201/6/949

[607] Am Acad Pediatrics. Toxic effects of indoor molds. Committee on Environ Health. *Pediatrics* 1998;101(4 Pt1):712-4 http://aappolicy.aappublications.org/cgi/content/full/pediatrics;101/4/712

[608] Noah PW. The role of microorganisms in psoriasis. *Semin Dermatol*. 1990 Dec;9(4):269-76

oil can be added to washing detergent to kill dust mites[609], as described in the following section. Buildings may have to be professionally and thoroughly remediated; on occasion, people will need to change to different work areas (ie, new office space, work from home, change jobs) or—if the home is affected—relocate to a new living space.

- o Building-associated neurological damage modeled in human cells (*Mycopathologia* 2010 Dec[610]): "Damage to human neurological system cells resulting from exposure to mycotoxins confirms a previously controversial public health threat for occupants of water-damaged buildings. ... Damage to the neurological system can result from exposure to trichothecene mycotoxins in the indoor environment. This study demonstrates that neurological system cell damage can occur from satratoxin H exposure to neurological cells at exposure levels that can be found in water-damaged buildings contaminated with fungal growth. The constant activation of inflammatory and apoptotic pathways at low levels of exposure in human brain capillary endothelial cells, astrocytes, and neural progenitor cells may amplify devastation to neurological tissues and lead to neurological system cell damage from indirect events triggered by the presence of trichothecenes."

- o Changes in pro-inflammatory cytokines in association with exposure to moisture-damaged building microbes (*Eur Respir J* 2001 Dec[611]): "In the present study, the authors compared the respiratory symptoms, the production of inflammatory mediators interleukin (IL)-1, IL-4, IL-6, tumour necrosis factor-alpha (TNF-alpha) and cell count in nasal lavage fluid and induced sputum samples of subjects working in moisture-damaged and control school buildings. ... The authors found a significant elevation of IL-1, TNF-alpha and IL-6 in nasal lavage fluid and IL-6 in induced sputum during the spring term in the subjects from the moisture-damaged school building compared to the subjects from the control building. The exposed workers reported sore throat, phlegm, eye irritation, rhinitis, nasal obstruction and cough in parallel with these findings. The present data suggests an association between microbial exposure, and symptoms as well as changes in pro-inflammatory mediators detected from both the upper and lower airways."

- o Co-cultivated damp building related microbes *Streptomyces californicus* and *Stachybotrys chartarum* induce immunotoxic and genotoxic responses via oxidative stress (*Inhal Toxicol* 2009 Aug[612]): "Oxidative stress has been proposed to be one mechanism behind the adverse health outcomes associated with living in a damp indoor environment. In the present study, the capability of damp building-related microbes *Streptomyces californicus* and *Stachybotrys chartarum* to induce oxidative stress was evaluated in vitro. In addition, the role of oxidative stress in provoking the detected cytotoxic, genotoxic, and inflammatory responses was studied by inhibiting the production of reactive oxygen species (ROS) using N-acetyl-l-cysteine (NAC). RAW264.7 macrophages were exposed in a dose- and time-dependent manner to the spores of co-cultivated *S. californicus* and *S. chartarum*, to their separately cultivated spore-mixture, or to the spores of these microbes alone. **... All the studied microbial exposures triggered oxidative stress and subsequent cellular damage in RAW264.7 macrophages**. The ROS scavenger, NAC, prevented growth arrest, apoptosis, DNA damage, and cytokine production induced by the co-culture since it reduced the intracellular level of ROS within macrophages. In contrast, the DNA damage and cell cycle arrest induced by the spores of *S. californicus* alone could not be prevented by NAC. Bioaerosol-induced oxidative stress in macrophages may be an important mechanism behind the frequent respiratory symptoms and diseases suffered by residents of moisture damaged buildings. Furthermore, microbial interactions during co-cultivation stimulate the production of highly toxic compound(s) which may significantly increase oxidative damage."

[609] Tovey ER, McDonald LG. A simple washing procedure with eucalyptus oil for controlling house dust mites and their allergens in clothing and bedding. *J Allergy Clin Immunol*. 1997 Oct;100(4):464-6

[610] Karunasena E, Larrañaga MD, Simoni JS, Douglas DR, Straus DC. Building-associated neurological damage modeled in human cells: a mechanism of neurotoxic effects by exposure to mycotoxins in the indoor environment. *Mycopathologia*. 2010 Dec;170(6):377-90

[611] Purokivi MK, Hirvonen MR, Randell JT, Roponen MH, Meklin TM, Nevalainen AL, Husman TM, Tukiainen HO. Changes in pro-inflammatory cytokines in association with exposure to moisture-damaged building microbes. *Eur Respir J*. 2001 Dec;18(6):951-8

[612] Markkanen Penttinen P, Pelkonen J, Tapanainen M, Mäki-Paakkanen J, Jalava PI, Hirvonen MR. Co-cultivated damp building related microbes Streptomyces californicus and Stachybotrys chartarum induce immunotoxic and genotoxic responses via oxidative stress. *Inhal Toxicol*. 2009 Aug;21(10):857-67

o <u>Chlamydophila pneumoniae antibodies in office workers with and without inflammatory rheumatic diseases in a moisture-damaged building</u> (*Eur J Clin Microbiol Infect Dis* 2005 Mar[613]): "In the study reported here, we evaluated the serum samples obtained from 18 of the office workers, both at work and following a vacation period of 2–4 weeks' duration. **Among the 18 employees, seven had rheumatic diseases and two had upper and lower respiratory symptoms**, while nine employees had no diseases or prolonged respiratory symptoms. All of the subjects were female and their mean age at the time of the study was about 50 years. ... The elevated antibody levels in the employees we tested might have been caused by prolonged exposure to *C. pneumoniae* or some immunologically active part(s) of the microbe. **The clustering of inflammatory rheumatic diseases among individuals in moisturedamaged buildings is rare and its causes are not known. We suggest that *C. pneumoniae* or some other microbe(s) capable of producing similar antibody reactions and living possibly within amoebae potentially cause these clusters.**"

o <u>Inflammatory mediators in nasal lavage, induced sputum and serum of employees with rheumatic and respiratory disorders</u> (*Eur Respir J 2001* Sep[614]): "Exposure to microbes present in mould-damaged buildings has been linked to increased frequency of various inflammatory diseases. The current study examined differences in inflammatory mediators in nasal lavage (NAL), induced sputum (IS) and serum of occupants with rheumatic or respiratory disorders and their controls, all working in the same moisture-damaged building. ... Concentrations of NO, interleukin (IL)-1, IL-4, IL-6 and tumour necrosis factor-alpha in NAL, IS and serum (excluding NO and IL-1) of the subjects were measured during an occupational exposure period and the vacation period without such exposure. **The concentrations of IL-4 in NAL fluid were significantly higher among all occupants during the working period (geometric mean 8.5 microg** x mL(-1), range 0-206.5 microg x mL(-1)), as **compared to that during vacation (0.4 microng** x mL(-1) range 0-3.7 pg x mL(-1)) (p = 0.008). Absence from the work environment also significantly diminished reporting of symptoms. IL-4 levels in the serum of case subjects were significantly higher than in controls. Moreover, employees with respiratory symptoms had markedly higher exhaled NO values than their controls (p = 0.028). In summary, these data suggest that mediators in nasal lavage samples reflect the occupational exposure to moulds, whereas possible indicators of existing disorders are detectable in serum."

o <u>Joint symptoms and diseases associated with moisture damage in a health center</u> (*Clin Rheumatol* 2003 Dec[615]): "Rheumatic diseases do not usually cluster in time and space. It has been proposed that **environmental exposures may initiate autoimmune responses**. We describe a cluster of rheumatic diseases among a group of health center employees who began to complain of symptoms typically related to moldy houses, including mucocutaneous symptoms, nausea and fatigue, within a year of moving into a new building. Dampness was found in the insulation space of the concrete floor below ground level. **Microbes indicating mold damage and actinobacteria were found in the flooring material and in the outer wall insulation.** ... All 34 subjects working at the health center had at least some rheumatic complaints. Two fell ill with a typical rheumatoid factor (RF)-positive **rheumatoid arthriti**s (RA), and 10 had **arthritis that did not conform to any definite arthritic syndrome** (three met the classification criteria for RA). Prior to moving into the problem building one subject had suffered **reactive arthritis**, which had then recurred. Another employee had undiagnosed **ankylosing spondylitis** and later developed **psoriatic arthritis**, and another developed **undifferentiated vasculitis**. A total of 16 subjects developed **joint pains**, 11 of these after beginning work at the health center. Three subjects developed **Raynaud's symptom.**

[613] Seuri M, Paldanius M, Leinonen M, Roponen M, Hirvonen MR, Saikku P. Chlamydophila pneumoniae antibodies in office workers with and without inflammatory rheumatic diseases in a moisture-damaged building. *Eur J Clin Microbiol Infect Dis*. 2005 Mar;24(3):236-7

[614] Roponen M, Kiviranta J, Seuri M, Tukiainen H, Myllykangas-Luosujärvi R, Hirvonen MR. Inflammatory mediators in nasal lavage, induced sputum and serum of employees with rheumatic and respiratory disorders. *Eur Respir J*. 2001 Sep;18(3):542-8

[615] Luosujärvi RA, Husman TM, Seuri M, Pietikäinen MA, Pollari P, Pelkonen J, Hujakka HT, Kaipiainen-Seppänen OA, Aho K. Joint symptoms and diseases associated with moisture damage in a health center. *Clin Rheumatol*. 2003 Dec;22(6):381-5

Fourteen cases had elevated levels of **circulating immune complexes** in 1998, 17 in 1999, but there were only three cases in 2001, when the health center had been closed for 18 months. **The high incidence of joint problems among these employees suggests a common triggering factor for most of the cases. As some of the symptoms had tended to subside while the health center was closed, the underlying causes are probably related to the building itself** and possibly to the abnormal microbial growth in its structures."

Cleaning the home/work/recreational environment of microbial contaminants

Household "dust" is actually a complex mixture of microscopic particles such as fabric fragments (from bedding, carpet, clothing, etc.), pollen (from outdoor plants), dirt (which has settled from the air), dead skin cells (from humans and pets), bacteria and mold, and the feces of dust mites and other insects. Since dust, especially the feces from dust mites, is very allergenic, particularly for patients with eczema, we are wise to take effective steps to reduce the amount of dust/contaminants to which we are exposed. Reducing the amount of "dust" in a home environment involves 3 general steps:

1. **Dust, mold, and chemical removal**
   - <u>Cleaning</u>: Periodically, use a damp cloth on furniture to remove dust that accumulates.
   - <u>Vacuuming</u>: Vacuum the floors/carpet and ensure that the vacuum is equipped with an *allergy filter* or HEPA filter to ensure that the dust is not simply transposed from the floor back into the air and onto furniture, bedding, and clothes. In severe cases, patients with inflammatory disorders, allergies/eczema, and environmental sensitivity may choose to have carpets removed and replaced either with a low-offgassing/outgassing flooring such as bamboo hardwoods or ceramic tile.
   - <u>Exclude pollen/mold</u>: Close doors and windows on days the pollen/mold count is high.
   - <u>Pet control</u>: If you have pets, it is often helpful to 1) wash them regularly, 2) keep them off the bedding, and/or 3) allow them to stay outdoors as much as is possible and practical.
   - <u>Using air filters for the central cooling/heating unit</u>: Consider the "Filterete Allergen Reducing Filter" from 3M (comes with a purple label). Other, more expensive and effective options are available for complicated cases.
   - <u>Vinyl/hypoallergenic mattress cover</u>: Buy and use a simple hypoallergenic or vinyl mattress cover to eliminate exposure to years of accumulated dust inside the mattress which is slept on for 8 hours each night. The goal is create an airtight seal around the mattress to contain the dust and antigens. Vinyl mattress covers are inexpensive and widely available.
2. **Reducing the amount of moisture in the air**. Ideally, the steam from bathing and cooking areas should be vented outdoors so that moisture does not accumulate inside the living area. Moisture is necessary for dust mites and mold to live and to create allergens; if the air is very moist then the inflammation-producing activities of the dust mites and mold are stimulated. Conversely, by reducing the humidity in the air, we are able to impair the microbes and thus reduce the amount of antigens. Reducing the amount of moisture in the air by use of an electric dehumidifier may be necessary to help reduce the amount of both dust allergen and mold in a home.
3. **Wash clothes/linens with eucalyptus oil to eliminate dust mites:** The combination of 1) hot water, 2) detergent, and 3) eucalyptus oil is an effective and natural way to get rid of dust mites and dust allergens. As validated by research published in *Journal of Allergy and Clinical Immunology*[616], this is an effective technique for killing and eliminating dust mites from clothing and bed sheets. "Bi-O-Klean Hand Dishwashing Liquid" available at Whole Foods Market or "Kit liquid dishwashing detergent concentrate" meet the criteria for the selection of a detergent for this purpose. Eucalyptus oil must never be applied to the skin or taken internally.

Metric measurements from the original study	*"American" unit translation*	*One-half recipe*
1. **Eucalyptus oil**: 100 mL	6 tablespoons or 3.4 oz.	3 tablespoons or 1½ oz.
2. **Detergent**: 25 mL liquid concentrated dishwashing detergent	1 ½ tablespoons or 0.8 oz.	¾ tablespoons or 0.4 oz.
3. **Warm water** (30°C): 50 Liters	86°F water: 13 gallons	86°F water: 6 gallons
4. **Soak clothing/bedding in hot detergent-eucalyptus solution for 15-30 minutes, then wash in machine as usual.**		

---

[616] 1) When mixed, the oil-detergent mixture should dissolve to form a clear homogenous solution, and 2) five mL (1 teaspoon) of the mixture stirred with 200 mL (6 oz.) of water should form a "milky, opaque solution that is stable (does not "break oil") for at least 10 minutes." Tovey ER, McDonald LG. A simple washing procedure with eucalyptus oil for controlling house dust mites and their allergens in clothing and bedding. *J Allergy Clin Immunol*. 1997 Oct;100(4):464-6

Problematic Bacteria, Yeast, and Parasites: A Listing of Commonly Encountered Dysbiotic Microorganisms
All of the following yeast, bacteria, and "parasites" have been observed in various patients in my private practice of chiropractic and naturopathic medicine. Even though several of these microbes are considered nonpathogenic by outdated medical paradigms[617,618,619] that are still hypnotized by Pasteur and Koch (ie, the "external invader paradigm"), their presence is generally inconsistent with optimal health and their eradication is rewarding for both doctor and patient. In other words, **even if a microbe is not a true pathogen and is thus not a therapeutic target from a *disease-oriented paradigm*, we as clinicians are still justified in eradicating it from our chronically ill patient from a *wellness-oriented paradigm* because we know that 1) eradicating potentially harmful bacteria will do no harm to the patient, and 2) in many cases—indeed *the majority* of cases—patients experience a significant and sustained clinical improvement regardless of their presenting complaint, thus implying a causal relationship between the microbe and the non-infectious illness.**

The following microbes are commonly detected with stool testing performed by a specialty laboratory. **One of the benefits of specialized stool testing is that it allows the presence of microbes to be determined within a context that evaluates the patient's individualized response.** For example, the finding of a mild degree of *Candida albicans* ("+1" on a 0-4 scale) might be considered insignificant; however if no other pathogens are identified, and the secretory IgA, lactoferrin, and lysozyme levels are elevated, then the clinician is justified in determining that the patient is having a hypersensitivity reaction to an otherwise "benign" yeast. **Remember, we are not looking for classic "infection" here; we are looking to determine which underlying disruptions may be exacerbating inflammation and the patient's symptomatology.** We have to look beyond the *disease-associated characteristics of the microbe* to see *the patient's individualized response to the microbe*. **Often what we find when working with autoimmune/inflammatory patients is that they are having a *pathogenic inflammatory response* to a *nonpathogenic* microbe.** When reading the following table, rather than focusing on the details, readers should read the information with due dilligance with the final goal being not the memorization of microb-disease associations but rather the concept that microbial colonization is a sufficient trigger for induction of inflammation and the clinical appearance of many "autoimmune disorders." The distinguishing characteristic that differentiates "an idiopathic autoimmune disease" from "microbe-triggered reactive arthritis" is not the biochemistry of the inflammatory cascade nor the pathohistologic findings; but rather, the defining characteristic of reactive arthritis is the presence of an idenfiied microbial exposure. Therefore, the practical distinction is made by the clinician—not the disease entity itself. If the physician searches for and emprically treats the microbial triggers for most "idiopathic inflammatory disorders" and "autoimmune diseases", then that clinician will—in the words of Henry David Thoreau in <u>Walden</u>—"meet with a success unexpected in common hours."

Commonly Encountered Dysbiotic Microorganisms—*alphabetized listing*

Dysbiotic microbe	Pathophysiology and clinical manifestations
Aeromonas hydrophila	• *Aeromonas hydrophila* can cause colitis and should therefore be eradicated immediately upon detection.[620]
Blastocystis hominis	• Commonly asymptomatic; can cause abdominal pain, nausea, vomiting, diarrhea, weight loss[621,622], fever, chills, malaise, anorexia, flatus, eosinophilia[623] • Fecal leukocytes are occasionally seen[624]; can cause colitis[625]

[617] "...standard of care in developed countries is to maintain schizophrenia patients on neuroleptics, this practice is not supported by the 50-year research record for the drugs. ...this paradigm of care worsens long-term outcomes, ... 40% of all schizophrenia patients would fare better if they were not so medicated." Whitaker R. The case against antipsychotic drugs: a 50-year record of doing more harm than good. *Med Hypotheses*. 2004;62:5-1 psychrights.org/Research/Digest/Chronicity/50yearecord.pdf
[618] Hyman M. Paradigm shift: the end of "normal science" in medicine understanding function in nutrition, health, and disease. *Altern Ther Health Med*. 2004 Sep-Oct;10(5):10-5, 90-4
[619] Heaney RP. Vitamin D, nutritional deficiency, and the medical paradigm. *J Clin Endocrinol Metab*. 2003 Nov;88(11):5107-8 http://jcem.endojournals.org/cgi/content/full/88/11/5107
[620] Farraye FA, Peppercorn MA, Ciano PS, Kavesh WN. Charles A. Segmental colitis associated with Aeromonas hydrophila. *Am J Gastroenterol*. 1989 Apr;84(4):436-8
[621] O'Gorman MA, Orenstein SR, Proujansky R, Wadowsky RM, Putnam PE, Kocoshis SA. Prevalence and characteristics of Blastocystis hominis infection in children. *Clin Pediatr* (Phila) 1993 Feb;32(2):91-6
[622] Telalbasic S, Pikula ZP, Kapidzic M. Blastocystis hominis may be a potential cause of intestinal disease. *Scand J Infect Dis* 1991;23(3):389-90
[623] Sheehan DJ, Raucher BG, McKitrick JC. Association of Blastocystis hominis with signs and symptoms of human disease. *J Clin Microbiol*. 1986;24(4):548-50
[624] Diaczok BJ, Rival J. Diarrhea due to Blastocystis hominis: an old organism revisited. *South Med J* 1987 Jul;80(7):931-2
[625] Russo AR, Stone SL, Taplin ME, Snapper HJ, Doern GV. Presumptive evidence for Blastocystis hominis as a cause of colitis. *Arch Intern Med*. 1988 May;148(5):1064

Commonly Encountered Dysbiotic Microorganisms—*alphabetized listing,* continued

Microbe	Pathophysiology and clinical manifestations
Candida albicans and other yeasts	• Although normal in small amounts ("+1"), excess *Candida* in the intestines is never a sign of optimal health. Patients may have mild general symptoms such as fatigue and dyscognition ("brain fog"); gas and intestinal bloating following consumption of carbohydrates are common. • *Candida* produces an immunosuppressive myotoxin called gliotoxin as well as an IgA-destroying protease and can cause watery diarrhea, particularly in elderly, ill, and immunosuppressed patients.[626] • *Candida* is always present in the gastrointestinal tract of women with recurrent yeast vaginitis.[627] • Some people have an inflammatory hypersensitivity to *Candida,* as it can cause **local allergic dermatitis/mucositis**[628], **colitis**[629], and **pulmonary inflammation (hypersensitivity alveolitis** from gastrointestinal colonization).[630] • Other yeasts such as *Candida parapsilosis* and *Geotrichum capitatum* are occasionally seen and should be eradicated.
Citrobacter rodentium *Citrobacter freundii*	• *Citrobacter freundii* is a gram-negative anaerobe; it produces pro-inflammatory endotoxin • *Citrobacter* species may cause **gastroenteritis** in humans[631] • Most strains of *Citrobacter freundii* produce hydrogen sulfide[632] which interferes with mitochondrial function and energy production and may be a major causative molecule in **ulcerative colitis**.[633] • Animal studies have shown that this bacterium can induce an intense inflammatory response in the gastrointestinal tract that resembles **inflammatory bowel disease**.[634] • Gastrointestinal dysbiosis with *Citrobacter freundii* may be causative in so-called "rheumatoid arthritis" in some patients.[author's experience]
Dientamoeba fragilis	• *Dientamoeba fragilis* is a flagellate protozoan that can cause **diarrhea, abdominal pain, nausea, vomiting, fatigue, malaise, eosinophilia, urticaria, pruritus and/or weight loss**. It is commonly associated with pinworm infection and may produce a clinical picture that mimics **food allergy, colitis, or eosinophilic enteritis**.[635]

[626] Gupta TP, Ehrinpreis MN. Candida-associated diarrhea in hospitalized patients. *Gastroenterology* 1990 Mar;98(3):780-5

[627] Miles MR, Olsen L, Rogers A. Recurrent vaginal candidiasis. Importance of an intestinal reservoir. *JAMA.* 1977 Oct 24;238(17):1836-7

[628] Ramirez De Knott HM, McCormick TS, et al. Cutaneous hypersensitivity to Candida albicans in idiopathic vulvodynia. *Contact Dermatitis.* 2005 Oct;53(4):214-8

[629] Doby T. Monilial esophagitis and colitis. *J Maine Med Assoc.* 1971 May;62(5):109-14

[630] "We conclude that the disease was induced by C.a.-antigen reaching the lungs from the intestinal tract via the bloodstream." Schreiber J, Struben C, Rosahl W, Amthor M. Hypersensitivity alveolitis induced by endogenous candida species. *Eur J Med Res.* 2000 Mar 27;5(3):126

[631] "Members of this genus can cause neonatal meningitis and, perhaps, gastroenteritis in both children and adults." Lipsky BA, Hook EW 3rd, Smith AA, Plorde JJ. Citrobacter infections in humans: experience at the Seattle Veterans Administration Medical Center and a review of the literature. *Rev Infect Dis.* 1980 Sep-Oct;2:746-60

[632] Lennette EH (editor in chief). Manual of Clinical Microbiology. Fourth Edition. Washington DC; American Society for Microbiology: 1985, page 269. See also http://web.indstate.edu/thcme/micro/GI/general/sld038.htm Accessed 10/27/2005

[633] "CONCLUSIONS: Metabolic effects of sodium hydrogen sulfide on butyrate oxidation along the length of the colon closely mirror metabolic abnormalities observed in active ulcerative colitis, and the increased production of sulfide in ulcerative colitis suggests that the action of mercaptides may be involved in the genesis of ulcerative colitis." Roediger WE, Duncan A, Kapaniris O, Millard S. Reducing sulfur compounds of the colon impair colonocyte nutrition: implications for ulcerative colitis. *Gastroenterology.* 1993 Mar;104(3):802-9

[634] Higgins LM, Frankel G, Douce G, Dougan G, MacDonald TT. Citrobacter rodentium infection in mice elicits a mucosal Th1 cytokine response and lesions similar to those in murine inflammatory bowel disease. *Infect Immun.* 1999 Jun;67(6):3031-9 http://iai.asm.org/cgi/reprint/67/6/3031.pdf

[635] Cuffari C, Oligny L, Seidman EG. Dientamoeba fragilis masquerading as allergic colitis. *J Pediatr Gastroenterol Nutr.* 1998 Jan;26(1):16-20

Commonly Encountered Dysbiotic Microorganisms—*alphabetized listing, continued*

Dysbiotic microbe	Pathophysiology and clinical manifestations
Endolimax nana	<ul><li>*Endolimax nana*, a protozoa, has a world-wide distribution and is commonly considered an harmless commensal of the intestine.[636]</li><li>Intestinal infection with *Endolimax nana* can cause a **peripheral arthropathy** that is clinically similar to **rheumatoid arthritis** and which remits with effective parasite eradication.[637]</li><li>In my own clinical practice, I have seen several cases of intestinal colonization with *Endolimax nana* in patients who presented with **chronic fatigue, myalgia, eczema**, and especially refractory **chronic vaginitis.**</li></ul>
Entamoeba histolytica	<ul><li>Induces tissue damage, **amebic colitis**, and **liver abscess.**[638]</li><li>Associated with **Henoch Schonlein purpura** in a single case report[639]</li><li>**Amebic colitis** may be misdiagnosed as **ulcerative colitis.**[640]</li><li>May contribute to **irritable bowel syndrome, rheumatoid arthritis, fibromyalgia, food allergy**, or **multiple chemical sensitivity** and can **exacerbate HIV infection.**[641]</li><li>Hepatic infection is associated with induction of antineutrophil cytoplasmic antibodies (ANCA) such as seen with the vasculitic disease Wegener's granulomatosis.[642]</li></ul>
Gamma strep *Enterococcus*	<ul><li>"Gamma strep", *Enterococcus faecalis*, and *Streptococcus faecalis* are somewhat interchangeable terms.[643,644,645] These terms refer to gram-positive *Enterococcus* species such as *Enterococcus faecalis*, which cause **urinary tract infections, bacteremia, intra-abdominal infections, and endocarditis.**</li><li>Enterococci produce **lipoteichoic acid** which is proinflammatory in a manner similar to endotoxin from gram-negative bacteria, and these gram-positive bacteria also appear to produce a superantigen.[646]</li><li>"Gamma strep" is commonly identified in stool tests of patients with **chronic unwellness and fatigue.**</li></ul>
Giardia lamblia *"Beaver fever"*	<ul><li>Causatively associated with **abdominal pain, diarrhea, constipation, bloating, chronic fatigue, and food allergy/intolerance.**[647]</li><li>May contribute to **irritable bowel syndrome, rheumatoid arthritis, food allergy, or multiple chemical sensitivity.**[648]</li><li>Extraintestinal symptoms of gastrointestinal *Giardia* infection can include **fever, maculopapular rashes, geographic tongue, pulmonary infiltrates, lymphadenopathy, <u>polyarthritis</u>, aphthous ulcers, and urticaria.**[649]</li></ul>

[636] Information available at http://www2.provlab.ab.ca/bugs/webbug/parasite/artifact/enana.htm as of December 26, 2003

[637] "Endolimax nana grew on stool culture. Both the patient's diarrhea and arthritis responded effectively to therapy with metronidazole. The diagnosis of parasitic rheumatism was made in retrospect." Burnstein SL, Liakos S. Parasitic rheumatism presenting as rheumatoid arthritis. *J Rheumatol*. 1983 Jun;10(3):514-5

[638] Huston CD. Parasite and host contributions to the pathogenesis of amebic colitis. *Trends Parasitol*. 2004 Jan; 20(1): 23-6

[639] Demircin G, Oner A, Erdogan O, Bulbul M, Memis L. Henoch Schonlein purpura and amebiasis. *Acta Paediatr Jpn*. 1998 Oct; 40(5): 489-91

[640] Galland L. Intestinal protozoan infection is a common unsuspected cause of chronic illness. *J Advancement Med*. 1989;2: 539-552

[641] Galland L. Intestinal protozoan infection is a common unsuspected cause of chronic illness. *J Advancement Med*. 1989;2: 539-552

[642] George J, Levy Y, Kallenberg CG, Shoenfeld Y. Infections and Wegener's granulomatosis--a cause and effect relationship? *QJM*. 1997 May;90(5):367-73 http://qjmed.oxfordjournals.org/cgi/reprint/90/5/367

[643] "Figure 38: "Gamma *Streptococcus*" : *Enterococcus faecalis*" and "The genus *Enterococcus* was once a part of the *Streptococcus* genus, was considered a "gamma *Streptococcus* species." http://www.microbelibrary.org/asmonly/details_print.asp?id=1986&lang

[644] "Enterococcus faecalis. Synonyms: group D strep, Streptococcus faecalis. Classification: facultative anaerobic, gram+ bacteria, cocci." http://medinfo.ufl.edu/year2/mmid/bms5300/bugs/strfaeca.html

[645] "Microscopically, Gram-positive cocci occurring in chains or pairs with individual cells being somewhat elongated can be presumed to be streptococci or enterococci." http://members.tripod.com/piece_de_resistance/SAARS/bugs/menteroc.htm

[646] Lynn E. Hancock and Michael S. Gilmore. Department of Microbiology and Immunology, University of Oklahoma Health Sciences Center. Pathogenicity of Enterococci published in "Gram-Positive Pathogens" edited by Fischetti V et al. http://w3.ouhsc.edu/enterococcus/lynn_revirew.asp

[647] Galland L, Lee M. #170 High frequency of giardiasis in patients with chronic digestive complaints. *Am J Gastroenterol* 1989;84:1181

[648] Galland L. Intestinal protozoan infection is a common unsuspected cause of chronic illness. *J Advancement Med*. 1989;2: 539-552

[649] Corsi A, Nucci C, Knafelz D, Bulgarini D, Di Iorio L, Polito A, De Risi F, Ardenti Morini F, Paone FM. Ocular changes associated with Giardia lamblia infection in children. *Br J Ophthalmol*. 1998 Jan;82(1):59-62 http://bjo.bmjjournals.com/cgi/content/full/82/1/59

Microbe	Pathophysiology and clinical manifestations
Giardia lamblia [continued from previous page]	• **Ocular complications** from gastrointestinal infection include iridocyclitis, choroiditis, retinal hemorrhages, anterior and posterior uveitis, retinal vasculitis, and "salt and pepper" retinal degeneration. These complications are most likely due to deposition of **immune complexes** in the retinal epithelium.[650] • Reported to have caused numerous cases of **reactive arthritis (peripheral arthritis and/or sacroiliitis)** in patients who are either positive or negative for HLA-B27[651]; "beaver fever" is a cause of reactive arthritis.[652] • Antigen detection appears superior to microscopic examination for detection.[653]
Hafnia alvei	• *Hafnia alvei* is a gram-negative bacterium capable of causing **reactive arthritis** from gastrointestinal infection; the reactive arthritis associated with *Hafnia alvei* occurs without association with HLA-B27.[654]
Helicobacter pylori	• *H. pylori* is a gram-negative endotoxin-producing rod that causes stomach ulcers and appears to cause **reactive arthritis** in some patients.[655] • *H. pylori* colonization is increased in patients with **scleroderma.**[656] • *H. pylori* is commonly found in the middle ear of patients with acute otitis media.[657] • Strongly and causatively associated with Raynaud's syndrome/phenomenon.
Klebsiella pneumoniae	• Many cases of gastrointestinal colonization with this microorganism produce no acute gastrointestinal symptoms such as nausea, vomiting, constipation, or diarrhea. Patients may have mild general symptoms such as fatigue and dyscognition ("brain fog"). • Can cause **diarrhea**[658] and **acute gastroenteritis.**[659] • Associated with **reactive arthritis** such as **ankylosing spondylitis.**[660] • Gram-negative bacteria, produces endotoxin/lipopolysaccharide that is capable of impairing cytochrome p-450 and **reducing hepatic clearance and urinary/biliary excretion of drugs.**[661]

[650] "The retinal changes associated with giardiasis are more than likely caused by immune mechanisms. Wania reported that circulating immune complexes were found in all of the patients with ocular complications he examined." Corsi A, Nucci C, Knafelz D, Bulgarini D, Di Iorio L, Polito A, De Risi F, Ardenti Morini F, Paone FM. Ocular changes associated with Giardia lamblia infection in children. *Br J Ophthalmol*. 1998 Jan;82(1):59-62 http://bjo.bmjjournals.com/cgi/content/full/82/1/59

[651] Layton MA, Dziedzic K, Dawes PT. Sacroiliitis in an HLA B27-negative patient following giardiasis. *Br J Rheumatol*. 1998 May;37(5):581-3 http://rheumatology.oxfordjournals.org/cgi/reprint/37/5/581

[652] "Giardia lamblia infection is rarely associated with adult reactive arthritis. We report the first North American case and review the pediatric and adult literature to date. Antimicrobial treatment is essential to eradicate the parasite and control the arthritis." Tupchong M, Simor A, Dewar C. Beaver fever--a rare cause of reactive arthritis. *J Rheumatol*. 1999 Dec;26(12):2701-2

[653] "For all patients, microscopy was uniformly negative, but 6 of 13 patients were antigen positive... Giardiasis, an increasing problem in family practice, should be considered early in patients with GI disturbances. New, sensitive immunodiagnostic tests that usually require a single specimen are more useful than microscopy." Chappell CL, Matson CC. Giardia antigen detection in patients with chronic gastrointestinal disturbances. *J Fam Pract*. 1992 Jul;35(1):49-53

[654] Toivanen P, Toivanen A. Two forms of reactive arthritis? *Ann Rheum Dis*. 1999 Dec;58(12):737-41 http://ard.bmjjournals.com/cgi/content/full/58/12/737 See also: Newmark JJ, Hobbs WN, Wilson BE. Reactive arthritis associated with Hafnia alvei enteritis. *Arthritis Rheum*. 1994 Jun;37(6):960

[655] "Our findings suggest that HP may be included in the list of possible arthritis triggering microbes." Melby KK, Kvien TK, Glennas A. Helicobacter pylori--a trigger of reactive arthritis? *Infection*. 1999;27(4-5):252-5

[656] "Patients with SSc have H. pylori infection at a higher prevalence than the general population." Yazawa N, Fujimoto M, Kikuchi K, Kubo M, Ihn H, Sato S, Tamaki T, Tamaki K. High seroprevalence of Helicobacter pylori infection in patients with systemic sclerosis: association with esophageal involvement. *J Rheumatol*. 1998 Apr;25(4):650-3

[657] "Twelve of 15 smears for MEE were positive for HP by immunohistochemistry and 14 by Giemsa that were Gram-negative." Morinaka S, Tominaga M, Nakamura H. Detection of Helicobacter pylori in the middle ear fluid of patients with otitis media with effusion. *Otolaryngol Head Neck Surg*. 2005 Nov;133(5):791-4

[658] Niyogi SK, Pal A, Mitra U, Dutta P. Enteroaggregative Klebsiella pneumoniae in association with childhood diarrhoea. *Indian J Med Res* 2000 Oct;112:133-4

[659] Ananthan, Raju S, Alavandi S. Enterotoxigenicity of Klebsiella pneumoniae associated with childhood gastroenteritis in Madras, India. *Jpn J Infect Dis* 1999 Feb;52(1):16-7

[660] Ahmadi K, Wilson C, Tiwana H, Binder A, Ebringer A. Antibodies to Klebsiella pneumoniae lipopolysaccharide in patients with ankylosing spondylitis. *Br J Rheumatol*. 1998 Dec;37(12):1330-3

[661] Hasegawa T, Takagi K, Kitaichi K. Effects of bacterial endotoxin on drug pharmacokinetics. *Nagoya J Med Sci* 1999 May;62(1-2):11-28

Commonly encountered dysbiotic microorganisms—*alphabetized listing, continued*

Dysbiotic microbe	Pathophysiology and clinical manifestations
Proteus mirabilis	• Gram-negative bacteria, produces endotoxin/lipopolysaccharide.[662] • Gastrointestinal and urinary tract colonization is associated with **rheumatoid arthritis**[663,664] and **ankylosing spondylitis.**[665] • In one of my patients, GI dysbiosis with *Proteus* incited "**idiopathic inflammatory polyneuropathy**" that disappeared within one month of parasite eradication and which coincided with normalization of hsCRP.
Pseudomonas aeruginosa	• *Pseudomonas aeruginosa* is a gram-negative bacterium, produces endotoxin[666] and can cause antibiotic-associated diarrhea.[667,668] • Many cases of gastrointestinal colonization with this microorganism produce no acute gastrointestinal symptoms such as nausea, vomiting, constipation, or diarrhea. Patients may have mild general symptoms such as fatigue and dyscognition ("brain fog"). • Patients with **multiple sclerosis** show evidence of a heightened immune response against *Pseudomonas aeruginosa*, consistent with cross-reactivity.[669]

Comprehensive Stool Analysis / Parasitology x3

MICROBIOLOGY

Bacteriology Culture

Beneficial flora		Imbalances		Dysbiotic flora	
Bifidobacter	4+	Haemolytic E. coli	4+	Pseudomonas sp.	4+
E. coli	4+	Gamma strep	2+		
Lactobacillus	2+				

Mycology (Yeast) Culture

Normal flora		Dysbiotic flora
Candida glabrata	1+	
Rhodotorula sp.	1+	

Stool culture results showing overgrowth of *Pseudomonas* in a patient with sensorimotor peripheral neuropathy—immunorestoration, immunomolulation, and antimicrobial therapy resulted in sustained remission of fatigue, periodic fever, and neuropathy: *Psuedomonas aeruginosa* shows cross-reactivity with human neuronal tissues.[670,671] Note also the abnormal yeast, consistent with GI immunosuppression.

---

[662] Kondakova et al. Structural and serological studies of the O-antigen of Proteus mirabilis O-9. *Carbohydr Res* 2003 May 23;338(11):1191-6

[663] Ebringer A, Rashid T, Wilson C. Rheumatoid arthritis: proposal for the use of anti-microbial therapy in early cases. *Scand J Rheumatol* 2003;32(1):2-11

[664] Rashid T, Darlington G, Kjeldsen-Kragh J, Forre O, Collado A, Ebringer A. Proteus IgG antibodies and C-reactive protein in English, Norwegian and Spanish patients with rheumatoid arthritis. *Clin Rheumatol* 1999;18(3):190-5

[665] Wilson C, Rashid T, Tiwana H, et al. Cytotoxicity responses to Peptide antigens in rheumatoid arthritis and ankylosing spondylitis. *J Rheumatol* 2003 May;30(5):972-8

[666] Bergan T. Pathogenetic factors of Pseudomonas aeruginosa. *Scand J Infect Dis Suppl.* 1981;29:7-12

[667] Kim et al. Pseudomonas aeruginosa as a potential cause of antibiotic-associated diarrhea. *J Korean Med Sci.* 2001 Dec;16(6):742-4

[668] Porco FV, Visconte EB. Pseudomonas aeruginosa as a cause of infectious diarrhea successfully treated with oral ciprofloxacin. *Ann Pharmacother.* 1995 Nov;29(11):1122-3

[669] Hughes LE, Bonell S, Natt RS, et al. Antibody responses to Acinetobacter spp. and Pseudomonas aeruginosa in multiple sclerosis: prospects for diagnosis using the myelin-acinetobacter-neurofilament antibody index. *Clin Diagn Lab Immunol.* 2001 Nov;8(6):1181-8

[670] Hughes LE, Bonell S, Natt RS, et al. Antibody responses to Acinetobacter spp. and Pseudomonas aeruginosa in multiple sclerosis: prospects for diagnosis using the myelin-acinetobacter-neurofilament antibody index. *Clin Diagn Lab Immunol.* 2001 Nov;8(6):1181-8 http://cvi.asm.org/content/8/6/1181.full.pdf

[671] Hughes LE, Smith PA, Bonell S, Natt RS, Wilson C, Rashid T, Amor S, Thompson EJ, Croker J, Ebringer A. Cross-reactivity between related sequences found in Acinetobacter sp., Pseudomonas aeruginosa, myelin basic protein and myelin oligodendrocyte glycoprotein in multiple sclerosis. *J Neuroimmunol.* 2003 Nov;144:105-15

Commonly encountered dysbiotic microorganisms—*alphabetized listing,* *continued*

Dysbiotic microbe	Pathophysiology and clinical manifestations
Staphylococcus aureus *Staphylococcus epidermidis*	• **Any and all *Staphylococcus aureus* should be eradicated immediately due to the well-known inflammatory consequences of the toxins and superantigens this bacterium produces.** *Staphylococcus aureus* is a gram-positive bacterium, certain strains of which produce the toxic shock syndrome toxin-1 (TSST-1) that produces scalded skin syndrome, toxic shock syndrome, and food poisoning; other strains of *Staphylococcus aureus* that do not produce TSST-1 are also capable of causing toxic shock syndrome from colonization of bone, vagina, wounds, or rectum.[672] • Gastrointestinal colonization with *Staphylococcus aureus* is a known cause of **acute colitis**[673], and nasal carriage of this bacterium is documented in patients with several autoimmune disorders, including **Wegener's granulomatosis**[674], **systemic lupus erythematosus**[675] and **psoriasis.**[676, 677] • *Staphylococcus aureus* can trigger **reactive arthritis.**[678] • *Staphylococcus epidermidis* can trigger **reactive arthritis and sacroiliitis.**[679] • Patients with **Behcet's syndrome** commonly have skin lesions that are colonized by *Staphylococcus aureus*.[680] • Most (57%) of patients with **atopic dermatitis** show evidence of IgE-mediated histamine release (i.e., "allergy") to exotoxins secreted from *Staphylococcus aureus*, which commonly colonizes eczematous skin[681]; in other words: most eczema patients are allergic to their own dermal bacteria and can thus be said to have *hypersensitivity dermal dysbiosis*.

---

[672] Shandera WX, Moran A. "Infectious diseases: viral and rickettsial." In Tierney LM, McPhee SJ Papadakis MA (eds). Current Medical Diagnosis and Treatment. 44th edition. New York: Lange; 2005, page 1356-8

[673] Watanabe H, Masaki H, Asoh N, Watanabe K, Oishi K, Kobayashi S, Sato A, Nagatake T. Enterocolitis caused by methicillin-resistant Staphylococcus aureus: molecular characterization of respiratory and digestive tract isolates. *Microbiol Immunol.* 2001;45(9):629-34 http://www.jstage.jst.go.jp/article/mandi/45/9/629/_pdf

[674] Popa ER, Stegeman CA, Kallenberg CG, Tervaert JW. Staphylococcus aureus and Wegener's granulomatosis. *Arthritis Res.* 2002;4(2):77-9 http://arthritis-research.com/content/4/2/077

[675] Medline abstract from Polish research: "In 9 from 14 patients with (64.3%) a.b. very massive growth of Staphylococcus aureus in culture from vestibulae of the nose swab was, in other cultures very massive growth of physiological flora was seen. ...clinical significance of asymptomatic bacteriuria and pathogenic bacteria colonisation of nostrils as a precedence to symptomatic infections needs further investigations." Koseda-Dragan M, Hebanowski M, Galinski J, Krzywinska E, Bakowska A. [Asymptomatic bacteriuria in women diagnosed with systemic lupus erythematosus (SLE)] *Pol Arch Med Wewn.* 1998 Oct;100(4):321-30.

[676] "The nasal carriage rate of Staphylococcus aureus in psoriatics was higher than the control groups." Singh G, Rao DJ. Bacteriology of psoriatic plaques. *Dermatologica.* 1978;157(1):21-7

[677] "In this study, S aureus was present in more than 50% of patients with AD and PS. We found that the severity of AD and PS significantly correlated to enterotoxin production of the isolated S aureus strains." Tomi NS, Kranke B, Aberer E. Staphylococcal toxins in patients with psoriasis, atopic dermatitis, and erythroderma, and in healthy control subjects. *J Am Acad Dermatol.* 2005 Jul;53(1):67-72

[678] "CONCLUSION--Reactive arthritis may rarely follow Staph aureus infection. HLA-B27 negativity may be associated with a self limited arthritis in these cases." Siam AR, Hammoudeh M. Staphylococcus aureus triggered reactive arthritis. *Ann Rheum Dis.* 1995 Feb;54(2):131-3

[679] "We report an unusual case of a patient with SE bacteriaemia, who developed elbow arthritis, asymmetrical sacroiliitis, keratoderma and restrictive cardiomyopathy." Giordano N, Senesi M, Battisti E, Palumbo F, Mondillo S, Bargagli G, Palazzuoli V, Nardi P, Gennari C. Reactive arthritis by staphylococcus epidermidis: report of an unusual case. *Clin Rheumatol.* 1996;15(1):59-61

[680] "At least one type of microorganism was grown from each pustule. Staphylococcus aureus (41/70, 58.6%, p = 0.008) and Prevotella spp (17/70, 24.3%, p = 0.002) were significantly more common in pustules from BS patients, and coagulase negative staphylococci (17/37, 45.9%, p = 0.007) in pustules from acne patients. CONCLUSIONS: The pustular lesions of BS are not usually sterile." Hatemi G, Bahar H, Uysal S, Mat C, Gogus F, Masatlioglu S, Altas K, Yazici H. The pustular skin lesions in Behcet's syndrome are not sterile. *Ann Rheum Dis.* 2004 Nov;63(11):1450-2

[681] "These data indicate that a subset of patients with AD mount an IgE response to SEs that can be grown from their skin." Leung DY, Harbeck R, Bina P, Reiser RF, Yang E, Norris DA, Hanifin JM, Sampson HA. Presence of IgE antibodies to staphylococcal exotoxins on the skin of patients with atopic dermatitis. Evidence for a new group of allergens. *J Clin Invest.* 1993 Sep;92(3):1374-80 http://www.pubmedcentral.gov/articlerender.fcgi?tool=pubmed&pubmedid=7690780

Commonly encountered dysbiotic microorganisms—*alphabetized listing,* *continued*

Dysbiotic microbe	Pathophysiology and clinical manifestations
Streptococcus pyogenes *Group A streptococci*	• Intestinal overgrowth of this bacterium, which produces peptidoglycans, can cause **dermatosis, <u>inflammatory polyarthritis</u>, tenosynovitis, malaise, fever, and cryoglobulinemia.**[682] • Non-infectious manifestations precipitated by infection with *S. pyogenes* include **autoimmune neuropsychiatric disorders** (including obsessive-compulsive disorder and Sydenham's chorea), **dystonia, glomerulonephritis, and reactive arthritis.**[683] • Group A streptococci can cause **reactive arthritis** in humans.[684] • *Streptococcus pyogenes* is a very likely trigger of **psoriasis**[685]; chronic penicillin treatment leads to clinical improvement of recalcitrant psoriasis.[686] • Certain strains of *S. pyogenes* produce an exotoxin that can cause toxic shock syndrome.[687]

Clinical Benefits of Identifying and Eradicating Dysbiosis

In the previous section, I described the biochemical/physiologic mechanisms by which microorganisms can contribute to disease *without causing a classic "infection"* and promote systemic inflammation and human disease. Thus having developed the precept that **microorganisms can cause inflammatory disease by noninfectious means**, I will (re)state here that the cure of human disease by eradication of harmful microbes is not a requirement to prove the validity of this thesis. Inflammation and autoimmunity are self-perpetuating phenomena that can persist despite the effective eradication of the principle cause, and research has demonstrated that microbial antigens can remain present in synovial fluid for several years after the eradication of the primary infection.[688] With that said, we are fortunate to observe that **many patients with autoimmunity are indeed benefited and occasionally "cured" by removal of instigating microbes**. I have seen this on numerous occasions in my clinical practice, and this phenomenon has also been documented in the research literature. Examples published in the research include the amelioration of one patient's scleroderma with the eradication of intestinal bacterial overgrowth[689], the amelioration of Wegener's granulomatosis with antimicrobial therapy against *Staphylococcus aureus*[690,691], and the alleviation of inflammatory arthritis following the use of antibiotics against genitourinary *Chlamydia trachomatis* and gastrointestinal *Salmonella enteritidis, Yersinia enterocolitica, Shigella flexneri* or *Campylobacter jejuni*.[692] Treatments for addressing dysbiosis and its numerous sequelae are described in the pages/sections that follow.

> **Landmark work by Dr Patricia Noah**
>
> "We have repeatedly observed psoriatic flares associated with microbial infection, sequestered antigen, and colonization. **Removal of these microbial foci results in clearing of the disease.**"
>
> Patricia Noah PhD from University of Tennessee College of Medicine. *Semin Dermatol.* 1990

---

[682] Ely PH. The bowel bypass syndrome: a response to bacterial peptidoglycans. *J Am Acad Dermatol.* 1980 Jun;2(6):473-87

[683] Hahn RG, Knox LM, Forman TA. Evaluation of poststreptococcal illness. *Am Fam Physician.* 2005 May 15;71(10):1949-54 aafp.org/afp/20050515/1949.pdf

[684] "We present a patient whose clinical features are more consistent with post-streptococcal reactive arthritis than acute rheumatic fever." Howell EE, Bathon J. A case of post-streptococcal reactive arthritis. *Md Med J.* 1999 Nov-Dec;48(6):292-4

[685] "These findings justify the hypothesis that S pyogenes infections are more important in the pathogenesis of chronic plaque psoriasis than has previously been recognized, and indicate the need for further controlled therapeutic trials of antibacterial measures in this common skin disease." El-Rachkidy RG, Hales JM, Freestone PP, Young HS, Griffiths CE, Camp RD. Increased Blood Levels of IgG Reactive with Secreted Streptococcus pyogenes Proteins in Chronic Plaque Psoriasis. *J Invest Dermatol.* 2007 Mar 8

[686] "Total duration of the study was two years. Initially benzathine penicillin 1.2 million units, was given I.M. AST fortnightly. After 24 weeks benzathine penicillin was reduced to 1.2 million units once a month... Significant improvement in the PASI score was noted from 12 weeks onwards. All patients showed excellent improvement at 2 years." Saxena VN, Dogra J. Long-term use of penicillin for the treatment of chronic plaque psoriasis. *Eur J Dermatol.* 2005 Sep-Oct;15(5):359-62 http://www.john-libbey-eurotext.fr/en/revues/medecine/ejd/e-docs/00/04/10/A4/article.md?type=text.html

[687] Chikkamuniyappa S. Streptococcal toxic shock syndrome and sepsis manifesting in a patient with chronic rheumatoid arthritis. *Dermatol Online J.* 2004 Jul 15;10(1):7

[688] "Extensive bacterial cultures of the synovial fluid were negative... We conclude that in patients with reactive arthritis after yersinia infection, microbial antigens can be found in synovial-fluid cells from the affected joints." Granfors K, Jalkanen S, von Essen R, Lahesmaa-Rantala R, Isomaki O, Pekkola-Heino K, Merilahti-Palo R, Saario R, Isomaki H, Toivanen A. Yersinia antigens in synovial-fluid cells from patients with reactive arthritis. *N Engl J Med.* 1989 Jan 26;320(4):216-2

[689] Over KE, Bucknall RC. Regression of skin changes in a patient with systemic sclerosis following treatment for bacterial overgrowth with ciprofloxacin. *Br J Rheumatol.* 1998 Jun;37(6):696

[690] Popa et al. Staphylococcus aureus and Wegener's granulomatosis. *Arthritis Res.* 2002;4(2):77-9 http://arthritis-research.com/content/4/2/077

[691] George J, Levy Y, Kallenberg CG, Shoenfeld Y. Infections and Wegener's granulomatosis--a cause and effect relationship? *QJM.* 1997 May;90(5):367-73 http://qjmed.oxfordjournals.org/cgi/reprint/90/5/367

[692] Kobayashi et al. Reactive arthritis: recent advances and clinical manifestations. *Intern Med.* 2005 May;44:408-12 jstage.jst.go.jp/article/internalmedicine/44/5/408/_pdf

Natural Treatments for the Eradication of Dysbiosis and Related Immune-Complex Diseases

Although antimicrobial drugs may be used, these are not universally curative and are not necessarily "more powerful" or "more effective" than natural treatments. Treatments for gastrointestinal dysbiosis may be somewhat summarized as follows: "*Starve, Poison, Crowd, Purge, and Support Immunity.*" The following concepts and therapeutics are particularly—though not exclusively—relevant for the treatment of *gastrointestinal* dysbiosis.

1. **Diet modifications ("*starve the microbes*")**: The diet plan should ensure **avoidance of sugar**, grains, soluble fiber, gums, prebiotics, and dairy products since these contain **fermentable carbohydrates that promote overgrowth of bacteria and other microorganisms in the gut**. Short-term **fasting** starves intestinal microbes, temporarily eliminates dietary antigens, alleviates "autointoxication", and stimulates the humoral immune system in the gut to more effectively destroy local microbes.[693,694] Thus, implementation of the "**specific carbohydrate diet**" popularized by Gottschall[695] along with periodic fasting, which has obvious anti-inflammatory benefits[696], can be used therapeutically in patients with conditions associated with dysbiosis-induced inflammation. Plant-based low-carbohydrate diets can lead to favorable changes in the quality and quantity of intestinal microflora. Hypoallergenic diets are proven beneficial for the treatment of the **immune complex disease** called mixed cryoglobulinemia.[697,698]

2. **Antimicrobial treatments ("*poison the microbes, not the patient*")**: Anti-microbial herbs can be used which directly kill or strongly inhibit the intestinal microbes. The most commonly used and well-documented botanicals in this regard are listed in the section below. Antimicrobial treatment is frequently continued for 1-3 months, and co-administration of drugs can be utilized when appropriate. Sometimes antimicrobial drugs are necessary, especially for acute and severe infections; often nutritional and botanical interventions are safer and more effective. Although these herbs are generally taken orally, some of them can also be applied topically (in a cream or lotion), and nasally (in a saline water lavage, as detailed previously). Botanical medicines are generally used in combination, and lower doses of each can be used when used in combination compared to the doses that are necessary when the herbs are used in isolation.

   - **Oregano oil in an emulsified and time-released tablet**: Botanical oils that are not emulsified do not attain maximal dispersion in the gastrointestinal tract; products that are not time-released may be absorbed before reaching the colon in sufficient concentrations. Emulsified oil of oregano in a time-released tablet is proven effective in the eradication of harmful gastrointestinal microbes, including *Blastocystis hominis*, *Entamoeba hartmanni*, and *Endolimax nana*.[699] An in vitro study[700] and clinical experience support the use of emulsified oregano against *Candida albicans*. The common dose is 600 mg per day in divided doses for at least 6 weeks.[701]

   - **Berberine**: Berberine is an alkaloid extracted from plant such as *Berberis vulgaris,* and *Hydrastis canadensis*, and it shows effectiveness against *Giardia*, *Candida,* and *Streptococcus* in addition to its direct anti-inflammatory and antidiarrheal actions. Oral dose of 400 mg per day is common for adults.[702] Topical *Mahonia/Berberis aquifolium* is effective for dermal psoriasis[703] via its combined anti-inflammatory and antimicrobial benefits.

[693] Trollmo C, Verdrengh M, Tarkowski A. Fasting enhances mucosal antigen specific B cell responses in rheumatoid arthritis. *Ann Rheum Dis*. 1997 Feb;56(2):130-4
[694] Ramakrishnan T, Stokes P. Beneficial effects of fasting and low carbohydrate diet in D-lactic acidosis associated with short-bowel syndrome. *JPEN J Parenter Enteral Nutr*. 1985 May-Jun;9(3):361-3
[695] Gottschall E. Breaking the Vicious Cycle: Intestinal Health Through Diet. Kirkton Press; Rev edition (August 1, 1994)
[696] "The pooling of these studies showed a statistically and clinically significant beneficial long-term effect." Muller H, de Toledo FW, Resch KL. Fasting followed by vegetarian diet in patients with rheumatoid arthritis: a systematic review. *Scand J Rheumatol*. 2001;30(1):1-10
[697] "CONCLUSION: These data show that an LAC diet decreases the amount of circulating immune complexes in MC and can modify certain signs and symptoms of the disease." Ferri C, Pietrogrande M, Cecchetti R, et al. Low-antigen-content diet in the treatment of patients with mixed cryoglobulinemia. *Am J Med*. 1989 Nov;87:519-24
[698] Pietrogrande M, Cefalo A, Nicora F, Marchesini D. Dietetic treatment of essential mixed cryoglobulinemia. *Ric Clin Lab*. 1986 Apr-Jun;16(2):413-6
[699] Force M, Sparks WS, Ronzio RA. Inhibition of enteric parasites by emulsified oil of oregano in vivo. *Phytother Res*. 2000 May;14(3):213-4
[700] Stiles JC, Sparks W, Ronzio RA. The inhibition of Candida albicans by oregano. *J Applied Nutr* 1995;47:96–102
[701] Force M, Sparks WS, Ronzio RA. Inhibition of enteric parasites by emulsified oil of oregano in vivo. *Phytother Res*. 2000 May;14(3):213-4
[702] Berberine. *Altern Med Rev*. 2000 Apr;5(2):175-7 http://www.thorne.com/altmedrev/.fulltext/5/2/175.pdf
[703] "Taken together, these clinical studies conducted by several investigators in several countries indicate that Mahonia aquifolium is a safe and effective treatment of patients with mild to moderate psoriasis." Gulliver WP, Donsky HJ. A report on three recent clinical trials using Mahonia aquifolium 10% topical cream and a review of the worldwide clinical experience with Mahonia aquifolium for the treatment of plaque psoriasis. *Am J Ther*. 2005 Sep-Oct;12(5):398-406

- *__Artemisia annua__*: Artemisinin has been safely used for centuries in Asia for the treatment of malaria[704,705], and it also has **effectiveness against anaerobic bacteria** due to the pro-oxidative sesquiterpene endoperoxide. In a recent study treating patients with malaria, "the adult artemisinin dose was 500 mg; children aged < 15 years received 10 mg/kg per dose" and thus the dose for an 80-lb child would be 363 mg per day by these criteria.[706] I commonly use **artemisinin at 100 mg twice per day (with other antimicrobial botanicals such as berberine) in divided doses for adults with dysbiosis.** One of the additional benefits of artemisinin is its systemic bioavailability.

- **St. John's Wort (*Hypericum perforatum*)**: Best known for its antidepressant action, **hyperforin from *Hypericum perforatum* also shows impressive antibacterial action, particularly against gram-positive bacteria such as *Staphylococcus aureus*, *Streptococcus pyogenes* and *Streptococcus agalactiae*.** According to in vitro studies, the lowest effective hyperforin concentration is 0.1 mcg/mL against *Corynebacterium diphtheriae* with increasing effectiveness against multiresistant *Staphylococcus aureus* at higher concentrations of 100 mcg/mL.[707] Since oral dosing with hyperforin can result in serum levels of 500 nanogram /mL (equivalent to 0.5 microgram/mL) then it is possible that high-dose hyperforin will have systemic antibacterial action. Regardless of its possible systemic antibacterial effectiveness, **hyperforin should clearly have antibacterial action when applied "topically" such as when it is taken orally against gastric and upper intestinal colonization.** Extracts from St. John's Wort hold particular promise against multidrug-resistant *Staphylococcus aureus*[708] and perhaps *Helicobacter pylori.*[709]

- **Myrrh (*Commiphora molmol*)**: Myrrh is remarkably effective against parasitic infections.[710] A recent clinical trial against **schistosomiasis**[711] showed "The parasitological cure rate after three months was 97.4% and 96.2% for *S. haematobium* and *S. mansoni* cases with the marvelous clinical cure without any side-effects."[712]

- **Bismuth**: Bismuth is commonly used in the empiric treatment of diarrhea (e.g., "Pepto-Bismol") and is commonly combined with other antimicrobial agents to reduce drug resistance and increase antibiotic effectiveness.[713]

- **Peppermint *(Mentha piperita)***: Peppermint shows antimicrobial and antispasmodic actions and has demonstrated clinical effectiveness in patients with bacterial overgrowth of the small bowel.

- **Uva Ursi**: Uva ursi can be used against gastrointestinal pathogens on a limited basis per culture and sensitivity findings; its primary historical and modern use is as a urinary antiseptic which is effective only when the urine pH is alkaline.[714] Components of uva ursi potentiate antibiotics.[715] **This herb has some ocular and neurologic toxicity and should be used with professional supervision for low-dose and/or short-term administration only**.[716]

---

[704] Dien TK, de Vries PJ, Khanh NX, Koopmans R, Binh LN, Duc DD, Kager PA, van Boxtel CJ. Effect of food intake on pharmacokinetics of oral artemisinin in healthy Vietnamese subjects. *Antimicrob Agents Chemother*. 1997 May;41(5):1069-72

[705] Giao PT, Binh TQ, Kager PA, Long HP, Van Thang N, Van Nam N, de Vries PJ. Artemisinin for treatment of uncomplicated falciparum malaria: is there a place for monotherapy? *Am J Trop Med Hyg*. 2001 Dec;65(6):690-5

[706] Giao PT, Binh TQ, Kager PA, Long HP, Van Thang N, Van Nam N, de Vries PJ. Artemisinin for treatment of uncomplicated falciparum malaria: is there a place for monotherapy? *Am J Trop Med Hyg*. 2001 Dec;65(6):690-5 http://www.ajtmh.org/cgi/reprint/65/6/690

[707] Schempp CM, Pelz K, Wittmer A, Schopf E, Simon JC. Antibacterial activity of hyperforin from St John's wort, against multiresistant Staphylococcus aureus and gram-positive bacteria. *Lancet*. 1999 Jun 19;353(9170):2129

[708] Gibbons S, Ohlendorf B, Johnsen I. The genus Hypericum--a valuable resource of anti-Staphylococcal leads. *Fitoterapia*. 2002 Jul;73(4):300-4

[709] "A butanol fraction of St. John's Wort revealed anti-Helicobacter pylori activity with MIC values ranging between 15.6 and 31.2 microg/ml." Reichling J, Weseler A, Saller R. A current review of the antimicrobial activity of Hypericum perforatum L. *Pharmacopsychiatry*. 2001 Jul;34 Suppl 1:S116-8

[710] El Baz MA, Morsy TA, El Bandary MM, Motawea SM. Clinical and parasitological studies on the efficacy of Mirazid in treatment of schistosomiasis haematobium in Tatoon, Etsa Center, El Fayoum Governorate. *J Egypt Soc Parasitol*. 2003 Dec;33(3):761-76

[711] Schistosomiasis. http://www.dpd.cdc.gov/dpdx/HTML/Schistosomiasis.htm

[712] Abo-Madyan AA, Morsy TA, Motawea SM. Efficacy of Myrrh in the treatment of schistosomiasis (haematobium and mansoni) in Ezbet El-Bakly, Tamyia Center, El-Fayoum Governorate, Egypt. *J Egypt Soc Parasitol*. 2004 Aug;34(2):423-46

[713] Veldhuyzen van Zanten SJ, Sherman PM, Hunt RH. Helicobacter pylori: new developments and treatments. *CMAJ*. 1997;156(11):1565-74 http://www.cmaj.ca/cgi/reprint/156/11/1565.pdf

[714] Yarnell E. Botanical medicines for the urinary tract. *World J Urol*. 2002 Nov;20(5):285-93

[715] Shimizu M, Shiota S, Mizushima T, Ito H, Hatano T, Yoshida T, Tsuchiya T. Marked potentiation of activity of beta-lactams against methicillin-resistant Staphylococcus aureus by corilagin. *Antimicrob Agents Chemother*. 2001 Nov;45(11):3198-201 http://aac.asm.org/cgi/reprint/45/11/3198

[716] "A 56-year-old woman who ingested uva ursi for 3 years noted a decrease in visual acuity within the past year. Ocular examination including fluorescein angiography revealed a typical bull's-eye maculopathy bilaterally." Wang L, Del Priore LV. Bull's-eye maculopathy secondary to herbal toxicity from uva ursi. *Am J Ophthalmol*. 2004 Jun;137(6):1135-7

- **Garlic**: Garlic shows *in vitro* antimicrobial action against numerous microorganisms, including *H. pylori, Pseudomonas aeruginosa,* and *Candida albicans*, and this effect is mediated *directly* via microbicidal actions as well as *indirectly* via dissolution of microbial biofilms[717] and inhibition of quorum sensing.[718] However, since the antimicrobial components of garlic are likely absorbed in the upper gastrointestinal tract, I propose that it is unlikely that garlic can exert a clinically significant anti-dysbiotic effect in the lower small intestine and colon. In fact, two studies in humans have shown that—despite its *in vitro* effectiveness against *H. pylori*—garlic is ineffective in the treatment of gastric *H. pylori* colonization.[719,720] While these studies argue against the use of garlic as antimicrobial monotherapy, the possibility remains that garlic may enhance the clinical effectiveness of other antimicrobial therapeutics via its aforementioned ability to weaken microbial biofilms and to impair quorum sensing, which otherwise serve to protect yeast/bacteria from immune attack and from antibacterial/antifungal therapeutics.
- **Cranberry**: Particularly effective for the prevention and adjunctive treatment of urinary tract infections, mostly by inhibiting adherence of *E. coli* to epithelial cells.[721]
- **Thyme (*Thymus vulgaris*)**: Thyme extracts have direct antimicrobial actions and also potentiate the effectiveness of tetracycline against drug-resistant *Staphylococcus aureus*.[722] Thyme also appears effective against *Aeromonas hydrophila*.[723]
- **Clove (*Syzygium* species)**: Clove's eugenol has been shown in animal studies to have a potent antifungal effect.[724]
- **Anise**: Although it has weak antibacterial action when used alone, anise does show in vitro activity against molds.[725]
- **Buchu/betulina**: Buchu has a long history of use against urinary tract infections and systemic infections.[726]
- **Caprylic acid and undecylenic acid**: Caprylic acid is a medium chain fatty acid that is commonly used in patients with dysbiosis, particularly that which has a fungal/yeast component. Beside empiric use, caprylic acid may be indicated by culture-sensitivity results provided with comprehensive parasitology. When bacterial/fungal sensitivity tests indicate caprylic acid, many clinicians prefer to use undecylenic acid which is reportedly up to six times more powerful than caprylic acid.[727] Commercial preparations delivering 50 mg undecylenic acid per gelcap can be taken orally in doses of 3-5 gelcaps three times per day. Anti-candidal action has been reported[728], and my impression is that undecylenic acid is among the more valuable therapeutics in the treatment of gastrointestinal dysbiosis.

---

[717] "Sub-MICs of allicin also diminished the biofilm formations by S. epidermidis." Perez-Giraldo C, Cruz-Villalon G, Sanchez-Silos R, Martinez-Rubio R, Blanco MT, Gomez-Garcia AC. In vitro activity of allicin against Staphylococcus epidermidis and influence of subinhibitory concentrations on biofilm formation. *J Appl Microbiol.* 2003;95(4):709-11

[718] "The results indicate that a QS-inhibitory extract of garlic renders P. aeruginosa sensitive to tobramycin, respiratory burst and phagocytosis by PMNs, as well as leading to an improved outcome of pulmonary infections." Bjarnsholt T, Jensen PO, Rasmussen TB, Christophersen L, Calum H, Hentzer M, Hougen HP, Rygaard J, Moser C, Eberl L, Hoiby N, Givskov M. Garlic blocks quorum sensing and promotes rapid clearing of pulmonary Pseudomonas aeruginosa infections. *Microbiology.* 2005 Dec;151(Pt 12):3873-80. The in vivo portion of this study was performed in animals, not humans.

[719] "This study did not support a role for either garlic or jalapenos in the treatment of H. pylori infection. Caution must be used when attempting to extrapolate data from in vitro studies to the in vivo condition." Graham DY, Anderson SY, Lang T. Garlic or jalapeno peppers for treatment of Helicobacter pylori infection. *Am J Gastroenterol.* 1999 May;94(5):1200-2

[720] "Five patients completed the study. There was no evidence of either eradication or suppression of H. pylori or symptom improvement whilst taking garlic oil." McNulty CA, Wilson MP, Havinga W, Johnston B, O'Gara EA, Maslin DJ. A pilot study to determine the effectiveness of garlic oil capsules in the treatment of dyspeptic patients with Helicobacter pylori. *Helicobacter.* 2001 Sep;6(3):249-53

[721] Lynch DM. Cranberry for prevention of urinary tract infections. *Am Fam Physician.* 2004 Dec 1;70(11):2175-7 http://www.aafp.org/afp/20041201/2175.pdf

[722] Fujita M, Shiota S, Kuroda T, Hatano T, Yoshida T, Mizushima T, Tsuchiya T. Remarkable synergies between baicalein and tetracycline, and baicalein and beta-lactams against methicillin-resistant Staphylococcus aureus. *Microbiol Immunol.* 2005;49(4):391-6

[723] "...thyme essential oil showed the greatest inhibition against A. hydrophila." Fabio A, Corona A, Forte E, Quaglio P. Inhibitory activity of spices and essential oils on psychrotrophic bacteria. *New Microbiol.* 2003 Jan;26(1):115-20

[724] Chami N, Chami F, Bennis S, Trouillas J, Remmal A. Antifungal treatment with carvacrol and eugenol of oral candidiasis in immunosuppressed rats. *Braz J Infect Dis.* 2004 Jun;8(3):217-26 http://www.scielo.br/pdf/bjid/v8n3/21619.pdf

[725] "Anise oil was not particularly inhibitory to bacteria (inhibition zone, approximately 25 mm); however, anise oil was highly inhibitory to molds." Elgayyar M, Draughon FA, Golden DA, Mount JR. Antimicrobial activity of essential oils from plants against selected pathogenic and saprophytic microorganisms. *J Food Prot.* 2001 Jul;64(7):1019-24

[726] "Buchu preparations are now used as a diuretic and for a wide range of conditions including stomach aches, rheumatism, bladder and kidney infections and coughs and colds." Simpson D. Buchu--South Africa's amazing herbal remedy. *Scott Med J* 1998 Dec;43(6):189-91

[727] Undecylenic acid. Monograph. *Altern Med Rev.* 2002 Feb;7(1):68-70 http://www.thorne.com/altmedrev/.fulltext/7/1/68.pdf

[728] McLain N, Ascanio R, Baker C, Strohaver RA, Dolan JW. Undecylenic acid inhibits morphogenesis of Candida albicans. *Antimicrob Agents Chemother.* 2000 Oct;44(10):2873-5 http://aac.asm.org/cgi/content/full/44/10/2873?view=long&pmid=10991877

- **Dill (_Anethum graveolens_)**: Dill shows activity against several types of mold and yeast.[729]
- **_Brucea javanica_**: Extract from _Brucea javanica_ fruit shows _in vitro_ activity against _Babesia gibsoni_, _Plasmodium falciparum_[730], _Entamoeba histolytica_[731] and _Blastocystis hominis_.[732,733]
- **_Acacia catechu_**: _Acacia catechu_ shows moderate _in vitro_ activity against _Salmonella typhi_.[734]

3. **_Oral administration of proteolytic enzymes_**: The use of polyenzyme therapy in patients with dysbiotic inflammation is justified for at least four reasons. First, orally administered proteolytic enzymes are efficiently absorbed by the gastrointestinal tract into the systemic circulation[735] to then provide a **clinically significant anti-inflammatory benefit** as I reviewed recently.[736] Second and more specifically, oral administration of proteolytic enzymes is generally believed to effect a **reduction in immune complexes and their clinical consequences**[737], and immune complexes are probably a major mechanism of dysbiosis-induced disease and are pathogenic in rheumatoid arthritis[738] and many other autoimmune diseases such as systemic lupus erythematosus, dermatomyositis, Sjogren's syndrome, and polyarteritis nodosa.[739] Third, proteolytic enzymes have been shown to **stimulate immune function**[740] and may thereby promote clearance of occult infections. Fourth, **proteolytic enzymes inhibit formation of microbial biofilms** and increase immune penetration and the effectiveness of antimicrobial therapeutics.[741] Although individual enzymes may be used in isolation, enzyme therapy is generally delivered in the form of polyenzyme preparations containing pancreatin, bromelain, papain, amylase, lipase, trypsin and alpha-chymotrypsin.[742]

4. **Probiotic supplementation ("_crowd out the bad with the good_")**: Given that "healthy" intestinal bacteria can alleviate disease and promote normal immune function[743], then it is conversely true that a condition of harmful or suboptimal intestinal bacteria could promote disease and lead to immune dysfunction. For patients with gastrointestinal and genitourinary dysbiosis, supplementation with _Bifidobacteria_, _Lactobacillus_, and perhaps _Saccharomyces_ and other beneficial strains is mandatory. The wide-ranging and well-documented benefits seen with probiotic supplementation provide direct support for the importance of microbial balance in health and disease. Supplementation with probiotics (live bacteria) is the best option, however prebiotics (such as fructooligosaccarides), and synbiotics (probiotics + prebiotics) may also be used. Synbiotic supplementation has been shown to reduce endotoxinemia and clinical symptoms

---

[729] "Antimicrobial testings showed high activity of the essential A. graveolens oil against the mold Aspergillus niger and the yeasts Saccharomyces cerevisiae and Candida albicans." Jirovetz L, Buchbauer G, Stoyanova AS, Georgiev EV, Damianova ST. Composition, quality control, and antimicrobial activity of the essential oil of long-time stored dill (Anethum graveolens L.) seeds from Bulgaria. _J Agric Food Chem_. 2003 Jun 18;51(13):3854-7

[730] Murnigsih T, Subeki, Matsuura H, et al. Evaluation of the inhibitory activities of the extracts of Indonesian traditional medicinal plants against Plasmodium falciparum and Babesia gibsoni. _J Vet Med Sci_. 2005 Aug;67(8):829-31 http://www.jstage.jst.go.jp/article/jvms/67/8/829/_pdf

[731] Wright CW, O'Neill MJ, Phillipson JD, Warhurst DC. Use of microdilution to assess in vitro antiamoebic activities of Brucea javanica fruits, Simarouba amara stem, and a number of quassinoids. _Antimicrob Agents Chemother_. 1988 Nov;32(11):1725-9
http://www.pubmedcentral.gov/articlerender.fcgi?tool=pubmed&pubmedid=2908094

[732] "Dichloromethane and methanol extracts from the Brucea javanica seed and a methanol extract from Quercus infectoria nut gall showed the highest activity." Sawangjaroen N, Sawangjaroen K. The effects of extracts from anti-diarrheic Thai medicinal plants on the in vitro growth of the intestinal protozoa parasite: Blastocystis hominis. _J Ethnopharmacol_. 2005 Apr 8;98(1-2):67-72

[733] "The crude extracts of Coptis chinensis (CC) and Brucea javanica (BJ) were found to be most active against B. hominis." Yang LQ, Singh M, Yap EH, Ng GC, Xu HX, Sim KY. In vitro response of Blastocystis hominis against traditional Chinese medicine. _J Ethnopharmacol_. 1996 Dec;55(1):35-42

[734] "Moderate antimicrobial activity was shown by Picorhiza kurroa, Acacia catechu, ..." Rani P, Khullar N. Antimicrobial evaluation of some medicinal plants for their anti-enteric potential against multi-drug resistant Salmonella typhi. _Phytother Res_. 2004 Aug;18(8):670-3

[735] Liebow C, Rothman SS. Enteropancreatic Circulation of Digestive Enzymes. _Science_ 1975; 189(4201): 472-474

[736] Vasquez A. Reducing pain and inflammation naturally - Part 3: Improving overall health while safely and effectively treating musculoskeletal pain. _Nutritional Perspectives_ 2005; 28: 34-38, 40-42

[737] Galebskaya LV, Ryumina EV, Niemerovsky VS, Matyukov AA. Human complement system state after wobenzyme intake. _VESTNIK MOSKOVSKOGO UNIVERSITETA. KHIMIYA_. 2000. Vol. 41, No. 6. Supplement. Pages 148-149

[738] Edwards JC, Cambridge G. Rheumatoid arthritis: the predictable effect of small immune complexes in which antibody is also antigen. _Br J Rheumatol_. 1998 Feb;37(2):126-30 http://rheumatology.oxfordjournals.org/cgi/reprint/37/2/126

[739] Jancar S, Sanchez Crespo M. Immune complex-mediated tissue injury: a multistep paradigm. _Trends Immunol_. 2005 Jan;26(1):48-55 http://www.i3u.org/i3u-papers/MSC-2005-TIMM.pdf

[740] Zavadova E, Desser L, Mohr T. Stimulation of reactive oxygen species production and cytotoxicity in human neutrophils in vitro and after oral administration of a polyenzyme preparation. _Cancer Biother_. 1995 Summer;10(2):147-52

[741] "The enzymes were shown to inhibit the biofilm formation. When applilied to the formed associations, the enzymes potentiated the effect of antibiotics on the bacteria located in them." Tets VV, Knorring Glu, Artemenko NK, Zaslavskaia NV, Artemenko KL. [Impact of exogenic proteolytic enzymes on bacteria][Article in Russian] _Antibiot Khimioter_. 2004;49(12):9-13

[742] Vasquez A. Reducing pain and inflammation naturally - Part 3: Improving overall health while safely and effectively treating musculoskeletal pain. _Nutritional Perspectives_ 2005; 28: 34-38, 40-42

[743] Isolauri E, Sutas Y, Kankaanpaa P, Arvilommi H, Salminen S. Probiotics: effects on immunity. _Am J Clin Nutr_. 2001 Feb;73(2 Suppl):444S-450S
http://www.ajcn.org/cgi/reprint/73/2/444S

in 50% of patients with minimal hepatic encephalopathy[744], and probiotic supplementation safely ameliorated the adverse effects of bacterial overgrowth in a clinical study of patients with renal failure.[745]

5. **Immunonutrition**: Obviously, the diet should be nutritious and free of sugars and other "junk foods" that promote inflammation and suppress immune function.[746] Especially in patients with gastrointestinal dysbiosis, vitamin and mineral supplementation should be used to counteract the effects of malabsorption, maldigestion, and hypermetabolism that accompany immune activation. Additionally, oral glutamine in doses of six grams three times daily can help normalize intestinal permeability, enhance immune function, and improve clinical outcomes in severely ill patients.[747] Zinc and vitamin A supplementation are each well known to support immune function against infection. Selenium has anti-inflammatory and antiviral actions.[748] Vitamin D supplementation reduces inflammation, protects against autoimmunity, and promotes immunity against viral and bacterial infections.[749] Supplementation with IgG from bovine colostrum can also provide benefit against chronic and acute infections.[750,751] Extracts from bovine thymus are safe for clinical use in humans and have shown anti-infective and anti-inflammatory benefits in elderly patients[752] as well as antirheumatic/anti-inflammatory benefits in patients with autoimmune diseases[753,754,755]; in an animal study of experimental dental disease, administration of thymus extract was shown to normalize immune function and reduce orodental dysbiosis.[756]

6. **Hepatobiliary stimulation for IgA-complex removal**: The binding of immunoglobuin A (IgA) with antigen creates IgA immune complexes that contribute to tissue destruction by complement activation (alternate pathway) and other pathomechanisms in IgA nephropathy[757], Henoch-Schonlein purpura[758], rheumatoid vasculitis[759], lupus[760], and Sjogren's syndrome.[761] Autoreactive IgA antibodies are a characteristic of lupus and Sjogren's syndrome[762] and correlate strongly with disease activity in rheumatoid arthritis.[763] **Immune complexes containing secretory IgA that has been reabsorbed from mucosal surfaces mediate many of the clinical phenomenon of dysbiosis-related musculoskeletal disease[764], and these same IgA-containing immune complexes are eliminated from the systemic**

[744] Liu Q, Duan ZP, Ha da K, et al. Synbiotic modulation of gut flora: effect on minimal hepatic encephalopathy in patients with cirrhosis. *Hepatology.* 2004 May;39(5):1441-9

[745] Simenhoff ML, Dunn SR, Zollner GP, Fitzpatrick ME, Emery SM, Sandine WE, Ayres JW. Biomodulation of the toxic and nutritional effects of small bowel bacterial overgrowth in end-stage kidney disease using freeze-dried Lactobacillus acidophilus. *Miner Electrolyte Metab.* 1996;22(1-3):92-6

[746] Seaman DR. The diet-induced proinflammatory state: a cause of chronic pain and other degenerative diseases? *J Manipulative Physiol Ther.* 2002 Mar-Apr;25:168-79.

[747] Miller AL. Therapeutic considerations of L-glutamine: a review of the literature. *Altern Med Rev.* 1999 Aug;4(4):239-48 http://www.thorne.com/altmedrev/.fulltext/4/4/239.pdf

[748] Beck MA. Nutritionally induced oxidative stress: effect on viral disease. *Am J Clin Nutr.* 2000 Jun;71(6 Suppl):1676S-81S http://www.ajcn.org/cgi/content/full/71/6/1676S

[749] Vasquez A, Manso G, Cannell J. The clinical importance of vitamin D (cholecalciferol): a paradigm shift with implications for all healthcare providers. *Altern Ther Health Med.* 2004 Sep-Oct;10(5):28-36 http://InflammationMastery.com/monograph04

[750] Mero A, Kahkonen J, Nykanen T, Parviainen T, Jokinen I, Takala T, Nikula T, Rasi S, Leppaluoto J. IGF-I, IgA, and IgG responses to bovine colostrum supplementation during training. *J Appl Physiol.* 2002 Aug;93(2):732-9 http://jap.physiology.org/cgi/content/full/93/2/732

[751] "The preparation has high antibacterial antibody titres, and a high capacity for the neutralization of bacterial toxins. It is well tolerated and highly effective in the treatment of severe diarrhoea, e.g. in AIDS patients." Stephan W, Dichtelmuller H, Lissner R. Antibodies from colostrum in oral immunotherapy. *J Clin Chem Clin Biochem.* 1990 Jan;28(1):19-23

[752] Pandolfi F, Quinti I, Montella F, Voci MC, Schipani A, Urasia G, Aiuti F. T-dependent immunity in aged humans. II. Clinical and immunological evaluation after three months of administering a thymic extract. *Thymus.* 1983 Apr;5(3-4):235-40

[753] Lavastida MT, Goldstein AL, Daniels JC. Thymosin administration in autoimmune disorders. *Thymus.* 1981 Feb;2(4-5):287-95

[754] Thrower PA, Doyle DV, Scott J, Huskisson EC. Thymopoietin in rheumatoid arthritis. *Rheumatol Rehabil.* 1982 May;21(2):72-7

[755] Malaise MG, Hauwaert C, Franchimont P, et al. Treatment of active rheumatoid arthritis with slow intravenous injections of thymopentin. A double-blind placebo-controlled randomised study. *Lancet.* 1985 Apr 13;1(8433):832-6

[756] Manti F, Kornman K, Goldschneider I. Effects of an immunomodulating agent on peripheral blood lymphocytes and subgingival microflora in ligature-induced periodontitis. *Infect Immun.* 1984 Jul;45(1):172-9 http://www.pubmedcentral.gov/articlerender.fcgi?tool=pubmed&pubmedid=6234232

[757] "...it is likely that the usual instance of IgA-associated glomerulonephritis is due to deposition of circulating immune complexes containing IgA." McPhaul JJ Jr. IgA-associated glomerulonephritis. *Annu Rev Med.* 1977;28:37-42

[758] "... it is generally considered to be an immune complex-mediated disease characterized by the presence of polymeric IgA1 (pIgA1)-containing immune complexes predominantly in dermal, gastrointestinal, and glomerular capillaries. ...also been observed in the kidneys of patients with liver cirrhosis, dermatitis herpetiformis, celiac disease, and chronic inflammatory disease of the lung. " Rai A, Nast C, Adler S. Henoch-Schonlein purpura nephritis. *J Am Soc Nephrol.* 1999 Dec;10(12):2637-44 http://jasn.asnjournals.org/cgi/content/full/10/12/2637

[759] Voskuyl AE, Hazes JM, Zwinderman AH, Paleolog EM, van der Meer FJ, Daha MR, Breedveld FC. Diagnostic strategy for the assessment of rheumatoid vasculitis. *Ann Rheum Dis.* 2003 May;62(5):407-13 http://ard.bmjjournals.com/cgi/reprint/62/5/407

[760] Sikander FF, Salgaonkar DS, Joshi VR. Cryoglobulin studies in systemic lupus erythematosus. *J Postgrad Med* 1989;35:139-43

[761] Pourmand N, Wahren-Herlenius M, Gunnarsson I, et al. Ro/SSA and La/SSB specific IgA autoantibodies in serum of patients with Sjogren's syndrome and systemic lupus erythematosus. *Ann Rheum Dis.* 1999 Oct;58(10):623-9 http://ard.bmjjournals.com/cgi/content/full/58/10/623

[762] Pourmand N, Wahren-Herlenius M, Gunnarsson I, et al. Ro/SSA and La/SSB specific IgA autoantibodies in serum of patients with Sjogren's syndrome and systemic lupus erythematosus. *Ann Rheum Dis.* 1999 Oct;58(10):623-9

[763] Jonsson T, Valdimarsson H. What about IgA rheumatoid factor in rheumatoid arthritis? *Ann Rheum Dis.* 1998 Jan;57(1):63-4 http://ard.bmjjournals.com/cgi/content/full/57/1/63

[764] Inman RD. Antigens, the gastrointestinal tract, and arthritis. *Rheum Dis Clin North Am.* 1991 May;17(2):309-21

circulation via the liver and biliary system[765,766], **thus providing the rationale for the use of botanicals and physiotherapeutics that promote liver function and bile flow in the treatment of IgA-mediated inflammatory disorders.** Numerous experimental studies in animals have shown that circulating IgA immune complexes are taken up by hepatocytes and then secreted into the bile for elimination.[767,768] The fact that bile duct obstruction retards systemic clearance of IgA immune complexes and that **normalization/optimization of bile flow reduces serum IgA levels by enhancing biliary excretion in animals**[769,770] **and humans**[771] proves the importance of ensuring optimal hepatobiliary function and supports the use of botanical and physiological therapeutics that facilitate bile flow. A 1929 clinical study with human patients published in *Archives of Internal Medicine* provided irrefutable radiographic documentation that **therapeutic enemas safely and effectively stimulate bile flow for 45-60 minutes following administration**[772], and this finding, along with the obvious quantitative reduction in intestinal microbes induced by such "cleansing", helps explain the reported benefits of colonics/enemas in patients with systemic illness[773,774,775,776] and other immune-complex associated diseases such as cancer.[777] Validation of this concept is demonstrated by the significant efficacy of immunoadsorption[778] and plasmapheresis[779,780] (techniques for removing immune complexes) in patients with lupus. Furthermore, this directly supports the naturopathic concept of "treating the liver" in patients with systemic disease by the use of dietary and botanical therapeutics that stimulate bile flow, such as beets, ginger[781], curcumin/turmeric[782], *Picrorhiza*[783], milk thistle[784], *Andrographis paniculata*[785], and *Boerhaavia diffusa*.[786] Investigation of an antirheumatic benefit from phytophysiotherapeutic hepatobiliary stimulation is worthy of clinical trials with pre- and post-intervention measurement of serum immune complexes and other clinical indexes.[787]

[765] Russell MW, Brown TA, Claflin JL, Schroer K, Mestecky J. Immunoglobulin A-mediated hepatobiliary transport constitutes a natural pathway for disposing of bacterial antigens. *Infect Immun*. 1983 Dec;42(3):1041-8 http://www.pubmedcentral.gov/articlerender.fcgi?tool=pubmed&pubmedid=6642659

[766] "The liver therefore appears to be singularly capable of transporting both free and complexed IgA into its secretion, the bile." Russell MW, Brown TA, Mestecky J. Preferential transport of IgA and IgA-immune complexes to bile compared with other external secretions. *Mol Immunol*. 1982 May;19(5):677-82

[767] "These results indicate that mouse hepatocytes are involved in the uptake and hepatobiliary transport of pIgA and pIgA-IC of low mol. wt." Phillips JO, Komiyama K, Epps JM, Russell MW, Mestecky J. Role of hepatocytes in the uptake of IgA and IgA-containing immune complexes in mice. *Mol Immunol*. 1988 Sep;25(9):873-9

[768] "Thus hepatobiliary transport appears to be the major pathway for the clearance of both IgA IC and free IgA from the circulation." Brown TA, Russell MW, Kulhavy R, Mestecky J. IgA-mediated elimination of antigens by the hepatobiliary route. *Fed Proc*. 1983 Dec;42(15):3218-21

[769] "Clearance of IgA immune complexes was delayed after bile duct ligation." Harmatz PR, Kleinman RE, Bunnell BW, McClenathan DT, Walker WA, Bloch KJ. The effect of bile duct obstruction on the clearance of circulating IgA immune complexes. *Hepatology*. 1984 Jan-Feb;4(1):96-100

[770] Lemaitre-Coelho I, Jackson GD, Vaerman JP. High levels of secretory IgA and free secretory component in the serum of rats with bile duct obstruction. *J Exp Med*. 1978 Mar 1;147(3):934-9 http://www.jem.org/cgi/reprint/147/3/934

[771] "CONCLUSIONS: Biliary obstruction secondary to both calculus or malignancy of the hepatobiliary system causes suppression of bile IgA secretion and elevated serum level of secretory IgA. Bile secretory IgA secretion recovers with endoscopic drainage of the obstructed system." Sung JJ, Leung JC, Tsui CP, Chung SS, Lai KN. Biliary IgA secretion in obstructive jaundice: the effects of endoscopic drainage. *Gastrointest Endosc*. 1995 Nov;42(5):439-44

[772] Garbat AL, Jacobi HG. Secretion of Bile in Response to Rectal Installations. *Arch Intern Med* 1929; 44: 455-462

[773] Crinnion WJ. Results of a decade of naturopathic treatment for environmental illnesses. *J Naturopathic Med* 1994;17:21-27

[774] Snyder RG. The value of colonic irrigations in countering auto-intoxication of intestinal origin. *Medical Clinics of North America* 1939; May: 781-788

[775] Marshall HK, Thomson CR. Colon irrigation in the treatment of mental disease. *N Engl J Med* 1932; 207 (Sept 8): 454-7

[776] Bastedo WA. Colon irrigations: their administration, therapeutic applications, and dangers. *Journal of the American Medical Association* 1932; 98(9): 734-6

[777] Gonzalez NJ, Isaacs LL. Evaluation of pancreatic proteolytic enzyme treatment of adenocarcinoma of the pancreas, with nutrition and detoxification support. *Nutr Cancer*. 1999;33(2):117-24

[778] Braun N, Erley C, Klein R, Kotter I, Saal J, Risler T. Immunoadsorption onto protein A induces remission in severe systemic lupus erythematosus. *Nephrol Dial Transplant*. 2000 Sep;15(9):1367-72 http://ndt.oxfordjournals.org/cgi/reprint/15/9/1367

[779] Santos-Ocampo AS, Mandell BF, Fessler BJ. Alveolar hemorrhage in systemic lupus erythematosus: presentation and management. *Chest*. 2000 Oct;118(4):1083-90 http://www.chestjournal.org/cgi/content/full/118/4/1083

[780] Choi BG, Yoo WH. Successful treatment of pure red cell aplasia with plasmapheresis in a patient with systemic lupus erythematosus. *Yonsei Med J*. 2002 Apr;43(2):274-8 http://www.eymj.org/2002/pdf/04274.pdf

[781] "Further analyses for the active constituents of the acetone extracts through column chromatography indicated that [6]-gingerol and [10]-gingerol, which are the pungent principles, are mainly responsible for the cholagogic effect of ginger." Yamahara J, Miki K, Chisaka T, Sawada T, Fujimura H, Tomimatsu T, Nakano K, Nohara T. Cholagogic effect of ginger and its active constituents. *J Ethnopharmacol*. 1985;13(2):217-25

[782] "On the basis of the present findings, it appears that curcumin induces contraction of the human gall-bladder." Rasyid A, Lelo A. The effect of curcumin and placebo on human gall-bladder function: an ultrasound study. *Aliment Pharmacol Ther*. 1999 Feb;13(2):245-9

[783] "Significant anticholestatic activity was also observed against carbon tetrachloride induced cholestasis in conscious rat, anaesthetized guinea pig and cat. Picroliv was more active than the known hepatoprotective drug silymarin." Saraswat B, Visen PK, Patnaik GK, Dhawan BN. Anticholestatic effect of picroliv, active hepatoprotective principle of Picrorhiza kurrooa, against carbon tetrachloride induced cholestasis. *Indian J Exp Biol*. 1993 Apr;31(4):316-8

[784] "We conclude that SIL counteracts TLC-induced cholestasis by preventing the impairment in both the BS-dependent and -independent fractions of the bile flow." Crocenzi FA, Sanchez Pozzi EJ, Pellegrino JM, Rodriguez Garay EA, Mottino AD, Roma MG. Preventive effect of silymarin against taurolithocholate-induced cholestasis in the rat. *Biochem Pharmacol*. 2003 Jul 15;66(2):355-64

[785] "Andrographolide from the herb Andrographis paniculata (whole plant) per se produces a significant dose (1.5-12 mg/kg) dependent choleretic effect (4.8-73%) as evidenced by increase in bile flow, bile salt, and bile acids in conscious rats and anaesthetized guinea pigs." Shukla B, Visen PK, Patnaik GK, Dhawan BN. Choleretic effect of andrographolide in rats and guinea pigs. *Planta Med*. 1992 Apr;58(2):146-9

[786] "The extract also produced an increase in normal bile flow in rats suggesting a strong choleretic activity." Chandan BK, Sharma AK, Anand KK. Boerhaavia diffusa: a study of its hepatoprotective activity. *J Ethnopharmacol*. 1991 Mar;31(3):299-307

[787] Vasquez A. Do the Benefits of Botanical and Physiotherapeutic Hepatobiliary Stimulation Result From Enhanced Excretion of IgA Immune Complexes? *Naturopathy Digest* 2006; January: http://www.naturopathydigest.com/archives/2006/jan/vasquez_immune.php

7. **Ensure generous bowel movements and consider therapeutic purgatives (*purge: to free from impurities*)**: Dysbiotic patients should consume a low-fermentation fiber-rich diet that allows for 1-2 very generous bowel movements per day. Constipation must absolutely be eliminated—pun intended; **for patients being treated for dysbiosis of any type, constipation is absolutely unacceptable, since the gastrointestinal tract provides the largest burden of pro-inflammatory (eg, endotoxin, bacterial DNA) and anti-metabolic (eg, D-lactate, H2S) microbial debris and metabolites.** Patients with severe or recalcitrant dysbiosis can start the day with a laxative dose of ascorbic acid (e.g., 20-60 grams with 4 cups of water) and should expect liquid diarrhea within 30-60 minutes. The goal here is purgative physical removal of enteric microbes; in high concentrations, ascorbic acid has a direct antibacterial effect. Magnesium in elemental doses of 500-1,500 mg also helps soften stool and promote laxation. One-two cups of coffee promotes the laxative effect and provides some sense of pleasure to an otherwise not-so-pleasant experience; however, dysbiosis-affected patients often feel impressively better following therapeutic laxation. Rapid-acting antimicrobials, such as iodine/iodide, can be coadministered. Electrolyte replacement, for example with salted vegetable juice, is advisable for patinets using therapeutic laxation on a regular basis.

The clinical implementation of an anti-dysbiosis program must be tailored to the patient's overall condition and his/her willingness to implement the above-mentioned treatment options. Some patients are only willing to take a few treatments, while empowered autonomous nonmasochistic patients are more willing to do **whatever is necessary** in order to regain their health, even if it means taking numerous supplements, improving diet, starting/ending the day with enemas, and making appropriate changes in lifestyle and relationships to improve immune function. To the extent that we *first, do no harm*, all of the above-mentioned therapeutic interventions are reasonable "alternatives" to life-long medicalization, surgery, and immune-system destroying high-dose chemotherapy, which is astoundingly expensive, highly hazardous, and incompletely effective. **Patients with autoimmune diseases have numerous, largely untapped options for the treatment of their autoimmune diseases**; therefore, (pseudo)justifying lethal and expensive and devastating medical interventions on the basis of a "lack of other treatment alternatives"[788] when reasonable, safe, and effective options have not been implemented is scientifically inaccurate, ethically untenable, and medicolegally questionable.

[788] Binks M, Passweg JR, Furst D, et al. Phase I/II trial of autologous stem cell transplantation in systemic sclerosis: procedure related mortality and impact on skin disease. *Ann Rheum Dis.* 2001 Jun;60(6):577-84 http://ard.bmjjournals.com/cgi/content/full/60/6/577

❸ Nutritional Immunomodulation:
Nutritional interventions to induce regulatory T-cells (Treg)

Major Concepts in this Section

"Inflammatory balance" is largely a biochemical endpoint whereas "immune balance" refers more directly to immunophenotypic predominance. In this section, I will outline a nutrition-based clinical protocol for the induction of active cell-mediated anti-inflammation via selective induction of regulatory T-cells ("Treg"). The goal with this component of the functional Inflammology protocol is to utilize the body's own immunomodulating ability by providing the appropriate nutritional climate for epigenetic upregulation of expression of the transcription factor FoxP3, which is the main identifier of the Treg phenotype. Components of this protocol are proven to provide clinical benefit; this nutritional immunomodulation protocol performs best when utilized within an intact functional inflammology protocol, as described throughout this chapter.

The earliest thymocytes, formed by cells originated in the bone marrow, are CD3(+)CD4(-)CD8(-) **double-negative** T cells; far from being benign, these double-negative cells contribute to autoimmunity (ANA formation), notably in the setting of mitochondrial dysfunction

Among the earliest cell types in the thymus, Th0 further mature in the thymus (and tonsils), avoid deletion if auto-reactive, and then circulate to the "periphery", which mostly means the GALT (gut-associated lymphoid tissue); therefore, nutritional status and gut milieu/climate are powerful factors determining the programming of Th0 cells into effector cell types

Undifferentiated T-cell (Th0-cell)

IL-4

IL-12, IL-27, prolactin

Nutritional deficiencies
Excess sodium
Inflammatory milieu
Dysbiosis

Treg suppression of Th1, Th2, and Th17 inflammation

Regulatory T-cell (Treg): Immunomodulation

Th1 cell: Cell-mediated inflammation

Th2 cell: Antibody formation, humoral inflammation

Th17-cell: Autoimmunity

Sustained/chronic cell-mediated inflammation, tissue injury, IFN-gamma production

Allergy, humoral (auto)immunity via ANA and other autoantibodies

Autoimmunity, Inflammation, tissue injury, IL-17 production

Tolerance, Anti-inflammation, IL-10 production

Immunophenotype determination per inflammatory/microbial/nutritional climate: The cytokine climate, nutritional status, and microbial balance determine which immunocyte phenotype will be selected. If the climate is "hostile" then pro-inflammatory immunocytes will be selected; if nutritional needs are met and the internal milieu is relatively un-inflamed and un-infected, then tolerogenic T-regulatory cells will predominate. Thus, when dealing with disorders of sustained inflammation/allergy/autoimmunity, the task of the physician is to create or re-create the conditions for immunotolerance to predominate.

Although the term "nutritional immunomodulation" can be used to include nearly any dietary pattern or nutrient intake that has a meaningful effect on immune function (in which case, the term would encompass the totality of all food and nutrient intake), in this section I will use the term to specifically denote epigenetic induction of regulatory T-cells (Treg) from their precursors—the undifferentiated (indicated by the number zero, or "0") naïve T-helper cells—known as Th0 cells. This is a new, exciting, and remarkably well-documented therapeutic tool that we now have in our food-based armamentarium in the battles against common immune diseases such as metabolic inflammation (eg, diabetes mellitus and the metabolic syndrome), allergy (eg, asthma) and autoimmunity eg, (psoriasis, rheumatoid arthritis, SLE, and multiple sclerosis). For this discussion of nutritional immunomodulation, readers need to gain progressive understanding of the following cell types and their nutritional influences and physiologic/pathologic effects:

- CD3(+)CD4(-)CD8(-) double negative T cells: These cells arrived from the bone marrow to the thymus, but have not yet been fully "programed" for their ultimate functions; however, these cells are not benign and appear to contribute to autoimmune-type inflammation via necrotic-inflammatory cell death via a mechanism that is activated by mitochondrial dysfunction: activation of mTOR.
- Th0—niave T-cells: These cells have been "partially programmed" to become effector cells, particularly Th1, Th2, Th17, or T-regulatory cells.
- Th1 cells: Contribute to cell-mediated "chronic inflammation."
- Th2 cells: Contribute to antibody-mediated inflammation, allergies, and formation of autoreactive antibodies such as ANA.
- Th17 cells: Contribute very significantly to autoimmune-type inflammation as seen in SLE and multiple sclerosis.
- T-regulatory cells: Dampen the activity of Th1, Th2, Th17 cells, and thereby promote active anti-inflammation and immune tolerance to self and environment.
- γδ T cells, gamma delta T cells: Gamma-delta T-cells are notorious for their promotion of autoimmunity and allergic inflammation; one animal study has shown that the population of gamma-delta T-cells is doubled by consumption of genetically modified food (corn).

The "reciepe" by which we optimize induction of the Treg phenotype is as follows:
1. Mitochondrial optimization: Recently, mitochondrial dysfunction in general and mTOR activation in particular has been shown to inhibit induction of Treg cells; inhibition of mTOR with NAC 4,800mg/d in divided doses was shown to inhibit mTOR and promote induction of the FoxP3 phenotype Treg cells and result in clinical alleviation of disease in patients with SLE.
2. Probiotics: Molecular signatures from probiotic bacteria synergize to promote epigenetic induction of Treg cells; probiotic metabolites—particularly butyrate—also promote the histone acetylation which is a common theme in FoxP3 induction.
3. Lipoic acid: Lipoic acid is an antioxidant and direct inhibitor of NF-kappaB; a clinical trial in humans with multiple sclerosis showed that lipoic acid 400mg PO TID reduced IL-17 levels by 35-50%—the clinical importance of this is massive, given that IL-17 is a major effector of tissue destruction in autoimmune diseases.
4. Vitamin A: Retinoic acid is required for Treg induction. Many patients have insufficient intake of preformed vitiamin A and must therefore use oral vitamin A supplementation; relatedly, 27-47% of women are "slow converters" of beta-carotene to vitamin A, and they must likewise supplement with vitamin A in order to meet physiologic needs. Hypothyroidism also impairs conversion of beta-carotene to vitamin A; zinc is also needed for this conversion. Women who are pregnant or might become pregnant are generally advised to keep vitamin A intake below 8,000-9,000 IU/day from all sources; otherwise, a time-limited loading dose of 100,000-300,000 IU/d for 7-10 days followed by a maintenance dose of 10,000-25,000 IU/d is reasonable for children and adults. Vitamin A toxicity is

monitored clinically with "two pains"—bone pain and headache, "two skins"—dry skin and chapped lips, and "two labs"—elevated GGT and triglycerides.

5. <u>Inflammation reduction</u>: Reducing inflammation in general and IL-6 in particular is important for decreasing induction of inflammatory phenotypes—Th1, Th2, Th17—and optimizing induction of Treg.

6. <u>Vitamin D3</u>: Three clinical trials in humans have shown that vitamin D3 supplementation (detailed previously in this textbook) induces higher number and function of Treg cells within approximately 1 month.

7. <u>Fatty acids—GLA and n3 fatty acids</u>: N3 fatty acids and GLA have shown the ability to reduce autoimmunity in general and to promote Treg in particular.

8. <u>Infection/dysbiosis clearance</u>: Gastrointestinal dysbiosis prompts formation of pro-inflammatory effector cells: Th1, Th2, Th17. Therefore, eliminating/reducing problematic microbes and promoting systemic eubiosis is important for inducing immunophenotype balance. I am particularly interested in and impressed by the role of segmented filamentous bacteria (SFB) in this regard.

9. <u>Green tea</u>: Green tea component EGCG induces Treg cells. Patients are recommended to have two cups per day and/or use standardized oral supplementation (caffeinated or decaffeinated).

10. <u>Sodium avoidance</u>: Sodium—independent from the chloride anion—induces Th17 cells.

Readers can recall this Treg-induction reciepe by the acronym "My plaid figs" as illustrated below.

<u>Nutritional Immunomodulation:</u> Induction of Treg at the expense/suppression of Th-1/2/17

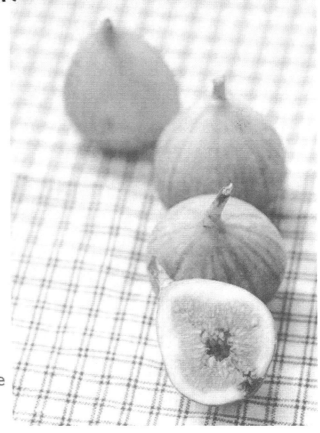

Organic/nonGMO

1. Mitochondrial optimization

2. Probiotics

3. Lipoic acid

4. A-vitamin

5. Infection/dysbiosis clearance

6. D-vitamin

7. Fatty acids: EPA-DHA and GLA

8. IL-6 reduction: create overall antiinflammatory milieu

9. Green tea

10. Sodium avoidance

Will someone please tell me the new acronym?

DrV's nutritional immunomodulation protocol: Easy to remember with the updated acronym, easy to implement clinically via supplementation and occasional use of antibiotics, whether nutritional, botanical, or pharmaceutical, and highly safe and efficacious.

Paradoxically, many of us in the clinical nutrition field have been employing this technique for many years without fully realizing the mechanisms behind the clinical benefits that we consistently observed. I recall the case of a young woman I treated in approximately 2003 for her then 18-year history of treatment-resistant full-body psoriasis; her recovery was so rapid and nearly complete that the case has always stood out in my memory. This case (included below) was published in print and on the internet in 2005 in the professional magazine *Nutritional Wellness*[789] in a discussion of my 5-part nutrition protocol (detailed in the previous section of this chapter); an updated version of the case is provided here:

A young woman with full-body psoriasis unresponsive to drug treatment

- <u>Case</u>: This is a 17-year-old woman with head-to-toe psoriasis since childhood. She wears long pants and long-sleeved shirts year-round to conceal her skin lesions, and the psoriasis is a major interference to her social life. Palliative medications have ceased to help. I recall the first time that I saw this patient, I either thought to myself or said aloud, "This psoriasis looks like a second-degree burn" because the inflammation was pervasive, extremely red/erythematous, and had caused thickening of the skin.
- <u>Treatment</u>: The Paleo-Mediterranean diet[790] was implemented, with an emphasis on food allergy identification. We used a multivitamin-mineral supplement with 200 mcg selenium to compensate for the nutritional insufficiencies and selenium deficiency common in patients with psoriasis; likewise, 10 mg of folic acid was added to address the relative vitamin deficiencies and elevated homocysteine common in these patients.[791] Combination fatty acid therapy with EPA and DHA from fish oil and GLA from borage oil was used for the anti-inflammatory and skin-healing benefits.[792] Vitamin E (1,200 IU of mixed tocopherols) and lipoic acid (1,000 mg per day) were added for their anti-inflammatory benefits and to combat the oxidative stress that is characteristic of psoriasis.[793] Of course, probiotics were used to modify gut flora, which is commonly deranged in patients with psoriasis.[794]
- <u>Results</u>: Within a few weeks, this patient's "lifelong psoriasis" was essentially gone. Food allergy identification and avoidance played a major role in the success of this case; in her case, the offending food was chicken broth. When I saw the patient again nine months later for her second visit, she had no visible evidence of psoriasis. Her "medically untreatable" condition was essentially cured by the use of my basic protocol, with the addition of a few extra nutrients. At the second visit—approximately 4-5 weeks after the first visit—I recall saying to the patient, "You no longer have findings consistent with the diagnosis of psoriasis anymore."
- <u>New perspective and mechanisms of effectiveness</u>: The success of this case was effected via nutritional immunomodulation. Without knowng I was doing so, I had implemented nearly a perfect recipe for induction of Treg cells for the endogenous suppression of unregulated and damaging (Th17-mediated) inflammation.

Treatments and rationale at the time	***Actual nutritional immunomodulation***
Cod liver oil for anti-inflammatory EPA and DHA	The ❶ vitamin A, ❷ vitamin D, ❸ EPA and DHA in the cod liver oil stimulated induction of Treg cells to provide endogenous cell-mediated anti-inflammation
Paleo diet for general health promotion, increased intake of potassium relative to sodium	Elimination of wheat, common allergens, and increased consumption of vegetables promoted ❹ antinflammatory climate and modified gastrointestinal bacteria; ❺sodium avoidance
Lipoic acid for antioxidant and anti-NFkB activity	❻ 35-50% reduction in IL-17; ❼ lipoic acid also helps to optimize mitochondrial function and suppresses mTOR, an effect which is expected to promote Treg
Probiotics for global benefit	❽ Probiotics promote Treg

---

[789] Vasquez A. Implementing the Five-Part Nutritional Wellness Protocol for the Treatment of Various Health Problems. *Nutritional Wellness* 2005 Nov

[790] Vasquez A. Revisiting the Five-Part Nutritional Wellness Protocol: The Supplemented Paleo-Mediterranean Diet. Nutritional Perspectives 2011 January

[791] Vanizor Kural B, et al. Plasma homocysteine and its relationships with atherothrombotic markers in psoriatic patients. *Clin Chim Acta* 2003;332(1-2):23-3.

[792] Vasquez A. New insights into fatty acid supplementation and its effect on eicosanoid production and genetic expression. *Nutritional Perspect* 2005: Jan: 5-16

[793] Kokcam I, Naziroglu M. Antioxidants and lipid peroxidation status in the blood of patients with psoriasis. *Clin Chim Acta* 1999;289(1-2):23-31

[794] Waldman A, et al. Incidence of Candida in psoriasis: a study on the fungal flora of psoriatic patients. *Mycoses* 2001;44(3-4):77-81.

The earliest thymocytes, formed by cells originated in the bone marrow, are CD3(+)CD4(-)CD8(-) **double-negative** T cells. Far from being benign, these double-negative cells contribute to autoimmunity (especially ANA formation, notably in the setting of mitochondrial dysfunction) via inflammatory necrosis and stimulation of DAMP (damage-associated molecular pattern) receptors.

Among the earliest cell types in the thymus, Th0 further mature in the thymus (and tonsils), avoid deletion if auto-reactive, and then circulate to the "periphery", which mostly means the GALT (gut-associated lymphoid tissue); therefore, nutritional status and gut milieu/climate are powerful factors determining the programming of Th0 cells into effector cell types

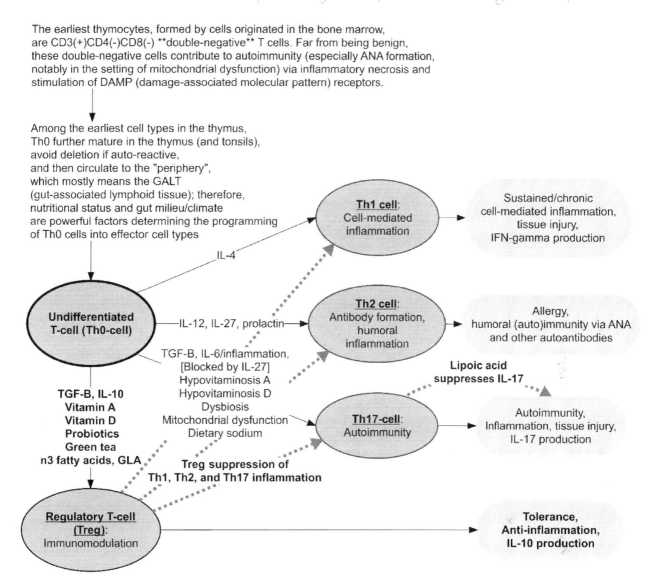

Nutritional immunomodulation of immunophenotype via induction of Treg phenotype from undifferentiated T-cells: Vitamin A, vitamin D3, probiotics, and an anti-inflammatory milieu promote immune tolerance and avoidance of allergic, inflammatory, and autoimmune diseases by several mechanisms, an important one illustrated here is that of induction of Treg phenotype for suppression of excess Th17 activity.

❹ Dysfunctional Mitochondria:

A Common Causative, Contributing, and Consequential Component of Cardiometabolic Syndrome, Hypertension, Neurodegeneration, Inflammation, Allergy and Autommunity

Major Concepts in this Section
Mitochondria do much more than simply produce ATP; they also sense and respond to nutritional status (not simply metabolize available carbon substrates), sense and respond to microbes, are vulnerable to the presence of bacteria and viruses, create reactive oxygen (ROS) and nitrogen species (RNS), are involved in the secretion and reception of insulin, and can promote inflammation and immune imbalance via elaboration of cytokines and Th-17 cells, respectively. Mitochondria are also key players in the determination of the timing and type of cell death, whether by apoptosis or necrosis. When mitochondria are functioning "normally" and "optimally", the various roles of mitochondria can be said to be mostly efficient and beneficent; however, when mitochondria become injured, impaired, or otherwise "dysfunctional" then the ATP-producing and other roles played by mitochondria are adversely affected to the detriment of the human host. The physiologic roles and consequences of dysfunction are outlined in the table below:

Physiologic roles of mitochondria	Consequences of mitochondrial dysfunction
1) Efficiently produce ATP	Inefficient production of ATP with reduced total output
2) Sense and respond to microbes	Exaggerated response to microbes with inefficient and excessive immune and inflammatory responses
3) Theoretically, mitochondria perform normal duties especially ATP production without regard for infectious disease status	Mitochondria can be destroyed by infectious agents, such as herpes simplex virus; other microbes and their products (such as bacterial endotoxin) cause mitochondrial dysfunction with the 3 most classic characteristics of mitochondrial dysfunction
4) Create ROS and RNS as a side-effect of metabolism	Produce excessive ROS and RNS which leads to damage at four levels: 1) mitochondrial—e.g., mitochondrial inner membrane (MIM) and mitochondrial DNA, 2) cellular—e.g., nuclear DNA, 3) tissue—e.g., substantia nigra in Parkinson's disease, 4) systemic—e.g., measureable alterations in oxidative markers, such as TBARS and GSH. Note that oxidative damage to the MIM causes increased oxidant production via dysfunction of the ETC, thereby creating a vicious cycle.
5) Secretion and reception of insulin	Mitochondrial dysfunction contributes to the "diabetic phenotype of hyperglycemia" via impaired pancreatic secretion of insulin and also by impaired peripheral reception of insulin.
6) Normally, mitochondria should not have an appreciable or adverse effect on immune and inflammatory balance	Mitochondrial dysfunction in general and mitochondrial hyperpolariziation in particular promote increased production of inflammatory cytokines, cyclooxygenase, and Th-17 cells.
7) Mitochondrial-triggered apoptosis needs to be appropriately timed per cell.	An excess of apoptosis leads to premature tissue failure, while a failure of cell-killing and relative immortalization of cells contributes to autoimmunity and also cancer. Inflammatory cell death—necrosis—promotes additional inflammation via DAMP-receptor activation.

The three most classic characteristics of mitochondrial dysfunction are ❶ impaired ATP production: reduced efficiency and reduced amount of ATP production, ❷ increased free radical production, and ❸ increased inflammatory tendency, via chemical and enzymatic mediators (such as cytokines and cyclooxygenase) and cellular effectors (especially Th-17 cells). Given the consequences (introduced above) and high prevalence of mitochondrial disorders in routine outpatient clinical practice, physicians need to appreciate the practical, efficient, and effective, clinical means by which mitochondrial function can be restored, protected, and optimized.

Mitochondria—Re-Introduction and New Perspectives:

- Production of cellular energy in the form of ATP: Mitochondria are organelles ("small organs") within each cell that produce the majority of cellular energy for biochemical reactions and cellular processes. The primary fuel used by cells of the body is ATP—adenosine triphosphate. Everyone who has studied mitochondria—ranging from high-school and undergraduate students of Biology all the way to doctorate-level medical/healthcare professionals—is familiar with the fact that mitochondria make ATP; in fact, for most people, whether they are general public or doctors, this is all they know about mitochondria. New research, however, has shown us that mitochondria have many roles in addition to their ability to produce cellular energy. Most importantly, mitochondria are now known to play important roles in perpetuating chronic inflammation, responding to microbial infections, triggering of cell death, and controlling various metabolic processes.[795,796]

- Perpetuation of chronic inflammation: Most relevant to the focus of this work on clinical conditions related to inflammation is the fact that mitochondria have the ability to trigger inflammatory responses via activation of the nuclear transcription factor kappa-B (NFkB). Transcription factors are intracellular molecules that bind to the genetic material (DNA) in the nucleus of the cell to influence the activation or transcription of specific genes; in this case the transcription factor kappaB is most notorious for its activation of genes that promote inflammatory responses—necessary for short-term responses to injury or infection, but harmful when protracted and nonspecific. In this way, certain types of mitochondrial stimulation/activation/dysfunction can contribute to "chronic inflammation"; conversely, interventions that restore/improve proper mitochondrial function have generally been shown to provide anti-inflammatory benefits.

- Responsiveness to microbial infections: Very interestingly, mitochondria have the ability to sense and respond to microbial infections, particularly infections due to viruses and Gram-negative bacteria. This may be related to the evolutionary origin of mitochondria, which is generally perceived to be that of aerobic bacteria that formed a symbiotic intercellular relationship with eukaryotic cells; the primitive bacteria would have needed the ability to respond to stresses in its environment, particularly potential invasion by or competition from infectious agents.

- Triggering of cell death via apoptosis and/or necrosis: Mitochondria are known to play a dual role in relation to a particular form of cell death called "apoptosis" which can be thought of as a peaceful/programmed/noninflammatory death of a cell (in contrast to "necrosis" which is inflammatory cellular death, and "autoschizis" which is cellular self-destruction through progressive fragmentation such as seen in cancer cells, for example, following administration of vitamins C and K3[797]). Mitochondria have a two-part function, either promoting or resisting cell death; stated more simply and clearly: mitochondria play a role in keeping healthy cells alive, while promoting the death/apoptosis of unhealthy/dysfunctional/malignant cells. Mitochondrial dysfunction, as should be expected, impairs normal function and thus leads to the opposite of what we normally expect from mitochondria. In mitochondrial dysfunction, instead of promoting the death of dysfunctional cells, these cells become immortal and resistant to death; examples of this are autoreactive cells and cancer cells, which should have been "killed off" by apoptosis before being allowed to accumulate to such an extent that they cause harm to the host, either by autoimmunity or malignancy, respectively. In mitochondrial dysfunction, instead of keeping healthy cells alive, mitochondria promote the death of otherwise healthy cells; an example of this is the loss of neurons that help control movement or which contribute to learning and thinking, thus resulting in Parkinson's disease or Alzheimer's disease, respectively.

- Contribution to control of various metabolic processes: Mitochondria play an integral role in several physiologic processes, including blood pressure control and blood glucose control. The release of insulin from the beta-cells in the pancreas is triggered by a cascade of events beginning with elevated levels of blood glucose and resulting in the entry of calcium into these cells with subsequent release of insulin into the blood; thus, mitochondrial dysfunction results in impaired pancreatic responsiveness to elevated glucose levels, thereby contributing to the complex condition we know as type-2 diabetes mellitus. Mild impairment of muscle contractility in the heart, which can be due to

---

[795] Pieczenik SR, Neustadt J. Mitochondrial dysfunction and molecular pathways of disease. *Exp Mol Pathol.* 2007 Aug;83(1):84-92

[796] Green DR, Galluzzi L, Kroemer G. Mitochondria and the autophagy-inflammation-cell death axis in organismal aging. *Science.* 2011 Aug 26;333(6046):1109-12

[797] Lasalvia-Prisco E, Cucchi S, Vázquez J, et al. Serum markers variation consistent with autoschizis induced by ascorbic acid-menadione in patients with prostate cancer. *Med Oncol.* 2003;20(1):45-52

mitochondrial dysfunction and nutrient deficiencies/imbalances, leads to reduced heart function, which causes reflex activation of the sympathetic nervous system—the "panic response" of the nervous system that causes the "fight or flight" phenomenon. Chronic low-level activation of the sympathetic nervous system promotes several adverse effects associated with stress/fight/flight/panic, including elevated blood pressure (hypertension), activation of the renin-aldosterone system (water retention), vasoconstriction (reduced peripheral circulation) and hypercoagulability (promotion of blood clots, thrombosis). Natural treatments that restore or support mitochondrial function generally lower blood pressure in hypertensives, reduce blood glucose levels in diabetics, and reduce markers of inflammation in healthy patients as well as patients with inflammatory diseases; these examples will be further detailed throughout the multivolume textbook of _Inflammation Mastery_ starting in 2014.

An accurate contemporary understanding of mitochondria in clinical medicine requires ❶ an updated conceptual appreciation of the roles of mitochondria in normal physiology and the consequences of mitochondrial dysfunction and the implications for various diagnoses and disease states, ❷ a "detailed familiarity" with ATP-producing processes and pathways, of which five are most important: 1) glycolysis, 2) pyruvate dehydrogenase, 3) Krebs cycle, citric acid cycle, 4) electron transport chain, and 5) alternate fuel (e.g., fructose, ketones, fatty acids, amino acids, ethanol) inputs into glycolysis and the citric acid cycle, and ❸ knowledge about how to improve/restore/optimize mitochondrial function—a customizable clinical strategy.

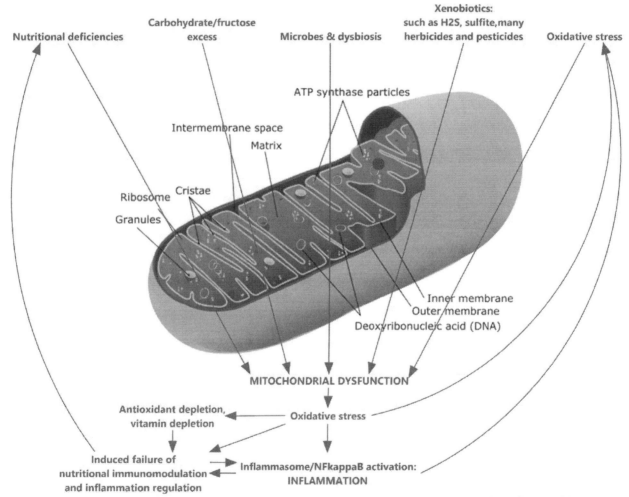

Vasquez, _Mitochondrial Nutrition_. 2014

Schematic overview of mitochondrial dysfunction's major causes and consequences: Notice the presence of vicious cycles whereby cause becomes consequence, and then consequence becomes cause. Several dietary, nutritional, botanical, pharmaceutical/microbiologic, and sociopolitical interventions are obvious from the diagram.

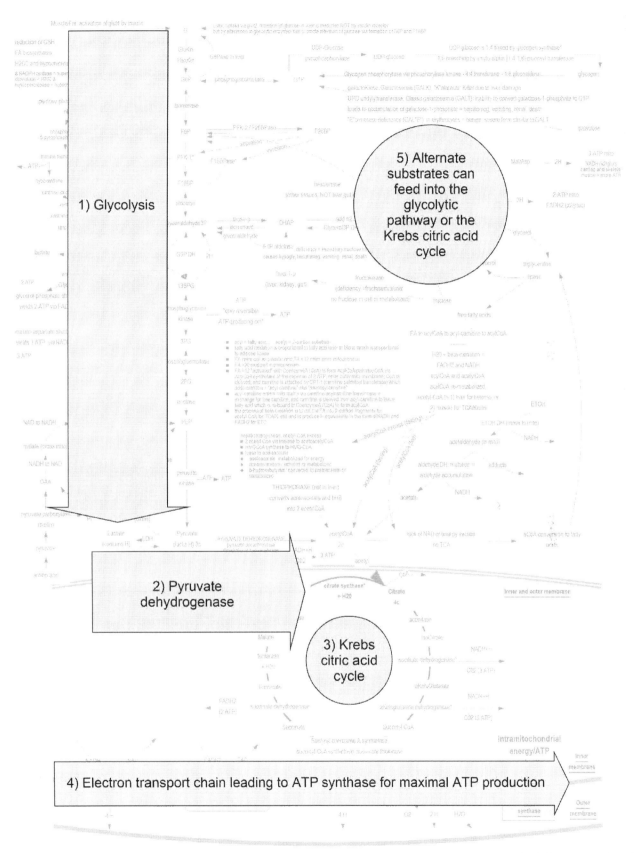

Conceptual overview of 1) glycolysis, 2) pyruvate dehydrogenase complex/shuttle, 3) Krebs' citric acid cycle, 4) electron transport chain, and 5) the accessory pathways that feed into the glycolysis or Krebs' cycle: Clinical implications are discussed in the text.

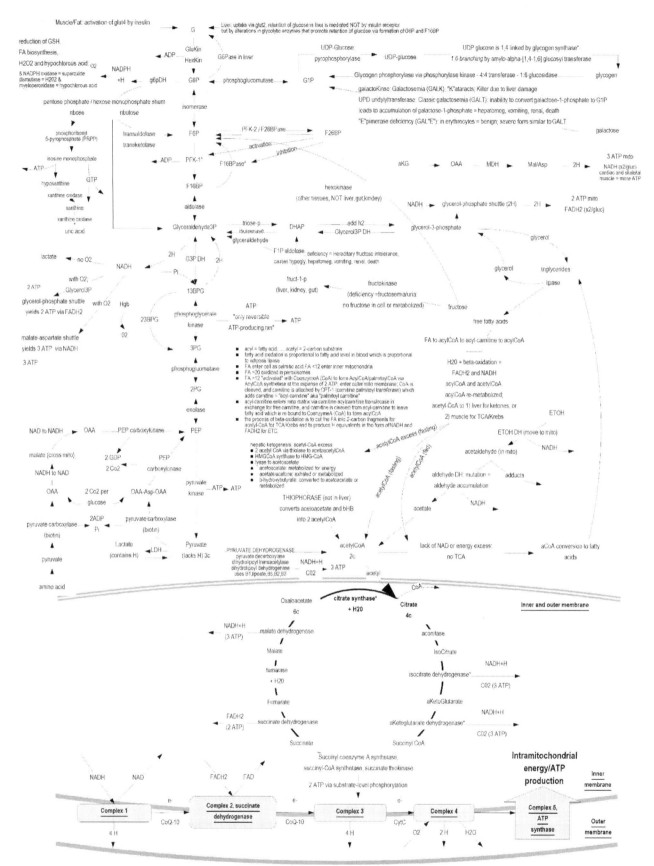

Detailed overview of 1) glycolysis, 2) pyruvate dehydrogenase complex/shuttle, 3) Krebs' citric acid cycle, 4) electron transport chain, and 5) the accessory pathways that feed into the glycolysis or Krebs' cycle: Clinical implications are discussed in the text.

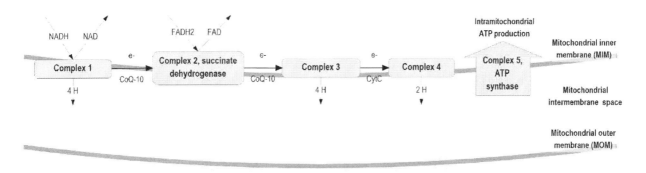

Vasquez A. Integrative Rheumatology and Inflammation Mastery. 3rd ed. Seattle, WA: CreateSpace, 2014. In press.

Electron transport chain (ETC) structure, with additional emphasis on the "nonstructure" of the innermembrane space created by the inner and outer mitochondrial membranes, permeability of both of which must be tightly regulated for optimal mitochondrial performance, including but not limited to ATP production: The semi-contained mitochondrial intermembrane space allows the accumulation of protons from the electron transport chain (ETC) to concentrate into a "pressurized" electromechanical gradient that powers ETC Complex #5, also called ATP synthase. ATP synthase is powered via the transmittal of protons from their high concentration gradient in the intermembrane space through the structure of the ATP synthase enzyme, which acts as a "pore" or "pressure valve" allowing protons to move to an area of lesser concentration inside the mitochondria. If the ATP synthase enzyme is bypassed due to a defective or "leaky" inner membrane that allows protons to leak back into the mitochondria, then the production of cellular energy will be reduced, leading to metabolic impairments such as increased free radical production (as the ETC works harder to compensate for reduced efficiency) and clinical manifestations such as fatigue, dyscognition, and muscle (e.g., heart) impairment including body aches and pains consistent with clinical presentations of fibromyalgia and chronic fatigue syndrome. Transmembrane potential of the mitochondrial inner membrane (MIM) is essential for the electromechanical gradient that drives ATP synthase; compromise of this membrane due to dietary faults (e.g., fatty acid deficiency, antioxidant deficiency) or biochemical faults (e.g., overproduction of free radicals which damage the MIM) will lead to hyperpermeability of the MIM ("leaky mitochondria") and reduced ATP synthesis. Clinical implications and interventions are discussed in the text; most of the clinical work in this regard has been lead by Professor Garth Nicolson PhD.

A Practical, Cost-Effective, Safe, Ethical Clinical Approach to Improving Mitochondrial Function—DrV's Strategy Suitable for Most Cases of Mitochondrial Dysfunction Seen in General Outpatient Practice

Mitochondrial disorders can be categorized based on the underlying etiology or combination of etiologies:

1) <u>Primary/genotropic mitochondrial disorders</u>: These can range from mild to severe, from occult to life-threatening, and although usually apparent in infancy-childhood, these primary/genotropic disorders can present later in adult life. Manifestations can be generalized affecting multiple organ systems or specific to one system—most commonly either the heart or central nervous system. Due to their rarity, severity, and need for specialist management, these primary/genotropic disorders are not the focus of the following section, although much of the information will be relevant, and conceptually and clinically applicable. For example, the rather common *and notably mild* primary/genotropic mitochondrial disorders associated with migraine headaches are a clear example of a heritable/primary/genotropic mitochondriopathy that responds very well to the interventions described below, especially nutrients that support the electron transport chain (ETC), namely coenzyme Q10 (CoQ-10), riboflavin, magnesium as discussed and cited below. In the main, primary/genotropic mitochondrial disorders are relatively rare.

2) <u>Secondary/acquired mitochondrial disorders</u>: Mitochondrial performance can be severely impaired by secondary/acquired conditions, such as exposure to certain pharmaceutical drugs, toxic industrial chemicals, toxic metals, and bacterial or viral infections; these types of mitochondrial disorders have been previously underappreciated but are progressively gaining a foothold in the consciousness of researchers and clinicians worldwide. These secondary/acquired mitochondrial disorders can affect anyone at any time. The clinical strategy for these conditions should be obvious, focusing on the support of optimal mitochondrial function (outlined below) while eliminating the problematic infection and/or toxic exposure (customized per patient's exposure). Importantly, secondary/acquired mitochondrial disorders are increasingly recognized as common (as more physicians become aware

of the clinical frequency and implications of mitochondrial dysfunction) and are becoming more common (as our environment becomes more polluted with herbicides, pesticides, and other persistent organic pollutants as a result of governmental-political failure to regulate industry and protect humanity from unfettered corporate profiteering.

3) <u>Mixed-etiology (perhaps also called tertiary) mitochondrial disorders</u>: Of course, a patient could have both a primary/genotropic disorder along with a secondary/acquired mitochondrial disorder. The classic example of this combination is migranogenic mitochondrial impairment (primary disorder) exacerbated by one or more secondary disorders such as microbial colonization, a pro-inflammatory diet, or nutrient (e.g., magnesium) deficiency; this model helps explain—and place into perspective—the hereditary and environmental contributions to such mixed-etiology mitochondrial disorders.

When possible, the cause of the mitochondrial dysfunction should be treated directly; however, in practical reality of clinical practice, we often have to use an empirical and eclectic approach. Note that eclecticism and empiricism are not the same as random and illogical; even when using an empirical and eclectic approach, we clinicians can choose among the more efficacious and applicable interventions per research and nuances of patient history and assessment. For more complicated or severe cases, we can use laboratory assessments, depending on the problem suspected clinically; however, more skilled and experienced clinicians tend to find that laboratory tests for the assessment of mitochondrial function are not needed on a routine basis. On the contrary, the vast majority of mitochondrial dysfunction

2013 INTERNATIONAL CONFERENCE ON
HUMAN NUTRITION AND **FUNCTIONAL MEDICINE**
PORTLAND OREGON CONVENTION CENTER · SEPTEMBER 25-29, 2013

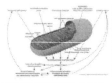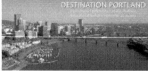

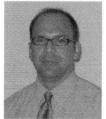

Mitochondrial Nutrition and Beyond:
Mitochondrial Optimization for Optimal Health
> **Brief introduction and review**
> **Mitochondrial interventions**

Alex Vasquez D.C., N.D., D.O., F.A.C.N.

<u>Video presentation and slides</u>: Dr Vasquez's presentation is available online at www.Vimeo.com/ICHNFM and the accompanying slides are available in printed book format at www.CreateSpace.com/4478800

observed or suspected in routine outpatient clinical practice can be treated without mitochondria-specific, time-consuming, resource-depleting, and treatment-delaying laboratory assessments.

Interventions that support/improve mitochondrial function: As a group of intracellular organelles numbering from—for example, and not including the zero per erythrocyte—200 per cell in the biceps to 3,500 per cardiomyocyte, **mitochondria are a heterogenous group**, populated by those with a theoretical optimal performance ("Olympians") down to those with cell-threatening and body-damaging effects ("misfits"). The mitochondrial population must therefore be occasionally culled for the health of the cell and of the larger organism.[798] Generally, the interconnected eliminative and regenerative processes can be described with the following terminology; additional terms are also listed here for convenience.

1) <u>Fusion</u>: The binding of two mitochondria into one single mitochondria,

2) <u>Reallocation/partitioning</u>: The redistribution of "better" and "worse" mitochondrial components into regions that will eventually split to generate progeny.

3) <u>Fission</u>: The splitting of the large mitochondrion into two daughter mitochondria: 90% of the time, both offspring will be sufficiently healthy and will have benefitted from the reallocation of genetic and structural material, while approximately 10% of the time, one mitochondrion will have received the better components and thus has significantly improved function, and the other ("the runt") will have been allocated a disproportionate share of the damaged/expended/oxidized mitochondrial goods and will therefore have severely impaired function, which targets it for destruction.

---

[798] Twig G, Hyde B, Shirihai OS. Mitochondrial fusion, fission and autophagy as a quality control axis: the bioenergetic view. *Biochimica et Biophysica Acta* 2008 May; 1777: 1092–1097

4) <u>Mitophagy/autophagy</u>: Targeted destruction of dysfunctional mitochondria; this can occur following the fusion-fission cycle or likely—in the case of a severely dysfunctional *misfit* mitochondria—directly, i.e., without preceding fusion and fission. Although destruction/removal often has a negative connotation (perhaps mostly in Western cultures unconsciously dominated by the Greek-Roman Apollonian ideal without the balancing Dionysian construct), readers should appreciate that mitophagy is necessary for sustaining cellular and organismal health; defects in mitophagy are inconsistent with health and survival. As discussed below, some of the benefits of carbohydrate restriction, fasting, and exercise are mediated by the promotion of mitophagy, because mild cellular stresses prompt the fusion/fission/mitophagy process, which generally leads to enhanced health and performance of the remaining mitochondrial mass. Obviously, if mitophagy proceeds unchecked, then cells will lose the mitochondria's ability to form sufficient ATP and carry out other functions, and cell death will result. Insufficient mitophagy is damaging to the organism because it promotes oxidative and inflammatory injury, while excess mitophagy depletes ATP and causes cell death and resultant tissue/organism failure.

5) <u>Biogenesis</u>: Just as mitophagy can occur without a preceding fusion-fission cycle, so can fission; if a mitochondrion is a reasonably robust *Olympian* and if it is stimulated by intracellular signals indicating sufficient nutrients and need are present, it can split, accumulate nutrients, and grow, thus contributing directly to an enhanced mitochondrial population and expanded mitochondrial biomass.

6) <u>Δψm, MIM transmembrane potential (MIMtmp)</u>: MIM transmembrane potential (MIMtmp) is a quantification of proton concentration in the intermembrane space. For optimal mitochondrial performance, MIMtmp needs to be conceptually "in the middle"—niether too high nor too low.

- <u>Excessive MIM transmembrane potential—mitochondrial hyperpolarization—essentially turns off ETC flow and "shuts down" or "hibernates" the mitochondria, which is now resistant to triggering of apoptosis, promoting cell immortalization seen in cancer, autoimmunity, and vascular smooth muscle hyperproliferation</u>: Excessive polarization of the transmembrane potential (MIM hyperpolarization, MIMhp) can be caused by LPS activation of TLR, and it can also be caused by immune activation itself, with the latter resulting in a vicious cycle because immune activation causes MIMhp which then triggers activation of mTOR, which promotes additional inflammation and autoimmunity as well as resistance to apoptosis, allowing autoreactive lymphocytes to evade deletion. While mitochondrial hyperpolarization impairs apoptosis, cell death via necrosis is enhanced, and this "inflammatory death" of immunocytes contributes to total inflammatory load since necrotic debris from cells and mitochondria activates damage associated molecular pattern (DAMP) receptors which promote inflammation.

> **MIM hyperpolarization is characteristic of cancer and autoimmunity, with the latter secondary to mTOR activation and its inhibition of FoxP3+ Treg generation**
>
> - "Maximal hyperpolarization stalls respiration and oxidative phosphorylation, essentially "shutting off mitochondria" and shifting energy production to the cytoplasm, with glycolysis becoming the primary source of ATP. A glycolytic phenotype is associated with resistance to apoptosis, in part because the "inactive" hyperpolarized mitochondria cannot induce apoptosis. The majority of human cancers are characterized by hyperpolarized mitochondria, and this metabolic remodeling might be the basis of the Warburg effect in cancer."*
> - "Mitochondrial hyperpolarization and the resultant ATP depletion sensitize T cells for necrosis, which may significantly contribute to inflammation in patients with SLE."**
>
> *Michelakis ED. Mitochondrial medicine: a new era in medicine opens new windows and brings new challenges. *Circulation*. 2008 May
> **Gergely P Jr, Grossman C, Niland B, et al. Mitochondrial hyperpolarization and ATP depletion in patients with systemic lupus erythematosus. *Arthritis Rheum*. 2002 Jan

- <u>Reduced MIM transmembrane potential "deflates" the proton gradient that is needed to drive ATP synthase; an excessive reduction triggers MTP-mediated apoptosis</u>: A reduction in MIMtmp can be caused by 1) reduced Krebs' and/or ETC performance causing reduced proton generation, or by leakage of protons back through the MIM via 2) unregulated *basal* transmembrane permeability ("leaky mitochondria") due to oxidative damage to the MIM or dietary lack of appropriate fatty acids and phospholipids for MIM structure and maintenance, 3) heightened *augmented physiologic* channel-mediated transmembrane conductance via UPC (uncoupling proteins) or the dreaded MTP (mitochondrial transition pore) which is activated by reduced MIMtmp and leads to further rapid "deflating" of the mitochondria, spewing of apoptotic mediators to the cytoplasm and resultant cell death, 4) artificial *pharmacologic/xenobiotic* ionophore-mediated transmembrane conductance via substances such as salycilate and 2,4-dinitrophenol, and/or possibily 5) leakiness of the MOM, which is generally incompatable with mitochondrial and cell survival. **When MIMtmp is reduced by whatever means, then ATP synthase's rotary catalysis of ATP production will be reduced, thus severely compromising the generation of cellular energy.**

Conceptually and therefore practically, clinicians benefit from organizing information into categories that can then be subdivided into individual therapeutics; the three main categories of "interventional mitochondrial medicine" as I am defining it are ❶ therapeutic mitophagy—interventions which support therapeutic mitophagy such as carbohydrate/calorie restriction and physical exercise, ❷ mitochondrial support and stimulation—nutritional/phytonutritional support of biochemical processes (e.g., Kreb's cycle and ETC) and physiologic processes (e.g., biogenesis), and ❸ therapeutic disinhibition—removing the obstacles to mitochondrial performance such as xenobiotics and infections. Practically and respectively, these three steps are applied as 1) lifestyle, 2) supplementation, and 3) removal; skilled clinicians should be able to address each of these components simultaneously, prioritizing each particular treatment plan per the needs and responses of the patient. Students/clinicians implementing these protocols should already be familiar with dosing and administration and therefore such information is not included here; further, doses have to be modified per patient not simply based on age, weight, renal function, and (poly)pharmacy, but also per the level of need for and engagement with the overall treatment plan. With regard to the latter two considerations, the dose, duration, and variety of interventions is determined by severity of the illness(es) and the willingness vs resistance of the patient to do the whole program or simply a fewer parts of it. Indeed, doing every aspect of every component of the FINDSEX protocol would be prohibitively expensive and impractically time-consuming for most patients; here, physicians will have to guide patients to the most effective and necessary components of the protocol to customize the plan for the needs, abilities, and nuances of each patient.

❶ **Therapeutic mitophagy *via lifestyle*:** My concept of "therapeutic mitophagy" is this: the intentional induction/promotion of mitopaghy—for either/both of the following: reduction in mitochondrial mass for a reduction in inflammatory signaling and oxidant production, and the "culling of the mitochondrial herd" to eliminate the lower-performing mitochondria. Carbohydrate restriction and moderate exercise are two safe and universally available and affordable means to therapeutically/intentionally induce mitophagy and achive its numerous anti-oxidant and anti-inflammatory benefits.

1. **Carbohydrate restriction/avoidance, fasting, ketogenic diet**:
    - Mitochondrial mechanism(s): High dietary loads of carbohydrates overwhelm the nonregulated enzymatic systems involved in substrate conversion, leading to what can be described as a short-term "mitochondrial burnout" due to excess subsequent free radical generation; evidence of this appears quite clear, with an irrefutable collection of data from human trials showing that 100g glucose leads to oxidative stress, antioxidant depletion, a measurable inflammatory response, and immune/phagocytic suppression. Conversely, carbohydrate restriction promotes mitochondrial function generally by allowing mitochondria to adapt to being fueled by a variety of sources (leading to structural reorganization of ETC supercomplex assembly[799]), rather than the "easy currency" and "quick fix" of carbohydrate; specifically, carbohydrate restriction promotes ketogenesis and resultant endogenous production of beta-hydroxy-butyrate (bHB) which stimulates complexes 3 and 4 of the ETC. Whereas consumption/provision of "simple" carbohydrates appears to overwhelm mitochondria and lead to oxidative stress and inflammation; carbohydrate avoidance and promotion of a mildly

---

[799] Lapuente-Brun E, Moreno-Loshuertos R, Acín-Pérez R, et al. Supercomplex assembly determines electron flux in the mitochondrial electron transport chain. *Science*. 2013 Jun 28;340(6140):1567-70

ketotic state have the opposite effects—anti-inflammatory and antioxidant benefits. The mild stress of caloric/carbohydrate restriction prompts a wide range of physiologic adaptations, one of which is mitophagy, which has the overall effect of reducing oxidant stress and pro-inflammatory signaling.

- <u>Clinical benefits</u>: Carbohydrate avoidance—and its physiologic converse of ketogenesis promotion—demonstrates an unsurpassed cure rate of hypertension and diabetes mellitus type-2. Carbohydrate avoidance promotes endogenous antioxidant defenses, systemic anti-inflammation, longevity in multiple species, and a rejuvanitive phenotype via—among several other means—histone acetylation.

2. **Exercise**:
   - <u>Mitochondrial mechanism(s)</u>: Improves oxygen delivery via vasodilation and increased cardiovascular output (heart rate X stroke volume). Promotes mito-availability of magnesium due to systemic alkalinization secondary to physiologic hyperventilation and resultant respiratory alkalosis; alkalinity promotes renal retention of magnesium and increases intracellular uptake of magnesium thereby increasing magnesium's availability to various enzymes, including the phosphorylating ATP synthase. The stress of exercise prompts a wide range of physiologic adaptations, one of which is mitophagy, which has the overall effect of reducing oxidant stress and pro-inflammatory signaling; exercise also promotes mitochondrial biogenesis and induction/upregulation of ATP-producing substrate-converting enzymes.
   - <u>Clinical benefits</u>: Weight loss, anti-inflammation via elaboration of myokines and via reduction in (visceral) adopose), enhanced insulin responsiveness via muscle uptake of glucose as well as increased elaboration of GLUT-4 receptors, reduced mental depression and psychological dependency, enhanced appearance and self-esteem, likely increased competence and intelligence via skill-building and exercise-induced neurogenesis assuming that one is in [has created for oneself] an environment conducive to intellectual optimization; obviously, this requires more than simply the provision of exercise for neurogenesis and synaptic plactisity; one must give these new neuroconnections something to ponder and perform.

❷ **Mitochondrial support *via supplementation***: Many interventions are available which serve to either support or stimulate mitochondrial function. Simply "stimulating" mitochondrial function would be a pretty stupid idea if a sizeable portion of the individual's mitochondrial population is dysfunctional; stimulating dysfunctional mitochondria would be expected to promote inflammation and oxidative stress. Clinicians should seek to—as we say in naturopathic medicine—*reestablish the foundation for* (mitochondrial) *health* before employing attempts at mitochondrial stimulation or interventions that promote biogenesis. Thus, in this second category, I will list—in somewhat of a prioritized sequence—those therapeutics which generally support and can later be used to optimize mitochondrial function generally and ATP production specifically. The prioritization of these is somewhat—but not entirely—conceptual; the actual "priority" is the one-many that will best benefit the individual patient.

3. **<u>Healthy diet and broad-spectrum high-potency vitamin and mineral supplementation, eg, a professional-quality six-per-day multivitamin/mineral supplement (note that these are parts of the foundational plan for essentially all patients per my "5-Part Supplemented Paleo-Mediteranean Diet"[800])</u>:**
   - <u>Mitochondrial mechanism(s)</u>: Vitamins (coenzymes) and minterals (cofactors) must be present in sufficient amounts in order for biochemical reactions to proceed with health-optimizing efficiency; nutritional deficiencies impair biochemical efficiency and initiate the progressive reductions in cellular function that initiates/promotes/mimicks and contributes to various disease states. Most people (eg, Americans) are nutrient deficient and should take a multivitamin and multimineral supplement[801,802], and people with metabolic impairments such as those due to single nucleotide polymorphisms (SNPs) will need to use "high-dose vitamin therapy" for the duration of their lives in order to stimulate their

[800] Vasquez A. Revisiting the Five-Part Nutritional Wellness Protocol: The Suppplemented Paleo-Mediterranean Diet. *Nutritional Perspectives* 2011 Jan: 19-25 http://www.ichnfm.org/faculty/vasquez/pdf/vasquez_2011_five-part_protocol_revisited.pdf
[801] Fletcher RH, Fairfield KM. Vitamins for chronic disease prevention in adults: clinical applications. *JAMA*. 2002 Jun 19;287(23):3127-9
[802] Heaney RP. Long-latency deficiency disease: insights from calcium and vitamin D. *Am J Clin Nutr*. 2003 Nov;78(5):912-9

variant enzymes[803] and—speaking casually—push sluggish enzymes to complete their reactions. More specifically, B1 (thiamine), B2 (riboflavin), B3 (niacin), B5 (pantothenate), and lipoic acid are required components for the pyruvate dehydrogenase complex[804] which transfers/converts pyruvate made in the cytoplasm into acetyl-CoA in the mitochondria. B2 is required for the formation of flavin adenine dinucleotide (FAD), and B3 is required for the formation of niacinamide adenine dinucleotide (NAD)—both of these constituents are absolutely required for mitochondrial production of ATP. Further, B2 is a cofactor for glutamate dehydrogenase which converts glutamate to alpha-ketoglutarate for use in the Kreb's cycle. Magnesium is required for phosphorylation reactions, e.g., phosphorylation of ADP to ATP by Complex 5—ATP synthase. Antioxidants, such as tocopherols in general (especially gamma) and tocopherol succinate in particular, help to protect oxidation-vulnerable phospholipids and nuclear and mitochondrial DNA. For general biochemical and antioxidant "support" of mitochondrial function, and for the prevention and treatment of mitochondrial disorders—regardless of cause—routine use of a high-quality broad-spectrum multivitamin and multimineral supplement is reasonable.

- Clinical benefits: B1 improves renal function in DM. B2 improves mood, especially in women, and doses of 400mg daily are remarkably effective for migraine prophylaxis with the most likely effect being mediated via improved function of ETC Complex #2. B3 is also effective against migraine, perhaps partly via vasodilation, but more likely via stimulation of ETC Complex #1. The vitamin CoQ-10 is necessary for ETC Complexes #1-3. These and other nutrient-specific locations are illustrated in the diagram below of the ETC.

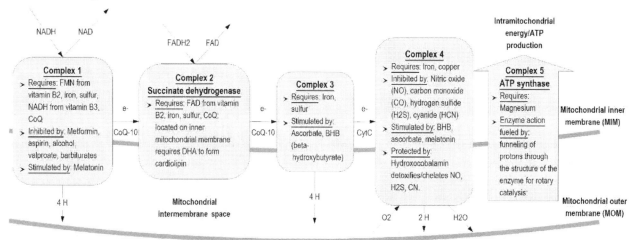

Reduce mitochondrial protein synthesis: Tetracyclines, chloramphenicol
Cause mtDNA depletion: Adriamycin/doxorubicin, zidovudine, herpes simplex virus

Vasquez A. Integrative Rheumatology and Inflammation Mastery. 3rd ed. Seattle, WA: CreateSpace, 2014.

Electron transport chain (ETC) with some requirements, inhibitors, stimulators, and protectors: Clinical implications are obvious from the diagram and are additionally discussed in the text.

4. **Coenzyme-Q10**: CoQ-10 would have received better public acceptance if Folkers had named it "vitamin Q" instead of "coenzyme Q", per his own admission.
   - Mitochondrial mechanism(s): Transfers electrons between complexes 1,2,3. Funtions as lipid-soluble antioxidant. Direct anti-inflammatory effect via inhibition of NFkB.
   - Clinical benefits: The single most effective "vitamin" treatment for hypertension; alleviates hypertension and insulin resistance probably via improvement of mitochondrial function. Remarkably effective for migraine prophylaxis in adults and children; clinical benefits also shown for Parkinson's disease and Huntington's disease (delayed progression) and asthma (reduced medication

---

[803] Ames BN, Elson-Schwab I, Silver EA. High-dose vitamin therapy stimulates variant enzymes with decreased coenzyme binding affinity (increased K(m)): relevance to genetic disease and polymorphisms. *Am J Clin Nutr.* 2002 Apr;75(4):616-58

[804] My source of information on this list of coenzymes is my professor in medical school at UNTHSC, Ladislav Dory PhD. I realize some might debate this list of cofactors; but likewise my professor—based on his intimate work with mitochondria—would likely refute those debates. So, I think this list is reasonable for purposes presented here.

dependency). One of the best treatments for renal insufficiency; CoQ-10 100-300mg/d and thiamine 100mg TID (along with other nutrients) should be combined for this use.

5. **"Vitamin E"**: What is meant by "vitamin E" here is mixed tocopherols with at least 40% gamma-tocopherol; additionally, alpha-tocopherol succinate has been described as being somewhat "mitochondria specific" and might be used alongside mixed tocopherols.
    - Mitochondrial mechanism(s): Generalized anti-inflammatory and anti-oxidant effects; specifically helps to protect cell membranes in general and mitochondrial membranes in particular.
    - Clinical benefits: Anti-inflammatory and immune-modulating effects (e.g., reductions in IgE in patients with eczema, and reductions in ANA in patients with various autoimmune diseases). Alleviates pain in osteoarthritis; can help to restore/normalize mitochondrial function in pateints with mitochondrial disease.

6. **Lipoic acid**:
    - Mitochondrial mechanism(s): Coenzyme for various enzymatic reactions, including pyruvate dehydrogenase. Water-soluble and lipid-soluble antioxidant. Anti-inflammatory benefits via direct inhibition of NFkB as well as via reductions in IL-17.
    - Clinical benefits: Diabetic neuropathy, hypertension, diabetes mellitus type-2. Lipoic acid and acetyl-L-carnitine function additively/synergistically and should generally be used together. Lipoic acid has a short half-life and should therefore be administered in divided doses throughout the day, e.g., 300-400mg TID-QID.

7. **Acetyl-L-carnitine**:
    - Mitochondrial mechanism(s): L-carnitine is required for mitochondrial beta-oxidation of long-chain fatty acids for ATP production; long-chain fatty acids must be in the form of esters of L-carnitine (acylcarnitines) in order to enter the mitochondrial matrix where beta-oxidation occurs.[805]
    - Clinical benefits: Alzhemer's disease, hypertension, insulin resistance, Peyrone's disease. Lipoic acid and acetyl-L-carnitine function additively/synergistically and should generally be used together.

8. **Magnesium (Mg)**:
    - Mitochondrial mechanism(s): Magnesium plays a pivotal role in formation of the transition state of the ATP synthase enzyme (complex 5) where ATP is synthesized from ADP and inorganic phosphate.[806]
    - Clinical benefits: Hypertension, seizures/epilepsy, migraine and all types of headaches, insulin resistance, heart failure, depression, anxiety, bruxism and muscle cramps. Mg alleviates neurogenic inflammation in animal models.

9. **Medium-chain triglycerides (MTC)**:
    - Mitochondrial mechanism(s): MTC and the ketone bodies (KB) into which they are converted are clearly the preferred fuel source for most mitochondria under normal conditions. MTC and KB actually improve mitochondrial function via upregulation/induction of key enzymes and ETC complexes 3 and 4; in contrast to CHO such as fructose which cause mitochondrial damage, MTC and KB improve and restore mitochondrial function while serving as a fuel source. Beta-hydroxybutyrate (bHB) bolsters antioxidant defenses and promotes histone acetylation for induction of a rejuvenative phenotype.
    - Clinical benefits: Administration of MTC (eg, coconut oil), caprylic acid and relative derrivatives, and/or fasting—which promotes endogenous bHB production—leads to clinical improvements in and alleviation of Alzheimer's disease, asthma and various inflammatory disorders. Note that ketogenic diet thereapy is among one of the best and safest treatments for both chronic epilepsy and status epilepticus.

[805] Linus Pauling Institute Micronutrient Information Center. L-Carnitine. lpi.oregonstate.edu/infocenter/othernuts/carnitine/
[806] Ko YH, Hong S, Pedersen PL. Chemical mechanism of ATP synthase. *J Biol Chem.* 1999 Oct 8;274(41):28853-6

11. **Resveratrol**:
   - Mitochondrial mechanism(s): Resveratrol promotes mitochondrial biogenesis, hence is reputation for being the botanical mimic of exercise. Additionally, resveratrol also has some anti-oxidant and anti-inflammatory actions; paradoxically, resveratrol may have an estrogenic effect at the level of the estrogen receptor while also suppressing activity of aromatase.
   - Clinical benefits: Improvement in endothelial function; cardioprotective benefits.
12. **DHA (docosahexaenoic acid) from fish oil or blue-green algae**:
   - Mitochondrial mechanism(s): DHA becomes integrated into the phospholipid phosphatidylserine, which is the structural anchor for succinate dehydrogenase—a key enzyme in both the Krebs' cycle and the ETC (complex 2).
   - Clinical benefits: Antiinflammatory, cardioprotective, neuroprotective, improves cardiovascular health, improves brain function in various neuropsychiatric disorders such as depression, anxiety, bipolar, schizophrenia.
13. **Optimization of iron status—avoiding iron deficiency (both systemic and cerebral) while also avoiding iron overload**: Iron deficiency impairs mitochondrial function because iron is needed for several biochemical reactions in the electron transport chain; conversely, iron overload also impairs mitochondrial function due to free radical damage. The amount of iron in the body can be accurately determined by the blood test "serum ferritin." Per my publications on this topic and review of the literature (more than 300 papers read), optimal iron status correlates with a serum ferritin of 40-70 ng/ml; the only exception to this rule appears to be a subset of patients with restless leg syndrome (RLS) who have a defect in the transport of iron into the brain, such that they need higher levels of iron correlating with a serum ferritin up to 120 ng/ml. Stated again and differently, some patients with RLS have a defect in the transport of iron into the brain, and this defect can be overcome by allowing the patient to have higher-than-normal levels of iron, up to 120 ng/ml. Iron overload is a common problem, too, either due to lifestyle factors such as overconsumption of alcohol and/or iron-rich foods such as beef and liver, or due to diseases such as type-2 diabetes, metabolic syndrome, or the genetic iron-accumulation disorder hemochromatosis, which is one of the most common genetic diseases seen in humans with a frequency of approximately 1 per 200-250 in the general population. Hereditary iron overload disorders are seen in people of all genetic backgrounds and ethnicities; they appear most common in persons of African descent (perhaps as high as 1 per 80 persons). Serum ferritin levels higher than 200 ng/ml in a woman or 300 ng/ml in a man strongly suggest the probability of excess iron and warrant evaluation and treatment, even in the absence of clinical pathology[807]; overt pathologic damage caused by iron is generally seen with ferritin values greater than 1,000 mcg/L. [Note: when discussing ferritin, the measurement units mcg/L and ng/ml are equivalent.]

> **Optimal iron status is necessary for optimal mitochondrial function**
> - Measure serum ferritin: For most patients, optimal iron status correlates with a serum ferritin of 40-70 ng/ml.
> - Avoid iron deficiency: Iron is a required component of cytochrome C in the electron transport chain (ETC) that produces ATP.
> - Avoid iron overload: Excess iron causes free radical damage that impairs mitochondrial function.

   - Mitochondrial mechanism(s): Iron is necessary for ETC complexes 3 and 4; iron deficiency causes ETC dysfunction, which generally results in reduced ATP formation and increased oxidant formation. Iron overload promotes lipid oxidation and DNA damage, both of which can contribute to mitochondrial impairment. Iron obviously plays other roles, such as formation of hemoglobin, synthesis of dopamine, function of thyroid hormones, fatty acid metabolism, etc.
   - Clinical benefits: Patients generally feel better when their iron status is optimized so that they are neither iron-deficient nor iron-overloaded. For most patients, optimal iron status correlates with a serum ferritin of 40-70 ng/ml.

---

[807] Barton JC, McDonnell SM, Adams PC,et al. Management of hemochromatosis. *Ann Intern Med.* 1998 Dec 1;129(11):932-9

15. **N-Acetyl-Cysteine (NAC)**:

- Mitochondrial mechanism(s): NAC provides cysteine for GSH production. NAC also inhibits NFkB. NAC inhibits viral replication (eg, HIV) more effectively than and independently from its conversion to GSH. Recently, NAC at relatively high doses of 4,800mg/d in divided doses was shown to modulate mitochondrial hyperpolarization (by dissociating the generally resultant mTOR activation) and lead to very important clinical and immunological improvements in patients with SLE; NAC was shown to be safe and well-tolerated by all SLE patients up to 2.4g/d with reversible nausea in 33% of patients receiving 4.8g/d. This study by Lai, Hanczko, Bonilla, et al[808] is truly a landmark contribution and advance in the field of rheumatology and immunology because it proves 1) that mitochondrial dysfunction directly leads to an autoimmune phenotype, and 2) that inhibition of mTOR by NAC is safe and effective in patients with SLE; important insights from this remarkable work are as follows:

  o NAC 4,800mg/d proved safe and clinically beneficial in patients with SLE, leading to reductions in disease activity and ANA levels.

  o Mitochondrial hyperpolarization (MHP) causes mTOR activation which in turn suppresses the expression of the FoxP3 transcription factor necessary for induction of T-regulatory cells. Note that the mTOR activation is the cause of the FoxP3 suppression; ironically, NAC actually increases MHP but dissociates it from mTOR by having a greater effect on and via mTOR suppression. The nutritional supplement NAC works in a similar manner as does the immunosuppressive drug rapamycin, with a mechanism of suppression of mTOR and the effect of enhancing endogenous anti-inflammatory immunomodulation via CD4+ CD25+ FoxP3+ T-regulatory cells. Stated again and differently, NAC paradoxically worsens

> **Mechanistic and clinical proof that mitochondrial dysfunction directly contributes to autoimmunity**
>
> "Similar to the effect of rapamycin, **suppression of mTOR by NAC was accompanied by increased FoxP3 expression in CD4+/CD25+ T cells**. These results suggest that the effect of NAC on the immune system is 1) cell type-specific and 2) it occurs through disconnecting the activation of mTOR from the elevation of Δψm in lupus T cells, similar to the effect of rapamycin."
>
> Lai ZW, Hanczko R, Bonilla E, et al. N-acetylcysteine reduces disease activity by blocking mammalian target of rapamycin in T cells from systemic lupus erythematosus patients. *Arthritis Rheum.* 2012 Sep

  mitochondrial hyperpolarization in patients with SLE but does so at the same time that it has a more significant impact on mTOR; NAC's rapamycin-like targeting of mTOR dissociates mitochondrial hyperpolarization from mTOR activation. The reduction in mTOR activity (which is of greater consequence than the increase in MIM polarization) allows enhanced expression of FoxP3 for increased elaboration of T-regulatory cells, thereby providing endogenous immunoregulation.

  o "MHP of lupus T cells, which most prominently affects DN [double-negative, autoimmunity-promoting] T cells, was associated with resistance to activation-induced apoptosis. In 27 SLE patients receiving daily NAC doses of 1.2 g, 2.4 g, and 4.8 g considered together, both **spontaneous and CD3/CD28-induced apoptosis of DN T cells were markedly increased** and the **expansion of these cells was effectively reversed**. The **elimination of DN T cells, which are known promote anti-DNA autoantibody production by B cells**, is likely to contribute to reduced anti-DNA titers and to the efficacy of NAC.

  o "The therapeutic importance of NAC for SLE is reflected by: 1) achieving clinical improvement in two validated disease activity scores within 3 months; 2) diminishing fatigue (21), which is considered the most disabling symptom in a majority of SLE patients (22); 3) absence of significant side-effects; and 4) affordability of this medication. A monthly supply of 600-mg NAC capsules (120–240 capsules) costs $15–$30 on the retail market. This sharply contrasts with average annual direct medical costs estimated to be ~$22,580 per patient in 2009.Thus,

---

[808] Lai ZW, Hanczko R, Bonilla E, et al. N-acetylcysteine reduces disease activity by blocking mammalian target of rapamycin in T cells from systemic lupus erythematosus patients: a randomized, double-blind, placebo-controlled trial. *Arthritis Rheum.* 2012 Sep;64(9):2937-46
http://www.ncbi.nlm.nih.gov/pmc/articles/PMC3411859/

the cost of NAC at \$180–\$360/year would be negligible in comparison to the overall expenditures to society and the expected benefit in reducing the need for vastly more expensive medications burdened with potentially serious side-effects."

16. **General antioxidant support**: Naturally-derived antioxidants in general tend to have anti-inflammatory, disease-alleviating, and health-promoting benefits; much of the benefit from eating a complex plant-based diet is derived from the additive and synergistic biochemical and physiologic benefits provided by phytonutrients, of which 5,000-8,000 exist.[809] Hence, as I have stated and published for many years, the best approach is a plant-based diet that provides adequate protein, reduces intake of starchy phytonutrient-deficient carbohydrates, completely avoids wheat and syrups, and atop which is added a broad-spectrum high-potency multivitamin and multimineral supplement for nutrient provision and additional antioxidant support.[810]

- Mitochondrial mechanism(s): Speaking generally, broadly, and accurately, we can estimate that antiinflammatory and antioxidant therapeutics/diets/interventions/supplements will tend to improve mitochondrial function; sophomores will argue against this by stating that oxidative stress induces hormesis to which I'll reply that chronic/sustained/long-term minute-by-minute adaptation is not possible because adaptive mechanisms are not long to be depleted. A better approach is to provide sufficient and perhaps supraphysiologic antioxidant support via diet and supplements and to then punctuate that biochemical bliss reasonable bouts of hormetic shock such as fasting, exercise, and ethanol to which defensive/adaptive mechanisms can respond—this is the best of both words, to which a few exceptions are noted, such as blunting of physiologic responsiveness to exercise with antioxidant supplementation in patients with DM-2/MetSyn.

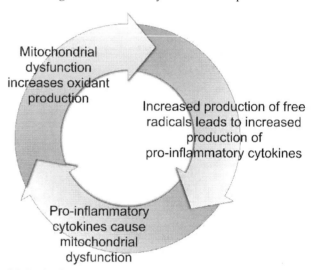

Mitochondrial dysfunction as cause and consequence of oxidative stress and inflammation: Clinical implications are obvious from the diagram and are additionally discussed in the text.

Identical arguments are valid or invalid within different clinical contexts, and the argument in favor of high(er) dosing of antioxidants is—as logically anticipated—more easily made when treating *autoimmue* patients with more severe oxidant and inflammatory stress

- Clinical benefits: Paraphrasing Dr Bruce Ames: Mitochondrial oxidative decay is a major contributor to aging and is accelerated by many common micronutrient deficiencies; an optimum intake of micronutrients can "tune-up mitochondrial metabolism" and give a marked increase in health, particularly for the poor, elderly, and obese, at little cost.[811]

17. **General anti-inflammatory support**:
- Mitochondrial mechanism(s): Pro-inflammatory cytokines such as interferon (IFN)-gamma, interleukin (IL)-1b, and tumor necrosis factor (TNF)-alpha impair mitochondrial function via cytokine-stimulated iNOS-induced nitric oxide (NO) production[812], and mitochondrial dysfunction increases elaboration of ROS which act as signaling molecules to increase the production of pro-

---

[809] Liu RH. Health benefits of fruit and vegetables are from additive and synergistic combinations of phytochemicals. *Am J Clin Nutr.* 2003 Sep;78(3 Suppl):517S-520S
[810] Vasquez A. Revisiting the Five-Part Nutritional Wellness Protocol: The Suppplemented Paleo-Mediterranean Diet. *Nutritional Perspectives* 2011 Jan: 19-25 http://www.ichnfm.org/faculty/vasquez/pdf/vasquez_2011_five-part_protocol_revisited.pdf
[811] Ames BN, Atamna H, Killilea DW. Mineral and vitamin deficiencies can accelerate the mitochondrial decay of aging. *Mol Aspects Med.* 2005 Aug-Oct;26(4-5):363-78
[812] "These data suggest that IL-1b–induced NO production in cardiac myocytes lowers energy production and myocardial contractility through a direct attack on the mitochondria, rather than through cGMP-mediated pathways." Tatsumi T, Matoba S, Kawahara A, et al. Cytokine-induced nitric oxide production inhibits mitochondrial energy production and impairs contractile function in rat cardiac myocytes. *J Am Coll Cardiol.* 2000 Apr;35(5):1338-46

inflammatory cytokines[813]; adding to this, mitochondrial dysfunction also increases cellular sensitivity to pro-inflammatory cytokines. [814] Obviously, the stage is thus set for a self-perpetuating cycle.

- Clinical benefits: Vitamin D3 supplementation, low-carbohydrate diets, and multivitamin-multimineral supplementation are excellent examples of anti-inflammatory interventions that are safe and effective. Additional anti-inflammatory benefit can be obtained by eradicating dysbiotic infections, correcting hormone imbalances, reducing obesity, etc.

18. **High-salycilate diet and/or low-dose aspirin to provide salycilate for ionophore alleviation of mitochondrial hyperpolarization — hypothesis**:
    - Mitochondrial mechanism(s): To the best of my knowledge, I am the first to propose that the well-documented benefits of plant-based diets against cancer and autoimmunity may stem in part from the ionophore action of salysilate against mitochondrial hyperpolarization which is common both in cancer and autoimmunity.
    - Clinical benefits: High-plant diets and low-dose aspirin have shown benefit against inflammatory states; what I propose here is that part of the mechanism may be that of alleviation of mitochondrial hyperpolarization by the ionophore action of salicylic acid, a well-absorbed phytochemical that is believed to be signficinatly responsible for the health-promoting and anticancer benefits of plant-based diets.

19. **Alkalinization, acid-base balance, pH**: Several general statements can be made on this topic that are true and which will serve as an introduction to the topic of acid-base balance in the body. Although I initially approached this topic of acid-base balance with some skepticism and disregard, I have come to have profound and deep respect for this simple concept and intervention that provides numerous very important clinical benefits. Overall, the human body produces and excess of acidic substances that require balancing via internal buffering systems and also via dietary consumption of alkaline base-forming substances. The *internal* buffering systems succeed at keeping the acid-base balance within a range compatible for survival; *internal* buffering systems include control of respiratory rate, and the adaptations of the kidneys. The *external* buffering system of dietary consumption of foods that have an alkalinizing effect help to fine-tune the pH of the body in very important ways. My description is: *internal* acid-base buffering via respiration and renal adaptation sustains *life*, while the *external* acid-base buffering of dietarily consumed alkalinizing substances sustains *health*. The Western diet promotes diet-induced metabolic acidosis, while a plant-based Paleolithic diet or vegetarian diet promotes alkalinization.
    - Mitochondrial mechanism(s): Alkalinizaiton promotes renal retention and cellular uptake of magnesium, which is an essential nutrient for efficient action of complex 5, ATP synthase. In neurons, magnesium along with zinc also provide partial blockade of NMDA receptor channeling of calcium; high-levels of intracellular calcium ("intrcellular hypercalcinosis"[815]) promote inflammation and cause mitochondrial stress.
    - Clinical benefits: In sum, the benefits of slight alkalinization to achieve a urine pH of 7.5-8.5 include:
        - Increased renal retention of potassium, calcium, and magnesium,
        - Increased (11%) intracellular uptake and retention of magnesium,
        - Increased excretion of toxins and xenobiotics, per the 2004 Position Paper on Urine Alkalinization by Proudfoot, et al.
        - Reduction in serum cortisol,
        - Improved markers of bone health: reduced bone breakdown,
        - Increased production of endorphins, which elevate mood and alleviate pain.

---

[813] Naik E, Dixit VM. Mitochondrial reactive oxygen species drive proinflammatory cytokine production. *J Exp Med*. 2011 Mar 14;208(3):417-20
[814] "Our findings indicate that mitochondrial dysfunction could amplify the responsiveness to cytokine-induced chondrocyte inflammation through ROS production and NF-κB activation." Vaamonde-García C, Riveiro-Naveira RR, Valcárcel-Ares MN, et al. Mitochondrial dysfunction increases inflammatory responsiveness to cytokines in normal human chondrocytes. *Arthritis Rheum*. 2012 Sep;64(9):2927-36
[815] Vasquez A. Intracellular Hypercalcinosis. A Functional Nutritional Disorder with Implications Ranging From Myofascial Trigger Points to Affective Disorders, Hypertension and Cancer. *Naturopathy Digest* 2006 http://www.naturopathydigest.com/archives/2006/sep/vasquez.php

21. **Melatonin support, including 5HTP and sleep**:
   - Mitochondrial mechanism(s): Melatonin stimulates complexes 1 and 4 of the ETC; melatonin is also a powerful antioxidant.
   - Clinical benefits: Physiologic dose is 200 mcg/night; clinical doses range from 200mcg-40mg taken before night bedtime. Benefits are noted in cancer, fibromyalgia, migraine, hypertension, and of course jet-lag and insomnia. With regard to improving sleep, some patients respond better to lower doses <3mg/night while higher doses >6mg/night have a paradoxic effect of impairing sleep.
22. **Oxygen, deep breathing, exercise, hyperbaric oxygen**:
   - Mitochondrial mechanism(s): Oxygen is the molecular "magnet" which pulls protons through the ETC for the formation of water. Without oxygen to receive mitochondrial protons, mammalian cellular respiration ceases. Mild/moderate exercise promotes physiologic hyperventilation and increased cardiac output, increasing blood/nutrent and oxygen delivery to issues while also promoting systemic alkalinization via respiratory alkalosis. Hyperbaric oxygen can be used to "force" oxygen into underperfused tissues and to maximize oxygen-to-cell delivery thereby promoting mitochondrial function; excess oxygen therapy can have a detrimental effect via increased free radical production and also via promotion of vascular hyperproliferation, as noted in the treatment of the retinopathy of prematurity.
   - Clinical benefits: People feel better when they exercise and breathe deeply; doing so regularly improves mitochondrial performance.

❸ **Mitochondrial disinhibition *via elimination of infections and xenobiotics***: If a patient has mitochondrial dysfunction not caused mostly by genetic mutations (eg, low likelihood of inherited or spontaneous mitochondrial disease) nor by the biochemical impairment caused by coenzyme and cofactor deficiencies (eg, let's assume the patient is well-nourished and is taking a high-potency broad-spectrum multivitamin and multimineral supplement), then we must ask, "What *exogenous* factors can cause mitochondrial impairment?" Beyond the temporary (1-3 hours) impairment of mitochondrial function via consumption of simple carbohydrates such as glucose and fructose (400 calories or more at a time), the most common causes of sustained mitochondrial impairment are microbes and xenobiotics.

23. **Detoxification, avoidance of toxins (xenobiotics) that impair mitochondrial function**:
   - Mitochondrial mechanism(s): Many persistent organic pollutants (POPs) such as pesticides (eg, dielderin) and dioxin-related compounds cause mitochondrial impairment.
   - Clinical benefits: Xenobiotic mitochondriopathy is noted in Parkinson's disease, as well as insulin resistance and metabolic syndrome. Detoxification can be promoted by chlorella, exercise, nutritional supplementation (e.g., NAC for GSH protection and conjugation) as discussed in this textbook.
24. **Eradication of gastrointestinal dysbiosis & small intestine bacterial overgrowth**:
   - Mitochondrial mechanism(s): Dysbiotic bacteria in the intestines impair systemic mitochondrial function via gut-to-systemic absorption of D-lactic acid, hydrogen sulfide, and endotoxin/LPS.
   - Clinical benefits: Chronic fatigue syndrome, fibromyalgia, migraine headaches. Pathophysiology, assessments, and treatments for dysbiosis are detailed elsewhere in this textbook.
25. **Eradication/suppression of any peristent "internal" infections**: Essentially any chronic infection will be associated with immune activation and thus inflammation and elaboration of cytokines; both inflammation as a general process and the elaboration of specific cytokines are known to impair mitochondrial function. Furthermore, some microorganism capable of causing chronic infections such as *Chlamydophila pneumoniae* (*CP*) are called "obligate intracellular bacteria/parasites" because these microbes are incapable of producing their own energy in the form of ATP and thus they must siphon cellular fuel from the host they have infected. Chronic viral infections—particularly those persistent infections caused by members of the herpes family of viruses—should be tested for with blood tests from a standard medical lab; assertive non-drug treatment to suppress viral replication should be implemented for 2-6 months and then serologic (blood) tests can be repeated to determine success of viral suppression. Pathophysiology, assessments, and treatments for dysbiosis are detailed throughout this textbook; note the section on laboratory assessments in Chapter 1. The following table provides examples of pathogens, assessments, and interventions.

Microbial Mitochondriopathy—Introduction to key examples of common clinical relevance

Microbes capable of contributing to fatigue, mitochondrial dysfunction, and energy impairment due to chronic occult/silent infections in humans	*Sample interventions*
• <u>HSV—herpes simplex viruses types 1 and 2</u>: Although infection with HSV is common, higher antibody titers correlate with higher levels of viral replication; thus [nutritional] treatments should be implemented to reduce viral replication in order to improve energy levels and avoid illness associated with HSV-1 (and to a lesser extent HSV-2) such as Alzheimer's disease, risk of which correlates with IgM antibodies to HSV.[816] Generally, testing IgG antibodies is sufficient. **HSV infection kills mitochondria by destroying mitochondrial DNA.**[817]	<u>DrV's antiviral protocol:</u> • <u>Vitamin A</u>: 100,000 international units limited to 10 days only • <u>Vitamin D3</u>: 10,000 IU/d for 10 days • <u>Selenium</u>: 600 mcg per day • <u>Lipoic acid</u>: 200 to 400 mg three times per day • <u>NAC</u>: 1,000 mg 2 to 3 times per day between meals • <u>Melatonin</u>: taken at night: 3-20 mg • <u>Licorice</u>: tea or capsules; monitor for hypertension and hypokalemia with extended use. • <u>CoQ-10</u>: 100-300mg to protect mitochondria and avoid virus-induced fatigue
• <u>CMV—cytomegalovirus</u>: Another member of the herpes family of viruses, chronic low-grade CMV infection is very common in humans; IgG antibodies or more direct tests (no perfect test exists) should be performed, nutritional viral suppression implemented, and antibodies are then retested. **CMV infection causes mitochondrial dysfunction.**[818]	
• <u>HHV-6—Human herpes virus type-6</u>: Associated with chronic fatigue syndrome, a condition known to be associated with mitochondrial dysfunction. **Proteins of HHV-6 infection alter mitochondrial membrane potential and cause mitochondrial dysfunction.** Generally, testing IgG antibodies is sufficient.	
• <u>EBV—Epstein Barr virus</u>: EBV is the cause of infectious mononucleosis, a common illness experienced by most people throughout the world. While most patients recover uneventfully from the infection, some patients appear to harbor a chronic ongoing infection with EBV as evidenced by a combination of several laboratory tests available for antibodies and antigens. **Patients who develop chronic fatigue following EBV infection show evidence of alterations in mitochondrial function.**[819]	
• <u>CP—*Chlamydophila pneumoniae*</u>: Although infection with *CP* initially causes increased production of ATP, the ultimate outcome is cell death; **"Chlamydiae are obligate intracellular gram-negative bacteria and are dependent on the host cell for ATP.** Thus, chlamydial infection may alter the intracellular levels of ATP and affect all energy-dependent processes within the cell."[820] IgG antibody titers can be measured with levels >1:60 indicative of chronic infection and consideration for treatment.	• <u>NAC</u>: 1,000 mg 2 to 3 times per day between meals • <u>Long-term azithromycin</u>: 250-500mg every-other-day for 4-6 months then retest titer

---

[816] Letenneur L, Pérès K, Fleury H, et al. Seropositivity to herpes simplex virus antibodies and risk of Alzheimer's disease: a population-based cohort study. *PLoS One*. 2008;3(11):e3637

[817] "Mitochondria have crucial roles in the life and death of mammalian cells, and help to orchestrate host antiviral defences. Here, we show that the ubiquitous human pathogen herpes simplex virus (HSV) induces rapid and complete degradation of host mitochondrial DNA during productive infection of cultured mammalian cells." Saffran HA, Pare JM, Corcoran JA, Weller SK, Smiley JR. Herpes simplex virus eliminates host mitochondrial DNA. *EMBO Rep*. 2007 Feb;8(2):188-9 http://www.nature.com/embor/journal/v8/n2/full/7400878.html and http://www.ncbi.nlm.nih.gov/pmc/articles/PMC1796774/pdf/7400878.pdf

[818] McCormick AL, Smith VL, Chow D, Mocarski ES. Disruption of mitochondrial networks by the human cytomegalovirus UL37 gene product viral mitochondrion-localized inhibitor of apoptosis. *J Virol*. 2003 Jan;77(1):631-41

[819] "A comparison of gene expression profiles early and late following EBV infection revealed that those who did not recover had differentially expressed genes implicating mitochondrial perturbations with fatty acid metabolism, mitochondrial function and apoptosis pathways." Vernon SD, Whistler T, Cameron B, et al. Preliminary evidence of mitochondrial dysfunction associated with post-infective fatigue after acute infection with Epstein Barr virus. *BMC Infect Dis*. 2006 Jan 31;6:15

[820] Yaraei K, Campbell LA, Zhu X, et al. Effect of Chlamydia pneumoniae on cellular ATP content in mouse macrophages: role of Toll-like receptor 2. *Infect Immun*. 2005 Jul;73(7):4323-6

26. **Avoidance of dietary sulfite, eradication of H2S-producing dysbiosis, and/or chelation/detoxification of sulfite and H2Swith hydroxocobalamin**: Sulfite is a substance found naturally and in significant amounts in some foods such as dried fruit and red wine; it is also added to some foods and drugs as a preservative/antimicrobial/bleaching agent. Sulfite is also produced internally/endogenously from the metabolism of sulfur-containing substances such as amino acids. Sulfite is well-known to trigger asthma and migraine headaches in some patients; of note, both asthma and migraine are complex disorders characterized in part by mitochondrial dysfunction. In 2004 Zhang and coworkers[821] showed that the cellular toxicity of sulfite in brain cells is mediated (at least in part) by inhibition mitochondrial glutamate dehydrogenase, which converts the amino acid and neurotransmitter glutamate into the fuel source alpha-keto-glutarate (AKG); the addition of sulfite increased production of ROS and reduced production of ATP

(ATP production was reduced by ~ 50%)—increased ROS and decreased ATP is the classic dyad of mitochondrial impairment. Therefore, sulfite is a mitochondrial toxin; this explains its ability to exacerbate asthma and migraine, two conditions strongly associated with preexisting mitochondrial dysfunction. Vitamin B-12 is available in several different forms—cyanocobalamin, hydroxocobalamin, adenosylcobalamin, methylcobalamin; of these, only the hydroxocobalamin form has been shown to bind to sulfite and neutralize or "detoxify" it in a clinically significant manner with benefits for patients with sulfite-induced asthma as well as migraines. Further, an indirect mechanism by which sulfur/sulfite-containing foods and drugs may trigger asthma is via the conversion of sulfur/sulfite to sulfur dioxide in the gastrointestinal tract by intestinal bacteria[822]; the sulfur dioxide can then be either absorbed into the

> ### Vitamin B12 in the form of hydroxocobalamin can be used clinically to neutralize sulfite and hydrogen sulfide (H2S)
>
> "Serum concentrations of sulfide before and after administration of hydroxocobalamin were 0.22 and 0.11 µg/mL, respectively; serum concentrations of thiosulfate before and after hydroxocobalamin administration were 0.34 and 0.04 µmol/mL, respectively. **Hydroxocobalamin is believed to form a complex with H2S in detoxification pathways of H2S.** …The decreased sulfide concentration suggests that hydroxocobalamin therapy may be effective for acute H2S poisoning. The decreased thiosulfate concentration seems to be associated with formation of a thiosulfate/hydroxocobalamin complex, because hydroxocobalamin can form a complex with thiosulfate. …Therefore, prompt administration of hydroxocobalamin after H2S exposure may be effective for H2S poisoning."
>
> Fujita et al. A fatal case of acute hydrogen sulfide poisoning caused by hydrogen sulfide: hydroxocobalamin therapy for acute H2S poisoning. *J Analytical Toxicol* 2011 Mar

intestine and/or released from the gastrointestinal tract via regurgitation (i.e., "burping") to reach the lungs, where it may trigger asthma or be readily absorbed into the systemic circulation. Lastly and very importantly, sulfur-containing substances can be converted by some intestinal bacteria into the potent mitochondrial toxin hydrogen sulfide, which poisons the ETC more powerfully than does cyanide.

- Mitochondrial mechanism(s): Sulfite is a mitochondrial toxin, especially in brain cells; therefore avoidance or neutralization of sulfite helps avoid interference with normal mitochondrial respiration. Hydrogen sulfide (H2S) poisons the mitochondrial ETC more powerfully than does cyanide. Sulfite and H2S are both chelated and neutralized by hydroxocobalamin.
- Clinical benefits: Sulfite avoidance helps some patients avoid exacerbations of asthma and migraine. Clinical trials have demonstrated that administration of the sulfite-binding nutrient vitamin B-12 in the form of hydroxocobalamin helps alleviate/prevent migraine and asthma in some patients. Oral administration of hydroxocobalamin 2,000-4,000mcg per exposure (ie, taken before exposure to sulfite-containing foods or medications) or daily doses of 4,000-8,000mcg/day is reasonable; orally administered vitamin B12 at doses of 2,000mcg/day can achieve higher serum levels than can a routine medical protocol of intramuscular vitamin B12.

---

[821] Zhang X, Vincent AS, Halliwell B, Wong KP. A mechanism of sulfite neurotoxicity: direct inhibition of glutamate dehydrogenase. *J Biol Chem*. 2004 Oct 8;279(41):43035-45

[822] "Inhalation of sulfur dioxide (SO2) generated in the stomach following ingestion of sulfite-containing foods or beverages..." Lester MR. Sulfite sensitivity: significance in human health. *J Am Coll Nutr*. 1995 Jun;14(3):229-32

PERSPECTIVES

Mitochondrial Medicine Arrives to Prime Time in Clinical Care: Nutritional Biochemistry and Mitochondrial Hyperpermeability ("Leaky Mitochondria") Meet Disease Pathogenesis and Clinical Interventions

Alex Vasquez, DC, ND, DO, FACN

Alex Vasquez, DC, ND, DO, FACN, is director of programs at the International College of Human Nutrition and Functional Medicine in Barcelona, Spain and online at ICHNFM.org. (*Altern Ther Health Med.* 2014;20(suppl 1):26-30.)

Corresponding author: Alex Vasquez, DC, ND, DO, FACN
E-mail address: ichnfm@gmail.com

MITOCHONDRIAL MEDICINE ARRIVES TO GENERAL PRACTICE AND ROUTINE PATIENT CARE

Mitochondrial disorders were once relegated to "orphan" status as topics for small paragraphs in pathology textbooks and the hospital-based practices of subspecialists. With the increasing appreciation of the high frequency and ease of treatment of mitochondrial dysfunction, this common cause and consequence of many conditions seen in both primary and specialty care deserves the attention of all practicing clinicians.

We all know that mitochondria are the intracellular organelles responsible for the production of the currency of cellular energy in the form of the molecule adenosine triphosphate (ATP); by this time, contemporary clinicians should be developing an awareness of the other roles that mitochondria play in (patho)physiology and clinical practice. Beyond being simple organelles that make ATP, mitochondria play clinically significant roles in autoimmunity, inflammation, cancer, insulin resistance, cardiometabolic disease such as hypertension and heart failure, and neurologic disorders such as Alzheimer's and Parkinson's diseases. As I stated during the recent International Conference on Human Nutrition and Functional Medicine[1] in Portland, Oregon, in September 2013, we have collectively arrived at a time when mitochondrial therapeutics and the contribution of mitochondrial dysfunction to clinical diseases must be considered on a routine basis in clinical practice. *Mitochondrial medicine* is no longer an orphan topic, nor is it a superfluous consideration relegated to boutique practices. Mitochondrial medicine is ready for prime time—now—both in the general practice of primary care as well as in specialty and subspecialty medicine. What I describe here as the "new" mitochondrial medicine is the application of assessments and treatments to routine clinical practice primarily for the treatment of secondary/acquired forms of mitochondrial impairment that contribute to common conditions such as fatigue, depression, fibromyalgia, diabetes mellitus, hypertension, neuropsychiatric and neurodegenerative conditions, and other inflammatory and dysmetabolic conditions such as allergy and autoimmunity.

BEYOND BIOCHEMISTRY

Structure and function are of course intimately related and must be appreciated before clinical implications can be understood and interventions thereafter applied with practical precision. The 4 main structures and spaces of the mitochondria are (1) intramitochondrial matrix—the innermost/interior aspect of the mitochondria containing various proteins, enzymes of the Krebs cycle, and mitochondrial DNA; (2) inner membrane—the largely impermeable lipid-rich convoluted/invaginated membrane that envelopes and defines the matrix and which is the structural home of many enzymes, transport systems, and important structures such as cardiolipin and the electron transport chain (ETC); (3) intermembrane space—contains noteworthy molecules: creatine-phosphokinase and cytochrome c; and (4) outer membrane—comparatively more permeable (to molecules <10 000 Dalton) and—like the inner membrane—very lipid-rich and with active and passive transport systems for select molecules that need to enter and exit the mitochondria. Clinicians need to appreciate that mitochondrial membrane integrity is of the highest importance; just as we have come to appreciate the

❺ Stress, Sleep, Style of Living, and Everything Else that Starts with the Letter "S": Social and pSychological Influences, Self-Esteem, Spinal Health, Specialized Supplementation, Surgery

Major Concepts in this Section
Originally this section started with stress modulation/reduction/master and sleep optimization/deprivation, and it has since expanded to include additional considerations, as described below.

- Style of living—lifestyle: Includes the considerations below, as well as one's general approach to thinking, problem-solving, and living. Lifestyle is of course powerfully and inextricably connected with culture and thus geography.
- Stress: Eustress is generally considered beneficial; but eventually even eustress can be detrimental if prolonged without respit. Dys-stress or distress impairs would healing, promotes nutrient loss, and promotes microbial pathogenicity via what is generally described as "microbial endocrinology."
- Sleep: Sleep deprivation/inrerruption promotes immune dysregulation and a pro-inflammatory response.
- Social influences: Social influences on inflammatory and immune status are mediated via food, social connection (eg, Spain) vs isolation (eg, United States), xenobiotic pollution, and the level of sociopolitical chaos to which one is exposed.
- pSychology: One's mental outlook, self-perception, and psychoepistimology, etc.
- Self-esteem: Brilliantly articulated by Dr Nathaniel Branden to include the following: ❶ Living Consciously, ❷ Self-Acceptance, ❸ Self-Responsibility, ❹ Self-Assertiveness, ❺ Living Purposefully, ❻ Personal Integrity.
- Spinal health: Spinal manipulative therapy is remarkably effective for certain health problems, for which no pharmaceutical/nutritional/botanical treatment is equally effective.
- Specialized supplementation: Atop the nutritional considerations discussed in this text, patients often benefit from additional custom-tailored supraphysiologic supplementation, such as pyridoxine 250-500mg/d for the treatment of premenstrual problems, edema, and excess glutaminergic neurotransmission.
- Surgery: Surgery is an important treatment consideration not simply for trauma and the removal of strucrual and gross pathologies, but also for functional problems such as migraine headaches associated with patent foramen ovale.
- Sweat: Metaphor for daily exercise and exertion (not simply activity).
- Stamp your passport: Conscious and periodic implementation of "geographic cure" is reasonable, and is a great way to renew, recharge, and see amazing things in the world that are inspiring for our lives.

Recreation is Re-creation
• "Truth, however, must meet with opposition and be able to fight, and we must be able to rest from it at times in falsehood otherwise truth will grow tiresome, powerless, and insipid, and will render us equally so." *Friedrich Nietzsche* • "Take a break from the work before the work breaks you." *Hernando Vasquez* • "I should mention that a purposeful, self-disciplined life does not mean a life without time or space for rest, relaxation, recreation, random or even frivolous activity. It merely means that such activities are chosen consciously, with the knowledge that it is safe and appropriate to engage in them. And in any event, the temporary abandonment of purpose also serves a purpose, whether consciously intended or not: that of regeneration." *Nathaniel Branden*

❶ Food ❷ Infections ❸ Nutri-immunomod ❹ Dys mito ❺ Stress/Sleep/Socio/Surg/Sup ❻ <u>Endo</u> ❼ Xeno

❻ Endocrine Imbalances:
Hormonal Evaluations and Interventions:
Anti-inflammatory Orthoendocrinology

Major Concepts in this Section

Hormones affect and are affected by inflammatory status. In this section, I will focus on the seven hormones of greatest signicance to inflammatory homeodynamics. Readers should mentally organize this information in the following way:

❶ <u>Hormones that are commonly **elevated** and **need to be reduced** in inflammatory states</u>:
    1.   Prolactin
    2.   Insulin
    3.   Estrogen
❷ <u>Hormones that are commonly **reduced** and **need to be elevated** in inflammatory states</u>:
    4.   Cortisol
    5.   DHEA
    6.   Testosterone
❸ <u>Thyroid status is considered separately</u>: See Chapter 1 for discussion of a novel way (contrasted to the standard allopathic viewpoint) of assessing and treating hypothyroidism in general and functional/peripheral/metabolic hypothyroidism in particular. Thyroid status is less potent as an influence on inflammatory balance when compared to the 6 other hormones listed above; however, occasionally a patient will have severe musculoskeletal inflammation (eg, bilateral adhesive capsulitis, oligoarthritis, proximal myopathy[823]) responsive solely to thyroid hormone monotherapy.

<u>*Introduction*</u>: Steroidal and peptide hormones have significant immunomodulating properties, and a characteristic pattern of disruption is commonly seen in patients with autoimmunity. Relatively simple natural and/or pharmacologic interventions can be used to safely and effectively correct hormonal disturbances with the dual benefits of improved overall health and the amelioration of autoimmunity. I have coined the term "orthoendocrinology"[824] to describe this technique of addressing numerous disturbances in endocrine function by using the "right hormones" based on a similar conceptual model to Linus Pauling's suggestion that health might be optimized by the use of the "right molecules" (orthomolecular medicine, orthomolecular nutrition) rather than endless reliance on the cyclical prescriptions of what he called "toximolecular" substances. I will keep this overview and application straightforward, simple, and clinically relevant.

> **Hormones affect inflammation**
>
> "The altered hormonal status could result in relative immunological hyperactivity contributing to enhance tissue damage and disease severity."
>
> Mirone, Barini, Barini. Androgen and prolactin levels in systemic sclerosis: relationship to disease severity. *Ann N Y Acad Sci* 2006

<u>The typical hormonal pattern (partial is more common than complete) that is seen in patients with systemic autoimmunity is described here</u>:

- High prolactin
- High insulin
- High estrogen

- Low cortisol
- Low DHEA
- Low testosterone

<u>Additional considerations</u>:
- <u>Growth hormone</u>: Variable and apparently less important; can be assessed per patient.

---

[823] Bowman CA, et al. Bilateral adhesive capsulitis, oligoarthritis and proximal myopathy as presentation of hypothyroidism. *Br J Rheumatol*. 1988 Feb;27(1):62-4
[824] As of November 15, 2005 the word "orthoendocrinology" cannot be found either on Pubmed/Medline or Internet search using Google, Yahoo, or MSN search engines.

- Progesterone: Variable and apparently less important; can be assessed per patient.
- Pregnenolone: Less potent with regard to inflammation than are prolactin, estrogen, cortisol, DHEA, and testosterone; can be measured by laboratory and treated per patient need. Earlier studies showed antinflammatory benefit with supplementation.
- Thyroid: Hypothyroidism and/or thyroid autoimmunity; see Chapter 1 for a few considerations and case reports.

Testing and treatment hormonal status in patients with autoimmunity: Patients with autoimmune disorders commonly have deficiencies and imbalances in their hormones, particularly steroid and "sex" hormones, which are potent immunomodulators. The classic pattern which may be expressed incompletely in an individual patient, is that of excess prolactin and estrogen, and insufficient cortisol, testosterone, and DHEA. The role of progesterone seems less clear, with some patients showing normal, excess, or insufficient amounts; obviously, this can be tested in an individual patient (random serum test in men or 21st-day/midluteal serum sample from a premenopausal woman). All testing methods—via serum, saliva, or urine—have their individual advantages and disadvantages. Generally however, serum is considered the standard; following this I prefer polyhormonal assessment with 24-hour urine collections, and the last resort is saliva testing, which is the most controversial and least reliable. Thyroid autoimmunity and hypothyroidism are both common in autoimmune/inflammatory patients; comprehensive thyroid assessment with TSH, T4, and anti-TPO antibodies can be justified in nearly any rheumatic patient.

- **Hyperprolactinemia and latent hyperprolactinemia**: Besides its obvious role in lactation, prolactin is a polyfunctional hormone that, at the very least, stimulates the liver to produce excess sex-hormone-binding globulin (SHBG) which adsorbs sex hormones, rendering them less effective due to reduced bioavailability; the resultant *functional hypogonadism* deprives the immune system of the modulation/suppression normally effected by these hormones. Beyond these well-known physiologic roles, **prolactin is now known to be powerfully proinflammatory.**[825] **Patients with RA and SLE have higher basal and stress-induced levels of prolactin compared with normal controls.**[826,827] **Patients with scleroderma have relatively high prolactin**[828] **and low DHEA.**[829] **Patients with polymyalgia rheumatica have elevated prolactin that correlates with increased symptomatology.**[830] Elevated prolactin levels may further exacerbate immune dysfunction by increasing hepatic production of sex-hormone binding globulin and reducing bioavailability of testosterone, thus depriving cells and tissues of testosterone's potent anti-inflammatory and immunoregulatory properties. Prolactin is routinely measured in serum; high values should be reduced with effective treatment, whether nutritional, botanical, or pharmacologic.

  > **Prolactin is pro-inflammatory, and anti-prolactin interventions provide an anti-inflammatory benefit**
  >
  > "Multiple lines of evidence support the concept that the anterior pituitary hormone **prolactin** has a pathogenic role in rheumatic and autoimmune diseases including, but not limited to, rheumatoid arthritis (RA), systemic lupus erythematosus (SLE), Reiter's syndrome, psoriatic arthritis, and uveitis."
  >
  > McMurray RW. *Semin Arthritis* Rheum. 2001

  - Thyroid hormone: **Hypothyroidism frequently causes hyperprolactinemia** that is reversible upon effective treatment of hypothyroidism. Conversely, due to its immunodysregulating

[825] "Multiple lines of evidence support the concept that the anterior pituitary hormone prolactin has a pathogenic role in rheumatic and autoimmune diseases including, but not limited to, rheumatoid arthritis (RA), systemic lupus erythematosus (SLE), Reiter's syndrome, psoriatic arthritis, and uveitis." McMurray RW. Bromocriptine in rheumatic and autoimmune diseases. *Semin Arthritis Rheum*. 2001 Aug;31(1):21-32

[826] Dostal C, Moszkorzova L, Musilova L, Lacinova Z, Marek J, Zvarova J. Serum prolactin stress values in patients with systemic lupus erythematosus. *Ann Rheum Dis*. 2003 May;62(5):487-8 http://ard.bmjjournals.com/cgi/content/full/62/5/487

[827] "RESULTS: A significantly higher rate of elevated PRL levels was found in SLE patients (40.0%) compared with the healthy controls (14.8%). No proof was found of association with the presence of anti-ds-DNA or with specific organ involvement. Similarly, elevated PRL levels were found in RA patients (39.3%)." Moszkorzova L, Lacinova Z, Marek J, Musilova L, Dohnalova A, Dostal C. Hyperprolactinaemia in patients with systemic lupus erythematosus. *Clin Exp Rheumatol*. 2002 Nov-Dec;20(6):807-12

[828] Straub RH, Zeuner M, Lock G, Scholmerich J, Lang B. High prolactin and low dehydroepiandrosterone sulphate serum levels in patients with severe systemic sclerosis. *Br J Rheumatol*. 1997 Apr;36(4):426-32 http://rheumatology.oxfordjournals.org/cgi/reprint/36/4/426

[829] "CONCLUSION: Our data show that, as in other autoimmune diseases, low serum DHEAS is a feature of premenopausal SSc patients. More extensive prospective studies are needed to define the exact role of DHEAS dysregulation in SSc." La Montagna G, Baruffo A, Buono G, Valentini G. Dehydroepiandrosterone sulphate serum levels in systemic sclerosis. *Clin Exp Rheumatol*. 2001 Jan-Feb;19(1):21-6

[830] Straub RH, Georgi J, Helmke K, Vaith P, Lang B. In polymyalgia rheumatica serum prolactin is positively correlated with the number of typical symptoms but not with typical inflammatory markers. *Rheumatology* (Oxford). 2002 Apr;41(4):423-9 http://rheumatology.oxfordjournals.org/cgi/content/full/41/4/423

effects, elevated prolactin appears capable of inducing hypothyroidism and autoimmune thyroiditis.[831] Assessing hyperprolactinemic patients for thyroid disturbances with TSH, T4, T3, and anti-TPO antibodies is strongly advised. Thyroid status should be evaluated in all patients with hyperprolactinemia.

- o <u>High-dose pyridoxine</u>: B6 (250 mg qd-bid with food) is used by some doctors to lower prolactin despite the lack of consistently demonstrated benefit in the research literature.
- o <u>*Vitex astus-cagnus* and other supporting botanicals and nutrients</u>: **Vitex lowers serum prolactin in humans**[832,833] **via a dopaminergic effect.**[834] Vitex is considered safe for clinical use; mild and reversible adverse effects possibly associated with Vitex include nausea, headache, gastrointestinal disturbances, menstrual disorders, acne, pruritus and erythematous rash. No drug interactions are known, but given the herb's dopaminergic effect it should probably be used with some caution in patients treated with dopamine antagonists such as the so-called antipsychotic drugs (most of which do not work very well and/or carry intolerable adverse effects[835,836]). In a recent review, Bone[837] stated that daily doses can range from 500 mg to 2,000 mg DHE (dry herb equivalent) and can be tailored to the suppression of prolactin. Due at least in part to its content of L-dopa, ***Mucuna pruriens* shows clinical dopaminergic activity** as evidenced by its effectiveness in Parkinson's disease[838]; up to 15-30 gm/d of mucuna has been used clinically but doses will be dependent on preparation and phytoconcentration. Triptolide and other **extracts from *Tripterygium wilfordii* Hook F** exert clinically significant anti-inflammatory action in patients with rheumatoid arthritis[839,840] and also offer protection to dopaminergic neurons.[841,842] Ironically, even though tyrosine is the nutritional precursor to dopamine with evidence of clinical effectiveness (e.g., narcolepsy[843], enhancement of

[831] "...PRL level is higher in SLE patients and that in the presence of hyperPRL there is increased prevalence of antithyroid antibodies, evidencing the association of PRL and autoimmunity and pointing to the appropriateness of assessing and monitoring the progress of these markers in patients affected by these disorders." Kramer CK, Tourinho TF, de Castro WP, da Costa Oliveira M. Association between systemic lupus erythematosus, rheumatoid arthritis, hyperprolactinemia and thyroid autoantibodies. *Arch Med Res.* 2005 Jan-Feb;36(1):54-8

[832] "Since AC extracts were shown to have beneficial effects on premenstrual mastodynia serum prolactin levels in such patients were also studied in one double-blind, placebo-controlled clinical study. Serum prolactin levels were indeed reduced in the patients treated with the extract." Wuttke W, Jarry H, Christoffel V, Spengler B, Seidlova-Wuttke D. Chaste tree (Vitex agnus-castus)--pharmacology and clinical indications. *Phytomedicine.* 2003 May;10(4):348-57

[833] German abstract from Medline: "The prolactin release was reduced after 3 months, shortened luteal phases were normalised and deficits in the luteal progesterone synthesis were eliminated." Milewicz A, Gejdel E, Sworen H, Sienkiewicz K, Jedrzejak J, Teucher T, Schmitz H. [Vitex agnus castus extract in the treatment of luteal phase defects due to latent hyperprolactinemia. Results of a randomized placebo-controlled double-blind study] *Arzneimittelforschung.* 1993 Jul;43(7):752-6

[834] "Our results indicate a dopaminergic effect of Vitex agnus-castus extracts and suggest additional pharmacological actions via opioid receptors." Meier B, Berger D, Hoberg E, Sticher O, Schaffner W. Pharmacological activities of Vitex agnus-castus extracts in vitro. *Phytomedicine.* 2000 Oct;7(5):373-81

[835] "The majority of patients in each group discontinued their assigned treatment owing to inefficacy or intolerable side effects or for other reasons." Lieberman JA, Stroup TS, McEvoy JP, Swartz MS, Rosenheck RA, Perkins DO, Keefe RS, Davis SM, Davis CE, Lebowitz BD, Severe J, Hsiao JK; Clinical Antipsychotic Trials of Intervention Effectiveness (CATIE) Investigators. Effectiveness of antipsychotic drugs in patients with chronic schizophrenia. *N Engl J Med.* 2005 Sep 22;353(12):1209-23

[836] Whitaker R. The case against antipsychotic drugs: a 50-year record of doing more harm than good. *Med Hypotheses.* 2004;62(1):5-13

[837] "In conditions such as endometriosis and fibroids, for which a significant estrogen antagonist effect is needed, doses of at least 2 g/day DHE may be required and typically are used by professional herbalists." Bone K. New Insights into Chaste Tree. *Nutritional Wellness* 2005 November http://www.nutritionalwellness.com/archives/2005/nov/11_bone.php

[838] "CONCLUSIONS: The rapid onset of action and longer on time without concomitant increase in dyskinesias on mucuna seed powder formulation suggest that this natural source of L-dopa might possess advantages over conventional L-dopa preparations in the long term management of PD." Katzenschlager R, Evans A, Manson A, Patsalos PN, Ratnaraj N, Watt H, Timmermann L, Van der Giessen R, Lees AJ. Mucuna pruriens in Parkinson's disease: a double blind clinical and pharmacological study. *J Neurol Neurosurg Psychiatry.* 2004 Dec;75(12):1672-7

[839] "The ethanol/ethyl acetate extract of TWHF shows therapeutic benefit in patients with treatment-refractory RA. At therapeutic dosages, the TWHF extract was well tolerated by most patients in this study." Tao X, Younger J, Fan FZ, Wang B, Lipsky PE. Benefit of an extract of Tripterygium Wilfordii Hook F in patients with rheumatoid arthritis: a double-blind, placebo-controlled study. *Arthritis Rheum.* 2002 Jul;46(7):1735-43

[840] "CONCLUSION: The EA extract of TWHF at dosages up to 570 mg/day appeared to be safe, and doses > 360 mg/day were associated with clinical benefit in patients with RA." Tao X, Cush JJ, Garret M, Lipsky PE. A phase I study of ethyl acetate extract of the Chinese antirheumatic herb Tripterygium wilfordii hook F in rheumatoid arthritis. *J Rheumatol.* 2001 Oct;28(10):2160-7

[841] "Our data suggests that triptolide may protect dopaminergic neurons from LPS-induced injury and its efficiency in inhibiting microglia activation may underlie the mechanism." Li FQ, Lu XZ, Liang XB, Zhou HF, Xue B, Liu XY, Niu DB, Han JS, Wang XM. Triptolide, a Chinese herbal extract, protects dopaminergic neurons from inflammation-mediated damage through inhibition of microglial activation. *J Neuroimmunol.* 2004 Mar;148(1-2):24-31

[842] "Moreover, tripchlorolide markedly prevented the decrease in amount of dopamine in the striatum of model rats. Taken together, our data provide the first evidence that tripchlorolide acts as a neuroprotective molecule that rescues MPP+ or axotomy-induced degeneration of dopaminergic neurons, which may imply its therapeutic potential for Parkinson's disease." Li FQ, Cheng XX, Liang XB, Wang XH, Xue B, He QH, Wang XM, Han JS. Neurotrophic and neuroprotective effects of tripchlorolide, an extract of Chinese herb Tripterygium wilfordii Hook F, on dopaminergic neurons. *Exp Neurol.* 2003 Jan;179(1):28-37

[843] "Of twenty-eight visual analogue scales rating mood and arousal, the subjects' ratings in the tyrosine treatment (9 g daily) and placebo periods differed significantly for only three (less tired, less drowsy, more alert)." Elwes RD, Crewes H, Chesterman LP, Summers B, Jenner P, Binnie CD, Parkes JD. Treatment of narcolepsy with L-tyrosine: double-blind placebo-controlled trial. *Lancet.* 1989 Nov 4;2(8671):1067-9

memory[844] and cognition[845]), **supplementation with tyrosine appears to actually increase rather than decrease prolactin levels[846]; therefore tyrosine should be used cautiously if at all in patients with systemic inflammation.** Furthermore, the finding that **high-protein meals stimulate prolactin release[847]** may partly explain the benefits of vegetarian diets in the treatment of systemic inflammation; since vegetarian diets are comparatively low in protein compared to omnivorous diets, they may lead to a relative reduction in prolactin production due to lack of stimulation.

- o Bromocriptine: Bromocriptine has long been considered the pharmacologic treatment of choice for elevated prolactin.[848] Typical dose is 2.5 mg per day (effective against lupus[849]); gastrointestinal upset and sedation are common.[850] **Clinical intervention with bromocriptine appears warranted in patients with RA, SLE, Reiter's syndrome, psoriatic arthritis, and probably multiple sclerosis and uveitis.[851]**

- o Cabergoline/Dostinex: Cabergoline/Dostinex is a newer dopamine agonist with few adverse effects; typical dose starts at 0.5 mg per week (0.25 mg twice per week).[852] Several studies have indicated that cabergoline is safer and more effective than bromocriptine for reducing prolactin levels[853] and the dose can often be reduced after successful prolactin reduction, allowing for reductions in cost and adverse effects.[854] Although fewer studies have been published supporting the antirheumatic benefits of cabergoline than bromocriptine, the scientific rationale for its use is derived from the success of bromocriptine in various rheumatic/autoimmune diseases. Erb et al[855] published a case report of a woman with unremitting rheumatoid arthritis who achieved remarkable clinical improvement and who was able to reduce her need for other antirheumatic drugs with the use of cabergoline 0.5 mg per day.

- **Insulin, hyperinsulinemia:** As a marker for insulin resistance and perhaps xenobiotic exposure, fasting serum insulin is a surrogate marker for an inflammatory state. A challenge exists in determining the accurate pro- or anti-inflammatory effect of insulin itself, because the net effect of the hormone *in vivo* is inflammation-lowering via glucose-lowering. Although major medical labs such as LabCorp (website reviewed January 2014) use a reference range of 2.6-24.9 µIU/mL, such a range is clinically ridiculous except for screening for overt pathology and should be replaced with the following:

  - o **Healthy** fasting serum insulin: <5 µIU/mL
  - o **Mild-moderate insulin resistance** fasting serum insulin: 5-15 µIU/mL
  - o **Marked-severe insulin resistance** fasting fasting serum insulin: 15 µIU/mL

---

[844] "Ten men and 10 women subjects underwent these batteries 1 h after ingesting 150 mg/kg of l-tyrosine or placebo. Administration of tyrosine significantly enhanced accuracy and decreased frequency of list retrieval on the working memory task during the multiple task battery compared with placebo." Thomas JR, Lockwood PA, Singh A, Deuster PA. Tyrosine improves working memory in a multitasking environment. *Pharmacol Biochem Behav.* 1999 Nov;64(3):495-500

[845] "Ten subjects received five daily doses of a protein-rich drink containing 2 g tyrosine, and 11 subjects received a carbohydrate rich drink with the same amount of calories (255 kcal)." Deijen JB, Wientjes CJ, Vullinghs HF, Cloin PA, Langefeld JJ. Tyrosine improves cognitive performance and reduces blood pressure in cadets after one week of a combat training course. *Brain Res Bull.* 1999 Jan 15;48(2):203-9

[846] "Tyrosine (when compared to placebo) had no effect on any sleep related measure, but it did stimulate prolactin release." Waters WF, et al. A comparison of tyrosine against placebo, phentermine, caffeine, and D-amphetamine during sleep deprivation. *Nutr Neurosci.* 2003;6(4):221-35

[847] "Whereas carbohydrate meals had no discernible effects, high protein meals induced a large increase in both PRL and cortisol; high fat meals caused selective release of PRL."Ishizuka, et al. Pituitary hormone release in response to food ingestion. *J Clin Endocrinol Metab* 1983Dec;57:1111-6

[848] Beers MH, Berkow R (eds). The Merck Manual. Seventeenth Edition. Whitehouse Station; Merck Research Laboratories 1999 Page 77-78

[849] "A prospective, double-blind, randomized, placebo-controlled study compared BRC at a fixed daily dosage of 2.5 mg with placebo... Long term treatment with a low dose of BRC appears to be a safe and effective means of decreasing SLE flares in SLE patients." Alvarez-Nemegyei J, Cobarrubias-Cobos A, Escalante-Triay F, Sosa-Munoz J, Miranda JM, Jara LJ. Bromocriptine in systemic lupus erythematosus: a double-blind, randomized, placebo-controlled study. *Lupus.* 1998;7(6):414-9

[850] Serri O, Chik CL, Ur E, Ezzat S. Diagnosis and management of hyperprolactinemia. *CMAJ.* 2003 Sep 16;169(6):575-81 http://www.cmaj.ca/cgi/content/full/169/6/575

[851] "...clinical observations and trials support the use of bromocriptine as a nonstandard primary or adjunctive therapy in the treatment of recalcitrant RA, SLE, Reiter's syndrome, and psoriatic arthritis and associated conditions unresponsive to traditional approaches." McMurray RW. Bromocriptine in rheumatic and autoimmune diseases. *Semin Arthritis Rheum.* 2001 Aug;31(1):21-32

[852] Serri O, Chik CL, Ur E, Ezzat S. Diagnosis and management of hyperprolactinemia. *CMAJ.* 2003 Sep 16;169(6):575-81 http://www.cmaj.ca/cgi/content/full/169/6/575

[853] "CONCLUSION: These data indicate that cabergoline is a very effective agent for lowering the prolactin levels in hyperprolactinemic patients and that it appears to offer considerable advantage over bromocriptine in terms of efficacy and tolerability." Sabuncu T, Arikan E, Tasan E, Hatemi H. Comparison of the effects of cabergoline and bromocriptine on prolactin levels in hyperprolactinemic patients. *Intern Med.* 2001 Sep;40(9):857-61

[854] "Cabergoline also normalized PRL in the majority of patients with known bromocriptine intolerance or -resistance. Once PRL secretion was adequately controlled, the dose of cabergoline could often be significantly decreased, which further reduced costs of therapy." Verhelst J, Abs R, Maiter D, van den Bruel A, Vandeweghe M, Velkeniers B, Mockel J, Lamberigts G, Petrossians P, Coremans P, Mahler C, Stevenaert A, Verlooy J, Raftopoulos C, Beckers A. Cabergoline in the treatment of hyperprolactinemia: a study in 455 patients. *J Clin Endocrinol Metab.* 1999 Jul;84(7):2518-22 http://jcem.endojournals.org/cgi/content/full/84/7/2518

[855] Erb N, Pace AV, Delamere JP, Kitas GD. Control of unremitting rheumatoid arthritis by the prolactin antagonist cabergoline. *Rheumatology* (Oxford). 2001 Feb;40(2):237-9 http://rheumatology.oxfordjournals.org/cgi/content/full/40/2/237

The goal when considering serum insulin within the context of alleviating inflammation is not to lower serum insulin per se, but rather to alleviate the causative insulin resistance. Stated perhaps more plainly, an elevation in fasting serum insulin is indicative of insulin resistance (except in the exceedingly rare case of insulinoma or exogenous insulin administration which can be distinguished by concomitant measurement of C-peptide) which is itself a proinflammatory state; thus, our goal is to reduce fasting serum insulin not because we are targeting insulin per se but rather because we are measuring serum insulin as a marker for insulin resistance and thus a particular type of *metabolic inflammation*. First-line therapy for insulin resistance is carbohydrate restriction via plant-based low-carohydrate Paleo diet, exercise and physical activity >60 minutes/day, vitamin and mineral supplementation, especially vitamin D3, chromium, magnesium, CoQ-10, and mixed tocopherols.

- **Estrogen:** Nearly all autoimmune disorders are more common in females than males, suggesting a possible immunodysregulation by estrogen. Despite the complex and multifaceted nature of the endocrine system, we may safely generalize that the estrogens are immunostimulatory and immunodysregulatory while androgens are immunosuppressive and immunoregulatory[856]; thus, elevated estrogen:androgen ratios promote/exacerbate autoimmunity. Furthermore, many chemical/pollutant xenobiotics have estrogen-like effects ("xenoestrogens") and are consistently associated with induction or exacerbation of autoimmunity. So-called **"estrogen-replacement therapy" used in postmenopausal women increases the risk for lupus and scleroderma.**[857] **Men with rheumatoid arthritis show an excess of estradiol** and a decrease in DHEA, and the **excess estrogen is proportional to the degree of inflammation.**[858] Estrogen(s) can be measured in serum and/or 24-hour urine samples. Beyond looking at estrogens from a *quantitative* standpoint, they can also be *qualitatively* analyzed with respect to the ratio of estrone:estradiol:estriol as well as the balance between the "good" 2-hydroxyestrone relative to the purportedly carcinogenic and proinflammatory 16-alpha-hydroxyestrone. Interventions to lower estrogen levels can include the following:

> **Estrogen is pro-inflammatory, and anti-estrogen interventions provide an anti-inflammatory benefit**
>
> "Using **antiestrogen** medication [tamoxifen or **anastrozole**] in women with dermatomyositis may result in a significant improvement in their rash, possibly via the inhibition of TNF-alpha production by immune or other cells."
>
> Sereda and Werth. *Arch Dermatol.* 2006

  - Weight loss and weight optimization: Excess adiposity and obesity raise estrogen levels due to high levels of aromatase (the hormone that makes estrogens from androgens) in adipose tissue; weight optimization and loss of excess fat helps normalize hormone levels and reduce inflammation. In overweight patients, *weight loss* is the means to attaining the goal of *weight optimization*; the task is not complete until the body mass index is normalized/optimized.
  - Avoidance of ethanol: Ethanol stimulates estrogen production, particularly in men.
  - Surgical correction of varicocele in affected men: Men with varicocele have higher estrogen levels due to temperature-induced alterations in enzyme function in the testes; surgical correction of the varicocele lowers estrogen levels.
  - "Anti-estrogen diet": Foods and supplements such as green tea, diindolylmethane (DIM), indole-3-carbinol (I3C), licorice, and a high-fiber crucifer-based "anti-estrogenic diet" can also be used; monitoring clinical status and serum estradiol will prove or disprove efficacy. Whereas **16-alpha-hydroxyestrone is pro-inflammatory and immunodysregulatory, 2-**

---

[856] "In general, androgens seem to inhibit immune activity, while oestrogen seems to have a more powerful effect on immune cells and to stimulate immune activity." Tanriverdi F, Silveira LF, MacColl GS, Bouloux PM. The hypothalamic-pituitary-gonadal axis: immune function and autoimmunity. *J Endocrinol.* 2003 Mar;176(3):293-304 http://joe.endocrinology-journals.org/cgi/content/abstract/176/3/293

[857] "These studies indicate that estrogen replacement therapy in postmenopausal women increases the risk of developing lupus, scleroderma, and Raynaud disease..." Mayes MD. Epidemiologic studies of environmental agents and systemic autoimmune diseases. *Environ Health Perspect.* 1999 Oct;107 Suppl 5:743-8

[858] "RESULTS: DHEAS and estrone concentrations were lower and estradiol was higher in patients compared with healthy controls. DHEAS differed between RF positive and RF negative patients. Estrone did not correlate with any disease variable, whereas estradiol correlated strongly and positively with all measured indices of inflammation." Tengstrand B, Carlstrom K, Fellander-Tsai L, Hafstrom I. Abnormal levels of serum dehydroepiandrosterone, estrone, and estradiol in men with rheumatoid arthritis: high correlation between serum estradiol and current degree of inflammation. *J Rheumatol.* 2003 Nov;30(11):2338-43

hydroxyestrone has anti-inflammatory action[859] and has been described as "the good estrogen"[860] due to its anticancer and comparatively health-preserving qualities. **In a recent short-term study using I3C in patients with SLE, I3C supplementation at 375 mg per day was well tolerated and resulted in modest treatment-dependent clinical improvement as well as favorable modification of estrogen metabolism away from 16-alpha-hydroxyestrone and toward 2-hydroxyestrone.[861]**

- o <u>Pharmacologic aromatase inhibition</u>: In our office, we commonly measure serum estradiol in men and administer the aromatase inhibitor anastrozole/Arimidex 1 mg (≥2-3 doses per week) to men whose estradiol level is greater than 32 picogram/mL. The Life Extension Foundation[862] advocates that the optimal serum estradiol level for a man is 10-30 picogram/mL. Clinical studies using anastrozole/arimidex in men have shown that aromatase blockade lowers estradiol and raises testosterone[863]; generally speaking, this is exactly the result that we want in patients with severe systemic autoimmunity. Whether using anastrozole/Arimidex, frequency of dosing is based on serum and clinical response. Letrozole/Femara is a newer pharmacologic aromatase inhibitor which appears to have slight superiority over anastrozole in terms of anti-estrogen efficacy; however, I am quite convinced that letrozole/Femara is also an androgen receptor agonist and therefore I generally avoid this drug like the plague. Relatedly, the botanical *Rhodiola rosea* can elevate testosterone and estradiol, making the latter particularly difficult to control. On occasion, we have seen some men make so much testosterone→estradiol that they require both anastrozole/Arimidex *and* letrozole/Femara along with licorice daily in order to control their testosterone and estradiol levels. Licorice lowers testosterone and thus the precursor to estradiol in both men and women within about four days of oral administration, whether by standardized capsules or by tea from the root. Of course, anastrozole/Arimidex can be administered to women in 1 mg doses ranging from once per week to 5-7 times per week depending on clinical and serologic response. **In two recent case reports, administration of anti-estrogen medication—either tamoxifen or anastrozole—resulted in clinical improvements in two women with dermatomyositis.[864]**

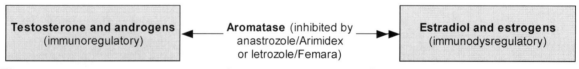

<u>The aromatase enzyme converts androgens to estrogens</u>: If estrogens are high and androgens are low, then estrogens can be lowered and androgens raised via inhibition of aromatase. If androgens are low and estrogens are low, then administration of androgens will raise both the androgens and the estrogens, possibly necessitating the coadministration of an aromatase inhibitor.

- **<u>Testosterone:</u>** Androgen deficiencies predispose to, are exacerbated by, and contribute to autoimmune/inflammatory disorders. **A large proportion of men with lupus or RA have low testosterone[865]** and suffer the effects of hypogonadism: fatigue, weakness, depression, slow healing, low libido, and difficulties with sexual performance. Particularly in men, blood samples should be

---

[859] "Micromolar concentrations of beta-estradiol, estrone, 16-alpha-hydroxyestrone and estriol enhance the oxidative metabolism of activated human PMNL's. The corresponding 2-hydroxylated estrogens 2-OH-estradiol, 2-OH-estrone and 2-OH-estriol act on the contrary as powerful inhibitors of cell activity." Jansson G. Oestrogen-induced enhancement of myeloperoxidase activity in human polymorphonuclear leukocytes--a possible cause of oxidative stress in inflammatory cells. *Free Radic Res Commun*. 1991;14(3):195-208

[860] "Even more dramatically, in the case of laryngeal papillomas induction of 2-hydroxylation with indole-3-carbinol (I3C) has resulted in inhibition of tumor growth during the time that the patients continue to take I3C or vegetables rich in this compound." Bradlow HL, Telang NT, Sepkovic DW, Osborne MP. 2-hydroxyestrone: the 'good' estrogen. *J Endocrinol*. 1996 Sep;150 Suppl:S259-65

[861] "Women with SLE can manifest a metabolic response to I3C and might benefit from its antiestrogenic effects." McAlindon TE, Gulin J, Chen T, Klug T, Lahita R, Nuite M. Indole-3-carbinol in women with SLE: effect on estrogen metabolism and disease activity. *Lupus*. 2001;10(11):779-83

[862] Male Hormone Modulation Therapy, Page 4 Of 7: http://www.lef.org/protocols/prtcl-130c.shtml Accessed October 30, 2005

[863] "These data demonstrate that aromatase inhibition increases serum bioavailable and total testosterone levels to the youthful normal range in older men with mild hypogonadism." Leder BZ, Rohrer JL, Rubin SD, Gallo J, Longcope C. Effects of aromatase inhibition in elderly men with low or borderline-low serum testosterone levels. *J Clin Endocrinol Metab*. 2004 Mar;89(3):1174-80 http://jcem.endojournals.org/cgi/reprint/89/3/1174

[864] "Using antiestrogen medication in women with DM may result in a significant improvement in their rash, possibly via the inhibition of TNF-alpha production by immune or other cells." Sereda D, Werth VP. Improvement in dermatomyositis rash associated with the use of antiestrogen medication. *Arch Dermatol*. 2006 Jan;142(1):70-2

[865] Karagiannis A, Harsoulis F. Gonadal dysfunction in systemic diseases. *Eur J Endocrinol*. 2005 Apr;152(4):501-13 http://www.eje-online.org/cgi/content/full/152/4/501

drawn for *free* and *total* testosterone along with serum estradiol. Since some labs accept ridiculously low levels of testosterone as "within normal limits" clinicians should not necessarily wait until the patient is pathologically hypogonadal before implementing treatment. Clinicians must appreciate the interrelationship of testosterone with estrogen in order to interpret the patient's status appropriately and implement proper treatment. Since testosterone is converted to estradiol by aromatase, a patient with low testosterone and high estradiol is properly treated with aromatase inhibition (e.g., Arimidex/anastrozole) rather than testosterone; administration of Arimidex/anastrozole to men simultaneously lowers estradiol and raises testosterone.[866] Conversely, low testosterone along with low estrogen indicates the appropriateness of testosterone replacement. The need for co-administration of testosterone and Arimidex/anastrozole is not uncommon in order to raise testosterone without leading to an iatrogenic increase in estrogen due to shunting by aromatase. Follow-up testing of testosterone and estradiol 4-8 weeks after the implementation of testosterone replacement is advised to ensure optimal hormone status and that the additional *immunoregulatory* testosterone is not being shunted into *immunodysregulatory* estradiol. Doses of Arimidex/anastrozole typically range from 1 mg administered 1-4 times per week; the drug appears to have a wide margin of safety, and doses of 10 mg per day are used in women with estrogen-responsive breast cancer. As with any modulation/administration of testosterone and estrogen, follow-up testing of hormones and serum lipids is recommended to ensure the attainment of optimal status and the avoidance of complications, such as suppression of HDL synthesis which would be expected to have adverse cardiovascular consequences. Assessing serum PSA is a prerequisite to testosterone administration in men. **Testosterone therapy improves clinical status and wellbeing in women with rheumatoid arthritis**.[867] Transdermal testosterone creams can be used with dose tailored to serum and clinical response.

- **Cortisol:** In physiologic doses cortisol is immunoregulatory and mildly yet significantly immunosuppressive ("*physiologic immunosuppression*"), while at higher doses the hormone becomes immunosuppressive ("*pharmacologic immunosuppression*") and brings additional adverse effects such as weight gain, truncal obesity, hypertension, glucose intolerance and increased susceptibility to infections—the classic manifestations of hypercortisolemia seen in Cushing's disease.[868] Insufficiencies of cortisol production contribute to the development and perpetuation of allergies, fatigue, inflammation, and autoimmunity.[869] The works of Drs. John Tintera and William Jefferies have remained important despite being ignored by most endocrinologists; Jefferies' books[870] and articles[871] are still widely available and provide concepts and clinically relevant applications. In a 1998 summary by Jefferies[872] on the etiology of rheumatoid arthritis, he reviewed evidence suggesting that subacute hypoadrenalism results in insufficiencies of cortisol and DHEA, both of which are necessary for immunomodulation and immunocompetence; insufficiencies of these hormones leaves the body

---

[866] "These data demonstrate that aromatase inhibition increases serum bioavailable and total testosterone levels to the youthful normal range in older men with mild hypogonadism. Serum estradiol levels decrease modestly but remain within the normal male range." Leder BZ, Rohrer JL, Rubin SD, Gallo J, Longcope C. Effects of aromatase inhibition in elderly men with low or borderline-low serum testosterone levels. *J Clin Endocrinol Metab.* 2004 Mar;89(3):1174-80 http://jcem.endojournals.org/cgi/content/full/89/3/1174

[867] "An improvement in ESR, Dutch health assessment questionnaire, and pain was noted. ...Testosterone may improve the general wellbeing of postmenopausal women with active rheumatoid arthritis." Booji A, Biewenga-Booji CM, Huber-Bruning O, Cornelis C, Jacobs JW, Bijlsma JW. Androgens as adjuvant treatment in postmenopausal female patients with rheumatoid arthritis. *Ann Rheum Dis.* 1996 Nov;55(11):811-5

[868] Kirk LF Jr, Hash RB, Katner HP, Jones T. Cushing's disease: clinical manifestations and diagnostic evaluation. *Am Fam Physician.* 2000 Sep 1;62(5):1119-27, 1133-4 http://www.aafp.org/afp/20000901/1119.html

[869] "Yet evidence that patients with rheumatoid arthritis improved with small, physiologic dosages of cortisol or cortisone acetate was reported over 25 years ago, and that patients with chronic allergic disorders or unexplained chronic fatigue also improved with administration of such small dosages was reported over 15 years ago..." Jefferies WM. Mild adrenocortical deficiency, chronic allergies, autoimmune disorders and the chronic fatigue syndrome: a continuation of the cortisone story. *Med Hypotheses.* 1994 Mar;42(3):183-9 http://www.thebuteykocentre.com/Irish_%20Buteykocenter_files/further_studies/med_hyp2.pdf and http://members.westnet.com.au/pkolb/med_hyp2.pdf

[870] Jefferies WMcK. Safe Uses of Cortisol. Second Edition. Springfield, CC Thomas, 1996

[871] "Yet evidence that patients with rheumatoid arthritis improved with small, physiologic dosages of cortisol or cortisone acetate was reported over 25 years ago, and that patients with chronic allergic disorders or unexplained chronic fatigue also improved with administration of such small dosages was reported over 15 years ago..." Jefferies WM. Mild adrenocortical deficiency, chronic allergies, autoimmune disorders and the chronic fatigue syndrome: a continuation of the cortisone story. *Med Hypotheses.* 1994 Mar;42(3):183-9 http://www.thebuteykocentre.com/Irish_%20Buteykocenter_files/further_studies/med_hyp2.pdf and http://members.westnet.com.au/pkolb/med_hyp2.pdf

[872] "The etiology of rheumatoid arthritis ...explained by a combination of three factors: (i) a relatively mild deficiency of cortisol, ..., (ii) a deficiency of DHEA, ...and (iii) infection by organisms such as mycoplasma,..." Jefferies WM. The etiology of rheumatoid arthritis. *Med Hypotheses.* 1998 Aug;51(2):111-4

vulnerable to chronic infections (i.e., multifocal dysbiosis, as detailed previously) and the systemic proinflammatory sequelae that result in so-called "autoimmunity." Differential diagnoses in patients with low adrenal function include congenital adrenal hypoplasia, adrenoleukodystrophy, autoimmune Addison disease, and chronic hypopituarism. A small short-term randomized crossover clinical trial published in *The Lancet* showed benefit of 5-10 mg/day of cortisol in patients with chronic fatigue syndrome.[873] Supplementation with up to 20 mg per day of cortisol/Cortef is physiologic; higher doses in the range of 40 mg per day may benefit patients, especially during times of stress, but are adrenosuppressive. My preference is to dose 10 mg first thing in the morning, then 5 mg in late morning and 5 mg in midafternoon in an attempt to replicate the diurnal variation and normal morning peak of cortisol levels. In patients with hypoadrenalism, administration of pregnenolone in doses of 10-60 mg in the morning may also be beneficial; DHEA supplementation is beneficial for patients with adrenal insufficiency.

Criteria for the diagnosis of adrenal insufficiency in children and adults

- <u>First-morning cortisol less than 8-10 mcg/dL</u>: An 8:00 am serum cortisol concentration less than 8-10 mcg/dL suggests adrenal insufficiency.
- <u>Serum cortisol less than 18 mcg/dL during illness or stress or with elevated ACTH</u>: Serum cortisol concentration less than 18 mcg/dL in a sick and stressed patient, or associated with an elevated ACTH, is highly suggestive of adrenal insufficiency.
- <u>Post-ACTH serum cortisol less than 18 mcg/dL</u>: Serum cortisol less than 18 mcg/dL obtained 30-60 minutes following ACTH injection is diagnostic of adrenal insufficiency.
- <u>Serum cortisol that fails to double within 30-60 minutes after ACTH injection</u>: This test involves three steps: 1) blood sample is taken for serum cortisol, 2) ACTH is injected, 3) blood sample for serum cortisol is taken again at 30-60 minutes. Cortisol production should double following injection of ACTH; this is a demonstration of adrenal reserve and the ability of the adrenal glands to respond to stress.
- <u>Low output of adrenal hormones measured in 24-hour urine samples</u>: This provides sufficient objective data to justify a clinical trial of cortisol replacement in patients with a suggestive clinical picture and lack of contraindications.
- <u>Proper dosing of cosyntropin/ACTH</u>: Injections of "ACTH" are generally performed with the intravenous or intramuscular injection of "Cosyntropin" which is a synthetic peptide fragment of ACTH used for adrenal stimulation. According to the review by Wilson, the **standard dose for adults is 250 mcg**. "For infants, the author suggests 50 mcg of cosyntropin (approximately 250 mg/m2)."

Jefferies WMcK. <u>Safe Uses of Cortisol. Second Edition</u>. Springfield, CC Thomas, 1996 page 39
http://www.medicinenet.com/cosyntropin-injectable/article.htm Accessed December 7, 2006
Wilson TA. Adrenal Hypoplasia. *eMedicine* http://www.emedicine.com/PED/topic45.htm Accessed November 18, 2005

- **DHEA (insufficiency and supraphysiologic supplementation):** Patients with autoimmunity should be tested for DHEA insufficiency by measurement of serum DHEA-sulfate; insufficiencies should generally be corrected except in cases of concomitant hormone-responsive cancer such as breast cancer or prostate cancer. Physiologic doses are approximately 15-25 mg for women and 25-50 mg for men. However, many patients with autoimmunity will respond favorably to supraphysiologic doses in the range of 200 mg per day. The rationale for using high-dose DHEA in patients with autoimmune diseases is supported by the following:
  1. DHEA is a natural metabolite/hormone of the human body made in the adrenal glands.
  2. Patients with autoimmune diseases are commonly treated with prednisone and other corticosteroids for months or years at a time. Use of prednisone causes adrenal suppression with resultant suppression of DHEA levels.[874]

---

[873] "In some patients with chronic fatigue syndrome, low-dose hydrocortisone reduces fatigue levels in the short term." Cleare AJ, Heap E, Malhi GS, Wessely S, O'Keane V, Miell J. Low-dose hydrocortisone in chronic fatigue syndrome: a randomised crossover trial. *Lancet*. 1999 Feb 6;353(9151):455-8

[874] "Basal serum DHEA and DHEAS concentrations were suppressed to a greater degree than was cortisol during both daily and alternate day prednisone treatments. ...Thus, adrenal androgen secretion was more easily suppressed than was cortisol secretion by this low dose of glucocorticoid, but there was no advantage to alternate day therapy." Rittmaster RS, Givner ML. Effect of daily and alternate day low dose prednisone on serum cortisol and adrenal androgens in hirsute women. *J Clin Endocrinol Metab*. 1988 Aug;67(2):400-3

3. As a consequence of prednisone treatment, many patients lose bone mass and develop osteoporosis. DHEA has been shown to reverse the osteoporosis and loss of bone mass induced by corticosteroid treatment.[875]

4. DHEA shows no acute or subacute toxicity even when used in supraphysiologic doses, even when used in sick patients. For example, in a study of 32 patients with HIV, DHEA doses of 750 mg – 2,250 mg per day were well tolerated and produced no dose-limiting adverse effects.[876] This lack of toxicity compares favorably with any and all so-called "antirheumatic" drugs, nearly all of which show alarming comparable toxicity.

5. DHEA is inexpensive. Even at the relatively high dose of 200 mg per day, the cost is less than $40 per month.

6. When used at doses of 200 mg per day, DHEA safely provides clinical benefit for patients with various autoimmune diseases, including ulcerative colitis, Crohn's disease[877], and SLE.[878]

7. 200 mg per day of DHEA allows SLE patients to reduce their dose of prednisone (thus avoiding its adverse effects) while achieving symptomatic improvement. In other words, it allows for improved health and reduced medication use and therefore fewer side effects.[879]

Thus, based on these financial, safety, and effectiveness considerations, the administration of DHEA is reasonable for patients with moderate or severe autoimmune disease. Furthermore, since optimal clinical response appears to correlate with serum levels that are supraphysiologic[880], treatment may be implemented with little regard for initial DHEA levels, particularly when 1) the dose of DHEA is kept as low as possible, 2) duration is kept as short as possible, 3) other interventions are used to address the underlying cause of the disease, 4) the patient is deriving benefit and the risk-to-benefit ratio is favorable.

- **Thyroid (insufficiency or autoimmunity):** Hypothyroidism is a common concomitant to many of the autoimmune diseases. Overt or imminent hypothyroidism is suggested by TSH greater than 2 mU/L[881] or 3 mU/L[882], low T4 or T3, and/or the presence of anti-thyroid peroxidase antibodies.[883] Specific treatment considerations include the following:
   o Selenium: Supplementation with either selenomethonine[884] or sodium selenite[885,886] can reduce thyroid autoimmunity and improve peripheral conversion of T4 to T3. Selenium may be

---

[875] "CONCLUSION: Prasterone treatment prevented BMD loss and significantly increased BMD at both the lumbar spine and total hip in female patients with SLE receiving exogenous glucocorticoids." Mease PJ, Ginzler EM, Gluck OS, Schiff M, Goldman A, Greenwald M, Cohen S, Egan R, Quarles BJ, Schwartz KE. Effects of prasterone on bone mineral density in women with systemic lupus erythematosus receiving chronic glucocorticoid therapy. *J Rheumatol*. 2005 Apr;32(4):616-21

[876] "Thirty-one subjects were evaluated and monitored for safety and tolerance. The oral drug was administered three times daily in doses ranging from 750 mg/day to 2,250 mg/day for 16 weeks. ... The drug was well tolerated and no dose-limiting side effects were noted." Dyner TS, Lang W, Geaga J, Golub A, Stites D, Winger E, Galmarini M, Masterson J, Jacobson MA. An open-label dose-escalation trial of oral dehydroepiandrosterone tolerance and pharmacokinetics in patients with HIV disease. *J Acquir Immune Defic Syndr*. 1993 May;6(5):459-65

[877] "CONCLUSIONS: In a pilot study, dehydroepiandrosterone was effective and safe in patients with refractory Crohn's disease or ulcerative colitis." Andus T, Klebl F, Rogler G, Bregenzer N, Scholmerich J, Straub RH. Patients with refractory Crohn's disease or ulcerative colitis respond to dehydroepiandrosterone: a pilot study. *Aliment Pharmacol Ther*. 2003 Feb;17(3):409-14

[878] "CONCLUSION: The overall results confirm that DHEA treatment was well-tolerated, significantly reduced the number of SLE flares, and improved patient's global assessment of disease activity." Chang DM, Lan JL, Lin HY, Luo SF. Dehydroepiandrosterone treatment of women with mild-to-moderate systemic lupus erythematosus: a multicenter randomized, double-blind, placebo-controlled trial. *Arthritis Rheum*. 2002 Nov;46(11):2924-7

[879] "CONCLUSION: Among women with lupus disease activity, reducing the dosage of prednisone to < or = 7.5 mg/day for a sustained period of time while maintaining stabilization or a reduction of disease activity was possible in a significantly greater proportion of patients treated with oral prasterone, 200 mg once daily, compared with patients treated with placebo." Petri MA, Lahita RG, Van Vollenhoven RF, Merrill JT, Schiff M, Ginzler EM, Strand V, Kunz A, Gorelick KJ, Schwartz KE; GL601 Study Group. Effects of prasterone on corticosteroid requirements of women with systemic lupus erythematosus: a double-blind, randomized, placebo-controlled trial. *Arthritis Rheum*. 2002 Jul;46(7):1820-9

[880] "CONCLUSION: The clinical response to DHEA was not clearly dose dependent. Serum levels of DHEA and DHEAS correlated only weakly with lupus outcomes, but suggested an optimum serum DHEAS of 1000 microg/dl." Barry NN, McGuire JL, van Vollenhoven RF. Dehydroepiandrosterone in systemic lupus erythematosus: relationship between dosage, serum levels, and clinical response. *J Rheumatol*. 1998 Dec;25(12):2352-6

[881] Weetman AP. Hypothyroidism: screening and subclinical disease. *BMJ*. 1997 Apr 19;314(7088):1175-8 http://bmj.bmjjournals.com/cgi/content/full/314/7088/1175

[882] "Now AACE encourages doctors to consider treatment for patients who test outside the boundaries of a narrower margin based on a target TSH level of 0.3 to 3.0. AACE believes the new range will result in proper diagnosis for millions of Americans who suffer from a mild thyroid disorder, but have gone untreated until now." American Association of Clinical Endocrinologists (AACE). 2003 Campaign Encourages Awareness of Mild Thyroid Failure, Importance of Routine Testing http://www.aace.com/pub/tam2003/press.php November 26, 2005

[883] Beers MH, Berkow R (eds). The Merck Manual. Seventeenth Edition. Whitehouse Station; Merck Research Laboratories 1999 Page 96

[884] Duntas LH, Mantzou E, Koutras DA. Effects of a six month treatment with selenomethionine in patients with autoimmune thyroiditis. *Eur J Endocrinol*. 2003 Apr;148(4):389-93 http://eje-online.org/cgi/reprint/148/4/389

[885] Gartner R, Gasnier BC, Dietrich JW, Krebs B, Angstwurm MW. Selenium supplementation in patients with autoimmune thyroiditis decreases thyroid peroxidase antibodies concentrations. *J Clin Endocrinol Metab*. 2002 Apr;87(4):1687-91 http://jcem.endojournals.org/cgi/content/full/87/4/1687

[886] "We recently conducted a prospective, placebo-controlled clinical study, where we could demonstrate, that a substitution of 200 wg sodium selenite for three months in patients with autoimmune thyroiditis reduced thyroid peroxidase antibody (TPO-Ab) concentrations significantly." Gartner R, Gasnier BC. Selenium in the treatment of autoimmune thyroiditis. *Biofactors*. 2003;19(3-4):165-70

started at 500-800 mcg per day (for 1-3 months) and tapered to 200-400 mcg per day for maintenance.[887]

- o L-thyroxine/levothyroxine/Synthroid—prescription synthetic T4: 25-50 mcg per day is a common starting dose which can be adjusted based on clinical and laboratory response. Thyroid hormone supplements must be consumed separately from soy products (by at least 1-2 hours) and preferably on an empty stomach to avoid absorption interference by food, fiber, and minerals, especially calcium. Doses are generally started at one-half of the daily dose for the first 10 days after which the full dose is used. Caution must be applied in patients with adrenal insufficiency and/or those with cardiovascular disease.

- o Liothyronine, Cytomel®: Cytomel is prescription synthetic T3. Except in patients with myxedema for whom the appropriate starting dose is 5 mcg per day, treatment generally starts with 25 mcg per day and can be increased to 75 mcg per day; dose is adjusted based on clinical and laboratory response. As stated previously, thyroid hormone supplements must be consumed separately from soy products (by at least 1-2 hours) and preferably on an empty stomach to avoid absorption interference by food, fiber, and minerals, especially calcium. Time-released T3 can be obtained from a compounding pharmacy.

- o Armour thyroid—prescription natural T4 and T3 from cow/pig thyroid gland: 60 mg (one grain) is a common starting and maintenance dose. Since administration of Armour thyroid frequently increases serum levels of anti-thyroid antibodies in patients with preexisting thyroid autoimmunity, **many doctors choose to not use Armour thyroid in patients with thyroid autoimmunity**. Some patients prefer to divide their daily dose to maintain constant serum levels of T3.

- o Thyrolar/Liotrix—prescription synthetic T4 with T3: Dosed incrementally as "1", "2", or "3." This product has been difficult to obtain for the past few years due to manufacturing problems (http://thyrolar.com/); previously it was my treatment of choice due to the combination of T4 and T3 and the lack of antigenicity compared to gland-derived products.

- o Thyroid glandular—nonprescription T3: Producers of nutritional products are able to distribute T3 because it is not listed by the FDA as a prescription item. Nutritional supplement companies may start with Armour thyroid, remove the T4, and sell the thyroid glandular with active T3 thereby providing a nonprescription source of active thyroid hormone. For many patients, one tablet per day is at least as effective as a prescription source of thyroid hormone. Since it is derived from a glandular and therefore potentially antigenic source, thyroid glandular is not used in patients with thyroid autoimmunity due to its ability to induce increased production of anti-thyroid antibodies.

- o L-tyrosine and iodine: Some patients with mild hypothyroidism respond to supplementation with L-tyrosine and iodine. Tyrosine is commonly used in doses of 4-9 grams per day in divided doses. According to Abraham and Wright[888], doses of iodine may be as high as 12.5 milligrams (12,500 micrograms), which is slightly less than the average daily intake in Japan at 13.8 mg per day.

- **Pregnenolone:** Several reviews and clinical trials from the early 1950s showed moderate clinical effectiveness and absence of adverse effects from oral administration of pregnenolone in doses as high as 500-1,000 mg/d in patients with rheumatoid arthritis and other rheumatic conditions.[889,890,891,892] Following oral administration of pregnenolone in doses of approximately 500 mg/d, beneficial results are noted in approximately 50-80% of patients. Responders will show reduced pain, swelling, and objective reductions in inflammation measured by ESR and will have increased strength and mobility. No important adverse effects have been reported, particularly with regard to pulse rate, blood

---

[887] Bruns F, Micke O, Bremer M. Current status of selenium and other treatments for secondary lymphedema. *J Support Oncol*. 2003 Jul-Aug;1(2):121-30 http://www.supportiveoncology.net/journal/articles/0102121.pdf

[888] Wright JV. Why you need 83 times more of this essential, cancer-fighting nutrient than the "experts" say you do. *Nutrition and Healing* 2005; volume 12, issue 4.

[889] Freeman H, Pincus G, Johnson CW, et al. Therapeutic efficacy of delta-5-pregnenolone in rheumatoid arthritis. *J American Medical Association* 1950; April 15: 1124-8

[890] Stock JP, McClure EC. Pregnenolone in the treatment of rheumatoid arthritis. *Lancet* 1950 Jul 22;2(4):125-8

[891] Dordick JR, Ehrlich ME, Alexander S, Kissin M. Pregnenolone in rheumatoid arthritis. *N Engl J Med*. 1951 Mar 1;244(9):324-6

[892] Freeman H, Pincus G, Bachrach S, et al. Oral steroid medication in rheumatoid arthritis. *J Clin Endocrinol Metab*. 1950 Dec;10(12):1523-32

pressure, or glucose homeostasis. In contrast to the adverse withdrawal effects noted with prednisone/prednisolone, discontinuance of pregnenolone does not immediately result in exacerbation of inflammation and has never been reported to incite adrenal insufficiency. Oral administration of pregnenolone produces better clinical response than does intramuscular administration, apparently due to the relative insolubility of parenteral pregnenolone. The low cost and absence of adverse effects makes pregnenolone a reasonable therapeutic intervention in patients with rheumatic disease because the treatment may provide benefit and/or mitigate the need for treatments with greater toxicity and cost. However, this treatment should not be relied upon as monotherapy and/or in patients with important inflammatory complications such as iritis, scleritis, or temporal arteritis. In contrast to the much higher doses of 500-1,000 mg/d reported in the studies cited above in this paragraph, I generally limit pregnenolone doses to 10-50 mg/d taken in the morning in patients who may derive benefit; some patients—generally those with hypoadrenalism—notice a marked improvement in energy (to the point of causing insomnia) with doses as low as 5-10 mg/d.

DrV's Summary and Practical Guide to Orthoendocrinology: Read preceeding discussions

Assessments	*Interventions and Notes*
Serum prolactin	• Reduce elevations or treat empirically regardless of serum prolactin level; cabergoline 0.25-0.5 mg twice weekly; also consider using pyridoxine 250-500 mg/d, *Vitex* to effect. • Many studies have now demonstrated that empiric cabergoline is a reasonable, safe, and effective treatment for the more severe inflammatory disorders; cabergoline produces is anti-inflammatory benefit via blocking prolactin signaling within the immune system and not by primarily affecting pituitary output of prolactin.
Serum fasting insulin as a marker of insulin resistance and metabolic inflammation	• Improve insulin sensitivity by reducing carbohydrate intake and improving insulin secretion and reception. Insulin resistance most commonly results from 1) systemic inflammation, 2) xenobiotic down-regulation of GLUT receptors via the aryl-hydrocarbon receptor, 3) micronutrient deficiencies, 4) cortisol excess, 5) physiologic and protective insulin resistance secondary to ceramide accumulation as a result of cellular carbohydrate overload.
Serum estradiol	• Reduce serum estradiol with weight loss, alcohol and caffeine avoidance, treatment for obesity, surgical correction of varicocele in men, anastrazole 1mg 2-3 times weekly is effective and safe in most cases, especially for men • Consider monitoring osteoporosis risk in cases of prolonged hypoestrogenemia, which should generally be avoided.
Serum DHEA sulfate	• Physiologic doses are 15 mg/d for women and 25 mg/d for men; supraphysiologic dosing up to 200mg/d is effective, safe, and well-represented in the rheumatology literature for the treatment of RA, SLE, and IBD.
Serum cortisol, preferably before and after ACTH	• See interpretive guide provided previously. • Physiolgic doses of ≤ 10-20 mg/d orally administered cortisol can be used empirically under appropriate supervision, with the first dose of 10mg administered upon waking in the moring and optional additional doses of 5 mg each administered in the late morning and early afternoon to mimic physiologic secrection.
Serum free and total testosterone	• If total testosterone is low, evaluate for primary or secondary hypogonadism. • If testosterone is low and estrogen is low, consider transdermal testosterone therapy. • If free testosterone is low and total testosterone is normal, likely due to elevated SHBG, generally due to excess estrogen or excess prolactin. • If testosterone is low and estrogen is high, then use aromatase inhibition and/or correct the hypogonadism resulting from obesity/inflammation. • Always assess free and total testosterone in conjunction with serum estradiol.

Always use the lowest dose of hormonal intervention necessary to achieve the desired result; lower doses of each intervention can be used when more interventions (e.g., nutritional, mitochondrial, antidysbiotic) are used.

❼ Xenobiotic Immunotoxicity:
Exposure, Accumulation, Detoxification

Major Concepts in this Section

Exposure to "foreign substances" such as toxic chemicals and toxic metals is inescapable in our polluted world and modern lives; exposure invariably results in some level of accumulation. Accumulation of toxic metals and chemicals produces additive and synergistic toxic effects on the entire organism, notably via endocrine disruption, immune imbalance and suppression, oxidative stress, immunogentic modification of endogenous antigens via xenobiotic haptenization, and mitochondrial dysfunction, which then leads to systemic inflammation, reduced cell/tissue performance, and additional oxidative stress. Despite these facts and the obvioius clinical implications, most doctorate-level physicians—except for naturopathic clinicians—receive no training in these topics and the clinical remediation via therapeutic detoxification. Thus, the naturopathic profession stands clearly preeminent in its profession-wide training in the appreciation, assessment and treatment of xenobiotic-induced illness.

Xenobiotic Immunotoxicity and Treatment by Therapeutic Detoxification: Ultracondensed Clinical Review

Chemicals such as pesticides, synthetic fertilizers, herbicides, fungicides, industrial pollution, car exhaust, solvents, and innumerable others are bioaccumulative and can alter immune function. The classic manifestation of xenobiotic immunotoxicity is the combination of reduced resistance to infections and increased allergic and autoimmune disorders. The subject of environmental medicine and detoxification is much to broad and complex to review completely in this textbook, and while naturopathic physicians are trained in these topics, other healthcare professionals are not unless they attend post-graduate training and take the time to read articles and textbooks on these topics. Readers for whom these topics are new are encouraged to access the following citations for additional information.[893,894,895,896,897] What follows here will be an ultracondensed clinical review focusing on major concepts and problem-specific solutions.

For the sake of simplicity and with recognition of the various nuances of different xenobiotics, I generalize toxicity into two categories, either *chemicals* or *heavy metals*. Most patients have an overlay of these two problems, so that the clinical manifestations and treatments have several commonalities.

- Chemical toxicity: Accumulation of xenobiotics can cause immune dysfunction and can contribute to the development of "autoimmunity." Examples of xenobiotic-induced autoimmunity include 1) the increased autoimmunity seen in farmers exposed to pesticides[898], 2) the scleroderma-like disease that results from exposure to vinyl chloride[899], 3) the association of mercury and pesticide exposure with lupus[900], and 4) the well-recognized connection between drug and chemical exposure and various autoimmune syndromes such as drug-induced lupus.[901] More than 40 pharmaceutical drugs are

---

[893] "Caffeine enemas cause dilation of bile ducts, which facilitates excretion of toxic cancer breakdown products by the liver and dialysis of toxic products from blood across the colonic wall. The therapy must be used as an integrated whole." Gerson M. The cure of advanced cancer by diet therapy: a summary of 30 years of clinical experimentation. *Physiol Chem Phys.* 1978;10(5):449-64

[894] "The writer has observed numerous cases suffering from such conditions as chronic arthritis, hypertension, coronary disease, chronic abdominal distention, constipation, and colitis, in which the element of constipation, auto-intoxication and possible colon infection seemed to play a prominent part, which responded very satisfactorily to colonic irrigations after failure to improve following the usual forms of medical treatment." Snyder RG. The value of colonic irrigations in countering auto-intoxication of intestinal origin. *Medical Clinics of North America* 1939; May: 781-788

[895] Gonzalez NJ, Isaacs LL. Evaluation of pancreatic proteolytic enzyme treatment of adenocarcinoma of the pancreas, with nutrition and detoxification support. *Nutr Cancer.* 1999;33(2):117-24

[896] Crinnion WJ. Results of a decade of naturopathic treatment for environmental illness: a review of clinical records. *J Naturopathic Med* 1997;7:21-27

[897] Sherman JD. *Chemical exposure and disease. Diagnostic and investigative techniques.* Princeton Scientific Publishing; 1994

[898] "IgG levels decreased with increasing p,p'-DDE levels, with a statistically significant decrease of approximately 50% in the highest two categories of exposure. Sixteen (12%) were positive for antinuclear antibodies... These analyses provide evidence that p,p'-DDE modulates immune responses in humans." Cooper GS, Martin SA, Longnecker MP, Sandler DP, Germolec DR. Associations between plasma DDE levels and immunologic measures in African-American farmers in North Carolina. *Environ Health Perspect.* 2004 Jul;112(10):1080-4

[899] "Vinyl chloride (VC) monomer can induce a scleroderma-like syndrome in a proportion of workers exposed to it during production of polyvinyl chloride." Black CM, Welsh KI, Walker AE, et al. Genetic susceptibility to scleroderma-like syndrome induced by vinyl chloride. *Lancet.* 1983 Jan 1;1(8314-5):53-5

[900] "...reported occupational exposure to mercury (OR 3.6), mixing pesticides for agricultural work (OR 7.4), and among dental workers (OR 7.1, 95% CI 2.2, 23.4). ...these associations were fairly strong and statistically significant..." Cooper GS, Parks CG, Treadwell EL, St Clair EW, Gilkeson GS, Dooley MA. Occupational risk factors for the development of systemic lupus erythematosus. *J Rheumatol.* 2004 Oct;31(10):1928-33

[901] Hess EV. Environmental chemicals and autoimmune disease: cause and effect. *Toxicology.* 2002 Dec 27;181-182:65-70

known to cause drug-induced lupus.[902] Every one of us is exposed to toxic chemicals every day, and every one of us has chemical accumulation and the potential for xenobiotic-induced disease. Except for denial (shown to be clinically ineffective), we cannot escape from the chemical consequences of living in a world with tens of thousands of synthetic chemicals. According to limited analyses, the average American has accumulated at least 18 different chemicals[903], and analyses that are more detailed show that even more chemicals and metals have been accumulated.[904] Common sources of these chemicals include pesticides, synthetic fertilizers, herbicides, fungicides, industrial pollution, car exhaust, solvents, paints, perfumes, plastic food/drink containers, non-stick cookware, Styrofoam, trichloroethylene from dry cleaning, rubber, carpet, plastics, glues, propellants, petroleum fuels such as gasoline, detergents, and other "cleaners." Clinical consequences of chemical toxicity are diverse, can affect nearly every organ system, and may be predicted to some extent by the pattern of chemical exposure since some chemicals have characteristic sequelae. Most chemicals, especially those which are fat-soluble, can readily enter the body via respiratory, gastrointestinal, and transdermal routes. Once in the bloodstream, chemicals are either detoxified (inactivated and/or solubilized) by the liver and then excreted via urine or bile, or to a lesser extent exhaled from the lungs or excreted via sweat. Chemicals which are not excreted from the body are stored in the tissues, particularly lipid-rich organs such as the liver, adipose, and brain. Molecular turnover and recycling (particularly lipolysis) liberates fat-stored xenobiotics for another opportunity for either detoxification or additional toxicity. The main route for detoxification is the liver, which hydrosolublizes xenobiotics via oxidation ("phase one") and conjugation ("phase two"). Generally speaking, oxidation reactions are dependent on the cytochrome P-450 system, which can be inhibited by various drugs (e.g., ketoconazole, erythromycin, ritonavir, cimetidine, omeprazole, ethanol), foods such as ethanol and grapefruit juice, bacterial endotoxin from bacterial overgrowth of the intestines, and/or by genetic defects known as single nucleotide polymorphisms ("SNiPs") which reduce xenobiotic clearance. Similarly, conjugation reactions can be inhibited by a low-vegetable diet, SNiPs, and insufficiencies of conjugation moieties such as glutathione, glycine, glutamine, taurine, ornithine, sulfur, and methyl groups. If oxidation is too slow, then xenobiotics are insufficiently detoxicated and insufficiently processed for conjugation, leading to xenobiotic accumulation. If oxidation is too fast relative to conjugation, then reactive intermediates are formed which are commonly more toxic than the original xenobiotic, and insufficient conjugation results in accumulation of reactive xenobiotics which are inherently prone to tissue haptenization (which can incite autoimmunity) and DNA intercalation (which promotes damage to DNA and the resultant mutation and oncogenesis). Optimally oxidized and conjugated xenobiotics are excreted in the urine (smaller molecules with molecular weight less than 400-600) or expelled in the bile (larger molecules with molecular weight greater than 400-600). Supranormal hydration and urinary alkalinization enhance renal clearance of weakly acidic xenobiotics and drugs, whereas dehydration and urinary acidity impair toxin excretion, generally speaking. Conjugated toxins expelled in the bile can be deconjugated by bacteria so that the toxin is reabsorbed, a phenomenon commonly referred to as "enterohepatic recycling"[905] or "enterohepatic recirculation."[906] Such recirculation is obviously less likely if gastrointestinal status and diet have been optimized to minimize the presence of deconjugating bacteria and to maximize fiber intake and laxation for the adsorption and expulsion of intraluminal toxins. Therapeutic colonics and enemas can be employed to stimulate bile flow from the

---

[902] "Drug-induced lupus has been reported as a side-effect of long-term therapy with over 40 medications... Several mechanisms for induction of autoimmunity will be discussed, including bystander activation of autoreactive lymphocytes due to drug-specific immunity or to non-specific activation of lymphocytes, direct cytotoxicity with release of autoantigens ..." Rubin RL. Drug-induced lupus. *Toxicology.* 2005;209(2):135-47

[903] Kristin S. Schafer, Margaret Reeves, Skip Spitzer, Susan E. Kegley. Chemical Trespass: Pesticides in Our Bodies and Corporate Accountability. Pesticide Action Network North America. May 2004 Available at http://www.panna.org/campaigns/docsTrespass/chemicalTrespass2004.dv.html on August 1, 2004

[904] Body Burden: The Pollution in People. http://ewg.org/issues/siteindex/issues.php?issueid=5004 Accessed February 6, 2006

[905] "Enterohepatic recycling occurs by biliary excretion and intestinal reabsorption of a solute, sometimes with hepatic conjugation and intestinal deconjugation. ... Of particular importance is the potential amplifying effect of enterohepatic variability in defining differences in the bioavailability, apparent volume of distribution and clearance of a given compound." Roberts MS, Magnusson BM, Burczynski FJ, Weiss M. Enterohepatic circulation: physiological, pharmacokinetic and clinical implications. *Clin Pharmacokinet.* 2002;41(10):751-90

[906] Liska DJ. The detoxification enzyme systems. *Altern Med Rev.* 1998 Jun;3(3):187-98

liver[907,908] and to remove bile-secreted toxins from the gut before deconjugation and re-absorption occur. Bile formation and expulsion are further stimulated by botanical medicines such as beets, ginger[909], curcumin/turmeric[910], *Picrorhiza*[911], milk thistle[912], *Andrographis paniculata*[913] and *Boerhaavia diffusa*.[914] Respiratory exhalation of toxins is enhanced by deep breathing and exercise, and hyperventilation promotes respiratory alkalosis which elevates urine pH and promotes excretion of weakly acidic drugs and xenobiotics as previously mentioned. Dermal excretion of toxins via sweat and expedited lipolysis are stimulated via low-temperature saunas and regular aerobic exercise. Xenobiotic oxidation can be promoted (cautiously) by reducing endotoxins from the gut and by the use of botanicals such as *Hypericum perforatum* which induce several isoforms of cytochrome P-450 via activation of the pregane X receptor. Xenobiotic conjugation is likewise promoted via nutrigenomic induction stimulated by cruciferous vegetables and their derivatives such as indole-3-carbinol (I3C) and dimethylindolylemethane (DIM). The plant-based diet is employed to provide fiber for bowel cleansing and the urinary alkalinization that is necessary for optimal urinary excretion of toxins, the majority of which are weak acids and are thus excreted more efficiently in alkaline urine. Sodium bicarbonate can also be used to induce urinary alkalinization. The diet must contain high-quality protein and can be supplemented with amino acids to support amino acid and glutathione conjugation. Serum, urine, and adipose samples can be analyzed to determine the intensity and diversity of chemical accumulation; I tend reserve such testing for patients who have been exposed to a specific chemical, particularly in occupational settings. For most patients, their chemical accumulation is so diverse that they may not display abnormally high levels of a specific chemical; their clinical manifestations are rather a manifestation of a wide plethora of different chemicals, which individually may be only modestly increased. Detoxification genotype can be determined by genomic testing for SNPs in oxidation and conjugation enzymes. Phenotype can be assessed by serum and urine measurements of post-challenge detoxification of benzoate, caffeine, acetylsalicylic acid, and acetaminophen. Amino acid status can be quantified and qualified via serum or urine amino acid analysis. Stool testing assesses digestion, absorption, and microflora status. Clinical implementation follows a screening physical examination and basic laboratory assessment (minimally including CBC, metabolic panel, and urinalysis). Stool testing is always reasonable when working with patients with fatigue and/or autoimmunity; however, this and the other detoxification-related tests can often be deferred and/or used selectively. The Paleo-Mediterranean diet provides ample high-quality protein, alkalinization, fiber, and phytonutrients to which may be added supplements of protein, amino acids (especially NAC, glycine, and glutamine), and vitamins and minerals. Antioxidant teas and fresh fruit and vegetable juices are consumed to increase frequency of urination and promote urinary alkalinization, due primarily to the content of potassium citrate. Exercise and low-temperature saunas promote sweating and xenobiotic-mobilizing lipolysis. Colonics and enemas cleanse the bowel and stimulate bile flow.[915,916] Bile flow is further stimulated by consumption of beets, ginger,

---

[907] Garbat, AL, Jacobi, HG: Secretion of Bile in Response to Rectal Installations. *Arch Intern Med* 1929; 44: 455-462

[908] "Caffeine enemas cause dilation of bile ducts, which facilitates excretion of toxic cancer breakdown products by the liver and dialysis of toxic products from blood across the colonic wall. The therapy must be used as an integrated whole." Gerson M. The cure of advanced cancer by diet therapy: a summary of 30 years of clinical experimentation. *Physiol Chem Phys*. 1978;10(5):449-64

[909] "Further analyses for the active constituents of the acetone extracts through column chromatography indicated that [6]-gingerol and [10]-gingerol, which are the pungent principles, are mainly responsible for the cholagogic effect of ginger." Yamahara J, Miki K, Chisaka T, Sawada T, Fujimura H, Tomimatsu T, Nakano K, Nohara T. Cholagogic effect of ginger and its active constituents. *J Ethnopharmacol*. 1985;13(2):217-25

[910] "On the basis of the present findings, it appears that curcumin induces contraction of the human gall-bladder." Rasyid A, Lelo A. The effect of curcumin and placebo on human gall-bladder function: an ultrasound study. *Aliment Pharmacol Ther*. 1999 Feb;13(2):245-9

[911] "Significant anticholestatic activity was also observed against carbon tetrachloride induced cholestasis in conscious rat, anaesthetized guinea pig and cat. Picroliv was more active than the known hepatoprotective drug silymarin." Saraswat B, Visen PK, Patnaik GK, Dhawan BN. Anticholestatic effect of picroliv, active hepatoprotective principle of Picrorhiza kurrooa, against carbon tetrachloride induced cholestasis. *Indian J Exp Biol*. 1993 Apr;31(4):316-8

[912] "We conclude that SIL counteracts TLC-induced cholestasis by preventing the impairment in both the BS-dependent and -independent fractions of the bile flow." Crocenzi FA, Sanchez Pozzi EJ, Pellegrino JM, Rodriguez Garay EA, Mottino AD, Roma MG. Preventive effect of silymarin against taurolithocholate-induced cholestasis in the rat. *Biochem Pharmacol*. 2003 Jul 15;66(2):355-64

[913] "Andrographolide from the herb Andrographis paniculata (whole plant) per se produces a significant dose (1.5-12 mg/kg) dependent choleretic effect (4.8-73%) as evidenced by increase in bile flow, bile salt, and bile acids in conscious rats and anaesthetized guinea pigs." Shukla B, Visen PK, Patnaik GK, Dhawan BN. Choleretic effect of andrographolide in rats and guinea pigs. *Planta Med*. 1992 Apr;58(2):146-9

[914] "The extract also produced an increase in normal bile flow in rats suggesting a strong choleretic activity." Chandan BK, Sharma AK, Anand KK. Boerhaavia diffusa: a study of its hepatoprotective activity. *J Ethnopharmacol*. 1991 Mar;31(3):299-307

[915] Garbat, AL, Jacobi, HG: Secretion of Bile in Response to Rectal Installations. *Arch Intern Med* 1929; 44: 455-462

[916] "Caffeine enemas cause dilation of bile ducts, which facilitates excretion of toxic cancer breakdown products by the liver and dialysis of toxic products from blood across the colonic wall. The therapy must be used as an integrated whole." Gerson M. The cure of advanced cancer by diet therapy: a summary of 30 years of clinical experimentation. *Physiol Chem Phys*. 1978;10(5):449-64

curcumin/turmeric, *Picrorhiza*, milk thistle, *Andrographis paniculata* and *Boerhaavia diffusa*. These interventions work in concert to enhance xenobiotic depuration ("The act or process of depurating or freeing from foreign or impure matter "[917]) and cleanse the tissues of accumulated toxins. Intervention can be acute or periodic, but must be maintained for the long-term in order to resist the re-accumulation that is destined to result from the chemical onslaught that is inescapable in our polluted world.

- <u>Heavy metal toxicity</u>: In contrast to chemical toxicity for which a generalized non-specific cleansing protocol is appropriate, toxic metals more commonly require specific interventions; treatment is determined by the identity of the metal. Metals which are considered toxic or which are linked to the induction of human diseases include aluminum, arsenic, cadmium, lead, and mercury. Other metals and minerals such as manganese, lithium, copper, and iron can be toxic when present in high amounts. In this section I will limit the discussion to mercury since this metal is 1) commonly elevated in chronically toxic patients, and 2) because this metal can contribute to autoimmunity.

  - <u>Mercury</u>: Chronic mercury toxicity is commonly discovered in clinical practice in patients with chronic unwellness, and a recent study published in *JAMA* showed that 8% of American women of childbearing age have sufficient levels of mercury in their bodies to produce neurologic damage in their children.[918] Accumulating evidence implicates mercury in the induction of immune dysfunction and the exacerbation of autoimmunity and allergy, and clinical trials indicate the benefit of mercury removal.

    - Mercury induces autoimmunity, immune complex formation and deposition, and the formation of antinuclear antibodies and antinucleolar antibodies in animal experiments.[919,920,921]

    - In a case-control study of 265 recently diagnosed lupus patients, occupational exposure to mercury increased the risk of developing lupus by 360%, while working in a dental office increased the risk by 710%.[922]

    - Patients with eczema have an increase body burden of mercury[923], suggesting the probability that mercury accumulation induces immune dysfunction and contributes to the clinical picture of immune-induced skin inflammation, to which is affixed the label of "eczema."

    - Leukocytes from autistic patients produce autoantigens when exposed to ethyl mercury (Thimerosal), thus clearly implicating mercury in the incitement and perpetuation of autoimmunity.[924]

    - A slight increase in risk for multiple sclerosis was noted among patients with many long-term mercury amalgam fillings.[925]

---

[917] "The act or process of depurating or freeing from foreign or impure matter." http://www.thefreedictionary.com/Depuration Verified March 11, 2007

[918] "However, approximately 8% of women had concentrations higher than the US Environmental Protection Agency's recommended reference dose (5.8 microg/L), below which exposures are considered to be without adverse effects. Women who are pregnant or who intend to become pregnant should follow federal and state advisories on consumption of fish." Schober SE, Sinks TH, Jones RL, Bolger PM, McDowell M, Osterloh J, Garrett ES, Canady RA, Dillon CF, Sun Y, Joseph CB, Mahaffey KR. Blood mercury levels in US children and women of childbearing age, 1999-2000. *JAMA*. 2003 Apr 2;289(13):1667-74

[919] "It is well established that in susceptible mouse strains, chronic treatment with subtoxic doses of mercuric chloride (HgCl2) induces a systemic autoimmune disease, which is characterized by increased serum levels of IgG1 and IgE antibodies, by the production of anti-nucleolar antibodies and by the development of immune complex-mediated glomerulonephritis." al-Balaghi S, Moller E, Moller G, Abedi-Valugerdi M. Mercury induces polyclonal B cell activation, autoantibody production and renal immune complex deposits in young (NZB x NZW)F1 hybrids. *Eur J Immunol*. 1996 Jul;26(7):1519-26

[920] "It is well demonstrated that mercury induces a systemic autoimmune disease in susceptible mouse strains... The dominant antibody in the kidney eluate of mercury-injected mice was of IgG1 isotype and found to be directed against double-stranded DNA, collagen, cardiolipin, phosphatidylethanolamine, and the hapten trinitrophenol, but not against nucleolar antigens." Abedi-Valugerdi M, Hu H, Moller G. Mercury-induced renal immune complex deposits in young (NZB x NZW)F1 mice: characterization of antibodies/autoantibodies. *Clin Exp Immunol*. 1997 Oct;110(1):86-91

[921] Abedi-Valugerdi M, Hu H, Moller G. Mercury-induced anti-nucleolar autoantibodies can transgress the membrane of living cells in vivo and in vitro. *Int Immunol*. 1999 Apr;11(4):605-15 http://intimm.oxfordjournals.org/cgi/content/full/11/4/605

[922] "...reported occupational exposure to mercury (OR 3.6), mixing pesticides for agricultural work (OR 7.4), and among dental workers (OR 7.1, 95% CI 2.2, 23.4). ...these associations were fairly strong and statistically significant..." Cooper GS, Parks CG, Treadwell EL, St Clair EW, Gilkeson GS, Dooley MA. Occupational risk factors for the development of systemic lupus erythematosus. *J Rheumatol*. 2004 Oct;31(10):1928-33

[923] Weidinger S, Kramer U, Dunemann L, Mohrenschlager M, Ring J, Behrendt H. Body burden of mercury is associated with acute atopic eczema and total IgE in children from southern Germany. *J Allergy Clin Immunol*. 2004 Aug;114(2):457-9

[924] Vojdani A, Pangborn JB, Vojdani E, Cooper EL. Infections, toxic chemicals and dietary peptides binding to lymphocyte receptors and tissue enzymes are major instigators of autoimmunity in autism. *Int J Immunopathol Pharmacol*. 2003 Sep-Dec;16(3):189-99

[925] "Although a suggestive elevated risk was found for those individuals with a large number of dental amalgams, and for a long period of time, the difference between cases and controls was not statistically significant." Bangsi D, Ghadirian P, Ducic S, Morisset R, Ciccocioppo S, McMullen E, Krewski D. Dental amalgam and multiple sclerosis: a case-control study in Montreal, Canada. *Int J Epidemiol*. 1998 Aug;27(4):667-71 http://ije.oxfordjournals.org/cgi/reprint/27/4/667

- It is highly probable that chronic mercury exposure, whether from diet or dental amalgams, alters gastrointestinal flora in favor of dysbiosis in general and antibiotic resistance in particular.[926] Thus, mercury may indirectly contribute to autoimmunity by promoting treatment-resistant dysbiosis, which then directly effects pro-inflammatory immune dysfunction.

- In a clinical trial with 35 patients, 71% experienced improvement in overall health following removal of mercury amalgams; the patients with the most improvement were patients with multiple sclerosis.[927] Whether this was due to reducing autoimmunity or to reducing neurotoxicity is not clear; certainly both mechanisms may explain the improvement. Mercury is directly neurotoxic independently from its almost certain ability to contribute to neuroautoimmunity; this is visually demonstrated in a video of brain neuron degeneration following exposure to mercury, available on-line from the University of Calgary at http://commons.ucalgary.ca/mercury/.[928]

Very interestingly, the patients most sensitive to mercury compounds appear to be those with a genotypic defect in phase-2 xenobiotic conjugation, specifically glutathione-S-transferase (GST).[929] What makes this even more interesting is the finding that mercury compounds can inhibit GST and produce a GST-deficient phenotype even when the original genotype was GST-normal.[930] Even though this latter finding was documented in *ex vivo* research with human erythrocytes, it correlates with the clinical experience of doctors who specialize in environmental medicine, namely that mercury accumulation appears to inhibit chemical xenobiotic detoxification. Thus mercury and chemical xenobiotics may work synergistically for the induction of immune dysfunction, with the former inhibiting the detoxification/conjugation of the latter. Regardless of the mechanisms involved, which are clearly numerous and synergistic, given that no safe level of mercury has been established, clinicians are justified in treating patients with evidence of mercury accumulation, chronic mercury toxicity. Based on numerous case reports documenting safety and efficacy of dimercaptosuccinic acid (DMSA), when used in children and adults[931,932,933,934,935], it is my chelating agent of choice for most patients with lead and mercury toxicity as I review in the DMSA monograph in the pages that follow. Clinical implementation of metal detoxification can be performed simultaneously with the chemical detoxification program described previously and outlined in the pages that follow. The difference is the addition of DMSA first

[926] Pike R, Lucas V, Stapleton P, Gilthorpe MS, Roberts G, Rowbury R, Richards H, Mullany P, Wilson M. Prevalence and antibiotic resistance profile of mercury-resistant oral bacteria from children with and without mercury amalgam fillings. *J Antimicrob Chemother*. 2002 May;49(5):777-83 http://jac.oxfordjournals.org/cgi/content/full/49/5/777 This seems to be a rather tragic article insofar as the researchers' conclusions are inconsistent with their findings; they state that mercury does not contribute to increased prevalence or numbers of antibiotic resistant bacteria, yet their data in Table 4 clearly demonstrate that patients with dental amalgams have more drug-resistant isolates than do patients without such toxic implantations. Note also that the bacteria studied here were from the oral cavity, not the gastrointestinal tract. A much better article on this topic is the following: "Our findings indicate that mercury released from amalgam fillings can cause an enrichment of mercury resistance plasmids in the normal bacterial floras of primates. Many of these plasmids also carry antibiotic resistance, implicating the exposure to mercury from dental amalgams in an increased incidence of multiple antibiotic resistance plasmids in the normal floras of nonmedicated subjects." Summers AO, Wireman J, Vimy MJ, Lorscheider FL, Marshall B, Levy SB, Bennett S, Billard L. Mercury released from dental "silver" fillings provokes an increase in mercury- and antibiotic-resistant bacteria in oral and intestinal floras of primates. *Antimicrob Agents Chemother*. 1993 Apr;37(4):825-34 pubmedcentral.gov/articlerender.fcgi?tool=pubmed&pubmedid=8280208
[927] "Out of 35 patients, 25 patients (71%) showed improvement of health... The highest rate of improvement was observed in patients with multiple sclerosis... Mercury-containing amalgam may be an important risk factor for patients with autoimmune diseases." Prochazkova J, Sterzl I, Kucerova H, Bartova J, Stejskal VD. The beneficial effect of amalgam replacement on health in patients with autoimmunity. *Neuro Endocrinol Lett*. 2004 Jun;25(3):211-8
[928] University of Calgary. How Mercury Causes Brain Neuron Degeneration. http://commons.ucalgary.ca/mercury/ Accessed November 24, 2005
[929] "The combined deletion (GSTT1-/GSTM1-) was markedly more frequent among thimerosal-sensitized patients than in healthy controls (17.6% vs. 6.5%, P = 0.0093) and in the "para-compound" group (17.6% vs. 6.1%, P =0.014), revealing a synergistic effect of these enzyme deficiencies." Westphal GA, Schnuch A, Schulz TG, Reich K, Aberer W, Brasch J, Koch P, Wessbecher R, Szliska C, Bauer A, Hallier E. Homozygous gene deletions of the glutathione S-transferases M1 and T1 are associated with thimerosal sensitization. *Int Arch Occup Environ Health*. 2000 Aug;73(6):384-8
[930] "Thus, sufficiently high doses of thimerosal may be able to change the phenotypic status of an individual--at least in vitro--by inhibition of the GST T1 enzyme." Muller M, Westphal G, Vesper A, Bunger J, Hallier E. Inhibition of the human erythrocytic glutathione-S-transferase T1 (GST T1) by thimerosal. Int *J Hyg Environ Health*. 2001 Jul;203(5-6):479-81
[931] Bradstreet J, Geier DA, Kartzinel JJ, Adams JB, Geier MR. A case-control study of mercury burden in children with autistic spectrum disorders. *Journal of American Physicians and Surgeons* 2003; 8: 76-79 http://www.jpands.org/vol8no3/geier.pdf
[932] Crinnion WJ. Environmental medicine, part three: long-term effects of chronic low-dose mercury exposure. *Altern Med Rev*. 2000 Jun;5(3):209-23 http://www.thorne.com/altmedrev/.fulltext/5/3/209.pdf
[933] Forman J, Moline J, Cernichiari E, et al. A cluster of pediatric metallic mercury exposure cases treated with meso-2,3-dimercaptosuccinic acid (DMSA). *Environ Health Perspect*. 2000 Jun;108(6):575-7 http://ehp.niehs.nih.gov/docs/2000/108p575-577forman/abstract.html
[934] Miller AL. Dimercaptosuccinic acid (DMSA), a non-toxic, water-soluble treatment for heavy metal toxicity. *Altern Med Rev*. 1998 Jun;3(3):199-207 http://www.thorne.com/altmedrev/.fulltext/3/3/199.pdf
[935] DMSA. *Altern Med Rev*. 2000 Jun;5(3):264-7 http://thorne.com/altmedrev/.fulltext/5/3/264.pdf

thing in the morning on an empty stomach at a dose of 10-30 mg per kg. Screening examination for overall health and kidney function should be performed before full-dose administration of DMSA, and sensitivity testing with <100 mg of DMSA is also reasonable to exclude allergy or idiosyncratic reactions to DMSA, which may indeed occur. DMSA is given in an "on and off" schedule, such as four days "on" and 3 days "off." Bile flow stimulation with botanicals and colonics for expulsion of mercury is the same as for xenobiotic detoxification. Two to four hours after consumption of DMSA, metal adsorbents such as phytochelatins and alginate can be used to bind metals in the gut and reduce enterohepatic recirculation. Antioxidants, especially selenium, are supplemented, and the diet is fresh, hypoallergenic, and Paleo-Mediterranean.

Problems and Solutions in Clinical Detoxification

Effects	Cause	Solutions
1) Toxicant exposure and accumulation	• Excess exposure in relation to genotypic/phenotypic detoxification capabilities	• Total load of all xenobiotics must be reduced because of the similar/identical pathways used for the elimination of chemicals. Avoid the following: paint fumes, perfume, varnish, new carpet, formaldehyde, food colors, food additives, artificial sweeteners, pesticides, herbicides, and industrial waste.[936] • Since the vast majority of toxicants originate from irresponsible corporations, social/political action is necessary to effect fundamental change.[937]
2) Phase 1 Oxidation inhibited, too slow	• SNiPs and genotypic variations • Certain drugs • Certain food components: arachidonate and flavonoids such as bergapten (67%), quercetin (55%), naringenin (39%) naringin (6%) • Viral infections • Heavy metals • Nutritional deficiencies • Gut-derived LPS/endotoxin	• Reduce drug need by restoring health and addressing underlying problems • Address viral infections and promote glutathione production, e.g., NAC[938] and lipoic acid[939] • Vitamin/mineral supplements to correct common deficiencies in American diet[940] and to induce activity of detoxifying enzymes[941] • Paleo[942]/Mediterranean diet[943] to provide foundational nutrition and improve health • Avoidance of excess arachidonate and grapefruit • Eliminate unfavorable microflora and reflorestate to reduce LPS/endotoxin load[944] • Chelate metals with chelating agent such as DMSA[945]

[936] Ross GH. Treatment options in multiple chemical sensitivity. *Toxicol Ind Health.* 1992 Jul-Aug;8(4):87-94

[937] Kristin S. Schafer, Margaret Reeves, Skip Spitzer, Susan E. Kegley. Chemical Trespass: Pesticides in Our Bodies and Corporate Accountability. Pesticide Action Network North America. May 2004 Available at http://www.panna.org/campaigns/docsTrespass/chemicalTrespass2004.dv.html on August 1, 2004

[938] "NAC treatment was well tolerated and resulted in a significant decrease in the frequency of influenza-like episodes, severity, and length of time confined to bed. Both local and systemic symptoms were sharply and significantly reduced in the NAC group." De Flora S, Grassi C, Carati L. Attenuation of influenza-like symptomatology and improvement of cell-mediated immunity with long-term N-acetylcysteine treatment. *Eur Respir J.* 1997 Jul;10(7):1535-41 Available on-line at http://erj.ersjournals.com/cgi/reprint/10/7/1535 on October 18, 2004

[939] "These findings confirm the involvement of ROI in NF-kappaB-mediated HIV gene expression as well as the efficacy of LA as a therapeutic regimen for HIV infection and acquired immunodeficiency syndrome (AIDS)." Merin JP, Matsuyama M, Kira T, Baba M, Okamoto T. Alpha-lipoic acid blocks HIV-1 LTR-dependent expression of hygromycin resistance in THP-1 stable transformants. *FEBS Lett.* 1996 Sep 23;394(1):9-13

[940] Fletcher RH, Fairfield KM. Vitamins for chronic disease prevention in adults: clinical applications. *JAMA.* 2002 Jun 19;287(23):3127-9

[941] Ames BN, Elson-Schwab I, Silver EA. High-dose vitamin therapy stimulates variant enzymes with decreased coenzyme binding affinity (increased K(m)): relevance to genetic disease and polymorphisms. *Am J Clin Nutr.* 2002 Apr;75(4):616-58

[942] O'Keefe JH Jr, Cordain L. Cardiovascular disease resulting from a diet and lifestyle at odds with our Paleolithic genome: how to become a 21st-century hunter-gatherer. *Mayo Clin Proc.* 2004 Jan;79(1):101-8

[943] Knoops KT, de Groot LC, Kromhout D, Perrin AE, Moreiras-Varela O, Menotti A, van Staveren WA. Mediterranean diet, lifestyle factors, and 10-year mortality in elderly European men and women: the HALE project. *JAMA.* 2004 Sep 22;292(12):1433-9

[944] Shedlofsky SI, Israel BC, Tosheva R, Blouin RA. Endotoxin depresses hepatic cytochrome P450-mediated drug metabolism in women. *Br J Clin Pharmacol.* 1997 Jun;43(6):627-32

[945] Miller AL. Dimercaptosuccinic Acid (DMSA), A Non-Toxic, Water-Soluble Treatment For Heavy Metal Toxicity. *Altern Med Rev* 1998;3(3):199-207

Problems and Solutions in Clinical Detoxification—*continued*

Effects	*Cause*	*Solutions*
3) Phase 1 Oxidation imbalanced, too fast relative to Phase 2	▪ Certain drugs or other toxicant exposure from endogenous or exogenous sources leads to upregulation of Phase 1	▪ Reduce drug need by restoring health and addressing underlying problems ▪ Suspect excess enterohepatic recirculation (via excess fecal β-glucuronidase): assess and optimize gastrointestinal flora by eliminating harmful bacteria and using probiotics[946] ▪ Upregulate phase 2 with diet and botanicals, such as cruciferous vegetables[947,948]
4) Phase 2 Conjugation too slow	▪ SNiPs: single nucleotide polymorphism defects in detoxification enzymes ▪ Fluoridated water: inhibits glucuronidation in some patients with Gilbert's syndrome[949] ▪ Lack of stimulation with diet and botanicals (i.e., insufficient intake of cruciferous vegetables)	▪ Avoid fluoridated water ▪ Upregulate phase 2 with diet and botanicals (citations above) ▪ Create balance by addressing the toxicant exposure that is upregulating phase 1
5) Phase 2 Conjugation Unsupported	▪ Insufficient protein for amino acids and sulfur; insufficient vitamins/minerals ▪ Poor digestion	▪ Paleo-Mediterranean diet with plenty of protein (this is not the time to be a *junkitarian* or *breaditarian*)[950] ▪ Cofactor supplementation: NAC, glutamine, glycine, taurine, sulfur, whey[951,952] ▪ Custom amino acid blend for recalcitrant cases[953]

[946] "Also they inhibited the harmful enzymes (beta-glucosidase, beta-glucuronidase, tryptophanase and urease) and ammonia production of intestinal microflora, and lowered pH of the culture media by increasing lactic acid bacteria of intestinal microflora." Park HY, Bae EA, Han MJ, Choi EC, Kim DH. Inhibitory effects of Bifidobacterium spp. isolated from a healthy Korean on harmful enzymes of human intestinal microflora. *Arch Pharm Res.* 1998 Feb;21(1):54-61

[947] "In conclusion, consumption of glucosinolate-containing Brussels sprouts for 1 week results in increased rectal GST-alpha and -pi isozyme levels. We hypothesize that these enhanced detoxification enzyme levels may partly explain the epidemiological association between a high intake of glucosinolates (cruciferous vegetables) and a decreased risk of colorectal cancer." Nijhoff WA, Grubben MJ, Nagengast FM, Jansen JB, Verhagen H, van Poppel G, Peters WH. Effects of consumption of Brussels sprouts on intestinal and lymphocytic glutathione S-transferases in humans. *Carcinogenesis.* 1995 Sep;16(9):2125-8

[948] "...human CYP1A2 and other CYP enzymes involved in oestrone 2-hydroxylation are induced by dietary broccoli." Kall MA, Vang O, Clausen J. Effects of dietary broccoli on human in vivo drug metabolizing enzymes: evaluation of caffeine, oestrone and chlorzoxazone metabolism. *Carcinogenesis.* 1996 Apr;17(4):793-9

[949] Lee J. Gilbert's disease and fluoride intake. *Fluoride* 1983; 16: 139-45

[950] O'Keefe JH Jr, Cordain L. Cardiovascular disease resulting from a diet and lifestyle at odds with our Paleolithic genome: how to become a 21st-century hunter-gatherer. *Mayo Clin Proc.* 2004 Jan;79(1):101-8 http://www.thepaleodiet.com/articles/Hunter-Gatherer%20Mayo.pdf

[951] "CONCLUSION: Supplementation with whey proteins persistently increased plasma glutathione levels in patients with advanced HIV-infection. The treatment was well tolerated." Micke P, Beeh KM, Buhl R. Effects of long-term supplementation with whey proteins on plasma glutathione levels of HIV-infected patients. *Eur J Nutr.* 2002 Feb;41(1):12-8

[952] "A significant increase in mononuclear cell glutathione was also observed in subjects receiving the WPI supplement following the 40 km simulated cycling trial." Middleton N, Jelen P, Bell G. Whole blood and mononuclear cell glutathione response to dietary whey protein supplementation in sedentary and trained male human subjects. *Int J Food Sci Nutr.* 2004 Mar;55(2):131-41

[953] Bralley JA. Lord RS. Treatment of chronic fatigue syndrome with specific amino acid supplementation. *Journal of Applied Nutrition* 1994; 46(3): 74-78

Problems and Solutions in Clinical Detoxification—*continued*

Effects	Cause	Solutions
6) Insufficient bile flow	• "Normal" bile flow appears too slow to keep pace with supraphysiologic toxicant exposure	• Stimulate bile flow with rectal instillations[954,955] and botanical medicines such as *Picrorhiza kurroa*[956] and *Andrographis paniculata*[957]
7) Urinary excretion insufficient due to insufficient hydration	• Subclinical dehydration is common and is exacerbated by diuretics such as ethanol and caffeine	• Drink water and antioxidant-rich teas and juices
8) Renal pH too acidic for optimal toxicant excretion	• Western/American diet promotes an acidic renal pH[958] which is known to reduce toxicant excretion[959]	• Vegetarian or Paleo-Mediterranean diet to alkalinize renal pH • Fruit/vegetable juices provide potassium and citrate for effective alkalinization of urine[960] • Use sodium bicarbonate[961] and/or potassium citrate as needed
9) Enterohepatic recirculation	• Constipation • Excess microflora (quantitative or qualitative) producing β-glucuronidase • Leaky gut	• Promote generous laxation: magnesium, fiber, vegetables, fruit, nuts, seeds • Optimize gastrointestinal microflora • Assess and normalize mucosal integrity • Rectal instillations may be used to cleanse the bowel and to increase bile flow as previously documented radiographically[962]; this appears to improve detoxification clinical results[963,964] presumably due to expedition of toxicant removal[965]

[954] Garbat, AL, Jacobi, HG: Secretion of Bile in Response to Rectal Installations. *Arch Intern Med* 1929; 44: 455-462

[955] "Caffeine enemas cause dilation of bile ducts, which facilitates excretion of toxic cancer breakdown products by the liver and dialysis of toxic products from blood across the colonic wall. The therapy must be used as an integrated whole." Gerson M. The cure of advanced cancer by diet therapy: a summary of 30 years of clinical experimentation. *Physiol Chem Phys.* 1978;10(5):449-64

[956] Vaidya AB, Antarkar DS, Doshi JC, Bhatt AD, Ramesh VV, Vora PV, Perissond DD, Baxi AJ, Kale PM. Picrorhiza kurroa (Kutaki) Royle ex Benth as a hepatoprotective agent--experimental & clinical studies. *J Postgrad Med* 1996;42:105-8 Available on October 18, 2004 at http://www.jpgmonline.com/article.asp?issn=0022-3859;year=1996;volume=42;issue=4;spage=105;epage=8;aulast=Vaidya

[957] "Andrographolide from the herb Andrographis paniculata (whole plant) per se produces a significant dose (1.5-12 mg/kg) dependent choleretic effect (4.8-73%) as evidenced by increase in bile flow, bile salt, and bile acids in conscious rats and anaesthetized guinea pigs." Shukla B, Visen PK, Patnaik GK, Dhawan BN. Choleretic effect of andrographolide in rats and guinea pigs. *Planta Med* 1992 Apr;58(2):146-9

[958] Cordain L: *The Paleo Diet: Lose weight and get healthy by eating the food you were designed to eat*. John Wiley & Sons Inc., New York 2002

[959] Proudfoot AT, Krenzelok EP, Vale JA. Position Paper on urine alkalinization. *J Toxicol Clin Toxicol*. 2004;42(1):1-26

[960] "New Guinean hunter-gatherer tribal group living in "the primitive feral condition" ...urine pH of adults was usually between 7.5 and 9.0." Sebastian A, Frassetto LA, Sellmeyer DE, Merriam RL, Morris RC Jr. Estimation of the net acid load of the diet of ancestral preagricultural Homo sapiens and their hominid ancestors. *Am J Clin Nutr*. 2002 Dec;76(6):1308-16

[961] "Urine alkalinization is a treatment regimen that increases poison elimination by the administration of intravenous sodium bicarbonate to produce urine with a pH > or = 7.5." Proudfoot AT, Krenzelok EP, Vale JA. Position Paper on urine alkalinization. *J Toxicol Clin Toxicol*. 2004;42(1):1-26

[962] "Caffeine enemas cause dilation of bile ducts, which facilitates excretion of toxic cancer breakdown products by the liver and dialysis of toxic products from blood across the colonic wall. The therapy must be used as an integrated whole." Gerson M. The cure of advanced cancer by diet therapy: a summary of 30 years of clinical experimentation. *Physiol Chem Phys.* 1978;10(5):449-64

[963] Snyder RG. The value of colonic irrigations in countering auto-intoxication of intestinal origin. *Medical Clinics of North America* 1939; May: 781-788

[964] Gonzalez NJ, Isaacs LL. Evaluation of pancreatic proteolytic enzyme treatment of adenocarcinoma of the pancreas, with nutrition and detoxification support. *Nutr Cancer*. 1999;33(2):117-24

[965] Crinnion WJ. Results of a decade of naturopathic treatment for environmental illness: a review of clinical records. *J Naturopathic Med* 1997;7:21-27

Problems and Solutions in Clinical Detoxification—*continued*

Effects	*Cause*	*Solutions*
10) Deconjugation by microflora	▪ Excess microflora (quantitative or qualitative) producing β-glucuronidase ▪ Constipation must be eliminated[966]	▪ Botanical and/or pharmaceutical antimicrobials/antifungals to reduce bacterial load in the intestines, similar to the use of antibiotics in the treatment of hepatic encephalopathy ▪ Prebiotics and probiotics to optimize gut flora ▪ Dietary fiber may be used to promote laxation and excretion of toxicants before enterohepatic recirculation; cholestyramine may be used in selected cases to augment fecal elimination of toxicants such as pesticides[967]
11) Heavy metal toxicity 12) Metal-induced alteration of detoxification (upregulation or downregulation of specific processes)	▪ Heavy metal exposure appears to inhibit Phase 1 oxidation (*in vitro*[968])	▪ Reduce exposure to toxicants ▪ Chelation, such as with DMSA which appears effective for mercury[969] and lead[970] ▪ Promote generous laxation: magnesium, fiber, vegetables, fruit, nuts, seeds ▪ Optimize gastrointestinal microflora ▪ Fruit/vegetable juices provide potassium and citrate for effective urinary alkalinization
13) Disease promotion via toxicants stored in body tissues, particularly adipose and brain	▪ Chemical toxicants are inherently biologically persistent ▪ Defective detoxification	▪ Sauna, hyperthermia, exercise to promote sweating and lipolysis[971,972] ▪ "Fat exchange" via low-fat diet to effect weight loss followed by supplementation of health-promoting uncontaminated fatty acids[973] ▪ Weight loss for obese patients only after detoxification program is well established

[966] "Enemas and suppositories stimulate colonic contractions and soften stools. Water, saline, soap suds, hypertonic sodium phosphate, and mineral oil are used as enemas. Acute water intoxication can occur with water enemas, especially in infants, children, and the elderly, if they have difficulty evacuating the water." Dosh SA. Evaluation and treatment of constipation. *J Fam Pract.* 2002 Jun;51(6):555-9 Available at http://www.jfponline.com/content/2002/06/jfp_0602_00541.asp on October 18, 2004

[967] "Output of chlordecone in bile was 10 to 20 times greater than in stool, suggesting that chlordecone is reabsorbed in the intestine. Cholestyramine, an anion-exchange resin that binds chlordecone, increased its fecal excretion by seven times." Cohn WJ, Boylan JJ, Blanke RV, Fariss MW, Howell JR, Guzelian PS. Treatment of chlordecone (Kepone) toxicity with cholestyramine. Results of a controlled clinical trial. *N Engl J Med.* 1978 Feb 2;298(5):243-8

[968] "All four of the metals investigated decreased the extent of CYP1A1 induction in HepG2 cells by at least one of the five PAHs, in some cases decreases were marked. The same order of effectiveness of metal-mediated decreases in CYP1A1 were cadmium > arsenic > lead > mercury for all the PAHs." Vakharia DD, Liu N, Pause R, Fasco M, Bessette E, Zhang QY, Kaminsky LS. Polycyclic aromatic hydrocarbon/metal mixtures: effect on PAH induction of CYP1A1 in human HEPG2 cells. Drug Metab Dispos. 2001 Jul;29(7):999-1006 Available at http://dmd.aspetjournals.org/cgi/content/full/29/7/999 on October 18, 2004

[969] "Thus, oral chelation with DMSA produced a significant mercury diuresis in these children. We observed no adverse side effects of treatment. DMSA appears to be an effective and safe chelating agent for treatment of pediatric overexposure to metallic mercury." Forman J, Moline J, Cernichiari E, Sayegh S, Torres JC, Landrigan MM, Hudson J, Adel HN, Landrigan PJ. A cluster of pediatric metallic mercury exposure cases treated with meso-2,3-dimercaptosuccinic acid (DMSA). *Environ Health Perspect.* 2000 Jun;108(6):575-7 Available at http://ehp.niehs.nih.gov/members/2000/108p575-577forman/108p575.pdf on October 18, 2004

[970] "To conclude, awareness and early diagnosis of lead toxicity is important. Succimer is an effective chelator in patients for lead toxicity. It can be administered orally and hospitalization eliminated. However, chelation therapy should never be used as a substitute for environmental assessment and lead abatement for lead poisoned children." Kalra V, Dua T, Kumar V, Kaul B. Succimer in symptomatic lead poisoning. *Indian Pediatr.* 2002 Jun;39(6):580-5 Available at http://www.indianpediatrics.net/june2002/june-580-585.htm on October 18, 2004

[971] Schnare DW, Ben M, Shields MG. Body Burden Reductions of PCBs, PBBs and Chlorinated Pesticide Residues in Human Subjects. *Ambio* 1984; 13 (5-6): 378-380

[972] Krop J. Chemical sensitivity after intoxication at work with solvents: response to sauna therapy. *J Altern Complement Med* 1998 Spring;4(1):77-86

[973] "Repeated fasting and refeeding with fish oil facilitated plasma exchange of n-3 for n-6 PUFA, improved BP, clinical metabolic parameters and lowered platelet reactivity in the vessel wall (primary hemostasis)." Yosefy C, Viskoper JR, Varon D, Ilan Z, Pilpel D, Lugassy G, Schneider R, Savyon N, Adan Y, Raz A. Repeated fasting and refeeding with 20:5, n-3 eicosapentaenoic acid (EPA): a novel approach for rapid fatty acid exchange and its effect on blood pressure, plasma lipids and hemostasis. *J Hum Hypertens* 1996 Sep;10 Suppl 3:S135-9

Toxicant Exposure: solvents, pesticides, herbicides, plastics, fire-proofing, dioxins, exhaust, PCB, mercury, lead, cadmium, and thousands of others; the ultimate causes and therefore solutions are found primarily in addressing corporate environmental policies and influence on government regulations, societal structure/expectations regarding materialism/independence/convenience/passivity

Biological Persistence: lipolysis/redistribution; detoxification/reabsorption

lipophilic chemicals are deposited in cell membranes/adipose

metals circulate and are deposited in tissues where they impair function and thereby contribute to 'disease'

Promote lipolysis with diet, exercise, sauna

some heavy metals may alter detoxification

treatment

DMSA chelation

Phase One: activation / oxidation
Rapidly inducible by toxicant exposure and some drugs; the main clinical problems here are
1) **inhibition** by SNiPs, nutrient deficiencies, drugs, LPS, heavy metals
2) **relative excess activity**: rapid phase one in relation to slow conjugation: the body is not making a mistake here; it is simply responding to exposure; the solutions are to reduce exposure and support conjugation

Clinical Solutions:
1) nutritional supplementation and diet improvement,
2) reduce exposure to drugs and other 'inducers' including enterohepatic recirculation (check increased permeability and fecal b-glucuronidase)
3) clean the gut to restore mucosal integrity and reduce LPS and b-glucuronidase

hydration/urination, bile formation/expulsion, maintenance of conjugation, botanical adsorbents, daily defecation

failure

excretion in urine, excretion via bile flow and defecation

enterohepatic recirculation

insufficient oxidation

sufficient oxidation

sufficient oxidation

chemical toxicant accumulation: increased disease risk: autoimmunity, Parkinson's disease, cancer, multiple chemical sensitivity, adverse drug reactions

a few chemicals are excreted following Phase 1 (without Conjugation)

Phase Two: conjugation
Insufficiently induced by toxicant exposure; failure of conjugation following oxidation is highly problematic; the main clinical problems here are
1) **slow action**: phase 2 is commonly slower than phase 1; slow action can be caused by nutritional deficiencies, insufficient intake of vegetables/crucifers, and SNiPs, which are surprisingly common and are consistently associated with increased risk for disease;
2) **insufficient nutrient intake for conjugation**: recall that most conjugation factors are, of course, derived from foods: amino acids and sulphur

Clinical Solutions:
1) general nutritional supplementation and diet improvement,
2) reduce exposure to all endogenous and exogenous toxicants: drugs, chemicals, enterohepatic recirculation, hyperabsorption due to increased permeability and fecal b-glucuronidase
3) induce conjugation with cruciferous vegetables and specific botanicals
4) stimulate bile flow and bowel cleansing

insufficient conjugation

successful conjugation

excretion in urine

hydration, healthy renal function (and alkalosis)

Toxicant is solublized for excretion in bile or urine

failure of bile formation, blockage in bile flow, dehydration, dysbiosis causing deconjugation constipation promoting reabsorption, insufficient fiber

bile formation, bile expulsion, maintenance of conjugation, daily defecation

excretion via bile flow and defecation

enterohepatic recirculation

Schematic Overview of Toxicant Exposure and Detoxification/Depuration: Graphic of pathways with clinical therapeutic implications

An Outline of the Use of Dimercaptosuccinic acid (DMSA)

Therapeutic: **Dimercaptosuccinic acid**

Common name: **DMSA**

Applications and mechanisms of action:

- DMSA is a well documented chelating agent that is FDA-approved for the treatment of lead poisoning.[974] It has been used safely and successfully in children and adults with lead and/or mercury toxicity, whether acute or chronic. The sulfur-containing moiety of the molecule binds to heavy metals, rendering them soluble, and then the metal-DMSA complex is excreted in urine or bile.

A few of the better articles on this topic are listed here:

- **DMSA-mercury testing in autistic children**: Two-hundred-twenty-one children with autism were challenged with 30 mg/kg of DMSA and showed significantly higher urinary mercury excretion compared to control subjects. The specific protocol is described as follows: "The Arizona State University Institutional Review Board approved our retrospective examination of cases and controls in this study. ... Informed consent was obtained from both cases and controls for DMSA chelation treatment. Controls and cases were both challenged with a three-day oral treatment of **DMSA (10 mg/kg per dose given three times daily).** After the ninth dose, the first voided morning urine was collected (when possible), or an overnight urine collection bag was worn. All laboratory analyses were performed by the Doctors Data, Inc., in Chicago, Ill."[975] No adverse effects were reported.

- **Mercury review by Dr. Walter Crinnion**: As one of the most experienced environmental medicine doctors in the US, Dr. Crinnion provides his perspective on the treatment of mercury toxicity, and states, "DMSA can be given to an adult at a dose of 500 mg tid... DMSA (30 mg/kg)... It is generally recommended that these agents be given in several day courses repeatedly, with rest periods in between."[976]

- **Nine cases of pediatric mercury poisoning safely treated with DMSA**: Nine mercury-poisoned children were treated with DMSA 30 mg/kg for 5 days followed by 20 mg/kg for 2 weeks; mercury levels declined in all children, and no adverse effects occurred.[977]

- **DMSA monographs**: monographs on the basic science and clinical applications of DMSA.[978,979]

- **Acute poisoning review**: A "nutshell" review of the management of acute poisoning.[980]

[974] "The Food and Drug Administration has recently licensed the drug DMSA (succimer) for reduction of blood lead levels >/= 45 micrograms/dl. This decision was based on the demonstrated ability of DMSA to reduce blood lead levels. An advantage of this drug is that it can be given orally." Goyer RA, Cherian MG, Jones MM, Reigart JR. Role of chelating agents for prevention, intervention, and treatment of exposures to toxic metals. *Environ Health Perspect.* 1995 Nov;103(11):1048-52 Http://ehp.niehs.nih.gov/docs/1995/103-11/meetingreport.html

[975] Bradstreet J, Geier DA, Kartzinel JJ, Adams JB, Geier MR. A case-control study of mercury burden in children with autistic spectrum disorders. *Journal of American Physicians and Surgeons* 2003; 8: 76-79 http://www.jpands.org/vol8no3/geier.pdf

[976] Crinnion WJ. Environmental medicine, part three: long-term effects of chronic low-dose mercury exposure. *Altern Med Rev.* 2000 Jun;5(3):209-23 http://www.thorne.com/altmedrev/.fulltext/5/3/209.pdf

[977] Forman J, Moline J, Cernichiari E, Sayegh S, Torres JC, Landrigan MM, Hudson J, Adel HN, Landrigan PJ. A cluster of pediatric metallic mercury exposure cases treated with meso-2,3-dimercaptosuccinic acid (DMSA). *Environ Health Perspect.* 2000 Jun;108(6):575-7 http://ehp.niehs.nih.gov/docs/2000/108p575-577forman/abstract.html

[978] Miller AL. Dimercaptosuccinic acid (DMSA), a non-toxic, water-soluble treatment for heavy metal toxicity. *Altern Med Rev.* 1998 Jun;3(3):199-207 http://www.thorne.com/altmedrev/.fulltext/3/3/199.pdf

[979] DMSA. *Altern Med Rev.* 2000 Jun;5(3):264-7 http://thorne.com/altmedrev/.fulltext/5/3/264.pdf

[980] Greene SL, Dargan PI, Jones AL. Acute poisoning: understanding 90% of cases in a nutshell. *Postgrad Med J.* 2005 Apr;81(954):204-16 http://pmj.bmjjournals.com/cgi/content/full/81/954/204

An Outline of the Use of Dimercaptosuccinic acid (DMSA)—*continued*

Toxicity:

- DMSA has a very favorable risk:benefit ratio when used in patients without renal/hepatic impairment and who are at average or greater-than-average risk for heavy metal accumulation/toxicity. Toxicity is very rare. Some articles make fleeting mention of bone marrow suppression, but this is almost never precipitated clinically and is practically never documented in the case reports and clinical studies using DMSA for the treatment of heavy metal toxicity. Patients should be tested for hematologic and metabolic status prior to DMSA administration; a CBC and metabolic/chemistry panel is sufficient.
- Allergic-type reactions to DMSA and/or the mobilization of heavy metals, especially mercury, are infrequent but not rare. To reduce the risk of precipitating such reactions, a trial dose of 100 mg (or less for children) should be used on a single occasion to ensure that IgE-mediated allergy or anaphylaxis does not occur with the higher doses used therapeutically. Like any drug, DMSA may precipitate idiosyncratic reactions, but these are by definition nearly impossible to predict. However, since idiosyncratic drug reactions appear to reflect imbalanced Phase 1 / Phase 2 detoxification, the likelihood of such a reaction can probably be reduced by ensuring that the patient is supplemented with antioxidants, fortified with sufficient protein for supporting Phase 2 conjugation reactions, and abstinent from other drugs which induce Phase 1 upregulation. Patients with adverse reactions to DMSA should either not use DMSA or should do so carefully, such as with a lower dose or after the underlying cause of the sensitivity has been addressed.

Dosage and administration:

- <u>Screening laboratory tests</u>: Urinalysis, CBC and chemistry panel with BUN, creatinine, and hepatic markers are sufficient for assessing renal, hepatic, and marrow status.
- <u>Empty stomach</u>: DMSA should be taken on an empty stomach, preferably 1-2 hours away from food. In particular, mineral supplements containing zinc and copper (etc) should be avoided for 4 hours before and after DMSA supplementation. Generally, first morning supplementation with a delayed or skipped breakfast is ideal.
- <u>The lowest therapeutic dose is generally 10 mg/kg per day, and the highest therapeutic dose is generally 30 mg/kg per day</u>. The 30 mg/kg dose is generally delivered in three divided doses (i.e., 10 mg/kg TID); however, a single-dose 30 mg/kg dose may be used provocatively for diagnostic purposes. Lower dosage schemes are appropriate for children or those with severe sensitivities. The highest scheme may also be appropriate for children but might otherwise be reserved for adult patients who are in otherwise good health. My clinical preference is to use 10mg/kg 3 days "on" and 4 days "off" with periodic monitoring of CBC and chemistry/metabolic parameters.

Body weight in lbs (kg)	10 mg/kg dose	30 mg/kg dose (bolus or divided)
40 lbs (18 kg)	180 mg	540 mg
80 lbs (36 kg)	360 mg	1080 mg
120 lbs (54 kg)	540 mg	1620 mg
160 lbs (72 kg)	720 mg	2,160 mg (limit to 2,000) mg
200 lbs (90 kg)	900 mg	2,700 (limit to 2,000) mg
240 lbs (108 kg)	1080 mg	3,240 (limit to 2,000) mg
280 lbs (126 kg)	1260 mg	3,780 (limit to 2,000) mg

An Outline of the Use of Dimercaptosuccinic acid (DMSA)—*continued*

Dosage and administration (continued):

- Cyclical dosing: DMSA is generally "cycled" which means that it is taken for a few days, the discontinued for a few days, then resumed, etc. This can be customized per patient for ease of compliance and variations in scheduling. For example, the patient might use DMSA for 5 days of the week, taking the weekends "off", or might use DMSA for 4 days on and 3 days off, etc. Every-other-day dosing is also reasonable. Treatment is generally continued for 1-2 months.

- Plenty of water: DMSA should be taken with 16 ounces of water. An additional 1-2 liters should be consumed over the next 2-4 hours.

Additional information:

- DMSA increases urinary excretion of copper in humans[981]; if treatment were excessively prolonged then theoretically this might lead to copper deficiency. Additionally, DMSA might be useful for people with excess copper. These areas require more research.

- Co-supplementation with the following can increase urinary metal excretion and/or reduce enterohepatic recycling of toxic metals. These can be used during DMSA treatment but should not be taken within 2-4 hours of DMSA supplementation so as not to bind with or otherwise interfere with DMSA absorption and utilization.

  - *Fruit and vegetable juices*: Potassium citrate has been shown to significantly increase mercury excretion in humans when used alone and/or with DMSA.[982,983] Fruit and vegetable juices are rich sources of potassium citrate and should be consumed liberally by patients undergoing detoxification. Furthermore, since urinary alkalinization greatly increases the urinary excretion of chemical/xenobiotics toxicants[984], essentially all patients undergoing detoxification programs should increase consumption of fruit and vegetable juices as well as fruits and vegetables.

  - *Phytochelatins*: Phytochelatins are metal-binding moieties from plants and algae.[985] Clinically, doctors use phytochelatin supplementation to bind metals in the gut for enhanced excretion, i.e., to prevent re-absorption of metals that have been detoxified into the gut lumen via the bile. High-fiber plant-based diets are beneficial for the same purpose.

  - *Selenium*: Selenium (Se) has many important actions in the body, one of which is that of an antioxidant. It is generally dosed at 200 mcg per day, but doses up to 800-1,000 mcg per day are generally safe for most adults. The study by Seppanen et al[986] showed 34% reduction in hair mercury following Se 100mcg/d.

---

[981] "The Food and Drug Administration has recently licensed the drug DMSA (succimer) for reduction of blood lead levels >/= 45 micrograms/dl. This decision was based on the demonstrated ability of DMSA to reduce blood lead levels. An advantage of this drug is that it can be given orally." Goyer RA, Cherian MG, Jones MM, Reigart JR. Role of chelating agents for prevention, intervention, and treatment of exposures to toxic metals. *Environ Health Perspect*. 1995 Nov;103(11):1048-52 Http://ehp.niehs.nih.gov/docs/1995/103-11/meetingreport.html

[982] "Based on the increase in urinary Hg concentrations after single doses, compared with controls, the order of efficacy was: DMPS plus K Cit., NAC plus K Cit. and DMSA (each producing an increase of 163%), then in descending order, DMSA plus K Cit., DMPS, NAC and K Cit." Hibberd AR, Howard MA, Hunnisett AG. Mercury from dental amalgam fillings studies on oral chelating agents for assessing and reducing mercury burdens in humans. *J Nutr Environ Med* 1998;8:219-231

[983] Crinnion WJ. Environmental medicine, part three: long-term effects of chronic low-dose mercury exposure. *Altern Med Rev*. 2000 Jun;5(3):209-23 http://www.thorne.com/altmedrev/.fulltext/5/3/209.pdf

[984] Proudfoot AT, Krenzelok EP, Vale JA. Position Paper on urine alkalinization. *J Toxicol Clin Toxicol*. 2004;42(1):1-26. This is a very important paper. Posted by the European Association of Poisons Centres and Clinical Toxicologists at http://www.eapcct.org/publicfile.php?folder=congress&file=PS_UrineAlkalinization.pdf

[985] Cobbett CS. Phytochelatins and their roles in heavy metal detoxification. *Plant Physiol*. 2000 Jul;123(3):825-32 http://www.plantphysiol.org/cgi/content/full/123/3/825 This is a basic science review with relevance for plant biology that discusses the use of phytochelatins to bind metals in the plant's environment. It does not discuss relevance of phytochelatins for the treatment of heavy metal exposure in humans.

[986] "The selenium supplementation group received daily 100 micrograms of selenomethionine. Selenium supplementation reduced pubic hair mercury level by 34% (p = 0.005) and elevated serum selenium by 73% and blood selenium by 59% in the supplemented group (p < 0.001 for both). The study indicates that mercury accumulation in pubic hair can be reduced by dietary supplementation with small daily amounts of organic selenium in a short range of time." Seppanen K, Kantola M, Laatikainen R, Nyyssonen K, Valkonen VP, Kaarlopp V, Salonen JT. Effect of supplementation with organic selenium on mercury status as measured by mercury in pubic hair. *J Trace Elem Med Biol*. 2000 Jun;14(2):84-7

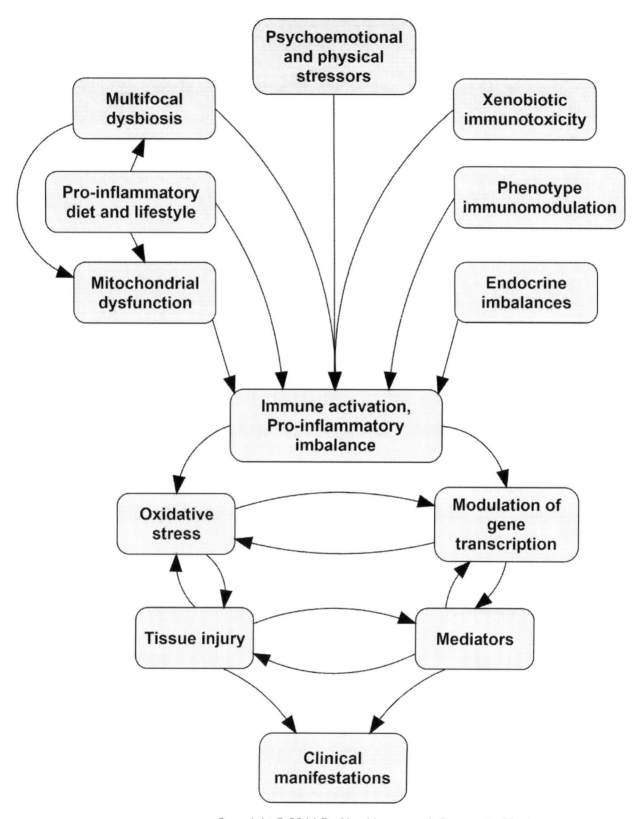

Copyright © 2014 Dr Alex Vasquez. InflammationMastery.com

Inflammation in a simple cause-and-effect diagram: The major causative factors amenable to clinical implementation are represented, along with the pathophysiologic consequences and clinical effects.

Outline the functional Inflammology protocol on this page to assess your ability to apply the information clinically:

_____

_____

_____

_____

_____

_____

Declarative knowledge: If you truly know it, you can articulate it. If you don't know it, you cannot articulate it. Conceptual knowledge must ultimately be translated into applicable and communicable knowledge; otherwise, it is not much more than "nice ideas."

"In order for a particular species to maintain itself and increase its power, its conception of reality must comprehend enough of the calculable and constant for it to base a scheme of behavior on it."

Nietzsche FW. *The Will to Power*, 1901, #480

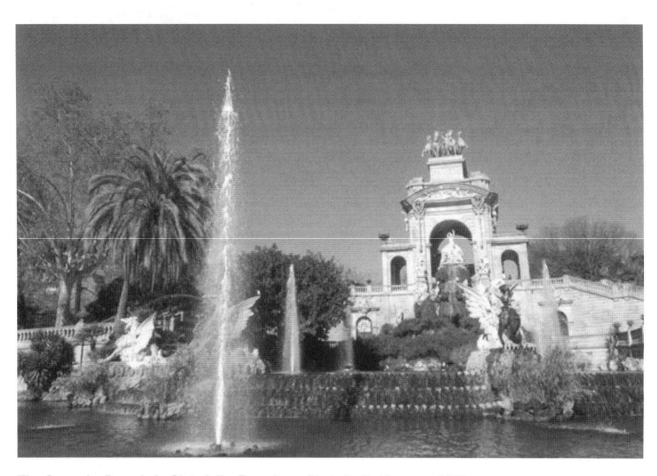

The Cascada, Parc de la Ciutadella, Barcelona: Photo by Dr Vasquez, 2013

Fibromyalgia

Introduction:
Fibromyalgia—also referred to as fibromyalgia syndrome (FMS)—is a clinical entity that has remained enigmatic to the medical profession despite the consistent publication of research that delineates its cause and its effective treatments. This chapter summarizes clinical assessments, treatments, and essential background information that should provide empowering knowledge for clinicians and for the patients suffering with this condition.

<u>Topics:</u>

- Introduction and Overview
- Clinical Presentation
- Prevalence, symptoms, and clinical findings
- Pathophysiology
- Diagnosis
- Standard Medical Treatment for Fibromyalgia
- Functional Medicine Considerations, Assessments, and Interventions
- Conditions that Mimic or Contribute to Symptoms of Fibromyalgia
- Small intestine bacterial overgrowth (SIBO) as the ultimate cause of and most logical explanation
- Therapeutic Interventions
- Conclusions and Clinical Approach

Fibromyalgia (FM)

Introduction

- **<u>Overview</u>**: Fibromyalgia (FM) is commonly described as an "idiopathic" (of unknown origin) syndrome principally characterized by widespread body pain and numerous myofascial tender points at specific locations. FM is most common in women 20-50 years of age, and the condition often presents with associated complaints of fatigue, headaches, subjective numbness, altered sleep patterns, and gastrointestinal disturbances. FM in children and adolescents presents similarly to FM in adults except for the comparatively higher prevalence of sleep disturbance and the finding of fewer tender points in children.[1] Until recently, fibromyalgia was considered a *diagnosis of exclusion* after infection, autoimmunity, or other primary causes of widespread pain were excluded by clinical and laboratory assessment. However, current criteria base the diagnosis on positive findings of chronic, widespread musculoskeletal pain in characteristic locations; these criteria will be described below. Fibromyalgia shares several clinical, demographic, and pathologic features with chronic fatigue syndrome (CFS) and irritable bowel syndrome (IBS); the reason for these overlaps is not generally understood by most clinicians and researchers but will be made plain in this writing.
- **<u>The common medical view—scientifically inaccurate, financially leveraged</u>**: The prevailing medical view, expressed by most medical doctors and the authors of widely cited articles, is that fibromyalgia is idiopathic—*of unknown origin*—with strong neuropsychogenic (*neuro*=nerves and brain, *psyche*=mind, *genic*=origin) influences (in other words, "It's all in your head.") and that, since the underlying causes of the condition have not been identified, the best therapeutic approach is symptom suppression via

---

[1] Siegel DM, Janeway D, Baum J. Fibromyalgia syndrome in children and adolescents: clinical features at presentation and status at follow-up. *Pediatrics* 1998;101:377-82

perpetual pharmacotherapy with adjunctive use of psychotherapy and limited exercise.[2,3,4] This prevailing medical view is unscientific (not based on science) and counterscientific (ignores and contradicts published and validated research), unethical (fails to provide effective treatment when such treatment is available; condemns patients to medicalization and suffering), and commercially leveraged (diagnostic criteria revision and many review articles discussing treatment are sponsored by drug companies; medical profession benefits financially by having many long-term drug-dependent patients).

- **Fibromyalgia is a disease, not a syndrome**: The term *syndrome* connotes that a cluster of symptoms is of a nonorganic, psychogenic, or idiopathic nature, whereas *disease* validates the organic and pathophysiological nature of an illness. This author advocates the use of *disease* rather than *syndrome* when describing fibromyalgia in appreciation of the real, organic, biochemical, and histopathological (*histo*=cells and tissues, *pathological*=disease) findings which clearly indicate that fibromyalgia is a specific disease entity and not simply a psychogenic or enigmatic cluster of symptoms. If fibromyalgia is a real, organic clinical entity (as will be documented here), then the appropriate designation is *fibromyalgia disease* (FMD) rather than *fibromyalgia syndrome* (FMS). For consistency and clarity within this section, the general term "fibromyalgia" will be used. Relatedly, the term "irritable bowel syndrome" (IBS) is also a misnomer that confuses professionals as well as the general public into thinking that the condition does not have identified causes and (nonpharmaceutical) treatments; despite promulgations to the contrary, the cause of IBS is well-known[5], and effective treatment is readily available.

Clinical Presentation

- **Prevalence, symptoms, and clinical findings**: Fibromyalgia is one of the most common chronic pain conditions, affecting an estimated 10 million people in the U.S. and an estimated 3-6% of people world-wide.[6] Approximately 10% of affected patients have severe symptoms resulting in partial or total disability. Affected patients report chronic aches, pains, and stiffness with a proclivity for localization near the neck, shoulders, low back, and hips. Pain and fatigue are typically exacerbated following physical exertion or psychological stress. Associated manifestations include fatigue, sleep disorders (including insomnia, unrefreshing sleep, and objective abnormalities such as an increase in stage 1 sleep, a reduction in delta sleep, and alpha-delta sleep anomaly), subjective numbness, headaches, and gastrointestinal disturbances consistent with a clinical diagnosis of irritable bowel syndrome (IBS). Clinical findings shared between FM and IBS include abdominal pain and discomfort, changed frequency of stool, diarrhea and/or constipation, abdominal bloating/distention/gas and flatulence, dyspepsia/heartburn, headaches especially migraine-type headaches), fatigue, myalgias, restless leg syndrome, anxiety, and depression. The **high prevalence (>50%) of migraine-type headaches in FM patients** suggests an underlying pathogenesis shared between cephalgia (*ceph*=head, *algia*=pain) and widespread myalgia (*myo*=muscle, *algia*=pain); one of the established and most likely causative abnormalities shared between migraine and FM is impaired mitochondrial function, which will be explained in greater detail later in this publication. Cognitive symptoms such as "brain fog" ("fibro-fog") and difficulty with memory and word retrieval, as well as **environmental intolerance (EI) and multiple chemical sensitivity (MCS)**, are seen in both FM and CFS[7]; again, this overlap of shared symptoms suggests a common etiopathogenesis (*etio*=cause, *patho*=disease, *genesis*=initiation). Routine physical examination and laboratory findings are generally normal, with the exception the physical examination finding of fibromyalgia tender points (described and diagrammed below in the section on Diagnosis per the 1990 diagnostic criteria).

[2] Chakrabarty S, Zoorob R. Fibromyalgia. *Am Fam Physician*. 2007 Jul 15;76(2):247-54
[3] Tierney ML. McPhee SJ, Papadakis MA (eds). Current Medical Diagnosis and Treatment 2006, 45th Edition. New York: Lange Medical Books, pages 820-821
[4] Simms RW. Nonarticular soft tissue disorders. In Andreoli TE, Carpenter CCJ, Griggs RC, and Benjamin IJ (eds). Cecil Essentials of Medicine. Seventh Edition. Philadelphia; Saunders Elsevier, 2007: 851-2
[5] Lin HC. Small intestinal bacterial overgrowth: a framework for understanding irritable bowel syndrome. *JAMA*. 2004 Aug 18;292(7):852-8
[6] "Fibromyalgia is one of the most common chronic pain conditions. The disorder affects an estimated 10 million people in the U.S. and an estimated 3-6% of the world population." National Fibromyalgia Association. http://fmaware.org/PageServera6cc.html?pagename=fibromyalgia_affected Accessed Sept 2012.
[7] Brown MM, Jason LA. Functioning in individuals with chronic fatigue syndrome: increased impairment with co-occurring multiple chemical sensitivity and fibromyalgia. *Dyn Med*. 2007 May 31;6:6 http://www.dynamic-med.com/content/6/1/6

Pathophysiology

- **<u>Abnormalities noted in muscle tissue of patients with FM</u>**: Muscle biopsies from patients with fibromyalgia show numerous histological, ultrastructural, and biochemical abnormalities, including defects in mitochondrial structure and function, reduced numbers of capillaries in skeletal muscle (leading to reduced blood supply to muscles), thickened capillary endothelium (thicker vessel walls), and ragged red fibers consistent with the development of **mitochondrial myopathy** (*myo*=muscle, *pathos*=disease). The histological finding of "rubber-band morphology" with reticular threads connecting neighboring cells in muscle biopsies of FM patients is associated with prolonged contractions in adjacent/neighboring muscle fibers; these abnormalities result in and perpetuate a low-energy state within myocytes (*myo*=muscle, *cytes*=cells).[8] Other studies have shown disorganization of actin filaments, accumulation of lipofuscin (cellular debris) consistent with premature muscle aging, accumulation of glycogen and lipid accumulation consistent with **mitochondrial impairment**, increased DNA fragmentation, **significant reductions in the number of mitochondria**, and focal areas of chronic muscle contraction.[9] These histological abnormalities are important and establish the fact that **fibromyalgia is a *disease of metabolic dysfunction*** rather than an *emotional disorder of psychogenic origin*; therefore, attributing the pain and fatigue of fibromyalgia to a mental-psychological cause or a central nervous system disorder such as central sensitization is unscientific and illogical.

- **<u>Biochemical abnormalities noted in patients with FM</u>**: Ultrastructural and biochemical abnormalities appear to be more pathologically significant and clinically relevant than the noted histological changes in skeletal muscle biopsy samples. Importantly, **the biochemical abnormalities *are the cause* of the histologic/tissue abnormalities**. Numerous **mitochondrial enzyme defects are seen**, including reduced activity of 3-hydroxy-CoA dehydrogenase, citrate synthase, and cytochrome oxidase. Levels of free magnesium are reduced by 31%, and levels of complexed ATP-magnesium are reduced by 12% in muscle from FM patients compared with levels seen in healthy controls; these biochemical and bioenergetic defects contribute to rapid-onset fatigue and muscle pain. From a neurophysiological perspective, magnesium can promote hypersensitivity to pain due to a reduction in the partial blockade of N-methyl-D-aspartate (NMDA) neurotransmitter receptor sites.[10] Reduced perfusion of muscle tissue during exercise results in relative tissue hypoxia, reduced muscle healing after the microtrauma of exercise, and promotion of muscle soreness due to accumulation of L-lactate (lactic acid).[11] **Increased oxidative stress** is also seen in FM patients,[12] providing additional objective evidence of the systemic, organic, and non-psychogenic nature of the illness. Evidence of hypothalamic-pituitary-adrenal disturbance and **increased cytokine production**

> ### Mitophagy: The body's inherent mechanism for the destruction of dysfunctional mitochondria
>
> <u>Concept</u>: Autophagic destruction of mitochondria is termed "mitophagy" and is the body's inherent mechanism for eliminating superfluous or dysfunctional mitochondria; this generally has a protective and life-sustaining effect. However, in the case of fibromyalgia wherein the mitochondrial dysfunction is persistent, prolonged mitophagy contributes to failure of adequate energy production and thereby contributes to clinical manifestations of fatigue, dyscognition, and impaired exercise/activity performance. Further, the consistent documentation of significant mitophagy in patients with fibromyalgia proves the biological/organic/real/pathophysiologic character of the illness and refutes the pharmacocentric paradigm which holds that the condition is of psychogenic or neurologic origin and thus to be treated with so-called "antidepressants" and/or analgesic drugs, respectively.
> - "The removal of damaged mitochondria that could contribute to cellular dysfunction or death is achieved through process of mitochondrial autophagy, i.e. mitophagy." Novak I. *Antioxid Redox Signal.* 2011
> - "Mitochondrial number and health are regulated by mitophagy, a process by which excessive or damaged mitochondria are subjected to autophagic degradation." Rambold. *Cell Cycle.* 2011
> - **"Autophagy can be beneficial for the cells by eliminating dysfunctional mitochondria, but massive autophagy can promote cell injury and may contribute to the pathophysiology of FM (fibromyalgia)."** Cordero. *Arthritis Res Ther.* 2010

---

[8] Olsen NJ, Park JH. Skeletal muscle abnormalities in patients with fibromyalgia. *Am J Med Sci.* 1998 Jun;315(6):351-8

[9] Sprott H, Salemi S, Gay RE, et al. Increased DNA fragmentation and ultrastructural changes in fibromyalgic muscle fibres. *Ann Rheum Dis.* 2004 Mar;63(3):245-51

[10] Park JH, Niermann KJ, Olsen N. Evidence for metabolic abnormalities in the muscles of patients with fibromyalgia. *Curr Rheumatol Rep.* 2000 Apr;2(2):131-40

[11] Elvin A, Siosteen AK, Nilsson A, Kosek E. Decreased muscle blood flow in fibromyalgia patients during standardised muscle exercise: a contrast media enhanced colour Doppler study. *Eur J Pain.* 2006 Feb;10(2):137-44

[12] Altindag O, Celik H. Total antioxidant capacity and the severity of the pain in patients with fibromyalgia. *Redox Rep.* 2006;11(3):131-5

(particularly interleukin-8, which promotes sympathetic pain, and interleukin-6, which induces hyperalgesia [increased perception of pain], fatigue, and depression[13]) further characterize the systemic and organic nature of this condition and are well documented in the research literature. **The majority of fibromyalgia patients demonstrate laboratory evidence of bacterial overgrowth in the small bowel**[14], and the details and important implications of this will be discussed below. **Vitamin D deficiency**—a recognized cause of chronic widespread pain as well as depression, muscle fatigue, and chronic low-grade inflammation—is also common in fibromyalgia patients.[15,16] FM patients have **significantly elevated blood levels of pentosidine**, which is an advanced glycation end-product (AGE) and marker of oxidative stress and glycosylation (sugar-protein binding); AGEs promote chronic inflammation and nociceptive sensitization leading to chronic pain.[17] Another AGE very similar to pentosidine, **carboxy-methyl-lysine (CML) is found in higher levels in the blood and muscle of FM patients**[18]; both pentosidine and CML cause expedited "muscle aging" and promote chronic pain and inflammation. These objective abnormalities of biochemical, histological, nutritional, and microbiological/gastrointestinal status force clinicians to appreciate the valid and organic nature of fibromyalgia. As previously stated, this evidence refutes promulgations espoused within standard allopathic/pharmaceutical medicine that fibromyalgia is an idiopathic condition warranting lifelong medicalization with expensive and potentially hazardous analgesic and antidepressant drugs; the focus on drug treatment to mask/suppress the pain of fibromyalgia detours doctors and patients away from focusing on the legitimate and validated causes of fibromyalgia and physiology-based (rather than pharmacology-based) means for alleviating the suffering and pain that these patients experience.

Objective "organic" abnormalities noted in patients with fibromyalgia
1. <u>Histologic and functional abnormalities in muscle tissue</u>: Disorganization of actin filaments, accumulation of lipofuscin bodies consistent with premature muscle aging, increased DNA fragmentation, and focal areas of chronic muscle contraction, reduced perfusion of muscle tissue during exercise (i.e., reduced blood flow to muscles).
2. <u>Mitochondrial defects</u>: Accumulation of glycogen (muscle sugar) and lipid (fat) indicate that intracellular energy production is impaired and that the cells are unable to efficiently convert fuel sources into energy in the form of ATP, adenosine triphosphate, which is the basic fuel source for cellular metabolism. Also noted are significant reductions in the number of mitochondria, reduced activity of important enzymes such as 3-hydroxy-CoA dehydrogenase, citrate synthase, and cytochrome oxidase. Nutritional deficiencies, such as CoQ-10 deficiency, promote mitochondrial dysfunction, thus leading to mitochondrial destruction (mitophagy) which ultimately results in reduced numbers of mitochondria and perpetuates and aggravates muscle fatigue, pain, and neurocognitive dysfunction (i.e., brain fog, difficulty thinking, depression).
3. <u>Oxidative stress</u>: Increased oxidative stress results from mitochondrial dysfunction and nutrient depletion.
4. <u>Neuroendocrine abnormalities</u>: Hypothalamic-pituitary-adrenal (HPA) disturbance indicates impaired function of the brain and endocrine system.
5. <u>Low-grade immune activation</u>: Increased cytokine production indicates a pro-inflammatory state.
6. <u>Bacterial overgrowth in the intestines</u>: FM patients nearly always have excess/overgrowth of bacteria in their intestines, referred to as SIBO—small intestine bacterial overgrowth.
7. <u>High prevalence of vitamin D deficiency</u>: Common in the general population but more common in patients with chronic pain; vitamin D deficiency causes chronic pain, depression/anxiety, and low-grade inflammation—all of these problems are seen in patients with fibromyalgia.
8. <u>Low blood levels of L-tryptophan</u>: FM patients have low levels of the amino acid tryptophan in their blood, despite adequate dietary intake. The most likely explanation for the deficiency of tryptophan is destruction of tryptophan by bacterial enzyme action. Several intestinal bacteria produce the enzyme tryptophanase, which destroys the amino acid tryptophan. Bacterial overgrowth results in more tryptophanase, resulting in tryptophan deficiency. Deficiency of tryptophan results in deficiencies of the hormones serotonin and melatonin, which result in anxiety, depression, food/sugar cravings, unrestful sleep, and mitochondrial dysfunction, since deficiency of melatonin causes reduced mitochondrial energy-production efficiency.

[13] Wallace DJ, Linker-Israeli M, Hallegua D, et al. Cytokines play an aetiopathogenic role in fibromyalgia. *Rheumatology* (Oxford). 2001 Jul;40(7):743-9

[14] Pimentel et al. A link between irritable bowel syndrome and fibromyalgia may be related to findings on lactulose breath testing. *Ann Rheum Dis*. 2004 Apr;63(4):450-2

[15] Huisman AM, White KP, Algra A, et al. Vitamin D levels in women with systemic lupus erythematosus and fibromyalgia. *J Rheumatol*. 2001 Nov;28(11):2535-9

[16] Armstrong DJ, Meenagh GK, Bickle I, et al. Vitamin D deficiency is associated with anxiety and depression in fibromyalgia. *Clin Rheumatol*. 2007 Apr;26(4):551-4

[17] Hein G, Franke S. Are advanced glycation end-product-modified proteins of pathogenetic importance in fibromyalgia? *Rheumatology* (Oxford). 2002 Oct;41(10):1163-7

[18] "In the interstitial connective tissue of fibromyalgic muscles we found a more intensive staining of the AGE CML, activated NF-kappaB, and also higher CML levels in the serum of these patients compared to the controls. RAGE was only present in FM muscle." Rüster M, Franke S, Späth M, Pongratz DE, Stein G, Hein GE. Detection of elevated N epsilon-carboxymethyllysine levels in muscular tissue and in serum of patients with fibromyalgia. *Scand J Rheumatol*. 2005 Nov-Dec;34(6):460-3

CONTROL

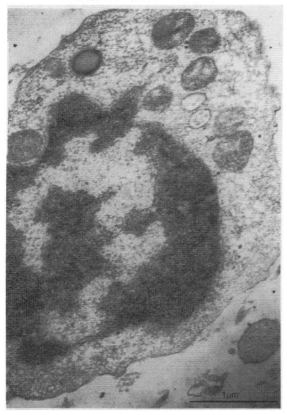

PATIENT

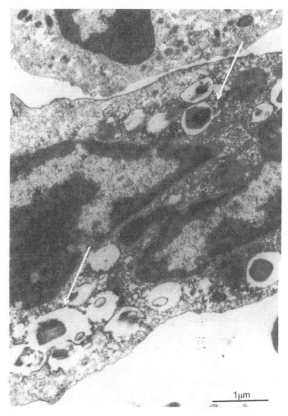

Blood cells in FM patients show mitochondrial destruction (mitophagy), as well as smaller size and lower number of mitochondria, indicating impaired mitochondrial function and reduced energy production: Structure of blood mononuclear cells (BMCs, cells of the immune system) from FM patients. The healthy/control BMCs show mitochondria with a normal structure. Autophagosomes (indicated by arrows), where mitochondria are destroyed (the process of mitophagy [*mito*=mitochondria, *phagy*=consumption], are noted in the BMCs of patients with FM. [Bar = 1 micrometer]. This open-access image is respectfully attributed to the brilliant research published by these researchers Cordero MD, De Miguel M, Moreno Fernández AM, Carmona López IM, Garrido Maraver J, Cotán D, Gómez Izquierdo L, Bonal P, Campa F, Bullon P, Navas P, Sánchez Alcázar JA. Mitochondrial dysfunction and mitophagy activation in blood mononuclear cells of fibromyalgia patients. *Arthritis Res Ther.* 2010;12(1):R17 arthritis-research.com/content/12/1/R17

Diagnosis

- **Clinical criteria—description and contrast of the 1990 criteria and the 2010 criteria**: Per guidelines published in 1990 by the American College of Rheumatology (ACR), a diagnosis of fibromyalgia can be made in a patient with inexplicable, widespread myofascial pain of at least 3 months' duration; *inexplicable* denotes normalcy of routine laboratory and physical examination findings and failure to find an alternate explanation or diagnosis, while *widespread* denotes bilateral pain above and below the waist not attributable to trauma or rheumatic disease and with pain at 11 of 18 classic tender point locations (see illustration below). FM tender points are assessed bilaterally at 9 paired sites: (sub)occiput (below the head at the neckline), low cervical spine (lower neck), trapezius and supraspinatus (two of the shoulder muscles), second rib (anterior, near costosternal [rib-breastbone] junction), lateral epicondyle, gluteal region, greater trochanter, and medial fat pad of the knees. Tender points are provoked by the clinician's application of approximately 9 pounds of fingertip pressure, which is sufficient to cause blanching of the clinician's nail bed. The tender points of fibromyalgia are distinguished from myofascial trigger points (MFTP, described by Travell[19]) and strain-counterstrain tender points (described in the osteopathic literature by Jones[20]). In contrast to MFTP, which are located toward the center of the muscle fiber and

---

[19] Simons DG, Travell JG, Simons LS. *Travell & Simons' Myofascial Pain and Dysfunction. The Trigger Point Manual*. Baltimore: Lippincott Williams & Wilkins; 1999
[20] Jones L, Kusunose R, Goering E. *Jones Strain-Counterstrain*. Carlsbad, Jones Strain Counterstrain Incorporated, 1995. [ISBN 0964513544]

which refer pain and show spontaneous electrocontractile activity[21], tender points of fibromyalgia are located near the tendinous insertions of muscle to bone and cause local pain only, without pain referral or contractile activity.

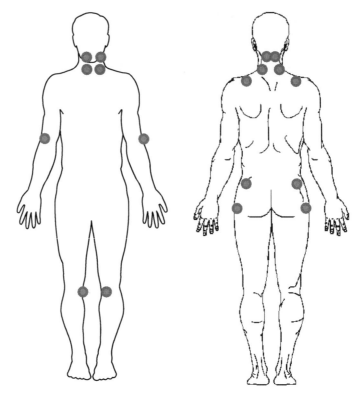

Clinical findings: Pain, on digital palpation, must be present in at least 11 of the following 18 tender point sites:

1. Occiput: at the suboccipital muscle insertions.
2. Low cervical: at the anterior aspects of the intertransverse spaces at C5-C7.
3. Trapezius: at the midpoint of the upper border.
4. Supraspinatus: at origins, above the scapula spine near the medial border.
5. Second rib: upper lateral to the second costochondral junction.
6. Lateral epicondyle: 2 cm distal to the epicondyles.
7. Gluteal: in upper outer quadrants of buttocks in anterior fold of muscle.
8. Greater trochanter: posterior to the trochanteric prominence.
9. Knee: at the medial fat pad proximal to the joint line.

Illustration of the 9 paired locations of FM tender points: Per 1990 ACR guidelines, the diagnosis of FM is supported when at least 11 out of 18 of these locations are painful. Digital palpation should be performed with an approximate force of 4 kg (9 lbs). A tender point has to be painful at palpation, not just "tender."[22]

In 2010, new ACR guidelines for the diagnosis and assessment of FM[23] were significantly changed from the 1990 guidelines. Very curiously, the authors state that one of their objectives was to create criteria that "do not require a tender point examination"; at first, this seems odd and clinically inconsistent considering that the tender point examination ❶ takes only about 60 seconds to perform, ❷ is noninvasive, ❸ was previously the standard by which the diagnosis was made, and ❹ is reasonable and responsible—physical examination of patients with pain is a reasonable standard of care. Oddly, the authors of the new guidelines note several "important problems" with the 1990 ACR criteria, such as "Patients who improved or whose symptoms and tender points decreased could fail to satisfy the ACR 1990 classification definition" and "there was little variation in symptoms among fibromyalgia patients." Clinicians should note that these so-called "problems" *are not problems at all* because patients who improve and thus no longer meet diagnostic criteria should not be considered to have an active disease/diagnosis, and that high-quality clinical criteria should indeed result in the specific definition of clinical disorder and thus in a well-defined cohort of patients; correcting these "problems" results in patients being diagnosed for longer periods of time (more *long-term* patients) and also results in more patients being diagnosed with fibromyalgia (more *total* patients). Perhaps even more curious is the fact that development of these new guidelines was sponsored by Lilly Research Laboratories, which is the "research" section of Eli Lilly and Company, one of the world's largest drug companies and the manufacturer of duloxetine/Cymbalta® which is one of the only drugs approved by the US Food and Drug Administration (FDA) for the treatment of fibromyalgia.[24] Among patients labeled with fibromyalgia, the new criteria increase the percentage of

[21] Hubbard DR, Berkoff GM. Myofascial trigger points show spontaneous needle EMG activity. *Spine*. 1993 Oct 1;18(13):1803-7
[22] The American College of Rheumatology 1990 Criteria for the Classification of Fibromyalgia. http://www.nfra.net/Diagnost.htm Accessed Nov 2011
[23] Wolfe F, et al. The ACR preliminary diagnostic criteria for fibromyalgia and measurement of symptom severity. *Arthritis Care Res*. 2010;62(5):600-10
[24] http://www.lilly.com/research/Pages/research.aspx and http://newsroom.lilly.com/ReleaseDetail.cfm?releaseid=316740 Accessed January 2012

patients diagnosable by criteria from 75% to 88%; whether the motivation to expand the patient population diagnosed with fibromyalgia is altruistic or financially motivated is subject to debate. The new criteria rely on a summation of two tallies—"widespread pain index" (WPI) and "symptom severity" (SS, parts 1 and 2)—with the diagnosis being supported by either **"WPI >7 and SS >5"** or **"WPI 3–6 and SS >9"**. Pain must have been consistent for at least three months and must not be attributable to another (obvious) cause.

Widespread pain index (WPI): Each positive location receives one point (max = 19)

1. Shoulder girdle, left
2. Shoulder girdle, right
3. Upper arm, left
4. Upper arm, right
5. Lower arm, left
6. Lower arm, right
7. Hip (buttock/trochanter), left
8. Hip (buttock/trochanter), right
9. Upper leg, left
10. Upper leg, right
11. Lower leg, left
12. Lower leg, right
13. Jaw, left
14. Jaw, right
15. Chest (sternum area)
16. Abdomen
17. Neck
18. Upper back
19. Lower back

Symptom severity (SS)—part 1: Each of the following three problems is quantified with the following scale (max = 9):

0 none: no problem
2 moderate: often present, considerable problems
1 mild: intermittent or mild problems
3 severe: continuous, life-disturbing problems

0 1 2 3 Fatigue   0 1 2 3 Waking unrefreshed   0 1 2 3 Cognitive symptoms

Symptom severity (SS)—part 2: The clinician considers the patient's "somatic symptoms in general" (listed below) and applies the following scale (max = 3):

0 no symptoms
2 a moderate number of symptoms
1 few symptoms
3 a great deal of symptoms

0 1 2 3 muscle pain	0 1 2 3 itching
0 1 2 3 irritable bowel syndrome	0 1 2 3 wheezing
0 1 2 3 fatigue/tiredness	0 1 2 3 Raynaud's phenomenon
0 1 2 3 thinking or remembering problems	0 1 2 3 hives/welts
0 1 2 3 muscle weakness	0 1 2 3 ringing in ears
0 1 2 3 headache	0 1 2 3 vomiting
0 1 2 3 pain/cramps in the abdomen	0 1 2 3 heartburn
0 1 2 3 numbness/tingling	0 1 2 3 oral ulcers
0 1 2 3 dizziness	0 1 2 3 loss of/change in taste
0 1 2 3 insomnia	0 1 2 3 seizures
0 1 2 3 depression	0 1 2 3 dry eyes
0 1 2 3 constipation	0 1 2 3 shortness of breath
0 1 2 3 pain in the upper abdomen	0 1 2 3 loss of appetite
0 1 2 3 nausea	0 1 2 3 skin rash
0 1 2 3 nervousness	0 1 2 3 sun sensitivity
0 1 2 3 chest pain	0 1 2 3 hearing difficulties
0 1 2 3 blurred vision	0 1 2 3 easy bruising
0 1 2 3 fever	0 1 2 3 hair loss
0 1 2 3 diarrhea	0 1 2 3 frequent urination
0 1 2 3 dry mouth	0 1 2 3 painful urination
	0 1 2 3 bladder spasms

Tally points from above; **patients may be diagnosed with FM if "WPI >7 and SS >5" or "WPI 3–6 and SS >9"**.
WPI = ____
SS1 + SS2 = ____

2010 Fibromyalgia diagnostic criteria—summary, chart for clinical use, discussion: Per the 2010 diagnostic criteria[25], patients may be diagnosed with fibromyalgia if "WPI >7 and SS >5" or "WPI 3–6 and SS >9". Of note, these new criteria reflect a major departure from the former criteria published and codified in 1990; of additional note, publication of these new criteria received sponsorship from a drug company which has an FDA-approved drug for this condition—this represents a massive conflict of interest, full manifestation of which would have the same for-profit entity influencing the criteria used by doctors for the diagnosis and then providing (i.e., selling for profit) one of the only approved drug treatment options. I have discussed these conundrums in video format at Vimeo.com/ICHNFM and Vimeo.com/DrVasquez.

---

[25] Wolfe F, et al. The ACR preliminary diagnostic criteria for fibromyalgia and measurement of symptom severity. *Arthritis Care Res.* 2010;62(5):600-10

- **Clinical profile and findings on common laboratory tests**: New-onset fibromyalgia is unlikely over age 50, and the condition never causes fever, significant weight loss, or other objective signs of acute or subacute illness. Hypothyroidism is common and can produce widespread myofascial pain along with depression and other complaints, resulting in a clinical picture that closely resembles FM; thus, a complete thyroid evaluation (detailed later) is essential during the initial evaluation of any fibromyalgia-like condition. Common rheumatic conditions such as rheumatoid arthritis (RA) and systemic lupus erythematosus (SLE) are excluded by the lack of other clinical manifestations (e.g., joint pain and swelling) and the lack of positive laboratory findings such as anti-cyclic citrullinated protein (CCP) antibodies and antinuclear antibodies (ANA), respectively. C-reactive protein (CRP) and erythrocyte sedimentation rate (ESR) are normal in FM patients; abnormalities with these or other common laboratory assessments suggest inflammatory disease, infection, or other concomitant illness. Hypophosphatemia (a low level of the electrolyte phosphate in the blood) can cause bone pain and muscle weakness; this condition is easily excluded by demonstration of normal serum phosphate level.

Standard Medical Treatment for Fibromyalgia

- **Overview**: Mild exercise, "patient education", and the use of pain-relieving drugs are mainstays of standard medical treatment delivered by most allopathic medical doctors (MDs), and osteopathic medical doctors (DOs) may add manual musculoskeletal treatments to enhance the benefits of drugs.[26] These interventions are only partially effective and offer no hope of actually curing the disease; thus, medical treatment relegates patients to a future of drug dependency, potential adverse effects (some of which can be fatal), and therapeutic inefficacy insofar as none of these treatments addresses the underlying cause of the disorder.

  - **Amitriptyline**: For many years, the most widely used drug for symptomatic treatment of fibromyalgia was amitriptyline (a tricyclic antidepressant), which has been used "off label"—without approval from the FDA—for this application. In the treatment of FM, the drug has low efficacy and high potential for adverse effects; up to 20% of patients suffer from weight gain, constipation, orthostatic hypotension, and/or agitation as a side-effect of the drug. Only 25% to 30% of fibromyalgia patients experience clinically significant improvement with amitriptyline.[27] According to recent research in rats, administration of amitriptyline causes deficiency of CoQ-10, impaired mitochondrial function, reduced ATP/energy production, and increased oxidative stress and free radical damage[28]; all of these drug-induced problems (discussed in detail later in this paper) are expected to worsen the pain and suffering experienced by FM patients. Thus, the use of amitriptyline cannot be considered to be consistent with the practice of good medicine due to its low efficacy and unacceptable risks for adverse effects.

  - **Pregabalin**: In 2007, the United States Food and Drug Administration (US FDA) approved pregabalin (Lyrica® sold/marketed by Pfizer) for symptomatic treatment of fibromyalgia[29]; however, because the drug does not address the primary cause(s) of the disease, patients must continue treatment indefinitely. Adverse effects of pregabalin include dizziness, sleepiness, blurred vision, **weight gain**, dry mouth, swelling of hands and feet, impairment of motor function, and problems with concentration and attention. Pregabalin when given at

> **Suicide and depression risk warning for pregabalin/Lyrica from the US FDA**
>
> "Antiepileptics drugs (AEDs), including Lyrica, increase the risk of suicidal thoughts or behavior in patients taking these drugs for any indication. Patients treated with any AED for any indication should be monitored for the emergence or worsening of depression, suicidal thoughts or behavior, and/or any unusual changes in mood or behavior."
>
> http://www.fda.gov/Safety/MedWatch/SafetyInformation/Safety-RelatedDrugLabelingChanges/ucm154524.htm
> Accessed September 2012

---

[26] Gamber RG, Shores JH, Russo DP, Jimenez C, Rubin BR. Osteopathic manipulative treatment in conjunction with medication relieves pain associated with fibromyalgia syndrome: results of a randomized clinical pilot project. *J Am Osteopath Assoc.* 2002 Jun;102(6):321-5 http://www.jaoa.org/content/102/6/321.full.pdf

[27] Leventhal LJ. Management of fibromyalgia. *Ann Intern Med.* 1999 Dec 7;131(11):850-8

[28] "Amitriptyline is a tricyclic antidepressant commonly prescribed for the treatment of several neuropathic and inflammatory illnesses. We have already reported that amitriptyline has cytotoxic effect in human cell cultures, increasing oxidative stress, and decreasing growth rate and mitochondrial activity." Bautista-Ferrufino MR, Cordero MD, Sánchez-Alcázar JA, et al. Amitriptyline induces coenzyme Q deficiency and oxidative damage in mouse lung and liver. *Toxicol Lett.* 2011 Jul 4;204(1):32-7

[29] FDA Approves First Drug for Treating Fibromyalgia. http://www.fda.gov/bbs/topics/NEWS/2007/NEW01656.html

the recommended dose of 150-225 mg twice per day for fibromyalgia costs $94-190 per month (pricing in 2013).

- **Duloxetine**: In 2008, the FDA announced duloxetine (Cymbalta® sold/marketed by Lilly) as the second approved drug for the treatment of fibromyalgia. Ironically, many physicians consider any "approved" drug to have scientific substantiation; however, in the case of duloxetine (as well as pregabalin) the exact mechanism of action is unknown[30] although duloxetine appears to inhibit reuptake of norepinephrine and serotonin, thereby increasing the action of these neurotransmitters in the synaptic cleft. Adverse effects from duloxetine include nausea, dry mouth, sleepiness, constipation, decreased appetite, and increased sweating; **duloxetine can also increase the risk of suicidal thinking and**

Black box warning for duloxetine/Cymbalta
"WARNING: Suicidality and Antidepressant Drugs: Antidepressants increased the risk compared to placebo of suicidal thinking and behavior (suicidality) in children, adolescents, and young adults in short-term studies of major depressive disorder (MDD) and other psychiatric disorders. Anyone considering the use of Cymbalta or any other antidepressant in a child, adolescent, or young adult must balance this risk with the clinical need. Short-term studies did not show an increase in the risk of suicidality with antidepressants compared to placebo in adults beyond age 24; there was a reduction in risk with antidepressants compared to placebo in adults aged 65 and older. Depression and certain other psychiatric disorders are themselves associated with increases in the risk of suicide. Patients of all ages who are started on antidepressant therapy should be monitored appropriately and observed closely for clinical worsening, suicidality, or unusual changes in behavior. Families and caregivers should be advised of the need for close observation and communication with the prescriber. Cymbalta is not approved for use in pediatric patients."
http://pi.lilly.com/us/cymbalta-pi.pdf Accessed January 2012

behavior and for this reason the drug carries a black box warning on the container. Duloxetine can cause serious and fatal adverse effects including the following: worsening depression and suicidality, serotonin syndrome, neuroleptic malignant syndrome, seizures, and Stevens-Johnson syndrome. Duloxetine given at the recommended dose of 60 mg per day for FM costs $170 per month (pricing in 2013).

- **Milnacipran**: Approved for the treatment of FM by the US FDA in 2009, milnacipran (Savella® sold/marketed by Forest Pharmaceuticals) inhibits norepinephrine and serotonin reuptake, i.e., it potentiates (increases the effect of) the neurotransmitters norepinephrine and serotonin, both of which decrease the experience of pain and elevate mood. Of course, other non-drug treatments (such as nutrients and dietary optimization) can have the same effect, but most medical doctors have no training in nondrug treatments[31,32,33,34] and thus habitually turn to drugs as the one-and-only answer

Black box warning for milnacipran/Savella
"Savella is a selective serotonin and norepinephrine reuptake inhibitor (SNRI), similar to some drugs used for the treatment of depression and other psychiatric disorders. Antidepressants increased the risk compared to placebo of suicidal thinking and behavior (suicidality) in children, adolescents, and young adults in short-term studies of major depressive disorder (MDD) and other psychiatric disorders."
http://www.frx.com/pi/Savella_pi.pdf, linked as "Full Prescribing Information" from http://www.savella.com/important-risk-information.aspx Accessed April 2012

to the patients' problems[35], especially when these are sanctified by FDA/government approval. Nondrug treatments that enhance serotonergic and noradrenergic neurotransmission include exercise, relaxation, massage, and nutritional supplementation with omega-3 fatty acids (as found in

---

[30] "exact mechanism of action unknown; inhibits norepinephrine and serotonin reuptake" https://online.epocrates.com; "Both Lyrica and Cymbalta reduce pain and improve function in people with fibromyalgia. While those with fibromyalgia have been shown to experience pain differently from other people, the mechanism by which these drugs produce their effects is unknown. http://www.fda.gov/ForConsumers/ConsumerUpdates/ucm107802.htm. Accessed January 2012

[31] "Internal medicine interns' perceive nutrition counseling as a priority, but lack the confidence and knowledge to effectively provide adequate nutrition education." Vetter ML, Herring SJ, Sood M, Shah NR, Kalet AL. What do resident physicians know about nutrition? An evaluation of attitudes, self-perceived proficiency and knowledge. *J Am Coll Nutr*. 2008 Apr;27(2):287-98 http://www.ncbi.nlm.nih.gov/pmc/articles/PMC2779722/

[32] "The amount of nutrition education that medical students receive continues to be inadequate." Adams KM, Kohlmeier M, Zeisel SH. Nutrition education in U.S. medical schools: latest update of a national survey. *Acad Med*. 2010 Sep;85(9):1537-42

[33] "Scientific advances on the relationship of dietary substances to the cellular mechanisms of disease occur with regularity and frequency. Yet, despite the prevalence of nutritional disorders in clinical medicine and increasing scientific evidence on the significance of dietary modification to disease prevention, present day practitioners of medicine are typically untrained in the relationship of diet to health and disease." Halsted CH. The relevance of clinical nutrition education and role models to the practice of medicine. *Eur J Clin Nutr*. 1999 May;53 Suppl 2:S29-34

[34] Vasquez A. Interventions need to be consistent with osteopathic philosophy. *J Am Osteopath Assoc*. 2006 Sep;106(9):528-9 http://www.jaoa.org/content/106/9/528.full.pdf

[35] Ely JW, Osheroff JA, Ebell MH, Bergus GR, Levy BT, Chambliss ML, Evans ER. Analysis of questions asked by family doctors regarding patient care. *BMJ*. 1999 Aug 7;319(7206):358-61 http://www.ncbi.nlm.nih.gov/pmc/articles/PMC28191/

fish oil), nutritional supplementation in general and vitamin D supplementation in particular. Adverse effects associated with use of milnacipran include seizures, suicidality, depression, worsening hypomania/mania, Stevens-Johnson syndrome (which is a medical emergency that can be fatal), serotonin syndrome, neuroleptic malignant syndrome, hypertensive (elevated blood pressure) crisis, tachycardia (rapid heart rate), hyponatremia (low sodium in the blood, which can occasionally result in permanent brain damage), abnormal bleeding (due to abnormal platelet function), glaucoma, and liver toxicity.[36] Treatment of fibromyalgia is the only FDA-approved use of this medication, which when used at the recommended dose of 50 mg twice daily costs $144 per month (pricing in April 2013). This drug is accompanied by a "black box warning" alerting physicians and patients to an increase in risk of suicide.

- **Cyclobenzaprine, Tramadol, and acetaminophen**: Cyclobenzaprine (a muscle-relaxing drug), Tramadol (a non-typical opioid, centrally-acting narcotic analgesic) and acetaminophen (centrally acting analgesic), show low efficacy and have little research supporting their use in the treatment of FM; these drugs also carry important risks for adverse effects, and they do not favorably alter the course of the disease over the long-term.[37] Per recent information from the American College of Rheumatology (ACR), treatment of FM with opioid drugs "may cause greater pain sensitivity or make pain persist."[38]

- **Exercise**: Low-intensity aerobic exercise may initially exacerbate symptoms but can result in very modest mental and physical improvement. Exercise alone cannot cure FM.

- **Cognitive-behavioral therapy (CBT)**: Cognitive-behavioral therapy helps patients deal with and adapt to the impact of the illness. Therapy alone cannot cure FM.

- **Patient (mis)education in standard medicine**: "Patient education" from a *medical* perspective generally means telling patients that ❶ they will probably have the condition forever, ❷ they will not immediately die from it, ❸ they need to take it seriously (i.e., comply with medical treatment), and ❹ they need to rely on drugs for alleviation of symptoms since no cause of the condition is known and therefore no direct treatment is available. From the medial perspective, these communications are considered "helpful" and "reassuring"; however, part of the effect that is created is **dependency** ("You need these drugs from me."), **passivity** ("There's nothing you can do about this, so don't even try to think for yourself or seek 'alternative' treatments."), and **co-victimization** ("We are both victims of our ignorance; I am in this with you in that we are both blind and dependent on drug management."). In the examples that follow, I will review and summarize patient educational materials from major medical journals; for efficiency, I will use quotes followed by my comments in *italics*:

  - Patient education from American Academy of Family Physicians accessed April 2012 from the website FamilyDoctor.org[39]:
    - "your muscles and organs are not being damaged." — *This is false/inaccurate information. Several primary research studies have demonstrated consistently pathologic and biochemical abnormalities in muscle tissue from patients with fibromyalgia; this research has been published in widely available peer-reviewed medical journals.*
    - "This condition is not life-threatening, but it is chronic (ongoing). Although there is no cure,..." — *This is false information (the condition is curable); the statement as it reads produces patient passivity and drug-dependency, which is exactly what the medical profession and the drug industry wants.*
    - "There isn't currently a cure for fibromyalgia. Your care will focus on helping you minimize the impact of fibromyalgia on your life and treating your symptoms. Your doctor can prescribe medicine to help with your pain,... The treatment recommendations your doctor makes won't do any good unless you follow them." — *Again, false information that promotes passivity and medical-drug dependency.*

---

[36] https://online.epocrates.com/noFrame/showPage.do?method=drugs&MonographId=4950 Accessed April 2012.
[37] Goldenberg DL, Burckhardt C, Crofford L. Management of fibromyalgia syndrome. *JAMA*. 2004 Nov 17;292(19):2388-95
[38] http://www.rheumatology.org/practice/clinical/patients/diseases_and_conditions/fibromyalgia.asp Accessed April 2012.
[39] American Academy of Family Physicians. http://familydoctor.org/familydoctor/en/diseases-conditions/fibromyalgia.html Accessed March 31, 2012

- Weak recommendations under the guise of "taking an active role in your healthcare" include 1) maintaining a healthy outlook, 2) support groups, 3) "**take medicines exactly as prescribed**", 4) moderate exercise, 5) stress management, 6) "establish healthy sleep habits", 7) make a routine daily schedule, 8) "make healthy lifestyle choices." *Most of these recommendations are blatantly passive, vague, and ineffective while fostering drug-dependency.*

- <u>"Patient Education—Fibromyalgia" from the American College of Rheumatology accessed in April 2012 from the website Rheumatology.org</u>[40]:
  - "Though there is no cure, medications can relieve symptoms."—*This is a commonly used statement within the medical community from doctors to patients to create passivity and drug/medical dependency.*
  - "There likely are certain genes that can make people more prone to getting fibromyalgia and the other health problems that can occur with it. Genes alone, though, do not cause fibromyalgia."—*These are common statements in the medical community, basically summed as "We don't know what we are doing but your only hope is to depend on us."*
  - "For the person with fibromyalgia, it is as though the "volume control" is turned up too high in the brain's pain processing centers."—*This promotes the concept of "primary central sensitization" (i.e., the brain has defied normal physiology and has somehow [without known cause, by itself] become too sensitive to pain); this "blame the brain" concept is used to leverage drug sales for pain-relieving and anti-depressant drugs as I have recently reviewed in video:* youtube.com/watch?v=41opevN87qs
  - "There is no cure for fibromyalgia. However, symptoms can be treated with both medication and non-drug treatments."—*This is the standard "party line" for the medical profession, whose chief goal is not to cure diseases but rather to drug them indefinitely, thereby creating a perpetual audience for their services and prescriptions. Honorable mention (more accurately: dishonorable mention) is generally given to "lifestyle modification" but is generally done so in a way that provides vague advice for ineffective interventions, thereby* **creating the illusion of options** *while undercutting any potential for these "options" to actually work.*
  - Non-drug treatments reviewed: relaxation, deep breathing, meditation, sleep, avoidance of nicotine and caffeine, exercise including such revelations as "take the stairs instead of the elevator, or park further [*sic*] away from the store", and "education" from other medical and special interest groups. *These are all essentially worthless suggestions, but they are effective distractions for patients and doctors so that effective treatments are marginalized and drug/medical dependency is fostered.*
  - Prescription drugs are given the primary emphasis in the treatment section. *Whether drugs are effective or not, the medical profession relies on drugs for its position in society and will therefore advocate their use.*

---

[40] http://www.rheumatology.org/practice/clinical/patients/diseases_and_conditions/fibromyalgia.asp Accessed March 31, 2012

The most common pattern in medical books and articles: components of the medical paradigm
1.	<u>Diseases are describable yet incomprehensible</u>: The condition generally is described as a complex interplay of genetic factors with numerous environmental factors; generally little or no intellectually worthwhile effort is made to understand these environmental factors, so the ultimate view that medical phycisians are taught is the the the disease is not understood and that drug therapy is the best available treatment.
2.	<u>Characteristics and diagnostic criteria are reviewed</u>: The medical profession is very good at defining and diagnosing problems, but the reliance on drugs often detours from the more effective nondrug treatments.
3.	<u>Nondrug treatments are marginalized</u>: Brief mention is made of diet and lifestyle and other non-drug treatments, but the information is nonspecific, very general, and almost always diluted to the point of inefficacy.
4.	<u>Authentic integrative and functional medicine approaches are essentially never mentioned</u>: Generally, the only nondrug treatments that are mentioned are weak or are mentioned so casually that no action can be taken from the information presented.
5.	<u>Nearly always the disease is described as chronic and incurable</u>: Even if a cure is known and published in available peer-reviewed research, most medical books and articles conclude that the causes are unknown and that drug treatment is warranted.
6.	<u>Drug treatments are emphasized</u>: Drug benefits are inflated and adverse effects are minimized if mentioned at all. Many review articles published in clinical journals are authored by consultants to the drug industry who profit from the sale of the drugs used to treat the condition about which they write; the general conclusion of these articles is that "Medical research is making considerable advances in our undersanding of Diseae X, which results from a complex interplay of genetic and environmental factors. The appropriate treatment for Disease X is Drug X, then others.
7.	<u>Hope for the future is always placed back in the hands of "more research" and "drug development"</u>: Often some mention of "hope for the future" is made, generally in the guise of "medical research" and "drug development"; all the while, safe and effective non-drug treatment approaches that go far beyond diet and lifestyle are virtually never mentioned.

Functional/Naturopathic Medicine Considerations, Assessments, and Interventions

- **Functional Medicine (FxMed) perspectives**: Two fundamental premises of Functional Medicine are: (1) chronic *diseases* are manifestations of chronic *dysfunctions*, and (2) dysfunction can result from a wide range of interconnected genotropic (gene-influenced), metabolic, nutritional, microbial, inflammatory, toxic, environmental, and psychological and social influences. **Many of these dysfunctions lie outside the narrow, pathology-based, pharmacocentric (drug-centered) view of standard allopathic medicine.** The functional medicine approach to each individual fibromyalgia patient is based on the presumption that the condition has an underlying primary cause (or several interconnected causes) and that the cause(s) can be identified and addressed. The cause(s) may be manifold and multifaceted and may differ among patients with the same diagnostic label. The FxMed approach includes the diagnostic and therapeutic considerations of standard medicine but extends far beyond these in assessment, treatment, and understanding. Clinicians trained in FxMed appreciate that as a diagnostic label, fibromyalgia is commonly applied to any patient with chronic, widespread pain and that the current trend to limit diagnostic evaluation in such patients will clearly result in failure to identify and address readily diagnosable and treatable problems that can result in a clinical picture that resembles FM. Clinicians must consider chronic infections (such as with hepatitis C virus, *Borrelia burgdorferi* [the bacteria strongly associated with Lyme disease], *Chlamydia/Chlamydophila pneumoniae*, and the protozoan parasite *Babesia*, which is also associated with Lyme disease and co-infection with *Borrelia burgdorferi*), cancerous conditions such as multiple myeloma and lymphoma, and autoimmune/rheumatic diseases such as polymyositis and polymyalgia rheumatica. A few of the other more exemplary conditions to consider in patients with widespread pain are vitamin D deficiency, hypothyroidism, iron overload, and chronic exposure to and accumulation of xenobiotics—perhaps most importantly mercury and lead.

Conditions that Mimic (or Contribute to) the Clinical Presentation of Fibromyalgia

- **Vitamin D deficiency**: A clinical picture nearly identical to fibromyalgia—chronic widespread pain, mental depression/anxiety, headaches, low-grade systemic inflammation—can result from vitamin D deficiency.[41] Fibromyalgia patients are commonly deficient in vitamin D, and indeed, **vitamin D deficiency—with its attendant pain, anxiety/depression, and normal lab values on routine laboratory**

[41] Plotnikoff GA, Quigley JM. Prevalence of severe hypovitaminosis D in patients with persistent, nonspecific musculoskeletal pain. *Mayo Clin Proc.* 2003;78(12):1463-70

testing—is often misdiagnosed as fibromyalgia, as reported by Holick.[42] Increased severity of the deficiency correlates with worsening depression and anxiety in these patients.[43] Correction of vitamin D deficiency by administration of vitamin D3 (cholecalciferol) in doses of 5,000-10,000 IU (international units) per day for several months has resulted in a dramatic alleviation of pain; such intervention among patients with low back pain has resulted in cure rates greater than 95%.[44] Other studies with vitamin D3 using doses 400-4,000 IU/day have shown that vitamin D3 supplementation for the correction of vitamin D deficiency alleviates depression and enhances sense of well-being. Vitamin D3 supplementation—or adequate endogenous production from ultraviolet light exposure (approximately 10-30 minutes per day of full-body exposure at midday, near the equator)—to meet physiological requirements of approximately 4,000 IU/day is safe and results in numerous major health benefits.[45,46,47] The only risk associated with vitamin D supplementation is hypercalcemia—too much calcium in the blood, mostly as a result of increased gastrointestinal absorption of calcium; hypercalcemia can cause abdominal pain, bone pain, fatigue, constipation, abnormal heart rhythm (arrhythmia), kidney stones, increased thirst and urination [additional details[48]]. Hypercalcemia caused solely by vitamin D3 supplementation is extremely rare; vitamin D supplementation in the range of 2,000 – 10,000 IU per day for adults is remarkably safe.[49,50] The main drug-nutrient interaction of relevance to vitamin D supplementation is with the drug hydrochlorothiazide, which is a diuretic drug used for the treatment of high blood pressure; this drug causes calcium retention by the kidney and when combined with vitamin D supplementation may lead to high levels of calcium in the blood (hypercalcemia). *Note from Dr Vasquez: I have only seen this occur one time in my clinical practice in a hypertensive patient taking hydrochlorothiazide who was vitamin D deficient; vitamin D supplementation at 2,000 IU/d caused a mild hypercalcemia within 10 days which was treated simply by discontinuing the vitamin D supplementation (also note that discontinuation of appropriate nutritional supplementation in favor of continuing a symptom-suppressing drug is generally not my preference but in this particular situation it was the best choice).* A group of conditions called granulomatous diseases—which can include lymphoma, sarcoidosis, and Crohn's disease—increase the risk for hypercalcemia; caution and more frequent laboratory monitoring must be employed when using physiological doses of vitamin D3 in patients with these conditions. Diagnosis of vitamin D3 deficiency is simple and is based upon measurement of serum 25-hydroxy vitamin D3 (25[OH]D) levels. Supplementation effectiveness and safety are monitored by measuring 25(OH)D levels and serum calcium, respectively. The two goals with supplementation of vitamin D3 are ❶ safety—avoidance of hypercalcemia or any calcium-related complications, and ❷ efficacy—serum 25[OH]D levels should enter into the optimal range of 50 – 100 ng/mL (125 - 250 nmol/L) per Vasquez[51,52] and Vasquez et al[53,54,55] as demonstrated in the illustration.

[42] Holick MF. Vitamin D: importance in the prevention of cancers, type 1 diabetes, heart disease, and osteoporosis. *Am J Clin Nutr.* 2004 Mar;79(3):362-71

[43] Armstrong DJ, et al. Vitamin D deficiency is associated with anxiety and depression in fibromyalgia. *Clin Rheumatol.* 2007 Apr;26(4):551-4

[44] Al Faraj S, Al Mutairi K. Vitamin D deficiency and chronic low back pain in Saudi Arabia. *Spine.* 2003;28:177-9

[45] Holick MF. Vitamin D: importance in the prevention of cancers, type 1 diabetes, heart disease, and osteoporosis. *Am J Clin Nutr.* 2004 Mar;79(3):362-71

[46] Vieth R. Vitamin D supplementation, 25-hydroxyvitamin D concentrations, and safety. *Am J Clin Nutr.* 1999 May;69(5):842-56

[47] Zittermann A. Vitamin D in preventive medicine: are we ignoring the evidence? *Br J Nutr.* 2003 May;89(5):552-72

[48] Mild hypercalcemia is not necessarily a problem by itself and must be evaluated within the patient's clinical context. When blood levels of calcium (normal range: 8.7-10.4 mg/dL) reach 12.0 mg/dL patients will start to develop symptoms; with levels of 14 mg/dL or higher, the patient is generally experiencing symptoms and complications and is in need of treatment (initially with administration of intravenous fluids and a loop diuretic such as furosemide).

[49] Vieth R. Vitamin D supplementation, 25-hydroxyvitamin D concentrations, and safety. *Am J Clin Nutr.* 1999 May;69(5):842-56

[50] Vasquez A, Manso G, Cannell J. The Clinical Importance of Vitamin D (Cholecalciferol): A Paradigm Shift with Implications for All Healthcare Providers. *Alternative Therapies in Health and Medicine* 2004; 10: 28-37 http://optimalhealthresearch.com/cholecalciferol.html

[51] Vasquez A. *Musculoskeletal Pain: Expanded Clinical Strategies.* Institute for Functional Medicine. 2008

[52] Vasquez A. Revisiting the Five-Part Nutritional Wellness Protocol: The Supplemented Paleo-Mediterranean Diet. *Nutritional Perspectives* 2011 January http://optimalhealthresearch.com/protocol.html

[53] Vasquez A, Manso G, Cannell J. The Clinical Importance of Vitamin D (Cholecalciferol): A Paradigm Shift with Implications for All Healthcare Providers. *Alternative Therapies in Health and Medicine* 2004; 10: 28-37 http://optimalhealthresearch.com/cholecalciferol.html

[54] Vasquez A, Cannell J. Calcium and vitamin D in preventing fractures: data are not sufficient to show inefficacy. [letter] *BMJ: British Medical Journal* 2005;331:108-9

[55] Vasquez A. Subphysiologic Doses of Vitamin D are Subtherapeutic: Comment on the Study by The Record Trial Group. *The Lancet* 2005 Published on-line May 6 http://optimalhealthresearch.com/cholecalciferol.html

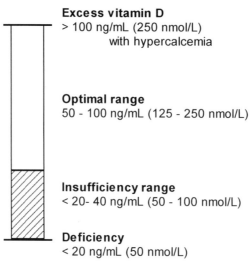

Excess vitamin D
> 100 ng/mL (250 nmol/L)
with hypercalcemia

Optimal range
50 - 100 ng/mL (125 - 250 nmol/L)

Insufficiency range
< 20- 40 ng/mL (50 - 100 nmol/L)

Deficiency
< 20 ng/mL (50 nmol/L)

Interpretation of serum 25(OH) vitamin D levels. Modified from Vasquez et al, *Alternative Therapies in Health and Medicine* 2004. Vasquez A. *Musculoskeletal Pain: Expanded Clinical Strategies* (Institute for Functional Medicine) 2008. Vasquez A. *Nutritional Perspectives* 2011 January

- **Functional/metabolic hypothyroidism**: Insufficient levels of thyroid hormone lead to an associated clinical condition called hypothyroidism (*hypo*=low, *thyroidism*=thyroid condition). Both mild and overt hypothyroidism are well known in the rheumatology literature as causes of diffuse body pain. As a cause of diffuse muscle pain, mild-moderate hypothyroidism can mimic fibromyalgia; more severe cases of hypothyroidism cause "hypothyroid myopathy" which typically manifests as polymyositis-like disease with proximal muscle weakness and an increased serum level of the enzyme creatine kinase, indicating muscle damage. In its most extreme, hypothyroid myopathy presents as muscle enlargement (pseudohypertrophy); in adults, this condition is called Hoffmann syndrome while in children it is known as Kocher-Debré-Sémélaigne syndrome.[56] Hypothyroidism is well known to cause depression and low-grade systemic inflammation; these are two findings common in FM. Another related problem commonly seen with both FM and hypothyroidism is IBS and small intestinal bacterial overgrowth (SIBO); hypothyroidism causes a slowing of intestinal motility, promoting stasis in the gastrointestinal tract which leads to an overgrowth of bacteria.[57] Detailed thyroid assessment should include measurements of thyroid stimulating hormone (TSH), free T4, free T3, total T3, reverse T3 (rT3), and antithyroid peroxidase (anti-TPO) and antithyroglobulin antibodies.

> **Terminology related to thyroid hormone production and metabolism**
>
> - <u>TSH—thyroid stimulating hormone</u>: Hormone secreted from the anterior pituitary gland to stimulate T4 and T3 production from the thyroid gland.
> - <u>T4</u>: The inactive form of thyroid hormone, accounting for about 80% of thyroid gland output.
> - <u>T3</u>: The active form of thyroid hormone produced from conversion of T4, accounts for about 20% of thyroid gland output. This is the form of thyroid hormone that is most important, because it is active and ready to stimulate metabolic processes.
> - <u>rT3—reverse T3</u>: During times of stress and also as a result of some drugs, T4 is preferentially converted to rT3, which is inactive and may actually impair the utilization of active T3. In some people, especially after a period of severe emotional stress, their thyroid hormone metabolism becomes skewed toward rT3 production, perhaps as an adaptive mechanism to conserve energy. However, increased rT3 production results in impaired thyroid hormone function and thereby promotes a clinical picture of hypothyroidism (low function of the thyroid gland) even when gland function is adequate; the problem is the hormone's peripheral metabolism, not its production from the gland.

- **Occult infections, especially with *Mycoplasma* species and *Chlamydia/Chlamydophila pneumoniae***: Clinicians are increasingly appreciating the role of occult intracellular infections in the genesis and/or perpetuation of chronic health problems, including some previously perplexing problems such as chronic

---

[56] Kedlaya D. Hypothyroid Myopathy. http://emedicine.medscape.com/article/313915-overview Accessed April 2012

[57] Lauritano EC, Bilotta AL, Gabrielli M, Scarpellini E, Lupascu A, Laginestra A, Novi M, Sottili S, Serricchio M, Cammarota G, Gasbarrini G, Pontecorvi A, Gasbarrini A. Association between hypothyroidism and small intestinal bacterial overgrowth. *J Clin Endocrinol Metab*. 2007 Nov;92(11):4180-4

fatigue syndrome (CFS), inflammatory arthritis, and multiple sclerosis (MS). For chronic *Chlamydophila* (previously *Chlamydia*) *pneumoniae* infection, testing for serum levels of antibodies is useful followed by treatment with antibacterial drugs such as azithromycin and nutritional supplements such as N-acetyl-cysteine (NAC) in appropriately selected patients; for chronic *Mycoplasma* infections, because of the various subspecies involved, polymerase chain reaction (PCR) testing appears to be preferred followed by treatment with doxycycline in adults.

- Clinical investigation: Prevalence of antibodies to *Chlamydophila pneumoniae* in persons without clinical evidence of respiratory infection (*Journal of Clinical Pathology* 2002 May[58]): The authors note that "Because there is as yet no standardization of serological criteria for persistent infection, we considered antibody titers of > 1/20 in the IgA fraction, together with **IgG titers of 1/64 to 1/256, to be indicative of persistent infection.**" This article supports clinical experience and post-graduate presentations[59] showing that in persons with fatigue and various other chronic health disorders characterized by pain and inflammation (such as chronic inflammatory arthritis[60] or spine[61] inflammation), the finding of IgG antibody levels >1:64 suggests that the patient has a persistent *Chlamydophila pneumoniae* infection which may be alleviated by the administration of—for example—the antibiotic **azithromycin** (adult dose 250 mg every other day due to the drug's long half-life, given for several weeks or months until symptoms are resolved and/or antibody titers are normalized) and **N-acetyl-cysteine** (NAC: 500-1,200 mg 1-3 times per day by mouth between meals). Positive antibody titers (levels) are common because the infection itself is common *as a transient condition*; the issue here is the determination of which patients have a *chronic* and *persistent* low-grade infection. The finding of an elevated antibody titer—that is a level greater than 1:64—indicates the need to consider long-term antimicrobial intervention.

08/29/11

```
Chlamydia pneumoniae IgG    >1:256   High      Neg:<1:16
Chlamydia pneumoniae IgM     <1:10             Neg:<1:10
```

Elevated titers to *Chlamydia/Chlamydophila pneumoniae* suggesting chronic persistent infection in a 40yo male physician *without pulmonary symptoms* but with a positive history of chronic sinus congestion and low-grade fatigue—improvement with azithromycin and NAC: This patient experienced years of severe psychologic and physiologic stress during a doctorate program and then had an acute upper respiratory illness onset in September 2010 while working in hospital emergency rooms and urgent care clinics; recurrent bouts of upper respiratory illness—attributed to viral infections—persisted for five months until February 2011. By the summer of 2011, the patient was relatively asymptomatic except for persistent sinus congestion and low-grade fatigue. No pulmonary symptoms such as shortness of breath were ever present. Following detection of the elevated antibody titer, the patient started on azithromycin and NAC as described above, which resulted in a short-term (12-hour) exacerbation of symptoms followed by complete and sustained resolution of sinus congestion and improved energy levels and exercise endurance.[62]

- Review: *Mycoplasma* blood infection in chronic fatigue and **fibromyalgia** syndromes (*Rheumatology International* 2003 Sep[63]): The author notes that "**Chronic fatigue syndrome (CFS) and fibromyalgia syndrome (FMS)** are characterized by a lack of consistent laboratory and clinical abnormalities. Although they are distinguishable as separate syndromes based on established criteria, a great number of patients are diagnosed with both." He goes on to say, "In studies using **polymerase chain reaction**

[58] Ben-Yaakov M, Eshel G, Zaksonski L, Lazarovich Z, Boldur I. Prevalence of antibodies to Chlamydia pneumoniae in an Israeli population without clinical evidence of respiratory infection. *J Clin Pathol*. 2002 May;55(5):355-8 http://jcp.bmj.com/content/55/5/355.long
[59] Stratton C. The Role of Chlamydophila in Autoimmune Disease. 2011 International Symposium -"The Challenge of Emerging Infections in the 21st Century: Terrain, Tolerance, and Susceptibility" hosted by The Institute for Functional Medicine www.functionalmedicine.org in Seattle, Washington in May 2011
[60] "This study was a 9-month, prospective, double-blind, triple-placebo trial assessing a 6-month course of combination antibiotics as a treatment for Chlamydia-induced ReA. Groups received 1) doxycycline and rifampin plus placebo instead of azithromycin; 2) azithromycin and rifampin plus placebo instead of doxycycline; or 3) placebos instead of azithromycin, doxycycline, and rifampin. ... These data suggest that a 6-month course of combination antibiotics is an effective treatment for chronic Chlamydia-induced ReA." Carter JD, Espinoza LR, Inman RD, et al. Combination antibiotics as a treatment for chronic Chlamydia-induced reactive arthritis: a double-blind, placebo-controlled, prospective trial. *Arthritis Rheum*. 2010 May;62(5):1298-307
[61] "The frequency of Chlamydia-positive ST samples, as determined by PCR, was found to be significantly higher in patients with uSpA than in patients with OA. Our results suggest that in many patients with uSpA, chlamydial infection, which is often occult, may be the cause." Carter JD, et al. Chlamydiae as etiologic agents in chronic undifferentiated spondylarthritis. *Arthritis Rheum*. 2009 May;60(5):1311-6
[62] Appreciation is given to Bill Beakey DOM of Professional Co-Op Services http://professionalcoop.com/ for provision of this laboratory assessment.
[63] Endresen GK. Mycoplasma blood infection in chronic fatigue and fibromyalgia syndromes. *Rheumatol Int*. 2003 Sep;23(5):211-5

[PCR] methods, **mycoplasma blood infection has been detected in about 50% of patients with CFS and/or FMS**, including patients with Gulf War illnesses and symptoms that overlap with one or both syndromes. **Such infection is detected in only about 10% of healthy individuals**, significantly less than in patients. Most patients with CFS/FMS who have mycoplasma infection appear to recover and reach their pre-illness state after **long-term antibiotic therapy with doxycycline**, and the infection cannot be detected after recovery. … It is not clear whether mycoplasmas are associated with CFS/FMS as causal agents, cofactors, or opportunistic infections in patients with immune disturbances."

- Clinical investigation: High prevalence of Mycoplasmal infections in symptomatic (chronic fatigue syndrome) family members of *Mycoplasma*-positive Gulf War illness patients (*Journal of Chronic Fatigue Syndrome* 2003[64]): The authors state, "…a relatively common finding in Gulf War Illness patients is a bacterial infection due to *Mycoplasma* species, we examined military families (149 patients: 42 veterans, 40 spouses, 32 other relatives and 35 children with at least one family complaint of illness) selected from a **group of 110 veterans with Gulf War Illness who tested positive (~41%) for at least one of four *Mycoplasma* species**: *M. fermentans, M. hominis, M. pneumoniae* or *M. genitalium*. Consistent with previous results, over 80% of Gulf War Illness patients who were positive for blood mycoplasmal infections had **only one *Mycoplasma* species, in particular *M. fermentans*** (Odds ratio = 17.9, P <0.001). In healthy control subjects the incidence of mycoplasmal infection was ~8.5% and none were found to have multiple mycoplasmal species."

- **Hemochromatosis and iron overload:** Genetic hemochromatosis is a common iron-accumulation disease that causes chronic persistent musculoskeletal pain, even while most routine laboratory tests are normal; thus, the clinical presentation of iron overload may be confused with that of fibromyalgia—both are common conditions commonly presenting with inexplicable (i.e., normal values of routine laboratory tests) nontraumatic musculoskeletal pain. Hemochromatosis is one of the most common hereditary disorders among Caucasians, with a homozygote (two of the same genes, results in more severe disease) frequency of approximately 1 in 200 to 250 persons and a heterozygote (only one affected gene, less severe disease) frequency of approximately 1 in 7 persons. Various other hereditary iron overload disorders affect all races, with the highest prevalence in persons of African descent (as high as 1 in 80 according to some small studies among hospitalized African-American patients).[65,66] Eighty percent of hemochromatosis patients have chronic musculoskeletal pain, which is commonly the earliest or only presenting complaint.[67] In contrast to the clinical presentation of FM, the musculoskeletal manifestations of iron overload are classically arthritic (i.e., in the joints) rather than muscular, with the joints of the hands, wrists, hips, and knees most commonly affected. However, due to the widespread distribution of pain and the normalcy of routine laboratory results, iron overload can mimic fibromyalgia. Given the high population prevalence of iron overload and the high frequency with which it presents with musculoskeletal manifestations, **all patients with chronic, nontraumatic musculoskeletal pain must be tested for iron overload.** Serum ferritin, which can be used alone or with transferrin saturation, is the best single laboratory test; confirmed results greater than 200 mcg/L in women and 300 mcg/L in men necessitate treatment with diagnostic and therapeutic phlebotomy (frequent "blood donation" is the most effective treatment for chronic iron overload).[68]

- **Accumulation of xenobiotics (including mercury and lead):** Xenobiotic (foreign chemical) accumulation may occasionally cause widespread pain resembling fibromyalgia, and xenobiotic detoxification (depuration) can alleviate pain in affected patients. Toxic chemical and toxic metal accumulation is common in humans worldwide and has been well-documented in Americans. Eight percent (8%) of American women of childbearing age have sufficiently high levels of mercury in their blood to increase

[64] Nicolson GL, Nasralla MY, Nicolson NL. High prevalence of Mycoplasmal infections in symptomatic (chronic fatigue syndrome) family members of *Mycoplasma*-positive Gulf War illness patients. *Journal of Chronic Fatigue Syndrome* 2003; 11(2): 21-36 http://www.immed.org/GulfWarIllness/10.01.11update/GWIfamilyJCFS_.pdf
[65] Wurapa RK, Gordeuk VR, Brittenham GM, Khiyami A, Schechter GP, Edwards CQ. Primary iron overload in African Americans. *Am J Med.* 1996 Jul;101(1):9-18
[66] Barton JC, Edwards CQ, Bertoli LF, Shroyer TW, Hudson SL. Iron overload in African Americans. *Am J Med.* 1995 Dec;99(6):616-23
[67] Vasquez A. Musculoskeletal disorders and iron overload disease: comment on the American College of Rheumatology guidelines for the initial evaluation of the adult patient with acute musculoskeletal symptoms. *Arthritis Rheum.* 1996 Oct;39(10):1767-8
[68] Barton JC, McDonnell SM, Adams PC, et al. Management of hemochromatosis. Hemochromatosis Management Working Group. *Ann Intern Med.* 1998 Dec 1;129(11):932-9

the risk of health problems such as neurological damage in their children.[69] Americans in general show alarmingly high concentrations and combinations of neurotoxic (nerve-damaging), carcinogenic (cancer-causing), diabetogenic (diabetes-causing), and immunotoxic (immune-poisoning) xenobiotics/toxins.[70] Adverse effects of toxic chemicals (e.g., pesticides, herbicides, solvents, plastics, formaldehyde, petroleum byproducts) and heavy metals (especially lead and mercury) are well described throughout the biomedical literature and have been clinically reviewed by Crinnion.[71,72,73,74] Among toxins with the ability to produce chronic muscle pain, mercury may deserve special recognition given its ubiquitous distribution in the human population and the scientific evidence detailing its numerous adverse effects.[75,76] Whether by metabolic, neurological, or endocrinologic means, occult mercury toxicity may manifest as a syndrome of widespread muscle pain that resembles fibromyalgia.[77]

Acrodynia is a subacute peripheral pain syndrome due to mercury toxicity classically seen in children.[78] Acute mercury intoxication can result in severe skeletal muscle damage (rhabdomyolysis).[79] Mercury in organic and inorganic forms interferes with acetylcholine reception and several crucial aspects of the sarcoplasmic reticulum, including calcium-magnesium-ATPase and calcium transport; these adverse effects establish a molecular basis for a

> **Potential benefits of reducing the body burden of mercury in patients with chronic pain and fatigue**
>
> "We suggest that **metal-driven inflammation** may affect the hypothalamic-pituitary-adrenal axis (HPA axis) and indirectly trigger psychosomatic multisymptoms characterizing **chronic fatigue syndrome, fibromyalgia,** and other diseases of unknown etiology."
>
> Sterzl I, et al. Mercury and nickel allergy: risk factors in fatigue and autoimmunity. *Neuro Endocrinol Lett.* 1999

mercurial myopathy (mercury-induced muscle disease).[80,81] The toxicity of mercury is greatly increased by simultaneous accumulation of lead, elevated levels of which are also common in the U.S. population. Demonstration of high mercury and lead levels in urine following administration of a chelating agent such as dimercaptosuccinic acid (DMSA) can be used to diagnose chronic mercury or lead overload, and orally administered DMSA is also used for treatment.[82,83,84,85] Failure to preadminister a chelating agent prior to measurement of urine mercury renders the test insensitive for chronic accumulation and can thus give the false impression that mercury is not contributory to fibromyalgia, as concluded by Kotter et al.[86] Orally administered selenium, phytochelatins (metal-binding peptides from plants[87]), a high-fiber diet, and potassium citrate can be used to augment mercury excretion.[88]

- Case report: Therapeutic detoxification to reduce the body burden of toxic metals (lead and mercury) in a woman diagnosed with FM leads to complete relief of FM symptoms: This 54-year-old athletic female with healthy diet, lifestyle, and supportive relationship presented with chronic diffuse musculoskeletal pain. Health history was significant for decades of environmental illness/intolerance (EI) also known as multiple chemical sensitivity (MCS). Family history was positive for maternal temporal (giant cell) arteritis, an autoimmune disease characterized by inflamed arteries in the neck,

[69] "However, approximately 8% of women had concentrations higher than the US Environmental Protection Agency's recom-mended reference dose (5.8 μg/L), below which exposures are considered to bewith-out adverse effects." Schober SE,et al. Blood mercury levels in US children and women of childbearing age,1999-2000.*JAMA*2003;289:1667-74

[70] Kristin S. Schafer, Margaret Reeves, Skip Spitzer, Susan E. Kegley. Chemical Trespass: Pesticides in Our Bodies and Corporate Accountability. Pesticide Action Network North America. May 2004 Available at http://www.panna.org/ on August 1, 2004 See also: Body Burden: The Pollution in People. http://ewg.org/ 2006 Feb

[71] Crinnion WJ. Environmental medicine, part one: the human burden of environmental toxins and their common health effects. *Altern Med Rev.* 2000 Feb;5(1):52-63

[72] Crinnion WJ. Environmental medicine, part 2 - health effects of and protection from ubiquitous airborne solvent exposure. *Altern Med Rev.* 2000 Apr;5(2):133-43

[73] Crinnion WJ. Environmental medicine, part three: long-term effects of chronic low-dose mercury exposure. *Altern Med Rev.* 2000 Jun;5(3):209-23

[74] Crinnion WJ. Environmental medicine, part 4: pesticides - biologically persistent and ubiquitous toxins. *Altern Med Rev.* 2000 Oct;5(5):432-47

[75] Elemental Mercury Vapor Poisoning -- North Carolina, 1988. http://www.cdc.gov/mmwr/preview/mmwrhtml/00001499.htm

[76] Shih H, Gartner JC Jr. Weight loss, hypertension, weakness, and limb pain in an 11-year-old boy. *J Pediatr.* 2001 Apr;138(4):566-9

[77] Sterzl I, Prochazkova J, Hrda P, et al. Mercury and nickel allergy: risk factors in fatigue and autoimmunity. *Neuro Endocrinol Lett.* 1999;20:221-8

[78] Padlewska KK. Acrodynia. Last Updated: February 15, 2007 eMedicine http://www.emedicine.com/derm/topic592.htm Accessed October 25, 2007

[79] Chugh KS, Singhal PC, Uberoi HS. Rhabdomyolysis and renal failure in acute mercuric chloride poisoning. *Med J Aust.* 1978 Jul 29;2(3):125-6

[80] Chiu VC, Mouring D, Haynes DH. Action of mercurials on the active and passive transport properties of sarcoplasmic reticulum. *J Bioenerg Biomembr.* 1983 Feb;15(1):13-25

[81] Shamoo AE, Maclennan DH, Elderfrawi ME. Differential effects of mercurial compounds on excitable tissues. *Chem Biol Interact.* 1976 Jan;12(1):41-52

[82] Kalra V, et al. Succimer in Symptomatic Lead Poisoning. *Indian Pediatrics* 2002; 39:580-585 http://www.indianpediatrics.net/june2002/june-580-585.htm

[83] Bradstreet J, Geier DA, Kartzinel JJ, Adams JB, Geier MR. A case-control study of mercury burden in children with autistic spectrum disorders. *Journal of American Physicians and Surgeons* 2003; 8: 76-79 http://www.jpands.org/vol8no3/geier.pdf

[84] Forman J, Moline J, Cernichiari E, et al. A cluster of pediatric metallic mercury exposure cases treated with meso-2,3-dimercaptosuccinic acid (DMSA). *Environ Health Perspect.* 2000 Jun;108(6):575-7 http://ehp.niehs.nih.gov/docs/2000/108p575-577forman/abstract.html

[85] Miller AL. Dimercaptosuccinic acid (DMSA), a non-toxic, water-soluble treatment for heavy metal toxicity. *Altern Med Rev.* 1998 Jun;3(3):199-207

[86] Kotter I, Durk H, Saal JG, et al. Mercury exposure from dental amalgam fillings in the etiology of primary fibromyalgia. *J Rheumatol.* 1995;22:2194-5

[87] Cobbett CS. Phytochelatins and their roles in heavy metal detoxification. *Plant Physiol.* 2000;123:825-32 plantphysiol.org/content/123/3/825

[88] Vasquez A. *Musculoskeletal Pain: Expanded Clinical Strategies:* published in 2008 by the Institute for Functional Medicine

head, and shoulders. Physical examination revealed numerous tender points consistent with fibromyalgia. The patient's history and stool analysis (comprehensive bacteriology and parasitology, tests for intestinal "infections") were unremarkable and unsupportive of either identifiable infection or nonspecific bacterial overgrowth. Laboratory investigations revealed normal results for hsCRP (high-sensitivity c-reactive protein, a marker for inflammation), CK (creatine kinase, a marker of muscle damage and myositis), ANA (anti-nuclear antibodies, elevated in many autoimmune diseases such as lupus/SLE), vitamin D, calcium, phosphorus, and comprehensive thyroid evaluation. The patient was then (defensively) referred to an excellent osteopathic medical internist who diagnosed the patient with fibromyalgia. The patient was unsatisfied with the diagnosis of FM and returned to the current author, who then performed urine heavy metal testing provoked with 10 mg per kilogram of dimercaptosuccinic acid (DMSA). Results revealed the highest levels of lead and mercury encountered in the author's practice at that time. As in the accompanying lab results, lead levels were 6x above the reference range and mercury levels were 7x above the reference range. The patient was commenced on DMSA 10 mg/kg/d three days "on" and 4 days "off" (cyclic dosing is used to avoid toxicity in general and bone marrow toxicity [neutropenia] in particular), selenium 800 mcg/d to promote excretion of toxic metals and to support renal and antioxidant protection, vegetable juices to provide potassium and citrate for urinary alkalinization and enhanced excretion of xenobiotics[89], and a proprietary phytochelatin (metal-binding peptides from plants) concentrate to bind toxic metals in the gut and thereby promote their fecal excretion by blocking enterohepatic recycling/recirculation. DMSA chelation is approved by the US Food and Drug Administration (FDA) for the treatment of lead toxicity in children.[90] The use of DMSA for children and adults is supported by peer-reviewed literature[91,92,93,94,95] and has been reviewed in more detail by this author in *Integrative Rheumatology*.[96] After approximately 8 months of treatment, the patient was completely free of pain, and the clinical improvement was associated with a reduction in both lead and mercury of approximately 50% as demonstrated by follow-up laboratory testing. This case was published in peer-reviewed literature for continuing education credits for physicians.[97]

Date Completed: 10/22/2005

Lead	30	<	5
Mercury	21	<	3

Date Completed: 6/30/2006

Lead	15	<	5
Mercury	8.2	<	4

Marked accumulation of lead and mercury in a patient diagnosed with FM—complete elimination of pain and stiffness following identification and reduction in the body burden of lead and mercury: *Presentation*: 54yo woman presents with nontraumatic widespread pain consistent with a diagnosis of fibromyalgia; the diagnosis of FM is confirmed by two clinicians. All laboratory test results were normal except for urine toxic metal testing which showed 6x elevations of lead and 7x elevations of mercury. Treatment for lead and mercury toxicity was started as described above and the patient experienced safe and effective alleviation of all pain after 8 months of treatment; reductions in pain correlated directly with reductions in body burden of lead and mercury.

[89] CrinnionWJ.Environmental medicine, part3:long-term effects of chronic low-dose mercury exposure.*AlternMedRev*2000Jun;5:209-23
[90] "The Food and Drug Administration has recently licensed the drug DMSA (succimer) for reduction of blood lead levels >/= 45 micrograms/dl. This decision was based on the demonstrated ability of DMSA to reduce blood lead levels. An advantage of this drug is that it can be given orally." Goyer RA, Cherian MG, Jones MM, Reigart JR. Role of chelating agents for prevention, intervention, and treatment of exposures to toxic metals. *Environ Health Perspect*. 1995 Nov;103(11):1048-52
[91] Bradstreet et al. A case-control study of mercury burden in children with autistic spectrum disorders. *Journal of American Physicians and Surgeons* 2003; 8: 76-79
[92] Crinnion WJ. Environmental medicine, part three: long-term effects of chronic low-dose mercury exposure. *Altern Med Rev*. 2000 Jun;5(3):209-23
[93] Forman J, Moline J, Cernichiari E, et al. A cluster of pediatric metallic mercury exposure cases treated with meso-2,3-dimercaptosuccinic acid (DMSA). *Environ Health Perspect*. 2000 Jun;108(6):575-7 http://ehp.niehs.nih.gov/docs/2000/108p575-577forman/abstract.html
[94] Miller AL. Dimercaptosuccinic acid (DMSA), a non-toxic, water-soluble treatment for heavy metal toxicity. *Altern Med Rev*. 1998 Jun;3(3):199-207
[95] DMSA. *Altern Med Rev*. 2000 Jun;5(3):264-7 http://thorne.com/altmedrev/.fulltext/5/3/264.pdf
[96] Vasquez A. *Integrative Rheumatology*. IBMRC 2006, 2007 and all future editions. http://optimalhealthresearch.com/rheumatology.html
[97] Vasquez A. *Musculoskeletal Pain: Expanded Clinical Strategies*. Institute for Functional Medicine. 2008

Small intestine bacterial overgrowth (SIBO) is the ultimate cause of and most logical explanation for FM:

- Small intestine bacterial overgrowth (SIBO)—also referred to as "intestinal bacterial overgrowth" or simply "bacterial overgrowth"—provides the single best model for explaining the clinical and pathophysiological manifestations of fibromyalgia. Although commonly underappreciated by many clinicians, SIBO is common in clinical practice, affecting for example approximately 40% of patients with rheumatoid arthritis, 84% of patients with IBS, and 90% to 100% of patients with fibromyalgia. **In a study of 42 fibromyalgia patients, all 42 FM patients showed laboratory evidence of SIBO, and the severity of the intestinal bacterial overgrowth correlated positively with the severity of the fibromyalgia**, thus indicating the plausibility of a causal relationship.[98] The links between fibromyalgia and IBS are also strong; **most IBS patients meet strict diagnostic criteria for fibromyalgia, and most fibromyalgia patients meet strict criteria for IBS**. Lubrano et al[99] showed that fibromyalgia severity correlated with IBS severity among patients who met strict diagnostic criteria for both conditions. The high degree of overlap between these two diagnostic labels suggests that these conditions are two variations of a common pathophysiological process—SIBO.[100] SIBO causes altered bowel function, immune activation, and visceral hypersensitivity, and it is the best causative explanation for the clinical and pathophysiological manifestations of IBS; for more details and citations, see the excellent review by Lin published in *Journal of the American Medical Association* in 2004.[101] IBS is characterized by *visceral* hyperalgesia (hypersensitivity to pain), just as fibromyalgia is characterized by *skeletal muscle* hyperalgesia. Given that strong evidence indicates that IBS is caused by SIBO and that IBS and fibromyalgia are variations of the same pathophysiological process, then fibromyalgia may therefore be caused by SIBO. However, these links and interconnections require substantiation, as provided below.

What is the evidence linking fibromyalgia with SIBO? What are the molecular mechanisms by which absorbed toxins and metabolites from SIBO can contribute to muscle pain and the mitochondrial/ATP/energy defects and the muscle tissue abnormalities seen in fibromyalgia patients?

1. <u>Small intestine bacterial overgrowth is highly prevalent in fibromyalgia</u>: Several studies have shown that 90% to 100% of fibromyalgia patients have evidence of SIBO; such a strong correlation and the dose-response relationship imply causality and must be integrated into any science-based model of fibromyalgia.

    - <u>Clinical study: Patients with FM have evidence of frequent and severe bacterial overgrowth in the intestines</u> (*Annals of the Rheumatic Diseases* 2004 Apr[102]): The **breath hydrogen test** is used for the detection of SIBO and involves orally administering a carbohydrate (such as lactulose, a source of sugar for bacteria) which is converted to hydrogen through bacterial fermentation; the exhaled hydrogen in the breath is measured as an indirect quantification of the amount of bacteria in the intestines. In this study, 20% of "healthy" control patients were found to have intestinal bacterial overgrowth via an abnormal hydrogen breath test compared with 93/111 (84%) subjects with IBS and **42/42 (100%) with fibromyalgia**. Subjects with fibromyalgia had higher hydrogen production (indicating more severe SIBO), peak hydrogen, and area under the curve than subjects with IBS. **The degree of somatic pain in fibromyalgia correlates significantly with the hydrogen level seen on the breath test.**

2. <u>Fibromyalgia is tightly correlated with irritable bowel syndrome, a condition caused by small intestine bacterial overgrowth</u>: Fibromyalgia and IBS are strongly convergent, and the evidence

---

[98] Pimentel M, Wallace D, Hallegua D, Chow E, Kong Y, Park S, Lin HC. A link between irritable bowel syndrome and fibromyalgia may be related to findings on lactulose breath testing. *Ann Rheum Dis.* 2004 Apr;63(4):450-2

[99] Lubrano E, et al. Fibromyalgia in patients with irritable bowel syndrome. An association with the severity of the intestinal disorder. *Int J Colorectal Dis.* 2001 Aug;16(4):211-5

[100] Veale D, Kavanagh G, Fielding JF, Fitzgerald O. Primary fibromyalgia and the irritable bowel syndrome: different expressions of a common pathogenetic process. *Br J Rheumatol.* 1991 Jun;30(3):220-2

[101] Lin HC. Small intestinal bacterial overgrowth: a framework for understanding irritable bowel syndrome. *JAMA.* 2004 Aug 18;292(7):852-8

[102] Pimentel M, Wallace D, Hallegua D, Chow E, Kong Y, Park S, Lin HC. A link between irritable bowel syndrome and fibromyalgia may be related to findings on lactulose breath testing. *Ann Rheum Dis.* 2004 Apr;63(4):450-2

indicates that IBS is caused largely or completely by SIBO; again, for more details and citations, see the brilliant article by Lin, cited previously.

3. <u>Small intestine bacterial overgrowth leads to systemic absorption of toxins that impair brain/nerve and muscle/mitochondrial function</u>: SIBO is associated with overproduction and absorption of bacterial cellular debris (e.g., lipopolysaccharide [LPS], bacterial DNA, peptidoglycans, teichoic acid, exotoxins) and antimetabolites—substances which are directly toxic to cellular energy/ATP production and muscle and nerve function—such as D-lactic acid, tyramine, tartaric acid, hydrogen sulfide. Intestinal gram-negative bacteria produce endotoxin (also known as lipopolysaccharide, LPS), which impairs skeletal muscle energy/ATP production (by stimulating skeletal muscle sodium-potassium-ATPase). Endotoxin also raises blood lactate (indicating impaired cellular energy production) under aerobic conditions in humans.[103] **Thus, via direct and indirect effects on cellular metabolism, chronic low-dose bacterial LPS/endotoxin exposure can result in impaired muscle metabolism and reduced ATP synthesis via impairment of mitochondrial function.** Intestinal bacteria also produce D-lactate, a well-known metabolic toxin in humans; SIBO often results in variable levels of D-lactate acidosis, severe cases of which can progress from fatigue and malaise to encephalopathy (e.g., confusion, ataxia, slurred speech, altered mental status) and death.[104] Supporting the proposal that bacterial overgrowth with D-lactate-producing bacteria is a contributor to the chronic fatigue syndromes including fibromyalgia is an excellent study published in 2009 showing that **patients with chronic fatigue syndrome have intestinal overgrowth of bacteria that produce the cellular toxin D-lactate**; specifically the research showed that these chronic fatigue patients have **a 7-fold increase in D-lactate producing *Enterococcus* and 1,100-fold increase in D-lactate producing *Streptococcus*.** Energy/ATP underproduction and lactate overproduction cause muscle fatigue and muscle pain. An additional cellular toxin produced by intestinal bacteria is hydrogen sulfide (H2S), which causes DNA damage[105] (noted previously to be increased in fibromyalgia patients) and which impairs cellular energy production, a finding relevant to *but not necessarily limited to* the pathogenesis of ulcerative colitis.[106,107] Bacteria and yeast in the intestines produce H2S, which can bind to the mitochondrial enzyme cytochrome c oxidase (part of Complex IV of the electron transport chain), thereby impairing oxidative phosphorylation and ATP production; this may partly explain the association of gastrointestinal dysbiosis and small intestine bacterial overgrowth (SIBO) with conditions such as chronic fatigue syndrome (CFS) and fibromyalgia.[108]

    ▫ <u>Experimental study: Effect of *E. coli* endotoxin on mitochondrial form and function. (*Annals of Surgery* 1971 Dec[109])</u>: Authors of this paper show that treatment of normal rat liver mitochondria with *E. coli* endotoxin results in mitochondrial impairment. They note previous research showing that animal exposure to *E. coli* endotoxin causes inhibition of mitochondrial respiration and uncoupling of oxidative phosphorylation. Near their conclusion, the authors write, "Thus we have evidence to show that topical ***E. coli* endotoxin has pathologic effects on both membrane integrity and internal mechanochemical systems of isolated mitochondria.**" Readers should appreciate that *E. coli* is a common inhabitant of the gastrointestinal tract of humans and that its population is quantitatively increased during states of bacterial overgrowth of the small bowel, as is commonly seen in most patients with fibromyalgia. More recently, research has shown that impairment of mitochondrial function (noted in patients with fibromyalgia) can lead to destruction of

[103] Bundgaard H, Kjeldsen K, Suarez Krabbe K, van Hall G, Simonsen L, Qvist J, Hansen CM, Moller K, Fonsmark L, Lav Madsen P, Klarlund Pedersen B. Endotoxemia stimulates skeletal muscle Na+-K+-ATPase and raises blood lactate under aerobic conditions in humans. *Am J Physiol Heart Circ Physiol.* 2003 Mar;284(3):H1028-34
[104] Vella A, Farrugia G. D-lactic acidosis: pathologic consequence of saprophytism. *Mayo Clin Proc.* 1998 May;73(5):451-6
[105] Attene-Ramos MS, Wagner ED, Gaskins HR, Plewa MJ. Hydrogen sulfide induces direct radical-associated DNA damage. *Mol Cancer Res.* 2007 May;5(5):455-9
[106] Magee EA, Richardson CJ, Hughes R, Cummings JH. Contribution of dietary protein to sulfide production in the large intestine: an in vitro and a controlled feeding study in humans. *Am J Clin Nutr.* 2000 Dec;72(6):1488-94
[107] Babidge W, Millard S, Roediger W. Sulfides impair short chain fatty acid beta-oxidation at acyl-CoA dehydrogenase level in colonocytes: implications for ulcerative colitis. *Mol Cell Biochem.* 1998 Apr;181(1-2):117-24
[108] Lemle MD. Hypothesis: chronic fatigue syndrome is caused by dysregulation of hydrogen sulfide metabolism. *Med Hypotheses.* 2009 Jan;72(1):108-9
[109] White RR 4th, Mela L, Miller LD, Berwick L. Effect of E. coli endotoxin on mitochondrial form and function: inability to complete succinate-induced condensed-to-orthodox conformational change. *Ann Surg.* 1971 Dec;174(6):983-90

mitochondria by a process termed "mitophagy" (noted in patients with fibromyalgia); over time, loss of mitochondria via mitophagy leads to reduced numbers of mitochondria in muscle and other tissues (noted in patients with fibromyalgia) and contributes to the fatigue and other symptoms which characterize FM.

▫ Clinical study: Increased D-lactic acid intestinal bacteria in patients with chronic fatigue syndrome (*In Vivo* 2009 Jul-Aug[110]): This excellent clinical research fully supports the pathoetiologic (disease causation) model presented in this chapter, which is derived and updated from a previous publication by this author: Vasquez A. *Musculoskeletal Pain: Expanded Clinical Strategies* published by the Institute for Functional Medicine in 2008. The authors of this 2009 study state in the summary of their research, "Patients with chronic fatigue syndrome (CFS) are affected by symptoms of cognitive dysfunction and neurological impairment, the cause of which has yet to be elucidated. However, these symptoms are strikingly similar to those of patients presented with D-lactic acidosis. A significant increase of Gram-positive facultative anaerobic fecal microorganisms in 108 CFS patients as compared to 177 control subjects is presented in this report. The viable count of D-lactic acid producing *Enterococcus* and *Streptococcus* spp. in the fecal samples from the CFS group ($3.5 \times 10^{(7)}$ cfu [colony forming units]/L and $9.8 \times 10^{(7)}$ cfu/L respectively) were significantly higher than those for the control group ($5.0 \times 10^{(6)}$ cfu/L and $8.9 \times 10^{(4)}$ cfu/L respectively). **[Note: This is approximately a 7x increase in D-lactate producing *Enterococcus* and 1,100x increase in D-lactate producing *Streptococcus*.]** Analysis of exometabolic profiles of *Enterococcus faecalis* and

> **Patients with "chronic fatigue syndrome" and the associated neurologic dysfunction and muscle dysfunction have intestinal overgrowth of bacteria that produce D-lactic acid, a known neurotoxin and metabolic poison**
>
> In 2007 and 2008, the current author (AV) wrote and published *Musculoskeletal Pain: Expanded Clinical Strategies** with the Institute for Functional Medicine; this chapter on fibromyalgia is derived and updated from that work. In that publication, I reviewed evidence that fibromyalgia—at that time considered mysterious, idiopathic, chronic, relentless, and treatable only by pain-relieving drugs—was most likely caused by small intestine bacterial overgrowth (SIBO) and the resultant absorption of metabolic toxins and immunogenic debris. This perspective has been supported by numerous publications, particularly the article published by Sheedy et al** in 2009, which showed for the first time that patients with chronic fatigue syndrome—a condition tightly correlated with and which often overlaps with fibromyalgia—have SIBO with various bacteria that are high-output producers of D-lactic acid, a known neurotoxin and metabolic poison which potentially contributes to many of the main clinical, biochemical, and histologic manifestations of FM, namely mental fatigue and dyscognition (difficulty thinking), muscle fatigue and pain, biochemical evidence of mitochondrial impairment, and histologic evidence of mitochondrial myopathy.
>
> *Vasquez A. *Musculoskeletal Pain: Expanded Clinical Strategies*. Institute for Functional Medicine, 2008.
> **Sheedy, et al. Increased d-lactic acid intestinal bacteria in patients with chronic fatigue syndrome. *In Vivo*. 2009 Jul

Streptococcus sanguinis, representatives of *Enterococcus* and *Streptococcus* spp. respectively, by NMR and HPLC showed that these organisms produced significantly more lactic acid from (13)C-labeled glucose, than the Gram negative *Escherichia coli*. Further, **both E. faecalis and S. sanguinis secrete more D-lactic acid than E. coli.** This study suggests a probable link between intestinal colonization of Gram-positive facultative anaerobic D-lactic acid bacteria and symptom expressions in a subgroup of patients with CFS. Given the fact that **this might explain not only neurocognitive dysfunction in CFS patients but also mitochondrial dysfunction, these findings may have important clinical implications.**"

---

[110] Sheedy JR, Wettenhall RE, Scanlon D, et al. Increased d-lactic acid intestinal bacteria in patients with chronic fatigue syndrome. *In Vivo*. 2009 Jul-Aug;23(4):621-8

5. <u>Bacterial LPS and other antigens absorbed from the intestine during SIBO contribute to a subclinical inflammatory state that results in pain hypersensitivity and increased cytokine release, both of which are characteristics of fibromyalgia</u>: In animal models and in human research studies, exposure to bacterial endotoxin/LPS has been shown to increase the brain's sensitivity to and perception of pain. Immune-mediated and inflammation-mediated pathways that promote pain sensitivity and pain perception include ❶ reduced production of nitric oxide with ❷ increased production of prostaglandins and cytokines, resulting in ❸ the sensitization of peripheral and/or central neurons to pain perception/transmission. In support of this concept, Lin[111] wrote in 2004, "**The immune response to bacterial antigen in SIBO provides a framework for understanding the hypersensitivity in both fibromyalgia and IBS.**" A later paper by Othmanm, Agüero, and Lin[112] in 2008 stated, "…a recent animal study demonstrated that exposure to endotoxin increased the production of prostaglandins and simultaneously decreased nitrous oxide production, resulting in inflammatory hyperalgesia" and "These observations suggest that SIBO is a common feature in both [IBS and FM] disorders and that altered gut microbiota in SIBO may play a role in the induction of somatic or visceral hypersensitivity, with affected patients meeting the diagnostic criteria for IBS, fibromyalgia or both disorders."

> **Exposure to the bacterial endotoxin lipopolysaccharide (LPS) causes increased sensitivity to painful stimuli (hyperalgesia) and a reduction in opioid analgesia (anti-analgesia)**
>
> "Intraperitoneal injection of toxins, such as the bacterial endotoxin lipopolysaccharide (LPS), is associated with a well-characterized increase in sensitivity to painful stimuli (hyperalgesia) and a longer-lasting reduction in opioid analgesia (anti-analgesia) when pain sensitivity returns to basal levels."
>
> Johnston IN, Westbrook RF. Inhibition of morphine analgesia by LPS: role of opioid and NMDA receptors and spinal glia. *Behav Brain Res.* 2005 Jan

6. <u>Central sensitization (enhanced and autonomous pain hypersensitivity) seen in FM can be caused by bacterial LPS</u>: Somewhat independent from the immune/inflammation-mediated hyperalgesia induced by LPS is the hyperalgesia mediated by central nervous system responses. The central sensitization seen with fibromyalgia[113] might be explained as being caused by intestinally-derived bacterial toxins. **Bacterial LPS/endotoxin promotes central sensitization via direct activation of NMDA receptors and by inducing hyperalgesia (elevated pain perception) and anti-analgesia (reduced response to pain inhibition).**[114] Accumulated evidence suggests that fibromyalgia may be a disorder of somatic hypersensitivity induced by bacterial toxins derived from quantitative excess or qualitative abnormalities in gut bacteria.[115]

7. <u>SIBO commonly causes nutrient malabsorption and thus predisposes to subclinical selective malnutrition, specifically micronutrient deficiency</u>: SIBO causes nutrient malabsorption[116] and can thereby contribute to the vitamin D and magnesium deficiencies that promote pain and mitochondrial dysfunction, respectively, and which are common in fibromyalgia. Intestinal bacterial overgrowth causes nutrient malabsorption via intestinal inflammation and villus atrophy (anatomic impairment) and impairment of digestion, specifically the enzymatic degradation of mucosal peptidases and disaccharidases by bacterial proteases (biochemical impairment). As reported by McEvoy and colleagues[117], bacterial contamination [overgrowth] of the small intestine is an important cause of occult malabsorption and malnutrition, especially in the elderly.

8. <u>SIBO can be triggered or exacerbated by emotional stress</u>: SIBO can be triggered in humans by reduced mucosal immunity following stressful life events, and this helps explain the link between

[111] Lin HC. Small intestinal bacterial overgrowth: a framework for understanding irritable bowel syndrome. *JAMA.* 2004 Aug 18;292(7):852-8
[112] Othman M, Agüero R, Lin HC. Alterations in intestinal microbial flora and human disease. *Curr Opin Gastroenterol.* 2008 Jan;24(1):11-6
[113] Meeus M, Nijs J. Central sensitization: a biopsychosocial explanation for chronic widespread pain in patients with fibromyalgia and chronic fatigue syndrome. *Clin Rheumatol.* 2007 Apr;26(4):465-73
[114] Johnston IN, Westbrook RF. Inhibition of morphine analgesia by LPS: role of opioid and NMDA receptors and spinal glia. *Behav Brain Res.* 2005;156(1):75-83
[115] Othman M, Agüero R, Lin HC. Alterations in intestinal microbial flora and human disease. *Curr Opin Gastroenterol.* 2008 Jan;24(1):11-6
[116] Elphick HL, Elphick DA, Sanders DS. Small bowel bacterial overgrowth. An underrecognized cause of malnutrition in older adults. Geriatrics. 2006 Sep;61(9):21-6
[117] McEvoy A, Dutton J, James OF. Bacterial contamination of the small intestine is an important cause of occult malabsorption in the elderly. *Br Med J* (Clin Res Ed). 1983 Sep 17;287(6395):789-93 http://www.ncbi.nlm.nih.gov/pmc/articles/PMC1549133/

psychoemotional stress and the SIBO-related conditions IBS and FM. Chronic mental-emotional stress causes reduced production of the antibody secretory IgA (sIgA) which is the primary line of defense against bacteria and other microorganisms in the gastrointestinal tract; thus, mental-emotional stress can reduce intestinal immunity and thereby promote SIBO. Further, stress in humans triggers enhanced microbial pathogenicity via microbial endocrinology.

9. <u>Oxidative stress triggers exaggerated pain perception—hyperalgesia (hypersensitivity to pain) and allodynia (perception of pain from normal stimuli)</u>: Patients with fibromyalgia show evidence of increased free radical (oxidant) production and reduced antioxidant defenses. Increased oxidative stress can be caused by immune activation and mitochondrial dysfunction; immune activation and mitochondrial dysfunction also promote oxidative stress and depletion of antioxidants, resulting in a vicious cycle, as illustrated. In the excellent review by Cordero et al[118], the authors note that recent studies have shown that oxidative stress causes peripheral and central sensitization and alters nerve sensitivity to pain (nociception), resulting in hyperalgesia—hypersensitivity to normal stimuli. The free radical (oxidant) superoxide promotes the development of pain through direct peripheral sensitization and the release of various cytokines (such as TNF-α, IL-1β, and IL-6), the formation of peroxynitrite (ONOO-), and PARP activation. PARP—poly-ADP-ribose-polymerase—is a nuclear enzyme activated by superoxide/peroxynitrite radicals; activation of PARP promotes the development of pain syndromes, including the components of small sensory fiber neuropathy, thermal and mechanical hyperalgesia, tactile allodynia, and exaggerated pain behavior in animal models of diabetic neuropathy.[119,120]

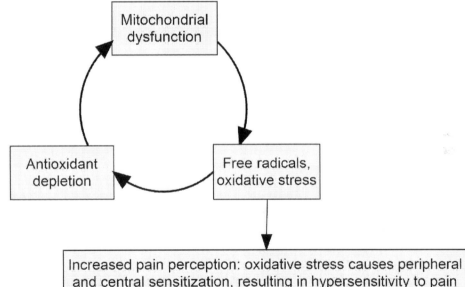

Mitochondrial dysfunction promotes central sensitization via oxidative stress and cytokine release: Mitochondrial dysfunction increases free radical production, which promotes "neurologic hypersensitivity" to pain, i.e., the pain in fibromyalgia is not simply due to muscle fatigue due to mitochondrial dysfunction although that is clearly a major component. The mitochondrial dysfunction also promotes central sensitization, which should be treated directly via alleviating the mitochondrial dysfunction and the causative dysbiosis, in addition to patient-specific factors.

---

[118] Cordero MD, et al. Mitochondrial dysfunction and mitophagy activation in blood mononuclear cells of fibromyalgia patients. *Arthritis Res Ther*. 2010;12(1):R17
[119] Wang ZQ, Porreca F, Cuzzocrea S et al. A newly identified role for superoxide in inflammatory pain. *J Pharmacol Exp Ther*. 2004 Jun;309(3):869-78
[120] Ilnytska O, et al. Poly(ADP-ribose) polymerase inhibition alleviates experimental diabetic sensory neuropathy. *Diabetes* 2006 Jun;55:1686-94

10. <u>Low plasma levels of L-tryptophan seen in fibromyalgia patients can be caused by degradation of dietary tryptophan by the bacterial enzyme tryptophanase</u>: Patients with fibromyalgia have low blood levels of the amino acid L-tryptophan[121], which is used in the body to make serotonin (important for mood maintenance and pain alleviation) and melatonin (important for normal sleep and for support of mitochondrial function and antioxidant protection). Bacteria such as *Escherichia coli, Proteus vulgaris,* and *Bacteroides* produce the enzyme tryptophanase[122], which destroys L-tryptophan in the gut before it is absorbed from ingested foods; thus, generalized bacterial overgrowth of the small intestine could reasonably be expected to exacerbate this phenomenon. In patients with fibromyalgia, higher tryptophan levels correlate positively with serotonin levels and with less pain and better sleep, while lower tryptophan levels are associated with sleep impairment, reduced serotonin levels, and higher levels of substance P, a neurotransmitter that promotes inflammation and pain perception.[123] Fibromyalgia patients produce 31% less melatonin than do healthy controls, and "this may contribute to impaired sleep at night, fatigue during the day, and changed pain perception."[124] Thus, a likely sequence of events is that, for example, a period of stressful life events can cause impair gastrointestinal immunity leading to intestinal bacterial overgrowth, which itself causes tryptophan degradation via elaboration of bacterial tryptophanase, causing tryptophan deficiency and resultant deficiencies of serotonin (leading to pain, depression, anxiety, and food/carbohydrate craving) and melatonin (leading to sleep disturbance, impaired antioxidant defense and mitochondrial function, and impaired immune responsiveness).

11. <u>The therapies that help fibromyalgia share mechanisms of action consistent with the model presented here</u>: As will be reviewed below under *Therapeutic Interventions,* essentially all of the most successful therapies for fibromyalgia have effects on intestinal flora, muscle perfusion/contractility, or mitochondrial bioenergetics (biological production of cellular energy/ATP). This is true for vegetarian diets (which favorably alter gut flora and improve antioxidant defenses), supplementation with tryptophan/melatonin (which preserve mitochondrial function during bacterial LPS/endotoxin exposure), physical treatments such as acupuncture (which improves tissue perfusion), and the use of nutrients such as magnesium, acetyl-L-carnitine, D-ribose, creatine, and coenzyme Q-10—all of which support or improve mitochondrial function.

12. <u>Restless leg syndrome and fibromyalgia commonly co-exist, and restless leg syndrome can be alleviated by eradication of SIBO</u>: Restless leg syndrome (RLS) occurs in approximately 30% of FM patients and can be effectively treated by addressing SIBO with a combination of antibiotics (drugs or botanical medicines that eradicate bacteria) and probiotics (products containing beneficial bacteria, which help restore "microbial balance" in the gastrointestinal tract).[125]

13. <u>Antimicrobial/antibiotic treatment alleviates fibromyalgia in most FM patients, just as it also alleviates gastrointestinal symptoms in patients with irritable bowel syndrome (IBS)</u>: Finally and most importantly, **antimicrobial therapy alleviates FM (and IBS) symptoms in direct proportion to the success of bacterial overgrowth eradication**, thus adding strong direct evidence in support of SIBO as a main cause of FM.[126,127] Recent clinical trials have shown that treatment of the

[121] "Plasma-free tryptophan is inversely related to the severity of subjective pain in 8 patients who fulfilled criteria for a variety of non-articular rheumatism, the "fibrositis syndrome". The observation is consistent with animal and human studies suggesting a relationship between reduced brain serotonin metabolism and pain reactivity." Moldofsky H, Warsh JJ. Plasma tryptophan and musculoskeletal pain in non-articular rheumatism ("fibrositis syndrome"). *Pain.* 1978 Jun;5(1):65-71
[122] Demoss RD, Moser K. Tryptophanase in Diverse Bacterial Species. *Journal of Bacteriology* 1969; 98: 167-171
[123] "A strong negative correlation between SP and 5-HIAA (P = .000) as well as between SP and TRP (P = .009) could be demonstrated. High serum concentrations of 5-HIAA and TRP showed a significant relation to low pain scores (5-HIAA: P = .030; TRP: P = .014). Moreover, 5-HIAA was strongly related to good quality of sleep (P = .000), while SP was related to sleep disturbance (P = .005)." Schwarz MJ, Späth M, Müller-Bardorff H, Pongratz DE, Bondy B, Ackenheil M. Relationship of substance P, 5-hydroxyindole acetic acid and tryptophan in serum of fibromyalgia patients. *Neurosci Lett.* 1999 Jan 15;259(3):196-8
[124] "The FMS patients had a 31% lower MT secretion than healthy subjects during the hours of darkness... Patients with fibromyalgic syndrome have a lower melatonin secretion during the hours of darkness than healthy subjects. This may contribute to impaired sleep at night, fatigue during the day, and changed pain perception." Wikner J, Hirsch U, Wetterberg L, Röjdmark S. Fibromyalgia--a syndrome associated with decreased nocturnal melatonin secretion. *Clin Endocrinol* (Oxf) 1998 Aug;49:179-83
[125] Weinstock LB, Fern SE, Duntley SP. Restless Legs Syndrome in Patients with Irritable Bowel Syndrome: Response to Small Intestinal Bacterial Overgrowth Therapy. *Dig Dis Sci.* 2007 May;53(5):1252-6
[126] Wallace DJ, Hallegua DS. Fibromyalgia: the gastrointestinal link. *Curr Pain Headache Rep.*2004 Oct;8(5):364-8
[127] Pimentel M, Hallegua DS, Wallace DJ, et al. Improvement of symptoms by eradication of small intestinal overgrowth in FM: a double-blind study. [Abstract] *Arthritis Rheum* 1999, 42:S343

fibromyalgia-related conditions IBS and SIBO by use of the nonabsorbed oral antibiotic rifaximin results in significant diminution of IBS-SIBO symptomatology with benefits lasting after the discontinuation of therapy.[128,129]

- Clinical trial: Rifaximin therapy for patients with irritable bowel syndrome without constipation (*New England Journal of Medicine* 2011 Jan[130]): Authors of this study evaluated rifaximin, a minimally absorbed antibiotic, as treatment for IBS. Subjects were given rifaximin at a dose of 550 mg or placebo, three times daily for 2 weeks and were followed for 10 weeks thereafter. "Significantly more patients in the rifaximin group than in the placebo group had adequate relief of global IBS symptoms during the first 4 weeks after treatment (40.8% vs. 31.2%). Similarly, more patients in the rifaximin group than in the placebo group had adequate relief of bloating (39.5% vs. 28.7%). In addition, significantly more patients in the rifaximin group had a response to treatment as assessed by daily ratings of IBS symptoms, bloating, abdominal pain, and stool consistency. The incidence of adverse events was similar in the two groups." Thus, among patients who had IBS without constipation, treatment with rifaximin for 2 weeks provided significant relief of IBS symptoms, bloating, abdominal pain, and loose or watery stools. *Comments by Dr Vasquez: Shortcomings of the intervention used in this IBS-rifaximin study include ❶ failure to use long-term treatment, which is often necessary in the treatment of chronic SIBO, ❷ failure to co-administer an antifungal agent to avert fungal growth in the intestines which commonly occurs as a result of antimicrobial/antibacterial drug treatment, ❸ failure to administer probiotics to re-establish beneficial flora, and ❹ failure to implement dietary modification to sustain the beneficial eradication of excess bacteria—allowing patients to continue their unhealthy diets and lifestyles is the most assured way to ensure that the condition (SIBO-IBS) will return.*

- Review of clinical trials: Rifaximin as treatment for SIBO and IBS (*Expert Opinion on Investigational Drugs* 2009 Mar[131]): A recognized expert in the treatment of SIBO-related conditions, Dr Pimentel writes, "**Rifaximin is a broad-range, gastrointestinal-specific antibiotic that demonstrates no clinically relevant bacterial resistance**. Therefore, rifaximin may be useful in the treatment of gastrointestinal disorders associated with altered bacterial flora, including irritable bowel syndrome (IBS) and small intestinal bacterial overgrowth (SIBO)." He also notes regarding the use of rifaximin in the treatment of IBS, "Rifaximin improved global symptoms in 33 - 92% of patients and eradicated SIBO in up to 84% of patients with IBS, with results sustained up to 10 weeks post-treatment. Rifaximin caused a lower number of adverse events compared with metronidazole or levofloxacin and may have a more favorable adverse event profile than systemic antibiotics, without clinically relevant antibiotic resistance."

- Results of two clinical trials of antibiotics in the treatment of fibromyalgia: Fibromyalgia—the gastrointestinal link (*Current Pain and Headache Reports* 2004 Oct[132]): This article discusses the results of two experiments using antibiotics in the treatment of FM: ❶ 96 patients with SIBO diagnosed by lactulose hydrogen breath testing (LHBT) were offered antibiotic treatment for the reduction of gastrointestinal bacteria; 25 of the 96 patients returned for a follow-up LHBT. Neomycin was the most commonly used antibiotic. Eleven of the 25 patients achieved complete transient eradication of SIBO after antibiotic treatment and experienced better improvement in more of their FM symptom scores when compared with the patients who did not achieve complete eradication. This indicates that **a direct relationship exists between the presence of SIBO and intestinal and extraintestinal**

[128] Pimentel M, Park S, Mirocha J, Kane SV, Kong Y. The effect of a nonabsorbed oral antibiotic (rifaximin) on the symptoms of the irritable bowel syndrome: a randomized trial. *Ann Intern Med.* 2006 Oct 17;145(8):557-63

[129] Sharara AI, Aoun E, Abdul-Baki H, Mounzer R, Sidani S, Elhajj I. A randomized double-blind placebo-controlled trial of rifaximin in patients with abdominal bloating and flatulence. *Am J Gastroenterol.* 2006 Feb;101(2):326-33

[130] Pimentel M, Lembo A, Chey WD, et al. Rifaximin therapy for patients with irritable bowel syndrome without constipation. *N Engl J Med.* 2011 Jan 6;364(1):22-32

[131] Pimentel M. Review of rifaximin as treatment for SIBO and IBS. *Expert Opin Investig Drugs.* 2009 Mar;18(3):349-58

[132] Wallace DJ, Hallegua DS. Fibromyalgia: the gastrointestinal link. *Curr Pain Headache Rep.* 2004 Oct;8(5):364-8

symptoms in fibromyalgia, and that FM can be alleviated by effective **antimicrobial/antibiotic treatment**. ❷ In this double-blind trial of eradication of SIBO in fibromyalgia, 46 patients fulfilling the established criteria for FM were tested for SIBO using LHBT. Forty-two of the 46 patients (91.3%) were positive for SIBO and were randomized to receive placebo or 500 mg of liquid neomycin (a minimally-absorbed gastrointestinal-specific antibiotic drug) twice daily for 10 days. Only six of the 20 patients (30%) in the neomycin group achieved eradication (indicating inefficacy of treatment); thus, no statistically significant difference between groups was available for analysis. Thereafter, 28 patients in the double-blind study testing positive for SIBO went on to receive open-label antibiotic treatment to eradicate SIBO, and this time 17 of the 28 patients (60.7%) achieved eradication of SIBO. When these 23 patients were compared with the 15 patients who failed to eradicate or did not undergo open-label treatment, significant improvement attributable to antibiotic treatment in the FM scores was detected. **Results show that eradication of bacterial overgrowth results in a clinically significant alleviation of FM symptoms.**

Thus, overall and when integrated together, the research literature provides compelling evidence linking intestinal bacterial overgrowth with the genesis and perpetuation of fibromyalgia. Chronic low-dose exposure to bacterial debris such as lipopolysaccharide/endotoxin and metabolic toxins such as hydrogen sulfide and D-lactic acid from SIBO is a plausible cause of impaired cellular energy production that results in chronic, widespread muscle fatigue and soreness and which may culminate in the clinical presentation of fibromyalgia. The individual components of this model have been substantiated by mechanistic studies in animals and/or research studies in humans. CFS also shares many epidemiological and clinical similarities with FM, and a similar pathophysiology is highly probable.

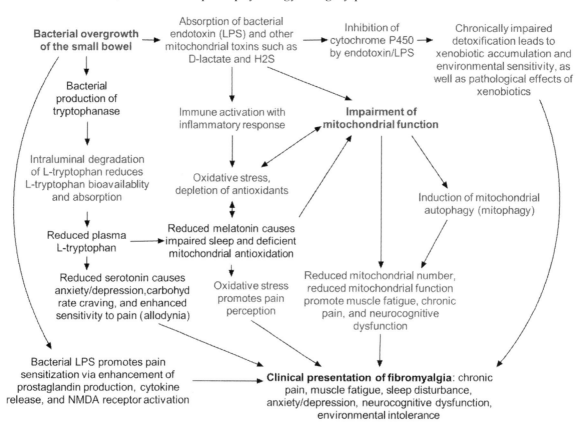

How small intestine bacterial overgrowth (SIBO) causes fibromyalgia: Bacterial overgrowth of the small bowel leads to chronic low-grade tryptophan insufficiency resulting in reduced endogenous production of serotonin (important for positive mood and relief from anxiety pain) and of melatonin (important for restful sleep and protection of mitochondria from oxidative stress). Bacterial mitochondrial toxins such as endotoxin, H2S, D-lactate cause impaired mitochondrial energy production, which leads to mitophagy, muscle fatigue, pain, and cognitive impairment.

A consistent report from many CFS and fibromyalgia patients is that of environmental intolerance (EI) and multiple chemical sensitivity (MCS), often grouped together as EI-MCS; these are complex disorders that the medical profession has failed to appreciate and which are characterized by adverse physiological responses to ambient levels of toxic chemicals and other environmental exposures. EI-MCS can be plausibly explained by SIBO because bacterial LPS/endotoxin impairs hepatic cytochrome P450 detoxification enzymes, resulting in reduced drug metabolism and impaired clearance of xenobiotics/toxins.[133] Accumulation of xenobiotics in CFS patients[134] might therefore be explained in part by LPS-induced inhibition of xenobiotic clearance secondary to SIBO. Further, the metabolic and immunologic effects of LPS can also account for the immune activation, neurological dysfunction, and musculoskeletal complaints noted in patients with CFS, IBS, and FM. A simplified yet accurate model of fibromyalgia which accounts for the major clinical and objective abnormalities seen with this condition is presented in the diagram that follows. Following the exclusion of diagnosable and treatable conditions that can contribute to or mimic fibromyalgia, and by using an integrated model of functional medicine clinicians can design treatment plans based on the previously reviewed pathogenesis and on the therapeutic considerations detailed in the following section.

Therapeutic Interventions

- **Overview**: Treatments for FM should be ❶ science-based and should ❷ directly address the cause(s) of the disorder; treatments should be ❹ safe (generally) and ❺ effective and ❻ without potential for serious adverse effects. Drug treatment of FM does not meet these criteria; the integrative, nutritional, and functional medicine approaches outlined below can—when properly employed by a skilled clinician—address the cause(s) of FM in a way that is scientific, direct, safe, effective, and well tolerated by essentially all patients. **Treatments for FM must emphasize eradication of SIBO, prevention of SIBO recurrence, the restoration/establishment of optimal nutritional status, and specific support for optimal mitochondrial function; anything less than this will fail to be effective.** Clinical interventions for the treatment of SIBO include dietary carbohydrate restriction, normalization of slow gastrointestinal transit time (e.g., correction of hypothyroidism), selective use of probiotic supplements to normalize intestinal flora, support of mucosal immunity (with nutrients such as vitamin A, zinc, and L-glutamine), and eradication of bacterial overgrowth with drugs (such as ciprofloxacin, rifaximin, amoxicillin/Augmentin[135], metronidazole) and/or natural products (such as berberine[136], *Artemisia annua*, peppermint oil[137], and emulsified time-released oil of oregano[138])—each of these have been reviewed in greater detail elsewhere by this author.[139] Failure of any monotherapeutic approach to immediately resolve the clinical manifestations of FM can explained by the secondary metabolic, immune, and neurophysiological effects that have generally persisted over periods ranging from years to decades for most patients; in other words, the treatment program must be multifaceted in order to address the numerous major problems that cause FM, and the treatment plan must also be sustained long enough to correct the abnormal physiologic patterns that have been established by the body's response/adaptation to the disease process. The treatment program (examples provided) must be complete in order to facilitate correction of systemic oxidative damage (broad-spectrum antioxidant support), resultant nutritional deficiencies (diet optimization, vitamin and mineral supplementation), immune sensitization and

[133] Shedlofsky SI, Israel BC, McClain CJ, Hill DB, Blouin RA. Endotoxin administration to humans inhibits hepatic cytochrome P450-mediated drug metabolism. *J Clin Invest*. 1994 Dec;94(6):2209-14

[134] Dunstan RH, Donohoe M, Taylor W, Roberts TK, Murdoch RN, Watkins JA, McGregor NR. A preliminary investigation of chlorinated hydrocarbons and chronic fatigue syndrome. *Med J Aust*. 1995 Sep 18;163(6):294-7

[135] Malik BA, Xie YY, Wine E, Huynh HQ. Diagnosis and pharmacological management of small intestinal bacterial overgrowth in children with intestinal failure. *Can J Gastroenterol*. 2011 Jan;25(1):41-5. This is a remarkable article and probably one of the most brilliant articles on the treatment of SIBO with drugs.

[136] [No authors listed] Berberine. *Altern Med Rev*. 2000 Apr;5(2):175-7

[137] "A case report of a patient with SIBO who showed marked subjective improvement in IBS-like symptoms and significant reductions in hydrogen production after treatment with ECPO is presented. While further investigation is necessary, the results in this case suggest one of the mechanisms by which ECPO improves IBS symptoms is antimicrobial activity in the small intestine." Logan AC, Beaulne TM. The treatment of small intestinal bacterial overgrowth with enteric-coated peppermint oil: a case report. *Altern Med Rev*. 2002 Oct;7(5):410-7

[138] Force M, Sparks WS, Ronzio RA. Inhibition of enteric parasites by emulsified oil of oregano in vivo. *Phytother Res*. 2000 May;14(3):213-4

[139] Vasquez A. Reducing Pain and Inflammation Naturally. Part 6: Nutritional and Botanical Treatments Against "Silent Infections" and Gastrointestinal Dysbiosis, Commonly Overlooked Causes of Neuromusculoskeletal Inflammation and Chronic Health Problems. *Nutr Perspect* 2006; Jan: 5-21. For more updated information, see: Vasquez A. *Integrative Rheumatology*

induction of proinflammatory cycles (anti-inflammatory nutrition), alterations in neurotransmission and membrane receptor function (amino acid and fatty acid supplementation), and the inflammation-induced disturbances in pain reception and hypothalamic-pituitary-endocrine function (assess/correct hormonal imbalances; supplement with n-3 fatty acids and olive oil to reduce hypothalamic inflammation[140], etc.). Further, patients treated for SIBO who do not positively change their diets and lifestyles (which probably promoted the genesis and perpetuation of the disease-causing SIBO in the first place) are subject to continual recurrence until such changes are implemented and faithfully maintained.

- **FOOD AND NUTRITION**: As with many rheumatologic/painful/inflammatory conditions with a strong component of gastrointestinal dysbiosis, the single best diet is a vegan or pesco-vegetarian diet free of gluten and most grains (judicious use of brown rice excepted); clearly the diet must emphasize vegetable intake and avoidance of fermentable substrate to induce quantitative reductions and qualitative improvements in microbial populations and metabolic activity. Beyond the gut, the benefits of minimized carbohydrate intake include weight loss (generally beneficial in this patient population), alleviation of physiologic and psychologic dependence on carbohydrate (over)consumption, and increased endogenous production of beta-hydroxy-butyrate which stimulates the terminal complexes of the mitochondrial electron transport chain while also promoting histone acetylation (via inhibition of histone deacetylase) for enhanced DNA transcription resulting in what has been referred to as a rejuvenative phenotype. My foundational diet-nutritional program—the 5-part "supplemented Paleo-Mediterranean Diet"—can easily be modified to pesco-vegetarian or lacto-pesco-vegetarian variants to enhance high-quality protein intake while continuing to emphasize vegetable, nut, and seed intake to maximize fiber and micronutrient intake. In particular, whey protein isolate is attractive in this patient population due to the high content of tryptophan (to correct the common tryptophan deficiency), the glutathione precursors (to alleviate oxidative stress and enhance mitochondrial function), immunoglobulins (to support mucosal defenses against bacterial overgrowth), and growth factors including whey's insulotrophic effect to promote anabolism with resultant improvements in muscle function and gut mucosal integrity. Systemic alkalinization supported by plant-based potassium citrate promotes xenobiotic excretion (reduction in total load of persistent organic pollutants and toxic metals such as lead and mercury) and endogenous production of endorphins (enhanced mood, pain relief). The increased intake of vitamins (including physiologic doses of vitamin D3), minerals, ALA, GLA, EPA, DHA, and probiotics all synergize to alleviate SIBO, oxidative stress, pain and inflammation while also promoting optimal immune and mitochondrial functions. Allergy identification and avoidance is easily achieved via the very practical and no-cost elimination-and-challenge technique. In particular for patients with fibromyalgia, magnesium intake is increased via consumption of dark green vegetables and nutritional supplements while magnesium

> **Patients with migraine headaches—noted in 50% of patients with fibromyalgia—often have food allergies/sensitivities/intolerances**
>
> "The commonest foods causing reactions were wheat (78%), orange (65%), eggs (45%), tea and coffee (40% each), chocolate and milk (37%) each), beef (35%), and corn, cane sugar, and yeast (33% each). When an average of ten common foods were avoided there was a dramatic fall in the number of headaches per month, 85% of patients becoming headache-free."
>
> Grant EC. Food allergies and migraine. *Lancet*. 1979 May

absorption is promoted by optimized vitamin D status while renal retention of magnesium is promoted with urinary alkalinization. The consistent and pathologic secondary tryptophan deficiency is foremost corrected by eradicating the causative SIBO and the resultant intraintestinal bacterial tryptophanase-catalyzed degradation of ingested tryptophan and via dietary supplementation with L-tryptophan, 5-hydroxytryptophan, and/or whey protein isolate.

- Diet optimization with the five-part "supplemented Paleo-Mediterranean Diet" (*Nutr Perspect* 2011 Jan[141]): The "supplemented Paleo-Mediterranean Diet" (SPMD)—the 5-part nutritional wellness protocol—as described in most of my textbooks in "chapter 2" and also in my articles available on-

---

[140] Milanski M, et al. Saturated fatty acids produce an inflammatory response predominantly through the activation of TLR4 signaling in hypothalamus: implications for the pathogenesis of obesity. *J Neurosci.* 2009 Jan 14;29(2):359-70
[141] Vasquez A. Revisiting the Five-Part Nutritional Wellness Protocol: Supplemented Paleo-Mediterranean Diet. *Nutr Perspect* 2011 Jan optimalhealthresearch.com/protocol.html

line at http://optimalhealthresearch.com/protocol.html should be implemented for most FM patients; exceptions to this general rule might include patients with renal insufficiency due to the risk for potassium excess (hyperkalemia[Note 142]). Because any patient might have an allergy or intolerance to any food (even a healthy food like citrus fruit, chicken or eggs), patients and doctors must be aware of the potential for food allergies and will therefore have to customize the Paleo-Mediterranean diet *for each individual patient* to exclude foods to which the patient might be allergic or sensitive/intolerant. Otherwise, this 5-part nutrition protocol is based on ❶ vegetables, nuts, seeds, (berries, fruits, and juices generally have to be avoided during treatment for SIBO due to the high content of sugars and—with juice—the rapid passage through the gastrointestinal tract) and lean sources of protein, ❷ high-potency multivitamin and multimineral supplementation, ❸ physiologic doses of vitamin D3 to optimize blood levels of vitamin D3 (measured as 25-OH-vitamin D), ❹ combination fatty acid supplementation (with flax oil [for ALA], fish oil [for EPA and DHA], and borage oil [for GLA] with oleic acid from olive oil incorporated into the diet), and ❺ probiotics—foods or supplements that contain living bacteria with beneficial qualities. The diet should emphasize strict avoidance of grains in general and gluten-containing grains *especially wheat* in particular. This diet is essential for the provision of sufficient protein, fiber, phytonutrients, and alkalinization—potassium citrate is most concentrated in vegetables and helps the body maintain proper acid-alkaline balance.[143] The diet should be low in carbohydrates to reduce fermentable substrate to intestinal bacteria. The most important books for patients to read in support of this diet are *The Paleo Diet* by Dr Loren Cordain and *Breaking the Vicious Cycle* by Elaine Gottschall; an open-access summary of the diet plan is available at OptimalHealthResearch.com/spmd.html.

- Vegetarian diet: Fibromyalgia syndrome improved using a mostly raw vegetarian diet (*BMC Complementary and Alternative Medicine* 2001 Sep[144]): Diets high in fruits, vegetables, nuts, berries, and seeds provide ample fiber to promote laxation and can be useful as adjunctive treatment for gastrointestinal dysbiosis in general and SIBO in particular (i.e., *quantitative* reduction in GI dysbiosis). Perhaps more importantly, plant-based diets result in *qualitative* benefits by changing microbial behavior and reducing production of irritants, toxins, and bacterial metabolites, including the mitochondrial poisons D-lactate and hydrogen sulfide. Fibromyalgia patients who consume a mostly vegetarian diet have experienced significant improvements in function and reductions in FM symptomatology. Poorly designed dietary interventions that allow abundant intake of whole-grain bread, pasta, rice, and fruit juice[145] would be expected to fail because such high-carbohydrate diets feed intestinal bacteria with an abundance of substrate and would therefore be expected to sustain or exacerbate SIBO. Another advantage to a plant-based mostly-raw diet is the avoidance of dietary advanced glycation end-products (AGEs) which are inflammation-promoting chemical combinations of proteins with sugars, which can be consumed in the diet (e.g., baked deserts) or formed endogenously/internally as a result of oxidative stress and elevated blood sugar levels (e.g., diabetes mellitus). As discussed previously, FM patients show higher levels of AGEs in blood cells and muscle tissue; AGEs promote chronic pain and inflammation[146], and therefore dietary and nutritional

---

[142] Because the kidneys are responsible for excreting potassium, reduced kidney function (kidney failure, renal insufficiency) implies that the kidneys may not be able to perform the function of excreting potassium; thus, consumption of a potassium-rich diet could contribute to a dangerous situation of excess potassium in the blood known as hyperkalemia (*hyper*=too much, *kal*=potassium, *emia*=blood disorder). For patients with renal insufficiency, consumption of an otherwise health-promoting diet rich in fruits and vegetables might cause a problem if potassium accumulates in the blood due to impaired excretion. Blood tests can assess renal function as well as the blood potassium level. This is one example of why a clinician/doctor should be employed by patients before implementing diet modification and nutritional supplementation. Dr Vasquez can be contacted via his websites http://HealGrowThriveMedicine.com/ (for patients) and http://OptimalHealthResearch.com/ (for doctors and students).

[143] "The modern Western-type diet is deficient in fruits and vegetables and contains excessive animal products, generating the accumulation of non-metabolizable anions and a lifespan state of overlooked metabolic acidosis, whose magnitude increases progressively with aging due to the physiological decline in kidney function." Adeva MM, Souto G. Diet-induced metabolic acidosis. *Clin Nutr.* 2011 Aug;30(4):416-21

[144] Donaldson MS, Speight N, Loomis S. Fibromyalgia syndrome improved using a mostly raw vegetarian diet: an observational study. *BMC Complement Altern Med.* 2001;1:7 http://www.biomedcentral.com/1472-6882/1/7

[145] Michalsen A, Riegert M, Lüdtke R, Bäcker M, Langhorst J, Schwickert M, Dobos GJ. Mediterranean diet or extended fasting's influence on changing the intestinal microflora, immunoglobulin A secretion and clinical outcome in patients with rheumatoid arthritis and fibromyalgia: an observational study. *BMC Complement Altern Med.* 2005 Dec 22;5:22

[146] "In the interstitial connective tissue of fibromyalgic muscles we found a more intensive staining of the AGE CML, activated NF-kappaB, and also higher CML levels in the serum of these patients compared to the controls. RAGE was only present in FM muscle." Rüster M, Franke S, Späth M, Pongratz DE, Stein G, Hein GE. Detection of elevated N epsilon-carboxymethyllysine levels in muscular tissue and in serum of patients with fibromyalgia. *Scand J Rheumatol.* 2005 Nov-Dec;34(6):460-3

strategies that reduce AGE intake and/or AGE formation are 1) without risk, and 2) likely to provide manifold health benefits, including but not limited to reductions in pain and inflammation.

Dr Vasquez's Five-part Nutrition Protocol: The "Supplemented Paleo-Mediterranean Diet"

1. **Diet: Emphasize vegetables, nuts, seeds, berries, and lean sources of protein** (fish, grass-fed lamb/beef). Minimize fruit intake due to higher sugar content while treating SIBO; the goal is to deprive the bacteria and yeast in the intestines of their preferred food source (carbohydrates, sugars). Make modifications for patient-specific food allergies and sensitivities; this is especially important for patients with known allergy-related conditions such as migraine headaches. Patients with kidney disease should use caution when consuming a potassium-rich diet. (Vasquez A. Revisiting the Five-Part Nutritional Wellness Protocol: The Supplemented Paleo-Mediterranean Diet. *Nutritional Perspectives* 2011 Jan)
2. **Multivitamin and multimineral supplement**: Nutrient deficiencies are common and are easily treated with nutritional supplementation. (Fletcher and Fairfield. Vitamins for chronic disease prevention in adults. *JAMA* 2002 Jun)
3. **Vitamin D dosed at 2,000-10,000 IU per day**: The adult requirement for vitamin D3 is approximately 4,000 IU per day; some patients may achieve optimal blood levels with lower doses, but generally daily doses of 4,000-10,000 IU are necessary. (Vasquez A, et al. The Clinical Importance of Vitamin D. *Alternative Therapies in Health and Medicine* 2004 Sep)
4. **Combination fatty acid supplementation**: A combination of flax oil, borage oil, and fish oil provides the health-promoting fatty acids (ALA, GLA, EPA, DHA). Patients should consume organic virgin olive oil liberally with foods. (Vasquez A. New Insights into Fatty Acid Supplementation and Its Effect on Eicosanoid Production and Genetic Expression. *Nutritional Perspectives* 2005; Jan)
5. **Probiotics**: Health-promoting bacteria can be consumed in the form of powders, pills, and fermented foods such as yogurt and kefir.

- **Tryptophan and 5-hydroxytryptophan (5-HTP):** Tryptophan is an amino acid found in many foods and is essential for human health and survival. Tryptophan is available as a nutritional supplement only by a doctor's prescription; it is available over-the-counter in a nonprescription supplement in the form of 5-hydroxytryptophan (5-HTP), which is commonly sourced from the seeds of *Griffonia simplicifolia*, a woody climbing shrub native to West and Central Africa. Tryptophan is the precursor to the neurotransmitter serotonin, which has antidepressant, anti-anxiety, and analgesic properties. Patients with FM are known to have low blood levels (i.e., functional nutritional insufficiency) of tryptophan, and the severity of the deficiency correlates with the severity of pain.[147,148,149] Blood levels of serotonin are often below normal in FM patients.[150] The accepted *medical-pharmacological* use of selective serotonin reuptake inhibitors (SSRI) drugs to treat the pain, depression, and anxiety associated with FM supports the use of 5-HTP to raise serotonin levels *naturally* by correcting the underlying nutritional insufficiency. As an over-the-counter nutritional supplement, the 5-hydroxylated form of tryptophan (5-HTP) has been used clinically and in numerous research studies. **Supplementation with 5-HTP has been shown to significantly alleviate symptoms of fibromyalgia.**[151] Commonly used doses range from 50 to 300 mg/d, with larger doses divided throughout the day. If tryptophan rather than 5-HTP is used, results are improved when taken on an empty stomach with carbohydrate (such as honey or fruit juice) to induce insulin secretion, which preferentially promotes uptake of tryptophan into the brain. Deficiency of either magnesium or vitamin B6 impairs conversion of 5-HTP into serotonin, and therefore the interventional program must ensure nutritional supra-sufficiency.
  - <u>Primary fibromyalgia syndrome and 5-hydroxy-L-tryptophan: a 90-day open study (*Journal of Internal Medicine Research* 1992 Apr[152]):</u> An open 90-day study in 50 fibromyalgia patients showed significant improvement in all measured parameters (number of tender points, anxiety, pain

[147] Moldofsky H, Warsh JJ. Plasma tryptophan and musculoskeletal pain in non-articular rheumatism ("fibrositis syndrome"). *Pain*. 1978 Jun;5(1):65-71
[148] Yunus MB, Dailey JW, Aldag JC, Masi AT, Jobe PC. Plasma tryptophan and other amino acids in primary fibromyalgia: a controlled study. *J Rheumatol*. 1992 Jan;19(1):90-4
[149] Russell IJ, Michalek JE, Vipraio GA, Fletcher EM, Wall K. Serum amino acids in fibrositis/fibromyalgia syndrome. *J Rheumatol* Suppl. 1989 Nov;19:158-63
[150] Wolfe F, Russell IJ, Vipraio G, Ross K, Anderson J. Serotonin levels, pain threshold, and fibromyalgia symptoms in the general population. *J Rheumatol*. 1997;24(3):555-9
[151] Caruso I, Sarzi Puttini P, Cazzola M, Azzolini V. Double-blind study of 5-hydroxytryptophan versus placebo in the treatment of primary fibromyalgia syndrome. *J Int Med Res*. 1990 May-Jun;18(3):201-9
[152] Sarzi Puttini P, Caruso I. Primary fibromyalgia syndrome and 5-hydroxy-L-tryptophan: a 90-day open study. *J Int Med Res*. 1992 Apr;20(2):182-9

intensity, quality of sleep, fatigue) after treatment with 5-HTP; global clinical improvement assessed by the patient and the investigator indicated a "good" or "fair" response in nearly 50% of the patients during the treatment period.

- □ Double-blind study of 5-hydroxytryptophan versus placebo in the treatment of primary fibromyalgia syndrome (*Journal of Internal Medicine Research* 1990 May-Jun[153]): A double-blind, placebo-controlled study using 5-HTP in 50 fibromyalgia patients showed significant improvement in all measured parameters, with only mild and transient side effects. *Note by Dr Vasquez: Again, the common dose range for 5-HTP is 50 to 300 mg per day with doses greater than 100 mg generally best divided throughout the day (e.g., 50 mg thrice per day). I generally recommend starting with 50-100 mg about one hour before bedtime, then adding incremental additions of 50 mg throughout the day for a maximum daily dose of 300 mg. Effectiveness is increased with additional supplementation with magnesium, vitamin B6 (pyridoxine), and the fatty acids found in fish oil (EPA and DHA).*

- **Magnesium:** Magnesium deficiency is epidemic in industrialized societies due to insufficient dietary intake (e.g., from mineral water and leafy green vegetables) and concomitant metabolic-urinary acidosis, which increases urinary magnesium loss.[154,155] Additional causes of magnesium deficiency in fibromyalgia patients include vitamin D deficiency, malabsorption due to SIBO, and the stress of chronic illness. Magnesium deficiency exacerbates the symptoms of fibromyalgia by contributing to impairment of energy/ATP production in skeletal muscle, increased muscle tone and spasms (hypomagnesemic tetany), and anxiety and increased pain sensitivity—hyperalgesia via NMDA receptor overstimulation and neurocortical hyperexcitability. Magnesium deficiency also promotes constipation and intestinal stasis, which exacerbates SIBO. Magnesium supplementation (600 mg or to bowel tolerance to a limit of 1,500 mg in divided doses [bowel tolerance is defined as the dose—commonly of magnesium or vitamin C—that produces slightly loose stools due to the osmotic laxative effect]) should be used routinely in fibromyalgia patients; the primary cautions with magnesium use are renal insufficiency and the use of magnesium-sparing drugs such as the diuretic drug spironolactone. Modest benefits demonstrated in clinical trials with magnesium and malic acid[156] can easily be exceeded with concomitant interventions to address vitamin D deficiency, SIBO, and mitochondrial dysfunction.

- **S-adenosylmethionine (SAMe):** Studies using oral or intravenous administration of the nutritional supplement SAMe have reported conflicting results; however, the overall trend seems to indicate that SAMe (800 mg/d orally) is safe and beneficial in the treatment of fibromyalgia.[157] SAMe helps maintain mitochondrial function by preserving glutathione, and its contribution of methyl groups is important for the regulation of gene expression and neurotransmitter synthesis. *Comment by Dr Vasquez: I do not regularly use this supplement, and I would only use it as a last resort if nothing else had worked or if a particular patient had a specific indication for this supplement.*

- **INFECTIONS/DYSBIOSIS:** As reviewed in a previous section, fibromyalgia patients have a remarkably high prevalence of occult SIBO, the severity of which directly correlates with the severity of FM symptomatology and the eradication of which directly correlates with alleviation of FM. SIBO is the single primary pathoetiologic mechanism that explains each and every abnormality seen in this condition; the response of fibromyalgia patients to gastrointestinal-specific nonabsorbable antimicrobial treatments such as rifaximin provides diagnostic proof of effective treatment of the causative SIBO. Jejunal aspiration is expensive, inconvenient, cumbersome, invasive, and not completely sensitive, while breath hydrogen and methane testing is also cumbersome and relatively expensive (especially when compared to making a clinical diagnosis and confirmatory treatment) and is likewise not completely reliable. Post-prandial gas

[153] Caruso I, Sarzi Puttini P, Cazzola M, Azzolini V. Double-blind study of 5-hydroxytryptophan versus placebo in the treatment of primary fibromyalgia syndrome. *J Int Med Res*. 1990 May-Jun;18(3):201-9

[154] Cordain L, Eaton SB, Sebastian A, Mann N, Lindeberg S, Watkins BA, O'Keefe JH, Brand-Miller J. Origins and evolution of the Western diet: health implications for the 21st century. *Am J Clin Nutr*. 2005 Feb;81(2):341-54

[155] Rylander R, Remer T, Berkemeyer S, Vormann J. Acid-base status affects renal magnesium losses in healthy, elderly persons. *J Nutr*. 2006 Sep;136(9):2374-7

[156] Russell IJ, Michalek JE, Flechas JD, Abraham GE. Treatment of fibromyalgia syndrome with Super Malic: a randomized, double blind, placebo controlled, crossover pilot study. *J Rheumatol*. 1995 May;22(5):953-8

[157] Leventhal LJ. Management of fibromyalgia. *Ann Intern Med*. 1999 Dec 7;131(11):850-8

and bloating is a reliable clinical indicator of SIBO, and empiric treatment of SIBO with a low-carbohydrate diet (LCD) and antimicrobial agents that results in clinical improvement (which may include alleviation of musculoskeletal pain, improved cognition, alleviation of fatigue, and—especially in elderly patients—alleviation of malabsorption and malnutrition) confirms the diagnosis. Stated more plainly, effective implementation of LCD with antimicrobial treatment is both diagnostic and therapeutic; this allows the diagnosis to be made efficiently and with high specificity, (sensitivity depends upon efficacy) and bypassing expensive/insensitive/nontherapeutic/cumbersome diagnostic methods expedites physicians' efficacy and patients' relief in a manner that is safe and cost-effective, especially when compared to perpetual nontherapeutic symptomatic polypharmacy.

- Low-carbohydrate diet, specific-carbohydrate diet: Patients can follow a diet that emphasizes consumption of low-carbohydrate vegetables, nuts, and seeds and excludes grains (especially wheat, which is very highly fermentable), starches from foods such as potatoes, and disaccharides such as lactose and sucrose; most of the characteristics of a competent low-carbohydrate diet can be achieved within a "Paleo diet" such as described and popularized by Cordain. Alternatively or additionally, patients can follow the specific-carbohydrate diet described and popularized by Gottschall.

- Probiotics: Probiotics are beneficial bacteria that can be consumed in foods or as nutritional supplements to populate the gut, particularly following antibiotic use or long-term dietary neglect. In addition to their availability in capsules and powders, probiotics are widely consumed in the form of yogurt, kefir, and other cultured foods, and they have an excellent record of safety. Probiotic supplements are available in different strengths (quantity), potencies (viability), and combinations of bacteria (diversity). Some probiotics also contain fermentable carbohydrates (prebiotics) such as fructooligosaccharides (FOS) and inulin, which are substrates to nourish the beneficial bacteria. From a practical clinical perspective, the clinician can choose probiotic foods and supplements and instruct the patient

A practical summary of SIBO: small intestine bacterial overgrowth
1. <u>Definition</u>: Generalized nonspecific overpopulation of bacteria (commonly with other microbes such as yeast) in the small intestine (and large intestine, too).
2. <u>Frequency</u>: Very common in clinical practice and the general population.
3. <u>Primary symptoms</u>: Gas and bloating, especially after carbohydrate consumption; may also have constipation and/or diarrhea.
4. <u>Secondary symptoms</u>: Fatigue, muscle aches, difficulty with concentration and cognition ("brain fog"), nutritional deficiencies due to malabsorption, immune activation due to absorption of microbial debris and metabolites, muscle pain due to dysbiotic mitochondropathy and LPS- and cytokine-induced central sensitization.
5. <u>Diagnosis</u>: ❶ Based on the symptoms above, ❷ jejunal aspiration is the gold standard but is expensive, cumbersome, and potentially hazardous, ❸ measurement of fermentation products (hydrogen and methane) in breath following consumption of a carbohydrate such as glucose, sucrose, or lactulose; the amount of "gas" produced is proportional to the bacterial population, ❹ may find elevated short chain fatty acids (SCFA) in stool or elevated folate in blood, but not all cases of SIBO produce high levels of SCFA or folate, ❺ clinical response to low-carbohydrate diet and/or antibiotic drugs or antimicrobial herbs. The current author (AV) uses #1 in conjunction with #5 most commonly.
6. <u>Treatments</u>: Low-carbohydrate diet with antibiotic drugs (e.g., rifamixin (200 or 550 mg each) 400-550 mg tid po [1,200-1,650 mg daily] for 10-30 days) or antimicrobial herbs (e.g., time-released emulsified oregano oil 600 mg daily for 4-6 weeks, and/or berberine 400-1,500 mg daily for 4 weeks).

to use these on an ongoing, periodic, or rotational basis. Probiotics (i.e., bacteria only) may have a therapeutic advantage over prebiotics or synbiotics (probiotics+prebiotics) when treating SIBO because the fermentable carbohydrate in prebiotics and synbiotics may exacerbate the preexisting bacterial overgrowth by providing already overpopulated bacteria with additional substrate. The benefits of probiotic supplementation have been demonstrated in patients with IBS, rotavirus infection, eczema and increased intestinal permeability, and SIBO associated with renal failure. To date, no studies using probiotics in the treatment of fibromyalgia have been published.

- Antimicrobial agents: Antimicrobial agents can be categorized as either natural or pharmaceutical, and as absorbable and systemic or nonabsorbable and gastrointestinal-specific. These can be used empirically, as such treatment for suspected SIBO is well documented in the peer-reviewed clinical medicine literature; however, clinicians must always consider risk-to-benefit ratios especially when using the pharmaceutical antimicrobials which can induce systemic adverse effects (e.g., drug allergy or Stevens-Johnson syndrome or quinolone tendonopathy) or gastrointestinal adverse effects (e.g., nonspecific diarrhea, yeast overgrowth, *Clostridium difficile* diarrhea). Clinicians must always determine the proper choice and dose of therapeutic agents per patient. Two of the best and most important articles on the subject of SIBO are "Lin HC. Small intestinal bacterial overgrowth: a framework for understanding irritable bowel syndrome. *JAMA* 2004 Aug" (concepts and system-wide pathophysiology) and "Malik et al. Diagnosis and pharmacological management of small intestinal bacterial overgrowth in children with intestinal failure. *Can J Gastroenterol* 2011 Jan" (excellent sections on clinical diagnosis and pharmacologic management emphasizing rotational implementation of gut-specific antimicrobials). I prefer to use natural antimicrobial agents continuously for an extended period of time either alone or in conjunction with pharmaceutical antibacterial drugs, which I tend to use on a rotating basis of 7-14 days. Occasionally I will use a short course of an antiparasitic drug such as metronidazole or tinidazole, and I nearly always implement an extended course of antifungal treatment—either oregano oil or nystatin as nonabsorbable agents—punctuated by fluconazole/Diflucan if I suspect treatment resistant gastrointestinal yeast or any dermatologic or sinorespiratory yeast. Clinicians should appreciate that *yeast* colonization of the intestines promotes *bacterial* colonization of the intestines via—for example—elaboration by *Candida albicans* of a sIgA-protease and gliotoxin, an appreciated immunosuppressant. The following list emphasizes the antimicrobial agents I most commonly utilize, always in conjunction with nutritional supplementation (to restore immune function and mucosal defenses) and reduction in dietary carbohydrate intake (to reduce fermentable substrate and thereby "starve the microbes"). Although some dosage and duration suggestions are provided, the clinical reality is that patients need to be treated with "*dose and duration to effect*" or "*titrate to effect*"—meaning that the milligram dose per day and the duration of treatment can and should be customized per the patient's response to treatment. Combination therapy (i.e., more than one treatment at a time), prolonged therapy (treatment of chronic [poly]dysbiosis generally requires longer duration of treatment than does treatment of acute monomicrobial infections), and periodic/punctual treatment (for exacerbations and recurrences).

▫ Clinical support favoring "open label" empiric antimicrobial treatment of SIBO in patients with fibromyalgia (*Current Pain and Headache Reports* 2004 Oct[158]): This article discusses the results of two experiments using antibiotics in the treatment of FM: ❶ 96 patients with SIBO diagnosed by lactulose hydrogen breath testing (LHBT) were offered **antibiotic treatment** for the reduction of gastrointestinal bacteria; 25 of the 96 patients returned for a follow-up LHBT. **Neomycin** was the most commonly used antibiotic. Eleven of the 25 patients achieved complete transient eradication of SIBO after antibiotic treatment and experienced better improvement in more of their FM symptom scores when compared with the patients who did not achieve complete eradication. This indicates that a direct relationship exists between the presence of SIBO and intestinal and extraintestinal symptoms in fibromyalgia, and that FM can be alleviated by effective antimicrobial/antibiotic treatment. ❷ In this double-blind trial of eradication of SIBO in fibromyalgia, 46 patients fulfilling the established criteria for FM were tested for SIBO using LHBT. Forty-two of the 46 patients (91.3%) were positive for SIBO and were randomized to receive placebo or 500 mg of **liquid neomycin** (a minimally-absorbed gastrointestinal-specific antibiotic drug) twice daily for 10 days. Only six of the 20 patients (30%) in the neomycin group achieved eradication (indicating inefficacy of treatment); thus, no statistically significant difference between groups was available for analysis. Thereafter, 28 patients in the double-blind study testing positive for SIBO went on to receive **open-label antibiotic treatment** to eradicate SIBO, and this time 17 of the 28 patients (60.7%) achieved eradication of SIBO. When these 23 patients were compared with the 15 patients who failed to eradicate or did not undergo open-label treatment, significant

[158] Wallace DJ, Hallegua DS. Fibromyalgia: the gastrointestinal link. *Curr Pain Headache Rep*. 2004 Oct;8(5):364-8

improvement attributable to antibiotic treatment in the FM scores was detected. Results suggest that eradication of bacterial overgrowth results in a statistically and clinically significant alleviation of FM symptoms.

▫ <u>Nonprescription antimicrobial agents—examples</u>: Most of the agents listed below have their primary or exclusive area of effectiveness within the lumen of the gastrointestinal tract. These agents are generally broad-spectrum and nonspecific, which is perfectly appropriate when treating nonspecific SIBO.

  ◦ <u>Oregano oil (time-released emulsified preparation named "ADP" from Biotics Research Corporation) 600 mg/d generally given as 200 mg/d PO TID for 6 weeks</u>: Oil of Mediterranean oregano *Oreganum vulgare* was orally administered to 14 adult patients whose stools tested positive for enteric parasites, *Blastocystis hominis*, *Entamoeba hartmanni* and *Endolimax nana*. Six weeks of supplementation with 600 mg emulsified oil of oregano daily resulted in complete disappearance of *Entamoeba hartmanni* (four cases), *Endolimax nana* (one case), and *Blastocystis hominis* in eight cases. *Blastocystis hominis* scores declined in three additional cases.[159] Many clinicians use ADP as a standard treatment for gastrointestinal dysbiosis due to bacteria, yeast, and/or other microbes; it is very safe and has a wide range of antimicrobial action.

  ◦ <u>Berberine (generally available as generic berberine hydrochloride or as a plant-based standardized extract with synergistic phytochemicals[160]) 1,000 mg/d in divided doses PO for up to 3 months</u>: Berberine is a botanical alkaloid with millennia of clinical use for various conditions and also specifically for the treatment of infectious diseases, such as those caused by *E coli*, *Giardia lamblia* (comparable to metronidazole), *Entamoeba histolytica*, and *Chlamydia trachomatis*.[161] Many clinicians use berberine as a standard treatment for gastrointestinal dysbiosis due to bacteria, yeast, and/or other microbes; it is very safe and has a wide range of antimicrobial action. Berberine 1,000-1,5000 mg/d for three months provides major clinical benefits and is effective treatment for dyslipidemia, insulin resistance, diabetes mellitus type-2 (comparable to metformin), and overweight/obesity.[162,163,164,165] Berberine is available in a "generic" form from many nutraceutical companies.

  ◦ <u>Undecylenic acid (also known as 10-undecenoic acid, available as "Formula SF722" from Thorne Research, each gelcap contains 10-undecenoic acid 50 mg) dosed at "450-750 mg undecylenic acid daily in three divided doses"[166] equates to 10-15 capsules per day, or 5 capsules 2-3 times per day</u>: An eleven-carbon monounsaturated fatty acid found naturally in the body (occurring in sweat) and produced commercially by the vacuum distillation of castor bean oil, undecylenate shows laboratory and clinical human-trial effectiveness against

[159] Force M, Sparks WS, Ronzio RA. Inhibition of enteric parasites by emulsified oil of oregano in vivo. *Phytother Res*. 2000 May;14(3):213-4

[160] Stermitz FR, Lorenz P, Tawara JN, Zenewicz LA, Lewis K. Synergy in a medicinal plant: antimicrobial action of berberine potentiated by 5'-methoxyhydnocarpin, a multidrug pump inhibitor. *Proc Natl Acad Sci U S A*. 2000 Feb 15;97(4):1433-7

[161] [No authors listed]. Berberine. *Altern Med Rev*. 2000 Apr;5(2):175-7

[162] Kong W, Wei J, Abidi P, Lin M, Inaba S, Li C, Wang Y, Wang Z, Si S, Pan H, Wang S, Wu J, Wang Y, Li Z, Liu J, Jiang JD. Berberine is a novel cholesterol-lowering drug working through a unique mechanism distinct from statins. *Nat Med*. 2004 Dec;10(12):1344-51

[163] "In this pilot study, obese human subjects (Caucasian) were given 500 mg berberine orally three times a day for twelve weeks. The efficacy and safety of berberine treatment was determined by measurements of body weight, comprehensive metabolic panel, blood lipid and hormone levels, expression levels of inflammatory factors, complete blood count, and electrocardiograph. A Sprague-Dawley rat experiment was also performed to identify the anti-obesity effects of berberine treatment. The results demonstrate that berberine treatment produced a mild weight loss (average 5 lb/subject) in obese human subjects. But more interestingly, the treatment significantly reduced blood lipid levels (23% decrease of triglyceride and 12.2% decrease of cholesterol levels) in human subjects." Hu Y, Ehli EA, Kittelsrud J, et al. Lipid-lowering effect of berberine in human subjects and rats. *Phytomedicine*. 2012 Jul 15;19(10):861-7

[164] "In study A, 36 adults with newly diagnosed type 2 diabetes mellitus were randomly assigned to treatment with berberine or metformin (0.5 g 3 times a day) in a 3-month trial. The hypoglycemic effect of berberine was similar to that of metformin. Significant decreases in hemoglobin A1c (from 9.5%+/-0.5% to 7.5%+/-0.4%, P<.01), fasting blood glucose (from 10.6+/-0.9 mmol/L to 6.9+/-0.5 mmol/L, P<.01), postprandial blood glucose (from 19.8+/-1.7 to 11.1+/-0.9 mmol/L, P<.01), and plasma triglycerides (from 1.13+/-0.13 to 0.89+/-0.03 mmol/L, P<.05) were observed in the berberine group. In study B, 48 adults with poorly controlled type 2 diabetes mellitus were treated supplemented with berberine in a 3-month trial. Berberine acted by lowering fasting blood glucose and postprandial blood glucose from 1 week to the end of the trial. Hemoglobin A1c decreased from 8.1%+/-0.2% to 7.3%+/-0.3% (P<.001)." Yin J, Xing H, Ye J.Efficacy of berberine in patients with type 2 diabetes mellitus. *Metabolism*. 2008 May;57(5):712-7

[165] "One hundred sixteen patients with type 2 diabetes and dyslipidemia were randomly allocated to receive berberine (1.0 g daily) and the placebo for 3 months. ... In the berberine group, fasting and postload plasma glucose decreased from 7.0 +/- 0.8 to 5.6 +/- 0.9 and from 12.0 +/- 2.7 to 8.9 +/- 2.8 mm/liter, HbA1c from 7.5 +/- 1.0% to 6.6 +/- 0.7%, triglyceride from 2.51 +/- 2.04 to 1.61 +/- 1.10 mm/liter, total cholesterol from 5.31 +/- 0.98 to 4.35 +/- 0.96 mm/liter, and low-density lipoprotein-cholesterol from 3.23 +/- 0.81 to 2.55 +/- 0.77 mm/liter,..." Zhang Y, Li X, Zou D, Liu W, et al. Treatment of type 2 diabetes and dyslipidemia with the natural plant alkaloid berberine. *J Clin Endocrinol Metab*. 2008 Jul;93(7):2559-65

[166] [No authors listed] Undecylenic acid. Monograph. *Altern Med Rev*. 2002 Feb;7(1):68-70

Herpes Simplex, *Candida albicans*, and tinea pedis caused by *Trychophyton rubrumor* and *Trychophyton mentagrophytes*.

- ◦ Combination botanical antimicrobials ("Tricycline" from Allergy Research Group): Contains black walnut, artemesinin, berberine, and citrus seed extract; in the early days of my clinical practice, I used this product routinely with a standard dosing of "2 capsules twice per day until the bottle [n=90] is empty."
- ◦ Ascorbate-mannitol powder (""Mixed ascorbate powder" from Biotics Research Corporation containing per one teaspoon [5 grams] ascorbate 2,800 mg, calcium 200 mg, magnesium 100 mg, and mannitol): The current author—Dr Vasquez—has used this treatment empirically with great success in achieving rapid quantitative reductions in gastrointestinal microbes. For many years plain ascorbic acid was used at doses of 30-60 grams (30,000-60,000 mg) to induce therapeutic laxation (occasionally described as "do-it-yourself top-to-bottom gastrointestinal lavage") with onset of action generally within 30-60 minutes following consumption of powered ascorbate in approximately 1-2 liters of water, preferably *and often necessarily* with a bowel peristalsis stimulant such as coffee. The goal and purpose are to achieve a cleansing water bolus that purges the bowels of dysbiotic microbes and their proinflammatory debris and mitochondria-impairing metabolites. The use of therapeutic laxatives for the treatment of intestinal parasitic disease is well represented in the Infectous Disease and Tropical Medicine literature; for this instance, we are using ascorbic acid as an osmotic laxative. In high concentrations, ascorbic acid is directly microbicidal. Additional agents can be ingested simultaneously for additional antimicrobial effect (e.g., iodine-iodide 12-48 mg [given that the standard antimicrobial dose for systemic/dermal infections usually starts at 1,000mg/d]) or intraluminal adsorption (e.g., activated charcoal).

- ▫ Prescription-restricted antimicrobial agents—examples: In this section specific for the SIBO of fibromyalgia, nonabsorbable agents (rifaximin, vancomycin, nystatin) are appropriate; agents with systemic absorption (Augmentin and fluconazole) are listed here due to their high efficacy and frequent clinical utilization.
  - ◦ Rifaximin/Xifaxan: Rifaximin (gut-specific antibacterial drug) should not be confused with rifampin (systemic antibacterial drug, often used in the treatment of mycobacterium infections such as tuberculosis but also used for other bacterial infections); remember to "get your **facts/fax** right by using ri**fax**imin/Xi**fax**an" while you "use rif**amp**in **to amp**lify the effectiveness of systemic antibiotics in the treatment of chronic infections but it also **amps up** cytochrome p450 and adverse drug effects."
  - ◦ Vancomycin orally administered: Clinicians should consider this non/poorly-absorbed antibiotic which is effective against Gram-positive bacteria. Human studies have shown effectiveness in the treatment of IBS, constipation, and primary sclerosing cholangitis. In one particularly remarkable case of a patient with rheumatoid arthritis, I prescribed 125mg/d with great success with the intention to target Gram-positive Th17-inducing segmented filamentous bacteria.
  - ◦ Augmentin 1-2g BID: This combination of amoxicillin and clavulanate shows efficacy against more than 90% of gastrointestinal bacteria which contribute to SIBO.
  - ◦ Nystatin 500,000 units BID-TID PO duration as needed (e.g., 1-6 months empirically or with any use of antibacterial drugs: Nystatin is a safe nonabsorbable gentle and commonly effective antifungal agent originally derived from a natural source of soil microorganisms. Its lack of significant intestinal absorption reduces the incidence of adverse effects while also prohibiting systemic antifungal effectiveness, except for reducing the total microbial load (TML) by reducing gastrointestinal fungal population. Nystatin is safe for long-term use, is inexpensive, and should generally be used anytime that antibiotic/antibacterial drugs are employed.

- Fluconazole/Diflucan 100-150-200 mg every other day for 4-5 doses over 8-10 days: The long half-life of 30 hours allows discontinuous alternate-day dosing without loss of efficacy for most routine outpatient applications. This drug is absorbed systemically with excellent tissue penetration for the delivery of multifocal antifungal effectiveness (e.g., alleviation of sinus and genitourinary fungal infections/colonization)

- **NUTRITIONAL IMMUNOMODULATION:** My coinage of the term and technique "nutritional immunomodulation" refers to a specific protocol designed to induce epigenetic modifications in undifferentiated Th-0 cells for their preferential promotion into the T-regulatory (Treg) FOXp3+ phenotype while shifting immune (im)balance away from the proinflammatory Th-1, Th-2, and Th-17 phenotypes. The primary components of this protocol can be safely implemented in essentially any and all patients without adverse effect; these fundamental components include low-carbohydrate plant-based diet to promote a systemic anti-inflammatory state, vitamin D3, combination fatty acid supplementation for n-3 fatty acids and GLA, probiotics (note that the first four components of the protocol are already represented in the foundational five-part nutritional protocol), vitamin A, lipoic acid, green tea, and a low-sodium diet. More assertive antidysbiotic interventions to promote healthy microbial balance in the gastrointestinal lumen may include botanical/nutritional/pharmacologic antimicrobial interventions, with some preferential utilization of orally administered vancomycin based on research supporting its effectiveness against segmented filamentous bacteria which are specific inducers of the Th-17 phenotype. Since fibromyalgia in its pure form is not directly due to an immune imbalance in the way considered here, this component of the functional inflammology protocol is not specifically relevant; however, for the many patients with concomitant diagnoses of fibromyalgia with another systemic/inflammatory/autoimmune disease (such as diabetes mellitus, rheumatoid arthritis, multiple sclerosis, or psoriasis) then of course this nutritional immunomodulation protocol should be implemented.

- **DYSFUNCTIONAL MITOCHONDRIA:** The basic view that mitochondria are the "powerhouses" of the cell responsible for the formation of cellular energy in the form of ATP is what most people learn in high school biology, and little if any additional knowledge is added to medical physicians' appreciation of the diversity of mitchondria's biologic roles in medical school. Lack of appreciation of the importance of the role of mitochondrial in general and mitochondrial dysfunction in particular in health and disease has left a huge blind spot in the therapeutic vision of most clinicians; by failing to appreciate and correct mitochondrial dysfunction, clinicians have missed a valuable component to the treatment plans of many and probably most of their patients. In addition to the well-known role that mitochondria have in the formation of energy-ATP, mitochondria also play major roles in pancreatic insulin secretion, peripheral insulin reception, microbial surveillance, and maintenance of inflammatory balance, insofar as mitochondrial dysfunction clearly contributes to a pro-diabetic and insulin-insulin resistant state, as well as enhanced pro-inflammatory responsiveness to microbial (including viral) stimuli. Fibromyalgia is clearly identified with mitochondrial dysfunction, and while the secondary mitochondrial dysfunction is one of the major causes of fibromyalgic muscle pain and fatigue, the mitochondrial dysfunction does not itself cause fibromyalgia, the primary cause of which is SIBO. Thus, SIBO's generation of LPS, D-lactate, and other mitochondrial toxins is the primary/direct cause of the mitochondrial dysfunction; effective treatment must emphasize SIBO eradication and mitochondrial resuscitation. We can compartmentalize major components of mitochondrial structure and function into these three main components: ❶ citric acid cycle, ❷ electron transport chain, ❸ and the structural integrity of the inner and outer mitochondrial membranes. The main area of clinical importance can be discussed within a conversation of the electron transport chain (ETC) since this is fed by the citric acid cycle and is structurally interwoven into the inner mitochondrial membrane and fully dependent upon the nonpermeability of the outer mitochondrial membrane for the maintenance of the electromechanical proton gradient. Primary treatment must always be directed at the primary cause of any disease—not its secondary complications; in the case of FM, the SIBO must always be treated. Among mitochondria-specific treatments for fibromyalgia, supplementation with CoQ-10, melatonin, and acetyl-carnitine (preferably with lipoic acid) are the best studied and most efficacious.

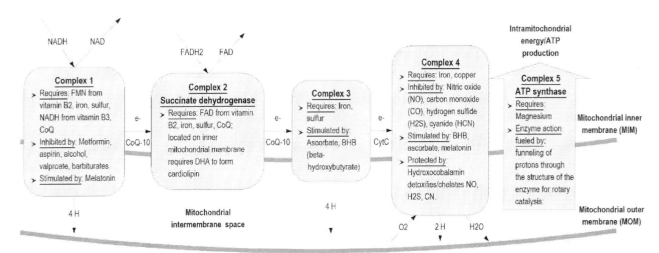

Reduce mitochondrial protein synthesis: Tetracyclines, chloramphenicol
Cause mtDNA depletion: Adriamycin/doxorubicin, zidovudine, herpes simplex virus

Vasquez A. Integrative Rheumatology and Inflammation Mastery. 3rd ed. Seattle, WA: CreateSpace, 2014.

Each step of the mitochondrial electron transport chain requires specific nutrients, without which energy/ATP production cannot proceed: Complex 1 requires vitamin B2 (riboflavin), vitamin B3 (niacin), and CoQ-10. Complex 2 requires vitamin B2 (riboflavin), iron, CoQ-10, and the fatty acid DHA for the function of succinate dehydrogenase. Complex 3 requires iron. Complex 4 requires vitamin C and copper. Step 4 is the enzyme ATP synthase, which produces cellular energy in the form of ATP.

- **Coenzyme Q10 (CoQ-10):** An endogenous antioxidant, vitamin-like substance, and essential component of the mitochondrial electron transport chain, oral supplementation with CoQ-10 has been used therapeutically in numerous studies for the successful treatment of migraine, heart failure, hypertension, and renal failure. Additional data have shown immunomodulatory roles for CoQ-10, and many clinicians employ it as adjunctive treatment for viral infections, cancer, and allergies.[167,168] The electron transport chain is the terminal step in mitochondrial energy/ATP production; as readers can see in the following diagram, each step or "complex" of the electron transport chain requires nutrients, without which energy/ATP production will be impaired, and provision of which (via supplementation) will generally enhance mitochondrial energy/ATP production. Per Cordero et al[169] in 2012, **CoQ-10 levels are 40% lower in blood cells of patients with FM compared with levels in healthy persons**, and reduced levels of CoQ-10 correlate with markers associated with expedited destruction of mitochondria (mitophagy).
  - Clinical investigation: Mitochondrial dysfunction and mitophagy activation in blood mononuclear cells of fibromyalgia patients (*Arthritis Research Therapy* 2010 Jan[170]): The authors studied 2 male and 18 female FM patients and 10 healthy controls. They evaluated mitochondrial function in blood mononuclear cells from FM patients measuring CoQ-10 levels with high-performance liquid chromatography (HPLC) and measuring mitochondrial membrane potential with flow cytometry. Oxidative stress was determined by measuring mitochondrial superoxide production and lipid peroxidation in blood mononuclear cells and plasma from FM patients. Autophagy activation was evaluated in blood mononuclear cells; mitophagy was confirmed by measuring citrate synthase activity and electron microscopy examination of blood mononuclear cells. The authors **found reduced levels of CoQ-10, decreased mitochondrial membrane**

[167] Gaby AR. The role of Coenzyme Q10 in clinical medicine: Part 1. *Altern Med Rev* 1996;1:11-17
[168] Gaby AR. The role of Coenzyme Q10 in clinical medicine: Part 2. *Altern Med Rev* 1996;1: 168-175
[169] Cordero MD, De Miguel M, Moreno Fernández AM, et al. Mitochondrial dysfunction and mitophagy activation in blood mononuclear cells of fibromyalgia patients: implications in the pathogenesis of the disease. *Arthritis Res Ther*. 2010;12(1):R17. Epub 2010 Jan 28.
[170] Cordero MD, De Miguel M, Moreno Fernández AM, Carmona López IM, Garrido Maraver J, Cotán D, Gómez Izquierdo L, Bonal P, Campa F, Bullon P, Navas P, Sánchez Alcázar JA. Mitochondrial dysfunction and mitophagy activation in blood mononuclear cells of fibromyalgia patients: implications in the pathogenesis of the disease. *Arthritis Res Ther*. 2010;12(1):R17. Epub 2010 Jan 28.

potential, **increased levels of mitochondrial superoxide in blood mononuclear cells (indicating increased oxidative stress and reduced antioxidant defense),** and increased levels of lipid peroxidation in both blood mononuclear cells and plasma from FM patients. Importantly, the authors note that "mitochondrial dysfunction was also associated with increased expression of autophagic genes and the elimination of dysfunctional mitochondria with mitophagy." *Comment by Dr Vasquez: What this means in practical terms is that the **biochemical aberrations that cause mitochondrial dysfunction lead to destruction of mitochondria via "mitophagy"** which literally means "mitochondrial consumption", a process by which dysfunctional mitochondria are eliminated by degradative processes.*

▫ Clinical trial using a combination of <u>*Ginkgo biloba* and CoQ-10 (*Journal of Internal Medicine Research* 2002 Mar[171]):</u> In an open trial of 23 fibromyalgia patients, the combination of 200 mg CoQ-10 and 200 mg *Ginkgo biloba* (for a total dose of 48 mg flavone glycosides and 12 mg terpene lactones) daily for 84 days was shown to provide clinical benefit in 64% of patients. CoQ-10 is often deficient in FM patients, and this deficiency both *causes* and *results from* mitochondrial dysfunction; stated differently, CoQ-10 depletion and mitochondrial dysfunction form a vicious cycle, a relationship of reciprocal causality. *Ginkgo biloba* extract is an extensively researched botanical medicine with a long history of safe and effective clinical use for various conditions, especially those associated with reduced blood flow and impaired mitochondrial function. *Ginkgo biloba* is a botanical/herbal medicine with a long history of human use; the three most important physiologic effects of *Ginkgo biloba* are ❶ vasodilation—improves blood circulation (which is often compromised in FM patients), ❷ improves mitochondrial function and ATP/energy production, and ❸ antioxidant benefits—quenches/absorbs free radicals, which are oxygen-containing molecules that cause damage to cell structures and body tissues. Given these therapeutic benefits, *Ginkgo* would appear to be a reasonable therapeutic agent to address the secondary pathophysiology in fibromyalgia. *Ginkgo biloba* products are generally standardized for the content of flavone glycosides (approximately 24%) and terpene lactones (approximately 6%) with adult doses ranging from 60-240 mg/d and generally 120 mg/d. *Comment by Dr Vasquez: Ginkgo biloba and CoQ-10 are very safe and appropriate for use by nearly all FM patients.*

▫ <u>Case series of FM patients treated with CoQ-10 (*Mitochondrion* 2011 Jul[172]):</u> The authors note that CoQ-10 is an essential electron carrier in the mitochondrial respiratory chain and a strong antioxidant and that **low CoQ-10 levels have been detected in patients with FM.** The authors found that "**FM patients with CoQ-10 deficiency showed a statistically significant reduction in symptoms after CoQ-10 treatment during 9 months (300 mg/day).** Determination of deficiency and consequent supplementation in FM may result in clinical improvement." *Comment by Dr Vasquez: This is a small but important study documenting 1) that CoQ-10 deficiency is common in FM patients, and 2) that CoQ-10 supplementation alleviates the clinical manifestations/symptoms of FM, consistent with the integrated model of FM presented in this book, which includes the components of nutrient deficiency and mitochondrial dysfunction. Although standardized blood testing for CoQ-10 levels is widely available, testing for and documentation of CoQ-10 deficiency is not necessary before the use of CoQ-10 supplementation.*

▫ <u>Clinical investigation and clinical trial: Oxidative stress, headache symptoms in fibromyalgia and the role of CoQ-10 in clinical improvement (*PLoS One* 2012 Apr[173]):</u> The authors introduce this study by noting that FM is a chronic pain syndrome with "unknown etiology" and a wide spectrum of symptoms such as allodynia (perception of pain from stimuli that are not normally painful), debilitating fatigue, joint stiffness, and migraine headaches. The authors note a link between oxidative stress and the clinical symptoms in FM. In this study, the researchers examined oxidative stress and bioenergetic status in blood mononuclear cells (BMCs) and the association

[171] Lister RE. An open, pilot study to evaluate the potential benefits of coenzyme Q10 combined with Ginkgo biloba extract in fibromyalgia syndrome. *J Int Med Res.* 2002 Mar-Apr;30(2):195-9

[172] Cordero MD et al. Coenzyme Q(10): a novel therapeutic approach for Fibromyalgia? case series with 5 patients. *Mitochondrion.* 2011 Jul;11(4):623-5

[173] Cordero MD, Cano-Garcia FJ, Alcocer-Gómez E, et al. Oxidative stress correlates with headache symptoms in fibromyalgia: coenzyme Q10 effect on clinical improvement. *PLoS One.* 2012;7(4):e35677 http://www.ncbi.nlm.nih.gov/pmc/articles/PMC3330812/

with headache symptoms in FM patients. Following this correlative analysis, the authors assessed the effects of oral CoQ-10 supplementation on biochemical markers and clinical improvements. In 20 FM patients and 15 healthy controls, a variety of validated clinical and biochemical parameters was assessed; specifically for the biochemical component, measurements were performed for serum CoQ-10, catalase, lipid peroxidation (LPO) levels and ATP levels in BMCs. In patients with FM, the authors found lower CoQ-10 (CoQ-10 deficiency), lower catalase (reduced antioxidant defenses) and lower ATP levels (reduced energy production) in BMCs while FM patients also showed elevated LPO (evidence of free-radical damage) in BMCs. Lower levels of CoQ-10 and catalase levels in BMCs correlated with greater severity-frequency of headache. **In this clinical trial using CoQ-10 300 mg/d for 3 months, CoQ-10 supplementation caused significant reductions in pain and tender points, significant reductions in headache impact, significant elevations in cellular levels of CoQ-10, a reduction in malondialdehyde (marker of lipid peroxidation) from 30nmol to 5 nmol (normal 6 nmol), an increase in catalase levels from 35 U/mg to 85 U/mg (normal 96 U/mg), and an increase in BMC production of ATP/energy from 61 nmol/mg to 191 nmol/mg (normal 202 nmol/mg).** Supplementation with CoQ-10 300 mg/day divided in three doses for 3 months "restored biochemical parameters and induced a significant improvement in clinical and headache symptoms." *Note by Dr Vasquez: The dose of CoQ-10 used clinically is generally approximately 100 mg per day, and occasionally a patient or doctor might decide to use a higher dose, which might be up to 300 mg per day.*

- **Melatonin:** Melatonin is a hormone produced in the pineal gland of the brain; melatonin is synthesized from the neurotransmitter serotonin, and production of both serotonin and melatonin are dependent on the nutritional availability of tryptophan and/or 5-HTP as discussed above. Patients with FM show decreased nocturnal secretion of melatonin.[174] Melatonin benefits FM patients through a wide range of mechanisms, including promotion of restful sleep and reduction in LPS-induced mitochondrial impairment. As a powerful antioxidant, melatonin scavenges oxygen and nitrogen-based reactants generated in mitochondria and thereby limits the loss of intramitochondrial glutathione, the most important component of antioxidant defense; this prevents damage to mitochondrial protein and DNA. **Melatonin increases the activity of Complexes 1 and 4 of the mitochondrial electron transport chain, improving mitochondrial respiration and increasing ATP synthesis** under various physiological and experimental conditions.[175] Successful treatment with melatonin or its precursor tryptophan/5-HTP should not deter the clinician from addressing other contributing or causative problems such as vitamin D deficiency, gastrointestinal dysbiosis including SIBO, magnesium deficiency, and chronic psychoemotional stress. The adult physiologic dose which mimics natural internal (endogenous) production is approximately 200-500 mcg [micrograms] nightly. In adults, supplementation with melatonin has a wide therapeutic index and has been used safely and effectively in doses up to 20 to 40 mg [milligrams] nightly.

  - Case series (n=4): Melatonin therapy in fibromyalgia (*Journal of Pineal Research* 2006 Jan[176]): Melatonin (3–6 mg per night, administered orally 1 hour before bedtime) has been reported to normalize sleep, alleviate pain and fatigue, and resolve many other clinical manifestations of FM. The authors report, "After 15 days of treatment with melatonin, all patients developed a sleep/wake cycle that was considered normal. They also mentioned a significant reduction of pain. At this time, the patients were taken off hypnotics. Thirty days after the initiation of melatonin, other medications were withdrawn and thereafter they only took melatonin." *Comment by Dr Vasquez: These results are impressive, but—again—the other components of FM such as SIBO and CoQ-10 deficiency should also be treated assertively to reduce the risk of relapse and to treat the underlying problems; good healthcare and good self-care should extend beyond mere symptom alleviation.*

---

[174] Wikner J, et al. Fibromyalgia--a syndrome associated with decreased nocturnal melatonin secretion. *Clin Endocrinol* (Oxf). 1998 Aug;49(2):179-83
[175] León J, Acuña-Castroviejo D, Escames G, Tan DX, Reiter RJ. Melatonin mitigates mitochondrial malfunction. *J Pineal Res*. 2005 Jan;38(1):1-9
[176] Acuna-Castroviejo D, Escames G, Reiter RJ. Melatonin therapy in fibromyalgia. *J Pineal Res*. 2006 Jan;40(1):98-9

- Clinical trial (n=101): Adjuvant use of melatonin for treatment of fibromyalgia (*Journal of Pineal Research*. 2011 Apr[177]): group A (24 patients) treated with 20 mg/day fluoxetine alone; group B (27 patients) treated with melatonin 5 mg alone; group C (27 patients) treated with 20 mg fluoxetine plus 3 mg melatonin; group D (23 patients) treated with 20 mg fluoxetine plus 5 mg melatonin for 8 weeks. "Using melatonin (3 mg or 5 mg/day) in combination with 20 mg/day fluoxetine resulted in significant reduction in both total and different components of Fibromyalgia Impact Questionnaire score compared to the pretreatment values. In conclusion, **administration of melatonin, alone or in a combination with fluoxetine, was effective in the treatment of patients with FMS.**"

- **Acetyl-L-carnitine (ALC):** Acetyl-L-carnitine is a form of the amino acid L-carnitine, most notable for its critical role in supporting mitochondrial energy/ATP production by supporting the metabolism (beta oxidation) of fatty acids in the mitochondria. A large study with 102 patients showed that ALC (administered by oral and parenteral routes, 1500 mg/d) was beneficial in patients with fibromyalgia.[178] Given the role of ALC in supporting and improving mitochondrial function, this supplement probably benefits fibromyalgia patients by compensating for LPS-induced skeletal muscle dysfunction.

- **D-ribose:** D-ribose is a naturally occurring pentose carbohydrate available as a dietary supplement. When administered orally (5 g thrice daily), it safely provides numerous benefits to fibromyalgia patients, according to a recent pilot study with 41 patients.[179] Improvements are seen in energy, sleep, mental clarity, pain intensity, and well-being, as well as global assessment. Among its beneficial mechanisms of action is enhancement of mitochondrial ATP production. Thus, the benefits of D-ribose supplementation may be mediated by restoration or preservation of mitochondrial impairment caused by LPS in fibromyalgia patients.

- **Creatine monohydrate:** Skeletal muscle levels of phosphocreatine and ATP are reduced in patients with fibromyalgia compared with normal controls; thus, oral supplementation with creatine would appear to be an obvious intervention to restore these depressed levels to normal. Although no formal trials have been conducted, Artimal et al[180] reported that a patient with severe refractory fibromyalgia attained sustained alleviation of depression and pain, as well as improvements in sleep and quality of life, following oral administration of creatine monohydrate for 4 weeks (3 grams daily in the first week, then 5 grams daily). Creatine supplementation has been shown to improve ATP production and oxygen utilization in brain and skeletal muscle in humans.[181]

- **SOCIOLOGY/PSYCHOLOGY, SLEEP, STRESS, SPINAL HEALTH, SOMATIC TREATMENTS, SWEAT/EXERCISE**: Common clinical and lifestyle considerations are listed in the following sections.
  - **Sociology/psychology, and stress management/reduction**: Everyone—patients as well as clinicians—can benefit from developing self-awareness, emotional intelligence, and other core life skill and insights; since much of our perception of stress has a psycho-epistemological basis, enhanced self-awareness in this key area can help to deconstruct the phenomenon of stress and its secondary consequences. Because this consideration is self-evident in terms of safety, efficacy, broad applicability, and life-enhancement, specific literature will not be reviewed here.
  - **Sleep**: Sleep deprivation induces immune suppression, enhanced sensitivity to pain, and an objectively documentable proinflammatory state evidenced by increases in serum hsCRP. Patients should be encouraged to optimize sleep by avoiding late-in-the-day exercise, overstimulation, caffeine (which generally has a half-life of six hours), and overuse of bright lights following nightfall; items that are conducive to sleep are having a dark and quiet room, relaxing music or reading, and using

---

[177] Hussain SA, Al-Khalifa II, Jasim NA, Gorial FI. Adjuvant use of melatonin for treatment of fibromyalgia. *J Pineal Res*. 2011 Apr;50(3):267-71

[178] Rossini M, Di Munno O, Valentini G, Bianchi G, Biasi G, Cacace E, Malesci D, La Montagna G, Viapiana O, Adami S. Double-blind, multicenter trial comparing acetyl l-carnitine with placebo in the treatment of fibromyalgia patients. *Clin Exp Rheumatol*. 2007 Mar-Apr;25(2):182-8

[179] Teitelbaum JE, Johnson C, St Cyr J. The use of D-ribose in chronic fatigue syndrome and fibromyalgia: a pilot study. *J Altern Complement Med*. 2006 Nov;12(9):857-62

[180] Amital D, Vishne T, Rubinow A, Levine J. Observed effects of creatine monohydrate in a patient with depression and fibromyalgia. *Am J Psychiatry*. 2006 Oct;163(10):1840-1

[181] Watanabe A, Kato N, Kato T. Effects of creatine on mental fatigue and cerebral hemoglobin oxygenation. *Neurosci Res*. 2002 Apr;42(4):279-85

melatonin. Enhancement of sleep quality and duration have been shown to alleviate systemic inflammation, tendency toward insulin resistance, and pain perception/sensitivity.

- **Sweating and exercise**: Obesity/overweight and physical inactivity are consistently associated with elevated risk for and experience of depression, low self-esteem, social isolation, systemic inflammation, cardiometabolic disease and diabetes mellitus type-2, cancers of various types, and inflammatory disorders such as asthma and psoriasis. Weight optimization and physical activity promote enhanced self-confidence, self-efficacy, skill-building, social interaction, and reductions in cause-specific and all-cause mortality. Mechanistically, exercise—defined here as physical activity of sustained duration and intensity to promote diaphoresis/sweating—promotes lipolysis (for mobilization of adipose-stored toxins, weight reduction, and enhanced BHB production for induction of histone acetylation and ECT stimulation), promotes glycolysis (to promote induction of enhanced mitochondrial function and insulin sensitivity), and hyperventilation which results in respiratory alkalosis and secondary urinary alkalinization (which promotes mineral retention, xenobiotic excretion, endorphin elevation, and cortisol reduction). Commonly accepted international guidelines as well as common sense advocate 30-60 minutes of daily exercise that should globally include components such as aerobic training, resistance training, skill-building, balance, and flexibility; intensity, duration, and variety are tailored to patient needs and preferences. Because this consideration is self-evident in terms of safety, efficacy, broad applicability, and life-enhancement, specific literature will not be reviewed here.

- **Somatic treatments (chiropractic, acupuncture, osteopathic manipulation, qigong, balneotherapy)**: Chiropractic treatment (including spinal manipulation, stretching, soft tissue treatments, and therapeutic ultrasound) has shown benefit in several fibromyalgia case series and clinical trials.[182,183] Acupuncture (including traditional, nontraditional, and electrical stimulation) also has been found beneficial for fibromyalgia patients.[184,185,186] Acupuncture may relieve fibromyalgia pain by improving regional blood flow, in addition to other mechanisms.[187,188] Because specific needle placement does not appear to be important[189], the conclusion that true acupuncture is ineffective because it may not differ markedly from the results obtained by sham acupuncture[190] may not be logical. A similar conundrum is seen in other clinical trials involving physical interventions such as manual osseous manipulation, wherein authentic treatments and sham treatments may both be effective by virtue of common physiological responses.[191] A short-term trial showed that osteopathic manipulative therapy with standard medical care was superior to medical care alone for FM patients.[192] Qigong was found helpful for 10 fibromyalgia patients, and benefits were still apparent at 3 months' follow-up.[193] In a randomized, controlled clinical trial among 24 female fibromyalgia patients, balneotherapy (bath therapy) in daily 20-minute sessions 5 days per week for 3 weeks (total of 15 sessions; water temperature: 96.8°F = 36°C), resulted in statistically significant reductions in measured inflammatory

---

[182] Citak-Karakaya I, Akbayrak T, Demirturk F, Ekici G, Bakar Y. Short and long-term results of connective tissue manipulation and combined ultrasound therapy in patients with fibromyalgia. *J Manipulative Physiol Ther*. 2006 Sep;29(7):524-8

[183] Blunt KL, Rajwani MH, Guerriero RC. The effectiveness of chiropractic management of fibromyalgia patients: a pilot study. *J Manipulative Physiol Ther*. 1997 Jul-Aug;20(6):389-99

[184] Martin DP, Sletten CD, Williams BA, Berger IH. Improvement in fibromyalgia symptoms with acupuncture: results of a randomized controlled trial. *Mayo Clin Proc*. 2006 Jun;81(6):749-57

[185] Singh BB, Wu WS, Hwang SH, Khorsan R, Der-Martirosian C, Vinjamury SP, Wang CN, Lin SY. Effectiveness of acupuncture in the treatment of fibromyalgia. *Altern Ther Health Med*. 2006 Mar-Apr;12(2):34-41

[186] Deluze C, Bosia L, Zirbs A, Chantraine A, Vischer TL. Electroacupuncture in fibromyalgia: results of a controlled trial. *BMJ*. 1992 Nov 21;305(6864):1249-52

[187] Sandberg M, Larsson B, Lindberg LG, Gerdle B. Different patterns of blood flow response in the trapezius muscle following needle stimulation (acupuncture) between healthy subjects and patients with fibromyalgia and work-related trapezius myalgia. *Eur J Pain*. 2005 Oct;9(5):497-510

[188] Sandberg M, Lindberg LG, Gerdle B. Peripheral effects of needle stimulation (acupuncture) on skin and muscle blood flow in fibromyalgia. *Eur J Pain*. 2004 Apr;8(2):163-71

[189] Harris RE, Tian X, Williams DA, Tian TX, Cupps TR, Petzke F, Groner KH, Biswas P, Gracely RH, Clauw DJ. Treatment of fibromyalgia with formula acupuncture: investigation of needle placement, needle stimulation, and treatment frequency. *J Altern Complement Med*. 2005 Aug;11(4):663-71

[190] Assefi NP, Sherman KJ, Jacobsen C, Goldberg J, Smith WR, Buchwald D. A randomized clinical trial of acupuncture compared with sham acupuncture in fibromyalgia. *Ann Intern Med*. 2005 Jul 5;143(1):10-9

[191] Mein EA, Greenman PE, McMillin DL, Richards DG, Nelson CD. Manual medicine diversity: research pitfalls and the emerging medical paradigm. *J Am Osteopath Assoc*. 2001 Aug;101(8):441-4

[192] Gamber RG, Shores JH, Russo DP, Jimenez C, Rubin BR. Osteopathic manipulative treatment in conjunction with medication relieves pain associated with fibromyalgia syndrome: results of a randomized clinical pilot project. *J Am Osteopath Assoc*. 2002 Jun;102(6):321-5

[193] Chen KW, Hassett AL, Hou F, Staller J, Lichtbroun AS. A pilot study of external qigong therapy for patients with fibromyalgia. *J Altern Complement Med*. 2006 Nov;12(9):851-6

mediators (PGE2, interleukin-1, LTB4) and amelioration of clinical symptoms among treated FM patients.[194] The symptomatic benefits of balneotherapy for FM patients have been corroborated in other trials.[195,196,197]

- **ENDOCRINE OPTIMIZATION:** Peptide-based and steroid-based hormones have wide-ranging effects beyond those with which they are classically and thus simplistically associated. The "main" hormones that we consider in most chronic inflammatory disorders are the three pro-inflammatory hormones (prolactin, estradiol, and insulin) and the three anti-inflammatory hormones (DHEA, cortisol, and testosterone); each of these hormones can be objectively assessed with serologic testing and modulated with therapeutic intervention. A full thyroid evaluation—including history, physical examination (with particular scrutiny for cold extremities [DDX: hypothyroidism, hypogonadism, vasoconstriction/vaso-obstruction, Raynaud's disorder, peripheral vascular disease, H2S-producing GI dysbiosis], relative bradycardia [DDX, hypothyroidism, heart block, beta-blocker medications], and delayed Achilles reflex return [considered diagnostic of hypothyroidism]), and laboratory evaluation (including TSH, free T4, total or free T3, rT3, and antithyroid antibodies) is warranted in any patient whose concerns include fatigue, depression, systemic inflammation and chronic pain; musculoskeletal manifestations of hypothyroidism include muscle pain, weakness, myopathy, and adhesive capsulitis. The pineal hormone melatonin was discussed in a previous section.

- **XENOBIOTIC ACCUMULATION/DETOXIFICATION:** The term "xenobiotics" is generally used to refer to carbon-based foreign chemicals such as persistent organic pollutants (POPs) including herbicides, pesticides, phthalates, parabens, dioxin-related chemicals, and many others; used more casually, the term may also be used to include noncarbon-based foreign substances such as toxic metals like lead, mercury, cadmium, and arsenic. Thus, "xenobiotics" has become somewhat synonymous with "toxins" in both professional-level and vernacular conversations. Laboratory assessments for chemical and metal toxins are commercially available through specialized medical laboratories and are based on analysis of blood and urine. The many biochemical and physiologic components of detoxification/depuration have been reviewed in chapter 4 of this book. Essentially everyone—all humans on the planet worldwide—have biochemical evidence of xenobiotic chemical/metal accumulation, generally with numerous xenobiotics, which have additive and synergistic adverse effects on physiology and health. Thus, scientifically, since xenobiotic accumulation is pandemic, consideration of and treatment for xenobiotic accumulation via therapeutic detoxification programs and lifestyle interventions should be routine. Easy and effective means for promoting detoxification of chemicals and metals include plant-based diet to promote bowel and renal excretion of toxins (via reduced enterohepatic recycling [better microflora, more fiber for adsorption, more frequent fecal excretion] and reduced renal resorption [urinary alkalinization], respectively), NAC for arsenic chelation and GSH production, sweating/exercise (lipolysis promotes mobilization of lipophilic toxins from adipose tissue, diaphoresis promotes direct toxin excretion), sufficient micronutrient and protein intake supports phase 1 and phase 2 of the oxidation and conjugation processes in the liver. Chemical xenobiotics can be bound in the gut during the normal process of enterohepatic recycling/recirculation with periodic or rotational use of activated charcoal, cholestyramine, and chlorella; anecdotal reports from clinical practices support the use of phytochelatin (metal-binding peptides from plants, used by plants for protection from metal toxicity) in the prevention/treatment of metal toxicity in humans but no formal clinical studies have been performed to document the effectiveness of this approach although its safety is clinically appreciated.

  - Pilot study: Chlorella pyrenoidosa for patients with fibromyalgia syndrome (Phytother Res 2000 May[198]): Chlorella pyrenoidosa is a unicellular green alga that grows in fresh water. It is a dense source of nutrients, particularly vitamin D (500 IU vitamin D per 1.35 g Chlorella). Chlorella may have value in treating some fibromyalgia patients, but overall the efficacy is low. Thus, Chlorella should not be used as monotherapy for fibromyalgia, although it may be a useful adjunct either as a source of vitamin D,

---

[194] Ardiç F, Ozgen M, Aybek H, et al. Effects of balneotherapy on serum IL-1, PGE2 and LTB4 levels in fibromyalgia patients. *Rheumatol Int.* 2007 Mar;27(5):441-6
[195] Evcik D, Kizilay B, Gökçen E. The effects of balneotherapy on fibromyalgia patients. *Rheumatol Int.* 2002 Jun;22(2):56-9
[196] Fioravanti A, Perpignano G, Tirri G, et al. Effects of mud-bath treatment on fibromyalgia patients: a randomized clinical trial. *Rheumatol Int.* 2007 Oct;27(12):1157-61
[197] Dönmez A, Karagülle MZ, Tercan N, et al. SPA therapy in fibromyalgia: a randomised controlled clinic study. *Rheumatol Int.* 2005 Dec;26(2):168-72
[198] Merchant RE, et al. Nutritional supplementation with Chlorella pyrenoidosa for patients with fibromyalgia syndrome: a pilot study. *Phytother Res* 2000 May;14:167-73

as a means to help modify gut flora, or as an aid in the detoxification of xenobiotics due to its ability to bind ingested and bile-excreted toxins and prevent their absorption and reabsorption in a manner similar to that of cholestyramine, a drug used to bind cholesterol in the gut, promote its excretion, and thereby lower blood cholesterol levels.[199,200,201] This "detoxifying" effect of *Chlorella* in humans is supported by 2 clinical trials showing that nursing mothers who supplement with *Chlorella* during lactation transfer less dioxin in their breast milk compared to nursing mothers who do not consume *Chlorella*.[202,203]

- Clinical investigation: Reduced exposure to xenobiotics (cosmetics) alleviates fibromyalgia (*Journal of Women's Health* 2004 Mar[204]): Women use more cosmetic products than do men, and fibromyalgia is more common in women. Cosmetic products generally contain skin-absorbable xenobiotics with potentially adverse effects; therefore this study was conducted to determine if avoidance of cosmetics would alleviate symptoms of FM. The author of this report describes a prospective, randomized, controlled trial of 48 women with FM (some of whom had a rheumatic condition) who were regular users of cosmetics was carried out to investigate if a reduced use of cosmetics would reduce the symptoms. The patients were told to avoid or completely abstain from using all ointments, creams, skin lotions, pain-relieving liniments, cleaning lotions, oil treatments, hair-coloring chemicals, and tanning lotion; they were also advised to reduce their use of soap and shampoo, both of which—like skin creams—are generally formulated with perfumes and other chemicals and applied to large regions of the body. This research showed that, after 2 years, FM patients who reduced their exposure to chemicals/xenobiotics/cosmetics experienced significant reductions in pain, sleep disturbances, and musculoskeletal stiffness (p < 0.02), together with better physical function and improved sense of well-being as measured by the Fibromyalgia Impact Questionnaire (FIQ). Thus, avoiding chemical exposure appears to provide no-cost no-risk therapeutic benefit to FM patients by alleviating pain and improving several indicators of overall health.

Conclusions and Therapeutic Approach

- In sum, current research indicates that fibromyalgia results from impairment of cellular energy/ATP production (mitochondrial dysfunction) and induction of pain hypersensitivity (peripheral and central sensitization) due to absorbed metabolic toxins from bacterial/microbial overgrowth of the gastrointestinal tract; this is complicated by induction of tryptophan deficiency which is most likely caused by tryptophan degradation by bacterial tryptophanase activity and which leads to serotonin and melatonin insufficiencies, which lead to associated biochemical and clinical consequences, discussed previously. Available studies have shown that SIBO is ubiquitous among fibromyalgia patients and that antimicrobial interventions—whether pharmaceutical or nutritional—are efficacious. Secondary physiological effects such as mitochondrial impairment, pain sensitization, nutritional deficiencies, oxidative stress, and reduced tissue perfusion are treated with combined use of select therapeutics as reviewed previously. Patients presenting with widespread pain should be screened for causative underlying disease; if no other explanation can be found, then the diagnosis of fibromyalgia should be made, and the condition should be treated with the nondrug therapeutics discussed above. The first visit can include history, physical examination, and laboratory tests; initial laboratory assessment should include complete blood count (CBC), metabolic/chemistry panel, serum 25-hydroxyvitamin D, C-reactive protein (CRP), anti-nuclear antibodies (ANA), antibodies against cyclic citrullinated proteins (anti-CCP antibodies), ferritin, muscle enzymes aldolase and creatine kinase, and a complete thyroid assessment including TSH, free T4, free T3, total T3, reverse T3 (rT3), and antithyroid peroxidase and antithyroglobulin antibodies. First-day

[199] Pore RS. Detoxification of chlordecone poisoned rats with chlorella and chlorella derived sporopollenin. *Drug Chem Toxicol.* 1984;7(1):57-71
[200] Morita K, Ogata M, Hasegawa T. Chlorophyll derived from Chlorella inhibits dioxin absorption from the gastrointestinal tract and accelerates dioxin excretion in rats. *Environ Health Perspect.* 2001 Mar;109(3):289-94
[201] Morita K, Matsueda T, Iida T, Hasegawa T. Chlorella accelerates dioxin excretion in rats. *J Nutr.* 1999 Sep;129(9):1731-6
[202] Nakano S, Noguchi T, Takekoshi H, Suzuki G, Nakano M. Maternal-fetal distribution and transfer of dioxins in pregnant women in Japan, and attempts to reduce maternal transfer with Chlorella (Chlorella pyrenoidosa) supplements. *Chemosphere.* 2005 Dec;61(9):1244-55
[203] Nakano S, Takekoshi H, Nakano M. Chlorella (Chlorella pyrenoidosa) supplementation decreases dioxin and increases immunoglobulin a concentrations in breast milk. *J Med Food.* 2007 Mar;10(1):134-42
[204] Sverdrup B. Use less cosmetics--suffer less from fibromyalgia? *J Womens Health* (Larchmt). 2004 Mar;13(2):187-94

interventions can include dietary optimization, multivitamin-multimineral supplementation (including vitamin D3 and magnesium), tryptophan/5-HTP, CoQ10, mixed tocopherols, and combination fatty acids including gamma-linolenic acid (GLA), eicosapentaenoic acid (EPA) and docosahexaenoic acid (DHA). SIBO can be treated empirically, or it can be objectively assessed with breath hydrogen and methane testing, stool analysis, culture, microscopy, and parasitology. At follow-up visits, additional assessments and interventions (such as for toxic metals and chronic occult infections) can be used to fine-tune the diagnosis and further discover and define its contributors in order to maximize the patient's response to treatment and promote optimal recovery and health.

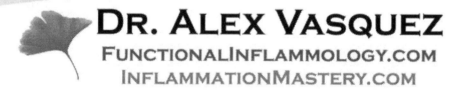

MIGRAINE HEADACHES, HYPOTHYROIDISM, AND FIBROMYALGIA:

ASSESSMENTS AND THERAPEUTIC APPROACHES USING INTEGRATIVE CHIROPRACTIC, NATUROPATHIC, OSTEOPATHIC, AND FUNCTIONAL MEDICINE

Is "central sensitization" in fibromyalgia a bunch of c.r.a.p. (Commercial Rationalization Advocating Pharmaceuticals)?

DR. ALEX VASQUEZ
FUNCTIONALINFLAMMOLOGY.COM
INFLAMMATIONMASTERY.COM

Video reviews by Dr Vasquez: Please see vimeo.com/DrVasquez and vimeo.com/ICHNFM for many videos by Dr Vasquez and colleagues.

Rheumatoid Arthritis

> **Introduction:**
> Rheumatoid arthritis (RA) is one of the most common and "most classic" systemic autoimmune diseases. Despite its name, RA affects much more than the musculoskeletal system: rheumatoid lung, rheumatoid kidney disease, and other systemic, vasculitic, and (sub)cutaneous complications are not uncommon. Readers should begin to recognize the "patterns of inflammation" that result in distinct diagnostic labels are simply "variations on a theme" based on a finite number of identifiable and modifiable factors, which are largely amenable to nonpharmacologic interventions.

<u>Topics</u>:
- Introduction and Overview
- Clinical Presentation
- Prevalence, Symptoms, and Clinical Findings
- Pathophysiology
- Differential Diagnosis
- Diagnosis
- Standard Medical Treatment
- Therapeutic Interventions—Clinical Application of the Functional Inflammology Protocol via FINDSEX™ acronym

Rheumatoid Arthritis
"RA"

<u>Description/pathophysiology</u>:
- <u>Description in a nutshell</u>: RA is a relatively common, persistent, symmetric, destructive, systemic inflammatory "autoimmune" disease chiefly characterized by peripheral arthritis but which may also affect the proximal joints (e.g., hips and shoulders), the axial skeleton (e.g., spine—notably the atlantoaxial joint—as well as the sacroiliac joints), and internal organs (e.g., "rheumatoid lung") and vascular system (e.g., rheumatoid vasculitis).
- <u>Basic pathology</u>: A pathogenic hallmark of the disease is immune complex formation and intra-articular deposition with resultant release of cytokines and other pro-inflammatory mediators. Immune complexes are important instigators of rheumatoid arthritis and vasculitis, and rheumatoid factor (RF) antibodies are important contributors to these immune complexes.[1,2] The chronic/sustained inflammation leads to synovial thickening, villous hypertrophy (pannus formation), and intraarticular colonization with activated lymphocytes and plasma cells. The localized immunocytes cause inflammation and tissue destruction via elaboration of matrix metalloproteinases (including collagenases), prostaglandins, and cytokines such as IL-1.
- <u>Prevalence</u>: Affects 0.8-1% of all populations: considered the second most common rheumatic diagnosis[3] after "osteoarthritis", many cases of which are actually genetic hemochromatosis, one of the most common hereditary conditions in humans (heterozygote frequency: 1:7; homozygote frequency 1:200-250).

---

[1] Beers MH, Berkow R (eds). <u>The Merck Manual. Seventeenth Edition.</u> Whitehouse Station; Merck Research Laboratories: 1999, page 416
[2] Jonsson T, Valdimarsson H. What about IgA rheumatoid factor in rheumatoid arthritis? *Ann Rheum Dis.* 1998 Jan;57(1):63-4
http://ard.bmjjournals.com/cgi/content/full/57/1/63
[3] Hardin JG, Waterman J, Labson LH. Rheumatic disease: Which diagnostic tests are useful? *Patient Care* 1999; March 15: 83-102

- o Musculoskeletal disorders and iron overload disease (*Arthritis Rheum* 1996 Oct[4]—full text provided within this textbook): "Arthropathy affects up to 80% of iron-overloaded patients and is often the only manifestation of the disease. ... Thus, since iron overload affects such a large portion of the population and arthropathy is a common manifestation of this disorder, patients with musculoskeletal symptoms should be screened for iron overload."
- Introduction to standard allopathic medical perspective and treatment: From the allopathic perspective, RA is seen as a chronic "idiopathic" inflammatory disorder primarily affecting the peripheral joints but also affecting the axial skeleton and internal organs; it is generally treated with NSAIDs and other "anti-inflammatory" and immunosuppressive drugs, which are palliative and have no chance of providing cure. The standard sequential protocol is as follows: NAIDs and acetaminophen, prednisone, methotrexate, (perhaps sulfasalazine and hydroxychloroquine), then—ever more commonly prescribed—the "biologics", which may be followed by newer experimental and immunoparalytic drugs; this routine protocol has value in the acute suppression of inflammation, but it is notoriously expensive, wrought with adverse effects, and ineffective for the authentic treatment of rheumatoid arthritis, as noted in the landmark 2012 article cited here:
  - o Sustained rheumatoid arthritis remission is uncommon in clinical practice (*Arthritis Res Ther* 2012 Mar[5]): "This study shows that in clinical practice, a minority of RA patients are in sustained remission. ... Other studies have described sustained remission in daily practice as uncommon, being reached by only 17% to 36% of RA patients for up to 6 months. These studies did not evaluate time in remission beyond 6 months. A recent study investigated the probability of remaining in remission up to 24 months, according to the ACR/EULAR, SDAI, and CDAI remission criteria in two different cohorts. They also concluded that long-term remission is rare, considering that the probability of a remission lasting 2 years was 6% to 14%."
- Introduction to naturopathic medicine and functional medicine perspective and treatment: From the perspective of naturopathic medicine and functional medicine, the condition is considered highly amenable to treatment provided that such treatment is multifaceted and addresses the allergic, dysbiotic, nutritional, mitochondrial, endocrinologic, and immunophenotypic components of this multifaceted phenomenon.
- Etiological considerations include:
  - o Genetic predisposition and HLA-DR: HLA-DR4 is positive in 70% of RA patients, compared to 28% of control patients. "Genetic risk factors do not fully account for the incidence of RA, suggesting that environmental factors also play a role in the etiology of the disease. ...[C]limate and urbanization have a major impact on the incidence and severity of RA in groups of similar genetic background."[6]
  - o Urbanization / Western lifestyle: Urbanization is a risk factor for the development of rheumatic disease.[7,8] Urbanization is associated with increased risk of vitamin D deficiency and increased exposure to nutritionally-depleted multiallergenic genetically-modified AGE-laden phytonutrient-deficient prohyperglycemic "convenience foods", sleep disturbances, and exposure to particulate debris (i.e., pollution from diesel and other petrochemical combustion); each of these factors has been shown in animal models or human trials to promote systemic inflammation.
  - o Female gender / estrogen: Women are affected 2-3x more often than men. Male RA patients tend to have relative reductions in DHEA and testosterone and relative excess of estrogen and prolactin. Predisposing factors for women include vitamin D deficiency, dysestrogenism, and the anatomically shorter urethra which predisposes the female urinary tract to recurrent microbial colonization.

[4] Vasquez A. Musculoskeletal disorders and iron overload disease: comment on the American College of Rheumatology guidelines for the initial evaluation of the adult patient with acute musculoskeletal symptoms. *Arthritis Rheum*. 1996 Oct;39(10):1767-8
[5] Prince FH, Bykerk VP, Shadick NA, Lu B, Cui J, Frits M, Iannaccone CK, Weinblatt ME, Solomon DH. Sustained rheumatoid arthritis remission is uncommon in clinical practice. *Arthritis Res Ther*. 2012 Mar 19;14(2):R68 http://arthritis-research.com/content/14/2/R68
[6] Fauci AS, Braunwald E, Isselbacher KJ, et al., eds. Harrison's Principles of Internal Medicine. 14th ed. New York, NY: McGraw-Hill; 1998, page 1881
[7] "In particular, a significantly lower prevalence of RA in rural areas compared with urban cohorts has led to the hypothesis that environmental factors associated with urbanization may be involved in disease pathogenesis." Adebajo A, Davis P. Rheumatic diseases in African blacks. *Semin Arthritis Rheum*. 1994 Oct;24(2):139-53
[8] "The general impression is that rheumatoid arthritis (RA) has a lower prevalence and a milder course in developing countries. Epidemiological studies from different regions show that varying prevalence is possibly related to urbanization." Kalla AA, Tikly M. Rheumatoid arthritis in the developing world. *Best Pract Res Clin Rheumatol*. 2003 Oct;17(5):863-75

- o Tobacco/cigarette smoke: Habitual tobacco/cigarette smoking increases exposure to reactive oxygen species, vasoactive/vasoconstrictive substances, carcinogens, and bacterial endotoxin. Tobacco leaves are noted for their high surface area which—unfortunately for smokers—serves as a deposition reservoir for both ambient radioactive particles[9,10] as well as Gram-negative bacteria, Gram-positive bacteria, and fungi[11]; thereby, tobacco smoking increases exposure to radioactive particles as well as microbial debris (e.g., endotoxin, exotoxin, and bacterial DNA). Thus, the finding that tobacco smoking—particularly from cigarette smoke which is inhaled deeply into the lungs in contrast with cigar smoke which is generally inhaled only into the mouth and pharynx—is a major risk factor for the development of rheumatoid arthritis and other systemic inflammatory/autoimmune/autoinflammatory disorders is consistent with the microbial/dysbiotic model discussed later in this section.
  - ▪ Cigarette smoking and inflammation (*J Dent Res* 2012 Feb[12]): **"CS [cigarette smoking] impairs innate defenses against pathogens, modulates antigen presentation, and promotes autoimmunity.** … Potential mechanisms by which CS promotes rheumatoid arthritis include the release of intracellular proteins from ROS-activated or injured cells, augmentation of auto-reactive B-cell function, altered presentation of antigens by CS-impaired antigen-presenting cells, altered regulatory T-cell functions, and T-cell activation by antigens found in CS."
- o Occult viral, bacterial or parasitic infections:
  - ▪ Viral: **"Cytomegalovirus and rubella viruses have been cultured from the synovium in patients with rheumatoid arthritis…"** "Some evidence suggests hepatitis C virus as a possible trigger to rheumatoid arthritis."[13] The implications of this data are unclear; however, possibilities include: 1) virus *directly* provoking joint destruction, 2) virus *indirectly* provoking joint destruction, such as via immune complexes, 3) noncausal, coincidental finding, 4) inability of RA patients to clear this infection due to immunologic deficits which accompany immune dysfunction. Remember, "Unhealthy people are unhealthy", and an *associated* abnormality does not imply a *causal* relationship. Sick people tend to get sicker and enter vicious cycles that can amplify the original illness and lead to the genesis of new, additive health problems. Additionally, given that nutritional

"Classic" multifocal dysbiosis in RA
• Nasopharynx: *Streptococcus pyogenes*
• Gastrointestinal: *Eubacterium aerofaciens*
• Genitourinary: *Proteus mirabilis*

    deficiencies—pandemic in the general population and even more common in patients with chronic illness (due to malabsorption, hypermetabolism of immune activation, and nutrient losses and malabsorption due to pharmaceutical drugs, etc)—promote viral mutagenesis and replication, the possibility exists that enhanced viral replication in patients with RA/autoimmunity is a surrogate marker for nutritional deficiency; relatedly, enhanced viral replication might be a surrogate marker for enhanced activity of the NFkB pathway, which is upregulated in inflammatory responses and which promotes viral replication. More likely from this author's perspective is the probability that increased viral replication/presence is—regardless of primary etiology—a likely contributor to the total microbial load (TML) and total

---

[9] "Tobacco leaves are large and have sticky exudates that retain the radon decay products once they deposit on the leaves." Savidou A, Kehagia K, Eleftheriadis K. Concentration levels of 210Pb and 210Po in dry tobacco leaves in Greece. *J Environ Radioact.* 2006;85(1):94-102

[10] "Leaf tobacco contains minute amounts of lead 210 (210Pb) and polonium 210 (210Po), both of which are radioactive carcinogens and both of which can be found in smoke from burning tobacco. Tobacco smoke also contains carcinogens that are nonradioactive. People who inhale tobacco smoke are exposed to higher concentrations of radioactivity than nonsmokers. Deposits of 210Pb and alpha particle-emitting 210Po form in the lungs of smokers, generating localized radiation doses far greater than the radiation exposures humans experience from natural sources. This radiation exposure, delivered to sensitive tissues for long periods of time, may induce cancer both alone and synergistically with nonradioactive carcinogens." Kilthau GF. Cancer risk in relation to radioactivity in tobacco. *Radiol Technol.* 1996 Jan-Feb;67(3):217-22

[11] "Cured tobacco in diverse types of cigarettes is known to harbor a plethora of bacteria (Gram-positive and Gram-negative), fungi (mold, yeast), spores, and is rich in endotoxin (lipopolysaccharide). Reviewed herein are recent observations of the authors' team and other investigators that support the hypothesis that lung inflammation of long-term smokers may be attributed in part to tobacco-associated bacterial and fungal components that have been identified in tobacco and tobacco smoke." Pauly JL, Smith LA, Rickert MH, Hutson A, Paszkiewicz GM. Review: Is lung inflammation associated with microbes and microbial toxins in cigarette tobacco smoke? *Immunol Res.* 2010 Mar;46(1-3):127-36

[12] Lee J, Taneja V, Vassallo R. Cigarette smoking and inflammation: cellular and molecular mechanisms. *J Dent Res.* 2012 Feb;91(2):142-9
http://www.ncbi.nlm.nih.gov/pmc/articles/PMC3261116/

[13] Siegel LB, Gall EP. Viral infection as a cause of arthritis. *Am Fam Physician* 1996 Nov 1;54(6):2009-15

inflammatory/antigenic load (TIL, TAL) that perpetuates chronic/sustained immune activation and which thus drives systemic inflammation and the clinical manifestation of autoimmunity.

- Bacterial (specific species and generalized SIBO—small intestine bacterial overgrowth): **RA is associated with gastrointestinal and genitourinary colonization with** *Proteus mirabilis*.[14,15] **Approximately 40% of patients with rheumatoid arthritis have bacterial overgrowth of the small bowel, and the severity of bacterial overgrowth correlates positively with the severity of the musculoskeletal inflammation,** suggesting the probability of a causal relationship.[16] Relatedly, clinicians should recall that peptidoglycans, bacterial cell wall debris, endotoxins, indole, skatole and numerous other gut-derived "toxins" can promote joint inflammation.[17,18] **Animal models have demonstrated that gut-derived metabolites can cause inflammatory degenerative arthritis that resembles rheumatoid arthritis.**[19,20] **The dysbiotic contribution to rheumatoid arthritis is likely to be both** *qualitative* **(related to specific inciting microbes) and** *quantitative* **(related to total, nonspecific bacterial overgrowth of the gut and multifocal mucosal colonization).** Accordingly, research published in 2007 showed that dietary modification was comparable in benefit to prednisolone, supporting the model that gastrointestinal dysfunction—namely, food allergic reactions (and probably intestinal dysbiosis)—is a major etiologic component of rheumatoid arthritis, at least in its initial stages; the authors concluded, "**This study supports the concept that rheumatoid arthritis may be a reaction to a food antigen(s) and that the disease process starts within the intestine.**"[21]
  - Cell wall fragments from major residents of the human intestinal flora induce chronic arthritis in rats. (*J Rheumatol* 1989 Aug[22]): "A single intraperitoneal injection of cell wall fragments from *Eubacterium aerofaciens* or *Bifidobacterium* species induced persistent chronic arthritis, in contrast to those from *Eubacterium rectale*, *Clostridium species* and *Lactobacillus leichmanii*. The results show that cell wall fragments of major residents from the human fecal flora can induce chronic arthritis in the rat and support the hypothesis that normal human intestinal flora plays a role in the induction of arthritis in man."
  - Normal intestinal microbiota in the etiopathogenesis of rheumatoid arthritis (*Ann Rheum Dis* 2003 Sep[23]): The ability of bacterial cell walls to induce chronic, erosive arthritis was first described in the rat by using *Streptococcus pyogenes*. Self-perpetuating arthritis, closely resembling human rheumatoid arthritis by histological criteria, develops in susceptible rat strains after a single intraperitoneal injection of the bacterial cell wall. In addition to *Streptococcus pyogenes*, several bacterial species representing *Lactobacillus*, *Bifidobacterium*, *Eubacterium*, *Collinsella*, and *Clostridium* have been observed to have a similar ability.
- Parasitic: Gastrointestinal parasite infections, such as with *Endolimax nana*[24] and other microbes such a *Giardia lamblia*, can induce a systemic inflammatory response that mimics rheumatoid arthritis and is cured with parasite eradication.

[14] Ebringer A, Rashid T, Wilson C. Rheumatoid arthritis: proposal for the use of anti-microbial therapy in early cases. *Scand J Rheumatol* 2003;32(1):2-11

[15] Rashid T, Darlington G, Kjeldsen-Kragh J, Forre O, Collado A, Ebringer A. Proteus IgG antibodies and C-reactive protein in English, Norwegian and Spanish patients with rheumatoid arthritis. *Clin Rheumatol* 1999;18(3):190-5

[16] "Eight (32%) of the patients with RA had hypochlorhydria or achlorhydria... A high frequency of small intestinal bacterial overgrowth was found in patients with RA; it was associated with a high disease activity and observed in patients with hypochlorhydria or achlorhydria and in those with normal acid secretion." Henriksson AE, Blomquist L, Nord CE, Midtvedt T, Uribe A. Small intestinal bacterial overgrowth in patients with rheumatoid arthritis. *Ann Rheum Dis.* 1993 Jul;52(7):503-10

[17] Simelyte E, Rimpilainen M, Lehtonen L, Zhang X, Toivanen P. Bacterial cell wall-induced arthritis: chemical composition and tissue distribution of four Lactobacillus strains. *Infect Immun.* 2000 Jun;68(6):3535-40 http://iai.asm.org/cgi/reprint/68/6/3535

[18] Toivanen P. Normal intestinal microbiota in the aetiopathogenesis of rheumatoid arthritis. *Ann Rheum Dis.* 2003 Sep;62(9):807-11 http://ard.bmjjournals.com/cgi/reprint/62/9/807

[19] Nakoneczna I, Forbes JC, Rogers KS. The arthritogenic effect of indole, skatole and other tryptophan metabolites in rabbits. *Am J Pathol.* 1969 Dec;57(3):523-38

[20] Rogers KS, Forbes JC, Nakoneczna I. Arthritogenic properties of lipophilic, aryl molecules. *Proc Soc Exp Biol Med.* 1969 Jun;131(2):670-2

[21] Podas T, Nightingale JM, Oldham R, Roy S, Sheehan NJ, Mayberry JF. Is rheumatoid arthritis a disease that starts in the intestine? A pilot study comparing an elemental diet with oral prednisolone. *Postgrad Med J.* 2007 Feb;83(976):128-31

[22] Severijnen AJ, van Kleef R, Hazenberg MP, van de Merwe JP. Cell wall fragments from major residents of the human intestinal flora induce chronic arthritis in rats. *J Rheumatol.* 1989 Aug;16(8):1061-8

[23] Toivanen P. Normal intestinal microbiota in the aetiopathogenesis of rheumatoid arthritis. *Ann Rheum Dis.* 2003 Sep;62(9):807-11

[24] "Endolimax nana grew on stool culture. Both the patient's diarrhea and arthritis responded effectively to therapy with metronidazole. The diagnosis of parasitic rheumatism was made in retrospect." Burnstein SL, Liakos S. Parasitic rheumatism presenting as rheumatoid arthritis. *J Rheumatol.* 1983 Jun;10(3):514-5

Clinical presentations:

- <u>Course</u>: Variable course with exacerbations and remissions; the general trend is one of progressive joint destruction and systemic inflammation-induced damage.
- <u>Presentation</u>: The disease begins slowly in 2/3 of patients and can be slow to reach a diagnostic threshold—generally takes 9 months between initial onset and diagnosis; may affect only one joint initially. 10% have acute-onset polyarthritis. RA can affect any age, either gender, and clinical presentations will vary.
    - o 2-3x more common in women than men.
    - o Age of onset is typically 25-50 years of age.
    - o "Peripheral symmetric polyarthropathy" is a classic description for RA; but this same description can be applied to many cases of hemochromatosis and SLE as well.
    - o Palpable joint swelling with synovitis and effusion.
    - o Morning stiffness > 1 hour.
    - o <u>Typical autoimmune systemic manifestations</u>: fatigue, malaise, low-grade fever, anorexia, and weight loss—note that all of these clinical presentations are manifestations of immune activation in general and increased cytokine production in particular.
- <u>Musculoskeletal</u>:
    - o The joints most commonly affected are the wrists, MCP, PIP, MTP (metatarsophalangeal) joints, and knees (Baker's cyst is common). In severe or advanced disease, essentially any joint in the body—including the TMJ and upper cervical spine—can be involved.
    - o Most common at PIP, MCP joints, wrists (i.e., "knuckles and wrists").
    - o Upper cervical spine involvement can lead to atlantoaxial instability—upper cervical spine manipulation is contraindicated until atlantoaxial instability has been excluded clinically or radiographically.
    - o Periarticular muscle atrophy and osteoporosis—due to inflammation and disuse.
    - o Generalized osteoporosis is common due to inflammation, disuse/deconditioning, hypogonadism, and drug effects.
    - o Advanced complications include radial deviation of the wrists and ulnar deviation of the fingers, swan neck deformity (PIP hyperextension with DIP hyperflexion), and boutonniere deformity (PIP hyperflexion with DIP hyperextension).
- <u>Skin</u>: Rheumatoid nodules (subcutaneous inflammatory granulomas) are seen in up to 30% of patients. These are also rarely seen in patients with hemochromatoic arthropathy mimicking RA.[25]
- <u>Arteries and vessels</u>: Rheumatoid vasculitis leads to impaired circulation, causing necrosis of affected tissues/organs: fingers, skin, internal organs, and nerves (peripheral neuropathy).
- <u>Pulmonary manifestations</u>: Dyspnea, pulmonary nodules, fibrosis; more common in men.
- <u>Eye</u>: Complications are seen in 1% of patients but can lead to rapid blindness.
- <u>Other autoimmune diseases</u>: Up to 20% of patients with RA develop Sjogren's syndrome. SLE, MS, Hashimoto's thyroiditis, and mixed connective tissue disease can easily co-exist beside a primary clinical presentation of RA.

Major differential diagnoses:

- <u>Osteoarthritis (OA)</u>: OA tends to be monoarticular or oligoarticular rather than polyarticular; OA is generally only minimally inflammatory (except after the progression of joint destruction) whereas RA is clearly more inflammatory as assessed clinically and serologically (with ESR or CRP). OA is more likely to be asymmetric whereas RA is nearly always symmetric (except in cases of stroke, paralysis, or peripheral nerve lesion due to interference with neurogenic inflammation). Lab tests such as ANA, RF, and CCP antibodies are expected to be normal in OA; CRP and ESR may be moderately elevated in severe OA but inflammatory markers are generally much lower than the levels seen in RA.

---

[25] "These manifestations which are common to rheumatoid arthritis may be seen in hemochromatotic arthropathy." Bensen WG, Laskin CA, Little HA, Fam AG. Hemochromatotic arthropathy mimicking rheumatoid arthritis. A case with subcutaneous nodules, tenosynovitis, and bursitis. *Arthritis Rheum*. 1978 Sep-Oct;21(7):844-8.

- <u>SLE</u>: Differentiated by nonerosive arthritis, anti-DS-DNA antibodies, anti-Smith antibodies, low serum complement, the classic "butterfly rash", and an earlier and more frequent development of mucosal, serosal, vasculitic and renal complications.
- <u>Septic arthritis</u>: Differentiated by monoarthritis, fever, and purulent joint aspiration.
  - <u>**Septic arthritis may complicate pre-existing rheumatoid arthritis**</u>**,** <u>and patients with RA appear to be predisposed to septic arthritis</u>: Reasons for this septic predisposition include immune dysfunction, use of prednisone or other immunosuppressant medications, and concomitant obesity and/or diabetes. **Patients may lack the classic systemic manifestations of septic arthritis (fever, chills, leukocytosis) due to age, disease, or pharmaceutical immunosuppression.**[26,27] Patients may have concomitant respiratory or urinary tract infections, which makes the clinical presentation even more unclear. Treatment may require systemic antibiotics (oral or intravenous) and joint lavage with antibiotics.[28] **Failure to diagnose and treat septic arthritis promptly may result in deformity, disability, or death.**
- <u>Hemochromatosis and iron overload</u>: Given its high frequency and multifarious clinical presentations, iron overload is an essential diagnostic consideration in patients with rheumatic disease.[29,30] Doctors must test serum ferritin and transferrin saturation (along with CRP) as discussed in Chapter 1 in the section dealing with laboratory assessments.
- <u>Reactive arthritis</u>: Differentiated by the recent history of infection, greatly increased prevalence of HLA-B27, and the presence of uveitis/iritis, sacroiliac and lumbar involvement, predominant acute/subacute-onset inflammation of the heels, knees, hips.[31]
- <u>Gout and other crystal-induced arthropathy</u>: Asymmetric arthritis, negatively birefringent crystals demonstrated with joint aspiration.
- <u>Arthritis related to viral infection</u>: Such as parvovirus and hepatitis C[32]; clinical correlation with appropriate serologies are warranted.
- <u>Psoriatic arthritis</u>: Skin lesions, nail pitting, asymmetric arthritis, negative RF and CCP. Rarely, the joint inflammation of psoriatic arthritis precedes the expected dermatologic lesions: well-demarcated erythematous patches covered with silvery scales.
- <u>Adult Still's disease</u>: Diagnosis relies on *all of the following*: high fevers (>102.2°F), arthralgia/arthritis, RF<80, ANA<1:100, *plus two of the following*: skin rash (generalized and confluent red papules and plaques), pleuritis/pericarditis, WBC count >15,000 cells/mm[3], and hepatomegally/spenomegally/lymphadenopathy.
- <u>Ewing's sarcoma</u>: An aggressive bone malignancy that typically presents in children and young adults with periarticular bone pain and fever which can mimic inflammatory monoarthritis.

<u>Clinical assessment</u>:
- **History/subjective**:
  - Systemic manifestations with symmetric peripheral polyarthropathy.
  - Morning stiffness lasting more than 30-60 minutes is common.
- **Physical examination/objective**:
  - Assess joints, especially the distal/peripheral joints of the wrists/hands and ankles/feet. Remember that the initial manifestation of RA, like all inflammatory arthropathies, can affect any

[26] "Many patients lacked distinctive features of joint sepsis (fever, chills) and only one half had leukocytosis." Blackburn WD Jr, Dunn TL, Alarcon GS. Infection versus disease activity in rheumatoid arthritis: eight years' experience. *South Med J.* 1986 Oct;79(10):1238-41

[27] "Pain and loss of motion in the affected joint were prominent, but toxic features of pyogenic infections--hectic fever, chills, sweats, local warmth, or erythema--were conspicuously absent. Two patients had moderate fever and three patients had mild leukocytosis." Kraft SM, Panush RS, Longley S. Unrecognized staphylococcal pyarthrosis with rheumatoid arthritis. *Semin Arthritis Rheum.* 1985 Feb;14(3):196-201

[28] Septic arthritis complicating rheumatoid arthritis was due to Staphylococcus aureus (12 cases) and Escherichia coli (1 case). Recommended treatment: "The authors recommend as the treatment of choice: systemic antibiotic therapy and immediate arthrotomy followed by through-and-through irrigation with fluid containing the appropriate antibiotics." Gristina AG, Rovere GD, Shoji H. Spontaneous septic arthritis complicating rheumatoid arthritis. *J Bone Joint Surg Am.* 1974 Sep;56(6):1180-4

[29] **Vasquez A. Musculoskeletal disorders and iron overload disease: comment on the American College of Rheumatology guidelines for the initial evaluation of the adult patient with acute musculoskeletal symptoms. *Arthritis Rheum.* 1996 Oct;39(10):1767-8**

[30] "These manifestations which are common to rheumatoid arthritis may be seen in hemochromatotic arthropathy." Bensen WG, Laskin CA, Little HA, Fam AG. Hemochromatotic arthropathy mimicking rheumatoid arthritis. A case with subcutaneous nodules, tenosynovitis, and bursitis. *Arthritis Rheum.* 1978 Sep-Oct;21(7):844-8

[31] Author's note: I think rheumatoid arthritis should be considered a variant of reactive arthritis, with RA being triggered by multifocal dysbiosis (several subclinical infections) whereas the latter is triggered by a single true infection.

[32] Siegel LB, Gall EP. Viral infection as a cause of arthritis. *Am Fam Physician* 1996 Nov 1;54(6):2009-15

joint in the body, including the atlantoaxial joint. Flexion contractures and ulnar deviation of the fingers are common, classic findings of developed disease.

- o Clinically assess patient for exclusion of other diseases. Some patients with RA will develop other autoimmune diseases, especially hypothyroidism and Sjogren's syndrome.

- **Laboratory assessments**: Goals of laboratory testing are 1) exclude serious life-threatening conditions (e.g., septic arthritis), 2) quantitatively and qualitatively assess patient's health status, 3) determine nature and severity of underlying diseases and disorders for which correction can contribute to an overall improvement in immune function and reduction in total inflammatory load.

- o **CCP: Cyclic citrullinated protein antibody; Citrullinated protein antibodies (CPA); anti-CCP antibodies: anti-cyclic citrullinated peptide antibody**: Anti-CCP antibodies have 95-98% specificity for RA[33] and has become the laboratory standard for evaluating the diagnosis and prognosis of RA.[34] The best current data indicates that anti-CCP antibodies are sensitive and specific for RA[35], and clinicians should use this test in the diagnosis of RA.[36] Anti-CCP antibodies with a positive rheumatoid factor (RF) is termed "composite/conjugate seropositivity" and appears to be more specific than isolated anti-CCP or RF positivity.[37]

> **CCP antibodies: the single best laboratory test for the early detection, diagnosis, and monitoring of RA**
>
> "The anti-CCP test is more specific than the commonly used RF test (95% versus less than 90%) and has a comparable sensitivity (more than 70%). ... In conclusion, testing for anti-CCP autoantibodies is widely accepted as an indispensable tool for diagnosis and early treatment in the management of rheumatoid arthritis patients."
>
> van Venrooij WJ, van Beers JJ, Pruijn GJ. Anti-CCP Antibody, a Marker for the Early Detection of Rheumatoid Arthritis. *Ann N Y Acad Sci* 2008 Nov

- o C-reactive protein: CRP can be used to support the diagnosis (as it indicates inflammation) and can be used to monitor the disease and the response to treatment.[38]

- o Erythrocyte sedimentation rate: ESR is elevated in 90% of patients and can be used to support the diagnosis (as it indicates inflammation) and can be used to monitor the disease and the response to treatment.[39]

- o Complete blood count: CBC may reveal anemia of chronic disease, anemia due to NSAID-related gastrointestinal bleeding, or suggest nutritional deficiencies (namely B12 and folic acid as discussed in Chapter 1); elevated WBC suggests infection and requires clinical correlation.

- o Ferritin: As an acute phase reactant, serum ferritin is elevated by inflammation; as a marker for iron status, serum ferritin is elevated by iron overload and lowered by iron deficiency. Transferrin saturation and serum iron should be low in RA due to inflammation, whereas they are commonly elevated in patients with iron overload. In order to determine the acute phase contribution to an elevated ferritin level, an independent marker of inflammation such as CRP or ESR should be tested simultaneously. When in doubt, iron overload can be excluded with diagnostic phlebotomy, liver MRI, liver biopsy (especially if liver enzymes are elevated), or the response to therapeutic phlebotomy.[40]

---

[33] Hill J, Cairns E, Bell DA. The joy of citrulline: new insights into the diagnosis, pathogenesis, and treatment of rheumatoid arthritis. *J Rheumatol*. 2004 Aug;31(8):1471-3
[34] "We conclude that, at present, the antibody response directed to citrullinated antigens has the most valuable diagnostic and prognostic potential for RA." van Boekel MA, Vossenaar ER, van den Hoogen FH, van Venrooij WJ. Autoantibody systems in rheumatoid arthritis: specificity, sensitivity and diagnostic value. *Arthritis Res*. 2002;4(2):87-93 http://arthritis-research.com/content/4/2/87
[35] "Serum antibodies reactive with citrullinated proteins/peptides are a very sensitive and specific marker for rheumatoid arthritis." Migliorini P, Pratesi F, Tommasi C, Anzilotti C. The immune response to citrullinated antigens in autoimmune diseases. *Autoimmun Rev*. 2005 Nov;4(8):561-4
[36] "The anti-CCP test is more specific than the commonly used RF test (95% versus less than 90%) and has a comparable sensitivity (more than 70%). ... In conclusion, testing for anti-CCP autoantibodies is widely accepted as an indispensable tool for diagnosis and early treatment in the management of rheumatoid arthritis patients." van Venrooij WJ, van Beers JJ, Pruijn GJ. Anti-CCP Antibody, a Marker for the Early Detection of Rheumatoid Arthritis. *Ann N Y Acad Sci*. 2008 Nov;1143:268-85
[37] "...our findings suggest that a positive anti-CCP antibody result does not necessarily exclude SLE in African American patients presenting with inflammatory arthritis. In such patients, the additional assessment of IgA-RF or IgM-RF isotypes may be of added value since composite seropositivity appears to be nearly exclusive to patients with RA." Mikuls TR, Holers VM, Parrish L, Kuhn KA, Conn DL, Gilkeson G, Smith EA, Kamen DL, Jonas BL, Callahan LF, Alarcon GS, Howard G, Moreland LW, Bridges SL Jr. Anti-cyclic citrullinated peptide antibody and rheumatoid factor isotypes in African Americans with early rheumatoid arthritis. *Arthritis Rheum*. 2006 Sep;54(9):3057-9
[38] Gabay C, Kushner I. Acute-phase proteins and other systemic responses to inflammation. *N Engl J Med*. 1999 Feb 11;340(6):448-54
[39] Klippel JH (ed). Primer on the Rheumatic Diseases. 11th Edition. Atlanta: Arthritis Foundation. 1997 page 94
[40] "Therapeutic phlebotomy is used to remove excess iron and maintain low normal body iron stores, and it should be initiated in men with serum ferritin levels of 300 microg/L or more and in women with serum ferritin levels of 200 microg/L or more, regardless of the presence or absence of symptoms." Barton JC, McDonnell SM,

- Rheumatoid factor: RF is positive in 70-80% of patients with RA but is not specific and is not necessary for the diagnosis of RA. RF provides "supportive evidence" for the diagnosis of RA only in the presence of corresponding clinical manifestations. High RF levels indicate more severe disease and worse prognosis. IgA-RF appears to have clinical superiority over other forms of RF.[41] RF is seen in 5% of apparently healthy people, and it is present in some patients with iron overload, thus making the distinction between RA and hemochromatoic arthropathy all the more difficult.[42] Diseases (other than RA) associated with RF positivity include iron overload, chronic infections, hepatitis, sarcoidosis, and bacterial endocarditis.

- Thyroid assessment: Hypothyroidism can mimic systemic rheumatic disease by causing an inflammatory oligoarthropathy and myopathy, complete with elevations of CRP and ESR.[43] Overt or imminent hypothyroidism is suggested by TSH greater than 2 mU/L[44] or 3 mU/L[45], low T4 or T3, and/or the presence of anti-thyroid peroxidase antibodies (anti-TPO).[46] This author's current practice is—for the laboratory evaluation of hypothyroidism—to assess the full spectrum of thyroid indexes: THS, free T4, free or total T3, reverse T3 (rT3), and the antithyroid antibodies anti-thyroglobulin and anti-thyroid peroxidase (anti-TPO).

- Complete hormone assessment: Patients with RA commonly show elevations of prolactin and estradiol along with insufficiencies of testosterone, cortisol, and DHEA. These can be tested in serum, and early-morning serum cortisol is more accurate than late-day cortisol. Other options and details are provided in the following section under *Treatments* and in the section in Chapter 4 on *Orthoendocrinology*.

- Lactulose-mannitol assay for "leaky gut": Increased intestinal permeability (IP) is a common contributor to and complication of many inflammatory/rheumatic/chronic diseases including psoriasis[47], Behcet's disease[48], ankylosing spondylitis[49] and seronegative spondyloarthritis[50], enteropathic spondyloarthropathy and oligoarticular juvenile idiopathic arthritis[51], lupus[52], and chronic congestive heart failure.[53] This test may be used for the evaluation of gastrointestinal mucosal integrity, which simultaneously serves as a barometer of overall health and when elevated can indicate the presence of a variety of intestinal disorders, including celiac disease, food allergies, and GI dysbiosis. Thus, an elevated lactulose:mannitol ratio is *sensitive* but not *specific* for the presence of intestinal disorders. An elevated lactulose:mannitol ratio correlates with ❶ malnutrition, ❷ inflammatory bowel disease, ❸ NSAID or ethanol enterotoxicity, ❹ food allergies including celiac disease, and/or ❺ gastrointestinal dysbiosis, the latter of which then needs to be characterized with comprehensive stool testing and comprehensive parasitology; astute clinicians can generally exclude items 1-3 with appropriate history, physical examination, and routine

Adams PC, Brissot P, Powell LW, Edwards CQ, Cook JD, Kowdley KV. Management of hemochromatosis. Hemochromatosis Management Working Group. *Ann Intern Med.* 1998 Dec 1;129(11):932-9

[41] Jonsson T, Valdimarsson H. What about IgA rheumatoid factor in rheumatoid arthritis? *Ann Rheum Dis.* 1998 Jan;57(1):63-4 http://ard.bmjjournals.com/cgi/content/full/57/1/63

[42] "These manifestations which are common to rheumatoid arthritis may be seen in hemochromatotic arthropathy." Bensen WG, Laskin CA, Little HA, Fam AG. Hemochromatotic arthropathy mimicking rheumatoid arthritis. A case with subcutaneous nodules, tenosynovitis, and bursitis. *Arthritis Rheum.* 1978;21(7):844-8

[43] Bowman CA, Jeffcoate WJ, Pattrick M, Doherty M. Bilateral adhesive capsulitis, oligoarthritis and proximal myopathy as presentation of hypothyroidism. *Br J Rheumatol.* 1988;27(1):62-4

[44] Weetman AP. Hypothyroidism: screening and subclinical disease. *BMJ.* 1997 Apr 19;314(7088):1175-8 http://bmj.bmjjournals.com/cgi/content/full/314/7088/1175

[45] "Now AACE encourages doctors to consider treatment for patients who test outside the boundaries of a narrower margin based on a target TSH level of 0.3 to 3.0. AACE believes the new range will result in proper diagnosis for millions of Americans who suffer from a mild thyroid disorder, but have gone untreated until now." American Association of Clinical Endocrinologists (AACE). 2003 Campaign Encourages Awareness of Mild Thyroid Failure, Importance of Routine Testing http://www.aace.com/pub/tam2003/press.php November 26, 2005

[46] Beers MH, Berkow R (eds). The Merck Manual. Seventeenth Edition. Whitehouse Station; Merck Research Laboratories 1999 Page 96

[47] Humbert P, Bidet A, Treffel P, Drobacheff C, Agache P. Intestinal permeability in patients with psoriasis. *J Dermatol Sci.* 1991 Jul;2(4):324-6

[48] Fresko I, Hamuryudan V, Demir M, Hizli N, Sayman H, Melikoglu M, Tunc R, Yurdakul S, Yazici H. Intestinal permeability in Behcet's syndrome. *Ann Rheum Dis.* 2001 Jan;60(1):65-6

[49] Vaile JH, Meddings JB, Yacyshyn BR, Russell AS, Maksymowych WP. Bowel permeability and CD45RO expression on circulating CD20+ B cells in patients with ankylosing spondylitis and their relatives. *J Rheumatol.* 1999 Jan;26(1):128-35

[50] Di Leo V, D'Inca R, Bettini MB, Podswiadek M, Punzi L, Mastropaolo G, Sturniolo GC. Effect of Helicobacter pylori and eradication therapy on gastrointestinal permeability. Implications for patients with seronegative spondyloarthritis. *J Rheumatol.* 2005 Feb;32(2):295-300

[51] Picco P, Gattorno M, Marchese N, Vignola S, Sormani MP, Barabino A, Buoncompagni A. Increased gut permeability in juvenile chronic arthritides. A multivariate analysis of the diagnostic parameters. *Clin Exp Rheumatol.* 2000 Nov-Dec;18(6):773-8

[52] "Fourteen cases of primary lupus-associated protein-losing enteropathy have now been reported in the English-language literature." Perednia DA, Curosh NA. Lupus-associated protein-losing enteropathy. *Arch Intern Med.* 1990 Sep;150(9):1806-10

[53] "Chronic heart failure patients had a 35% increase of small intestinal permeability (lactulose/mannitol ratio: 0.023 vs. 0.017 ..., p = 0.006), a 210% increase of large intestinal permeability (sucralose excretion: 0.62 ... vs. 0.20), and a 29% decrease of D-xylose absorption, indicating bowel ischemia (26.7% vs. 37.4%, p = 0.003)." Sandek A, Bauditz J, Swidsinski A, et al. Altered intestinal function in patients with chronic heart failure. *J Am Coll Cardiol.* 2007 Oct 16;50(16):1561-9

laboratory assessments, thus leaving an abnormal IP test to be attributed to food allergies or GI parasites/dysbiosis, the former of which is assessed serologically or with elimination-challenge protocol (reviewed in Chapter 4) while the latter is assessed with comprehensive stool testing (including fecal sIgA and inflammatory markers such as lactoferrin and lysozyme) and comprehensive parasitology, which includes microscopic, culture, and antigen/toxin detection techniques.

o Comprehensive stool analysis and comprehensive parasitology with bacterial and fungal culture and sensitivity: **All patients with rheumatoid arthritis should be considered to have gastrointestinal dysbiosis until proven otherwise** by ❶ **dysbiosis laboratory assessment (including comprehensive stool testing with parasitology** *performed by a specialty laboratory*), and ❷ response to anti-dysbiosis treatment **which minimally includes the combination of anti-dysbiosis dietary modification (nutritional supplementation, plant-based diet, low-fermentation, high-fiber, superadequate protein and phytonutrients)** with antimicrobial drugs or botanicals, **commonly including berberine (500mg BID-TID for 3 months), emulsified time-released oil of oregano (200mg TID for 6 weeks[54]), Augmentin (2,000mg BID for variable durations of days to months to years—supportively, note successful use of long-term penicillin in the treatment of psoriasis[55]), azithromycin (500mg every other day for variable durations of days to months to years[56]), ciprofloxacin (short course only to avoid exacerbation/induction of tendonopathy), and metronidazole. Recently, I've become impressed by the efficacy of low-dose oral vancomycin 125-250mg PO QD; as a nonabsorbed antibiotic, the drug remains in the gut and is effective against segmented filamentous bacteria (SFB) which have been shown in several animal experiments to induce Th-17 effector cells which promote chronic arthritis/autoimmunity—for recent discussion, see my notes and videos from the 2013 International Conference on Human Nutrition and Functional Medicine: https://vimeo.com/ondemand/ichnfm.** A three-sample comprehensive parasitology examination performed by a **specialty laboratory** is strongly recommended as a minimal component of basic care. In lieu of *or preferably in addition to* a comprehensive parasitology test, patients can be treated for 4-8 weeks with broad-spectrum antimicrobial treatment (including an anti-dysbiosis diet) that is effective against gram-positive and gram-negative bacteria, aerobes and anaerobes, yeast, protozoa and amebas. For additional details, see the Section on *Multifocal Dysbiosis* in Chapter 4.

- **Imaging**:
  - o Radiographic changes are not seen in early disease and only have utility for clarifying diagnostic uncertainty later in the disease, screening for complications such as atlantoaxial instability, or for pre-operative assessment in patients who are candidates for joint repair or replacement.
  - o Radiographic findings when clustered are relatively specific in developed disease: soft tissue swelling, periarticular osteoporosis, joint space narrowing due to loss of cartilage, **marginal erosions**, ulnar/lateral deviation of the fingers, and subluxation and dislocation may occur.

- **Establishing the diagnosis**:
  - o The diagnosis is established by pattern recognition of the typical clinical manifestations and laboratory abnormalities and reasonable exclusion of protean diseases such as hepatitis C, SLE, and iron overload.

---

[54] "Oil of Mediterranean oregano *Oreganum vulgare* was orally administered to 14 adult patients whose stools tested positive for enteric parasites, *Blastocystis hominis*, *Entamoeba hartmanni* and *Endolimax nana*. After 6 weeks of supplementation with 600 mg emulsified oil of oregano daily, there was complete disappearance of *Entamoeba hartmanni* (four cases), *Endolimax nana* (one case), and *Blastocystis hominis* in eight cases. Also, *Blastocystis hominis* scores declined in three additional cases. Gastrointestinal symptoms improved in seven of the 11 patients who had tested positive for *Blastocystis hominis*." Force M, Sparks WS, Ronzio RA. Inhibition of enteric parasites by emulsified oil of oregano in vivo. *Phytother Res.* 2000 May;14(3):213-4

[55] Saxena VN, Dogra J. Long-term use of penicillin for the treatment of chronic plaque psoriasis. *Eur J Dermatol.* 2005 Sep-Oct;15(5):359-6

[56] Saxena VN, Dogra J. Long-term oral azithromycin in chronic plaque psoriasis: a controlled trial. *Eur J Dermatol.* 2010 May-Jun;20(3):329-33

2010 American College of Rheumatology/European League against Rheumatism classification criteria

Screening: Patients with at least 1 joint and definite clinical synovitis which is not explained by another disease.

A score of ≥6 is needed for the classification of definite RA:
- Score 1 large joint: 0
- 2–10 large joints: 1
- 1–3 small joints (with or without large joints): 2
- 4–10 small joints (with or without large joints): 3
- >10 joints (at least 1 small joint): 5

Serology: At least 1 test is needed:
- Negative RF (rheumatoid factor) and negative ACPA (anticitrullinated protein antibody): 0
- Low positive RF or low positive ACPA: 2
- High positive RF or high positive ACPA: 3

Acute phase reactants: At least 1 result is needed.
- Normal CRP (C-reactive protein) and normal ESR: 0
- Abnormal CRP or ESR: 1

Duration of symptoms: (self-reported)
- <6 weeks: 0
- ≥6 weeks: 1

Although patients with a score <6/10 are not classifiable as having RA, their status can be reassessed and the criteria might be fulfilled cumulatively over time.

http://onlinelibrary.wiley.com/doi/10.1002/art.27580/pdf
http://www.ncbi.nlm.nih.gov/pmc/articles/PMC3077961/pdf/nihms266537.pdf
http://www.unboundmedicine.com/5minute/view/5-Minute-Clinical-Consult/116053/all/Arthritis_Rheumatoid__RA

Complications:

- Disease complications are common and range from the inconveniences of pain and inflammation for patients with milder disease to the major complications of joint deformity, occupational and social disability, serious cardiovascular/renal/pulmonary/cerebral complications (due mostly to inflammation, fibrosis, and vasculitis), infections (especially septic arthritis), depression, and suicide. Adding drug side-effects atop these manifold disease complications makes managing the disease more difficult for doctors, and enduring the disease more difficult for patients.
- Mild disease results in mild symptoms and manageable impact on ADL (activities of daily living) and QOL (quality of life). Severe disease is painful, less responsive to treatment, disfiguring and generally devastating. Treatments that are inefficacious, unavailable, prohibitively expensive, or complicated by significant side effects contribute to despair. **RA patients are at increased risk for social isolation, depression, and suicide**[57]; these sociopsychiatric complications can be attributed to chronic pain, neuropsychiatric effects of inflammatory cytokines, therapeutic nihilism, adverse drug effects (e.g., NSAID- and steroid-induced psychosis), cerebral vasculitis, and nutritional deficiencies (e.g., EPA, DHA, vitamin D, zinc) in patients not cared for by competent integrative clinicians.
- Decreased life expectancy by 3-7 years, mostly due to infection, gastrointestinal bleeding, and cardiorenal complications.
- Patients with systemic inflammatory diseases are at increased risk for cardiovascular disorders (including hypertension, accelerated atherosclerosis, vasculitis) and renal complications (secondary to hypertension, vasculitis, immune complex deposition, NSAIDs and other drugs).

---

[57] "Rheumatoid arthritis (RA) is a somatic disorder, which is known to be associated with major depression, and prevalences exceeding even 40% have been reported [5, 6]. Recently, Treharne et al. [7] showed that 11% of hospital out-patients with RA had experienced suicidal ideation." Timonen M, Viilo K, Hakko H, Särkioja T, Ylikulju M, Meyer-Rochow VB, Väisänen E, Räsänen P. Suicides in persons suffering from rheumatoid arthritis. *Rheumatology* (Oxford). 2003 Feb;42(2):287-91

Clinical management:

- Routine assessment, surveillance for complications, compliance, consultation, laboratory follow-up, access to treatments: Clinical visits should include surveillance for subjective and objective indicators of disease progression/remission, treatment compliance (including overzealous compliance with its risk of adverse toxic effects or unnecessary expense, or undercompliance with attendant hazards of inefficacy and disease exacerbation), and overall health status. Questions are answered, and problems addressed. Necessary consultations are scheduled as needed; the referring provider sends a narrative letter and ensures that the patient has a scheduled appointment. Review and anticipatory scheduling of laboratory tests should be performed. Access to treatments should be verified. Appropriate documentation is mandatory.

- Standard medical treatments:
  - Discouraging the discouragement of "nutritional quackery": According to the *Merck Manual* (1999), "Food and diet quackery is common and should be discouraged."[58] In contrast to this allopathic rhetoric, the biomedical literature strongly supports the use of nutritional interventions for **direct benefits** (e.g., anti-inflammatory, analgesic, immunomodulatory, and drug-sparing effects) and **indirect benefits** (e.g., cardiorenal protection, alleviation of depression).

  - NSAIDs as first-line treatment: NSAIDS provide temporary pain relief while contributing to increased intestinal permeability, gastrointestinal hemorrhage, liver toxicity (dose-response relationship), renal toxicity (dose-response relationship) possible exacerbation of food allergies[59], and accelerated destruction of articular structures (especially indomethacin).[60,61,62]

  - Immunosuppression with prednisone, methotrexate, or other DMARD (disease-modifying antirheumatic drugs): **Despite the clinical drawbacks, philosophical inadequacies, and steep financial consequences, pharmacologic immunosuppression has a role in the management of patients with autoimmunity when their disease flares and threatens vital structures, particularly the heart, kidneys, and nervous system.** A common sequence of medicalization used by rheumatologists is:

    ❶ Begin first-visit treatment with daily/PRN low-dose prednisone (5-7.5 mg/day) and weekly methotrexate (7.5-15 mg/week, with daily folic acid to improve efficacy and reduce toxicity),

    ❷ Eventually add hydroxychloroquine and/or sulfasalazine as disease progresses,

    ❸ When the patient becomes "resistant to treatment" add either an oral immunosuppressant or one of the "biologics" such as the parenterally-administered TNF/cytokine blockers: etanercept, infliximab, adalimumab, etc.

    Such a drug protocol might easily cost $50,000 per year and carry complications such as increased risk and severity of opportunistic infections (especially tuberculosis), exacerbation of heart failure, and increased risk for lymphoma and—less commonly—SLE and CNS demyelination similar to multiple sclerosis. Immunosuppression with

---

[58] Beers MH, Berkow R (eds). The Merck Manual. Seventeenth Edition. Whitehouse Station; Merck Research Laboratories: 1999, page 419

[59] Abbreviations: cow's milk beta-lactoglobulin absorption (BLG), acetylsalicylic acid (ASA), disodium chromoglycate (DSCG). "ASA administration strongly increased BLG absorption, not prevented by DSCG pretreatment. … Our results suggest that prolonged treatment with nonsteroidal anti-inflammatory drugs induces an increase of food antigen absorption, apparently not related to anaphylaxis mediator release, with possible clinical effects." Fagiolo U, Paganelli R, Ossi E, Quinti I, Cancian M, D'Offizi GP, Fiocco U. Intestinal permeability and antigen absorption in rheumatoid arthritis. Effects of acetylsalicylic acid and sodium chromoglycate. *Int Arch Allergy Appl Immunol.* 1989;89(1):98-102

[60] "At…concentrations comparable to those… in the synovial fluid of patients treated with the drug, several NSAIDs suppress proteoglycan synthesis… These NSAID-related effects on chondrocyte metabolism … are much more profound in osteoarthritic cartilage than in normal cartilage, due to enhanced uptake of NSAIDs by the osteoarthritic cartilage." Brandt KD. Effects of nonsteroidal anti-inflammatory drugs on chondrocyte metabolism in vitro and in vivo. *Am J Med.* 1987 Nov 20; 83: 29-34

[61] "The case of a young healthy man, who developed avascular necrosis of head of femur after prolonged administration of indomethacin, is reported here." Prathapkumar KR, Smith I, Attara GA. Indomethacin induced avascular necrosis of head of femur. *Postgrad Med J.* 2000 Sep; 76(899): 574-5

[62] "This highly significant association between NSAID use and acetabular destruction gives cause for concern, not least because of the difficulty in achieving satisfactory hip replacements in patients with severely damaged acetabula." Newman NM, Ling RS. Acetabular bone destruction related to non-steroidal anti-inflammatory drugs. *Lancet.* 1985 Jul 6; 2(8445): 11-4

corticosteroids/prednisone promotes bacterial overgrowth of the small bowel in humans[63], and animal studies have demonstrated increased bacterial translocation following prednisone administration[64]; recall that intestinal bacterial overgrowth/translocation are both pro-inflammatory and arthritogenic. Prednisone also causes mitochondrial dysfunction, which exacerbates fatigue and inflammation.

- o Surgery: Surgery is used for deformities and other orthopedic complications, including atlantoaxial instability and protrusio acetabuli.

Functional Inflammology protocol via the FINDSEX™ acronym
1. Food, basic supplementation, allergy identification via elimination and challenge,
2. Infections and dysbiosis
3. Nutritional immunomodulation: nutritional induction of Treg cells at the reciprocal expense of Th-17 cells
4. Dysfunctional mitochondria: elimination, disinhibition, stimulation
5. Style of living: stress, sleep, sweat/exercise, spinal manipulation, surgery, stamp your passport and go
6. Endocrine balance and optimization
7. Xenobiotic immunotoxicity

- Food—diet, basic nutritional supplementation, food allergen avoidance: The diet should be plant-based, but not necessarily vegan or vegetarian; I refer to this diet at "plant-based Paleo" since "the Paleo diet" as commonly discussed is simply a diet of whole natural foods which can generally be consumed without cooking or processing. For purposes of meeting physiologic expectations and attaining the highest satiety, weight optimization, and nutrient density with a phytonutrient-dense low-fermentation diet, the diet should primarily consist of fruits, vegetables, nuts, seeds, berries, and lean sources of protein; carbohydrate intake is modulated per caloric and carbohydrate needs while protein intake is tailored to lean body mass, exercise and healing/recuperation needs. Preferred sources of protein are grass-fed land animals as well as wild-caught cold-water fish, both of which are low in total fat and high in the anti-inflammatory and immunomodulatory omega-3 fatty acids, especially EPA and DHA. Whey protein isolate can also be used as it is an inexpensive convenient source of high-quality protein well-tolerated for most patients and as it also contains many functional components such as glutathione precursors, tryptophan, immunoglobulins, and growth factors anti-gastrin effects which help to heal/protect damaged intestinal mucosa. Plant-based diets, which can be further phyto-supplemented with food concentrates and fruit/vegetable smoothies/juices, provide the greatest dietary density and diversity of phytonutrients which generally have antioxidant and anti-inflammatory effects; also very important is the highly important modulation of gastrointestinal flora by plant-based diets which serves as a major mechanism by which such diets exert their clinically significant systemic anti-inflammatory benefits. I have detailed this diet—"the Supplemented Paleo-Mediterranean diet" as a combination of the "Paleolithic" or "Paleo diet" and the well-known "Mediterranean diet", both of which are well described in peer-reviewed journals and the lay press. (See Chapter 2 and my other publications[65,66] for details). This diet is the most nutrient-dense diet available, and its benefits are further enhanced by supplementation with vitamins, minerals, and the health-promoting fatty acids: ALA, GLA, EPA, DHA, and oleic acid. Vitamin and mineral supplementation is warranted in the general population and even more so among patients[67], who are more likely to be nutrient deficient due to their disease processes, mediations, and concomitant

---

[63] "A 63-year-old man with systemic lupus erythematosus and selective IgA deficiency developed intractable diarrhoea the day after treatment with prednisone, 50 mg daily, was started. The diarrhoea was considered to be caused by bacterial overgrowth and was later successfully treated with doxycycline." Denison H, Wallerstedt S. Bacterial overgrowth after high-dose corticosteroid treatment. *Scand J Gastroenterol.* 1989 Jun;24(5):561-4

[64] "These bacteria also translocated to the mesenteric lymph nodes in mice injected with cyclophosphamide or prednisone." Berg RD, Wommack E, Deitch EA. Immunosuppression and intestinal bacterial overgrowth synergistically promote bacterial translocation. *Arch Surg.* 1988 Nov;123(11):1359-64

[65] Vasquez A. A Five-Part Nutritional Protocol that Produces Consistently Positive Results. *Nutritional Wellness* 2005 September Available in the printed version and on-line at http://www.nutritionalwellness.com/archives/2005/sep/09_vasquez.php and http://www.ichnfm.org/faculty/vasquez/profile.html

[66] Vasquez A. Implementing the Five-Part Nutritional Wellness Protocol for the Treatment of Various Health Problems. *Nutritional Wellness* 2005 November. Available on-line at http://www.nutritionalwellness.com/archives/2005/nov/11_vasquez.php and http://www.ichnfm.org/faculty/vasquez/profile.html

[67] "However, suboptimal intake of some vitamins, above levels causing classic vitamin deficiency, is a risk factor for chronic diseases and common in the general population, especially the elderly. ... Most people do not consume an optimal amount of all vitamins by diet alone. Pending strong evidence of effectiveness from randomized trials, it appears prudent for all adults to take vitamin supplements. ... Physicians should make specific efforts to learn about their patients' use of vitamins to ensure that they are taking vitamins they should, ..." Fletcher RH, Fairfield KM. Vitamins for chronic disease prevention in adults: clinical applications. *JAMA.* 2002 Jun 19;287(23):3127-9

problems such as mild metabolic acidosis, malabsorption, and drug-induced nutrient depletions. Beyond routine vitamin-mineral supplementation, additional vitamin D3 supplementation is generally needed to meet the physiologic requirement of approximately 4,000 IU per day and to achieve the physiologic and clinical benefits including prevention/alleviation of depression, chronic pain, diabetes mellitus, hypertension, immunosuppression, immune activation, and cancer.[68] Likewise, absolute or relative deficiencies/insufficiencies of health-promoting anti-inflammatory fatty acids—namely: ALA, GLA, EPA, DHA, and oleic acid—are common and clinically consequential

insofar as these deficiencies/insufficiencies promote chronic/sustained inflammation, pain, and neuroemotional impairment; thus, combination fatty acid therapy/replacement/supplementation (CFAT) is indicated based on its physiological effects and clinical benefits. Probiotics, especially when consumed in conjunction with a plant-based diet which promotes an enhanced milieu for their growth and effect, provide clear clinical benefits which are both local to the gut (e.g., reduced incidence of opportunistic infections/colonizations, prevention/amelioration of increased intestinal permeability) and systemic via the anti-inflammatory benefits of enhanced induction of Treg cells at the reciprocal expense of Th-17 cells. This "supplemented Paleo-Mediterranean diet" obviates overconsumption of chemical preservatives, artificial sweeteners, and carbohydrate-dominant foods such as candies, pastries, breads, potatoes, grains, and other foods with a high glycemic load and high glycemic index (from a practical and conceptual standpoint: glycemic load × glycemic index = glycemic impact = more oxidative

> **Nutritional deficiencies are common, and a nutritionally deficient state promotes depression, hyperphagia, inflammation, immune dysfunction/suppression/activation, and mitochondrial dysfunction; therefore, routine supplementation with vitamins and minerals is indicated.**
>
> "However, suboptimal intake of some vitamins, above levels causing classic vitamin deficiency, is a risk factor for chronic diseases and common in the general population, especially the elderly. … Most people do not consume an optimal amount of all vitamins by diet alone. Pending strong evidence of effectiveness from randomized trials, it appears prudent for all adults to take vitamin supplements. … Physicians should make specific efforts to learn about their patients' use of vitamins to ensure that they are taking vitamins they should, …."
>
> Fletcher and Fairfield. Vitamins for chronic disease prevention in adults: clinical applications. *JAMA* 2002 Jun

stress, antioxidant depletion, immunosuppression, and mitochondrial impairment). Additional details are provided in the subsections that follow:

- o Avoidance of pro-inflammatory foods: Pro-inflammatory foods act *directly* and *indirectly* to promote and exacerbate systemic inflammation. *Direct* mechanisms include the activation of Toll-like receptors and NF-kappaB, while *indirect* mechanisms include depleting the body of anti-inflammatory nutrients and dietary displacement of more nutrient-dense anti-inflammatory foods. Arachidonic acid (found in cow's milk, beef, liver, pork, and lamb) is the direct precursor to pro-inflammatory prostaglandins and leukotrienes[69] and pain-promoting isoprostanes.[70] Saturated fats promote inflammation by activating/enabling pro-inflammatory Toll-like receptors, which are otherwise "specific" for inducing pro-inflammatory responses to microorganisms.[71] Consumption of saturated fat in the form of cream creates marked oxidative stress and lipid peroxidation that lasts for at least 3 hours postprandially.[72] Corn oil rapidly activates NF-kappaB (in hepatic Kupffer cells) for a pro-

---

[68] Vasquez A, Manso G, Cannell J. The clinical importance of vitamin D (cholecalciferol): a paradigm shift with implications for all healthcare providers. *Altern Ther Health Med.* 2004 Sep-Oct;10(5):28-36 http://www.ichnfm.org/faculty/vasquez/profile.html

[69] Vasquez A. Reducing Pain and Inflammation Naturally. Part 2: New Insights into Fatty Acid Supplementation and Its Effect on Eicosanoid Production and Genetic Expression. *Nutritional Perspectives* 2005; January: 5-16 http://www.ichnfm.org/faculty/vasquez/profile.html

[70] Evans AR, Junger H, Southall MD, Nicol GD, Sorkin LS, Broome JT, Bailey TW, Vasko MR. Isoprostanes, novel eicosanoids that produce nociception and sensitize rat sensory neurons. *J Pharmacol Exp Ther.* 2000 Jun;293(3):912-20

[71] Lee JY, Sohn KH, Rhee SH, Hwang D. Saturated fatty acids, but not unsaturated fatty acids, induce the expression of cyclooxygenase-2 mediated through Toll-like receptor 4. *J Biol Chem.* 2001 May 18;276(20):16683-9. Epub 2001 Mar 2 http://www.jbc.org/cgi/content/full/276/20/16683

[72] "CONCLUSIONS: Both fat and protein intakes stimulate ROS generation. The increase in ROS generation lasted 3 h after cream intake and 1 h after protein intake. Cream intake also caused a significant and prolonged increase in lipid peroxidation." Mohanty P, Ghanim H, Hamouda W, Aljada A, Garg R, Dandona P. Both lipid and protein intakes stimulate increased generation of reactive oxygen species by polymorphonuclear leukocytes and mononuclear cells. *Am J Clin Nutr.* 2002 Apr;75(4):767-72 http://www.ajcn.org/cgi/content/full/75/4/767

inflammatory effect[73]; similarly, consumption of PUFA and linoleic acid promotes antioxidant depletion and may thus promote oxidation-mediated inflammation via activation of NF-kappaB. Linoleic acid causes intracellular oxidative stress and calcium influx and results in increased NF-kappaB-stimulated transcription of pro-inflammatory genes.[74] High glycemic foods cause oxidative stress[75,76] and inflammation via activation of NF-kappaB and other mechanisms—e.g., *white bread causes inflammation*[77] as does *a high-fat high-carbohydrate fast-food-style breakfast.*[78] High glycemic foods suppress immune function[79,80] and thus promote the perpetuation of microbial colonization and dysbiosis. Delivery of a high carbohydrate load to the gastrointestinal lumen promotes bacterial overgrowth[81,82], which is inherently pro-inflammatory[83,84] and which appears to be myalgenic

> **Systemic inflammatory diseases almost always have a major gastrointestinal component**
>
> "This study supports the concept that rheumatoid arthritis may be a reaction to a food antigen(s) and that the disease process starts within the intestine."
>
> Podas T, et al. Is rheumatoid arthritis a disease that starts in the intestine? A pilot study comparing an elemental diet with oral prednisolone. *Postgrad Med J.* 2007 Feb;83(976):128-31

in humans[85] at least in part due to the ability of endotoxin to impair muscle function.[86] Overconsumption of high-carbohydrate low-phytonutrient grains, potatoes, and manufactured foods displaces phytonutrient-dense foods such as fruits, vegetables, nuts, seeds, and berries which contain more than 8,000 phytonutrients, many of which have antioxidant and thus anti-inflammatory actions.[87,88]

- ○ Avoidance of allergenic foods: **Gluten-free vegetarian diets benefit patients with rheumatoid arthritis.**[89] Any patient may be allergic to any food, even if the food is generally considered a health-promoting food. Generally speaking, the most notorious allergens are wheat, citrus (especially citrus *juice* due to the industrial use of fungal hemicellulases), cow's milk, eggs, peanuts, chocolate, and yeast-containing foods. According to a study in patients

---

[73] Rusyn I, Bradham CA, Cohn L, Schoonhoven R, Swenberg JA, Brenner DA, Thurman RG. Corn oil rapidly activates nuclear factor-kappaB in hepatic Kupffer cells by oxidant-dependent mechanisms. *Carcinogenesis*. 1999 Nov;20(11):2095-100 http://carcin.oxfordjournals.org/cgi/content/full/20/11/2095

[74] "Exposing endothelial cells to 90 micromol linoleic acid/L for 6 h resulted in a significant increase in lipid hydroperoxides that coincided wih an increase in intracellular calcium concentrations." Hennig B, Toborek M, Joshi-Barve S, Barger SW, Barve S, Mattson MP, McClain CJ. Linoleic acid activates nuclear transcription factor-kappa B (NF-kappa B) and induces NF-kappa B-dependent transcription in cultured endothelial cells. *Am J Clin Nutr*. 1996 Mar;63(3):322-8 http://www.ajcn.org/cgi/reprint/63/3/322

[75] Mohanty P, Hamouda W, Garg R, Aljada A, Ghanim H, Dandona P. Glucose challenge stimulates reactive oxygen species (ROS) generation by leucocytes. *J Clin Endocrinol Metab*. 2000 Aug;85(8):2970-3 http://jcem.endojournals.org/cgi/content/full/85/8/2970 Glucose/carbohydrate and saturated fat consumption appear to be the two biggest offenders in the food-stimulated production of oxidative stress. The effect by protein is much less. "CONCLUSIONS: Both fat and protein intakes stimulate ROS generation. The increase in ROS generation lasted 3 h after cream intake and 1 h after protein intake. Cream intake also caused a significant and prolonged increase in lipid peroxidation." Mohanty P, Ghanim H, Hamouda W, Aljada A, Garg R, Dandona P. Both lipid and protein intakes stimulate increased generation of reactive oxygen species by polymorphonuclear leukocytes and mononuclear cells. *Am J Clin Nutr*. 2002 Apr;75(4):767-72 http://www.ajcn.org/cgi/content/full/75/4/767

[76] Koska J, Blazicek P, Marko M, Grna JD, Kvetnansky R, Vigas M. Insulin, catecholamines, glucose and antioxidant enzymes in oxidative damage during different loads in healthy humans. *Physiol Res*. 2000;49 Suppl 1:S95-100 http://www.biomed.cas.cz/physiolres/pdf/2000/49_S95.pdf

[77] "Conclusion - The present study shows that high GI carbohydrate, but not low GI carbohydrate, mediates an acute proinflammatory process as measured by NF-kappaB activity." Dickinson S, Hancock DP, Petocz P, Brand-Miller JC..High glycemic index carbohydrate mediates an acute proinflammatory process as measured by NF-kappaB activation. *Asia Pac J Clin Nutr*. 2005;14 Suppl:S120

[78] Aljada A, Mohanty P, Ghanim H, Abdo T, Tripathy D, Chaudhuri A, Dandona P. Increase in intranuclear nuclear factor kappaB and decrease in inhibitor kappaB in mononuclear cells after a mixed meal: evidence for a proinflammatory effect. *Am J Clin Nutr*. 2004 Apr;79(4):682-90 http://www.ajcn.org/cgi/content/full/79/4/682

[79] Sanchez A, Reeser JL, Lau HS, et al. Role of sugars in human neutrophilic phagocytosis. *Am J Clin Nutr*. 1973 Nov;26(11):1180-4

[80] "Postoperative infusion of carbohydrate solution leads to moderate fall in the serum concentration of inorganic phosphate. ... The hypophosphatemia was associated with significant reduction of neutrophil phagocytosis, intracellular killing, consumption of oxygen and generation of superoxide during phagocytosis." Rasmussen A, Segel E, Hessov I, Borregaard N. Reduced function of neutrophils during routine postoperative glucose infusion. *Acta Chir Scand*. 1988 Jul-Aug;154(7-8):429-33

[81] Ramakrishnan T, Stokes P. Beneficial effects of fasting and low carbohydrate diet in D-lactic acidosis associated with short-bowel syndrome. *JPEN J Parenter Enteral Nutr*. 1985 May-Jun;9(3):361-3

[82] Gottschall E. Breaking the Vicious Cycle: Intestinal Health Through Diet. Kirkton Press; Rev edition (August 1, 1994)

[83] Lin HC. Small intestinal bacterial overgrowth: a framework for understanding irritable bowel syndrome. *JAMA*. 2004 Aug 18;292(7):852-8

[84] Lichtman SN, Wang J, Sartor RB, Zhang C, Bender D, Dalldorf FG, Schwab JH. Reactivation of arthritis induced by small bowel bacterial overgrowth in rats: role of cytokines, bacteria, and bacterial polymers. *Infect Immun*. 1995 Jun;63(6):2295-301

[85] Pimentel M, et al. A link between irritable bowel syndrome and fibromyalgia may be related to findings on lactulose breath testing. *Ann Rheum Dis*. 2004 Apr;63:450-2

[86] Bundgaard H, Kjeldsen K, Suarez Krabbe K, van Hall G, Simonsen L, Qvist J, Hansen CM, Moller K, Fonsmark L, Lav Madsen P, Klarlund Pedersen B. Endotoxemia stimulates skeletal muscle Na+-K+-ATPase and raises blood lactate under aerobic conditions in humans. *Am J Physiol Heart Circ Physiol*. 2003 Mar;284(3):H1028-34. Epub 2002 Nov 21 http://ajpheart.physiology.org/cgi/reprint/284/3/H1028

[87] "We propose that the additive and synergistic effects of phytochemicals in fruit and vegetables are responsible for their potent antioxidant and anticancer activities, and that the benefit of a diet rich in fruit and vegetables is attributed to the complex mixture of phytochemicals present in whole foods." Liu RH. Health benefits of fruit and vegetables are from additive and synergistic combinations of phytochemicals. *Am J Clin Nutr*. 2003 Sep;78(3 Suppl):517S-520S

[88] Seaman DR. The diet-induced proinflammatory state: a cause of chronic pain and other degenerative diseases? *J Manipulative Physiol Ther*. 2002;25(3):168-79

[89] "The immunoglobulin G (IgG) antibody levels against gliadin and beta-lactoglobulin decreased in the responder subgroup in the vegan diet-treated patients, but not in the other analysed groups." Hafstrom I, Ringertz B, Spangberg A, von Zweigbergk L, Brannemark S, Nylander I, Ronnelid J, Laasonen L, Klareskog L. A vegan diet free of gluten improves the signs and symptoms of rheumatoid arthritis: the effects on arthritis correlate with a reduction in antibodies to food antigens. *Rheumatology* (Oxford). 2001 Oct;40(10):1175-9 http://rheumatology.oxfordjournals.org/cgi/content/abstract/40/10/1175

with migraine, some patients will have to avoid as many as 10 specific foods in order to become symptom-free.[90] **Celiac disease can present with inflammatory oligoarthritis that resembles rheumatoid arthritis and which remits with avoidance of wheat/gluten.** The inflammatory arthropathy of celiac disease has preceded bowel symptoms and/or an accurate diagnosis by as many as 3-15 years.[91,92] Clinicians must explain to their patients that celiac disease and wheat allergy are two different clinical entities and that exclusion of one does not exclude the other, and in neither case does mutual exclusion obviate the promotion of intestinal bacterial overgrowth (i.e., pro-inflammatory dysbiosis) by indigestible wheat oligosaccharides.

- o Gluten-free vegetarian/vegan diet: **Gluten-free vegetarian diets benefit patients with rheumatoid arthritis.**[93] Vegetarian/vegan diets have a place in the treatment plan of all patients with autoimmune/inflammatory disorders[94,95,96]; this is also true for patients for whom long-term exclusive reliance on a meat-free vegetarian diet is either not appropriate or not appealing. No scientist or clinician familiar with the research literature doubts the antirheumatic power and anti-inflammatory advantages of vegetarian diets, whether used short-term or long term.[97] The benefits of gluten-free vegetarian diets are well documented, and the mechanisms of action are well elucidated, including reduced intake of pro-inflammatory linoleic[98] and arachidonic acids[99], iron[100], common food antigens[101], gluten[102] and gliadin[103,104], pro-inflammatory sugars[105] and increased intake of omega-3 fatty acids, micronutrients[106], and anti-inflammatory and antioxidant phytonutrients.[107] Vegetarian diets

[90] Grant EC. Food allergies and migraine. *Lancet*. 1979 May 5;1(8123):966-9

[91] "We report six patients with coeliac disease in whom arthritis was prominent at diagnosis and who improved with dietary therapy. Joint pain preceded diagnosis by up to three years in five patients and 15 years in one patient." Bourne JT, Kumar P, Huskisson EC, Mageed R, Unsworth DJ, Wojtulewski JA. Arthritis and coeliac disease. *Ann Rheum Dis*. 1985 Sep;44(9):592-8

[92] "A 15-year-old girl, with synovitis of the knees and ankles for 3 years before a diagnosis of gluten-sensitive enteropathy, is described." Pinals RS. Arthritis associated with gluten-sensitive enteropathy. *J Rheumatol*. 1986 Feb;13(1):201-4

[93] "The immunoglobulin G (IgG) antibody levels against gliadin and beta-lactoglobulin decreased in the responder subgroup in the vegan diet-treated patients, but not in the other analysed groups." Hafstrom I, Ringertz B, Spangberg A, von Zweigbergk L, Brannemark S, Nylander I, Ronnelid J, Laasonen L, Klareskog L. A vegan diet free of gluten improves the signs and symptoms of rheumatoid arthritis: the effects on arthritis correlate with a reduction in antibodies to food antigens. *Rheumatology* (Oxford). 2001 Oct;40(10):1175-9 http://rheumatology.oxfordjournals.org/cgi/content/abstract/40/10/1175

[94] "After four weeks at the health farm the diet group showed a significant improvement in number of tender joints, Ritchie's articular index, number of swollen joints, pain score, duration of morning stiffness, grip strength, erythrocyte sedimentation rate, C-reactive protein, white blood cell count, and a health assessment questionnaire score." Kjeldsen-Kragh J, Haugen M, Borchgrevink CF, Laerum E, Eek M, Mowinkel P, Hovi K, Forre O. Controlled trial of fasting and one-year vegetarian diet in rheumatoid arthritis. *Lancet*. 1991 Oct 12;338(8772):899-902

[95] "During fasting, arthralgia was less intense in many subjects. In some types of skin diseases (pustulosis palmaris et plantaris and atopic eczema) an improvement could be demonstrated during the fast. During the vegan diet, both signs and symptoms returned in most patients, with the exception of some patients with psoriasis who experienced an improvement." Lithell H, Bruce A, Gustafsson IB, Hoglund NJ, Karlstrom B, Ljunghall K, Sjolin K, Venge P, Werner I, Vessby B. A fasting and vegetarian diet treatment trial on chronic inflammatory disorders. *Acta Derm Venereol*. 1983;63(5):397-403

[96] Tanaka T, Kouda K, Kotani M, Takeuchi A, Tabei T, Masamoto Y, Nakamura H, Takigawa M, Suemura M, Takeuchi H, Kouda M. Vegetarian diet ameliorates symptoms of atopic dermatitis through reduction of the number of peripheral eosinophils and of PGE2 synthesis by monocytes. *J Physiol Anthropol Appl Human Sci*. 2001 Nov;20(6):353-61 http://www.jstage.jst.go.jp/article/jpa/20/6/20_353/_article/-char/en

[97] "For the patients who were randomised to the vegetarian diet there was a significant decrease in platelet count, leukocyte count, calprotectin, total IgG, IgM rheumatoid factor (RF), C3-activation products, and the complement components C3 and C4 after one month of treatment." Kjeldsen-Kragh J, Mellbye OJ, Haugen M, Mollnes TE, Hammer HB, Sioud M, Forre O. Changes in laboratory variables in rheumatoid arthritis patients during a trial of fasting and one-year vegetarian diet. *Scand J Rheumatol*. 1995;24(2):85-93

[98] Rusyn I, Bradham CA, Cohn L, Schoonhoven R, Swenberg JA, Brenner DA, Thurman RG. Corn oil rapidly activates nuclear factor-kappaB in hepatic Kupffer cells by oxidant-dependent mechanisms. *Carcinogenesis*. 1999 Nov;20(11):2095-100 http://carcin.oxfordjournals.org/cgi/content/full/20/11/2095

[99] Vasquez A. Reducing Pain and Inflammation Naturally. Part 2: New Insights into Fatty Acid Supplementation and Its Effect on Eicosanoid Production and Genetic Expression. *Nutritional Perspectives* 2005; January: 5-16 http://www.ichnfm.org/faculty/vasquez/profile.html

[100] Dabbagh AJ, Trenam CW, Morris CJ, Blake DR. Iron in joint inflammation. *Ann Rheum Dis*. 1993 Jan;52(1):67-73

[101] Hafstrom I, Ringertz B, Spangberg A, von Zweigbergk L, Brannemark S, Nylander I, Ronnelid J, Laasonen L, Klareskog L. A vegan diet free of gluten improves the signs and symptoms of rheumatoid arthritis: the effects on arthritis correlate with a reduction in antibodies to food antigens. *Rheumatology* (Oxford). 2001 Oct;40(10):1175-9 http://rheumatology.oxfordjournals.org/cgi/reprint/40/10/1175

[102] "The data provide evidence that dietary modification may be of clinical benefit for certain RA patients, and that this benefit may be related to a reduction in immunoreactivity to food antigens eliminated by the change in diet." Hafstrom I, Ringertz B, Spangberg A, von Zweigbergk L, Brannemark S, Nylander I, Ronnelid J, Laasonen L, Klareskog L. A vegan diet free of gluten improves the signs and symptoms of rheumatoid arthritis: the effects on arthritis correlate with a reduction in antibodies to food antigens. *Rheumatology* (Oxford). 2001 Oct;40(10):1175-9

[103] "Despite the increased AGA [antigliadin antibodies] positivity found distinctively in patients with recent-onset RA, none of the RA patients showed clear evidence of coeliac disease." Paimela L, Kurki P, Leirisalo-Repo M, Piirainen H. Gliadin immune reactivity in patients with rheumatoid arthritis. Clin Exp Rheumatol. 1995 Sep-Oct;13(5):603-7

[104] "The median IgA antigliadin ELISA index was 7.1 (range 2.1-22.4) for the RA group and 3.1 (range 0.3-34.9) for the controls (p = 0.0001)." Koot VC, Van Straaten M, Hekkens WT, Collee G, Dijkmans BA. Elevated level of IgA gliadin antibodies in patients with rheumatoid arthritis. *Clin Exp Rheumatol*. 1989 Nov-Dec;7(6):623-6

[105] Seaman DR. The diet-induced proinflammatory state: a cause of chronic pain and other degenerative diseases? *J Manipulative Physiol Ther*. 2002 Mar-Apr;25(3):168-79

[106] Hagfors L, Nilsson I, Skoldstam L, Johansson G. Fat intake and composition of fatty acids in serum phospholipids in a randomized, controlled, Mediterranean dietary intervention study on patients with rheumatoid arthritis. *Nutr Metab* (Lond). 2005 Oct 10;2:26 http://www.nutritionandmetabolism.com/content/2/1/26

[107] Liu RH. Health benefits of fruit and vegetables are from additive and synergistic combinations of phytochemicals. *Am J Clin Nutr* 2003;78(3 Suppl):517S-520S http://www.ajcn.org/cgi/content/full/78/3/517S

also effect subtle yet biologically and clinically important changes—both *qualitative* and *quantitative*—in intestinal flora[108,109] that correlate with clinical improvement.[110] Patients who rely on the Paleo-Mediterranean diet (which is inherently omnivorous) can use vegetarian *meals* on a daily basis or for days at a time—for example, by having a daily vegetarian meal, or one week per month of vegetarianism. Some (not all) patients can use a purely vegetarian diet long-term provided that nutritional needs (especially protein and cobalamin) are consistently met.

- o **Routine carbohydrate restriction, periodic short-term fasting**: Whether the foundational diet is Paleo-Mediterranean, vegetarian, vegan, or a combination of all of these, autoimmune/inflammatory patients will still benefit from periodic fasting, whether on a weekly (e.g., every Saturday), monthly (every first week or weekend of the month, or every other month), or yearly (1-2 weeks of the year) basis. The diet should generally be low in carbohydrates in order to promote ketogenesis and to retard SIBO. Since consumption of food—particularly "unhealthy" (i.e., high-fat, high-sugar, allergenic, nutritionally depleted, AGE-laden) foods—induces an inflammatory effect[111], abstinence from food provides a relative anti-inflammatory effect. Fasting indeed provides a distinct anti-inflammatory benefit and may help "re-calibrate" metabolic and homeostatic mechanisms by breaking self-perpetuating "vicious cycles"[112] that autonomously promote inflammation independent of pro-inflammatory stimuli. Water-only fasting is completely hypoallergenic (assuming that the patient is not sensitive to chlorine, fluoride, or other contaminants), and subsequent re-introduction of foods provides the ideal opportunity to identify offending foods. Fasting deprives intestinal microbes of substrate[113], stimulates intestinal B-cell immunity[114], improves the bactericidal action of neutrophils[115], reduces lysozyme release and leukotriene formation[116], and ameliorates intestinal hyperpermeability.[117] Fasting and carbohydrate avoidance also promote endogenous production of beta-hydroxybutyrate (bHB) which promotes histone acetylation for induction of a rejuvenative phenotype while bHB also stimulates complexes 3 and 4 of the mitochondrial electron transport chain (mETC) for enhanced mitochondrial function and efficiency. **In case reports and clinical trials, short-term fasting (or protein-sparing fasting) has been documented as safe and effective treatment**

---

[108] "Significant alteration in the intestinal flora was observed when the patients changed from omnivorous to vegan diet. ... This finding of an association between intestinal flora and disease activity may have implications for our understanding of how diet can affect RA." Peltonen R, Kjeldsen-Kragh J, Haugen M, Tuominen J, Toivanen P, Forre O, Eerola E. Changes of faecal flora in rheumatoid arthritis during fasting and one-year vegetarian diet. *Br J Rheumatol*. 1994 Jul;33(7):638-43

[109] Toivanen P, Eerola E. A vegan diet changes the intestinal flora. *Rheumatology* (Oxford). 2002 Aug;41(8):950-1 http://rheumatology.oxfordjournals.org/cgi/reprint/41/8/950

[110] "We conclude that a vegan diet changes the faecal microbial flora in RA patients, and changes in the faecal flora are associated with improvement in RA activity." Peltonen R, Nenonen M, Helve T, Hanninen O, Toivanen P, Eerola E. Faecal microbial flora and disease activity in rheumatoid arthritis during a vegan diet. *Br J Rheumatol*. 1997 Jan;36(1):64-8 http://rheumatology.oxfordjournals.org/cgi/reprint/36/1/64

[111] Aljada A, Mohanty P, Ghanim H, Abdo T, Tripathy D, Chaudhuri A, Dandona P. Increase in intranuclear nuclear factor kappaB and decrease in inhibitor kappaB in mononuclear cells after a mixed meal: evidence for a proinflammatory effect. *Am J Clin Nutr*. 2004 Apr;79(4):682-90 http://www.ajcn.org/cgi/content/full/79/4/682

[112] "The ability of therapeutic fasts to break metabolic vicious cycles may also contribute to the efficacy of fasting in the treatment of type 2 diabetes and autoimmune disorders." McCarty MF. A preliminary fast may potentiate response to a subsequent low-salt, low-fat vegan diet in the management of hypertension - fasting as a strategy for breaking metabolic vicious cycles. *Med Hypotheses*. 2003 May;60(5):624-33

[113] Ramakrishnan T, Stokes P. Beneficial effects of fasting and low carbohydrate diet in D-lactic acidosis associated with short-bowel syndrome. *JPEN J Parenter Enteral Nutr*. 1985 May-Jun;9(3):361-3

[114] Trollmo C, Verdrengh M, Tarkowski A. Fasting enhances mucosal antigen specific B cell responses in rheumatoid arthritis. *Ann Rheum Dis*. 1997 Feb;56(2):130-4 http://ard.bmjjournals.com/cgi/content/full/56/2/130

[115] "An association was found between improvement in inflammatory activity of the joints and enhancement of neutrophil bactericidal capacity. Fasting appears to improve the clinical status of patients with RA." Uden AM, Trang L, Venizelos N, Palmblad J. Neutrophil functions and clinical performance after total fasting in patients with rheumatoid arthritis. *Ann Rheum Dis*. 1983 Feb;42(1):45-51

[116] "We thus conclude that a reduced ability to generate cytotaxins, reduced release of enzyme, and reduced leukotriene formation from RA neutrophils, together with an altered fatty acid composition of membrane phospholipids, may be mechanisms for the decrease of inflammatory symptoms that results from fasting." Hafstrom I, Ringertz B, Gyllenhammar H, Palmblad J, Harms-Ringdahl M. Effects of fasting on disease activity, neutrophil function, fatty acid composition, and leukotriene biosynthesis in patients with rheumatoid arthritis. *Arthritis Rheum*. 1988 May;31(5):585-92

[117] "The results indicate that, unlike lactovegetarian diet, fasting may ameliorate the disease activity and reduce both the intestinal and the non-intestinal permeability in rheumatoid arthritis." Sundqvist T, Lindstrom F, Magnusson KE, Skoldstam L, Stjernstrom I, Tagesson C. Influence of fasting on intestinal permeability and disease activity in patients with rheumatoid arthritis. *Scand J Rheumatol*. 1982;11(1):33-8

for SLE[118], RA[119], and non-rheumatic diseases such as chronic severe hypertension[120], moderate hypertension[121], obesity[122,123], type-2 diabetes[124], and epilepsy.[125]

○ <u>Broad-spectrum fatty acid therapy with ALA, EPA, DHA, GLA and oleic acid:</u> Fatty acid supplementation should be delivered in the form of combination therapy with ALA, GLA, DHA, and EPA. Given at doses of 3,000 – 9,000 mg per day, ALA from flaxseed oil has impressive anti-inflammatory benefits demonstrated by its ability to halve prostaglandin production in humans.[126] **Numerous studies have demonstrated the benefit of GLA in the treatment of rheumatoid arthritis when used at doses between 500 mg – 4,000 mg per day.[127,128] Fish oil provides EPA and DHA which have well-proven anti-inflammatory benefits in rheumatoid arthritis[129,130,131] and lupus.[132,133]** ALA, EPA, DHA, and GLA need to be provided in the form of supplements; when using high doses of therapeutic oils, *liquid* supplements that can be mixed in juice or a smoothie are generally more convenient and palatable than are *capsules*. For example, at the upper end of oral fatty acid administration, the patient may be consuming as much as one-quarter cup per day of fatty acid supplementation; this same dose administered in the form of pills would require at least 72 capsules to attain the equivalent doses of ALA, EPA, DHA, and GLA. Therapeutic amounts of oleic acid can be obtained from generous use of olive oil, preferably on fresh vegetables. Supplementation with polyunsaturated fatty acids warrants increased intake of antioxidants from diet, from fruit and vegetable juices, and from properly formulated supplements. Since patients with systemic inflammation are generally in a pro-oxidative state, consideration must be given to the timing and starting dose of fatty acid supplementation and the need for antioxidant protection; some patients should start with a low dose of fatty acid supplementation until inflammation and the hyperoxidative state have been reduced. Clinicians must realize that fatty acids are not clinically or biochemically interchangeable and that one fatty acid does not substitute for another; each of the health-promoting fatty acids—ALA, GLA, EPA, DHA, and oleic acid—must be supplied in order for its benefits to be

---

[118] Fuhrman J, Sarter B, Calabro DJ. Brief case reports of medically supervised, water-only fasting associated with remission of autoimmune disease. *Altern Ther Health Med.* 2002 Jul-Aug;8(4):112, 110-1

[119] "An association was found between improvement in inflammatory activity of the joints and enhancement of neutrophil bactericidal capacity. Fasting appears to improve the clinical status of patients with RA." Uden AM, Trang L, Venizelos N, Palmblad J. Neutrophil functions and clinical performance after total fasting in patients with rheumatoid arthritis. *Ann Rheum Dis.* 1983 Feb;42(1):45-51

[120] "The average reduction in blood pressure was 37/13 mm Hg, with the greatest decrease being observed for subjects with the most severe hypertension. Patients with stage 3 hypertension (those with systolic blood pressure greater than 180 mg Hg, diastolic blood pressure greater than 110 mg Hg, or both) had an average reduction of 60/17 mm Hg at the conclusion of treatment." Goldhamer A, Lisle D, Parpia B, Anderson SV, Campbell TC. Medically supervised water-only fasting in the treatment of hypertension. *J Manipulative Physiol Ther.* 2001 Jun;24(5):335-9 http://www.healthpromoting.com/335-339Goldhamer115263.QXD.pdf

[121] "RESULTS: Approximately 82% of the subjects achieved BP at or below 120/80 mm Hg by the end of the treatment program. The mean BP reduction was 20/7 mm Hg, with the greatest decrease being observed for subjects with the highest baseline BP." Goldhamer AC, Lisle DJ, Sultana P, Anderson SV, Parpia B, Hughes B, Campbell TC. Medically supervised water-only fasting in the treatment of borderline hypertension. *J Altern Complement Med.* 2002 Oct;8(5):643-50 http://www.healthpromoting.com/Articles/articles/study%202/acmpaper5.pdf

[122] Vertes V, Genuth SM, Hazelton IM. Supplemented fasting as a large-scale outpatient program. *JAMA.* 1977 Nov 14;238(20):2151-3

[123] Bauman WA, Schwartz E, Rose HG, Eisenstein HN, Johnson DW. Early and long-term effects of acute caloric deprivation in obese diabetic patients. *Am J Med.* 1988 Jul;85(1):38-46

[124] Goldhamer AC. Initial cost of care results in medically supervised water-only fasting for treating high blood pressure and diabetes. *J Altern Complement Med.* 2002 Dec;8(6):696-7 http://www.healthpromoting.com/Articles/pdf/Study%2032.pdf

[125] "The ketogenic diet should be considered as alternative therapy for children with difficult-to-control seizures. It is more effective than many of the new anticonvulsant medications and is well tolerated by children and families when it is effective." Freeman JM, Vining EP, Pillas DJ, Pyzik PL, Casey JC, Kelly LM. The efficacy of the ketogenic diet-1998: a prospective evaluation of intervention in 150 children. *Pediatrics.* 1998 Dec;102(6):1358-63 http://pediatrics.aappublications.org/cgi/reprint/102/6/1358

[126] Adam O, Wolfram G, Zollner N. Effect of alpha-linolenic acid in the human diet on linoleic acid metabolism and prostaglandin biosynthesis. *J Lipid Res.* 1986 Apr;27(4):421-6 http://www.jlr.org/cgi/reprint/27/4/421

[127] "Other results showed a significant reduction in morning stiffness with gamma-linolenic acid at 3 months and reduction in pain and articular index at 6 months with olive oil." Brzeski M, Madhok R, Capell HA. Evening primrose oil in patients with rheumatoid arthritis and side-effects of non-steroidal anti-inflammatory drugs. *Br J Rheumatol.* 1991 Oct;30(5):370-2

[128] Rothman D, DeLuca P, Zurier RB. Botanical lipids: effects on inflammation, immune responses, and rheumatoid arthritis. *Semin Arthritis Rheum.* 1995 Oct;25(2):87-96

[129] Adam O, Beringer C, Kless T, Lemmen C, Adam A, Wiseman M, Adam P, Klimmek R, Forth W. Anti-inflammatory effects of a low arachidonic acid diet and fish oil in patients with rheumatoid arthritis. *Rheumatol Int.* 2003 Jan;23(1):27-36

[130] Lau CS, Morley KD, Belch JJ. Effects of fish oil supplementation on non-steroidal anti-inflammatory drug requirement in patients with mild rheumatoid arthritis--a double-blind placebo controlled study. *Br J Rheumatol.* 1993 Nov;32(11):982-9

[131] Kremer JM, Jubiz W, Michalek A, Rynes RI, Bartholomew LE, Bigaouette J, Timchalk M, Beeler D, Lininger L. Fish-oil fatty acid supplementation in active rheumatoid arthritis. A double-blinded, controlled, crossover study. *Ann Intern Med.* 1987 Apr;106(4):497-503

[132] Walton AJ, Snaith ML, Locniskar M, Cumberland AG, Morrow WJ, Isenberg DA. Dietary fish oil and the severity of symptoms in patients with systemic lupus erythematosus. *Ann Rheum Dis.* 1991 Jul;50(7):463-6

[133] Duffy EM, Meenagh GK, McMillan SA, Strain JJ, Hannigan BM, Bell AL. The clinical effect of dietary supplementation with omega-3 fish oils and/or copper in systemic lupus erythematosus. *J Rheumatol.* 2004 Aug;31(8):1551-6

obtained; imbalanced supplementation causes or exacerbates biochemical imbalances and produces suboptimal results.[134]

- o Vitamin D3 supplementation with physiologic doses and/or tailored to serum 25(OH)D levels: Vitamin D deficiency is common in the general population and is even more common in patients with chronic illness and chronic musculoskeletal pain.[135] Correction of vitamin D deficiency supports normal immune function against infection and provides a clinically significant anti-inflammatory[136] and analgesic benefit in patients with back pain[137] and limb pain.[138] Reasonable daily doses for children and adults are 1,000-2,000 and 4,000 IU, respectively.[139] Deficiency and response to treatment are monitored with serum 25(OH)vitamin D while safety is monitored with serum calcium; inflammatory granulomatous diseases and certain drugs such as hydrochlorothiazide greatly increase the propensity for hypercalcemia and warrant increment dosing and frequent monitoring of serum calcium. Vitamin D2 (ergocalciferol) is not a human nutrient and should not be used in clinical practice.

- **Infections/colonizations/dysbiosis:** **All patients with rheumatoid arthritis have gastrointestinal dysbiosis until proven otherwise by the combination of 1) three-sample comprehensive parasitology examinations performed by a specialty laboratory and 2) clinical response to at least two 2-4 week courses of broad-spectrum antimicrobial treatment.** Yeast, bacteria, and parasites are treated as indicated based on identification and sensitivity results from comprehensive parasitology assessments. Patients taking immunosuppressant drugs such as corticosteroids/prednisone have increased risk of intestinal bacterial overgrowth and translocation.[140,141] Other dysbiotic loci should be investigated as discussed in Chapter 4 in the section on *Multifocal Dysbiosis*.

  - o Orodental dysbiosis: The systemic inflammatory response triggered by subclinical oral/dental "infections" is now believed to exacerbate conditions associated with inflammation, such as cardiovascular disease and diabetes mellitus.[142] Patients with RA have heightened antibody levels against common oral bacteria. IgG levels against *Porphyromonas gingivalis*, *Prevotella melaninogenica*, *Bacteroides forsythus*, and *Prevotella intermedia* were found to be significantly higher in RA patients when compared with those of controls.[143] In the first human clinical trial to test the hypothesis that treatment of orodental dysbiosis would provide subjective and objective clinical benefits for patients with RA, AlKatma et al[144] showed that **periodontal treatment consisting of scaling/root planing and oral hygiene instruction reduced symptom scores and ESR levels in patients with RA.**

[134] Vasquez A. Reducing Pain and Inflammation Naturally. Part 2: New Insights into Fatty Acid Supplementation and Its Effect on Eicosanoid Production and Genetic Expression. *Nutritional Perspectives* 2005; January: 5-16 http://www.ichnfm.org/faculty/vasquez/profile.html

[135] Plotnikoff GA, Quigley JM. Prevalence of severe hypovitaminosis D in patients with persistent, nonspecific musculoskeletal pain. *Mayo Clin Proc.* 2003 Dec;78(12):1463-70

[136] Timms PM, Mannan N, Hitman GA, Noonan K, Mills PG, Syndercombe-Court D, Aganna E, Price CP, Boucher BJ. Circulating MMP9, vitamin D and variation in the TIMP-1 response with VDR genotype: mechanisms for inflammatory damage in chronic disorders? *QJM.* 2002 Dec;95(12):787-96 http://qjmed.oxfordjournals.org/cgi/content/full/95/12/787

[137] Al Faraj S, Al Mutairi K. Vitamin D deficiency and chronic low back pain in Saudi Arabia. *Spine.* 2003 Jan 15;28(2):177-9

[138] Masood H, Narang AP, Bhat IA, Shah GN. Persistent limb pain and raised serum alkaline phosphatase the earliest markers of subclinical hypovitaminosis D in Kashmir. *Indian J Physiol Pharmacol.* 1989 Oct-Dec;33(4):259-61

[139] Vasquez A, Manso G, Cannell J. The clinical importance of vitamin D (cholecalciferol): a paradigm shift with implications for all healthcare providers. *Altern Ther Health Med.* 2004 Sep-Oct;10(5):28-36 http://www.ichnfm.org/faculty/vasquez/profile.html

[140] "A 63-year-old man with systemic lupus erythematosus and selective IgA deficiency developed intractable diarrhoea the day after treatment with prednisone, 50 mg daily, was started. The diarrhoea was considered to be caused by bacterial overgrowth and was later successfully treated with doxycycline." Denison H, Wallerstedt S. Bacterial overgrowth after high-dose corticosteroid treatment. *Scand J Gastroenterol.* 1989 Jun;24(5):561-4

[141] "These bacteria also translocated to the mesenteric lymph nodes in mice injected with cyclophosphamide or prednisone." Berg RD, Wommack E, Deitch EA. Immunosuppression and intestinal bacterial overgrowth synergistically promote bacterial translocation. *Arch Surg.* 1988 Nov;123(11):1359-64

[142] Amar S, Han X. The impact of periodontal infection on systemic diseases. *Med Sci Monit.* 2003 Dec;9(12):RA291-9 http://www.medscimonit.com/pub/vol_9/no_12/3776.pdf

[143] Ogrendik M, Kokino S, Ozdemir F, Bird PS, Hamlet S. Serum antibodies to oral anaerobic bacteria in patients with rheumatoid arthritis. *MedGenMed.* 2005 Jun 16;7(2):2

[144] "There was a statistically significant difference in DAS28 (4.3 +/- 1.6 vs. 5.1 +/- 1.2) and erythrocyte sedimentation rate (31.4 +/- 24.3 vs. 42.7 +/- 22) between the treatment and the control groups." Al-Katma MK, Bissada NF, Bordeaux JM, Sue J, Askari AD. Control of periodontal infection reduces the severity of active rheumatoid arthritis. *J Clin Rheumatol.* 2007 Jun;13(3):134-7

- o Genitourinary dysbiosis: Microbial contamination of the genitourinary tract can cause a systemic pro-inflammatory arthritogenic response in susceptible individuals; **in a study of 234 patients with inflammatory arthritis, 44% of patients had subclinical genitourinary colonization, mostly due to *Chlamydia, Mycoplasma,* or *Ureaplasma.*** [145]
- o Gastrointestinal dysbiosis: As discussed above in the section on *Laboratory Assessments,* microbiologic testing for GI dysbiosis is followed by specific or empiric treatment:
  - ▪ Oregano oil: Emulsified oil of oregano in a time-released tablet (A.D.P.®, patented by Biotics Research Corporation) is proven effective in the eradication of harmful gastrointestinal microbes, including *Blastocystis hominis, Entamoeba hartmanni,* and *Endolimax nana.* [146] An *in vitro* study [147] and clinical experience support the use of emulsified oregano against *Candida albicans* and various bacteria. The common dose is 600 mg per day in divided doses for 6 weeks. [148]

    > **Urogenital swab culture is the only useful diagnostic method for the detection of the arthritogenic infection**
    >
    > "Urogenital swab culture is a sensitive diagnostic method to identify the triggering infection in reactive arthritis."
    >
    > Erlacher L, et al. Reactive arthritis: urogenital swab culture is the only useful diagnostic method for the detection of the arthritogenic infection in extra-articularly asymptomatic patients with undifferentiated oligoarthritis. *Br J Rheumatol.* 1995 Sep

  - ▪ Berberine: Berberine is an alkaloid extracted from plants such as *Berberis vulgaris,* and *Hydrastis canadensis,* and it shows effectiveness against *Giardia, Candida,* and *Streptococcus* in addition to its direct anti-inflammatory and antidiarrheal actions. Oral dose of 400 mg per day has been traditionally common for adults [149]; newer clinical research using human patients has shown short-term safety and efficacy of berberine: 1,000 mg per day showed very impressive cholesterol-lowering benefits in hypercholesterolemic patients [150], and 1,500 mg per day showed hypoglycemic benefits for patients with type-2 diabetes mellitus. [151]
  - ▪ *Artemisia annua:* Artemisinin has been safely used for centuries in Asia for the treatment of malaria, and it also has effectiveness against anaerobic bacteria due to the pro-oxidative sesquiterpene endoperoxide. [152,153] This author has commonly used artemisinin at 200 mg per day in divided doses for adults with dysbiosis. Given its pro-oxidative mechanism, treatment should probably be of limited duration, i.e., 1-2 months; concomitant neuroprotection with CoQ-10 (et al) would be reasonable.
  - ▪ St. John's Wort (*Hypericum perforatum*): Hyperforin from *Hypericum perforatum* shows impressive antibacterial action *in vitro*, particularly against gram-positive bacteria such as *Staphylococcus aureus, Streptococcus pyogenes, Streptococcus agalactiae* [154] and

---

[145] "Urogenital swab cultures showed a microbial infection in 44% of the patients with oligoarthritis (15% Chlamydia, 14% Mycoplasma, 28% Ureaplasma), whereas in the control group only 26% had a positive result (4% Chlamydia, 7% Mycoplasma, 21% Ureaplasma)." Erlacher L, Wintersberger W, Menschik M, Benke-Studnicka A, Machold K, Stanek G, Soltz-Szots J, Smolen J, Graninger W. Reactive arthritis: urogenital swab culture is the only useful diagnostic method for the detection of the arthritogenic infection in extra-articularly asymptomatic patients with undifferentiated oligoarthritis. *Br J Rheumatol.* 1995 Sep;34(9):838-42 http://rheumatology.oxfordjournals.org/cgi/content/abstract/34/9/838

[146] Force M, Sparks WS, Ronzio RA. Inhibition of enteric parasites by emulsified oil of oregano in vivo. *Phytother Res.* 2000 May;14(3):213-4

[147] Stiles JC, Sparks W, Ronzio RA. The inhibition of Candida albicans by oregano. *J Applied Nutr* 1995;47:96–102

[148] Force M, Sparks WS, Ronzio RA. Inhibition of enteric parasites by emulsified oil of oregano in vivo. *Phytother Res.* 2000 May;14(3):213-4

[149] Berberine. Altern Med Rev. 2000 Apr;5(2):175-7 http://www.thorne.com/altmedrev/.fulltext/5/2/175.pdf

[150] "Oral administration of BBR in 32 hypercholesterolemic patients for 3 months reduced serum cholesterol by 29%, triglycerides by 35% and LDL-cholesterol by 25%." Kong W, Wei J, Abidi P, Lin M, Inaba S, Li C, Wang Y, Wang Z, Si S, Pan H, Wang S, Wu J, Wang Y, Li Z, Liu J, Jiang JD. Berberine is a novel cholesterol-lowering drug working through a unique mechanism distinct from statins. *Nat Med.* 2004 Dec;10(12):1344-51

[151] "In conclusion, this pilot study indicates that berberine is a potent oral hypoglycemic agent with beneficial effects on lipid metabolism." Yin J, Xing H, Ye J. Efficacy of berberine in patients with type 2 diabetes mellitus. *Metabolism.* 2008 May;57(5):712-7

[152] Dien TK, de Vries PJ, Khanh NX, Koopmans R, Binh LN, Duc DD, Kager PA, van Boxtel CJ. Effect of food intake on pharmacokinetics of oral artemisinin in healthy Vietnamese subjects. *Antimicrob Agents Chemother.* 1997 May;41(5):1069-72

[153] Giao PT, Binh TQ, Kager PA, Long HP, Van Thang N, Van Nam N, de Vries PJ. Artemisinin for treatment of uncomplicated falciparum malaria: is there a place for monotherapy? *Am J Trop Med Hyg.* 2001 Dec;65(6):690-5

[154] Schempp CM, Pelz K, Wittmer A, Schopf E, Simon JC. Antibacterial activity of hyperforin from St John's wort, against multiresistant Staphylococcus aureus and gram-positive bacteria. *Lancet.* 1999 Jun 19;353(9170):2129

perhaps gram-negative *Helicobacter pylori*.[155] Up to 600 mg three times per day of a 3% hyperforin standardized extract is customary in the treatment of depression.

- <u>Bismuth</u>: Bismuth is commonly used in the empiric treatment of diarrhea (e.g., "Pepto-<u>Bis</u>mol") and is commonly combined with other antimicrobial agents to reduce drug resistance and increase antibiotic effectiveness.[156]

- <u>Undecylenic acid</u>: Derived from castor bean oil, undecylenic acid has antifungal properties and is commonly indicated by sensitivity results obtained by stool culture. Common dosages are 150-250 mg tid (up to 750 mg per day).[157]

- <u>Peppermint *(Mentha piperita)*</u>: Peppermint shows antimicrobial and antispasmodic actions and has demonstrated clinical effectiveness in patients with bacterial overgrowth of the small bowel.

- <u>Commonly used antibiotic/antifungal drugs</u>: The most commonly employed drugs for intestinal bacterial overgrowth are described here.[158] Treatment duration is generally at least 2 weeks and up to 8 weeks, depending on clinical response and the severity and diversity of the intestinal overgrowth. With all anti*bacterial* treatments, use empiric anti*fungal* treatment to prevent yeast overgrowth; some patients benefit from antifungal treatment that is continued for *months* and occasionally *years*. Probiotic yeast and bacteria are generally appropriate except in patients with hypersensitivity, severe immunosuppression, or extreme or recalcitrant bacterial overgrowth of the intestines. Drugs can generally be co-administered with natural antibiotics/antifungals for improved efficacy.   Treatment can be guided by identification of the dysbiotic microbes and the results of culture and sensitivity tests. Examples of doses are provided below, but clinicians must choose dose and duration per their judgment, experience, and the patient's situation, comorbidity, age, hepatic and renal function, and accompanying polypharmacy; the use of dosing and drug-interaction data (e.g., *Epocrates*) is strongly recommended.

  ⇒ <u>Metronidazole</u>: 250-500 mg BID-QID (generally limit to 1.5-2 g/d); metronidazole has systemic bioavailability and effectiveness against a wide range of dysbiotic microbes, including protozoans, amebas/Giardia, *H. pylori*, *Clostridium difficile* and most anaerobic gram-negative bacilli.[159] Adverse effects are generally limited to stomatitis, nausea, diarrhea, and—rarely and/or with long-term use—peripheral neuropathy, dizziness, and metallic taste; the drug must not be consumed with alcohol. Metronidazole resistance by *Blastocystis hominis* and other parasites has been noted.

  ⇒ <u>Erythromycin</u>: 250-500 mg TID-QID; this drug is a widely used antibiotic that also has intestinal promotility benefits (thus making it an ideal treatment for intestinal bacterial overgrowth associated with or caused by intestinal dysmotility/hypomotility such as seen in scleroderma[160,161]). Do not combine erythromycin with the promotility drug **cisapride** due to risk for serious cardiac arrhythmia.

  ⇒ <u>Tetracycline</u>: 250-500 mg QID

  ⇒ <u>Ciprofloxacin</u>: 500 mg BID, caution: tendonopathy

---

[155] "A butanol fraction of St. John's Wort revealed anti-Helicobacter pylori activity with MIC values ranging between 15.6 and 31.2 microg/ml." Reichling J, Weseler A, Saller R. A current review of the antimicrobial activity of Hypericum perforatum L. *Pharmacopsychiatry*. 2001 Jul;34 Suppl 1:S116-8

[156] Veldhuyzen van Zanten SJ, Sherman PM, Hunt RH. Helicobacter pylori: new developments and treatments. *CMAJ*. 1997;156(11):1565-74 http://www.cmaj.ca/cgi/reprint/156/11/1565.pdf

[157] "Adult dosage is usually 450-750 mg undecylenic acid daily in three divided doses." Undecylenic acid. Monograph. *Altern Med Rev*. 2002 Feb;7(1):68-70 http://www.thorne.com/altmedrev/.fulltext/7/1/68.pdf

[158] Saltzman JR, Russell RM. Nutritional consequences of intestinal bacterial overgrowth. *Compr Ther*. 1994;20(9):523-30

[159] Tierney ML. McPhee SJ, Papadakis MA. <u>Current Medical Diagnosis and Treatment 2006</u>. 45th edition. New York; Lange Medical Books: 2006, pages 1578-1577

[160] "Prokinetic agents effective in pseudoobstruction include metoclopramide, domperidone, cisapride, octreotide, and erythromycin. ... The combination of octreotide and erythromycin may be particularly effective in systemic sclerosis." Sjogren RW. Gastrointestinal features of scleroderma. *Curr Opin Rheumatol*. 1996 Nov;8(6):569-75

[161] "CONCLUSIONS: Erythromycin accelerates gastric and gallbladder emptying in scleroderma patients and might be helpful in the treatment of gastrointestinal motor abnormalities in these patients." Fiorucci S, Distrutti E, Bassotti G, Gerli R, Chiucchiu S, Betti C, Santucci L, Morelli A. Effect of erythromycin administration on upper gastrointestinal motility in scleroderma patients. *Scand J Gastroenterol*. 1994 Sep;29(9):807-13

⇒ <u>Cephalexin/Keflex</u>: 250 mg QID

⇒ <u>Minocycline</u>: Minocycline (200 mg/day)[162] has received the most attention in the treatment of rheumatoid arthritis due to its superior response (65%) over placebo (13%)[163]; in addition to its antibacterial action, the drug is also immunomodulatory and anti-inflammatory. Ironically, minocycline can cause drug-induced autoimmunity, especially lupus.[164,165]

⇒ <u>Nystatin</u>: Nystatin 500,000 units BID-TID with food; duration of treatment begins with a minimum duration of 2-4 weeks and may continue as long as the patient is deriving benefit.

⇒ <u>Ketoconazole</u>: As a systemically bioavailable antifungal drug, ketoconazole has inherent anti-inflammatory benefits which may be helpful; however the drug inhibits androgen formation and may lead to exacerbation of the hypoandrogenism that is commonly seen in autoimmune patients and which contributes to the immune dysfunction.

▪ <u>Probiotics</u>: Live cultures in the form of tablets, capsules, yogurt, or kefir can be used per patient preference and tolerance. Obviously, dairy-based products should be avoided by patients with dairy allergy.

▪ *Saccharomyces boulardii*: A non-colonizing, non-pathogenic yeast that increases sIgA production and can aid in the elimination of pathogenic/dysbiotic yeast, bacteria, and parasites. It is particularly useful during antibiotic treatment to help prevent secondary *Candida* and *Clostridium difficile* infections. Common dose is 250 mg thrice daily.

▪ <u>Supplemented Paleo-Mediterranean diet / Specific Carbohydrate Diet</u>: The specifications of the *specific carbohydrate diet* (SCD) detailed by Gottschall[166] are met with adherence to the Paleo diet by Cordain.[167] The combination of both approaches and books will give patients an excellent combination of informational understanding and culinary versatility.

● <u>Nutritional immunomodulation</u>: The goal with this component of the protocol is to maximize induction of anti-inflammatory tolerogenic T-regulatory cells (Treg) at the reciprocal expense of pro-inflammatory pro-autoimmune Th-17 cells. Mechanisms for this process are manifold and reasonably well described via molecular mechanisms that culminate in the induction of FOXp3 transcription factor via epigenetic mechanisms; these will be detailed in an upcoming monograph and presentation by this author. A summary of the "plaid figs" protocol is as follows:

○ <u>Probiotics</u>: Probiotics promote immunotolerance (generally anti-inflammatory and specifically anti-allergy) in human and animal studies. Mechanisms are mostly epigenetic, via either living or dead probiotic microbes (i.e., molecular pattern recognition) and via metabolites—specifically: butyrate—which culminate in optimal induction of Treg.

○ <u>Lipoic acid</u>: 300mg TID-QID to suppress IL-17 in humans by 35-50% thereby shifting the balance of effector phenotypes away from Th-17 and toward tolerance and relative enhancement of Treg effect.

[162] "...48-week trial of oral minocycline (200 mg/d) or placebo." Tilley BC, Alarcon GS, Heyse SP, Trentham DE, Neuner R, Kaplan DA, Clegg DO, Leisen JC, Buckley L, Cooper SM, Duncan H, Pillemer SR, Tuttleman M, Fowler SE. Minocycline in rheumatoid arthritis. A 48-week, double-blind, placebo-controlled trial. MIRA Trial Group. *Ann Intern Med*. 1995 Jan 15;122(2):81-9

[163] "In patients with early seropositive RA, therapy with minocycline is superior to placebo." O'Dell JR, Haire CE, Palmer W, Drymalski W, Wees S, Blakely K, Churchill M, Eckhoff PJ, Weaver A, Doud D, Erikson N, Dietz F, Olson R, Maloley P, Klassen LW, Moore GF. Treatment of early rheumatoid arthritis with minocycline or placebo: results of a randomized, double-blind, placebo-controlled trial. *Arthritis Rheum*. 1997 May;40(5):842-8

[164] "...many cases of drug-induced lupus related to minocycline have been reported. Some of those reports included pulmonary lupus..." Christodoulou CS, Emmanuel P, Ray RA, Good RA, Schnapf BM, Cawkwell GD. Respiratory distress due to minocycline-induced pulmonary lupus. *Chest*. 1999 May;115(5):1471-3 http://www.chestjournal.org/cgi/content/full/115/5/1471

[165] Lawson TM, Amos N, Bulgen D, Williams BD.Minocycline-induced lupus: clinical features and response to rechallenge. *Rheumatology* (Oxford). 2001 Mar;40(3):329-35 http://rheumatology.oxfordjournals.org/cgi/content/full/40/3/329

[166] Gotschall E. Breaking the Vicious Cycle: Intestinal health though diet. Kirkton Press; Rev edition (August, 1994) http://www.scdiet.com/

[167] Cordain L: The Paleo Diet: Lose weight and get healthy by eating the food you were designed to eat. John Wiley & Sons Inc., New York 2002 http://thepaleodiet.com/

- A—vitamin A: Retinoic acid is essential for optimal induction of FOXp3 Treg. 27-47% of women (and likely a large proportion of men, as well) are unable to efficiently convert beta-carotene into vitamin A, and therefore these people/patients need preformed vitamin A. A loading dose of 100,000-300,000 IU/d for 7-10 days followed by a maintenance dose of 10,000-25,000 IU/d is reasonable except in women who are pregnant or might become pregnant in whom the total vitamin A dose should be kept below 9,000 IU/d to avoid purported risks for fetal malformations / birth defects.
- Inflammation reduction: Anti-inflammatory interventions such as weight loss / adipose reduction/minimization, moderate exercise, carbohydrate avoidance.
- D—vitamin D3: Three studies among normal, SLE, and MS patients have each shown that vitamin D3 supplementation induces greater number and function of Treg cells in adult humans following approximately one month of oral supplementation. The adult requirement for vitamin D is approximately 4,000 IU/d with optimal benefit obtained when serum 25-OH-D levels enter the optimal range as discussed elsewhere in this book.
- Fatty acid supplementation: N3 fatty acids and GLA have been shown to activate pathways involved in the maximal induction of anti-inflammation in general and Treg in particular.
- Infection/dysbiosis elimination: Dysbiosis in general—especially of the gastrointestinal tract—and especially colonization with segmented filamentous bacteria (SFB), which per animal studies, strongly promote induction of Th-17 cells, which are a major effector phenotype in the chronic/sustained inflammation of autoimmunity/auto-inflammation.
- Green tea: Epigallocatechin gallate (EGCG) induces Treg *in vitro*.
- Sodium avoidance: Sodium induces Th-17 proinflammatory effector cells.

- Dysfunctional mitochondria: Mitochondrial dysfunction has recently become well-established as a major contributor to chronic/sustained inflammation, diabetes mellitus and insulin resistance, hypertension, migraine headaches, neurodegeneration (Parkinson's and Alzheimer's diseases), fibromyalgia and chronic fatigue syndrome. Per my recent reviews and presentations[168], treatment of mitochondrial dysfunction has three major components: ❶ elimination, mitophagy, ❷ disinhibition, liberation, ❸ support, stimulation, biogenesis. Although my complete protocol has approximately 30 components, the most readily-utilized components suitable for most patients on the first day of treatment include:
  - Carbohydrate restriction:
  - Moderate exercise:
  - CoQ10 100-300 mg/d:
  - Acetyl-L-carnitine 1g BID IC:
  - Lipoic acid 300-400 mg TID:
  - Antiviral and antibacterial treatments as indicated per patient: Reviewed previously; antiviral protocol presented in Chapter 4.
- Style of living, spinal health, stress reduction/modulation, sweating/exercise: As reviewed in Chapter 2 on (Re)Establishing the Foundation for Health, components of "healthy living" and inflammation modulation/reduction include:
  - Sleep sufficiency:
  - Stress reduction/modulation:
  - "Sweating": A metaphor for exercise
  - Spinal health/adjusting/manipulation: As indicated.
  - Surgery—as needed:
  - Stamp your passport: Occasionally, we all need a break from the routine; travel to other cultures shows us different ways of living and makes clear how little we need to own/do in order to be happy.

---

[168] See: Createspace.com/4478800, Vimeo.com/ichnfm, and Ichnfm.org/events/MitochondrialMedicine/

- o <u>Self-expression and therapeutic writing</u>: Limited evidence indicates that self-expressive writing can significantly reduce symptomatology in patients with RA.[169]
- o <u>Sensory deprivation therapy, REST—reduced environmental stimulation therapy</u>:
- o <u>Specialized supplementation</u>: Several examples follow:
  - <u>Oral enzyme therapy with proteolytic/pancreatic enzymes</u>: Polyenzyme supplementation can be used to ameliorate the pathophysiology induced by immune complexes, as seen in rheumatoid arthritis.[170]
  - *Uncaria tomentosa, Uncaria guianensis*: Cat's claw has been safely and successfully used in the treatment of osteoarthritis[171] and **rheumatoid arthritis**.[172] High-quality extractions from reputable manufacturers used according to directions are recommended. Most products contain between 250-500 mg and are standardized to 3.0% alkaloids and 15% total polyphenols; QD-TID po dosing should be sufficient as *part* of a comprehensive plan.
  - *Harpagophytum procumbens*: Harpagophytum is a moderately effective botanical analgesic.[173,174,175,176,177] Products are generally standardized for the content of harpagosides, with a target dose of 60 mg harpagoside per day when used in isolation.[178]
  - <u>Willow bark</u>: Extracts from willow bark have proven safe and effective in the alleviation of moderate/severe low-back pain.[179,180] The mechanism of action appears to be inhibition of prostaglandin formation via inhibition of cyclooxygenase-2 gene transcription[181] by salicylates, phytonutrients which are widely present in fruits, vegetables, herbs and spices and which are partly responsible for the anti-cancer, anti-inflammatory, and health-promoting benefits of plant consumption.[182,183] According to a letter by Vasquez and Muanza[184], the only adverse effect that has been documented in association with willow bark was a single case of anaphylaxis in a patient previously sensitized to acetylsalicylic acid.

---

[169] "Rheumatoid arthritis patients in the experimental group showed improvements in overall disease activity (a mean reduction in disease severity from 1.65 to 1.19 [28%] on a scale of 0 [asymptomatic] to 4 [very severe] at the 4-month follow-up; P=.001), whereas control group patients did not change." Smyth JM, Stone AA, Hurewitz A, Kaell A. Effects of writing about stressful experiences on symptom reduction in patients with asthma or rheumatoid arthritis: a randomized trial. *JAMA*. 1999 Apr 14;281(14):1304-9

[170] Galebskaya LV, Ryumina EV, Niemerovsky VS, Matyukov AA. Human complement system state after wobenzyme intake. *VESTNIK MOSKOVSKOGO UNIVERSITETA. KHIMIYA*. 2000. Vol. 41, No. 6. Supplement. Pages 148-149

[171] Piscoya J, Rodriguez Z, Bustamante SA, Okuhama NN, Miller MJ, Sandoval M.Efficacy and safety of freeze-dried cat's claw in osteoarthritis of the knee: mechanisms of action of the species Uncaria guianensis. *Inflamm Res*. 2001 Sep;50(9):442-8

[172] "This small preliminary study demonstrates relative safety and modest benefit to the tender joint count of a highly purified extract from the pentacyclic chemotype of UT in patients with active RA taking sulfasalazine or hydroxychloroquine." Mur E, Hartig F, Eibl G, Schirmer M. Randomized double blind trial of an extract from the pentacyclic alkaloid-chemotype of uncaria tomentosa for the treatment of rheumatoid arthritis. *J Rheumatol*. 2002 Apr;29(4):678-81

[173] Chrubasik S, Thanner J, Kunzel O, Conradt C, Black A, Pollak S. Comparison of outcome measures during treatment with the proprietary Harpagophytum extract doloteffin in patients with pain in the lower back, knee or hip. *Phytomedicine* 2002 Apr;9(3):181-94

[174] Chantre P, Cappelaere A, Leblan D, Guedon D, Vandermander J, Fournie B. Efficacy and tolerance of Harpagophytum procumbens versus diacerhein in treatment of osteoarthritis. *Phytomedicine* 2000 Jun;7(3):177-83

[175] Leblan D, Chantre P, Fournie B. Harpagophytum procumbens in the treatment of knee and hip osteoarthritis. Four-month results of a prospective, multicenter, double-blind trial versus diacerhein. *Joint Bone Spine* 2000;67(5):462-7

[176] "...subgroup analyses suggested that the effect was confined to patients with more severe and radiating pain accompanied by neurological deficit. ...a slightly different picture, with the benefits seeming, if anything, to be greatest in the H600 group and in patients without more severe pain, radiation or neurological deficit." Chrubasik S, Junck H, Breitschwerdt H, Conradt C, Zappe H. Effectiveness of Harpagophytum extract WS 1531 in the treatment of exacerbation of low back pain: a randomized, placebo-controlled, double-blind study. *Eur J Anaesthesiol* 1999 Feb;16(2):118-29

[177] Chrubasik S, Model A, Black A, Pollak S. A randomized double-blind pilot study comparing Doloteffin and Vioxx in the treatment of low back pain. *Rheumatology* (Oxford). 2003 Jan;42(1):141-8

[178] "They took an 8-week course of Doloteffin at a dose providing 60 mg harpagoside per day... Doloteffin is well worth considering for osteoarthritic knee and hip pain and nonspecific low back pain." Chrubasik S, Thanner J, Kunzel O, Conradt C, Black A, Pollak S. Comparison of outcome measures during treatment with the proprietary Harpagophytum extract doloteffin in patients with pain in the lower back, knee or hip. *Phytomedicine* 2002 Apr;9(3):181-94

[179] Chrubasik S, Eisenberg E, Balan E, Weinberger T, Luzzati R, Conradt C. Treatment of low-back pain exacerbations with willow bark extract: a randomized double-blind study. *Am J Med*. 2000;109:9-14

[180] Chrubasik S, Kunzel O, Model A, Conradt C, Black A. Treatment of low-back pain with a herbal or synthetic anti-rheumatic: a randomized controlled study. Willow bark extract for low-back pain. *Rheumatology* (Oxford). 2001;40:1388-93

[181] Hare LG, Woodside JV, Young IS. Dietary salicylates. *J Clin Pathol* 2003 Sep;56(9):649-50

[182] Lawrence JR, Peter R, Baxter GJ, Robson J, Graham AB, Paterson JR. Urinary excretion of salicyluric and salicylic acids by non-vegetarians, vegetarians, and patients taking low dose aspirin. *J Clin Pathol*. 2003 Sep;56(9):651-3

[183] Paterson JR, Lawrence JR. Salicylic acid: a link between aspirin, diet and the prevention of colorectal cancer. *QJM*. 2001 Aug;94(8):445-8

[184] **Vasquez A, Muanza DN. Evaluation of Presence of Aspirin-Related Warnings with Willow Bark: Comment on the Article by Clauson et al.** ***Ann Pharmacotherapy*** **2005 Oct;39(10):1763**

- *Boswellia serrata*: *Boswellia* shows clear anti-inflammatory and analgesic action via inhibition of 5-lipoxygenase[185] and clinical benefits have been demonstrated in patients with osteoarthritis of the knees[186] as well as asthma[187] and ulcerative colitis.[188] Products are generally standardized to contain 37.5–65% boswellic acids, with a target dose is approximately 150 mg of boswellic acids TID; dose and number of capsules/tablets will vary depending upon the concentration found in differing products. A German study showing that *Boswellia* was ineffective for rheumatoid arthritis[189] was poorly conducted, with inadequate follow-up, inadequate controls, and abnormal dosing of the herb.

- Topical *Capsicum annuum, Capsicum frutescens* (Cayenne pepper, hot chili pepper): Controlled clinical trials have conclusively demonstrated capsaicin's ability to deplete sensory fibers of the neuropeptide substance P and to thus reduce pain. Topical capsaicin has been proven effective in relieving the pain associated with diabetic neuropathy[190], chronic low back pain[191], chronic neck pain[192], osteoarthritis[193], and **rheumatoid arthritis.**[194] Given the important role of neurogenic inflammation in chronic arthritis[195,196], **the use of topical *Capsicum* should not be viewed as merely symptomatic; by depleting neurons of substance P it may have the ability to help break the vicious cycle of neurogenic-immunogenic inflammation.**

- Phytonutritional modulation of NF-kappaB: As a stimulator of pro-inflammatory gene transcription, NF-kappaB is almost universally activated in conditions associated with inflammation.[197,198] As we would expect, **NF-kappaB plays a central role in the pathogenesis of synovitis and joint destruction seen in RA.**[199] Nutrients and botanicals which either directly or indirectly inhibit NF-kappaB for an anti-inflammatory benefit include vitamin D[200,201], curcumin[202] (requires piperine for

[185] Wildfeuer A, Neu IS, Safayhi H, Metzger G, Wehrmann M, Vogel U, Ammon HP. Effects of boswellic acids extracted from a herbal medicine on the biosynthesis of leukotrienes and the course of experimental autoimmune encephalomyelitis. *Arzneimittelforschung* 1998 Jun;48(6):668-74

[186] Kimmatkar N, Thawani V, Hingorani L, Khiyani R. Efficacy and tolerability of Boswellia serrata extract in treatment of osteoarthritis of knee--a randomized double blind placebo controlled trial. *Phytomedicine.* 2003 Jan;10(1):3-7

[187] Gupta I, Gupta V, Parihar A, Gupta S, Ludtke R, Safayhi H, Ammon HP. Effects of Boswellia serrata gum resin in patients with bronchial asthma: results of a double-blind, placebo-controlled, 6-week clinical study. *Eur J Med Res.* 1998 Nov 17;3(11):511-4

[188] Gupta I, Parihar A, Malhotra P, Singh GB, Ludtke R, Safayhi H, Ammon HP. Effects of Boswellia serrata gum resin in patients with ulcerative colitis. *Eur J Med Res.* 1997 Jan;2(1):37-43

[189] Sander O, Herborn G, Rau R. [Is H15 (resin extract of Boswellia serrata, "incense") a useful supplement to established drug therapy of chronic polyarthritis? Results of a double-blind pilot study] [Article in German] *Z Rheumatol.* 1998 Feb;57(1):11-6

[190] Treatment of painful diabetic neuropathy with topical capsaicin. A multicenter, double-blind, vehicle-controlled study. The Capsaicin Study Group. [No authors listed] *Arch Intern Med.* 1991 Nov;151(11):2225-9

[191] Keitel W, Frerick H, Kuhn U, Schmidt U, Kuhlmann M, Bredehorst A. Capsicum pain plaster in chronic non-specific low back pain. *Arzneimittelforschung.* 2001 Nov;51(11):896-903

[192] Mathias BJ, Dillingham TR, Zeigler DN, Chang AS, Belandres PV. Topical capsaicin for chronic neck pain. A pilot study. *Am J Phys Med Rehabil* 1995 Jan-Feb;74(1):39-44

[193] McCarthy GM, McCarty DJ. Effect of topical capsaicin in the therapy of painful osteoarthritis of the hands. *J Rheumatol.* 1992;19(4):604-7

[194] Deal CL, Schnitzer TJ, Lipstein E, Seibold JR, Stevens RM, Levy MD, Albert D, Renold F. Treatment of arthritis with topical capsaicin: a double-blind trial. *Clin Ther.* 1991 May-Jun;13(3):383-95

[195] Gouze-Decaris E, Philippe L, Minn A, Haouzi P, Gillet P, Netter P, Terlain B. Neurophysiological basis for neurogenic-mediated articular cartilage anabolism alteration. *Am J Physiol Regul Integr Comp Physiol.* 2001;280(1):R115-22 http://ajpregu.physiology.org/cgi/content/full/280/1/R115

[196] Decaris E, Guingamp C, Chat M, Philippe L, Grillasca JP, Abid A, Minn A, Gillet P, Netter P, Terlain B. Evidence for neurogenic transmission inducing degenerative cartilage damage distant from local inflammation. *Arthritis Rheum.* 1999;42(9):1951-60

[197] Tak PP, Firestein GS. NF-kappaB: a key role in inflammatory diseases. *J Clin Invest.* 2001 Jan;107(1):7-11 http://www.jci.org/cgi/content/full/107/1/7

[198] D'Acquisto F, May MJ, Ghosh S. Inhibition of Nuclear Factor KappaB (NF-B): An Emerging Theme in Anti-Inflammatory Therapies. *Mol Interv.* 2002 Feb;2(1):22-35 http://molinterv.aspetjournals.org/cgi/content/abstract/2/1/22

[199] "NF-B plays a central role in the pathogenesis of synovitis in RA and PsA." Foell D, Kane D, Bresnihan B, Vogl T, Nacken W, Sorg C, Fitzgerald O, Roth J. Expression of the pro-inflammatory protein S100A12 (EN-RAGE) in rheumatoid and psoriatic arthritis. *Rheumatology* (Oxford). 2003 Nov;42(11):1383-9 http://rheumatology.oxfordjournals.org/cgi/content/full/42/11/1383

[200] "1Alpha,25-dihydroxyvitamin D3 (1,25-(OH)2-D3), the active metabolite of vitamin D, can inhibit NF-kappaB activity in human MRC-5 fibroblasts, targeting DNA binding of NF-kappaB but not translocation of its subunits p50 and p65." Harant H, Wolff B, Lindley IJ. 1Alpha,25-dihydroxyvitamin D3 decreases DNA binding of nuclear factor-kappaB in human fibroblasts. *FEBS Lett.* 1998 Oct 9;436(3):329-34

[201] "Thus, 1,25(OH)2D3 may negatively regulate IL-12 production by downregulation of NF-kB activation and binding to the p40-kB sequence." D'Ambrosio D, Cippitelli M, Cocciolo MG, Mazzeo D, Di Lucia P, Lang R, Sinigaglia F, Panina-Bordignon P. Inhibition of IL-12 production by 1,25-dihydroxyvitamin D3. Involvement of NF-kappaB downregulation in transcriptional repression of the p40 gene. *J Clin Invest.* 1998 Jan 1;101(1):252-62

[202] "Curcumin, EGCG and resveratrol have been shown to suppress activation of NF-kappa B." Surh YJ, Chun KS, Cha HH, Han SS, Keum YS, Park KK, Lee SS. Molecular mechanisms underlying chemopreventive activities of anti-inflammatory phytochemicals: down-regulation of COX-2 and iNOS through suppression of NF-kappa B activation. *Mutat Res.* 2001 Sep 1;480-481:243-68

absorption[203]), lipoic acid[204], green tea[205], rosemary[206], grape seed extract[207], propolis[208], zinc[209], high-dose selenium[210], indole-3-carbinol[211,212], N-acetyl-L-cysteine[213], resveratrol[214,215], isohumulones[216], GLA via PPAR-gamma[217] and EPA via PPAR-alpha.[218] I have reviewed the phytonutritional modulation of NF-kappaB later in this text and elsewhere.[219] Several phytonutritional products targeting NF-kappaB are available.

- ▪ <u>Glucosamine sulfate and chondroitin sulfate</u>: Glucosamine sulfate and chondroitin sulfate are well tolerated and well documented for effective treatment of osteoarthritis.[220,221,222,223] Since these serve as substrate for the "rebuilding" and preservation of joint cartilage, they help shift the balance toward anabolism and away from catabolism within articular tissues. Many studies (of which few exist specifically in the treatment of RA) have used less-effective forms of glucosamine (hydrochloride

[203] Shoba G, Joy D, Joseph T, Majeed M, Rajendran R, Srinivas PS. Influence of piperine on the pharmacokinetics of curcumin in animals and human volunteers. *Planta Med*. 1998 May;64(4):353-6

[204] "ALA reduced the TNF-alpha-stimulated ICAM-1 expression in a dose-dependent manner, to levels observed in unstimulated cells. Alpha-lipoic acid also reduced NF-kappaB activity in these cells in a dose-dependent manner." Lee HA, Hughes DA.Alpha-lipoic acid modulates NF-kappaB activity in human monocytic cells by direct interaction with DNA. *Exp Gerontol*. 2002 Jan-Mar;37(2-3):401-10

[205] "In conclusion, EGCG is an effective inhibitor of IKK activity. This may explain, at least in part, some of the reported anti-inflammatory and anticancer effects of green tea." Yang F, Oz HS, Barve S, de Villiers WJ, McClain CJ, Varilek GW. The green tea polyphenol (-)-epigallocatechin-3-gallate blocks nuclear factor-kappa B activation by inhibiting I kappa B kinase activity in the intestinal epithelial cell line IEC-6. *Mol Pharmacol*. 2001 Sep;60(3):528-33

[206] "These results suggest that carnosol suppresses the NO production and iNOS gene expression by inhibiting NF-kappaB activation, and provide possible mechanisms for its anti-inflammatory and chemopreventive action." Lo AH, Liang YC, Lin-Shiau SY, Ho CT, Lin JK. Carnosol, an antioxidant in rosemary, suppresses inducible nitric oxide synthase through down-regulating nuclear factor-kappaB in mouse macrophages. *Carcinogenesis*. 2002 Jun;23(6):983-91

[207] "Constitutive and TNFalpha-induced NF-kappaB DNA binding activity was inhibited by GSE at doses > or =50 microg/ml and treatments for > or =12 h." Dhanalakshmi S, Agarwal R, Agarwal C. Inhibition of NF-kappaB pathway in grape seed extract-induced apoptotic death of human prostate carcinoma DU145 cells. *Int J Oncol*. 2003 Sep;23(3):721-7

[208] "Caffeic acid phenethyl ester (CAPE) is an anti-inflammatory component of propolis (honeybee resin). CAPE is reportedly a specific inhibitor of nuclear factor-kappaB (NF-kappaB)." Fitzpatrick LR, Wang J, Le T. Caffeic acid phenethyl ester, an inhibitor of nuclear factor-kappaB, attenuates bacterial peptidoglycan polysaccharide-induced colitis in rats. *J Pharmacol Exp Ther*. 2001 Dec;299(3):915-20

[209] "Our results suggest that zinc supplementation may lead to downregulation of the inflammatory cytokines through upregulation of the negative feedback loop A20 to inhibit induced NF-kappaB activation." Prasad AS, Bao B, Beck FW, Kucuk O, Sarkar FH. Antioxidant effect of zinc in humans. *Free Radic Biol Med*. 2004 Oct 15;37(8):1182-90

[210] Note that the patients in this study received a very high dose of selenium: 960 micrograms per day. This is at the top—and some would say over the top—of the safe and reasonable dose for long-term supplementation. In this case, the study lasted for three months. "In patients receiving selenium supplementation, selenium NF-kappaB activity was significantly reduced, reaching the same level as the nondiabetic control group. CONCLUSION: In type 2 diabetic patients, activation of NF-kappaB measured in peripheral blood monocytes can be reduced by selenium supplementation, confirming its importance in the prevention of cardiovascular diseases." Faure P, Ramon O, Favier A, Halimi S. Selenium supplementation decreases nuclear factor-kappa B activity in peripheral blood mononuclear cells from type 2 diabetic patients. *Eur J Clin Invest*. 2004 Jul;34(7):475-81

[211] Takada Y, Andreeff M, Aggarwal BB. Indole-3-carbinol suppresses NF-{kappa}B and I{kappa}B{alpha} kinase activation causing inhibition of expression of NF-{kappa}B-regulated antiapoptotic and metastatic gene products and enhancement of apoptosis in myeloid and leukemia cells. *Blood*. 2005 Apr 5; [Epub ahead of print]

[212] "Overall, our results indicated that indole-3-carbinol inhibits NF-kappaB and NF-kappaB-regulated gene expression and that this mechanism may provide the molecular basis for its ability to suppress tumorigenesis." Takada Y, Andreeff M, Aggarwal BB. Indole-3-carbinol suppresses NF-kappaB and IkappaBalpha kinase activation, causing inhibition of expression of NF-kappaB-regulated antiapoptotic and metastatic gene products and enhancement of apoptosis in myeloid and leukemia cells. *Blood*. 2005 Jul 15;106(2):641-9. Epub 2005 Apr 5.

[213] "CONCLUSIONS: Administration of N-acetylcysteine results in decreased nuclear factor-kappa B activation in patients with sepsis, associated with decreases in interleukin-8 but not interleukin-6 or soluble intercellular adhesion molecule-1. These pilot data suggest that antioxidant therapy with N-acetylcysteine may be useful in blunting the inflammatory response to sepsis." Paterson RL, Galley HF, Webster NR. The effect of N-acetylcysteine on nuclear factor-kappa B activation, interleukin-6, interleukin-8, and intercellular adhesion molecule-1 expression in patients with sepsis. *Crit Care Med*. 2003 Nov;31(11):2574-8

[214] "Resveratrol's anticarcinogenic, anti-inflammatory, and growth-modulatory effects may thus be partially ascribed to the inhibition of activation of NF-kappaB and AP-1 and the associated kinases." Manna SK, Mukhopadhyay A, Aggarwal BB. Resveratrol suppresses TNF-induced activation of nuclear transcription factors NF-kappa B, activator protein-1, and apoptosis: potential role of reactive oxygen intermediates and lipid peroxidation. *J Immunol*. 2000 Jun 15;164(12):6509-19

[215] "Both resveratrol and quercetin inhibited NF-kappaB-, AP-1- and CREB-dependent transcription to a greater extent than the glucocorticosteroid, dexamethasone." Donnelly LE, Newton R, Kennedy GE, Fenwick PS, Leung RH, Ito K, Russell RE, Barnes PJ.Anti-inflammatory Effects of Resveratrol in Lung Epithelial Cells: Molecular Mechanisms. *Am J Physiol Lung Cell Mol Physiol*. 2004 Jun 4 [Epub ahead of print]

[216] Yajima H, Ikeshima E, Shiraki M, Kanaya T, Fujiwara D, Odai H, Tsuboyama-Kasaoka N, Ezaki O, Oikawa S, Kondo K. Isohumulones, bitter acids derived from hops, activate both peroxisome proliferator-activated receptor alpha and gamma and reduce insulin resistance. *J Biol Chem*. 2004 Aug 6;279(32):33456-62. Epub 2004 Jun 3. http://www.jbc.org/cgi/content/full/279/32/33456

[217] "Thus, PPAR gamma serves as the receptor for GLA in the regulation of gene expression in breast cancer cells. " Jiang WG, Redfern A, Bryce RP, Mansel RE. Peroxisome proliferator activated receptor-gamma (PPAR-gamma) mediates the action of gamma linolenic acid in breast cancer cells. *Prostaglandins Leukot Essent Fatty Acids*. 2000 Feb;62(2):119-27

[218] "...EPA requires PPARalpha for its inhibitory effects on NF-kappaB." Mishra A, Chaudhary A, Sethi S. Oxidized omega-3 fatty acids inhibit NF-kappaB activation via a PPARalpha-dependent pathway. *Arterioscler Thromb Vasc Biol*. 2004 Sep;24(9):1621-7. Epub 2004 Jul 1. http://atvb.ahajournals.org/cgi/content/full/24/9/1621

[219] "Indeed, the previous view that nutrients only interact with human physiology at the metabolic/post-transcriptional level must be updated in light of current research showing that nutrients can, in fact, modify human physiology and phenotype at the genetic/pre-transcriptional level." Vasquez A. Reducing pain and inflammation naturally - part 4: nutritional and botanical inhibition of NF-kappaB, the major intracellular amplifier of the inflammatory cascade. A practical clinical strategy exemplifying anti-inflammatory nutrigenomics. *Nutritional Perspectives*, July 2005:5-12 http://www.ichnfm.org/faculty/vasquez/profile.html

[220] Braham R, Dawson B, Goodman C. The effect of glucosamine supplementation on people experiencing regular knee pain. *Br J Sports Med*. 2003;37(1):45-9

[221] Nguyen P, Mohamed SE, Gardiner D, Salinas T. A randomized double-blind clinical trial of the effect of chondroitin sulfate and glucosamine hydrochloride on temporomandibular joint disorders: a pilot study. *Cranio*. 2001 Apr;19(2):130-9

[222] "...oral glucosamine therapy achieved a significantly greater improvement in articular pain score than ibuprofen, and the investigators rated treatment efficacy as 'good' in a significantly greater proportion of glucosamine than ibuprofen recipients. In comparison with piroxicam, glucosamine significantly improved arthritic symptoms after 12 weeks of therapy..." Matheson AJ, Perry CM. Glucosamine: a review of its use in the management of osteoarthritis. *Drugs Aging*. 2003; 20(14): 1041-60

[223] Muller-Fassbender H, Bach GL, Haase W, Rovati LC, Setnikar I. Glucosamine sulfate compared to ibuprofen in osteoarthritis of the knee. *Osteoarthritis Cartilage*. 1994 Mar;2(1):61-9

is less effective than sulfate) for insufficient durations (average 4-6 months, when the appropriate duration is 1-3 years) and have thus underestimated the clinical value of this treatment.

- **Endocrine imbalances, orthoendocrinology:** Assess prolactin, cortisol, DHEA, free and total testosterone, serum estradiol, and thyroid status (e.g., TSH, T4, *and* anti-thyroid peroxidase antibodies).

  - Prolactin (excess): **Patients with RA and SLE have higher basal and stress-induced levels of prolactin compared with normal controls.**[224,225] **Men with RA have higher serum levels of prolactin, and these levels correlate with the severity and duration of the disorder.**[226,227] Serum prolactin is the standard assessment of prolactin status. Since elevated prolactin may be a sign of pituitary tumor, assessment for headaches, visual deficits, and other abnormalities of pituitary hormones (e.g., GH and TSH) should be performed; CT or MRI must be considered. Patients with prolactin levels less than 100 ng/mL and normal CT/MRI findings can be managed conservatively with effective prolactin-lowering treatment and annual radiologic assessment (less necessary with favorable serum response).[228, see review 229] Specific treatment options include the following:

    - Thyroid hormone: Hypothyroidism frequently causes hyperprolactinemia which is reversible upon effective treatment of hypothyroidism. Obviously therefore, thyroid status should be evaluated in all patients with hyperprolactinemia. Thyroid assessment and treatment is reviewed in Chapter 4 and later in this section.

    - *Vitex astus-cagnus* and other supporting botanicals and nutrients: **Vitex lowers serum prolactin in humans**[230,231] **via a dopaminergic effect.**[232] Vitex is considered safe for clinical use; mild and reversible adverse effects possibly associated with Vitex include nausea, headache, gastrointestinal disturbances, menstrual disorders, acne, pruritus and erythematous rash. No drug interactions are known, but given the herb's dopaminergic effect it should probably be used with some caution in patients treated with dopamine antagonists such as the so-called antipsychotic drugs.[233,234] Bone[235] stated that daily doses can range from 500 mg to 2,000 mg DHE (dry herb equivalent) and can be tailored to the suppression of prolactin. Due at least in part to its content of L-dopa, *Mucuna pruriens* **shows clinical dopaminergic activity** as evidenced by its effectiveness in Parkinson's disease[236]; up to 15-30 gm/d of mucuna has been used

[224] Dostal C, Moszkorzova L, Musilova L, Lacinova Z, Marek J, Zvarova J. Serum prolactin stress values in patients with systemic lupus erythematosus. *Ann Rheum Dis.* 2003 May;62(5):487-8 http://ard.bmjjournals.com/cgi/content/full/62/5/487

[225] "RESULTS: A significantly higher rate of elevated PRL levels was found in SLE patients (40.0%) compared with the healthy controls (14.8%). No proof was found of association with the presence of anti-ds-DNA or with specific organ involvement. Similarly, elevated PRL levels were found in RA patients (39.3%)." Moszkorzova L, Lacinova Z, Marek J, Musilova L, Dohnalova A, Dostal C. Hyperprolactinaemia in patients with systemic lupus erythematosus. *Clin Exp Rheumatol.* 2002 Nov-Dec;20(6):807-12

[226] "CONCLUSION: Men with RA have high serum PRL levels and concentrations increase with longer disease evolution and worse functional stage." Mateo L, Nolla JM, Bonnin MR, Navarro MA, Roig-Escofet D. High serum prolactin levels in men with rheumatoid arthritis. *J Rheumatol.* 1998 Nov;25(11):2077-82

[227] "Male patients affected by RA showed high serum PRL levels. The serum PRL concentration was found to be increased in relation to the duration and the activity of the disease. Serum PRL levels do not seem to have any relationship with the BMD, at least in RA." Seriolo B, Ferretti V, Sulli A, Fasciolo D, Cutolo M. Serum prolactin concentrations in male patients with rheumatoid arthritis. *Ann N Y Acad Sci.* 2002 Jun;966:258-62

[228] Beers MH, Berkow R (eds). The Merck Manual. Seventeenth Edition. Whitehouse Station; Merck Research Laboratories 1999 Page 77-78

[229] Serri O, Chik CL, Ur E, Ezzat S. Diagnosis and management of hyperprolactinemia. *CMAJ.* 2003 Sep 16;169(6):575-81 http://www.cmaj.ca/cgi/content/full/169/6/575

[230] "Since AC extracts were shown to have beneficial effects on premenstrual mastodynia serum prolactin levels in such patients were also studied in one double-blind, placebo-controlled clinical study. Serum prolactin levels were indeed reduced in the patients treated with the extract." Wuttke W, Jarry H, Christoffel V, Spengler B, Seidlova-Wuttke D. Chaste tree (Vitex agnus-castus)--pharmacology and clinical indications. *Phytomedicine.* 2003 May;10(4):348-57

[231] German abstract from Medline: "The prolactin release was reduced after 3 months, shortened luteal phases were normalised and deficits in the luteal progesterone synthesis were eliminated." Milewicz A, Gejdel E, Sworen H, Sienkiewicz K, Jedrzejak J, Teucher T, Schmitz H. [Vitex agnus castus extract in the treatment of luteal phase defects due to latent hyperprolactinemia. Results of a randomized placebo-controlled double-blind study] *Arzneimittelforschung.* 1993 Jul;43(7):752-6

[232] "Our results indicate a dopaminergic effect of Vitex agnus-castus extracts and suggest additional pharmacological actions via opioid receptors." Meier B, Berger D, Hoberg E, Sticher O, Schaffner W. Pharmacological activities of Vitex agnus-castus extracts in vitro. *Phytomedicine.* 2000 Oct;7(5):373-81

[233] "The majority of patients in each group discontinued their assigned treatment owing to inefficacy or intolerable side effects or for other reasons." Lieberman JA, Stroup TS, McEvoy JP, Swartz MS, Rosenheck RA, Perkins DO, Keefe RS, Davis SM, Davis CE, Lebowitz BD, Severe J, Hsiao JK; Clinical Antipsychotic Trials of Intervention Effectiveness (CATIE) Investigators. Effectiveness of antipsychotic drugs in patients with chronic schizophrenia. *N Engl J Med.* 2005 Sep 22;353(12):1209-23

[234] Whitaker R. The case against antipsychotic drugs: a 50-year record of doing more harm than good. *Med Hypotheses.* 2004;62(1):5-13

[235] "In conditions such as endometriosis and fibroids, for which a significant estrogen antagonist effect is needed, doses of at least 2 g/day DHE may be required and typically are used by professional herbalists." Bone K. New Insights Into Chaste Tree. *Nutritional Wellness* 2005 November http://www.nutritionalwellness.com/archives/2005/nov/11_bone.php

[236] "CONCLUSIONS: The rapid onset of action and longer on time without concomitant increase in dyskinesias on mucuna seed powder formulation suggest that this natural source of L-dopa might possess advantages over conventional L-dopa preparations in the long term management of PD." Katzenschlager R, Evans A, Manson A, Patsalos PN, Ratnaraj N, Watt H, Timmermann L, Van der Giessen R, Lees AJ. Mucuna pruriens in Parkinson's disease: a double blind clinical and pharmacological study. *J Neurol Neurosurg Psychiatry.* 2004 Dec;75(12):1672-7

clinically but doses will be dependent on preparation and phytoconcentration. **Triptolide and other extracts from *Tripterygium wilfordii* Hook F exert clinically significant anti-inflammatory action in patients with rheumatoid arthritis**[237,238] **and also offer protection to dopaminergic neurons.**[239,240] Ironically, even though tyrosine is the nutritional precursor to dopamine with evidence of clinical effectiveness (e.g., narcolepsy[241], enhancement of memory[242] and cognition[243]), **supplementation with tyrosine appears to actually increase rather than decrease prolactin levels**[244]**; therefore tyrosine should be used cautiously (if at all) in patients with systemic inflammation and elevated prolactin.** Furthermore, the finding that **high-protein meals stimulate prolactin release**[245] may partly explain the benefits of vegetarian diets in the treatment of systemic inflammation; since vegetarian diets are comparatively low in protein compared to omnivorous diets, they may lead to a relative reduction in prolactin production due to lack of protein-induced prolactin stimulation.

- <u>Bromocriptine</u>: Bromocriptine has long been considered the pharmacologic treatment of choice for elevated prolactin.[246] Typical dose is 2.5 mg per day (effective against lupus[247]); gastrointestinal upset and sedation are common.[248] Clinical intervention with bromocriptine appears warranted in patients with RA, SLE, reactive arthritis, psoriatic arthritis, and probably multiple sclerosis and uveitis.[249]

- <u>Cabergoline/Dostinex</u>: Cabergoline/Dostinex is a newer dopamine agonist with few adverse effects; typical dose starts at 0.5 mg per week (0.25 mg twice per week).[250] Several studies have indicated that cabergoline is safer and more effective than bromocriptine for reducing prolactin levels[251] and the dose can often be reduced after successful prolactin reduction, allowing for reductions in cost and adverse effects.[252]

[237] "The ethanol/ethyl acetate extract of TWHF shows therapeutic benefit in patients with treatment-refractory RA. At therapeutic dosages, the TWHF extract was well tolerated by most patients in this study." Tao X, Younger J, Fan FZ, Wang B, Lipsky PE. Benefit of an extract of Tripterygium Wilfordii Hook F in patients with rheumatoid arthritis: a double-blind, placebo-controlled study. *Arthritis Rheum*. 2002 Jul;46(7):1735-43

[238] "CONCLUSION: The EA extract of TWHF at dosages up to 570 mg/day appeared to be safe, and doses > 360 mg/day were associated with clinical benefit in patients with RA." Tao X, Cush JJ, Garret M, Lipsky PE. A phase I study of ethyl acetate extract of the chinese antirheumatic herb Tripterygium wilfordii hook F in rheumatoid arthritis. *J Rheumatol*. 2001 Oct;28(10):2160-7

[239] "Our data suggests that triptolide may protect dopaminergic neurons from LPS-induced injury and its efficiency in inhibiting microglia activation may underlie the mechanism." Li FQ, Lu XZ, Liang XB, Zhou HF, Xue B, Liu XY, Niu DB, Han JS, Wang XM. Triptolide, a Chinese herbal extract, protects dopaminergic neurons from inflammation-mediated damage through inhibition of microglial activation. *J Neuroimmunol*. 2004 Mar;148(1-2):24-31

[240] "Moreover, tripchlorolide markedly prevented the decrease in amount of dopamine in the striatum of model rats. Taken together, our data provide the first evidence that tripchlorolide acts as a neuroprotective molecule that rescues MPP+ or axotomy-induced degeneration of dopaminergic neurons, which may imply its therapeutic potential for Parkinson's disease." Li FQ, Cheng XX, Liang XB, Wang XH, Xue B, He QH, Wang XM, Han JS. Neurotrophic and neuroprotective effects of tripchlorolide, an extract of Chinese herb Tripterygium wilfordii Hook F, on dopaminergic neurons. *Exp Neurol*. 2003 Jan;179(1):28-37

[241] "Of twenty-eight visual analogue scales rating mood and arousal, the subjects' ratings in the tyrosine treatment (9 g daily) and placebo periods differed significantly for only three (less tired, less drowsy, more alert)." Elwes RD, Crewes H, Chesterman LP, Summers B, Jenner P, Binnie CD, Parkes JD. Treatment of narcolepsy with L-tyrosine: double-blind placebo-controlled trial. *Lancet*. 1989 Nov 4;2(8671):1067-9

[242] "Ten men and 10 women subjects underwent these batteries 1 h after ingesting 150 mg/kg of l-tyrosine or placebo. Administration of tyrosine significantly enhanced accuracy and decreased frequency of list retrieval on the working memory task during the multiple task battery compared with placebo." Thomas JR, Lockwood PA, Singh A, Deuster PA. Tyrosine improves working memory in a multitasking environment. *Pharmacol Biochem Behav*. 1999 Nov;64(3):495-500

[243] "Ten subjects received five daily doses of a protein-rich drink containing 2 g tyrosine, and 11 subjects received a carbohydrate rich drink with the same amount of calories (255 kcal)." Deijen JB, Wientjes CJ, Vullinghs HF, Cloin PA, Langefeld JJ. Tyrosine improves cognitive performance and reduces blood pressure in cadets after one week of a combat training course. *Brain Res Bull*. 1999 Jan 15;48(2):203-9

[244] "Tyrosine (when compared to placebo) had no effect on any sleep related measure, but it did stimulate prolactin release." Waters WF, Magill RA, Bray GA, Volaufova J, Smith SR, Lieberman HR, Rood J, Hurry M, Anderson T, Ryan DH. A comparison of tyrosine against placebo, phentermine, caffeine, and D-amphetamine during sleep deprivation. *Nutr Neurosci*. 2003;6(4):221-35

[245] "Whereas carbohydrate meals had no discernible effects, high protein meals induced a large increase in both PRL and cortisol; high fat meals caused selective release of PRL." Ishizuka B, Quigley ME, Yen SS. Pituitary hormone release in response to food ingestion: evidence for neuroendocrine signals from gut to brain. *J Clin Endocrinol Metab*. 1983 Dec;57(6):1111-6

[246] Beers MH, Berkow R (eds). <u>The Merck Manual. Seventeenth Edition</u>. Whitehouse Station; Merck Research Laboratories 1999 Page 77-78

[247] "A prospective, double-blind, randomized, placebo-controlled study compared BRC at a fixed daily dosage of 2.5 mg with placebo... Long term treatment with a low dose of BRC appears to be a safe and effective means of decreasing SLE flares in SLE patients." Alvarez-Nemegyei J, Cobarrubias-Cobos A, Escalante-Triay F, Sosa-Munoz J, Miranda JM, Jara LJ. Bromocriptine in systemic lupus erythematosus: a double-blind, randomized, placebo-controlled study. *Lupus*. 1998;7(6):414-9

[248] Serri O, Chik CL, Ur E, Ezzat S. Diagnosis and management of hyperprolactinemia. *CMAJ*. 2003 Sep 16;169(6):575-81 http://www.cmaj.ca/cgi/content/full/169/6/575

[249] "...clinical observations and trials support the use of bromocriptine as a nonstandard primary or adjunctive therapy in the treatment of recalcitrant RA, SLE, Reiter's syndrome, and psoriatic arthritis and associated conditions unresponsive to traditional approaches." McMurray RW. Bromocriptine in rheumatic and autoimmune diseases. *Semin Arthritis Rheum*. 2001 Aug;31(1):21-32

[250] Serri O, Chik CL, Ur E, Ezzat S. Diagnosis and management of hyperprolactinemia. *CMAJ*. 2003 Sep 16;169(6):575-81 http://www.cmaj.ca/cgi/content/full/169/6/575

[251] "CONCLUSION: These data indicate that cabergoline is a very effective agent for lowering the prolactin levels in hyperprolactinemic patients and that it appears to offer considerable advantage over bromocriptine in terms of efficacy and tolerability." Sabuncu T, Arikan E, Tasan E, Hatemi H. Comparison of the effects of cabergoline and bromocriptine on prolactin levels in hyperprolactinemic patients. *Intern Med*. 2001 Sep;40(9):857-61

[252] "Cabergoline also normalized PRL in the majority of patients with known bromocriptine intolerance or -resistance. Once PRL secretion was adequately controlled, the dose of cabergoline could often be significantly decreased, which further reduced costs of therapy." Verhelst J, Abs R, Maiter D, van den Bruel A, Vandeweghe M,

Although fewer studies have been published supporting the antirheumatic benefits of cabergoline than bromocriptine, its antirheumatic benefits have been documented in a case report of a patient with unremitting RA.[253]

o Estrogen (excess): **Men with rheumatoid arthritis show an excess of estradiol** and a decrease in DHEA, and the **excess estrogen is proportional to the degree of inflammation**.[254] Serum estradiol is commonly used to assess estrogen status; estrogens can also be measured in 24-hour urine samples. Beyond looking at estrogens from a *quantitative* standpoint, they can also be *qualitatively* analyzed with respect to the ratio of estrone:estradiol:estriol as well as the balance between the "good" 2-hydroxyestrone relative to the purportedly carcinogenic and proinflammatory 16-alpha-hydroxyestrone. Interventions to combat high estrogen levels may include any effective combination of the following:

- Weight loss and weight optimization: In overweight patients, *weight loss* is the means to attaining the goal of *weight optimization*; the task is not complete until the body mass index is normalized/optimized. Excess adiposity and obesity raise estrogen levels due to high levels of aromatase (the hormone that makes estrogens from androgens) in adipose tissue; weight optimization and loss of excess fat helps normalize hormone levels and reduce inflammation.

- Avoidance of ethanol: Estrogen production is stimulated by ethanol intake.

- Consider surgical correction of varicocele in affected men: Men with varicocele have higher estrogen levels due to temperature-induced alterations in enzyme function in the testes; surgical correction of the varicocele lowers estrogen levels.

- "Anti-estrogen diet": Foods and supplements such as green tea, diindolylmethane (DIM), indole-3-carbinol (I3C), licorice, and a high-fiber crucifer-based "anti-estrogenic diet" can also be used; monitoring clinical status and serum estradiol will prove or disprove efficacy. Whereas 16-alpha-hydroxyestrone is pro-inflammatory and immunodysregulatory, 2-hydroxyestrone has anti-inflammatory action[255] and been described as "the good estrogen"[256] due to its anticancer and comparatively health-preserving qualities. **In a recent short-term study using I3C in patients with SLE, I3C supplementation at 375 mg per day was well tolerated and resulted in modest treatment-dependent clinical improvement as well as favorable modification of estrogen metabolism away from 16-alpha-hydroxyestrone and toward 2-hydroxyestrone.**[257]

- Pharmacologic aromatase inhibition: In our office, we commonly measure serum estradiol in men and administer the aromatase inhibitor anastrozole/Arimidex 1 mg (≥2-3 doses per week) to men whose estradiol level is greater than 32 picogram/mL. The Life Extension Foundation[258] advocates that the optimal serum estradiol level for a man is 10-30 picogram/mL. Clinical studies using anastrozole/Arimidex in men

Velkeniers B, Mockel J, Lamberigts G, Petrossians P, Coremans P, Mahler C, Stevenaert A, Verlooy J, Raftopoulos C, Beckers A. Cabergoline in the treatment of hyperprolactinemia: a study in 455 patients. *J Clin Endocrinol Metab*. 1999 Jul;84(7):2518-22 http://jcem.endojournals.org/cgi/content/full/84/7/2518

[253] Erb N, Pace AV, Delamere JP, Kitas GD. Control of unremitting rheumatoid arthritis by the prolactin antagonist cabergoline. *Rheumatology* (Oxford). 2001 Feb;40(2):237-9 http://rheumatology.oxfordjournals.org/cgi/content/full/40/2/237

[254] "RESULTS: DHEAS and estrone concentrations were lower and estradiol was higher in patients compared with healthy controls. DHEAS differed between RF positive and RF negative patients. Estrone did not correlate with any disease variable, whereas estradiol correlated strongly and positively with all measured indices of inflammation." Tengstrand B, Carlstrom K, Fellander-Tsai L, Hafstrom I. Abnormal levels of serum dehydroepiandrosterone, estrone, and estradiol in men with rheumatoid arthritis: high correlation between serum estradiol and current degree of inflammation. *J Rheumatol*. 2003 Nov;30(11):2338-43

[255] "Micromolar concentrations of beta-estradiol, estrone, 16-alpha-hydroxyestrone and estriol enhance the oxidative metabolism of activated human PMNL's. The corresponding 2-hydroxylated estrogens 2-OH-estradiol, 2-OH-estrone and 2-OH-estriol act on the contrary as powerful inhibitors of cell activity." Jansson G. Oestrogen-induced enhancement of myeloperoxidase activity in human polymorphonuclear leukocytes--a possible cause of oxidative stress in inflammatory cells. *Free Radic Res Commun*. 1991;14(3):195-208

[256] "Even more dramatically, in the case of laryngeal papillomas induction of 2-hydroxylation with indole-3-carbinol (I3C) has resulted in inhibition of tumor growth during the time that the patients continue to take I3C or vegetables rich in this compound." Bradlow HL, Telang NT, Sepkovic DW, Osborne MP. 2-hydroxyestrone: the 'good' estrogen. *J Endocrinol*. 1996 Sep;150 Suppl:S259-65

[257] "Women with SLE can manifest a metabolic response to I3C and might benefit from its antiestrogenic effects." McAlindon TE, Gulin J, Chen T, Klug T, Lahita R, Nuite M. Indole-3-carbinol in women with SLE: effect on estrogen metabolism and disease activity. *Lupus*. 2001;10(11):779-83

[258] Male Hormone Modulation Therapy, Page 4 Of 7: http://www.lef.org/protocols/prtcl-130c.shtml Accessed October 30, 2005

have shown that aromatase blockade lowers estradiol and raises testosterone[259]; generally speaking, this is exactly the result that we want in patients with severe systemic autoimmunity. When using anastrozole/Arimidex, frequency of dosing is based on serum and clinical response. On occasion, we have seen some men make so much testosterone→estradiol that they require anastrozole/Arimidex along with licorice daily in order to control their testosterone and estradiol levels. Licorice lowers testosterone and thus the precursor to estradiol in both men and women within about four days of oral administration, whether by standardized capsules or by tea from cut and sifted root. Letrozole/Femara is an effective aromatase inhibitor; however, it also appears to antagonize androgen receptors and should therefore generally be avoided.

- o <u>Cortisol (insufficiency)</u>: Cortisol has immunoregulatory and "immunosuppressive" actions at physiological concentrations. Low adrenal function is common in patients with chronic inflammation.[260,261,262] Assessment of cortisol production and adrenal function was detailed in Chapter 4 under the section of *Orthoendocrinology*. Supplementation with 20 mg per day of cortisol/Cortef is physiologic; this author's preference is to dose 10 mg immediately in the morning, then 5 mg in late morning and 5 mg in midafternoon in an attempt to replicate the diurnal variation and normal morning peak of cortisol levels. In patients with documented hypoadrenalism, administration of pregnenolone in doses of 10-60 mg in the morning may also be beneficial.

- o <u>Testosterone (insufficiency)</u>: Androgen deficiencies predispose to, are exacerbated by, and contribute to autoimmune/inflammatory disorders. **A large proportion of men with SLE or RA have low testosterone**[263,264] and suffer the effects of hypogonadism: fatigue, weakness, depression, slow healing, low libido, and difficulties with sexual performance. Testosterone levels may rise following DHEA supplementation (especially in women) and can be elevated in men by the use of anastrozole/Arimidex. Otherwise, transdermal testosterone such as Androgel, Testim, or custom-compounded formula can be applied as indicated.

- o <u>DHEA (insufficiency / supraphysiologic supplementation)</u>: DHEA is an anti-inflammatory and immunoregulatory hormone that is commonly deficient in patients with autoimmunity and inflammatory arthritis.[265] DHEA levels are suppressed by prednisone[266], and DHEA supplementation has been shown to reverse the osteoporosis and loss of bone mass induced by corticosteroid treatment.[267] DHEA shows no acute or subacute toxicity even when used in supraphysiologic doses, even when used in sick patients. For example, in a study of 32 patients with HIV, DHEA doses of 750 mg – 2,250 mg per day were well-tolerated and

[259] "These data demonstrate that aromatase inhibition increases serum bioavailable and total testosterone levels to the youthful normal range in older men with mild hypogonadism." Leder BZ, Rohrer JL, Rubin SD, Gallo J, Longcope C. Effects of aromatase inhibition in elderly men with low or borderline-low serum testosterone levels. *J Clin Endocrinol Metab*. 2004 Mar;89(3):1174-80 http://jcem.endojournals.org/cgi/reprint/89/3/1174

[260] "Yet evidence that patients with rheumatoid arthritis improved with small, physiologic dosages of cortisol or cortisone acetate was reported over 25 years ago, and that patients with chronic allergic disorders or unexplained chronic fatigue also improved with administration of such small dosages was reported over 15 years ago..." Jefferies WM. Mild adrenocortical deficiency, chronic allergies, autoimmune disorders and the chronic fatigue syndrome: a continuation of the cortisone story. *Med Hypotheses*. 1994 Mar;42(3):183-9 http://www.thebuteykocentre.com/Irish_%20Buteykocenter_files/further_studies/med_hyp2.pdf http://members.westnet.com.au/pkolb/med_hyp2.pdf

[261] "The etiology of rheumatoid arthritis ...explained by a combination of three factors: (i) a relatively mild deficiency of cortisol, ..., (ii) a deficiency of DHEA, ...and (iii) infection by organisms such as mycoplasma,..." Jefferies WM. The etiology of rheumatoid arthritis. *Med Hypotheses*. 1998 Aug;51(2):111-4

[262] Jefferies W McK. <u>Safe Uses of Cortisol. Second Edition</u>. Springfield, CC Thomas, 1996

[263] Karagiannis A, Harsoulis F. Gonadal dysfunction in systemic diseases. *Eur J Endocrinol*. 2005 Apr;152(4):501-13 http://www.eje-online.org/cgi/content/full/152/4/501

[264] "Using analysis of covariance, patients with rheumatoid arthritis showed significantly lower serum testosterone (p less than 0.05) and derived free testosterone (p less than 0.01) concentrations and significantly higher serum LH and FSH concentrations (p less than 0.05) compared with controls." Gordon D, Beastall GH, Thomson JA, Sturrock RD. Androgenic status and sexual function in males with rheumatoid arthritis and ankylosing spondylitis. *Q J Med*. 1986 Jul;60(231):671-9

[265] "DHEAS concentrations were significantly decreased in both women and men with inflammatory arthritis (IA) (P < 0.001)." Dessein PH, Joffe BI, Stanwix AE, Moomal Z. Hyposecretion of the adrenal androgen dehydroepiandrosterone sulfate and its relation to clinical variables in inflammatory arthritis. *Arthritis Res*. 2001;3(3):183-8. Epub 2001 Feb 21. http://arthritis-research.com/content/3/3/183

[266] "Basal serum DHEA and DHEAS concentrations were suppressed to a greater degree than was cortisol during both daily and alternate day prednisone treatments. ...Thus, adrenal androgen secretion was more easily suppressed than was cortisol secretion by this low dose of glucocorticoid, but there was no advantage to alternate day therapy." Rittmaster RS, Givner ML. Effect of daily and alternate day low dose prednisone on serum cortisol and adrenal androgens in hirsute women. *J Clin Endocrinol Metab*. 1988 Aug;67(2):400-3

[267] "CONCLUSION: Prasterone treatment prevented BMD loss and significantly increased BMD at both the lumbar spine and total hip in female patients with SLE receiving exogenous glucocorticoids." Mease PJ, Ginzler EM, Gluck OS, Schiff M, Goldman A, Greenwald M, Cohen S, Egan R, Quarles BJ, Schwartz KE. Effects of prasterone on bone mineral density in women with systemic lupus erythematosus receiving chronic glucocorticoid therapy. *J Rheumatol*. 2005 Apr;32(4):616-21

produced no dose-limiting adverse effects.[268] This lack of toxicity compares favorably with any and all so-called "antirheumatic" drugs, nearly all of which show impressive comparable toxicity. **When used at doses of 200 mg per day, DHEA safely provides clinical benefit for patients with various autoimmune diseases, including ulcerative colitis, Crohn's disease[269], and SLE.**[270] In patients with SLE, DHEA supplementation allows for reduced dosing of prednisone (thus avoiding its adverse effects) while providing symptomatic improvement.[271] Optimal clinical response appears to correlate with serum levels that are supraphysiologic[272], and therefore treatment may be implemented with little regard for initial/baseline DHEA levels provided that the patient is free of contraindications, particularly high risk for sex-hormone-dependent malignancy. Other than mild adverse effects predictable with any androgen (namely voice deepening, transient acne, and increased facial hair), DHEA supplementation does not cause serious adverse effects[273], and it is appropriate for routine clinical use particularly when 1) the dose of DHEA is kept as low as possible, 2) duration is kept as short as possible, 3) other interventions are used to address the underlying cause of the disease, 4) the patient is deriving benefit, and 5) the risk-to-benefit ratio is favorable. Astute clinicians should anticipate that DHEA supplementation can increase testosterone and estradiol levels—the former with benefit and the latter with detriment in patients with autoimmunity; thus, serum levels of DHEA, testosterone, and estradiol (and potentially other estrogen metabolites) need to be reevaluated if DHEA is added to the daily regimen. Commonly, rheumatic patients will show an increase in estradiol following use of DHEA, and these over-producers of estrogen ("rapid converters") should be co-treated with an aromatase inhibitor if DHEA supplementation elevates estrogen levels, especially if testosterone levels are low.

- o Thyroid (insufficiency or autoimmunity): Overt or imminent hypothyroidism is suggested by TSH greater than 2 mU/L[274] or 3 mU/L[275], low T4 or T3, and/or the presence of anti-thyroid peroxidase antibodies.[276] Hypothyroidism can cause an inflammatory myopathy that can resemble polymyositis, and hypothyroidism is a frequent complication of any and all autoimmune diseases. Specific treatment considerations include the following:
  - Selenium: Supplementation with either selenomethonine[277] or sodium selenite[278,279] can reduce thyroid autoimmunity and improve peripheral conversion of T4 to T3.

---

[268] "Thirty-one subjects were evaluated and monitored for safety and tolerance. The oral drug was administered three times daily in doses ranging from 750 mg/day to 2,250 mg/day for 16 weeks. ... The drug was well tolerated and no dose-limiting side effects were noted." Dyner TS, Lang W, Geaga J, Golub A, Stites D, Winger E, Galmarini M, Masterson J, Jacobson MA. An open-label dose-escalation trial of oral dehydroepiandrosterone tolerance and pharmacokinetics in patients with HIV disease. *J Acquir Immune Defic Syndr.* 1993 May;6(5):459-65

[269] "CONCLUSIONS: In a pilot study, dehydroepiandrosterone was effective and safe in patients with refractory Crohn's disease or ulcerative colitis." Andus T, Klebl F, Rogler G, Bregenzer N, Scholmerich J, Straub RH. Patients with refractory Crohn's disease or ulcerative colitis respond to dehydroepiandrosterone: a pilot study. *Aliment Pharmacol Ther.* 2003 Feb;17(3):409-14

[270] "CONCLUSION: The overall results confirm that DHEA treatment was well-tolerated, significantly reduced the number of SLE flares, and improved patient's global assessment of disease activity." Chang DM, Lan JL, Lin HY, Luo SF. Dehydroepiandrosterone treatment of women with mild-to-moderate systemic lupus erythematosus: a multicenter randomized, double-blind, placebo-controlled trial. *Arthritis Rheum.* 2002 Nov;46(11):2924-7

[271] "CONCLUSION: Among women with lupus disease activity, reducing the dosage of prednisone to < or = 7.5 mg/day for a sustained period of time while maintaining stabilization or a reduction of disease activity was possible in a significantly greater proportion of patients treated with oral prasterone, 200 mg once daily, compared with patients treated with placebo." Petri MA, Lahita RG, Van Vollenhoven RF, Merrill JT, Schiff M, Ginzler EM, Strand V, Kunz A, Gorelick KJ, Schwartz KE; GL601 Study Group. Effects of prasterone on corticosteroid requirements of women with systemic lupus erythematosus: a double-blind, randomized, placebo-controlled trial. *Arthritis Rheum.* 2002 Jul;46(7):1820-9

[272] "CONCLUSION: The clinical response to DHEA was not clearly dose dependent. Serum levels of DHEA and DHEAS correlated only weakly with lupus outcomes, but suggested an optimum serum DHEAS of 1000 microg/dl." Barry NN, McGuire JL, van Vollenhoven RF. Dehydroepiandrosterone in systemic lupus erythematosus: relationship between dosage, serum levels, and clinical response. *J Rheumatol.* 1998 Dec;25(12):2352-6

[273] Tierney ML. McPhee SJ, Papadakis MA. Current Medical Diagnosis and Treatment 2006. 45th edition. New York; Lange Medical Books: 2006, page 1721

[274] Weetman AP. Hypothyroidism: screening and subclinical disease. *BMJ.* 1997 Apr 19;314(7088):1175-8 http://bmj.bmjjournals.com/cgi/content/full/314/7088/1175

[275] "Now AACE encourages doctors to consider treatment for patients who test outside the boundaries of a narrower margin based on a target TSH level of 0.3 to 3.0. AACE believes the new range will result in proper diagnosis for millions of Americans who suffer from a mild thyroid disorder, but have gone untreated until now." American Association of Clinical Endocrinologists (AACE). 2003 Campaign Encourages Awareness of Mild Thyroid Failure, Importance of Routine Testing http://www.aace.com/pub/tam2003/press.php November 26, 2005

[276] Beers MH, Berkow R (eds). The Merck Manual. Seventeenth Edition. Whitehouse Station; Merck Research Laboratories 1999 Page 96

[277] Duntas LH, Mantzou E, Koutras DA. Effects of a six month treatment with selenomethionine in patients with autoimmune thyroiditis. *Eur J Endocrinol.* 2003 Apr;148(4):389-93 http://eje-online.org/cgi/reprint/148/4/389

[278] Gartner R, Gasnier BC, Dietrich JW, Krebs B, Angstwurm MW. Selenium supplementation in patients with autoimmune thyroiditis decreases thyroid peroxidase antibodies concentrations. *J Clin Endocrinol Metab.* 2002 Apr;87(4):1687-91 http://jcem.endojournals.org/cgi/content/full/87/4/1687

[279] "We recently conducted a prospective, placebo-controlled clinical study, where we could demonstrate, that a substitution of 200 wg sodium selenite for three months in patients with autoimmune thyroiditis reduced thyroid peroxidase antibody (TPO-Ab) concentrations significantly." Gartner R, Gasnier BC. Selenium in the treatment of autoimmune thyroiditis. *Biofactors.* 2003;19(3-4):165-70

Selenium may be started at 500-800 mcg per day and tapered to 200-400 mcg per day for maintenance.[280]

- L-thyroxine/levothyroxine/Synthroid—prescription synthetic T4: 25-50 mcg per day is a common starting dose which can be adjusted based on clinical and laboratory response. Thyroid hormone supplements must be consumed separately from soy products (by at least 1-2 hours) and preferably on an empty stomach to avoid absorption interference by food, fiber, and minerals, especially calcium. Doses are generally started at one-half of the daily dose for the first 10 days after which the full dose is used. Caution must be applied in patients with adrenal insufficiency and/or those with cardiovascular disease.

- Armour thyroid—prescription natural T4 and T3 from cow/pig thyroid gland: 60 mg (one grain) is a common starting and maintenance dose. Due to the exacerbating effect on thyroid autoimmunity, Armour thyroid is never used in patients with thyroid autoimmunity.

- Thyrolar/Liotrix—prescription synthetic T4 with T3: Dosed as "1" (low), "2" (intermediate), or "3" (high). Although this product has been difficult to obtain for the past few years due to manufacturing problems (http://thyrolar.com/), it has been my treatment of choice due to the combination of T4 and T3 and the lack of antigenicity compared to gland-derived products.

- Thyroid glandular—nonprescription T3: Producers of nutritional products are able to distribute T3 because it is not listed by the FDA as a prescription item. Nutritional supplement companies may start with Armour thyroid, remove the T4, and sell the thyroid glandular with active T3 thereby providing a nonprescription source of active thyroid hormone. For many patients, one tablet per day is at least as effective as a prescription source of thyroid hormone. Since it is derived from a glandular and therefore potentially antigenic source, thyroid glandular is not used in patients with thyroid autoimmunity due to its ability to induce increased production of anti-thyroid antibodies.

- L-tyrosine and iodine: Some patients with mild hypothyroidism respond to supplementation with L-tyrosine and iodine. Tyrosine is commonly used in doses of 4-9 grams per day in divided doses. According to Abraham and Wright[281], doses of iodine may be as high as 12.5 milligrams (12,500 micrograms), which is slightly less than the average daily intake in Japan at 13.8 mg per day. Supplementation with iodine/iodine combinations is likely to have an antimicrobial benefit against occult pro-inflammatory dysbiosis, but this benefit has not yet been tested in a human clinical trial.

- Xenobiotic accumulation, toxicant immunotoxicity, therapeutic detoxification: Humans in the general population have become living repositories for industrial pollutants and environmental contaminants, generally referred to in contemporary literature as POPs—persistent organic pollutants. POP retention/accumulation is causatively associated with induction of insulin resistance and the resulting hyperinsulinemia and hyperglycemia via suppression of GLUT-4 receptor expression via xenobiotic-induced activation of the aryl hydrocarbon receptor. The clinical work and published writings of Walter Crinnion ND are clearly preeminent in their detailing of the means and efficacy of clinical detoxification processes; a practical summary is provided in Chapter 4 of *Integrative Rheumatology* by Vasquez. Daily means of promoting/optimizing detoxification/depuration of immunotoxic xenobiotics are outlined below; the classic pattern of "xenobiotic immunotoxicity" is that of simultaneous/paradoxical immune

---

[280] Bruns F, Micke O, Bremer M. Current status of selenium and other treatments for secondary lymphedema. *J Support Oncol.* 2003 Jul-Aug;1(2):121-30 http://www.supportiveoncology.net/journal/articles/0102121.pdf
[281] Wright JV. Why you need 83 times more of this essential, cancer-fighting nutrient than the "experts" say you do. *Nutrition and Healing.* 2005; volume 12, issue 4.

suppression (e.g., increased frequency of infections and malignancy) along with immune activation/dysregulation (e.g. increased frequency of autoimmunity).

- o <u>Sweat/exercise/lipolysis</u>
- o <u>Supra-adequacy of dietary fiber</u>: to promote laxation and reduce xenobiotic enterohepatic recirculation; other factors that promote laxation such as exercise, magnesium, and thyroid (status) need to be considered.
- o <u>Chlorella</u>: Orally administered chlorella binds xenobiotics in the gastrointestinal tract and breaks the cycle of enterohepatic recirculation via adsorption (similar to that seen with cholestyramine) and enhanced fecal excretion
- o <u>Urinary alkalinization</u>: Urine pH of 7.5 enhances urinary elimination of xenobiotics per the landmark internationally-endorsed position paper by Proudfoot et al published in 2004.
- o <u>Disinhibition of phase-1 oxidation via cytochrome p450</u>: Elimination of drugs (such as omeprazole, cimetidine), foods (grapefruit, grapefruit juice), and Gram-negative microbes (SIBO) that impair activity of the CYP superfamily.
- o <u>Antioxidants and phase-2 conjugating agents</u>: NAC, glycine, sulfur, etc.

Psoriasis and Psoriatic Arthritis

Introduction:
Psoriasis is my favorite condition to treat; successful implementation of the Functional Inflammology protocol can lead to such rapid resolution of long-term skin lesions that objective improvement is clearly and objectively demonstrable—providing irrefutable proof of efficacy while immediately improving the patient's quality of life, sense of efficacy, and self-esteem.

From this chapter onward, readers should use the information in Chapter 4—detailing the concepts and implementation of the Functional Inflammology protocol—and apply those concepts and interventions to the clinical conditions in the book and encountered in clinical practice. |

Topics:

- Introduction and Overview
- Clinical Presentation
- Prevalence, Symptoms, and Clinical Findings
- Pathophysiology
- Differential Diagnosis
- Diagnosis
- Standard Medical Treatment
- Therapeutic Interventions

Psoriasis
Psoriatic Arthritis

Description/pathophysiology:

- Psoriatic arthritis is an inflammatory arthropathy seen in patients with psoriasis that can have both peripheral (e.g., hands and feet) and axial (i.e., spine and sacroiliac joints) manifestations. This condition has frequently been referred to as *psoriatic rheumatism* or *rheumatic psoriasis*.
- Similar to reactive arthritis and rheumatoid arthritis; strongly associated with streptococcal infections as well as staphylococcal infections.[1] Although many researchers have contributed to the literature which establishes psoriasis as a disease of multifocal dysbiosis, to the best of my knowledge the work of Patricia W. Noah PhD is exceptionally noteworthy; her 1990 review published in *Seminars in Dermatology*[2] is required reading for doctors wishing to gain independent *peer-reviewed* confirmation that **multifocal dysbiosis is the major initiator and perpetuator of this systemic autoimmune inflammatory disorder.** In this particular article, Dr

---

[1] Klippel JH (ed). <u>Primer on the Rheumatic Diseases.</u> 11th Edition. Atlanta: Arthritis Foundation. 1997 page 176
[2] Noah PW. The role of microorganisms in psoriasis. *Semin Dermatol*. 1990 Dec;9(4):269-76

Noah documents the experience of her group at the College of Medicine at the University of Tennessee, their anti-dysbiosis protocol, and its success in the treatment of psoriasis.

- **Psoriasis and psoriatic arthritis must be considered an autoimmune diseases** based on the findings of autoantibodies directed against dermal structures—stratum corneum[3] and keratinocytes[4]—and antibody-dependent and antibody-independent immune-mediated tissue destruction. Although stratum corneum antibodies are found in healthy patients without consequence, what makes them uniquely pathogenic in psoriasis is their tissue penetration in lesioned skin, their ability to bind with autoantigens, and their activation of complement.[5,6]

> **Active microbial colonization contributes to active psoriasis**
>
> "We have repeatedly observed psoriatic flares associated with microbial infection, sequestered antigen, and colonization.
>
> **Removal of these microbial foci results in clearing of the disease."**
>
> Noah P. The role of microorganisms in psoriasis. *Semin Dermatol.* 1990;9:269

> _**Commentary**_: Given the **overwhelming basic science and clinical research** implicating multifocal dysbiosis as the primary initiator of psoriasis—and by extension, psoriatic arthritis—it seems impossible that major allopathic textbooks such as *The Merck Manual*[7] and the widely read *Principles of Dermatology*[8] and *Current Medical Diagnosis and Treatment*[9] would perpetuate the myth that the condition is "idiopathic" so that no cure can be hoped for other than additive, endless, and perpetually "new" medicalization. This is clearly an example of medical practice being incongruent with biomedical research—at the patient's expense.

Clinical presentations:

- Dermal lesions are generally described as well demarcated erythematous patches with silvery scales. Lesions may be widespread or comparatively minor. Patients may have _hidden_ dermal lesions on scalp or in gluteal cleft; clinical examination in patients with oligoarthritis can search for dermal psoriatic lesions while assessing for cutaneous dysbiosis. Rarely, nail pitting is the only cutaneous lesion.
- Chronologic association of _dermal psoriasis_ with _psoriatic arthritis_:
  - 7-30% of patients with (dermal) psoriasis develop psoriatic arthritis
  - In 70% of patients, _dermal psoriasis_ precedes _psoriatic arthritis_ by several years

---

[3] "… titers of IgG anti-SC autoantibodies in psoriatic patients were not specifically higher than in normal controls but were more variable, indicating that their circulating levels are dependent on a delicate balance between consumption at inflammatory sites and a secondary increase due to SC-antigen release following inflammation." Tagami H, Iwatsuki K, Yamada M. Profile of anti-stratum corneum autoantibodies in psoriatic patients. *Arch Dermatol Res.* 1983;275(2):71-5

[4] "It seems that autoantibodies, although they do not appear to participate in the pathogenesis of psoriasis, are an important feature, and that skin antigens, which appear in lesional immature keratinocytes, cross-react with S. pyogenes and contribute to the autoimmune process in psoriasis." Perez-Lorenzo R, Zambrano-Zaragoza JF, Saul A, Jimenez-Zamudio L, Reyes-Maldonado E, Garcia-Latorre E. Autoantibodies to autologous skin in guttate and plaque forms of psoriasis and cross-reaction of skin antigens with streptococcal antigens. *Int J Dermatol.* 1998 Jul;37(7):524-31. The authors found that all psoriasis patients had dermal autoantibodies and that these antibodies reacted specifically with endogenous dermal antigens; thus their finding that "Deposits of immunoglobulin G (IgG) were not detected in the lesions" is unexpected and inexplicable. This statement from their research is inconsistent with the findings of other research groups, and—specifically—must be placed in a context of other articles, most notably "… titers of IgG anti-SC autoantibodies in psoriatic patients were not specifically higher than in normal controls but were more variable, indicating that their circulating levels are dependent on a delicate balance between consumption at inflammatory sites and a secondary increase due to SC-antigen release following inflammation." Tagami H, Iwatsuki K, Yamada M. Profile of anti-stratum corneum autoantibodies in psoriatic patients. *Arch Dermatol Res.* 1983;275(2):71-5.

[5] "The stratum corneum (SC) antibodies are present in all human sera as seen by indirect immunofluorescent (IF) staining… IF tests with proper controls showed that the SC antigen in psoriatic scales is coated not only with IgG but in a majority of the lesions also with complement." Beutner EH, Jarzabek-Chorzelska M, Jablonska S, Chorzelski TP, Rzesa G. Autoimmunity in psoriasis. A complement immunofluorescence study. *Arch Dermatol Res.* 1978 Apr 7;261(2):123-34

[6] "Indirect immunofluorescent (IF) tests on sections of normal human skin reveal the presence of antibodies to the stratum corneum in most normal human sera. ...Direct IF tests of psoriatic lesions revealed the presence of in vivo bound IgG as well as other immunoglobulins and complement in the stratum corneum." Beutner EH, Jablonska S, Jarzabek-Chorzelska M, Marciejowska E, Rzesa G, Chorzelski TP. Studies in immunodermatology. VI. IF studies of autoantibodies to the stratum corneum and of in vivo fixed IgG in stratum corneum of psoriatic lesions. *Int Arch Allergy Appl Immunol.* 1975;48(3):301-23

[7] Beers MH, Berkow R (eds). The Merck Manual. Seventeenth Edition. Whitehouse Station; Merck Research Laboratories 1999 pages 448 and 816

[8] Lookingbill DP, Marks JG, eds. Principles of dermatology. Philadelphia: W.B. Saunders, 1986: 138

[9] Tierney LM, McPhee SJ Papadakis MA (eds). Current Medical Diagnosis and Treatment. 35th edition. New York: Lange; 1996, page 101

- o In 15% of patients, *dermal psoriasis* and *psoriatic arthritis* occur at the same time
- o In 15% of patients, *psoriatic arthritis* precedes *dermal psoriasis*—this 'reverse presentation' is particularly common in children
- Onset may be gradual (70%) or acute (30%)
- In some patients the onset and disease can be of such severity that hospitalization is required.
- Peripheral joint involvement is more common in women; spinal involvement is more common in men, particularly in association with HLA-B27
- Peak onset age 30-55 years
- Musculoskeletal manifestations: prevalence: hands > feet > sacroiliac > spine
  - o Oligoarticular peripheral arthropathy—distal interphalangeal (DIP) joints are notably affected
  - o Peripheral polyarthritis: distribution may be symmetric or asymmetric
  - o Arthritis mutilans: total destruction of the phalanges and meta-tarsals/carpals
  - o Spinal and sacroiliac involvement: may affect any portion of the spine in a random fashion—lumbar spondylitis and sacroiliitis are more common than atlantoaxial instability; spinal involvement is more common in patients positive for HLA-B27
  - o Enthesitis: inflammation at the junction of tendons to bones, especially at the insertion of the Achilles tendon
- Systemic manifestations and complications
  - o Conjunctivitis, uveitis: seen in 30%
  - o Nail pitting may or may not be present; other findings may include transverse ridging, thickening, flaking and brittleness
  - o Aortic insufficiency
  - o Pulmonary fibrosis
  - o Swelling of the fingers and hands

Major differential diagnoses:

- Ankylosing spondylitis: does not occur with dermal psoriatic lesions
- Rheumatoid arthritis: differentiated from rheumatoid arthritis by 1) skin lesions, 2) absence of rheumatoid nodules, 3) negative rheumatoid factor
- Hemochromatosis: non-inflammatory peripheral arthropathy
- Reactive arthritis: does not classically occur with dermal psoriatic lesions
- Septic arthritis: e.g., infected psoriatic skin lesion predisposing to septicemia with resultant joint infection
- HIV infection: increased prevalence of psoriasis[10] especially associated with "an explosive onset of psoriasis and psoriatic arthritis" [11]

Clinical assessments:

- **History/subjective:**
  - o Inquire about the clinical presentations listed above
  - o Family and personal history of psoriasis is often positive

---

[10] Beers MH, Berkow R (eds). The Merck Manual. Seventeenth Edition. Whitehouse Station; Merck Research Laboratories 1999 page 448
[11] Klippel JH (ed). Primer on the Rheumatic Diseases. 11th Edition. Atlanta: Arthritis Foundation. 1997 page 176

- o Historical risk factors for psoriasis include bacterial pharyngitis and stressful life events[12]
- **Physical examination/objective**:
  - o Psoriasis—sharply demarcated erythematous plaque with silver scales
  - o Neuromusculoskeletal examination as indicated—see *Integrative Orthopedics*[13]
  - o Assess blood pressure and perform screening physical examination
- **Laboratory assessments**:
  - o <u>ANA</u>: Antinuclear antibodies are present in 47% of patients with psoriatic arthritis, further supporting the "autoimmune" description of this disease.[14]
  - o <u>Rheumatoid factor</u>: RF is negative: positive RF suggests concomitant RA along with psoriasis.
  - o <u>Chemistry/metabolic panel with uric acid</u>: Assess for overall status and elevated uric acid, the latter may be increased due to rapid skin turnover.
  - o <u>Ferritin</u>: Assess ferritin preferably with transferrin saturation and CRP to exclude iron overload.
  - o <u>CRP</u>: Generally elevated; can be used to track progression/remission of the disease
  - o <u>HLA-B27</u>: Present in 40% of patients with psoriatic arthritis; correlates with increased severity of disease, including increased CRP, increased propensity for sacroiliitis, and more extensive joint destruction.[15]
  - o <u>HIV serologic testing</u>: Especially for patients with severe disease and/or sudden onset.
  - o <u>Lactulose/mannitol assay for "leaky gut"</u>: Patients with psoriasis have increased intestinal permeability.[16]
  - o <u>Dysbiosis assessments</u>
    - ▪ <u>Gastrointestinal dysbiosis</u>: Comprehensive stool and parasitology testing must include bacterial/yeast culture; antigen or antibody testing for *H. pylori* is recommended; patients with psoriasis have shown a greatly increased prevalence of *H. pylori* compared with controls[17], and the authors of this study suggested a causal association; likewise intestinal colonization with yeasts including *Candida albicans* and *Geotrichum candidum* are found much more commonly in psoriatics than controls.[18] Stressing the importance of this association, Waldman et al[19] wrote, "Our results reinforce the hypothesis that *C. albicans* is one of the triggers to both exacerbation and persistence of psoriasis. We propose that in psoriatics with a significant quantity of

---

[12] "The study confirmed that recent pharyngeal infection is a risk factor for guttate psoriasis… Finally, the study added evidence to the belief that stressful life events may represent risk factors for the onset of psoriasis." Naldi L, Peli L, Parazzini F, Carrel CF; Psoriasis Study Group of the Italian Group for Epidemiological Research in Dermatology. Family history of psoriasis, stressful life events, and recent infectious disease are risk factors for a first episode of acute guttate psoriasis: results of a case-control study. *J Am Acad Dermatol.* 2001 Mar;44(3):433-8

[13] Vasquez A. <u>Integrative Orthopedics—The Art of Creating Wellness While Effectively Managing Acute and Chronic Musculoskeletal Disorders.</u> 2004: www.OptimalHealthResearch.com

[14] "RESULTS: 44/94 (47%) patients with PsA were ANA positive (>/=1/40); 13/94 (14%) had a clinically significant titre of >/=1/80. Three per cent had dsDNA antibodies, 2% had RF and anti-Ro antibodies, 1% had anti-RNP antibodies, and none had anti-La or anti-Smith antibodies." Johnson SR, Schentag CT, Gladman DD. Autoantibodies in biological agent naive patients with psoriatic arthritis. *Ann Rheum Dis.* 2005 May;64(5):770-2

[15] Tsai YG, Chang DM, Kuo SY, Wang WM, Chen YC, Lai JH. Relationship between human lymphocyte antigen-B27 and clinical features of psoriatic arthritis. *J Microbiol Immunol Infect.* 2003 Jun;36(2):101-4 http://www.jmii.org/content/abstracts/v36n2p101.php

[16] "The 24-h urine excretion of 51Cr-EDTA from psoriatic patients was 2.46 +/- 0.81%. These results differed significantly from controls (1.95 +/- 0.36%; P less than 0.05)." Humbert P, Bidet A, Treffel P, Drobacheff C, Agache P. Intestinal permeability in patients with psoriasis. *J Dermatol Sci.* 1991 Jul;2:324-6

[17] "In the current study, 20 (40%), psoriatic patients and 5 (10%) patients of control group demonstrated H. pylori antibodies... Although our study supports a causal role of H. pylori in the pathogenesis of psoriasis, a large scale study is needed to confirm the findings." Qayoom S, Ahmad QM. Psoriasis and helicobacter pylori. *Indian J Dermatol Venereol Leprol* 2003;69:133-134 http://www.ijdvl.com/

[18] Candida albicans (and other yeasts) was detected in 68% of psoriatics, 70% of eczematics, 54% of the controls. Qualitative analysis revealed a predominance of Candida albicans. Geotrichum candidum occurred in 22% of psoriatics, 10% of eczematics, and 3% of controls. Buslau M, Menzel I, Holzmann H. Fungal flora of human faeces in psoriasis and atopic dermatitis. *Mycoses.* 1990 Feb;33(2):90-4

[19] "Our results reinforce the hypothesis that C. albicans is one of the triggers to both exacerbation and persistence of psoriasis. We propose that in psoriatics with a significant quantity of Candida in faeces, an antifungal treatment should be considered as an adjuvant treatment of psoriasis." Waldman A, Gilhar A, Duek L, Berdicevsky I. Incidence of Candida in psoriasis--a study on the fungal flora of psoriatic patients. *Mycoses.* 2001 May;44(3-4):77-8

Candida in feces, an antifungal treatment should be considered as an adjuvant treatment of psoriasis."

- Dermal dysbiosis: Skin/nail culture, Giemsa staining, culture lesioned skin on blood agar, MacConkey agar, Sabouraud plates.[20]
- Sinorespiratory dysbiosis: Nasal swab and culture, throat culture for bacteria and yeasts.[21]
- Genitourinary dysbiosis: Culture and sensitivity testing for all organisms from clean catch specimens; assessment of sexual partners is advised.[22]
- Orodental dysbiosis: Culture of dentures and oral cavity for yeast and bacteria.
- Environmental dysbiosis: Examination, culture, and/or thorough cleaning of wigs, shoes, furniture, whirlpool/pool water.[23]

- **Imaging**:
  - Radiographic findings are characteristic and can aid in differential diagnosis; findings such as the osteolytic "pencil-in-cup" and "marginal erosions" are characteristic and differentiate psoriatic arthropathy from other conditions.
  - Radiographic changes in the spine may be severe even when the patient has mild or no symptoms—assess the spine radiographically before initiating spinal manipulative therapy. Note that inflammatory changes such as facet ankylosis and atlantoaxial instability may occur and could potentially complicate manipulative therapy.[24] Myelocompressive atlantoaxial subluxation has been reported as the presenting manifestation of psoriatic arthropathy.[25] Remarkably, Lee and Lui[26] published that, "...atlantoaxial subluxation without high cervical myelopathy has been reported in 45% of cases of psoriatic spondylitis."

- **Establishing the diagnosis**:
  - Pattern recognition: psoriasis with arthritis after the exclusion of RA, iron overload, AS, and HIV

Complications:

- Infection of skin lesions, may progress to septicemia or septic arthritis
- Atlantoaxial instability
- Cosmetic and functional deformity
- Pain
- Destructive and crippling arthritis
- Depression, social isolation, pain, reduced quality of life: **"Patients with psoriasis reported reduction in physical functioning and mental functioning comparable to that seen in cancer, arthritis, hypertension, heart disease, diabetes, and depression."[27]**

[20] Noah PW. The role of microorganisms in psoriasis. *Semin Dermatol.* 1990 Dec;9(4):269-76
[21] Noah PW. The role of microorganisms in psoriasis. *Semin Dermatol.* 1990 Dec;9(4):269-76
[22] Noah PW. The role of microorganisms in psoriasis. *Semin Dermatol.* 1990 Dec;9(4):269-76
[23] Noah PW. The role of microorganisms in psoriasis. *Semin Dermatol.* 1990 Dec;9(4):269-76
[24] Laiho K, Kauppi M. The cervical spine in patients with psoriatic arthritis. *Ann Rheum Dis.* 2002 Jul;6:650-2 ard.bmjjournals.com/cgi/content/full/61/7/650
[25] "We report severe upward axial dislocation and acquired basilar impression as a presenting manifestation of psoriatic arthropathy." Kaplan JG, Rosenberg RS, DeSouza T, Post KD, Freilich MD, Salamon O, Lantos G, Reinitz E. Atlantoaxial subluxation in psoriatic arthropathy. *Ann Neurol.* 1988 May;23(5):522-4
[26] "...atlantoaxial subluxation without high cervical myelopathy has been reported in 45% of cases of psoriatic spondylitis." Lee ST, Lui TN. Psoriatic arthritis with C-1-C-2 subluxation as a neurosurgical complication. *Surg Neurol.* 1986 Nov;26(5):428-30
[27] "Patients with psoriasis reported reduction in physical functioning and mental functioning comparable to that seen in cancer, arthritis, hypertension, heart disease, diabetes, and depression." Rapp SR, Feldman SR, Exum ML, Fleischer AB Jr, Reboussin DM. Psoriasis causes as much disability as other major medical diseases. *J Am Acad Dermatol* 1999 Sep;41(3 Pt 1):401-7

Clinical management:
- Referral if clinical outcome is unsatisfactory or if serious complications are evident.

Treatments:
- Medical treatments: The goal of medical treatment is to suppress inflammation and dermal proliferation; no consideration is given to searching for and addressing the underlying cause(s) of the disorder because the disease is considered idiopathic.[28] Medical textbooks describe the treatment as merely targeted toward the symptoms, e.g., "Treatment [of psoriatic arthritis] is symptomatic."[29] :
  - *For dermal psoriasis*:
    - Prescription topical steroids
    - Topical coal tars and hydrocarbons: carcinogenic
    - UV-B radiation
    - PUVA: psoralen with UV-A radiation; may result in cataracts and skin cancer
    - Methotrexate
    - Etretinate: a severely teratogenic retinoid
  - *For psoriatic arthritis*: Medical treatments for psoriatic arthritis are essentially the same as for rheumatoid arthritis[30] and are generally noncurative and "symptomatic."[31]
    - Etretinate: a severely teratogenic retinoid
    - PUVA: psoralen with UV-A radiation; may result in cataracts and skin cancer
    - Corticosteroids are not highly effective
    - Antimalarial drugs (commonly used against systemic lupus erythematosus) frequently exacerbate psoriasis
    - Methotrexate: Used for recalcitrant psoriatic arthritis.[32]
    - TNF inhibitors: Etanercept 25 mg subcutaneously twice weekly, or infliximab 5 mg/kg every other month. These drugs are clinically effective from the perspective of anti-inflammation, but they are associated with increased risks for lymphoma, infections, congestive heart failure, demyelinating diseases, and systemic lupus erythematosus.
- Avoidance of proinflammatory foods: Proinflammatory foods act *directly* or *indirectly*; direct mechanisms include activating Toll-like receptors or NF-kappaB or inducing oxidative stress, while indirect mechanisms include depleting the body of anti-inflammatory nutrients and displacing more nutritious anti-inflammatory foods. Arachidonic acid (found in beef, liver, pork, and cow's milk) is the direct precursor to proinflammatory prostaglandins and leukotrienes[33] and pain-promoting isoprostanes.[34] Saturated fats promote inflammation by activating/enabling proinflammatory Toll-like receptors.[35] Consumption of saturated fat in the form of cream creates marked oxidative stress and lipid peroxidation that lasts for at least 3

---

[28] Lookingbill DP, Marks JG, eds. Principles of dermatology. Philadelphia: W.B. Saunders, 1986: 138

[29] Tierney ML. McPhee SJ, Papadakis MA. Current Medical Diagnosis and Treatment 2006. 45th edition. New York; Lange Medical: 2006, pages 851-855

[30] Beers MH, Berkow R (eds). The Merck Manual. Seventeenth Edition. Whitehouse Station; Merck Research Laboratories 1999 page 448

[31] Tierney ML. McPhee SJ, Papadakis MA. Current Medical Diagnosis and Treatment 2006. 45th edition. New York; Lange Medical: 2006, pages 851-855

[32] Tierney ML. McPhee SJ, Papadakis MA. Current Medical Diagnosis and Treatment 2006. 45th edition. New York; Lange Medical: 2006, pages 851-855

[33] Vasquez A. Reducing Pain and Inflammation Naturally. Part 2: New Insights into Fatty Acid Supplementation and Its Effect on Eicosanoid Production and Genetic Expression. *Nutritional Perspectives* 2005; January: 5-16 www.optimalhealthresearch.com/part2

[34] Evans AR, Junger H, Southall MD, Nicol GD, Sorkin LS, Broome JT, Bailey TW, Vasko MR. Isoprostanes, novel eicosanoids that produce nociception and sensitize rat sensory neurons. *J Pharmacol Exp Ther.* 2000 Jun;293(3):912-20

[35] Lee JY, Sohn KH, Rhee SH, Hwang D. Saturated fatty acids, but not unsaturated fatty acids, induce the expression of cyclooxygenase-2 mediated through Toll-like receptor 4. *J Biol Chem.* 2001 May 18;276(20):16683-9. Epub 2001 Mar 2 http://www.jbc.org/cgi/content/full/276/20/16683

hours postprandially.[36] Corn oil rapidly activates NF-kappaB (in hepatic Kupffer cells) for a proinflammatory effect[37]; similarly, consumption of PUFA and linoleic acid promotes antioxidant depletion and may thus promote oxidation-mediated inflammation via activation of NF-kappaB; linoleic acid causes intracellular oxidative stress and calcium influx and results in increased transcription of NF-kappaB activated pro-inflammatory genes.[38] High glycemic foods cause oxidative stress[39,40] and inflammation via activation of NF-kappaB and other mechanisms—*white bread causes inflammation.*[41] High glycemic foods suppress immune function[42,43] and thus perpetuate and promote infection/dysbiosis. Delivery of a high carbohydrate load to the gastrointestinal lumen promotes bacterial overgrowth[44,45], which is inherently proinflammatory[46,47] and which appears to be myalgenic in humans.[48] Consumption of grains, potatoes, and manufactured foods displaces phytonutrient-dense foods such as fruits, vegetables, nuts, seeds, and berries which in sum contain more than 8,000 phytonutrients, many of which have anti-oxidant and thus anti-inflammatory actions.[49,50]

- <u>Avoidance of allergenic foods</u>: Any patient may be allergic to any food, even if the food is generally considered a health-promoting food. Generally speaking, the most notorious allergens are wheat, citrus (especially juice due to the industrial use of fungal hemicellulases), cow's milk, eggs, peanuts, chocolate, and yeast-containing foods; according to a study in patients with migraine, some patients will have to avoid as many as 10 specific foods in order to become symptom-free.[51] In 2005 I reported the remarkably successful treatment of a young

[36] "CONCLUSIONS: Both fat and protein intakes stimulate ROS generation. The increase in ROS generation lasted 3 h after cream intake and 1 h after protein intake. Cream intake also caused a significant and prolonged increase in lipid peroxidation." Mohanty P, Ghanim H, Hamouda W, Aljada A, Garg R, Dandona P. Both lipid and protein intakes stimulate increased generation of reactive oxygen species by polymorphonuclear leukocytes and mononuclear cells. *Am J Clin Nutr*. 2002 Apr;75(4):767-72 http://www.ajcn.org/cgi/content/full/75/4/767

[37] Rusyn I, Bradham CA, Cohn L, Schoonhoven R, Swenberg JA, Brenner DA, Thurman RG. Corn oil rapidly activates nuclear factor-kappaB in hepatic Kupffer cells by oxidant-dependent mechanisms. *Carcinogenesis*. 1999 Nov;20(11):2095-100 http://carcin.oxfordjournals.org/cgi/content/full/20/11/2095

[38] "Exposing endothelial cells to 90 micromol linoleic acid/L for 6 h resulted in a significant increase in lipid hydroperoxides that coincided with an increase in intracellular calcium concentrations." Hennig B, Toborek M, Joshi-Barve S, Barger SW, Barve S, Mattson MP, McClain CJ. Linoleic acid activates nuclear transcription factor-kappa B (NF-kappa B) and induces NF-kappa B-dependent transcription in cultured endothelial cells. *Am J Clin Nutr*. 1996 Mar;63(3):322-8 http://www.ajcn.org/cgi/reprint/63/3/322

[39] Mohanty P, Hamouda W, Garg R, Aljada A, Ghanim H, Dandona P. Glucose challenge stimulates reactive oxygen species (ROS) generation by leucocytes. *J Clin Endocrinol Metab*. 2000 Aug;85(8):2970-3 http://jcem.endojournals.org/cgi/content/full/85/8/2970 Glucose/carbohydrate and saturated fat consumption appear to be the two biggest offenders in the food-stimulated production of oxidative stress. The effect by protein is much less. "CONCLUSIONS: Both fat and protein intakes stimulate ROS generation. The increase in ROS generation lasted 3 h after cream intake and 1 h after protein intake. Cream intake also caused a significant and prolonged increase in lipid peroxidation." Mohanty P, Ghanim H, Hamouda W, Aljada A, Garg R, Dandona P. Both lipid and protein intakes stimulate increased generation of reactive oxygen species by polymorphonuclear leukocytes and mononuclear cells. *Am J Clin Nutr*. 2002 Apr;75(4):767-72 http://www.ajcn.org/cgi/content/full/75/4/767

[40] Koska J, Blazicek P, Marko M, Grna JD, Kvetnansky R, Vigas M. Insulin, catecholamines, glucose and antioxidant enzymes in oxidative damage during different loads in healthy humans. *Physiol Res*. 2000;49 Suppl 1:S95-100 http://www.biomed.cas.cz/physiolres/pdf/2000/49_S95.pdf

[41] "Conclusion - The present study shows that high GI carbohydrate, but not low GI carbohydrate, mediates an acute proinflammatory process as measured by NF-kappaB activity." Dickinson S, Hancock DP, Petocz P, Brand-Miller JC..High glycemic index carbohydrate mediates an acute proinflammatory process as measured by NF-kappaB activation. *Asia Pac J Clin Nutr*. 2005;14 Suppl:S120

[42] Sanchez A, Reeser JL, Lau HS, et al. Role of sugars in human neutrophilic phagocytosis. *Am J Clin Nutr*. 1973 Nov;26(11):1180-4

[43] "Postoperative infusion of carbohydrate solution leads to moderate fall in the serum concentration of inorganic phosphate. ... The hypophosphatemia was associated with significant reduction of neutrophil phagocytosis, intracellular killing, consumption of oxygen and generation of superoxide during phagocytosis." Rasmussen A, Segel E, Hessov I, Borregaard N. Reduced function of neutrophils during routine postoperative glucose infusion. *Acta Chir Scand*. 1988 Jul-Aug;154(7-8):429-33

[44] Ramakrishnan T, Stokes P. Beneficial effects of fasting and low carbohydrate diet in D-lactic acidosis associated with short-bowel syndrome. *JPEN J Parenter Enteral Nutr*. 1985 May-Jun;9(3):361-3

[45] Gottschall E. Breaking the Vicious Cycle: Intestinal Health Through Diet. Kirkton Press; Rev edition (August 1, 1994)

[46] Lin HC. Small intestinal bacterial overgrowth: a framework for understanding irritable bowel syndrome. *JAMA*. 2004 Aug 18;292(7):852-8

[47] Lichtman SN, Wang J, Sartor RB, Zhang C, Bender D, Dalldorf FG, Schwab JH. Reactivation of arthritis induced by small bowel bacterial overgrowth in rats: role of cytokines, bacteria, and bacterial polymers. *Infect Immun*. 1995 Jun;63(6):2295-301

[48] Pimentel M, et al. A link between irritable bowel syndrome and fibromyalgia may be related to findings on lactulose breath testing. *Ann Rheum Dis*. 2004 Apr;63(4):450-2

[49] "We propose that the additive and synergistic effects of phytochemicals in fruit and vegetables are responsible for their potent antioxidant and anticancer activities, and that the benefit of a diet rich in fruit and vegetables is attributed to the complex mixture of phytochemicals present in whole foods." Liu RH. Health benefits of fruit and vegetables are from additive and synergistic combinations of phytochemicals. *Am J Clin Nutr*. 2003 Sep;78(3 Suppl):517S-520S

[50] Seaman DR. The diet-induced proinflammatory state: a cause of chronic pain and other degenerative diseases? *J Manipulative Physiol Ther*. 2002;25(3):168-79

[51] Grant EC. Food allergies and migraine. *Lancet*. 1979 May 5;1(8123):966-9

woman with head-to-toe psoriasis who achieved complete and permanent remission of her "untreatable" "idiopathic" drug-resistant disease by diet modification, nutritional supplementation, and avoidance of offending allergens—in her case, chicken broth.[52] Patients with psoriasis and psoriatic arthritis show elevated frequency of occult celiac disease and "wheat allergy" (identified by anti-gliadin antibodies), and therefore the diet program for such patients should exclude wheat and other gluten-containing grains.[53] Celiac disease can present with inflammatory oligoarthritis that resembles rheumatoid arthritis and which remits with avoidance of wheat/gluten; the inflammatory arthropathy of celiac disease has preceded bowel symptoms and/or an accurate diagnosis by as many as 3-15 years.[54,55] Antibody patterns characteristic of celiac disease (IgG and IgA antigliadin antibodies, IgA antitransglutaminase antibody, IgA antiendomysial antibody) correlate with disease activity in patients with psoriasis[56], and gluten-free diets can lead to rapid resolution of skin lesions in patients with psoriasis.[57] Clinicians must explain to their patients that celiac disease and wheat allergy are two different clinical entities and that exclusion of one does not exclude the other, and in neither case does mutual exclusion obviate the promotion of intestinal bacterial overgrowth (i.e., proinflammatory dysbiosis) by indigestible wheat oligosaccharides.

- <u>Supplemented Paleo-Mediterranean diet</u>: The health-promoting diet of choice for the majority of people is a diet based on abundant consumption of fruits, vegetables, seeds, nuts, omega-3 and monounsaturated fatty acids, and lean sources of protein such as lean meats, fatty cold-water fish, soy and whey proteins. This diet obviates overconsumption of chemical preservatives, artificial sweeteners, and carbohydrate-dominant foods such as candies, pastries, breads, potatoes, grains, and other foods with a high glycemic load and high glycemic index. This "Paleo-Mediterranean Diet" is a combination of the "Paleolithic" or "Paleo diet" and the well-known "Mediterranean diet", both of which are well described in peer-reviewed journals and the lay press. (See Chapter 2 and my other publications[58,59] for details). Although this diet is the most-nutrient dense diet available, rational supplementation with vitamins, minerals, and health promoting fatty acids (i.e., ALA, GLA, EPA, DHA) makes this the best practical diet that can possibly be conceived and implemented.

- <u>Folic acid 5-20 mg per day</u>: Patients with psoriasis have reduced folate status and elevated homocysteine levels.[60] Wright and Gaby recommended 50-150 mg per day of folic acid for

[52] Vasquez A. Implementing the Five-Part Nutritional Wellness Protocol for the Treatment of Various Health Problems. *Nutritional Wellness* 2005 November. Available on-line at http://www.nutritionalwellness.com/archives/2005/nov/11_vasquez.php and http://optimalhealthresearch.com/protocol

[53] "Patients with PsoA have an increased prevalence of raised serum IgA [anti-gliadin antibodies] and of coeliac disease. Patients with raised IgA AGA seem to have more pronounced inflammation than those with a low IgA AGA concentration." Lindqvist U, Rudsander A, Bostrom A, Nilsson B, Michaelsson G. IgA antibodies to gliadin and coeliac disease in psoriatic arthritis. *Rheumatology* (Oxford). 2002 Jan;41(1):31-7 http://rheumatology.oxfordjournals.org/cgi/content/full/41/1/31

[54] "We report six patients with coeliac disease in whom arthritis was prominent at diagnosis and who improved with dietary therapy. Joint pain preceded diagnosis by up to three years in five patients and 15 years in one patient." Bourne JT, Kumar P, Huskisson EC, Mageed R, Unsworth DJ, Wojtulewski JA. Arthritis and coeliac disease. *Ann Rheum Dis.* 1985 Sep;44(9):592-8

[55] "A 15-year-old girl, with synovitis of the knees and ankles for 3 years before a diagnosis of gluten-sensitive enteropathy, is described." Pinals RS. Arthritis associated with gluten-sensitive enteropathy. *J Rheumatol.* 1986 Feb;13(1):201-4

[56] "The presence of CD-associated antibodies in psoriasis patients correlates with greater disease activity." Woo WK, McMillan SA, Watson RG, McCluggage WG, Sloan JM, McMillan JC. Coeliac disease-associated antibodies correlate with psoriasis activity. *Br J Dermatol.* 2004 Oct;151(4):891-4

[57] "The present case supports the association between CD and psoriasis and the concept that psoriasis in CD patients can be improved by GFD." Addolorato G, Parente A, de Lorenzi G, D'angelo Di Paola ME, Abenavoli L, Leggio L, Capristo E, De Simone C, Rotoli M, Rapaccini GL, Gasbarrini G. Rapid regression of psoriasis in a coeliac patient after gluten-free diet. A case report and review of the literature. *Digestion.* 2003;68(1):9-12. Epub 2003 Aug 29

[58] Vasquez A. A Five-Part Nutritional Protocol that Produces Consistently Positive Results. *Nutritional Wellness* 2005 September Available in the printed version and on-line at http://www.nutritionalwellness.com/archives/2005/sep/09_vasquez.php and http://optimalhealthresearch.com/protocol

[59] Vasquez A. Implementing the Five-Part Nutritional Wellness Protocol for the Treatment of Various Health Problems. *Nutritional Wellness* 2005 November. Available on-line at http://www.nutritionalwellness.com/archives/2005/nov/11_vasquez.php and http://optimalhealthresearch.com/protocol

[60] "The mean levels of serum tHcy, fibrinogen, fibronectin, sICAM, PAI-1 and AuAb-oxLDL were increased in patients whereas tPA, vitamin B(12) and folate levels were decreased significantly." Vanizor Kural B, Orem A, Cimsit G, Uydu HA, Yandi YE, Alver A. Plasma homocysteine and its relationships with atherothrombotic markers in psoriatic patients. *Clin Chim Acta.* 2003 Jun;332(1-2):23-30

psoriatics.[61] Folic acid has antiproliferative and anti-inflammatory effects mediated by nutrigenomic mechanisms. Folic acid, along with other vitamins and nutrients, may also help alleviate the biochemical aspect of the depression that is common in patients with psoriasis. Always supplement with vitamin B-12 in form of hydroxocobalamin or methylcobalamin (e.g., 2,000 mcg per day) when using high-dose folic acid.

- <u>Alcohol/ethanol avoidance</u>: Consumption of alcoholic beverages—even in low doses—increases intestinal permeability and exacerbates psoriasis. Psoriatics should avoid ethanol consumption[62]; wheat/grain antigens are immunogenic, ethanol exacerbates intestinal hyperpermeability, and some patients are sensitive to brewer's yeast.

- <u>Gluten-free vegetarian diet</u>: Vegetarian/vegan diets have a place in the treatment plan of all patients with autoimmune/inflammatory disorders[63]--including psoriasis and psoriatic arthritis[64]; this is also true for patients for whom long-term exclusive reliance on a meat-free vegetarian diet is either not appropriate or not appealing. No legitimate scientist or literate clinician doubts the antirheumatic power and anti-inflammatory advantages of vegetarian diets, whether used short-term or long term.[65] The benefits of gluten-free vegetarian diets are well documented, and the mechanisms of action are well elucidated, including reduced intake of proinflammatory linoleic[66] and arachidonic acids[67], iron[68], common food antigens[69], gluten[70] and gliadin[71,72], proinflammatory sugars[73] and increased intake of omega-3 fatty acids and micronutrients[74], and anti-inflammatory and anti-oxidant phytonutrients[75]; vegetarian diets

[61] Gaby A, Wright JV. <u>Nutritional Protocols</u>. 1998 Nutrition Seminars
[62] "We recommend that clinicians discourage patients with psoriasis from consuming alcohol, especially during periods of disease exacerbation." Behnam SM, Behnam SE, Koo JY. Alcohol as a risk factor for plaque-type psoriasis. *Cutis.* 2005 Sep;76(3):181-5
[63] "After four weeks at the health farm the diet group showed a significant improvement in number of tender joints, Ritchie's articular index, number of swollen joints, pain score, duration of morning stiffness, grip strength, erythrocyte sedimentation rate, C-reactive protein, white blood cell count, and a health assessment questionnaire score." Kjeldsen-Kragh J, Haugen M, Borchgrevink CF, Laerum E, Eek M, Mowinkel P, Hovi K, Forre O. Controlled trial of fasting and one-year vegetarian diet in rheumatoid arthritis. *Lancet.* 1991 Oct 12;338(8772):899-902
[64] "During the vegan diet, both signs and symptoms returned in most patients, with the exception of some patients with psoriasis who experienced an improvement." Lithell H, Bruce A, Gustafsson IB, Hoglund NJ, Karlstrom B, Ljunghall K, Sjolin K, Venge P, Werner I, Vessby B. A fasting and vegetarian diet treatment trial on chronic inflammatory disorders. *Acta Derm Venereol.* 1983;63(5):397-403
[65] "For the patients who were randomised to the vegetarian diet there was a significant decrease in platelet count, leukocyte count, calprotectin, total IgG, IgM rheumatoid factor (RF), C3-activation products, and the complement components C3 and C4 after one month of treatment." Kjeldsen-Kragh J, Mellbye OJ, Haugen M, Mollnes TE, Hammer HB, Sioud M, Forre O. Changes in laboratory variables in rheumatoid arthritis patients during a trial of fasting and one-year vegetarian diet. *Scand J Rheumatol.* 1995;24(2):85-93
[66] Rusyn I, Bradham CA, Cohn L, Schoonhoven R, Swenberg JA, Brenner DA, Thurman RG. Corn oil rapidly activates nuclear factor-kappaB in hepatic Kupffer cells by oxidant-dependent mechanisms. *Carcinogenesis.* 1999 Nov;20(11):2095-100 http://carcin.oxfordjournals.org/cgi/content/full/20/11/2095
[67] Vasquez A. Reducing Pain and Inflammation Naturally. Part 2: New Insights into Fatty Acid Supplementation and Its Effect on Eicosanoid Production and Genetic Expression. *Nutritional Perspectives* 2005; January: 5-16 http://optimalhealthresearch.com/part2
[68] Dabbagh AJ, Trenam CW, Morris CJ, Blake DR. Iron in joint inflammation. *Ann Rheum Dis.* 1993 Jan;52(1):67-73
[69] Hafstrom I, Ringertz B, Spangberg A, von Zweigbergk L, Brannemark S, Nylander I, Ronnelid J, Laasonen L, Klareskog L. A vegan diet free of gluten improves the signs and symptoms of rheumatoid arthritis: the effects on arthritis correlate with a reduction in antibodies to food antigens. *Rheumatology* (Oxford). 2001 Oct;40(10):1175-9 http://rheumatology.oxfordjournals.org/cgi/reprint/40/10/1175
[70] "The data provide evidence that dietary modification may be of clinical benefit for certain RA patients, and that this benefit may be related to a reduction in immunoreactivity to food antigens eliminated by the change in diet." Hafstrom I, Ringertz B, Spangberg A, von Zweigbergk L, Brannemark S, Nylander I, Ronnelid J, Laasonen L, Klareskog L. A vegan diet free of gluten improves the signs and symptoms of rheumatoid arthritis: the effects on arthritis correlate with a reduction in antibodies to food antigens. *Rheumatology* (Oxford). 2001 Oct;40(10):1175-9
[71] "Despite the increased AGA [antigliadin antibodies] positivity found distinctively in patients with recent-onset RA, none of the RA patients showed clear evidence of coeliac disease." Paimela L, Kurki P, Leirisalo-Repo M, Piirainen H. Gliadin immune reactivity in patients with rheumatoid arthritis. Clin Exp Rheumatol. 1995 Sep-Oct;13(5):603-7
[72] "The median IgA antigliadin ELISA index was 7.1 (range 2.1-22.4) for the RA group and 3.1 (range 0.3-34.9) for the controls (p = 0.0001)." Koot VC, Van Straaten M, Hekkens WT, Collee G, Dijkmans BA. Elevated level of IgA gliadin antibodies in patients with rheumatoid arthritis. *Clin Exp Rheumatol.* 1989 Nov-Dec;7(6):623-6
[73] Seaman DR. The diet-induced proinflammatory state: a cause of chronic pain and other degenerative diseases? *J Manipulative Physiol Ther.* 2002 Mar-Apr;25(3):168-79
[74] Hagfors L, Nilsson I, Skoldstam L, Johansson G. Fat intake and composition of fatty acids in serum phospholipids in a randomized, controlled, Mediterranean dietary intervention study on patients with rheumatoid arthritis. *Nutr Metab* (Lond). 2005 Oct 10;2:26 http://www.nutritionandmetabolism.com/content/2/1/26
[75] Liu RH. Health benefits of fruit and vegetables are from additive and synergistic combinations of phytochemicals. *Am J Clin Nutr* 2003;78(3 Suppl):517S-520S http://www.ajcn.org/cgi/content/full/78/3/517S

also effect profound changes—both *qualitative* and *quantitative*—in intestinal flora[76,77] that correlate with clinical improvement.[78] Patients who rely on the Paleo-Mediterranean Diet can use vegetarian meals, on a daily basis or for days at a time, for example, by having a daily vegetarian meal, or one week per month of vegetarianism. Of course, some (not all) patients can use a purely vegetarian diet long-term provided that nutritional needs (especially protein and cobalamin) are consistently met. One particular advantage to low-protein diets in psoriasis is that the relative reduction in amino acid availability should serve to reduce polyamine formation. Formed from amino acids via ornithine decarboxylase and other enzymes, polyamines stimulate dermal hyperproliferation and are elevated in patients with psoriasis.[79] Effective psoriasis treatments are associated with a reduction in dermal/urinary polyamine levels, and, conversely, reducing polyamine formation—via either dietary manipulation or antibiologic/pharmaceutical drugs—is associated with clinical improvements in patients with psoriasis.

- Short-term fasting: Whether the foundational diet is Paleo-Mediterranean, vegetarian, vegan, or a combination of all of these, autoimmune/inflammatory patients will still benefit from periodic fasting, whether on a weekly (e.g., every Saturday), monthly (every first week or weekend of the month, or every other month), or yearly (1-2 weeks of the year) basis. Since consumption of food—particularly unhealthy foods—induces an inflammatory effect[80], abstinence from food provides a relative anti-oxidative and anti-inflammatory benefit[81] with many of the antioxidant benefits beginning within 24 hours of the initiation of the fast.[82] Fasting indeed provides a distinct anti-inflammatory benefit and may help "re-calibrate" metabolic and homeostatic mechanisms by breaking self-perpetuating "vicious cycles"[83] that autonomously promote inflammation independent from proinflammatory stimuli. Of course, water-only fasting is completely hypoallergenic (assuming that the patient is not sensitive to chlorine, fluoride, or other contaminants), and subsequent re-introduction of foods provides the ideal opportunity to identify offending foods. Fasting deprives intestinal microbes of substrate[84], stimulates intestinal B-cell immunity[85], improves the bactericidal action of

---

[76] "Significant alteration in the intestinal flora was observed when the patients changed from omnivorous to vegan diet. ... This finding of an association between intestinal flora and disease activity may have implications for our understanding of how diet can affect RA." Peltonen R, Kjeldsen-Kragh J, Haugen M, Tuominen J, Toivanen P, Forre O, Eerola E. Changes of faecal flora in rheumatoid arthritis during fasting and one-year vegetarian diet. *Br J Rheumatol.* 1994 Jul;33(7):638-43

[77] Toivanen P, Eerola E. A vegan diet changes the intestinal flora. *Rheumatology* (Oxford). 2002 Aug;41(8):950-1 http://rheumatology.oxfordjournals.org/cgi/reprint/41/8/950

[78] "We conclude that a vegan diet changes the faecal microbial flora in RA patients, and changes in the faecal flora are associated with improvement in RA activity." Peltonen R, Nenonen M, Helve T, Hanninen O, Toivanen P, Eerola E. Faecal microbial flora and disease activity in rheumatoid arthritis during a vegan diet. *Br J Rheumatol.* 1997 Jan;36(1):64-8 http://rheumatology.oxfordjournals.org/cgi/reprint/36/1/64

[79] "Psoriasis lesions showed increased ornithine decarboxylase activity compared with uninvolved skin." Lowe NJ, Breeding J, Russell D. Cutaneous polyamines in psoriasis. *Br J Dermatol.* 1982 Jul;107(1):21-5

[80] Aljada A, Mohanty P, Ghanim H, Abdo T, Tripathy D, Chaudhuri A, Dandona P. Increase in intranuclear nuclear factor kappaB and decrease in inhibitor kappaB in mononuclear cells after a mixed meal: evidence for a proinflammatory effect. *Am J Clin Nutr.* 2004 Apr;79(4):682-90 http://www.ajcn.org/cgi/content/full/79/4/682

[81] "This is the first demonstration of ...a decrease in reactive oxygen species generation by leukocytes and oxidative damage to lipids, proteins, and amino acids after dietary restriction and weight loss in the obese over a short period." Dandona P, Mohanty P, Ghanim H, Aljada A, Browne R, Hamouda W, Prabhala A, Afzal A, Garg R. The suppressive effect of dietary restriction and weight loss in the obese on the generation of reactive oxygen species by leukocytes, lipid peroxidation, and protein carbonylation. *J Clin Endocrinol Metab.* 2001 Jan;86(1):355-62 http://jcem.endojournals.org/cgi/content/full/86/1/355

[82] "Thus, a 48h fast may reduce ROS generation, total oxidative load and oxidative damage to amino acids." Dandona P, Mohanty P, Hamouda W, Ghanim H, Aljada A, Garg R, Kumar V. Inhibitory effect of a two day fast on reactive oxygen species (ROS) generation by leucocytes and plasma ortho-tyrosine and meta-tyrosine concentrations. *J Clin Endocrinol Metab.* 2001 Jun;86(6):2899-902 http://jcem.endojournals.org/cgi/content/abstract/86/6/2899

[83] "The ability of therapeutic fasts to break metabolic vicious cycles may also contribute to the efficacy of fasting in the treatment of type 2 diabetes and autoimmune disorders." McCarty MF. A preliminary fast may potentiate response to a subsequent low-salt, low-fat vegan diet in the management of hypertension - fasting as a strategy for breaking metabolic vicious cycles. *Med Hypotheses.* 2003 May;60(5):624-33

[84] Ramakrishnan T, Stokes P. Beneficial effects of fasting and low carbohydrate diet in D-lactic acidosis associated with short-bowel syndrome. *JPEN J Parenter Enteral Nutr.* 1985 May-Jun;9(3):361-3

[85] Trollmo C, Verdrengh M, Tarkowski A. Fasting enhances mucosal antigen specific B cell responses in rheumatoid arthritis. *Ann Rheum Dis.* 1997 Feb;56(2):130-4 http://ard.bmjjournals.com/cgi/content/full/56/2/130

neutrophils[86], reduces lysozyme release and leukotriene formation[87], and ameliorates intestinal hyperpermeability.[88] In case reports and/or clinical trials, short-term fasting (or protein-sparing fasting) has been documented as safe and effective treatment for SLE[89], RA[90], and non-rheumatic diseases such as chronic severe hypertension[91], moderate hypertension[92], obesity[93,94], type-2 diabetes[95], and epilepsy.[96]

- Broad-spectrum fatty acid therapy with ALA, EPA, DHA, GLA and oleic acid: Fish oil supplementation (especially in combination with a low-fat, low-arachidonate diet[97]) has been shown to help alleviate dermal psoriasis.[98,99,100] Fish oil supplementation has also been shown to protect psoriasis patients against the iatrogenic nephrotoxicity of cyclosporin.[101] Fatty acid supplementation should be delivered in the form of combination therapy with ALA, GLA, DHA, and EPA. Given at doses of 3,000 – 9,000 mg per day, ALA from flax oil has impressive anti-inflammatory benefits demonstrated by its ability to halve prostaglandin production in humans.[102] Numerous studies have demonstrated the benefit of GLA in the treatment of

---

[86] "An association was found between improvement in inflammatory activity of the joints and enhancement of neutrophil bactericidal capacity. Fasting appears to improve the clinical status of patients with RA." Uden AM, Trang L, Venizelos N, Palmblad J. Neutrophil functions and clinical performance after total fasting in patients with rheumatoid arthritis. *Ann Rheum Dis.* 1983 Feb;42(1):45-51

[87] "We thus conclude that a reduced ability to generate cytotaxins, reduced release of enzyme, and reduced leukotriene formation from RA neutrophils, together with an altered fatty acid composition of membrane phospholipids, may be mechanisms for the decrease of inflammatory symptoms that results from fasting." Hafstrom I, Ringertz B, Gyllenhammar H, Palmblad J, Harms-Ringdahl M. Effects of fasting on disease activity, neutrophil function, fatty acid composition, and leukotriene biosynthesis in patients with rheumatoid arthritis. *Arthritis Rheum.* 1988 May;31(5):585-92

[88] "The results indicate that, unlike lactovegetarian diet, fasting may ameliorate the disease activity and reduce both the intestinal and the non-intestinal permeability in rheumatoid arthritis." Sundqvist T, Lindstrom F, Magnusson KE, Skoldstam L, Stjernstrom I, Tagesson C. Influence of fasting on intestinal permeability and disease activity in patients with rheumatoid arthritis. *Scand J Rheumatol.* 1982;11(1):33-8

[89] Fuhrman J, Sarter B, Calabro DJ. Brief case reports of medically supervised, water-only fasting associated with remission of autoimmune disease. *Altern Ther Health Med.* 2002 Jul-Aug;8(4):112, 110-1

[90] "An association was found between improvement in inflammatory activity of the joints and enhancement of neutrophil bactericidal capacity. Fasting appears to improve the clinical status of patients with RA." Uden AM, Trang L, Venizelos N, Palmblad J. Neutrophil functions and clinical performance after total fasting in patients with rheumatoid arthritis. *Ann Rheum Dis.* 1983 Feb;42(1):45-51

[91] "The average reduction in blood pressure was 37/13 mm Hg, with the greatest decrease being observed for subjects with the most severe hypertension. Patients with stage 3 hypertension (those with systolic blood pressure greater than 180 mg Hg, diastolic blood pressure greater than 110 mg Hg, or both) had an average reduction of 60/17 mm Hg at the conclusion of treatment." Goldhamer A, Lisle D, Parpia B, Anderson SV, Campbell TC. Medically supervised water-only fasting in the treatment of hypertension. *J Manipulative Physiol Ther.* 2001 Jun;24(5):335-9 http://www.healthpromoting.com/335-339Goldhamer115263.QXD.pdf

[92] "RESULTS: Approximately 82% of the subjects achieved BP at or below 120/80 mm Hg by the end of the treatment program. The mean BP reduction was 20/7 mm Hg, with the greatest decrease being observed for subjects with the highest baseline BP." Goldhamer AC, Lisle DJ, Sultana P, Anderson SV, Parpia B, Hughes B, Campbell TC. Medically supervised water-only fasting in the treatment of borderline hypertension. J Altern Complement Med. 2002 Oct;8(5):643-50 http://www.healthpromoting.com/Articles/articles/study%202/acmpaper5.pdf

[93] Vertes V, Genuth SM, Hazelton IM. Supplemented fasting as a large-scale outpatient program. *JAMA.* 1977 Nov 14;238(20):2151-3

[94] Bauman WA, Schwartz E, Rose HG, Eisenstein HN, Johnson DW. Early and long-term effects of acute caloric deprivation in obese diabetic patients. *Am J Med.* 1988 Jul;85(1):38-46

[95] Goldhamer AC. Initial cost of care results in medically supervised water-only fasting for treating high blood pressure and diabetes. J Altern Complement Med. 2002 Dec;8(6):696-7 http://www.healthpromoting.com/Articles/pdf/Study%2032.pdf

[96] "The ketogenic diet should be considered as alternative therapy for children with difficult-to-control seizures. It is more effective than many of the new anticonvulsant medications and is well tolerated by children and families when it is effective." Freeman JM, Vining EP, Pillas DJ, Pyzik PL, Casey JC, Kelly LM. The efficacy of the ketogenic diet-1998: a prospective evaluation of intervention in 150 children. *Pediatrics.* 1998 Dec;102(6):1358-63 http://pediatrics.aappublications.org/cgi/reprint/102/6/1358

[97] "Moderate or excellent improvement was observed in 58% of the patients, while mild improvement or no change was observed in 19% and 23%, respectively." Kragballe K, Fogh K. A low-fat diet supplemented with dietary fish oil (Max-EPA) results in improvement of psoriasis and in formation of leukotriene B5. *Acta Derm Venereol* 1989;69(1):23-8

[98] A clinical trial of 13 psoriatic patients: "Global clinical evaluation showed that eight patients demonstrated mild to moderate improvement in their psoriatic lesions. Improved clinical response correlated with high EPA/DCHA ratios attained in epidermal tissue specimens." Ziboh VA, Cohen KA, Ellis CN, Miller C, Hamilton TA, Kragballe K, Hydrick CR, Voorhees JJ. Effects of dietary supplementation of fish oil on neutrophil and epidermal fatty acids. Modulation of clinical course of psoriatic subjects. *Arch Dermatol* 1986 Nov;122(11):1277-82

[99] "Although its effects are modest, it is nontoxic and its favorable effect appears to continue for the duration of its usage, indicating that EPA could be beneficial for the long-term treatment of psoriasis." Kojima T, Terano T, Tanabe E, Okamoto S, Tamura Y, Yoshida S. Long-term administration of highly purified eicosapentaenoic acid provides improvement of psoriasis. *Dermatologica* 1991;182(4):225-30

[100] "In conclusion, modulation of eicosanoid metabolism by intravenous n-3 fatty acid supplementation appears to exert a rapid beneficial effect on inflammatory skin lesions in acute guttate psoriasis." Grimminger F, Mayser P, Papavassilis C, Thomas M, Schlotzer E, Heuer KU, Fuhrer D, Hinsch KD, Walmrath D, Schill WB, et al. A double-blind, randomized, placebo-controlled trial of n-3 fatty acid based lipid infusion in acute, extended guttate psoriasis. Rapid improvement of clinical manifestations and changes in neutrophil leukotriene profile. *Clin Investig* 1993 Aug;71(8):634-43

[101] "The results of this pilot study suggest that fish oil can reduce CyA-associated renal dysfunction in psoriasis patients." Stoof TJ, Korstanje MJ, Bilo HJ, Starink TM, Hulsmans RF, Donker AJ. Does fish oil protect renal function in cyclosporin-treated psoriasis patients? *J Intern Med* 1989 Dec;226(6):437-41

[102] Adam O, Wolfram G, Zollner N. Effect of alpha-linolenic acid in the human diet on linoleic acid metabolism and prostaglandin biosynthesis. *J Lipid Res.* 1986 Apr;27(4):421-6 http://www.jlr.org/cgi/reprint/27/4/421

rheumatoid arthritis when used at doses between 500 mg – 4,000 mg per day.[103,104] Fish oil provides EPA and DHA which have well-proven anti-inflammatory benefits in rheumatoid arthritis[105,106,107] and lupus.[108,109] ALA, EPA, DHA, and GLA need to be provided in the form of supplements; when using high doses of therapeutic oils, liquid supplements that can be mixed in juice or a smoothie are generally more convenient and palatable than capsules. Therapeutic amounts of oleic acid can be obtained from generous use of olive oil, preferably on fresh vegetables. Supplementation with polyunsaturated fatty acids warrants increased intake of antioxidants from diet, fruit and vegetable juices, and properly formulated supplements; since patients with systemic inflammation are generally in a pro-oxidative state, consideration must be given to the timing and starting dose of fatty acid supplementation and the need for anti-oxidant protection. See chapter on *Therapeutics* toward the end of this textbook for more details and biochemical pathways. Clinicians must realize that fatty acids are not clinically or biochemically interchangeable and that one fatty acid does not substitute for another; each of the fatty acids must be supplied in order for its benefits to be obtained.[110]

- <u>Vitamin D3 supplementation with physiologic doses and/or tailored to serum 25(OH)D levels</u>: Vitamin D deficiency is common in the general population and is even more common in patients with chronic illness and chronic musculoskeletal pain.[111] Vitamin D3 can be applied topically and is about as effective as topical steroids in the treatment of psoriatic skin lesions.[112] Correction of vitamin D deficiency supports normal immune function against infection and provides a clinically significant anti-inflammatory[113] and analgesic benefit in patients with back pain[114] and limb pain.[115] Reasonable daily doses for children and adults are 2,000 and 4,000 IU, respectively, as defined by Vasquez, et al.[116] Deficiency and response to treatment are monitored with serum 25(OH)vitamin D while safety is monitored with serum calcium; inflammatory granulomatous diseases and certain drugs such as hydrochlorothiazide greatly increase the propensity for hypercalcemia and warrant increment dosing and frequent monitoring of serum calcium.

[103] "Other results showed a significant reduction in morning stiffness with gamma-linolenic acid at 3 months and reduction in pain and articular index at 6 months with olive oil." Brzeski M, Madhok R, Capell HA. Evening primrose oil in patients with rheumatoid arthritis and side-effects of non-steroidal anti-inflammatory drugs. *Br J Rheumatol*. 1991 Oct;30(5):370-2

[104] Rothman D, DeLuca P, Zurier RB. Botanical lipids: effects on inflammation, immune responses, and rheumatoid arthritis. *Semin Arthritis Rheum*. 1995 Oct;25(2):87-96

[105] Adam O, Beringer C, Kless T, Lemmen C, Adam A, Wiseman M, Adam P, Klimmek R, Forth W. Anti-inflammatory effects of a low arachidonic acid diet and fish oil in patients with rheumatoid arthritis. *Rheumatol Int*. 2003 Jan;23(1):27-36

[106] Lau CS, Morley KD, Belch JJ. Effects of fish oil supplementation on non-steroidal anti-inflammatory drug requirement in patients with mild rheumatoid arthritis--a double-blind placebo controlled study. *Br J Rheumatol*. 1993 Nov;32(11):982-9

[107] Kremer JM, Jubiz W, Michalek A, Rynes RI, Bartholomew LE, Bigaouette J, Timchalk M, Beeler D, Lininger L. Fish-oil fatty acid supplementation in active rheumatoid arthritis. A double-blinded, controlled, crossover study. *Ann Intern Med*. 1987 Apr;106(4):497-503

[108] Walton AJ, Snaith ML, Locniskar M, Cumberland AG, Morrow WJ, Isenberg DA. Dietary fish oil and the severity of symptoms in patients with systemic lupus erythematosus. *Ann Rheum Dis*. 1991 Jul;50(7):463-6

[109] Duffy EM, Meenagh GK, McMillan SA, Strain JJ, Hannigan BM, Bell AL. The clinical effect of dietary supplementation with omega-3 fish oils and/or copper in systemic lupus erythematosus. *J Rheumatol*. 2004 Aug;31(8):1551-6

[110] Vasquez A. Reducing Pain and Inflammation Naturally. Part 2: New Insights into Fatty Acid Supplementation and Its Effect on Eicosanoid Production and Genetic Expression. *Nutritional Perspectives* 2005; January: 5-16 http://optimalhealthresearch.com/part2

[111] Plotnikoff GA, Quigley JM. Prevalence of severe hypovitaminosis D in patients with persistent, nonspecific musculoskeletal pain. *Mayo Clin Proc*. 2003 Dec;78(12):1463-70

[112] Lookingbill DP, Marks JG, eds. <u>Principles of dermatology</u>. Philadelphia: W.B. Saunders, 1986: 141

[113] Timms PM, Mannan N, Hitman GA, Noonan K, Mills PG, Syndercombe-Court D, Aganna E, Price CP, Boucher BJ. Circulating MMP9, vitamin D and variation in the TIMP-1 response with VDR genotype: mechanisms for inflammatory damage in chronic disorders? *QJM*. 2002 Dec;95(12):787-96 http://qjmed.oxfordjournals.org/cgi/content/full/95/12/787

[114] Al Faraj S, Al Mutairi K. Vitamin D deficiency and chronic low back pain in Saudi Arabia. *Spine*. 2003 Jan 15;28(2):177-9

[115] Masood H, Narang AP, Bhat IA, Shah GN. Persistent limb pain and raised serum alkaline phosphatase the earliest markers of subclinical hypovitaminosis D in Kashmir. *Indian J Physiol Pharmacol*. 1989 Oct-Dec;33(4):259-61

[116] Vasquez A, Manso G, Cannell J. The clinical importance of vitamin D (cholecalciferol): a paradigm shift with implications for all healthcare providers. *Altern Ther Health Med*. 2004 Sep-Oct;10(5):28-36 http://optimalhealthresearch.com/monograph04

- Assessment for dysbiosis: All dysbiotic loci should be investigated as discussed previously in this chapter and in greater detail in Chapter 4 of *Integrative Rheumatology* in the section on multifocal dysbiosis. In a very intensive investigation into the role of bacteria, yeast/fungi, and viruses in the pathogenesis of psoriasis, Noah[117] assessed microflora of 297 psoriasis patients by culture and serologic tests. Culture samples for aerobic bacteria, yeast, and dermatophytes were taken from the throat, urine, and skin surfaces from scalp, ears, chest, face, axillary, submammary, umbilical, upper back, inguinal crease, gluteal-fold, perirectal, vaginal, pubis, penis, scrotal, leg, hands, feet, finger, and toenail areas. More than 15 different microbes were causatively associated with exacerbation of psoriasis; this finding is entirely logical and is consistent with the 'idiopathic' nature of the illness and why Koch-indoctrinated researchers and clinicians have failed to understand the microbial contribution to autoimmune/inflammatory diseases. Given that each of the microbes listed (see shaded box on upcoming page) is a *common*—but not necessarily *optimal*—inhabitant of human surfaces and orifices, it is possible to see how their synergism *particularly in a genetically susceptible patient with hormonal imbalances*

Microorganisms causally associated with psoriasis:
1. Streptococcal groups A (including *Streptococcus pyogenes*), B, C, D, F, G, *S viridans*, *S pneumoniae*
2. *Klebsiella pneumoniae, oxytoca*
3. *Escherichia coli*
4. *Enterobacter cloacae, E aerogenes, E agglomerans*
5. *Proteus mirabilis, P vulgaris*
6. *Citrobacter freundii, C diversus*
7. *Morganella morganii*
8. *Pseudomonas aeruginosa, P maltiphilia, P putida*
9. *Serratia marcescens*
10. *Acinetobacter calbio aceticus, A luoffi*
11. *Flavobacterium* species
12. CDC groups Ve-1, Ve-2, E-o2
13. *Bacillus subtilis, B cereus*
14. *Staphylococcus aureus*
15. *Candida albicans, C parapsilosis*
16. *Torulopsis/Candida glabrata*
17. *Rhodotorula spp.*
18. *H. pylori**
See Noah P. The role of microorganisms in psoriasis. *Semin Dermatol.* 1990;9:269 * Qayoom S, Ahmad QM. Psoriasis and helicobacter pylori. *Indian J Dermatol Venereol Leprol* 2003;69:133-134

and a proinflammatory lifestyle/diet could tip the scales in favor of systemic inflammation and the picture/illusion of autoimmunity. Of the more than 15 categories/subspecies listed as causative microbes, what if only seven of these common "commensals" were present in a systemically-genetically-nutritionally-hormonally-emotionally predisposed patient, and each contributed only 5% to the pathophysiology of a patient's psoriasis? We would have already arrived at 35% of the psoriatic pathogenesis, leaving 10% each for hormones, diet, allergy, nutrition, xenobiotic accumulation (present in everyone[118,119]). While these numbers and percentages are purely speculative, I left 15% for "idiopathic" to keep researchers and clinicians alert to new possibilities and to placate the therapeutic and epidemiologic nihilists that have so far dominated the field of rheumatology with their "unknown cause" rhetoric. Each cause—each contributor to disease—may in itself be "clinically insignificant" but when additive and synergistic influences coalesce, we find ourselves confronted with an "idiopathic disease" and the decision to choose between the only two available options: 1) despair in the failure of our "one cause, one disease, one drug" paradigm, or 2) appreciate that numerous

---

[117] Noah PW. The role of microorganisms in psoriasis. *Semin Dermatol.* 1990 Dec;9(4):269-76
[118] "Although the use of HCB as a fungicide has virtually been eliminated, detectable levels of HCB are still found in nearly all people in the USA." Robinson PE, et al. An evaluation of hexachlorobenzene body-burden levels in the general population of the USA. *IARC Sci Publ* 1986;77:183-92
[119] "Many U.S. residents carry toxic pesticides in their bodies above government assessed "acceptable" levels." Pesticide Action Network North America (PANNA). Chemical Trespass: Pesticides in Our Bodies and Corporate Accountability. panna.org/campaigns/docsTrespass/chemicalTrespass2004.dv.html

influences work together to disrupt physiologic function and produce the biologic dysfunction that we experience as disease.

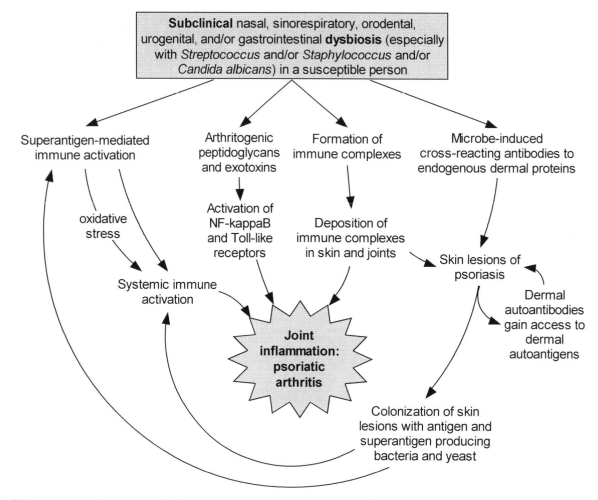

Microbes and Mechanistic Pathways in Psoriatogenic Multifocal Dysbiosis

    o   <u>Sinorespiratory/nasopharyngeal and dermal dysbiosis</u>: Sinorespiratory and dermal dysbiosis in patients with psoriasis is *qualitatively* (increased prevalence in psoriatics compared with healthy controls) and *quantitatively* (increased prevalence of toxin-producing strains compared to those found in controls) associated with the severity of the disease.[120] Patients with psoriasis show an increased rate of nasal/dermal colonization with *Staphylococcus aureus*[121,122], a microbe known to produce several powerfully inflammatory antigens, toxins, and superantigens, and nasal colonization

---

[120] "In this study, S aureus was present in more than 50% of patients with AD and PS. We found that the severity of AD and PS significantly correlated to enterotoxin production of the isolated S aureus strains." Tomi NS, Kranke B, Aberer E. Staphylococcal toxins in patients with psoriasis, atopic dermatitis, and erythroderma, and in healthy control subjects. *J Am Acad Dermatol.* 2005 Jul;53(1):67-72

[121] "In this study, S aureus was present in more than 50% of patients with AD and PS. We found that the severity of AD and PS significantly correlated to enterotoxin production of the isolated S aureus strains." Tomi NS, Kranke B, Aberer E. Staphylococcal toxins in patients with psoriasis, atopic dermatitis, and erythroderma, and in healthy control subjects. *J Am Acad Dermatol.* 2005 Jul;53(1):67-72

[122] "The nasal carriage rate of Staphylococcus aureus in psoriatics was higher than the control groups." Singh G, Rao DJ. Bacteriology of psoriatic plaques. *Dermatologica.* 1978;157(1):21-7

with which appears causally associated with the inflammatory/autoimmune disorder Wegener's granulomatosis.[123,124] A study by Bartenjev et al[125] showed that subclinical streptococcal/staphylococcal infections were detected in 68% of psoriasis patients and in only 11 % of the control group; these authors encouraged searching for and eliminating microbial infections as an important aspect of the management of psoriasis. Supportively, other researchers[126] have found that infection with *S pyogenes* can initiate and/or exacerbate guttate psoriasis; therefore streptococcal throat infections should be treated assertively and early to avoid triggering an exacerbation of psoriasis.[127] *Streptococcus pyogenes* is a very likely trigger of psoriasis[128]; chronic penicillin treatment leads to clinical improvement of recalcitrant psoriasis.[129] Patients with guttate psoriasis have increased oropharyngeal colonization with *Streptococcus hemolyticus* compared with controls.[130] Similar to Behcet's disease[131], the dermal lesions of psoriasis are commonly colonized by proinflammatory microbes including *Staphylococcus aureus*.[132] More conclusively, research by Villeda-Gabriel et al[133] and Perez-Lorenzo et al[134] has clearly shown that antibodies against *Streptococcus pyogenes* cross-react (perhaps via

---

[123] Brons RH, Bakker HI, Van Wijk RT, Van Dijk NW, Muller Kobold AC, Limburg PC, Manson WL, Kallenberg CG, Tervaert JW. Staphylococcal acid phosphatase binds to endothelial cells via charge interaction; a pathogenic role in Wegener's granulomatosis? *Clin Exp Immunol*. 2000 Mar;119(3):566-73 http://www.blackwell-synergy.com/doi/abs/10.1046/j.1365-2249.2000.01172.x

[124] Popa ER, Stegeman CA, Kallenberg CG, Tervaert JW. Staphylococcus aureus and Wegener's granulomatosis. *Arthritis Res*. 2002;4(2):77-9 http://arthritis-research.com/content/4/2/77

[125] "Subclinical streptococcal and/or staphylococcal infections were detected in 68 % of tested patients and in only 11 % of the control group. The results of this study indicate that subclinical bacterial infections of the upper respiratory tract may be an important factor in provoking a new relapse of chronic plaque psoriasis. Searching for, and eliminating, microbial infections could be of importance in the treatment of psoriasis." Bartenjev I, Rogl Butina M, Potocnik M. Subclinical microbial infection in patients with chronic plaque psoriasis. *Acta Derm Venereol Suppl* (Stockh). 2000;(211):17-8

[126] "CONCLUSIONS--This study confirms the strong association between prior infection with S pyogenes and guttate psoriasis but suggests that the ability to trigger guttate psoriasis is not serotype specific." Telfer NR, Chalmers RJ, Whale K, Colman G. The role of streptococcal infection in the initiation of guttate psoriasis. *Arch Dermatol*. 1992 Jan;128(1):39-42

[127] "CONCLUSIONS: This study confirms anecdotal and retrospective reports that streptococcal throat infections can cause exacerbation of chronic plaque psoriasis." Gudjonsson JE, Thorarinsson AM, Sigurgeirsson B, Kristinsson KG, Valdimarsson H. Streptococcal throat infections and exacerbation of chronic plaque psoriasis: a prospective study. *Br J Dermatol*. 2003 Sep;149(3):530-4

[128] "These findings justify the hypothesis that S pyogenes infections are more important in the pathogenesis of chronic plaque psoriasis than has previously been recognized, and indicate the need for further controlled therapeutic trials of antibacterial measures in this common skin disease." El-Rachkidy RG, Hales JM, Freestone PP, Young HS, Griffiths CE, Camp RD. Increased Blood Levels of IgG Reactive with Secreted Streptococcus pyogenes Proteins in Chronic Plaque Psoriasis. *J Invest Dermatol*. 2007 Mar 8; [Epub ahead of print]

[129] "Total duration of the study was two years. Initially benzathine penicillin 1.2 million units, was given I.M. AST fortnightly. After 24 weeks benzathine penicillin was reduced to 1.2 million units once a month... Significant improvement in the PASI score was noted from 12 weeks onwards. All patients showed excellent improvement at 2 years." Saxena VN, Dogra J. Long-term use of penicillin for the treatment of chronic plaque psoriasis. *Eur J Dermatol*. 2005 Sep-Oct;15(5):359-62 http://www.john-libbey-eurotext.fr/en/revues/medecine/ejd/e-docs/00/04/10/A4/article.md?type=text.html

[130] "A high incidence of Streptococcus hemolyticus culture was observed in the guttate psoriatic group compared with the plaque psoriasis and control groups." Zhao G, Feng X, Na A, Yongqiang J, Cai Q, Kong J, Ma H. Acute guttate psoriasis patients have positive streptococcus hemolyticus throat cultures and elevated antistreptococcal M6 protein titers. *J Dermatol*. 2005;32(2):91-6

[131] "At least one type of microorganism was grown from each pustule. Staphylococcus aureus (41/70, 58.6%, p = 0.008) and Prevotella spp (17/70, 24.3%, p = 0.002) were significantly more common in pustules from BS patients, and coagulase negative staphylococci (17/37, 45.9%, p = 0.007) in pustules from acne patients. CONCLUSIONS: The pustular lesions of BS are not usually sterile." Hatemi G, Bahar H, Uysal S, Mat C, Gogus F, Masatlioglu S, Altas K, Yazici H. The pustular skin lesions in Behcet's syndrome are not sterile. *Ann Rheum Dis*. 2004 Nov;63(11):1450-2

[132] "In this study, S aureus was present in more than 50% of patients with AD and PS. We found that the severity of AD and PS significantly correlated to enterotoxin production of the isolated S aureus strains." Tomi NS, Kranke B, Aberer E. Staphylococcal toxins in patients with psoriasis, atopic dermatitis, and erythroderma, and in healthy control subjects. *J Am Acad Dermatol*. 2005 Jul;53(1):67-72

[133] "The recognition by immunoblot of streptococcal antigens by serum of guttate psoriasis patients, the presence of autoantibodies against their own skin, and recognition of the same skin antigens by anti-streptococcal rabbit antibodies confirm the participation of the immune system and of streptococcal infections in guttate psoriasis." Villeda-Gabriel G, Santamaria-Cogollos LC, Perez-Lorenzo R, Reyes-Maldonado E, Saul A, Jurado-Santacruz F, Jimenez-Zamudio L, Garcia-Latorre E. Recognition of Streptococcus pyogenes and skin autoantigens in guttate psoriasis. *Arch Med Res*. 1998 Summer;29(2):143-8

[134] "It seems that autoantibodies, although they do not appear to participate in the pathogenesis of psoriasis, are an important feature, and that skin antigens, which appear in lesional immature keratinocytes, cross-react with S. pyogenes and contribute to the autoimmune process in psoriasis." Perez-Lorenzo R, Zambrano-Zaragoza JF, Saul A, Jimenez-Zamudio L, Reyes-Maldonado E, Garcia-Latorre E. Autoantibodies to autologous skin in guttate and plaque forms of psoriasis and cross-reaction of skin antigens with streptococcal antigens. *Int J Dermatol*. 1998 Jul;37(7):524-31. The authors found that all psoriais paitents had dermal autoantiboes and that these antibodies reacted specifically with endogenous dermal antigens; thus their finding that "Deposits of immunoglobulin G (IgG) were not detected in the lesions" is unexpected and inexplicable. This statement from their research is inconsistent with the findings of other research groups, and—specifically—must be placed in a context of other articles, most notably "... titers of IgG anti-SC autoantibodies in psoriatic patients were not specifically higher than in normal controls but were more variable, indicating that their circulating levels are dependent on a delicate balance between consumption at inflammatory sites and a secondary increase due to SC-antigen release following inflammation." Tagami H, Iwatsuki K, Yamada M. Profile of anti-stratum corneum autoantibodies in psoriatic patients. *Arch Dermatol Res*. 1983;275(2):71-5

molecular mimicry or epitope spreading) with dermal antigens; additionally, the work of Muto et al[135] showed that antibodies against streptococcal cell wall proteins could bind with nuclei and cytoplasm of cells from skin and synovium. Thus, psoriasis is indeed a microbe-induced autoimmune disease by virtue of these cross-reacting endogenous antibodies that bind with nuclear, dermal, and articular antigens. Patients with psoriasis have elevated serum levels of antibodies against streptococcal M12 protein[136], and patients with psoriatic arthritis have a heightened inflammatory response to staphylococcal superantigens.[137]

o Gastrointestinal dysbiosis: All patients with psoriatic arthritis should be considered to have gastrointestinal dysbiosis until proven otherwise. A three-sample comprehensive parasitology examination performed by a specialty laboratory is strongly recommended as a minimal component of basic care. In lieu of a comprehensive parasitology test, patients can be treated for 4-8 weeks with broad-spectrum antimicrobial treatment that is effective against gram-positive and gram-negative bacteria, aerobes and anaerobes, yeast, protozoa and amebas. For additional details, see the Section on *multifocal dysbiosis* in Chapter 4 of *Integrative Rheumatology*. Patients with psoriasis have shown a greatly increased prevalence of *H. pylori*[138] and *Candida albicans*[139] and *Geotrichum candidum*.[140]

o Antimicrobial treatments for (gastrointestinal) dysbiosis commonly include but are not limited to the following: Doses listed are for adults. Combination therapy generally allows for lower doses of each intervention to be used. Severe dysbiosis often requires weeks or months of treatment. Drugs are not necessarily more effective than natural treatments; in fact, often the botanicals work when the pharmaceuticals do not.

> ▪ Oregano oil: Emulsified oil of oregano in a time-released tablet is proven effective in the eradication of harmful gastrointestinal microbes, including *Blastocystis hominis*, *Entamoeba hartmanni*, and *Endolimax*

Emulsified time-released oil of oregano against gastrointestinal dysbiosis
"After 6 weeks of supplementation with 600 mg emulsified oil of oregano daily, there was complete disappearance of *Entamoeba hartmanni* (four cases), *Endolimax nana* (one case), and *Blastocystis hominis* in eight cases. Also, *Blastocystis hominis* scores declined in three additional cases. Gastrointestinal symptoms improved in seven of the 11 patients who had tested positive for *Blastocystis hominis*."
Force M, Sparks WS, Ronzio RA. Inhibition of enteric parasites by emulsified oil of oregano in vivo. *Phytother Res*. 2000 May

[135] "Monoclonal antibodies directed against type 12 Group A streptococcal cell wall antigens cross-react with nuclei and cytoplasm of cells from skin and synovium from controls, uninvolved skin of psoriatics and psoriatic plaques." Muto M, Fujikura Y, Hamamoto Y, Ichimiya M, Ohmura A, Sasazuki T, Fukumoto T, Asagami C. Immune response to Streptococcus pyogenes and the susceptibility to psoriasis. *Australas J Dermatol*. 1996 May;37 Suppl 1:S54-5
[136] "Patients with psoriasis had high serum titres of antibody against the M12 (C-region) streptococcal antigen compared to controls." Muto M, Fujikura Y, Hamamoto Y, Ichimiya M, Ohmura A, Sasazuki T, Fukumoto T, Asagami C. Immune response to Streptococcus pyogenes and the susceptibility to psoriasis. *Australas J Dermatol*. 1996 May;37 Suppl 1:S54-5
[137] "Our data raised the possibility that staphylococcal superantigens may also play an exacerbating role in PA." Yamamoto T, Katayama I, Nishioka K. Peripheral blood mononuclear cell proliferative response against staphylococcal superantigens in patients with psoriasis arthropathy. *Eur J Dermatol*. 1999 Jan-Feb;9(1):17-21 http://www.john-libbey-eurotext.fr/en/revues/medecine/ejd/e-docs/00/01/87/C8/resume.md
[138] "In the current study, 20 (40%), psoriatic patients and 5 (10%) patients of control group demonstrated H. pylori antibodies... Although our study supports a causal role of H. pylori in the pathogenesis of psoriasis, a large scale study is needed to confirm the findings." Qayoom S, Ahmad QM. Psoriasis and helicobacter pylori. *Indian J Dermatol Venereol Leprol* 2003;69:133-134 http://www.ijdvl.com/
[139] "Our results reinforce the hypothesis that C. albicans is one of the triggers to both exacerbation and persistence of psoriasis. We propose that in psoriatics with a significant quantity of Candida in faeces, an antifungal treatment should be considered as an adjuvant treatment of psoriasis." Waldman A, Gilhar A, Duek L, Berdicevsky I. Incidence of Candida in psoriasis--a study on the fungal flora of psoriatic patients. *Mycoses*. 2001 May;44(3-4):77-8
[140] Candida albicans (and other yeasts) was detected in 68% of psoriatics, 70% of eczematics, 54% of the controls. Qualitative analysis revealed a predominance of Candida albicans. Geotrichum candidum occurred in 22% of psoriatics, 10% of eczematics, and 3% of controls. Buslau M, Menzel I, Holzmann H. Fungal flora of human faeces in psoriasis and atopic dermatitis. *Mycoses*. 1990 Feb;33(2):90-4

nana.[141] An *in vitro* study[142] and clinical experience support the use of emulsified oregano against *Candida albicans* and various bacteria. The common dose is 600 mg per day in divided doses for 6 weeks.[143]

- Berberine: Berberine is an alkaloid found in *Hydrastis canadensis* (goldenseal), *Coptis chinensis* (Coptis, goldenthread), *Berberis/Mahonia aquifolium* (Oregon grape), *Berberis vulgaris* (barberry), and *Berberis aristata* (tree turmeric)[144], and it shows effectiveness against *Giardia, Candida,* and *Streptococcus* in addition to its direct anti-inflammatory and antidiarrheal actions. Oral dose of 400-800 mg per day in divided doses is common for adults.[145] Berberine-containing botanicals may provide additional benefit in the treatment of psoriatic disease due to the antiproliferative[146] and anti-inflammatory/antileukotriene[147] characteristics of berberine and other phytoconstituents. Berberine-containing plants have also been traditionally used for jaundice, an application supported by a recent animal study showing increased bilirubin excretion in rats following berberine administration.[148] Topical *Berberis/Mahonia* is effective for dermal psoriasis.[149]

- *Artemisia annua*: Artemisinin has been safely used for centuries in Asia for the treatment of malaria, and it also has effectiveness against anaerobic bacteria due to the pro-oxidative sesquiterpene endoperoxide.[150,151] I commonly use artemisinin at 200 mg per day in divided doses for adults with dysbiosis.

- St. John's Wort (*Hypericum perforatum*): *Hypericum* may prove to be an useful botanical for the treatment of psoriasis due to the combination of its antidepressant and antimicrobial benefits. Hyperforin from *Hypericum perforatum* also shows impressive antibacterial action, particularly against gram-positive bacteria such as *Staphylococcus aureus, Streptococcus pyogenes, Streptococcus agalactiae*[152] and perhaps *Helicobacter pylori*.[153] Up to 600 mg three times per day of a 3% hyperforin standardized extract is customary in the treatment of depression.

---

[141] Force M, Sparks WS, Ronzio RA. Inhibition of enteric parasites by emulsified oil of oregano in vivo. *Phytother Res*. 2000 May;14(3):213-4

[142] Stiles JC, Sparks W, Ronzio RA. The inhibition of Candida albicans by oregano. *J Applied Nutr* 1995;47:96–102

[143] Force M, Sparks WS, Ronzio RA. Inhibition of enteric parasites by emulsified oil of oregano in vivo. *Phytother Res*. 2000 May;14(3):213-4

[144] [No authors listed] Berberine. *Altern Med Rev*. 2000 Apr;5(2):175-7 http://www.thorne.com/altmedrev/.fulltext/5/2/175.pdf

[145] [No authors listed] Berberine. *Altern Med Rev*. 2000 Apr;5(2):175-7 http://www.thorne.com/altmedrev/.fulltext/5/2/175.pdf

[146] "The extract of the bark of Mahonia aquifolium is an inhibitor of keratinocyte growth with an IC50 of 35 microM. Of its main alkaloids tested, berberine inhibited cell growth to the same extent as did the Mahonia extract, while the benzylisoquinoline alkaloids berbamine and oxyacanthine were more potent inhibitors by a factor of three." Muller K, Ziereis K, Gawlik I. The antipsoriatic *Mahonia aquifolium* and its active constituents; II. Antiproliferative activity against cell growth of human keratinocytes. *Planta Med* 1995 Feb;61(1):74-

[147] "Inhibition of lipoxygenase by these compounds may contribute to the therapeutic effect of M. aquifolium extracts in the treatment of psoriasis." Misik V, Bezakova L, Malekova L, Kostalova D. Lipoxygenase inhibition and antioxidant properties of protoberberine and aporphine alkaloids isolated from Mahonia aquifolium. *Planta Med* 1995 Aug;61(4):372-3

[148] "Acute doses of berberine were found to increase the secretion of bilirubin in experimental hyperbilirubinemia without affecting the UDP-glucuronyltransferase activity and BSP clearance. Continuous treatment abolished this effect. This apparent tolerance could be attributed to the inhibitory action of chronic berberine treatment on UDP-glucuronyltransferase activity..." Chan MY. The effect of berberine on bilirubin excretion in the rat. *Comp Med East West*. 1977 Summer;5(2):161-8

[149] "Taken together, these clinical studies conducted by several investigators in several countries indicate that Mahonia aquifolium is a safe and effective treatment of patients with mild to moderate psoriasis." Gulliver WP, Donsky HJ. A report on three recent clinical trials using Mahonia aquifolium 10% topical cream and a review of the worldwide clinical experience with Mahonia aquifolium for the treatment of plaque psoriasis. *Am J Ther*. 2005 Sep-Oct;12:398-406

[150] Dien TK, de Vries PJ, Khanh NX, Koopmans R, Binh LN, Duc DD, Kager PA, van Boxtel CJ. Effect of food intake on pharmacokinetics of oral artemisinin in healthy Vietnamese subjects. *Antimicrob Agents Chemother*. 1997 May;41(5):1069-72

[151] Giao PT, Binh TQ, Kager PA, Long HP, Van Thang N, Van Nam N, de Vries PJ. Artemisinin for treatment of uncomplicated falciparum malaria: is there a place for monotherapy? *Am J Trop Med Hyg*. 2001 Dec;65(6):690-5

[152] Schempp CM, Pelz K, Wittmer A, Schopf E, Simon JC. Antibacterial activity of hyperforin from St John's wort, against multiresistant Staphylococcus aureus and gram-positive bacteria. *Lancet*. 1999 Jun 19;353(9170):2129

[153] "A butanol fraction of St. John's Wort revealed anti-Helicobacter pylori activity with MIC values ranging between 15.6 and 31.2 microg/ml." Reichling J, Weseler A, Saller R. A current review of the antimicrobial activity of Hypericum perforatum L. *Pharmacopsychiatry*. 2001 Jul;34 Suppl 1:S116-8

- **Bismuth**: Bismuth is commonly used in the empiric treatment of diarrhea (e.g., "Pepto-<u>Bis</u>mol") and is commonly combined with other antimicrobial agents to reduce drug resistance and increase antibiotic effectiveness.[154]
- <u>Undecylenic acid</u>: Derived from castor bean oil, undecylenic acid has antifungal properties and is commonly indicated by sensitivity results obtained by stool culture. Common dosages are 150-250 mg tid (up to 750 mg per day).[155]
- <u>Peppermint</u> *(Mentha piperita)*: Peppermint shows antimicrobial and antispasmodic actions and has demonstrated clinical effectiveness in patients with bacterial overgrowth of the small bowel.
- <u>Probiotics</u>: Live cultures in the form of tablets, capsules, yogurt, or kefir can be used per patient preference and tolerance. Obviously, dairy-based products should be avoided by patients with dairy allergy.
- <u>Supplemented Paleo-Mediterranean diet / specific carbohydrate diet</u>: The specifications of the specific carbohydrate diet detailed by Gottschall[156] are met with adherence to the Paleo diet by Cordain.[157] The combination of both approaches and books will give patients an excellent combination of informational understanding and culinary versatility. By now, clinicians should appreciate that part of any antimicrobial plan is immunorestoration via nutritional repletion

> **Microbial antigens evoke psoriasis and autoimmunity**
>
> "RESULTS: The predicted microbial product appeared heavily in lesional epidermis, but unexpectedly also as a thin deposit along the skin basement membrane zone (SBMZ) of apparently unaffected skin. Staining was negative for nonpsoriatic subjects. CONCLUSIONS: The findings support a direct effect of microbial antigen in psoriasis."
>
> Noah PW, Handorf CR, Skinner RB Jr, Mandrell TD, Rosenberg EW. Skin basement membrane zone: a depository for circulating microbial antigen evoking psoriasis and autoimmunity. *Skinmed.* 2006 Mar-Apr;5(2):72-9

and avoidance of diet-induced immunosuppression; as I have said many times in my seminars, "The most effective 'antibiotic' ever discovered is the human immune system; if you can restore its function, then the patient has a chance to clear the infection/dysbiosis that is triggering the systemic inflammation without the use of or with less reliance upon antibiotic drugs."

- <u>Topical antimicrobials</u>: Treating the dermal lesions of psoriatic arthritis may help break the vicious cycles of (super)antigen absorption which perpetuates immune dysfunction. A variety of botanical and pharmaceutical creams are available. *In vitro* evidence supports the use of equal parts honey, olive oil, and beeswax against *Staph aureus* and *Candida albicans*.[158] As mentioned previously, topical

---

[154] Veldhuyzen van Zanten SJ, Sherman PM, Hunt RH. Helicobacter pylori: new developments and treatments. *CMAJ.* 1997;156(11):1565-74 http://www.cmaj.ca/cgi/reprint/156/11/1565.pdf
[155] "Adult dosage is usually 450-750 mg undecylenic acid daily in three divided doses." Undecylenic acid. Monograph. *Altern Med Rev.* 2002 Feb;7(1):68-70 http://www.thorne.com/altmedrev/.fulltext/7/1/68.pdf
[156] Gotschall E. <u>Breaking the Vicious Cycle: Intestinal health though diet</u>. Kirkton Press; Rev edition (August, 1994) http://www.scdiet.com/ http://www.breakingtheviciouscycle.info/
[157] Cordain L: <u>The Paleo Diet: Lose weight and get healthy by eating the food you were designed to eat</u>. John Wiley & Sons Inc., New York 2002 http://thepaleodiet.com/
[158] "Honey, beeswax and olive oil mixture (1:1:1, v/v) is useful in the treatment of diaper dermatitis, psoriasis and eczema... CONCLUSIONS: Honey and honey mixture apparently could inhibit growth of S. aureus or C. albicans." Al-Waili NS. Mixture of honey, beeswax and olive oil inhibits growth of Staphylococcus aureus and Candida albicans. *Arch Med Res.* 2005 Jan-Feb;36(1):10-3

Mahonia/Berberis is effective for dermal psoriasis.[159] A topical gel containing artemesinin is also available for clinical use, and animal studies have demonstrated systemic absorption from topical application[160]; its use in humans with psoriasis has not been studied. Topical honey is better than acyclovir against oral and genital herpes; apply *qid* for 15 minutes.[161]

Antimicrobial treatment for psoriasis

"Patients are questioned, examined, and subjected to microbiologic laboratory investigations in an attempt to identify possibly relevant microorganisms, and then are treated with antibiotics. ... Results obtained with this approach compare favorably with those achieved with more usual anti-psoriasis treatments. We recommend that a microbiologic investigation and a trial of antimicrobial treatment should precede any plan to treat psoriasis patients with anything more than the simplest topical agents."

Rosenberg EW, Noah PW, Skinner RB Jr. Microorganisms and psoriasis. *J Natl Med Assoc.* 1994 Apr;86(4):305-10

- **Commonly used antibiotic/antifungal drugs**: The most commonly employed drugs for intestinal bacterial overgrowth are described here.[162] Treatment duration is generally at least 2 weeks and up to 8 weeks, depending on clinical response and the severity and diversity of the intestinal overgrowth. With all anti*bacterial* treatments, use empiric anti*fungal* treatment to prevent yeast overgrowth; some patients benefit from antifungal treatment that is continued for *months* and occasionally *years*. Drugs can generally be coadministered with natural antibiotics/antifungals for improved efficacy. Treatment can be guided by identification of the dysbiotic microbes and the results of culture and sensitivity tests.
  - Penicillin: Chronic penicillin treatment leads to clinical improvement of recalcitrant psoriasis; benefits are seen when treatment is continued for at least 12 weeks, according to a clinical trial of treatment lasting for two years.[163]
  - Metronidazole: 250-500 mg BID-QID (generally limit to 1.5 g/d); metronidazole has systemic bioavailability and effectiveness against a wide range of dysbiotic microbes, including protozoans, amebas/Giardia, *H. pylori*, *Clostridium difficile* and most anaerobic gram-negative bacilli.[164] Adverse effects are generally limited to stomatitis, nausea, diarrhea, and—rarely and/or with long-term use—peripheral neuropathy, dizziness, and metallic taste; the drug must not be consumed with alcohol. Metronidazole resistance by *Blastocystis hominis* and other parasites has been noted.

---

[159] "Taken together, these clinical studies conducted by several investigators in several countries indicate that Mahonia aquifolium is a safe and effective treatment of patients with mild to moderate psoriasis." Gulliver WP, Donsky HJ. A report on three recent clinical trials using Mahonia aquifolium 10% topical cream and a review of the worldwide clinical experience with Mahonia aquifolium for the treatment of plaque psoriasis. *Am J Ther.* 2005 Sep-Oct;12:398-406
[160] "This paper reports results of pharmacokinetic studies of this preparation when applied onto a fixed area of the shaved skin of mice and rabbits. ..The drug was found to be easily absorbed from the skin." Zhao KC, Xuan WY, Zhao Y, Song ZY. [The pharmacokinetics of a transdermal preparation of artesunate in mice and rabbits] [Article in Chinese] Yao Xue Xue Bao. 1989;24(11):813-6
[161] Al-Waili NS. Topical honey application vs. acyclovir for the treatment of recurrent herpes simplex lesions. *Med Sci Monit.* 2004 Aug;10(8):MT94-8. Epub 2004 Jul 23 http://www.medscimonit.com/pub/vol_10/no_8/4431.pdf
[162] Saltzman JR, Russell RM. Nutritional consequences of intestinal bacterial overgrowth. *Compr Ther.* 1994;20(9):523-30
[163] "Total duration of the study was two years. Initially benzathine penicillin 1.2 million units, was given I.M. AST fortnightly. After 24 weeks benzathine penicillin was reduced to 1.2 million units once a month... Significant improvement in the PASI score was noted from 12 weeks onwards. All patients showed excellent improvement at 2 years." Saxena VN, Dogra J. Long-term use of penicillin for the treatment of chronic plaque psoriasis. *Eur J Dermatol.* 2005 Sep-Oct;15(5):359-62 http://www.john-libbey-eurotext.fr/en/revues/medecine/ejd/e-docs/00/04/10/A4/article.md?type=text.html
[164] Tierney ML. McPhee SJ, Papadakis MA. Current Medical Diagnosis and Treatment 2006. 45th edition. New York; Lange Medical: 2006, pages 1578-1577

- ◆ Erythromycin: 250-500 mg TID-QID; this drug is a widely used antibiotic that also has intestinal promotility benefits (thus making it an ideal treatment for intestinal bacterial overgrowth associated with or caused by intestinal dysmotility/hypomotility such as seen in scleroderma[165,166]). Do not combine erythromycin with the promotility drug cisapride due to risk for serious cardiac arrhythmia.

Long-term penicillin for psoriasis
"Significant improvement in the PASI score was noted from 12 weeks onwards. All patients showed excellent improvement at 2 years. Patients tolerated the therapy well. Controlled studies are needed to further confirm the benefits of long-term use of benzathine penicillin in the treatment of psoriasis."   Saxena VN, Dogra J. Long-term use of penicillin for the treatment of chronic plaque psoriasis. *Eur J Dermatol.* 2005 Sep-Oct

- ◆ Tetracycline:
- ◆ Ciprofloxacin: An effective antimicrobial agent increasingly shunned due to its induction of tendonopathy.
- ◆ Cephalexin/Keflex:
- ◆ Minocycline: Minocycline (200 mg/day)[167] has received the most attention in the treatment of rheumatoid arthritis due to its superior response (65%) over placebo (13%)[168]; in addition to its antibacterial action, the drug is also immunomodulatory and anti-inflammatory. Ironically, minocycline can cause drug-induced autoimmunity, especially lupus.[169,170]
- ◆ Nystatin: Nystatin 500,000 units bid with food; duration of treatment begins with a minimum duration of 2-4 weeks and may continue as long as the patient is deriving benefit.
- ◆ Ketoconazole: As a systemically bioavailable antifungal drug, ketoconazole has inherent anti-inflammatory benefits which may be helpful; however the drug inhibits androgen formation and may lead to exacerbation of the hypoandrogenism that is commonly seen in autoimmune patients and which contributes to the immune dysfunction.

- • Orthoendocrinology: Assess melatonin, prolactin, cortisol, DHEA, free and total testosterone, serum estradiol, and thyroid status (e.g., TSH, T4, *and* anti-thyroid peroxidase antibodies).
  - ○ Melatonin: Melatonin is a pineal hormone with well-known sleep-inducing and immunomodulatory properties, and it is commonly administered in doses of 1-40 mg in the evening, before bedtime. Its exceptional safety is well documented. Although

---

[165] "Prokinetic agents effective in pseudoobstruction include metoclopramide, domperidone, cisapride, octreotide, and erythromycin. ... The combination of octreotide and erythromycin may be particularly effective in systemic sclerosis." Sjogren RW. Gastrointestinal features of scleroderma. *Curr Opin Rheumatol.* 1996 Nov;8(6):569-75

[166] "CONCLUSIONS: Erythromycin accelerates gastric and gallbladder emptying in scleroderma patients and might be helpful in the treatment of gastrointestinal motor abnormalities in these patients." Fiorucci S, Distrutti E, Bassotti G, Gerli R, Chiucchiu S, Betti C, Santucci L, Morelli A. Effect of erythromycin administration on upper gastrointestinal motility in scleroderma patients. *Scand J Gastroenterol.* 1994 Sep;29(9):807-13

[167] "...48-week trial of oral minocycline (200 mg/d) or placebo." Tilley BC, Alarcon GS, Heyse SP, Trentham DE, Neuner R, Kaplan DA, Clegg DO, Leisen JC, Buckley L, Cooper SM, Duncan H, Pillemer SR, Tuttleman M, Fowler SE. Minocycline in rheumatoid arthritis. A 48-week, double-blind, placebo-controlled trial. MIRA Trial Group. *Ann Intern Med.* 1995 Jan 15;122(2):81-9

[168] "In patients with early seropositive RA, therapy with minocycline is superior to placebo." O'Dell JR, Haire CE, Palmer W, Drymalski W, Wees S, Blakely K, Churchill M, Eckhoff PJ, Weaver A, Doud D, Erikson N, Dietz F, Olson R, Maloley P, Klassen LW, Moore GF. Treatment of early rheumatoid arthritis with minocycline or placebo: results of a randomized, double-blind, placebo-controlled trial. *Arthritis Rheum.* 1997 May;40(5):842-8

[169] "...many cases of drug-induced lupus related to minocycline have been reported. Some of those reports included pulmonary lupus..." Christodoulou CS, Emmanuel P, Ray RA, Good RA, Schnapf BM, Cawkwell GD. Respiratory distress due to minocycline-induced pulmonary lupus. *Chest.* 1999 May;115(5):1471-3 http://www.chestjournal.org/cgi/content/full/115/5/1471

[170] Lawson TM, Amos N, Bulgen D, Williams BD. Minocycline-induced lupus: clinical features and response to rechallenge. *Rheumatology* (Oxford). 2001 Mar;40(3):329-35 http://rheumatology.oxfordjournals.org/cgi/content/full/40/3/329

psoriatic patients appear to have lost the physiologic nocturnal peak of melatonin[171], the role of supplemental melatonin in the treatment of patients with psoriasis has not been researched; however clinicians may reasonably decide to add this to their patients' treatment plan as appropriate. In contrast to implementing treatment with high doses of 20-40 mg, starting with a relatively low dose (e.g., 1-5 mg) and increasing as tolerated is recommended. Melatonin (20 mg hs) appears to have cured two patients with drug-resistant sarcoidosis[172] and 3 mg provided immediate short-term benefit to a patient with multiple sclerosis.[173] Immunostimulatory anti-infective action of melatonin was demonstrated in a clinical trial wherein septic newborns administered 20 mg melatonin showed significantly increased survival over nontreated controls[174]; given that psoriasis is associated with many subclinical infections, melatonin may provide therapeutic benefit by virtue of its anti-infective properties.

o Prolactin (excess): According to clinical trials with small numbers of patients, whether prolactin levels are high or not, treatment with prolactin-lowering treatment (such as bromocriptine[175]) appears beneficial in patients with psoriatic arthritis. Serum prolactin is the standard assessment of prolactin status. Since elevated prolactin may be a sign of pituitary tumor, assessment for headaches, visual deficits, other abnormalities of pituitary hormones (e.g., GH and TSH) should be performed and CT or MRI must be considered. Patients with prolactin levels less than 100 ng/mL and normal CT/MRI findings can be managed conservatively with effective prolactin-lowering treatment and annual radiologic assessment (less necessary with favorable serum response).[176, see review 177] Patients with RA and SLE have higher basal and stress-induced levels of prolactin compared with normal controls.[178,179] A normal serum prolactin level does not necessarily exclude the use of prolactin-lowering intervention, especially since many autoimmune patients have latent hyperprolactinemia which may not be detected with random serum measurement of prolactin. Specific treatment options include the following:

▪ Thyroid hormone: Hypothyroidism frequently causes hyperprolactinemia which is reversible upon effective treatment of hypothyroidism. Obviously therefore,

[171] "Our results show that psoriatic patients had lost the nocturnal peak and usual circadian rhythm of melatonin secretion. Levels of melatonin were significantly lower than in controls at 2 a.m., and higher at 6 and 8 a.m. and at 12 noon." Mozzanica N, Tadini G, Radaelli A, Negri M, Pigatto P, Morelli M, Frigerio U, Esposti G, Rossi D, et al. Plasma melatonin levels in psoriasis. *Acta Derm Venereol.* 1988;68(4):312-6

[172] Cagnoni ML, Lombardi A, Cerinic MC, Dedola GL, Pignone A. Melatonin for treatment of chronic refractory sarcoidosis. *Lancet.* 1995 Nov 4;346(8984):1229-30

[173] "...administration of melatonin (3 mg, orally) at 2:00 p.m., when the patient experienced severe blurring of vision, resulted within 15 minutes in a dramatic improvement in visual acuity and in normalization of the visual evoked potential latency after stimulation of the left eye." Sandyk R. Diurnal variations in vision and relations to circadian melatonin secretion in multiple sclerosis. *Int J Neurosci.* 1995 Nov;83(1-2):1-6

[174] Gitto E, Karbownik M, Reiter RJ, Tan DX, Cuzzocrea S, Chiurazzi P, Cordaro S, Corona G, Trimarchi G, Barberi I. Effects of melatonin treatment in septic newborns. *Pediatr Res.* 2001 Dec;50(6):756-60 http://www.pedresearch.org/cgi/content/full/50/6/756

[175] "In 2 cases of psoriatic arthritis, adding bromocriptine to gold salts and nonsteroidal anti-inflammatory drug was followed by a drastic efficacy with spectacular improvement in clinical, biological and occupational status. Because none of the cases had hyperprolactinaemia, bromocriptine acted probably had an intrinic anti-inflammatory effect independent of its antiprolactinic effect." Eulry F, Mayaudon H, Bauduceau B, Lechevalier D, Crozes P, Magnin J, Claude-Berthelot C. [Blood prolactin under the effect of protirelin in spondylarthropathies. Treatment trial of 4 cases of reactive arthritis and 2 cases of psoriatic arthritis with bromocriptine] *Ann Med Interne* (Paris). 1996;147(1):15-9. French.

[176] Beers MH, Berkow R (eds). The Merck Manual. Seventeenth Edition. Whitehouse Station; Merck Research Laboratories 1999 Page 77-78

[177] Serri O, Chik CL, Ur E, Ezzat S. Diagnosis and management of hyperprolactinemia. *CMAJ.* 2003 Sep 16;169(6):575-81 http://www.cmaj.ca/cgi/content/full/169/6/575

[178] Dostal C, Moszkorzova L, Musilova L, Lacinova Z, Marek J, Zvarova J. Serum prolactin stress values in patients with systemic lupus erythematosus. *Ann Rheum Dis.* 2003 May;62(5):487-8 http://ard.bmjjournals.com/cgi/content/full/62/5/487

[179] "RESULTS: A significantly higher rate of elevated PRL levels was found in SLE patients (40.0%) compared with the healthy controls (14.8%). No proof was found of association with the presence of anti-ds-DNA or with specific organ involvement. Similarly, elevated PRL levels were found in RA patients (39.3%)." Moszkorzova L, Lacinova Z, Marek J, Musilova L, Dohnalova A, Dostal C. Hyperprolactinaemia in patients with systemic lupus erythematosus. *Clin Exp Rheumatol.* 2002 Nov-Dec;20(6):807-12

thyroid status should be evaluated in all patients with hyperprolactinemia. Thyroid assessment and treatment is reviewed later in this section.

- *Vitex astus-cagnus and other supporting botanicals and nutrients*: Vitex lowers serum prolactin in humans[180,181] via a dopaminergic effect.[182] Vitex is considered safe for clinical use; mild and reversible adverse effects possibly associated with Vitex include nausea, headache, gastrointestinal disturbances, menstrual disorders, acne, pruritus and erythematous rash. No drug interactions are known, but given the herb's dopaminergic effect it should probably be used with some caution in patients treated with dopamine antagonists such as the so-called antipsychotic drugs (most of which do not work very well and/or carry intolerable adverse effects[183,184]). In a recent review, Bone[185] stated that daily doses can range from 500 mg to 2,000 mg DHE (dry herb equivalent) and can be tailored to the suppression of prolactin. Due at least in part to its content of L-dopa, *Mucuna pruriens* shows clinical dopaminergic activity as evidenced by its effectiveness in Parkinson's disease[186]; up to 15-30 gm/d of mucuna has been used clinically but doses will be dependent on preparation and phytoconcentration. Triptolide and other extracts from *Tripterygium wilfordii* Hook F exert clinically significant anti-inflammatory action in patients with rheumatoid arthritis[187,188] and also offer protection to dopaminergic neurons.[189,190] Ironically, even though tyrosine is the nutritional precursor to dopamine with evidence of clinical effectiveness (e.g., narcolepsy[191],

[180] "Since AC extracts were shown to have beneficial effects on premenstrual mastodynia serum prolactin levels in such patients were also studied in one double-blind, placebo-controlled clinical study. Serum prolactin levels were indeed reduced in the patients treated with the extract." Wuttke W, Jarry H, Christoffel V, Spengler B, Seidlova-Wuttke D. Chaste tree (Vitex agnus-castus)--pharmacology and clinical indications. *Phytomedicine*. 2003 May;10:348-57

[181] German abstract from Medline: "The prolactin release was reduced after 3 months, shortened luteal phases were normalised and deficits in the luteal progesterone synthesis were eliminated." Milewicz A, Gejdel E, Sworen H, Sienkiewicz K, Jedrzejak J, Teucher T, Schmitz H. [Vitex agnus castus extract in the treatment of luteal phase defects due to latent hyperprolactinemia. Results of a randomized placebo-controlled double-blind study] *Arzneimittelforschung*. 1993 Jul;43(7):752-6

[182] "Our results indicate a dopaminergic effect of Vitex agnus-castus extracts and suggest additional pharmacological actions via opioid receptors." Meier B, Berger D, Hoberg E, Sticher O, Schaffner W. Pharmacological activities of Vitex agnus-castus extracts in vitro. *Phytomedicine*. 2000 Oct;7(5):373-81

[183] "The majority of patients in each group discontinued their assigned treatment owing to inefficacy or intolerable side effects or for other reasons." Lieberman JA, Stroup TS, McEvoy JP, Swartz MS, Rosenheck RA, Perkins DO, Keefe RS, Davis SM, Davis CE, Lebowitz BD, Severe J, Hsiao JK; Clinical Antipsychotic Trials of Intervention Effectiveness (CATIE) Investigators. Effectiveness of antipsychotic drugs in patients with chronic schizophrenia. *N Engl J Med*. 2005 Sep 22;353(12):1209-23

[184] Whitaker R. The case against antipsychotic drugs: a 50-year record of doing more harm than good. *Med Hypotheses*. 2004;62(1):5-13

[185] "In conditions such as endometriosis and fibroids, for which a significant estrogen antagonist effect is needed, doses of at least 2 g/day DHE may be required and typically are used by professional herbalists." Bone K. New Insights Into Chaste Tree. *Nutritional Wellness* 2005 November http://www.nutritionalwellness.com/archives/2005/nov/11_bone.php

[186] "CONCLUSIONS: The rapid onset of action and longer on time without concomitant increase in dyskinesias on mucuna seed powder formulation suggest that this natural source of L-dopa might possess advantages over conventional L-dopa preparations in the long term management of PD." Katzenschlager R, Evans A, Manson A, Patsalos PN, Ratnaraj N, Watt H, Timmermann L, Van der Giessen R, Lees AJ. Mucuna pruriens in Parkinson's disease: a double blind clinical and pharmacological study. *J Neurol Neurosurg Psychiatry*. 2004 Dec;75(12):1672-7

[187] "The ethanol/ethyl acetate extract of TWHF shows therapeutic benefit in patients with treatment-refractory RA. At therapeutic dosages, the TWHF extract was well tolerated by most patients in this study." Tao X, Younger J, Fan FZ, Wang B, Lipsky PE. Benefit of an extract of Tripterygium Wilfordii Hook F in patients with rheumatoid arthritis: a double-blind, placebo-controlled study. *Arthritis Rheum*. 2002 Jul;46(7):1735-43

[188] "CONCLUSION: The EA extract of TWHF at dosages up to 570 mg/day appeared to be safe, and doses > 360 mg/day were associated with clinical benefit in patients with RA." Tao X, Cush JJ, Garret M, Lipsky PE. A phase I study of ethyl acetate extract of the chinese antirheumatic herb Tripterygium wilfordii hook F in rheumatoid arthritis. *J Rheumatol*. 2001 Oct;28(10):2160-7

[189] "Our data suggests that triptolide may protect dopaminergic neurons from LPS-induced injury and its efficiency in inhibiting microglia activation may underlie the mechanism." Li FQ, Lu XZ, Liang XB, Zhou HF, Xue B, Liu XY, Niu DB, Han JS, Wang XM. Triptolide, a Chinese herbal extract, protects dopaminergic neurons from inflammation-mediated damage through inhibition of microglial activation. *J Neuroimmunol*. 2004 Mar;148(1-2):24-31

[190] "Moreover, tripchlorolide markedly prevented the decrease in amount of dopamine in the striatum of model rats. Taken together, our data provide the first evidence that tripchlorolide acts as a neuroprotective molecule that rescues MPP+ or axotomy-induced degeneration of dopaminergic neurons, which may imply its therapeutic potential for Parkinson's disease." Li FQ, Cheng XX, Liang XB, Wang XH, Xue B, He QH, Wang XM, Han JS. Neurotrophic and neuroprotective effects of tripchlorolide, an extract of Chinese herb Tripterygium wilfordii Hook F, on dopaminergic neurons. *Exp Neurol*. 2003 Jan;179(1):28-37

[191] "Of twenty-eight visual analogue scales rating mood and arousal, the subjects' ratings in the tyrosine treatment (9 g daily) and placebo periods differed significantly for only three (less tired, less drowsy, more alert)." Elwes RD, Crewes H, Chesterman LP, Summers B, Jenner P, Binnie CD, Parkes JD. Treatment of narcolepsy with L-tyrosine: double-blind placebo-controlled trial. *Lancet*. 1989 Nov 4;2(8671):1067-9

enhancement of memory[192] and cognition[193]), supplementation with tyrosine appears to actually increase rather than decrease prolactin levels[194]; therefore tyrosine should be used cautiously if at all in patients with systemic inflammation. Furthermore, the finding that high-protein meals stimulate prolactin release[195] may partly explain the benefits of vegetarian diets in the treatment of systemic inflammation; since vegetarian diets are comparatively low in protein compared to omnivorous diets, they may lead to a relative reduction in prolactin production due to lack of stimulation.

- <u>Bromocriptine</u>: Bromocriptine has long been considered the pharmacologic treatment of choice for elevated prolactin.[196] Bromocriptine appears to benefit most patients with psoriasis/psoriatic arthritis, according to a small Italian study[197] and three case reports in the French literature.[198] Typical dose is 2.5 mg per day (effective against lupus[199]); gastrointestinal upset and sedation are common.[200] Clinical intervention with bromocriptine appears warranted in patients with RA, SLE, Reiter's syndrome, psoriatic arthritis, and probably multiple sclerosis and uveitis.[201] A normal serum prolactin level does not necessarily exclude the use of prolactin-lowering intervention, especially since many autoimmune patients have latent hyperprolactinemia which may not be detected with random serum measurement of prolactin.

- <u>Cabergoline/Dostinex</u>: Cabergoline/Dostinex is a newer dopamine agonist with few adverse effects; typical dose starts at 0.5 mg per week (0.25 mg twice per week).[202] Several studies have indicated that cabergoline is safer and more effective than bromocriptine for reducing prolactin levels[203] and the dose can often be reduced after successful prolactin reduction, allowing for reductions in cost and adverse

[192] "Ten men and 10 women subjects underwent these batteries 1 h after ingesting 150 mg/kg of l-tyrosine or placebo. Administration of tyrosine significantly enhanced accuracy and decreased frequency of list retrieval on the working memory task during the multiple task battery compared with placebo." Thomas JR, Lockwood PA, Singh A, Deuster PA. Tyrosine improves working memory in a multitasking environment. *Pharmacol Biochem Behav.* 1999 Nov;64:495-500

[193] "Ten subjects received five daily doses of a protein-rich drink containing 2 g tyrosine, and 11 subjects received a carbohydrate rich drink with the same amount of calories (255 kcal)." Deijen JB, Wientjes CJ, Vullinghs HF, Cloin PA, Langefeld JJ. Tyrosine improves cognitive performance and reduces blood pressure in cadets after one week of a combat training course. *Brain Res Bull.* 1999 Jan 15;48(2):203-9

[194] "Tyrosine (when compared to placebo) had no effect on any sleep related measure, but it did stimulate prolactin release." Waters WF, Magill RA, Bray GA, Volaufova J, Smith SR, Lieberman HR, Rood J, Hurry M, Anderson T, Ryan DH. A comparison of tyrosine against placebo, phentermine, caffeine, and D-amphetamine during sleep deprivation. *Nutr Neurosci.* 2003;6(4):221-35

[195] "Whereas carbohydrate meals had no discernible effects, high protein meals induced a large increase in both PRL and cortisol; high fat meals caused selective release of PRL." Ishizuka B, Quigley ME, Yen SS. Pituitary hormone release in response to food ingestion: evidence for neuroendocrine signals from gut to brain. *J Clin Endocrinol Metab.* 1983 Dec;57(6):1111-6

[196] Beers MH, Berkow R (eds). <u>The Merck Manual. Seventeenth Edition</u>. Whitehouse Station; Merck Research Laboratories 1999 Page 77-78

[197] "Bromocriptin was shown to be effective in 13 of our 18 psoriatic patients." Valentino A, Fimiani M, Bilenchi R, Castelli A, Francini G, Gonnelli S, Gennari C, Andreassi L. [Therapy with bromocriptine and behavior of various hormones in psoriasis patients] *Boll Soc Ital Biol Sper.* 1984 Oct 30;60(10):1841-4. Italian.

[198] "All three were treated with bromocriptine (5 mg/d in 2 doses) after verification of normal baseline and protirelin-stimulation prolactin levels. There was a beneficial effect in nocturnal pain relief, morning stiffness, the Lee and Ritchie scores and biological markers of inflammation." Eulry F, Mayaudon H, Lechevalier D, Bauduceau B, Ariche L, Ouakil H, Crozes P, Magnin J. [Treatment of rheumatoid psoriasis with bromocriptine] *Presse Med.* 1995 Nov 18;24(35):1642-4. French.

[199] "A prospective, double-blind, randomized, placebo-controlled study compared BRC at a fixed daily dosage of 2.5 mg with placebo... Long term treatment with a low dose of BRC appears to be a safe and effective means of decreasing SLE flares in SLE patients." Alvarez-Nemegyei J, Cobarrubias-Cobos A, Escalante-Triay F, Sosa-Munoz J, Miranda JM, Jara LJ. Bromocriptine in systemic lupus erythematosus: a double-blind, randomized, placebo-controlled study. *Lupus.* 1998;7(6):414-9

[200] Serri O, Chik CL, Ur E, Ezzat S. Diagnosis and management of hyperprolactinemia. *CMAJ.* 2003 Sep 16;169(6):575-81 cmaj.ca/cgi/content/full/169/6/575

[201] "...clinical observations and trials support the use of bromocriptine as a nonstandard primary or adjunctive therapy in the treatment of recalcitrant RA, SLE, Reiter's syndrome, and psoriatic arthritis and associated conditions unresponsive to traditional approaches." McMurray RW. Bromocriptine in rheumatic and autoimmune diseases. *Semin Arthritis Rheum.* 2001 Aug;31(1):21-32

[202] Serri O, Chik CL, Ur E, Ezzat S. Diagnosis and management of hyperprolactinemia. *CMAJ.* 2003 Sep 16;169(6):575-81

[203] "CONCLUSION: These data indicate that cabergoline is a very effective agent for lowering the prolactin levels in hyperprolactinemic patients and that it appears to offer considerable advantage over bromocriptine in terms of efficacy and tolerability." Sabuncu T, Arikan E, Tasan E, Hatemi H. Comparison of the effects of cabergoline and bromocriptine on prolactin levels in hyperprolactinemic patients. *Intern Med.* 2001 Sep;40(9):857-61

effects.[204]   Although fewer studies have been published supporting the antirheumatic benefits of cabergoline than those supporting bromocriptine; its antirheumatic benefits have indeed been documented.[205]

- o Estrogen (excess): Although the classic pattern in patients with autoimmunity is elevated estrogen (generally considered immunodysregulatory) and reduced testosterone (generally considered anti-inflammatory and immunoregulatory), data in patients with psoriatic arthritis is inadequate to extend this otherwise consistent and successful generalization to this group. On the contrary, Stevens et al[206] published a case report of a woman with recalcitrant psoriasis and psoriatic arthritis who responded very well to anti-estrogen treatment. The small amount of data available actually suggests that estrogen may be beneficial (reduction in skin lesions with pregnancy) and that testosterone (in one woman who developed psoriasis following a testosterone-containing hormonal implant following oophorectomy) could exacerbate the disease. Estrogen and testosterone should be measured in serum and modulated appropriately as described in Chapter 4 of *Integrative Rheumatology* in the section on Orthoendocrinology on a *per patient* basis.

"Total estrogen load" correlates with inflammation
"We report a patient with severe psoriatic arthritis in whom the severity of both the arthritis and psoriasis fluctuated with the menstrual cycle. These features failed to improve with standard therapy, but there was a prompt response to treatment which suppressed estrogen secretion." Stevens HP, et al. Cyclical psoriatic arthritis responding to anti-oestrogen therapy. *Br J Dermatol.* 1993 Oct

- o Cortisol (insufficiency): Cortisol has immunoregulatory and "immunosuppressive" actions at physiological concentrations. Low adrenal function is common in patients with chronic inflammation[207,208,209] Assessment of cortisol production and adrenal function are detailed in Chapter 4 of *Integrative Rheumatology* under the section of Orthoendocrinology. Supplementation with 20 mg per day of cortisol/Cortef is physiologic; my preference is to dose 10 mg first thing in the morning, then 5 mg in late morning and 5 mg in midafternoon in an attempt to replicate the diurnal variation and normal morning peak of cortisol levels. In patients with hypoadrenalism, administration of pregnenolone in doses of 10-60 mg in the morning may also be beneficial.

---

[204] "Cabergoline also normalized PRL in the majority of patients with known bromocriptine intolerance or -resistance. Once PRL secretion was adequately controlled, the dose of cabergoline could often be significantly decreased, which further reduced costs of therapy." Verhelst J, Abs R, Maiter D, van den Bruel A, Vandeweghe M, Velkeniers B, Mockel J, Lamberigts G, Petrossians P, Coremans P, Mahler C, Stevenaert A, Verlooy J, Raftopoulos C, Beckers A. Cabergoline in the treatment of hyperprolactinemia: a study in 455 patients. *J Clin Endocrinol Metab*. 1999 Jul;84(7):2518-22 http://jcem.endojournals.org/cgi/content/full/84/7/2518

[205] Erb N, Pace AV, Delamere JP, Kitas GD. Control of unremitting rheumatoid arthritis by the prolactin antagonist cabergoline. *Rheumatology* (Oxford). 2001 Feb;40(2):237-9 http://rheumatology.oxfordjournals.org/cgi/content/full/40/2/237

[206] "We report a patient with severe psoriatic arthritis in whom the severity of both the arthritis and psoriasis fluctuated with the menstrual cycle. These features failed to improve with standard therapy, but there was a prompt response to treatment which suppressed oestrogen secretion." Stevens HP, Ostlere LS, Black CM, Jacobs HS, Rustin MH. Cyclical psoriatic arthritis responding to anti-oestrogen therapy. *Br J Dermatol*. 1993 Oct;129(4):458-60

[207] "Yet evidence that patients with rheumatoid arthritis improved with small, physiologic dosages of cortisol or cortisone acetate was reported over 25 years ago, and that patients with chronic allergic disorders or unexplained chronic fatigue also improved with administration of such small dosages was reported over 15 years ago..." Jefferies WM. Mild adrenocortical deficiency, chronic allergies, autoimmune disorders and the chronic fatigue syndrome: a continuation of the cortisone story. *Med Hypotheses*. 1994 Mar;42(3):183-9 http://www.thebuteykocentre.com/Irish_%20Buteykocenter_files/further_studies/med_hyp2.pdf http://members.westnet.com.au/pkolb/med_hyp2.pdf

[208] "The etiology of rheumatoid arthritis ...explained by a combination of three factors: (i) a relatively mild deficiency of cortisol, ..., (ii) a deficiency of DHEA, ...and (iii) infection by organisms such as mycoplasma,..." Jefferies WM. The etiology of rheumatoid arthritis. *Med Hypotheses*. 1998 Aug;51:111-4

[209] Jefferies W McK. Safe Uses of Cortisol. Second Edition. Springfield, CC Thomas, 1996

- o <u>Testosterone (insufficiency)</u>: Androgen deficiencies predispose to, are exacerbated by, and contribute to autoimmune/inflammatory disorders. Female patients with psoriasis have lower levels of testosterone compared to those seen in healthy controls.[210] A large proportion of men with lupus or RA have low testosterone[211] and suffer the effects of hypogonadism: fatigue, weakness, depression, slow healing, low libido, and difficulties with sexual performance. Testosterone levels may rise following DHEA supplementation (especially in women) and can be elevated in men by the use of anastrozole/Arimidex. Otherwise, transdermal testosterone such as Androgel or Testim can be applied as indicated.

- o <u>DHEA</u>: DHEA is an anti-inflammatory and immunoregulatory hormone that is commonly deficient in patients with autoimmunity and inflammatory arthritis.[212] However, the role of DHEA in psoriatic arthritis *en masse* is unclear due to conflicting data. One study showed that patients with psoriasis did not show evidence of DHEA insufficiency[213], while other studies—especially in the German literature—have consistently documented low serum and intracellular levels of DHEA.[214] DHEA levels should be measured in these patients—especially those with severe disease, deficiencies should be treated unless contraindicated, and therapeutic trials are not unreasonable. DHEA is an anti-inflammatory and immunoregulatory hormone which is commonly deficient in patients with autoimmunity, including polymyalgia rheumatica, lupus, and rheumatoid arthritis.[215] DHEA levels are suppressed by prednisone[216], and DHEA has been shown to reverse the osteoporosis and loss of bone mass induced by corticosteroid treatment.[217] DHEA shows no acute or subacute toxicity even when used in supraphysiologic doses, even when used in sick patients. For example, in a study of 32 patients with HIV, DHEA doses of 750 mg – 2,250 mg per day were well tolerated and produced no dose-limiting adverse effects.[218] This lack of toxicity compares favorably with any and all so-called "antirheumatic" drugs, nearly all of which show impressive

[210] "The testosterone levels and LH/FSH ratio were significantly lower in the psoriatic group." Pietrzak A, Lecewicz-Torun B, Jakimiuk A. Lipid and hormone profile in psoriatic females. *Ann Univ Mariae Curie Sklodowska* [Med]. 2002;57(2):478-83

[211] Karagiannis A, Harsoulis F. Gonadal dysfunction in systemic diseases. *Eur J Endocrinol*. 2005 Apr;152(4):501-13 http://www.eje-online.org/cgi/content/full/152/4/501

[212] "DHEAS concentrations were significantly decreased in both women and men with inflammatory arthritis (IA) (P < 0.001)." Dessein PH, Joffe BI, Stanwix AE, Moomal Z. Hyposecretion of the adrenal androgen dehydroepiandrosterone sulfate and its relation to clinical variables in inflammatory arthritis. *Arthritis Res*. 2001;3(3):183-8. Epub 2001 Feb 21. http://arthritis-research.com/content/3/3/183

[213] "Assessing the patients by group, the mean DHEAS level was markedly lower in the pemphigoid/pemphigus than in the psoriasis and OA patients (geometric mean 600 vs. 2130 and 2100 nmol/l, respectively; p < 0.001)." de la Torre B, Fransson J, Scheynius A. Blood dehydroepiandrosterone sulphate (DHEAS) levels in pemphigoid/pemphigus and psoriasis. *Clin Exp Rheumatol*. 1995 May-Jun;13(3):345-8

[214] "The effects of this dehydroepiandrosterone deficiency are changes in the humoral regulation of events in growth and proliferation in patients with psoriasis." Holzmann H, Benes P, Morsches B. [Dehydroepiandrosterone deficiency in psoriasis. Hypothesis on the etiopathogenesis of this disease] *Hautarzt*. 1980 Feb;31(2):71-5. Review. German.

[215] "The low levels found in patients with PM:TA are in accordance with those previously reported in immune-mediated diseases such as systemic lupus erythematosus (SLE) and rheumatoid arthritis, suggesting that diminution of DHEAS is a constant endocrinologic feature in these categories of patients." Nilsson E, de la Torre B, Hedman M, Goobar J, Thorner A. Blood dehydroepiandrosterone sulphate (DHEAS) levels in polymyalgia rheumatica/giant cell arteritis and primary fibromyalgia. *Clin Exp Rheumatol*. 1994 Jul-Aug;12(4):415-7

[216] "Basal serum DHEA and DHEAS concentrations were suppressed to a greater degree than was cortisol during both daily and alternate day prednisone treatments. ...Thus, adrenal androgen secretion was more easily suppressed than was cortisol secretion by this low dose of glucocorticoid, but there was no advantage to alternate day therapy." Rittmaster RS, Givner ML. Effect of daily and alternate day low dose prednisone on serum cortisol and adrenal androgens in hirsute women. *J Clin Endocrinol Metab*. 1988 Aug;67(2):400-3

[217] "CONCLUSION: Prasterone treatment prevented BMD loss and significantly increased BMD at both the lumbar spine and total hip in female patients with SLE receiving exogenous glucocorticoids." Mease PJ, Ginzler EM, Gluck OS, Schiff M, Goldman A, Greenwald M, Cohen S, Egan R, Quarles BJ, Schwartz KE. Effects of prasterone on bone mineral density in women with systemic lupus erythematosus receiving chronic glucocorticoid therapy. *J Rheumatol*. 2005 Apr;32(4):616-21

[218] "Thirty-one subjects were evaluated and monitored for safety and tolerance. The oral drug was administered three times daily in doses ranging from 750 mg/day to 2,250 mg/day for 16 weeks. ... The drug was well tolerated and no dose-limiting side effects were noted." Dyner TS, Lang W, Geaga J, Golub A, Stites D, Winger E, Galmarini M, Masterson J, Jacobson MA. An open-label dose-escalation trial of oral dehydroepiandrosterone tolerance and pharmacokinetics in patients with HIV disease. *J Acquir Immune Defic Syndr*. 1993 May;6(5):459-65

comparable toxicity. When used at doses of 200 mg per day, DHEA safely provides clinical benefit for patients with various autoimmune diseases, including ulcerative colitis, Crohn's disease[219], and SLE.[220] In patients with SLE, DHEA supplementation allows for reduced dosing of prednisone (thus avoiding its adverse effects) while providing symptomatic improvement.[221] Optimal clinical response appears to correlate with serum levels that are supraphysiologic[222], treatment may be implemented with little regard for initial DHEA levels, particularly when 1) the dose of DHEA is kept as low as possible, 2) duration is kept as short as possible, 3) other interventions are used to address the underlying cause of the disease, 4) the patient is deriving benefit and the risk-to-benefit ratio is favorable.

- Thyroid (insufficiency or autoimmunity): Overt or imminent hypothyroidism is suggested by TSH greater than 2 mU/L[223] or 3 mU/L[224], low T4 or T3, and/or the presence of anti-thyroid peroxidase antibodies.[225] Hypothyroidism can cause an inflammatory myopathy that can resemble polymyositis, and hypothyroidism is a frequent complication of any and all autoimmune diseases. Specific treatment considerations include the following:
  - Selenium: Supplementation with either selenomethonine[226] or sodium selenite[227,228] can reduce thyroid autoimmunity and improve peripheral conversion of T4 to T3. Selenium may be started at 500-800 mcg per day and tapered to 200-400 mcg per day for maintenance.
  - L-thyroxine/levothyroxine/Synthroid—prescription synthetic T4: 25-50 mcg per day is a common starting dose which can be adjusted based on clinical and laboratory response. All thyroid hormone supplements must be taken away from soy products and preferably on an empty stomach. Doses are generally started at one-half of the daily dose for the first 10 days after which the full dose is used. Caution must be applied in patients with adrenal insufficiency and/or those with cardiovascular disease.

---

[219] "CONCLUSIONS: In a pilot study, dehydroepiandrosterone was effective and safe in patients with refractory Crohn's disease or ulcerative colitis." Andus T, Klebl F, Rogler G, Bregenzer N, Scholmerich J, Straub RH. Patients with refractory Crohn's disease or ulcerative colitis respond to dehydroepiandrosterone: a pilot study. *Aliment Pharmacol Ther*. 2003 Feb;17(3):409-14

[220] "CONCLUSION: The overall results confirm that DHEA treatment was well-tolerated, significantly reduced the number of SLE flares, and improved patient's global assessment of disease activity." Chang DM, Lan JL, Lin HY, Luo SF. Dehydroepiandrosterone treatment of women with mild-to-moderate systemic lupus erythematosus: a multicenter randomized, double-blind, placebo-controlled trial. *Arthritis Rheum*. 2002 Nov;46(11):2924-7

[221] "CONCLUSION: Among women with lupus disease activity, reducing the dosage of prednisone to < or = 7.5 mg/day for a sustained period of time while maintaining stabilization or a reduction of disease activity was possible in a significantly greater proportion of patients treated with oral prasterone, 200 mg once daily, compared with patients treated with placebo." Petri MA, Lahita RG, Van Vollenhoven RF, Merrill JT, Schiff M, Ginzler EM, Strand V, Kunz A, Gorelick KJ, Schwartz KE; GL601 Study Group. Effects of prasterone on corticosteroid requirements of women with systemic lupus erythematosus: a double-blind, randomized, placebo-controlled trial. *Arthritis Rheum*. 2002 Jul;46(7):1820-9

[222] "CONCLUSION: The clinical response to DHEA was not clearly dose dependent. Serum levels of DHEA and DHEAS correlated only weakly with lupus outcomes, but suggested an optimum serum DHEAS of 1000 microg/dl." Barry NN, McGuire JL, van Vollenhoven RF. Dehydroepiandrosterone in systemic lupus erythematosus: relationship between dosage, serum levels, and clinical response. *J Rheumatol*. 1998 Dec;25(12):2352-6

[223] Weetman AP. Hypothyroidism: screening and subclinical disease. *BMJ*. 1997 Apr 19;314(7088):1175-8 http://bmj.bmjjournals.com/cgi/content/full/314/7088/1175

[224] "Now AACE encourages doctors to consider treatment for patients who test outside the boundaries of a narrower margin based on a target TSH level of 0.3 to 3.0. AACE believes the new range will result in proper diagnosis for millions of Americans who suffer from a mild thyroid disorder, but have gone untreated until now." American Association of Clinical Endocrinologists (AACE). 2003 Campaign Encourages Awareness of Mild Thyroid Failure, Importance of Routine Testing http://www.aace.com/pub/tam2003/press.php November 26, 2005

[225] Beers MH, Berkow R (eds). The Merck Manual. Seventeenth Edition. Whitehouse Station; Merck Research Laboratories 1999 Page 96

[226] Duntas LH, Mantzou E, Koutras DA. Effects of a six month treatment with selenomethionine in patients with autoimmune thyroiditis. *Eur J Endocrinol*. 2003 Apr;148(4):389-93 http://eje-online.org/cgi/reprint/148/4/389

[227] Gartner R, Gasnier BC, Dietrich JW, Krebs B, Angstwurm MW. Selenium supplementation in patients with autoimmune thyroiditis decreases thyroid peroxidase antibodies concentrations. *J Clin Endocrinol Metab*. 2002 Apr;87(4):1687-91 http://jcem.endojournals.org/cgi/content/full/87/4/1687

[228] "We recently conducted a prospective, placebo-controlled clinical study, where we could demonstrate, that a substitution of 200 wg sodium selenite for three months in patients with autoimmune thyroiditis reduced thyroid peroxidase antibody (TPO-Ab) concentrations significantly." Gartner R, Gasnier BC. Selenium in the treatment of autoimmune thyroiditis. *Biofactors*. 2003;19(3-4):165-70

- **Armour thyroid—prescription natural T4 and T3 from cow/pig thyroid gland:** 60 mg (one grain) is a common starting and maintenance dose. Due to the exacerbating effect on thyroid autoimmunity, Armour thyroid is never used in patients with thyroid autoimmunity.
- **Thyrolar/Liotrix—prescription synthetic T4 with T3:** Dosed as "1" (low), "2" (intermediate), or "3" (high). Although this product has been difficult to obtain for the past few years due to manufacturing problems (http://thyrolar.com/), it has been my treatment of choice due to the combination of T4 and T3 and the lack of antigenicity compared to gland-derived products.
- **Thyroid glandular—nonprescription T3:** Apparently, producers of nutritional products are able to distribute T3 because it is not listed by the FDA as a prescription item. A better nutritional company will start from Armour thyroid, remove the T4, and sell the thyroid glandular with active T3. For many patients, one tablet per day is at least as effective as a prescription source of thyroid hormone. Since it is derived from a glandular and therefore potentially antigenic source, thyroid glandular is not used in patients with thyroid autoimmunity.

- <u>Oral enzyme therapy with proteolytic/pancreatic enzymes</u>: Polyenzyme supplementation is used to ameliorate the pathophysiology induced by immune complexes, such as the related condition rheumatoid arthritis.[229]

- *Uncaria tomentosa, Uncaria guianensis*: Cat's claw has been safely and successfully used in the treatment of osteoarthritis[230] and rheumatoid arthritis.[231] Since serum nitric oxide levels are 5x higher in patients with psoriasis (157) than controls (32)[232], the nitric oxide inhibiting action of *Uncaria* may be particularly helpful, particularly if used with a low-arginine diet. However, the clinician must never waiver from attempts to identify the *cause* of the inflammation, rather than merely seeking to quench the *mediators* of inflammation. High-quality extractions from reputable manufacturers used according to directions are recommended. Most products contain between 250-500 mg and are standardized to 3.0% alkaloids and 15% total polyphenols; QD-TID po dosing should be sufficient as *part* of a comprehensive plan.

---

[229] Galebskaya LV, Ryumina EV, Niemerovsky VS, Matyukov AA. Human complement system state after wobenzyme intake. *VESTNIK MOSKOVSKOGO UNIVERSITETA. KHIMIYA.* 2000. Vol. 41, No. 6. Supplement. Pages 148-149

[230] Piscoya J, Rodriguez Z, Bustamante SA, Okuhama NN, Miller MJ, Sandoval M.Efficacy and safety of freeze-dried cat's claw in osteoarthritis of the knee: mechanisms of action of the species Uncaria guianensis. *Inflamm Res.* 2001 Sep;50(9):442-8

[231] "This small preliminary study demonstrates relative safety and modest benefit to the tender joint count of a highly purified extract from the pentacyclic chemotype of UT in patients with active RA taking sulfasalazine or hydroxychloroquine." Mur E, Hartig F, Eibl G, Schirmer M. Randomized double blind trial of an extract from the pentacyclic alkaloid-chemotype of uncaria tomentosa for the treatment of rheumatoid arthritis. *J Rheumatol.* 2002 Apr;29(4):678-81

[232] "The mean NO level in the psoriatic group was 157.7 with SD 50.4 while in the control group it was 32.8 with SD 4.03." Gokhale NR, et al. A study of serum nitric oxide levels in psoriasis. *Indian J Dermatol Venereol Leprol* 2005;71:175-178 http://www.ijdvl.com/

- _Harpagophytum procumbens_: Harpagophytum is a moderately effective botanical analgesic for musculoskeletal pain.[233,234,235,236,237] Products are generally standardized for the content of harpagosides, with a target dose of 60 mg harpagoside per day.[238]
- Willow bark: Extracts from willow bark have proven safe and effective in the alleviation of moderate/severe low-back pain.[239,240] The mechanism of action appears to be inhibition of prostaglandin formation via inhibition of cyclooxygenase-2 gene transcription[241] by salicylates, phytonutrients which are widely present in fruits, vegetables, herbs and spices and which are partly responsible for the anti-cancer, anti-inflammatory, and health-promoting benefits of plant consumption.[242,243] According to a letter by Vasquez and Muanza[244], the only adverse effect that has been documented in association with willow bark was a single case of anaphylaxis in a patient previously sensitized to acetylsalicylic acid.
- _Boswellia serrata_: _Boswellia_ shows clear anti-inflammatory and analgesic action via inhibition of 5-lipoxygenase[245] and clinical benefits have been demonstrated in patients with osteoarthritis of the knees[246] as well as asthma[247] and ulcerative colitis.[248] A German study showing that _Boswellia_ was ineffective for rheumatoid arthritis[249] was poorly conducted, with inadequate follow-up, inadequate controls, and abnormal dosing of the herb. Products are generally standardized to contain 37.5–65% boswellic acids, with a target dose is approximately 150 mg of boswellic acids TID; dose and number of capsules/tablets will vary depending upon the concentration found in differing products.
- Phytonutritional modulation of NF-kappaB: As a stimulator of pro-inflammatory gene transcription, NF-kappaB is almost universally activated in conditions associated with

[233] Chrubasik S, Thanner J, Kunzel O, Conradt C, Black A, Pollak S. Comparison of outcome measures during treatment with the proprietary Harpagophytum extract doloteffin in patients with pain in the lower back, knee or hip. _Phytomedicine_ 2002 Apr;9(3):181-94
[234] Chantre P, Cappelaere A, Leblan D, Guedon D, Vandermander J, Fournie B. Efficacy and tolerance of Harpagophytum procumbens versus diacerhein in treatment of osteoarthritis. _Phytomedicine_ 2000 Jun;7(3):177-83
[235] Leblan D, Chantre P, Fournie B. Harpagophytum procumbens in the treatment of knee and hip osteoarthritis. Four-month results of a prospective, multicenter, double-blind trial versus diacerhein. _Joint Bone Spine_ 2000;67(5):462-7
[236] "...subgroup analyses suggested that the effect was confined to patients with more severe and radiating pain accompanied by neurological deficit. ...a slightly different picture, with the benefits seeming, if anything, to be greatest in the H600 group and in patients without more severe pain, radiation or neurological deficit." Chrubasik S, Junck H, Breitschwerdt H, Conradt C, Zappe H. Effectiveness of Harpagophytum extract WS 1531 in the treatment of exacerbation of low back pain: a randomized, placebo-controlled, double-blind study. _Eur J Anaesthesiol_ 1999 Feb;16(2):118-29
[237] Chrubasik S, Model A, Black A, Pollak S. A randomized double-blind pilot study comparing Doloteffin and Vioxx in the treatment of low back pain. _Rheumatology_ (Oxford). 2003 Jan;42(1):141-8
[238] "They took an 8-week course of Doloteffin at a dose providing 60 mg harpagoside per day... Doloteffin is well worth considering for osteoarthritic knee and hip pain and nonspecific low back pain." Chrubasik S, Thanner J, Kunzel O, Conradt C, Black A, Pollak S. Comparison of outcome measures during treatment with the proprietary Harpagophytum extract doloteffin in patients with pain in the lower back, knee or hip. _Phytomedicine_ 2002 Apr;9(3):181-94
[239] Chrubasik S, Eisenberg E, Weinberger T, Luzzati R, Conradt C. Treatment of low-back pain exacerbations with willow bark extract: a randomized double-blind study. _Am J Med._ 2000;109:9-14
[240] Chrubasik S, Kunzel O, Model A, Conradt C, Black A. Treatment of low-back pain with a herbal or synthetic anti-rheumatic: a randomized controlled study. Willow bark extract for low-back pain. _Rheumatology_ (Oxford). 2001;40:1388-93
[241] Hare LG, Woodside JV, Young IS. Dietary salicylates. _J Clin Pathol_ 2003 Sep;56(9):649-50
[242] Lawrence JR, Peter R, Baxter GJ, Robson J, Graham AB, Paterson JR. Urinary excretion of salicyluric and salicylic acids by non-vegetarians, vegetarians, and patients taking low dose aspirin. _J Clin Pathol._ 2003 Sep;56(9):651-3
[243] Paterson JR, Lawrence JR. Salicylic acid: a link between aspirin, diet and the prevention of colorectal cancer. _QJM._ 2001 Aug;94(8):445-8
[244] Vasquez A, Muanza DN. Evaluation of Presence of Aspirin-Related Warnings with Willow Bark: Comment on the Article by Clauson et al. _Ann Pharmacotherapy_ 2005 Oct;39(10):1763
[245] Wildfeuer A, Neu IS, Safayhi H, Metzger G, Wehrmann M, Vogel U, Ammon HP. Effects of boswellic acids extracted from a herbal medicine on the biosynthesis of leukotrienes and the course of experimental autoimmune encephalomyelitis. _Arzneimittelforschung_ 1998 Jun;48(6):668-74
[246] Kimmatkar N, Thawani V, Hingorani L, Khiyani R. Efficacy and tolerability of Boswellia serrata extract in treatment of osteoarthritis of knee--a randomized double blind placebo controlled trial. _Phytomedicine._ 2003 Jan;10(1):3-7
[247] Gupta I, Gupta V, Parihar A, Gupta S, Ludtke R, Safayhi H, Ammon HP. Effects of Boswellia serrata gum resin in patients with bronchial asthma: results of a double-blind, placebo-controlled, 6-week clinical study. _Eur J Med Res._ 1998 Nov 17;3(11):511-4
[248] Gupta I, Parihar A, Malhotra P, Singh GB, Ludtke R, Safayhi H, Ammon HP. Effects of Boswellia serrata gum resin in patients with ulcerative colitis. _Eur J Med Res._ 1997 Jan;2(1):37-43
[249] Sander O, Herborn G, Rau R. [Is H15 (resin extract of Boswellia serrata, "incense") a useful supplement to established drug therapy of chronic polyarthritis? Results of a double-blind pilot study] [Article in German] _Z Rheumatol._ 1998 Feb;57(1):11-6

inflammation.[250,251]   As we would expect, NF-kappaB plays a central role in the pathogenesis of synovitis and joint destruction seen in RA and psoriatic arthritis.[252]   Nutrients and botanicals which either directly or indirectly inhibit NF-kappaB for an anti-inflammatory benefit include vitamin D[253,254], curcumin[255] (requires piperine for absorption[256]), lipoic acid[257], green tea[258], ursolic acid[259] from rosemary[260], grape seed extract[261], propolis[262], zinc[263], high-dose selenium[264], indole-3-carbinol[265,266], N-acetyl-L-cysteine[267], resveratrol[268,269],

[250] Tak PP, Firestein GS. NF-kappaB: a key role in inflammatory diseases. *J Clin Invest.* 2001 Jan;107(1):7-11 http://www.jci.org/cgi/content/full/107/1/7

[251] D'Acquisto F, May MJ, Ghosh S. Inhibition of Nuclear Factor KappaB (NF-B): An Emerging Theme in Anti-Inflammatory Therapies. *Mol Interv.* 2002 Feb;2(1):22-35 http://molinterv.aspetjournals.org/cgi/content/abstract/2/1/22

[252] "NF-B plays a central role in the pathogenesis of synovitis in RA and PsA." Foell D, et al. Expression of the pro-inflammatory protein S100A12 (EN-RAGE) in rheumatoid and psoriatic arthritis. *Rheumatology* (Oxford). 2003 Nov;42(11):1383-9 rheumatology.oxfordjournals.org/cgi/content/full/42/11/1383

[253] "1Alpha,25-dihydroxyvitamin D3 (1,25-(OH)2-D3), the active metabolite of vitamin D, can inhibit NF-kappaB activity in human MRC-5 fibroblasts, targeting DNA binding of NF-kappaB but not translocation of its subunits p50 and p65." Harant H, Wolff B, Lindley IJ. 1Alpha,25-dihydroxyvitamin D3 decreases DNA binding of nuclear factor-kappaB in human fibroblasts. *FEBS Lett.* 1998 Oct 9;436(3):329-34

[254] "Thus, 1,25(OH)₂D₃ may negatively regulate IL-12 production by downregulation of NF-kB activation and binding to the p40-kB sequence." D'Ambrosio D, Cippitelli M, Cocciolo MG, Mazzeo D, Di Lucia P, Lang R, Sinigaglia F, Panina-Bordignon P. Inhibition of IL-12 production by 1,25-dihydroxyvitamin D3. Involvement of NF-kappaB downregulation in transcriptional repression of the p40 gene. *J Clin Invest.* 1998 Jan 1;101(1):252-62

[255] "Curcumin, EGCG and resveratrol have been shown to suppress activation of NF-kappa B." Surh YJ, Chun KS, Cha HH, Han SS, Keum YS, Park KK, Lee SS. Molecular mechanisms underlying chemopreventive activities of anti-inflammatory phytochemicals: down-regulation of COX-2 and iNOS through suppression of NF-kappa B activation. *Mutat Res.* 2001 Sep 1;480-481:243-68

[256] Shoba G, Joy D, Joseph T, Majeed M, Rajendran R, Srinivas PS. Influence of piperine on the pharmacokinetics of curcumin in animals and human volunteers. *Planta Med.* 1998 May;64(4):353-6

[257] "ALA reduced the TNF-alpha-stimulated ICAM-1 expression in a dose-dependent manner, to levels observed in unstimulated cells. Alpha-lipoic acid also reduced NF-kappaB activity in these cells in a dose-dependent manner." Lee HA, Hughes DA.Alpha-lipoic acid modulates NF-kappaB activity in human monocytic cells by direct interaction with DNA. *Exp Gerontol.* 2002 Jan-Mar;37(2-3):401-10

[258] "In conclusion, EGCG is an effective inhibitor of IKK activity. This may explain, at least in part, some of the reported anti-inflammatory and anticancer effects of green tea." Yang F, Oz HS, Barve S, de Villiers WJ, McClain CJ, Varilek GW. The green tea polyphenol (-)-epigallocatechin-3-gallate blocks nuclear factor-kappa B activation by inhibiting I kappa B kinase activity in the intestinal epithelial cell line IEC-6. *Mol Pharmacol.* 2001 Sep;60(3):528-33

[259] Shishodia S, Majumdar S, Banerjee S, Aggarwal BB. Ursolic acid inhibits nuclear factor-kappaB activation induced by carcinogenic agents through suppression of IkappaBalpha kinase and p65 phosphorylation: correlation with down-regulation of cyclooxygenase 2, matrix metalloproteinase 9, and cyclin D1. *Cancer Res.* 2003 Aug 1;63(15):4375-83 http://cancerres.aacrjournals.org/cgi/content/full/63/15/4375

[260] "These results suggest that carnosol suppresses the NO production and iNOS gene expression by inhibiting NF-kappaB activation, and provide possible mechanisms for its anti-inflammatory and chemopreventive action." Lo AH, Liang YC, Lin-Shiau SY, Ho CT, Lin JK. Carnosol, an antioxidant in rosemary, suppresses inducible nitric oxide synthase through down-regulating nuclear factor-kappaB in mouse macrophages. *Carcinogenesis.* 2002 Jun;23(6):983-91

[261] "Constitutive and TNFalpha-induced NF-kappaB DNA binding activity was inhibited by GSE at doses > or =50 microg/ml and treatments for > or =12 h." Dhanalakshmi S, Agarwal R, Agarwal C. Inhibition of NF-kappaB pathway in grape seed extract-induced apoptotic death of human prostate carcinoma DU145 cells. *Int J Oncol.* 2003 Sep;23(3):721-7

[262] "Caffeic acid phenethyl ester (CAPE) is an anti-inflammatory component of propolis (honeybee resin). CAPE is reportedly a specific inhibitor of nuclear factor-kappaB (NF-kappaB)." Fitzpatrick LR, Wang J, Le T. Caffeic acid phenethyl ester, an inhibitor of nuclear factor-kappaB, attenuates bacterial peptidoglycan polysaccharide-induced colitis in rats. *J Pharmacol Exp Ther.* 2001 Dec;299(3):915-20

[263] "Our results suggest that zinc supplementation may lead to downregulation of the inflammatory cytokines through upregulation of the negative feedback loop A20 to inhibit induced NF-kappaB activation." Prasad AS, Bao B, Beck FW, Kucuk O, Sarkar FH. Antioxidant effect of zinc in humans. *Free Radic Biol Med.* 2004 Oct 15;37(8):1182-90

[264] Note that the patients in this study received a very high dose of selenium: 960 micrograms per day. This is at the top—and some would say over the top—of the safe and reasonable dose for long-term supplementation. In this case, the study lasted for three months. "In patients receiving selenium supplementation, selenium NF-kappaB activity was significantly reduced, reaching the same level as the nondiabetic control group. CONCLUSION: In type 2 diabetic patients, activation of NF-kappaB measured in peripheral blood monocytes can be reduced by selenium supplementation, confirming its importance in the prevention of cardiovascular diseases." Faure P, Ramon O, Favier A, Halimi S. Selenium supplementation decreases nuclear factor-kappa B activity in peripheral blood mononuclear cells from type 2 diabetic patients. *Eur J Clin Invest.* 2004 Jul;34(7):475-81

[265] Takada Y, Andreeff M, Aggarwal BB. Indole-3-carbinol suppresses NF-{kappa}B and I{kappa}B{alpha} kinase activation causing inhibition of expression of NF-{kappa}B-regulated antiapoptotic and metastatic gene products and enhancement of apoptosis in myeloid and leukemia cells. *Blood.* 2005 Apr 5; [Epub ahead of print]

[266] "Overall, our results indicated that indole-3-carbinol inhibits NF-kappaB and NF-kappaB-regulated gene expression and that this mechanism may provide the molecular basis for its ability to suppress tumorigenesis." Takada Y, Andreeff M, Aggarwal BB. Indole-3-carbinol suppresses NF-kappaB and IkappaBalpha kinase activation, causing inhibition of expression of NF-kappaB-regulated antiapoptotic and metastatic gene products and enhancement of apoptosis in myeloid and leukemia cells. *Blood.* 2005 Jul 15;106(2):641-9. Epub 2005 Apr 5.

[267] "CONCLUSIONS: Administration of N-acetylcysteine results in decreased nuclear factor-kappa B activation in patients with sepsis, associated with decreases in interleukin-8 but not interleukin-6 or soluble intercellular adhesion molecule-1. These pilot data suggest that antioxidant therapy with N-acetylcysteine may be useful in blunting the inflammatory response to sepsis." Paterson RL, Galley HF, Webster NR. The effect of N-acetylcysteine on nuclear factor-kappa B activation, interleukin-6, interleukin-8, and intercellular adhesion molecule-1 expression in patients with sepsis. *Crit Care Med.* 2003 Nov;31(11):2574-8

[268] "Resveratrol's anticarcinogenic, anti-inflammatory, and growth-modulatory effects may thus be partially ascribed to the inhibition of activation of NF-kappaB and AP-1 and the associated kinases." Manna SK, Mukhopadhyay A, Aggarwal BB. Resveratrol suppresses TNF-induced activation of nuclear transcription factors NF-kappa B, activator protein-1, and apoptosis: potential role of reactive oxygen intermediates and lipid peroxidation. *J Immunol.* 2000 Jun 15;164(12):6509-19

[269] "Both resveratrol and quercetin inhibited NF-kappaB-, AP-1- and CREB-dependent transcription to a greater extent than the glucocorticosteroid, dexamethasone." Donnelly LE, Newton R, Kennedy GE, Fenwick PS, Leung RH, Ito K, Russell RE, Barnes PJ.Anti-inflammatory Effects of Resveratrol in Lung Epithelial Cells: Molecular Mechanisms. *Am J Physiol Lung Cell Mol Physiol.* 2004 Jun 4 [Epub ahead of print]

isohumulones[270], GLA via PPAR-gamma[271] and EPA via PPAR-alpha.[272] I have reviewed the phytonutritional modulation of NF-kappaB later in this text and elsewhere.[273] Several phytonutritional products targeting NF-kappaB are available.

- Topical *Capsicum annuum, Capsicum frutescens* (Cayenne pepper, hot chili pepper): Topical capsaicin has proven beneficial for alleviating the pruritus of psoriasis, presumably by depleting cutaneous neurons of substance P.[274] Controlled clinical trials have conclusively demonstrated capsaicin's ability deplete sensory fibers of the neuropeptide substance P to thus reduce pain. Topical capsaicin is proven effective in relieving the pain associated with diabetic neuropathy[275], chronic low back pain[276], chronic neck pain[277], osteoarthritis[278], and rheumatoid arthritis.[279] Given the important role of neurogenic inflammation in chronic arthritis[280,281], the use of topical *Capsicum* should not be viewed as merely symptomatic; by depleting neurons of substance P it has the ability to help break the vicious cycle of neurogenic-immunogenic inflammation.

- Glucosamine sulfate and chondroitin sulfate: Glucosamine and chondroitin sulfates are well tolerated and well documented in the treatment of osteoarthritis.[282,283,284,285] Since these serve as substrate for the "rebuilding" and preservation of joint cartilage, they would clearly help shift the balance toward anabolism and away from catabolism within articular tissues.

- Carnitine fumarate: Fumaric acid 250-500 mg 3 times a day was advocated by Wright and Gaby[286], who advised beginning with a low dose and slowly increasing the dose over a period of weeks. Flushing and hypoglycemia may occur; serial measurements of liver and kidney function tests are mandatory since fumarate has been reported to cause liver and/or renal

[270] Yajima H, Ikeshima E, Shiraki M, Kanaya T, Fujiwara D, Odai H, Tsuboyama-Kasaoka N, Ezaki O, Oikawa S, Kondo K. Isohumulones, bitter acids derived from hops, activate both peroxisome proliferator-activated receptor alpha and gamma and reduce insulin resistance. *J Biol Chem*. 2004 Aug 6;279(32):33456-62. Epub 2004 Jun 3. http://www.jbc.org/cgi/content/full/279/32/33456

[271] "Thus, PPAR gamma serves as the receptor for GLA in the regulation of gene expression in breast cancer cells. " Jiang WG, Redfern A, Bryce RP, Mansel RE. Peroxisome proliferator activated receptor-gamma (PPAR-gamma) mediates the action of gamma linolenic acid in breast cancer cells. *Prostaglandins Leukot Essent Fatty Acids*. 2000 Feb;62(2):119-27

[272] "...EPA requires PPARalpha for its inhibitory effects on NF-kappaB." Mishra A, Chaudhary A, Sethi S. Oxidized omega-3 fatty acids inhibit NF-kappaB activation via a PPARalpha-dependent pathway. *Arterioscler Thromb Vasc Biol*. 2004 Sep;24(9):1621-7 http://atvb.ahajournals.org/cgi/content/full/24/9/1621

[273] "Indeed, the previous view that nutrients only interact with human physiology at the metabolic/post-transcriptional level must be updated in light of current research showing that nutrients can, in fact, modify human physiology and phenotype at the genetic/pre-transcriptional level." Vasquez A. Reducing pain and inflammation naturally - part 4: nutritional and botanical inhibition of NF-kappaB, the major intracellular amplifier of the inflammatory cascade. A practical clinical strategy exemplifying anti-inflammatory nutrigenomics. *Nutritional Perspectives*, July 2005:5-12. www.OptimalHealthResearch.com/part4

[274] "CONCLUSION: Topically applied capsaicin effectively treats pruritic psoriasis, a finding that supports a role for substance P in this disorder." Ellis CN, Berberian B, Sulica VI, Dodd WA, Jarratt MT, Katz HI, Prawer S, Krueger G, Rex IH Jr, Wolf JE. A double-blind evaluation of topical capsaicin in pruritic psoriasis. *J Am Acad Dermatol* 1993 Sep;29(3):438-42

[275] Treatment of painful diabetic neuropathy with topical capsaicin. A multicenter, double-blind, vehicle-controlled study. The Capsaicin Study Group. [No authors listed] *Arch Intern Med*. 1991 Nov;151(11):2225-9

[276] Keitel W, Frerick H, Kuhn U, Schmidt U, Kuhlmann M, Bredehorst A. Capsicum pain plaster in chronic non-specific low back pain. *Arzneimittelforschung*. 2001 Nov;51(11):896-903

[277] Mathias BJ, Dillingham TR, Zeigler DN, Chang AS, Belandres PV. Topical capsaicin for chronic neck pain. A pilot study. *Am J Phys Med Rehabil* 1995 Jan-Feb;74(1):39-44

[278] McCarthy GM, McCarty DJ. Effect of topical capsaicin in the therapy of painful osteoarthritis of the hands. *J Rheumatol*. 1992;19(4):604-7

[279] Deal CL, Schnitzer TJ, Lipstein E, Seibold JR, Stevens RM, Levy MD, Albert D, Renold F. Treatment of arthritis with topical capsaicin: a double-blind trial. *Clin Ther*. 1991 May-Jun;13(3):383-95

[280] Gouze-Decaris E, Philippe L, Minn A, Haouzi P, Gillet P, Netter P, Terlain B. Neurophysiological basis for neurogenic-mediated articular cartilage anabolism alteration. *Am J Physiol Regul Integr Comp Physiol*. 2001;280(1):R115-22 http://ajpregu.physiology.org/cgi/content/full/280/1/R115

[281] Decaris E, Guingamp C, Chat M, Philippe L, Grillasca JP, Abid A, Minn A, Gillet P, Netter P, Terlain B. Evidence for neurogenic transmission inducing degenerative cartilage damage distant from local inflammation. *Arthritis Rheum*. 1999;42(9):1951-60

[282] Braham R, Dawson B, Goodman C. The effect of glucosamine supplementation on people experiencing regular knee pain. *Br J Sports Med*. 2003;37(1):45-9

[283] Nguyen P, Mohamed SE, Gardiner D, Salinas T. A randomized double-blind clinical trial of the effect of chondroitin sulfate and glucosamine hydrochloride on temporomandibular joint disorders: a pilot study. *Cranio*. 2001 Apr;19(2):130-9

[284] "...oral glucosamine therapy achieved a significantly greater improvement in articular pain score than ibuprofen, and the investigators rated treatment efficacy as 'good' in a significantly greater proportion of glucosamine than ibuprofen recipients. In comparison with piroxicam, glucosamine significantly improved arthritic symptoms after 12 weeks of therapy..." Matheson AJ, Perry CM. Glucosamine: a review of its use in the management of osteoarthritis. *Drugs Aging*. 2003; 20(14): 1041-60

[285] Muller-Fassbender H, Bach GL, Haase W, Rovati LC, Setnikar I. Glucosamine sulfate compared to ibuprofen in osteoarthritis of the knee. *Osteoarthritis Cartilage*. 1994 Mar;2(1):61-9

[286] Gaby A, Wright JV. Nutritional Protocols. © 1998 by Nutrition Seminars

damage. **Carnitine appears to have anti-inflammatory action via its corticosteroid receptor agonist properties[287,288] and has been reported as beneficial in a case of psoriatic arthritis.[289]**

- <u>Spinal manipulation</u>: Many years ago I read a published case report of a female patient who experienced acute onset of psoriasis following trauma received during a skiing accident. Her psoriasis resolved promptly following a series of treatments of chiropractic spinal manipulative therapy.
- <u>Sarsaparilla (*Smilax* spp)</u>: A clinical trial published in the *New England Journal of Medicine* in 1942 documented benefit of a sarsaparilla compound.[290] The proposed mechanism of action includes the binding of bacterial endotoxins and preventing their local action and systemic absorption.
- <u>Hydrotherapy, local hyperthermia</u>: Hot bath hyperthermia (or heating pads[291]) improves skin lesions and lessens pruritus in the majority of patients with psoriasis.[292] The dermatologic improvements following hyperthermia can be objectively documented clinically and histologically/microscopically.[293]
- <u>Detoxification support</u>: Cytochrome P450 defects have been noted in patients with psoriasis and correlate with the severity of the disease.[294] See Chapter 4 of <u>Integrative Rheumatology</u> for discussion on Detoxification and Xenobiotic Immunotoxicity.

Notes:

_____

_____

_____

_____

_____

_____

_____

_____

---

[287] "Accumulating evidence from both animal and human studies indicates that pharmacologic doses of L-carnitine (LCAR) have immunomodulatory effects resembling those of glucocorticoids (GC)." Manoli I, De Martino MU, Kino T, Alesci S. Modulatory effects of L-carnitine on glucocorticoid receptor activity. *Ann N Y Acad Sci.* 2004 Nov;1033:147-57

[288] "Taken together, our results suggest that pharmacological doses of L-carnitine can activate GRalpha and, through this mechanism, regulate glucocorticoid-responsive genes, potentially sharing some of the biological and therapeutic properties of glucocorticoids."Alesci S, De Martino MU, Mirani M, Benvenga S, Trimarchi F, Kino T, Chrousos GP. L-carnitine: A nutritional modulator of glucocorticoid receptor functions. *FASEB J.* 2003 Aug;17(11):1553-5. Epub 2003 Jun 17 http://www.fasebj.org/cgi/reprint/02-1024fjev1

[289] Afeltra A, Amoroso A, Sgro P, Gandini L, Lenzi A. Clinical improvement in psoriatic arthritis symptoms during treatment for infertility with carnitine. *Clin Exp Rheumatol.* 2004 Jan-Feb;22(1):138

[290] Thurmon FM. The treatment of psoriasis with a sarsaparilla compound. *N Engl J Med* 1942; 227 (4): 128-33

[291] Urabe H, Nishitani K, Kohda H. Hyperthermia in the treatment of psoriasis. *Arch Dermatol.* 1981 Dec;117(12):770-4

[292] "These results indicate that simple repetitive water bath hyperthermia alone is effective in the treatment of psoriatic lesions in heatable locations." Boreham DR, Gasmann HC, Mitchel RE. Water bath hyperthermia is a simple therapy for psoriasis and also stimulates skin tanning in response to sunlight. *Int J Hyperthermia.* 1995 Nov-Dec;11(6):745-54

[293] "Electron microscopy of psoriatic skin prior to and after local hyperthermia revealed both temporary and gradual changes following treatment." Imayama S, Urabe H. Human psoriatic skin lesions improve with local hyperthermia: an ultrastructural study. *J Cutan Pathol.* 1984 Feb;11(1):45-52

[294] "Low CYP2C activity was associated with severe psoriasis, poor metaboliser status occurring in 50% of the severe group, but in none of the mild cases, p < 0.01." Helsby NA, Ward SA, Parslew RA, Friedmann PS, Rhodes LE. Hepatic cytochrome P450 CYP2C activity in psoriasis: studies using proguanil as a probe compound. *Acta Derm Venereol* 1998 Mar;78(2):81-3

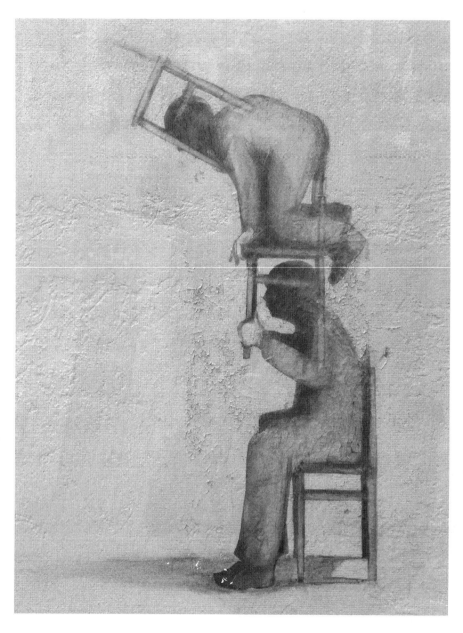

Anonymous art-quality graffiti in Paris, France—photo by Dr Vasquez in 2013: This image reminds me of the (common, American) educational process, which is often stupefying and *stupidifying*. Throughout most of my educational experience—including 12 years of doctorate-level study—I've found that most schools have impressively little commitment to *instruction* (Latin: *instruere*: to pack in, to load) and even less to *education* (Latin: *educare*: to lead out); in fact, most "professional" academicians and so-called "administrators" do not appreciate these words or concepts for their meanings nor their implications. In my experience as a Professor and Director at various schools, I frequently found so-called "senior administrators" to be completely incompetent in their roles, and completely corrupt in their willingness to literally sell-out quality faculty for personal gain and financial advantage, even at major cost to students, programs, courses, and the institution—I have seen this in various schools in various professions, including professions and some schools which I previously cherished. The pervasiveness and high level of incompetence and corruption in healthcare professions and institutions is bewildering. What I strive for with my books and courses is to resist the "dumbing down" of students and the dehumanization and eunuchification of academia in general and intellectuality in particular.

Systemic Lupus Erythematosus

Introduction:
As was said to me once by a Vice President of one of the largest hospital systems in Texas, SLE is a "big league" disease with numerous and potentially fatal complications; it is not to be taken lightly. Best interests of both doctor and patient are served by having a rheumatologist and/or internist as part of the care team. SLE is heterogeneous, multifactorial, and patient-specific in its pathology and clinical presentations.

Topics:

- Introduction and Overview
- Clinical Presentation
- Prevalence, Symptoms, and Clinical Findings
- Pathophysiology
- Differential Diagnosis
- Diagnosis
- Standard Medical Treatment
- Therapeutic Interventions

Systemic Lupus Erythematosus
"SLE" or "Lupus"

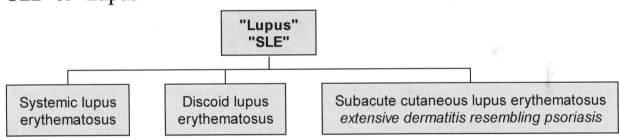

Description/pathophysiology:

- SLE is the prototype of multisystem autoimmune disease, characterized by a chronic progressive course with remissions and relapses. The skin, joints, kidneys, serosal membranes (pleura, pericardium, peritoneum), and vascular system are the most prominent targets of inflammatory attack; however, any cell and tissue may be damaged, either directly or indirectly. Autoantibodies (and resultant immune complexes) against a wide range of endogenous/self targets are pathogenic in SLE; however, **the current pathologic paradigm places ultimate responsibility on CD4+ helper T-cells—i.e., e.g., the Th1, Th2, Th17, a Treg cells discussed in Chapter 4**—rather than the antibody-producing B-cells/plasma cells. Tissue damage is largely mediated by **autoantibodies—particularly anti-nuclear antibodies (ANA)**—and the resulting **immune complexes**, cryoglobulins, and the subsequent inflammatory cascade.[1,2,3,4] **Patients**

[1] Tierney ML. McPhee SJ, Papadakis MA (eds). Current Medical Diagnosis and Treatment 2006. 45th edition. New York; Lange Medical Books: 2006, pages 833-837
[2] Suzuki N, Mihara S, Sakane T. Development of pathogenic anti-DNA antibodies in patients with systemic lupus erythematosus. *FASEB J.* 1997 Oct;11(12):1033-8 http://www.fasebj.org/cgi/reprint/11/12/1033
[3] "Pisetsky DS. Antibody responses to DNA in normal immunity and aberrant immunity. *Clin Diagn Lab Immunol.* 1998 Jan;5(1):1-6 http://cvi.asm.org/cgi/reprint/5/1/1
[4] Sikander FF, Salgaonkar DS, Joshi VR. Cryoglobulin studies in systemic lupus erythematosus. *J Postgrad Med* [serial online] 1989 [cited 2005 Nov 2];35:139-43

with SLE have impaired ability to clear immune complexes via hepatic and splenic routes[5,6]; therapeutic implications are discussed below. **SLE is considered a type-3 hypersensitivity disease because it is largely mediated by immune complex deposition** and secondary activation of the complement cascade and other inflammatory pathways.

- Allopathic perspective = "idiopathic": This condition is generally considered "idiopathic" in most cases, though in some patients the disease is induced by pharmaceutical drugs (especially hydralazine,

> **Immune complex pathophysiology**
>
> Consecutive linking of antigen and antibody results in formation of immune complexes which are predisposed for deposition in joints, skin, kidneys, and vasculature. Immune complex deposition results in focal and atopic (distant from site of antigen exposure) inflammatory damage of surrounding tissue via local activation of complement pathway and local inflammation, including recruitment of neutrophils and monocytes which release free radicals and autolytic lysosomal enzymes.

procainamide, D-penicillamine) and is then generally reversible upon discontinuation of the drug. Most people with complement deficiencies (a group of congenital immune defects) develop SLE. Other precipitating/contributing factors include ultraviolet light exposure, chemical exposure, and possibly consumption of alfalfa sprouts (based on animal data[7] and very little human data). Abnormal hormone metabolism has also been noted and may play a role in the pathogenesis as described in the section on *Orthoendocrinology*.

Clinical presentations:

- 85-90% of new patients are women in their childbearing years (frequency: 1 per 700 women); the ratio of women to men is 9:1 except among prepubertal children and older/postmenopausal men and women in which the ratio is 2:1.[8] The much higher prevalence of the disorder among women of childbearing age compared to men of the same age (11:1) implicates sex hormones and hormonal fluctuations as causative factors that predispose young women to this disorder.
- 4x more common in women of African descent (1 per 250) than Caucasian women (1 per 1000).[9]
  - *Comment and hypothesis*: The increased prevalence of SLE in dark-skinned women may be due at least in part to their higher prevalence of vitamin D deficiency, which unquestionably predisposes to inflammation, immune dysfunction, and the clinical manifestation of autoimmunity.[10] Although administration of vitamin D3 to cholecalciferol-deficient adults clearly has anti-inflammatory action[11,12], important windows of opportunity appear to occur *in utero* and within the first few postnatal months and years; for example, administration of vitamin D to **infants** reduces the subsequent incidence of type-1 *autoimmune-mediated* diabetes by 78%.[13] Vitamin D sufficiency appears to support immune function and thereby reduce the acquisition of infectious diseases[14]; thus, vitamin D may exert an anti-*rheumatic* benefit by exerting an anti-*infectious* benefit; i.e., by preventing the dysbiotic infections that may serve to trigger autoimmunity. Given the strength of evidence supporting the routine use of vitamin D3 supplementation in infants, children, and adults, healthcare providers should ensure adequate vitamin D status in their

[5] "These observations support the hypothesis that IC handling is abnormal in SLE." Davies KA, Peters AM, Beynon HL, Walport MJ. Immune complex processing in patients with systemic lupus erythematosus. In vivo imaging and clearance studies. *J Clin Invest*. 1992 Nov;90(5):2075-83 http://www.pubmedcentral.gov/articlerender.fcgi?tool=pubmed&pubmedid=1430231

[6] "These results indicate that Fc-mediated clearance of ICs is defective in patients with SLE and suggest that ligation of ICs by Fc receptors is critical for their efficient binding and retention by the fixed MPS in the liver." Davies KA, Robson MG, Peters AM, Norsworthy P, Nash JT, Walport MJ. Defective Fc-dependent processing of immune complexes in patients with systemic lupus erythematosus. *Arthritis Rheum*. 2002 Apr;46(4):1028-38

[7] "L-Canavanine sulfate, a constituent of alfalfa sprouts, was incorporated into the diet and reactivated the syndrome in monkeys in which an SLE-like syndrome had previously been induced by the ingestion of alfalfa seeds or sprouts." Malinow MR, Bardana EJ Jr, Pirofsky B, Craig S, McLaughlin P. Systemic lupus erythematosus-like syndrome in monkeys fed alfalfa sprouts: role of a nonprotein amino acid. *Science*. 1982 Apr 23;216(4544):415-7

[8] Manzi S. Epidemiology of systemic lupus erythematosus. *Am J Manag Care*. 2001 Oct;7(16 Suppl):S474-9 http://www.ajmc.com/files/articlefiles/A01_131_2001octManziS474_9.pdf

[9] Tierney ML. McPhee SJ, Papadakis MA. Current Medical Diagnosis and Treatment 2006. 45th edition. New York; Lange Medical Books: 2006, pages 833-837

[10] Cantorna MT. Vitamin D and autoimmunity: is vitamin D status an environmental factor affecting autoimmune disease prevalence? *Proc Soc Exp Biol Med*. 2000;223(3):230-3

[11] Timms PM, et al. Circulating MMP9, vitamin D and variation in the TIMP-1 response with VDR genotype: mechanisms for inflammatory damage in chronic disorders? *QJM*. 2002;95:787-96

[12] Van den Berghe G, et al. Bone turnover in prolonged critical illness: effect of vitamin D. *J Clin Endocrinol Metab*. 2003;88(10):4623-32

[13] "Children who regularly took the recommended dose of vitamin D (2000 IU daily) had a RR of 0.22 (0.05-0.89) compared with those who regularly received less than the recommended amount." Hypponen et al. Intake of vitamin D and risk of type 1 diabetes: a birth-cohort study. *Lancet*. 2001;358(9292):1500-3—one of the most important articles ever published.

[14] Wayse V, et al. Association of subclinical vitamin D deficiency with severe acute lower respiratory infection in Indian children under 5 y. *Eur J Clin Nutr*. 2004;58(4):563-7

patients[15,16,17] for the treatment and prevention of long-latency deficiency diseases[18] and alleviation of systemic inflammation.[19]

- Positive family history of the disease is common: daughters of a mother with SLE have a 1 in 40 prevalence of SLE, whereas sons have a 1 in 250 prevalence
- Clinical course may be slow or acute, involving many organ systems or only one, and is characterized by exacerbations and remissions
- **Classic autoimmune systemic manifestations: fatigue, malaise, low-grade fever, anorexia, weight loss, peripheral polyarthritis.** Septicemia and septic arthritis should always be considered in patients with SLE, especially those taking immunosuppressive drugs and those experiencing what appears to be an exacerbation of the disease.
  - Skin:
    - Malar "butterfly" rash over the cheeks and bridge of the nose: this is a classic manifestation of the disease but is seen in less than half of SLE patients.
    - Photosensitivity: erythematous skin rash develops readily on sun-exposed areas.
    - Hair loss.
    - Nail infarcts, periungual erythema, splinter hemorrhages.
    - Purpura.
  - Musculoskeletal:
    - 90% of patients have polyarthralgia—most commonly affecting the peripheral joints of the hands, wrists, knees, feet.
    - Polymyalgia, myositis, and myopathy; avascular necrosis due to corticosteroids.
  - Renal/kidney:
    - Immune complex-mediated glomerulonephritis: 50% of patients have clinical nephritis, hematuria, and proteinuria; renal function commonly declines during exacerbation of disease and then improves with disease remission.
    - **Renal failure is a leading cause of death in patients with SLE.**[20]
  - CNS:
    - 70% have EEG abnormalities
    - **Neuropsychiatric lupus is a medical emergency**[21]: characteristics include psychosis, seizures, transient ischemic attacks, severe depression, delirium, confusion. Exclude adverse drug effect (especially corticosteroid psychosis), infection, and hyponatremia.
    - Headaches, migraine, stroke
    - Peripheral and cranial neuropathies, transverse myelitis
    - Increased risk for meningitis when immunosuppressive therapy is used.
  - Cardiovascular and circulation:
    - Vasculitis
    - Thrombosis and **increased risk for myocardial infarction**
    - Pericarditis, myocarditis: may result in sudden death, heart failure, arrhythmias
    - Hypertension due to renal injury
    - Raynaud's phenomenon—periodic vasospasm affecting the hands and fingers
    - Antiphospholipid antibody syndrome—a major cause of complications
  - Lungs/pulmonary:
    - Pneumonitis: presents with fever, cough, dyspnea—important to **assess with radiographs and exclude infection**
    - Pleurisy, pleural effusion; **alveolar hemorrhage can be life-threatening**

[15] Vasquez A, Manso G, Cannell J. The clinical importance of vitamin D (cholecalciferol). *Altern Ther Health Med.* 2004 Sep-Oct;10(5):28-36
[16] Heaney RP. Vitamin D, nutritional deficiency, and the medical paradigm. *J Clin Endocrinol Metab.* 2003 Nov;88(11):5107-8
[17] Hollis BW, Wagner CL. Assessment of dietary vitamin D requirements during pregnancy and lactation. *Am J Clin Nutr.* 2004 May;79:717-26
[18] Heaney RP. Long-latency deficiency disease: insights from calcium and vitamin D. *Am J Clin Nutr.* 2003;78(5):912-9 jcem.endojournals.org/cgi/content/full/88/11/5107
[19] Timms et al. Circulating MMP9, vitamin D and variation in the TIMP-1 response with VDR genotype. *QJM.* 2002;95:787-96
[20] Suzuki et al. Development of pathogenic anti-DNA antibodies in patients with systemic lupus erythematosus. *FASEB J* 1997 Oct;11:1033-8
[21] McInnes I, Sturrock R. Rheumatological emergencies. *Practitioner.* 1994 Mar;238(1536):220-4

- o Hematologic/CBC abnormalities:
  - Leukopenia, lymphopenia
  - Thrombocytopenia
  - Anemia
  - Immune complexes: Immune complexes are elevated in patients with active SLE[22]
- o Gastrointestinal:
  - Nausea
  - Diarrhea
  - **Intestinal/mesenteric vasculitis and infarct—surgical emergency**—postprandial abdominal pain, cramps, vomiting, diarrhea
  - Pancreatitis
  - Increased intestinal permeability, occasionally of such severity that a protein-losing enteropathy results[23]
- o Eyes:
  - **Retinal vasculitis** (look for exudates with fundoscopic examination) can cause blindness in days—**treat as an emergency**
  - Other manifestations include conjunctivitis, photophobia, blurred vision
- o Other:
  - Edema—may be seen with cardiac or renal damage
  - Lymphadenopathy
  - Mucocutaneous ulcerations
  - Increased risk of miscarriage and congenital heart block

Major differential diagnoses:
- Infection
- Cancer, lymphoma
- RA or other autoimmune disease such as scleroderma, vasculitis, sarcoidosis
- Iron overload
- Fibromyalgia
- Porphyria cutanea tarda
- Drug hypersensitivity and drug-induced lupus: SLE is differentiated from drug-induced lupus by the following characteristics of drug-induced lupus: 1) temporal association with drug/medication use; remission of disease following drug discontinuation, and 2) lack of fully characteristic pattern of clinical and laboratory manifestations: lack of renal and CNS involvement, lack of hypocomplementemia and anti-native DNA antibodies. Clinicians must exclude drug-induced lupus before making diagnosis of SLE.

Clinical assessments:
- **History and physical examination**: consistent with the clinical presentations listed previously
- **Laboratory assessments**:
  - o Comprehensive laboratory evaluation: Use other tests (e.g. and especially, metabolic/chemistry panel, UA, CBC, etc.) to assess for complications and concomitant disease.
  - o **ANA: anti-nuclear antibodies**: **ANA is the best screening test and is now considered positive in 100% of patients.**[24] ANA levels correlate with disease activity. Previous editions of standard medical textbooks reported that this test was less than 100% sensitive for SLE; it may be that improvements in laboratory analysis now account for the 100% sensitivity. A positive ANA test result—even with a high titer—does not necessarily indicate that the patient has SLE, especially if no other signs or symptoms are present. ANA are directed against the following four targets: ❶ DNA, ❷ histones, ❸ non-histone proteins bound to RNA, ❹ nucleolar antigens.

---

[22] Suzuki N, Mihara S, Sakane T. Development of pathogenic anti-DNA antibodies in patients with systemic lupus erythematosus. *FASEB J.* 1997 Oct;11(12):1033-8
[23] "Fourteen cases of primary lupus-associated protein-losing enteropathy have now been reported in the English-language literature." Perednia DA, Curosh NA. Lupus-associated protein-losing enteropathy. *Arch Intern Med.* 1990 Sep;150(9):1806-10
[24] Tierney ML. McPhee SJ, Papadakis MA. Current Medical Diagnosis and Treatment 2006. 45th edition. New York; Lange Medical Books: 2006, pages 833-837

- Anti-double stranded (DS, native) DNA antibodies (anti-dsDNA): positive in ~60% of patients; specific (not sensitive) for SLE; when positive, anti-dsDNA levels correlate with disease activity.
- Anti-Sm (anti-Smith) antibodies: positive in ~30% of patients; specific (not sensitive) for SLE.[25]
- Anti-histone antibodies: seen in drug-induced lupus.
- Anti-Ro antibodies (SSA: Sjogren's syndrome antibodies): Seen with cutaneous SLE, Sjogren's syndrome, and neonatal lupus.[26]

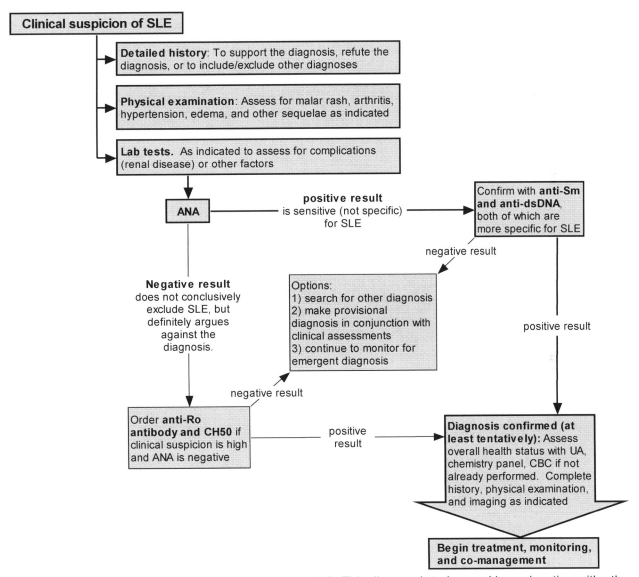

Algorithm for use of initial laboratory testing for SLE: This diagram is to be used in conjunction with other information presented in this book and any new published guidelines; however, this information will likely always remain clinically relevant and reasonably useful.

---

[25] Shojania K. Rheumatology: 2. What laboratory tests are needed? *CMAJ.* 2000 Apr 18;162(8):1157-63 http://www.cmaj.ca/cgi/content/full/162/8/1157
[26] Shojania K. Rheumatology: 2. What laboratory tests are needed? *CMAJ.* 2000 Apr 18;162(8):1157-63

- CRP is a sensitive indicator of inflammation, *except in SLE* where CRP levels can be normal even with severe active disease.[27,28]
- ESR is not useful in all patients with SLE.[29]
- Complement levels (CH50): Complement levels are lowered in accord with complement pathway activation by immune complexes; levels tend to normalize when disease is in remission.
  - Inherited complement deficiencies: 6% of SLE patients has an inherited/genetic deficiency in one or more complement proteins. Deficiency of C1q, C2, or **C4** appears to result in inability to clear immune complexes and thus results in exacerbation of disease manifestations due to immune complex deposition. C1q deficiency may impair clearance of apoptotic cells and thus promote antigenicity toward nuclear debris via—among many mechanisms—activation of DAMP (damage-associated molecular pattern) receptors.
- HLA-DR2 and HLA-DR3: These are more common in patients with SLE than in the general population.
- Serologic testing for syphilis (VDRL): A false-positive test for syphilis is characteristic of SLE and is a reflection of antiphospholipid antibodies.
- Antiphospholipid and Anticardiolipin antibodies: Antiphospholipid antibodies (directed against plasma proteins complexed to phospholipids) are seen in 40-50% of SLE patients. Antiphospholipid antibodies are associated with significantly increased risk for venous and arterial thrombosis. In SLE patients with antiphospholipid antibodies, treatment with anticoagulants such as warfarin/coumadin are commonly used (see INR below):
  - Anticardiolipin antibodies: This is one of several types of antiphospholipid antibodies; also used in syphilis serologic testing, and therefore SLE patients with anticardiolipin antibodies may have false positive result for syphilis. Anticardiolipin antibodies interfere with the PT (partial thromboplastin) test and are thus occasionally called "lupus anticoagulant"—this factitious anticoagulation is purely an *in vitro* phenomenon and is misleading since these same patients actually have a hypercoagulable state that predisposes them to arterial and venous thromboses. Readers attentive to the information on mitochondrial will have also noted that the phospholipid cardiolipin is located on the mitochondrial inner membrane, where it serves as an anchor for the enzyme succinate dehydrogenase; this data suggests an important role for mitochondrial dysfunction in SLE: a fact which is now very well proven, although not widely known by many practicing clinicians.
  - INR: International Normalized Ratio is a standardized quantification of Prothrombin Time (PT), which is a measure of clotting/bleeding tendency. INR is used to monitor dosing of warfarin/coumadin; generally the INR should be kept between 2.0-3.0.[30]
- Comprehensive testing for celiac disease and wheat allergy: Some patients diagnosed with "systemic lupus erythematosus" actually have autoimmunity and systemic inflammation due to occult celiac disease. These patients achieve clinical remission after avoiding gluten/gliadin-containing grains such as wheat.[31,32] **More than 23% of patients with SLE have anti-gliadin antibodies**.[33] In addition to IgA and IgG anti-gliadin antibodies, serologic testing for celiac disease includes IgA and IgG antiendomysial and anti-transglutaminase antibodies which should be

---

[27] Deodhar SD. C-reactive protein: the best laboratory indicator available for monitoring disease activity. *Cleve Clin J Med* 1989 Mar-Apr;56(2):126-30
[28] Gabay C, Kushner I. Acute-phase proteins and other systemic responses to inflammation. *N Engl J Med* 1999 Feb 11;340(6):448-54
[29] Klippel JH (ed). Primer on the Rheumatic Diseases. 11th Edition. Atlanta: Arthritis Foundation. 1997 page 94
[30] Tierney ML. McPhee SJ, Papadakis MA. Current Medical Diagnosis and Treatment 2006. 45th edition. New York; Lange Medical Books: 2006, pages 833-837
[31] "The immunological profile of IgA deficiency and/or raised double stranded DNA in the absence of antinuclear factor together with raised inflammatory markers and symptoms suggestive of an immune diathesis should alert the physician to the possibility of gluten sensitivity." Hadjivassiliou M, Sanders DS, Grunewald RA, Akil M. Gluten sensitivity masquerading as systemic lupus erythematosus. *Ann Rheum Dis.* 2004 Nov;63(11):1501-3 http://ard.bmjjournals.com/cgi/content/full/63/11/1501
[32] "Villous atrophy on duodenal biopsy specimens with a favorable response to a gluten-free diet was noted in all five patients." Zitouni M, Daoud W, Kallel M, Makni S. Systemic lupus erythematosus with celiac disease: a report of five cases. *Joint Bone Spine.* 2004 Jul;71(4):344-6
[33] "Twenty-four of 103 (23.3%) systemic lupus erythematosus patients tested positive for either antigliadin antibody, whereas none of the 103 tested positive for antiendomysial antibody." Rensch MJ, Szyjkowski R, Shaffer RT, Fink S, Kopecky C, Grissmer L, Enzenhauer R, Kadakia S. The prevalence of celiac disease autoantibodies in patients with systemic lupus erythematosus. *Am J Gastroenterol.* 2001 Apr;96(4):1113-5 For the authors to state that these patients did not have celiac disease simply because their intestinal biopsies were normal seems to indicate that the authors were ignorant of the modern paradigm of celiac disease which acknowledges that the disease can be present in the absence of gastrointestinal lesions.

interpreted along with a test for total serum IgA to identify those patients with selective IgA deficiency.

- **Imaging**:
    - o Imaging is used to in the assessment of complications and exclusion of concomitant diseases.
    - o The arthritis of SLE is typically mild (compared to rheumatoid arthritis) and is nondeforming.

Establishing the diagnosis: Clinical presentation and lab tests; more positives = more confident DX.
- **Qualification for a diagnosis of SLE requires at least four of the following eleven criteria**:
    1. Malar/cheek rash
    2. Discoid rash
    3. Photosensitivity
    4. Ulcerations of oral mucosa
    5. Joint pain and inflammation not attributable to other disease or trauma
    6. Serositis: Inflammation of the serous tissues, which line the lungs (pleura), heart (pericardium), and the inner lining of the abdomen (peritoneum) and associated organs
    7. Renal disease (any of the following): >3+ proteinuria measured by dipstick; cellular casts; proteinuria >0.5 grams per day
    8. CNS involvement: seizures or psychosis without other cause
    9. Hematologic abnormalities (any of the following): hemolytic anemia, leucopenia (45%), lymphopenia, thrombocytopenia (30%), anemia of chronic disease
    10. **Positive ANA**
    11. Additional serologic tests (any of the following):
        a. Positive LE cell prep
        b. Anti-native DNA antibody (50%)
        c. Anti-Sm antibody (20%)
        d. False-positive test for syphilis (25%)

Life-threatening complications and medical emergencies:
- **Infection—Infections are now the leading cause of death in patients with SLE**[34]
- **SLE complications: renal failure and CNS involvement**
- **Stroke, myocardial infarction**—Increased risk with male gender and antiphospholipid antibodies
- Septic arthritis
- Thromboembolism
- 10-year survival is >85%[35]

Overview of clinical management:
- **The clinical course of the disease is variable, marked by exacerbations and remissions. Life-threatening complications can develop rapidly and must be managed effectively to prevent patient morbidity and practitioner liability.**
- Treat patient safely and effectively. If you cannot get good results, refer them to someone who can. Refer if clinical outcome is unsatisfactory or if serious complications are possible. Stable patients are seen every 3-6 months for monitoring of disease activity, re-examination, and treatment recalibration.[36] Patients must understand that acute exacerbations and/or new symptoms—especially fever—must be evaluated promptly.
- Treatment must be customized to the patient and must be flexible to accommodate the natural exacerbations and remissions of the disease.

[34] Tierney ML. McPhee SJ, Papadakis MA. Current Medical Diagnosis and Treatment 2006. 45th edition. New York; Lange Medical Books: 2006, pages 833-837
[35] Tierney ML. McPhee SJ, Papadakis MA. Current Medical Diagnosis and Treatment 2006. 45th edition. New York; Lange Medical Books: 2006, pages 833-837
[36] Manzi S. Epidemiology of systemic lupus erythematosus. Am J Manag Care 2001 Oct;7(16Sup):S474-9 ajmc.com/files/articlefiles/A01_131_2001octManziS474_9.pdf

- To the extent possible, discourage use of NSAIDs since these drugs exacerbate joint destruction, renal impairment, and increased intestinal permeability which increases exposure to dietary and microbial antigens.

Treatments: The standard medical protocol centers on and starts with (new drugs are always being developed and added): prednisone, Plaquenil and immunoparalytic and immunosuppressive drugs.

1. **NSAIDs** are used for joint pain[37] despite adverse effects on the gut[38], joints[39,40,41], and kidneys.
2. **Antimalarial drug: hydroxychloroquine/Plaquenil**): Adverse effects include retinal damage, neuropathy, myopathy. As with anticonvulsant drugs, hydroxychloroquine/Plaquenil interferes with conversion of 25-hydroxycholecalciferol to the more active 1-25-dihydroxycholecalciferol[42]; this would be expected to exacerbate immune dysfunction, inflammation, hypertension, and depression.
3. **Danazol is an androgenic corticosteroid:** particularly used against thrombocytopenia
4. **Immunosuppression** with <u>prednisone</u> (promotes bacterial overgrowth and osteoporosis), <u>cyclophosphamide</u> (especially for renal involvement), <u>mycophenolate mofetil</u>, <u>azathioprine</u>, or other DMARD (disease-modifying antirheumatic drugs) is commonly used, particularly for the more serious complications of the disease such as those affecting the brain, heart, lungs, and kidneys. **Despite the clinical drawbacks and philosophical inadequacies, pharmacologic immunosuppression has a role in the management of patients with autoimmunity when their disease flares and threatens vital structures, particularly the heart, brain, and kidneys.**
5. **Anticoagulant drugs such as <u>warfarin</u>** are used for patients with antiphospholipid antibodies and resultant thrombotic complications.

Functional Inflammology protocol via the FINDSEX™ acronym
1. Food, basic supplementation, allergy identification via elimination and challenge,
2. Infections and dysbiosis
3. Nutritional immunomodulation: nutritional induction of Treg cells at the reciprocal expense of Th-17 cells
4. Dysfunctional mitochondria: elimination, disinhibition, stimulation
5. Style of living: stress, sleep, sweat/exercise, spinal manipulation, surgery, stamp your passport and go
6. Endocrine balance and optimization
7. Xenobiotic immunotoxicity

- <u>Avoidance of proinflammatory foods</u>: Pro-inflammatory foods act *directly* and *indirectly* to promote and exacerbate systemic inflammation. *Direct* mechanisms include the activation of Toll-like receptors and NF-kappaB, while *indirect* mechanisms include depleting the body of anti-inflammatory nutrients and dietary displacement of more nutrient-dense anti-inflammatory foods. Arachidonic acid (found in cow's milk, beef, liver, pork, and lamb) is the direct precursor to pro-inflammatory prostaglandins and leukotrienes[43] and pain-promoting isoprostanes.[44] Saturated fats promote inflammation by activating/enabling pro-inflammatory Toll-like receptors, which are otherwise "specific" for inducing

---

[37] Tierney ML. McPhee SJ, Papadakis MA. <u>Current Medical Diagnosis and Treatment 2006. 45th edition</u>. New York; Lange Medical Books: 2006, pages 833-837

[38] Abbreviations: cow's milk beta-lactoglobulin absorption (BLG), acetylsalicylic acid (ASA), disodium chromoglycate (DSCG). "ASA administration strongly increased BLG absorption, not prevented by DSCG pretreatment. In normal controls treated with a single dose of ASA we obtained similar results. Our results suggest that prolonged treatment with nonsteroidal anti-inflammatory drugs induces an increase of food antigen absorption, apparently not related to anaphylaxis mediator release, with possible clinical effects." Fagiolo U, Paganelli R, Ossi E, Quinti I, Cancian M, D'Offizi GP, Fiocco U. Intestinal permeability and antigen absorption in rheumatoid arthritis. Effects of acetylsalicylic acid and sodium chromoglycate. *Int Arch Allergy Appl Immunol*. 1989;89(1):98-102

[39] "At…concentrations comparable to those… in the synovial fluid of patients treated with the drug, several NSAIDs suppress proteoglycan synthesis…." Brandt KD. Effects of nonsteroidal anti-inflammatory drugs on chondrocyte metabolism in vitro and in vivo. *Am J Med*. 1987 Nov 20; 83(5A): 29-34

[40] "This highly significant association between NSAID use and acetabular destruction gives cause for concern, not least because of the difficulty in achieving satisfactory hip replacements in patients with severely damaged acetabula." Newman NM, Ling RS. Acetabular bone destruction related to non-steroidal anti-inflammatory drugs. *Lancet*. 1985 Jul 6; 2(8445): 11-4

[41] Vidal y Plana RR, et al. Articular cartilage pharmacology: I. In vitro studies on glucosamine and non steroidal anti-inflammatory drugs. *Pharmacol Res Commun*. 1978 Jun;10(6):557-69

[42] "CONCLUSION: Half the SLE and FM patients had 25(OH)-vitamin D levels < 50 nmol/l, a level at which PTH stimulation occurs. Our data suggest that in SLE patients HCQ might inhibit conversion of 25(OH)-vitamin D to 1,25(OH)2-vitamin D." Huisman AM, White KP, Algra A, Harth M, Vieth R, Jacobs JW, Bijlsma JW, Bell DA. Vitamin D levels in women with systemic lupus erythematosus and fibromyalgia. *J Rheumatol*. 2001 Nov;28(11):2535-9

[43] Vasquez A. Reducing Pain and Inflammation Naturally. Part 2: New Insights into Fatty Acid Supplementation and Its Effect on Eicosanoid Production and Genetic Expression. *Nutritional Perspectives* 2005; January: 5-16

[44] Evans AR, Junger H, Southall MD, Nicol GD, Sorkin LS, Broome JT, Bailey TW, Vasko MR. Isoprostanes, novel eicosanoids that produce nociception and sensitize rat sensory neurons. *J Pharmacol Exp Ther*. 2000 Jun;293(3):912-20

pro-inflammatory responses to microorganisms.[45] Consumption of saturated fat in the form of cream creates marked oxidative stress and lipid peroxidation that lasts for at least 3 hours postprandially.[46] Corn oil rapidly activates NF-kappaB (in hepatic Kupffer cells) for a pro-inflammatory effect[47]; similarly, consumption of PUFA and linoleic acid promotes antioxidant depletion and may thus promote oxidation-mediated inflammation via activation of NF-kappaB. Linoleic acid causes intracellular oxidative stress and calcium influx and results in increased NF-kappaB-stimulated transcription of pro-inflammatory genes.[48] High glycemic foods cause oxidative stress[49,50] and inflammation via activation of NF-kappaB and other mechanisms—e.g., *white bread causes inflammation*[51] as does *a high-fat high-carbohydrate fast-food-style breakfast.*[52] High glycemic foods suppress immune function[53,54] and thus promote the perpetuation of infection/dysbiosis. Delivery of a high carbohydrate load to the gastrointestinal lumen promotes bacterial overgrowth[55,56], which is inherently pro-inflammatory[57,58] and which appears to be myalgenic in humans[59] at least in part due to the ability of endotoxin to impair muscle function.[60] Overconsumption of high-carbohydrate low-phytonutrient grains, potatoes, and manufactured foods displaces phytonutrient-dense foods such as fruits, vegetables, nuts, seeds, and berries which contain more than 8,000 phytonutrients, many of which have antioxidant and thus anti-inflammatory actions.[61,62]

- <u>Avoidance of allergenic foods</u>: Any patient may be allergic to any food, even if the food is generally considered a health-promoting food. Generally speaking, the most notorious allergens are wheat, citrus (especially juice due to the industrial use of fungal hemicellulases), cow's milk, eggs, peanuts, chocolate, and yeast-containing foods; according to a study in patients with migraine, some patients will have to avoid as many as 10 specific foods in order to become symptom-free.[63] Celiac disease can present with inflammatory oligoarthritis that resembles rheumatoid arthritis and which remits with

[45] Lee JY, Sohn KH, Rhee SH, Hwang D. Saturated fatty acids, but not unsaturated fatty acids, induce the expression of cyclooxygenase-2 mediated through Toll-like receptor 4. *J Biol Chem*. 2001 May 18;276(20):16683-9. Epub 2001 Mar 2 http://www.jbc.org/cgi/content/full/276/20/16683

[46] "CONCLUSIONS: Both fat and protein intakes stimulate ROS generation. The increase in ROS generation lasted 3 h after cream intake and 1 h after protein intake. Cream intake also caused a significant and prolonged increase in lipid peroxidation." Mohanty P, Ghanim H, Hamouda W, Aljada A, Garg R, Dandona P. Both lipid and protein intakes stimulate increased generation of reactive oxygen species by polymorphonuclear leukocytes and mononuclear cells. *Am J Clin Nutr*. 2002 Apr;75(4):767-72 http://www.ajcn.org/cgi/content/full/75/4/767

[47] Rusyn I, Bradham CA, Cohn L, Schoonhoven R, Swenberg JA, Brenner DA, Thurman RG. Corn oil rapidly activates nuclear factor-kappaB in hepatic Kupffer cells by oxidant-dependent mechanisms. *Carcinogenesis*. 1999 Nov;20(11):2095-100 http://carcin.oxfordjournals.org/cgi/content/full/20/11/2095

[48] "Exposing endothelial cells to 90 micromol linoleic acid/L for 6 h resulted in a significant increase in lipid hydroperoxides that coincided wih an increase in intracellular calcium concentrations." Hennig B, Toborek M, Joshi-Barve S, Barger SW, Barve S, Mattson MP, McClain CJ. Linoleic acid activates nuclear transcription factor-kappa B (NF-kappa B) and induces NF-kappa B-dependent transcription in cultured endothelial cells. *Am J Clin Nutr*. 1996 Mar;63(3):322-8 http://www.ajcn.org/cgi/reprint/63/3/322

[49] Mohanty P, Hamouda W, Garg R, Aljada A, Ghanim H, Dandona P. Glucose challenge stimulates reactive oxygen species (ROS) generation by leucocytes. *J Clin Endocrinol Metab*. 2000 Aug;85(8):2970-3 http://jcem.endojournals.org/cgi/content/full/85/8/2970 Glucose/carbohydrate and saturated fat consumption appear to be the two biggest offenders in the food-stimulated production of oxidative stress. The effect by protein is much less. "CONCLUSIONS: Both fat and protein intakes stimulate ROS generation. The increase in ROS generation lasted 3 h after cream intake and 1 h after protein intake. Cream intake also caused a significant and prolonged increase in lipid peroxidation." Mohanty P, Ghanim H, Hamouda W, Aljada A, Garg R, Dandona P. Both lipid and protein intakes stimulate increased generation of reactive oxygen species by polymorphonuclear leukocytes and mononuclear cells. *Am J Clin Nutr*. 2002 Apr;75(4):767-72 http://www.ajcn.org/cgi/content/full/75/4/767

[50] Koska J, Blazicek P, Marko M, Grna JD, Kvetnansky R, Vigas M. Insulin, catecholamines, glucose and antioxidant enzymes in oxidative damage during different loads in healthy humans. *Physiol Res*. 2000;49 Suppl 1:S95-100 http://www.biomed.cas.cz/physiolres/pdf/2000/49_S95.pdf

[51] "Conclusion - The present study shows that high GI carbohydrate, but not low GI carbohydrate, mediates an acute proinflammatory process as measured by NF-kappaB activity." Dickinson S, Hancock DP, Petocz P, Brand-Miller JC..High glycemic index carbohydrate mediates an acute proinflammatory process as measured by NF-kappaB activation. *Asia Pac J Clin Nutr*. 2005;14 Suppl:S120

[52] Aljada A, Mohanty P, Ghanim H, Abdo T, Tripathy D, Chaudhuri A, Dandona P. Increase in intranuclear nuclear factor kappaB and decrease in inhibitor kappaB in mononuclear cells after a mixed meal: evidence for a proinflammatory effect. *Am J Clin Nutr*. 2004 Apr;79(4):682-90 http://www.ajcn.org/cgi/content/full/79/4/682

[53] Sanchez A, Reeser JL, Lau HS, et al. Role of sugars in human neutrophilic phagocytosis. *Am J Clin Nutr*. 1973 Nov;26(11):1180-4

[54] "Postoperative infusion of carbohydrate solution leads to moderate fall in the serum concentration of inorganic phosphate. ... The hypophosphatemia was associated with significant reduction of neutrophil phagocytosis, intracellular killing, consumption of oxygen and generation of superoxide during phagocytosis." Rasmussen A, Segel E, Hessov I, Borregaard N. Reduced function of neutrophils during routine postoperative glucose infusion. *Acta Chir Scand*. 1988 Jul-Aug;154(7-8):429-33

[55] Ramakrishnan T, Stokes P. Beneficial effects of fasting and low carbohydrate diet in D-lactic acidosis associated with short-bowel syndrome. *JPEN J Parenter Enteral Nutr*. 1985 May-Jun;9(3):361-3

[56] Gottschall E. Breaking the Vicious Cycle: Intestinal Health Through Diet. Kirkton Press; Rev edition (August 1, 1994)

[57] Lin HC. Small intestinal bacterial overgrowth: a framework for understanding irritable bowel syndrome. *JAMA*. 2004 Aug 18;292(7):852-8

[58] Lichtman SN, Wang J, Sartor RB, Zhang C, Bender D, Dalldorf FG, Schwab JH. Reactivation of arthritis induced by small bowel bacterial overgrowth in rats: role of cytokines, bacteria, and bacterial polymers. *Infect Immun*. 1995 Jun;63(6):2295-301

[59] Pimentel M, et al. A link between irritable bowel syndrome and fibromyalgia may be related to findings on lactulose breath testing. *Ann Rheum Dis*. 2004 Apr;63(4):450-2

[60] Bundgaard H, Kjeldsen K, Suarez Krabbe K, van Hall G, Simonsen L, Qvist J, Hansen CM, Moller K, Fonsmark L, Lav Madsen P, Klarlund Pedersen B. Endotoxemia stimulates skeletal muscle Na+-K+-ATPase and raises blood lactate under aerobic conditions in humans. *Am J Physiol Heart Circ Physiol*. 2003 Mar;284(3):H1028-34. Epub 2002 Nov 21 http://ajpheart.physiology.org/cgi/reprint/284/3/H1028

[61] "We propose that the additive and synergistic effects of phytochemicals in fruit and vegetables are responsible for their potent antioxidant and anticancer activities, and that the benefit of a diet rich in fruit and vegetables is attributed to the complex mixture of phytochemicals present in whole foods." Liu RH. Health benefits of fruit and vegetables are from additive and synergistic combinations of phytochemicals. *Am J Clin Nutr*. 2003 Sep;78(3 Suppl):517S-520S

[62] Seaman DR. The diet-induced proinflammatory state: a cause of chronic pain and other degenerative diseases? *J Manipulative Physiol Ther*. 2002;25(3):168-79

[63] Grant EC. Food allergies and migraine. *Lancet*. 1979 May 5;1(8123):966-9

avoidance of wheat/gluten; the inflammatory arthropathy of celiac disease has preceded bowel symptoms and/or an accurate diagnosis by as many as 3-15 years.[64,65] **Some patients diagnosed with "systemic lupus erythematosus" actually have autoimmunity and systemic inflammation due to occult celiac disease, and they achieve remarkable improvement—complete remission of systemic inflammation and the ability to discontinue all anti-inflammatory drugs—after avoiding gluten/gliadin-containing grains—most notoriously, wheat.**[66] In a study of 103 SLE patients, **more than 23% of SLE patients had anti-gliadin antibodies.**[67] Clinicians must explain to their patients that celiac disease and wheat allergy are two different clinical entities and that exclusion of one does not exclude the other, and in neither case does mutual exclusion obviate the promotion of intestinal bacterial overgrowth (i.e., proinflammatory dysbiosis) by indigestible wheat oligosaccharides.

- Cardiovascular disease (CVD) risk reduction: **Patients with SLE have an increased risk of cardiovascular disease due to the synergistic effects of inflammation, oxidative stress, antiphospholipid antibodies, and elevated homocysteine.** Obviously, the risk for CVD will be exacerbated if the SLE patient has other risk factors such as tobacco use, diabetes, obesity, hypertension, or physical inactivity. Therapeutic and interventional considerations specific to the prevention of cardiovascular disease include but are not limited to the following:
  - Cardioprotective diet: Paleo-Mediterranean diet
  - Fatty acid supplementation: Combination fatty acid supplementation with ALA, GLA, EPA, DHA[68,69]
  - Magnesium supplementation: > 200 mg up to bowel tolerance
  - Treatments to lower homocysteine: Doses given here for various treatments are for adults:
    - Folic acid: 5-10 mg, should be used with high-dose vitamin B-12
    - Hydroxocobalamin: 2,000-6,000 mcg/d orally, or 1,000-4,000 mcg/wk by injection
    - Pyridoxine: 250 mg/day with meals, co-administered with magnesium (e.g., >200 mg/d)
    - NAC: 600 mg tid
    - Betaine/ trimethylglycine: 1-2 grams tid (>6 grams daily when used alone)
    - Lecithin: 2.6 g choline/d (as phosphatidylcholine) decreased mean fasting plasma homocysteine by 18%.[70] Attaining this high dose might require as many as 45 capsules of commercially available supplements; an equivalent dose in the form of powdered lecithin granules delivered in a smoothie may be better tolerated than the capsules.
    - Thyroid hormone: as indicated
  - Policosanol—conflicting research (despite some impressive clinical results), this supplement has largely fallen out of favor: Policosanol (20 mg per day)[71,72] is derived from sugar cane,

[64] "We report six patients with coeliac disease in whom arthritis was prominent at diagnosis and who improved with dietary therapy. Joint pain preceded diagnosis by up to three years in five patients and 15 years in one patient." Bourne JT, Kumar P, Huskisson EC, Mageed R, Unsworth DJ, Wojtulewski JA. Arthritis and coeliac disease. *Ann Rheum Dis*. 1985 Sep;44(9):592-8

[65] "A 15-year-old girl, with synovitis of the knees and ankles for 3 years before a diagnosis of gluten-sensitive enteropathy, is described." Pinals RS. Arthritis associated with gluten-sensitive enteropathy. *J Rheumatol*. 1986 Feb;13(1):201-4

[66] "The immunological profile of IgA deficiency and/or raised double stranded DNA in the absence of antinuclear factor together with raised inflammatory markers and symptoms suggestive of an immune diathesis should alert the physician to the possibility of gluten sensitivity." Hadjivassiliou M, Sanders DS, Grunewald RA, Akil M. Gluten sensitivity masquerading as systemic lupus erythematosus. *Ann Rheum Dis*. 2004 Nov;63(11):1501-3 http://ard.bmjjournals.com/cgi/content/full/63/11/1501

[67] "Twenty-four of 103 (23.3%) systemic lupus erythematosus patients tested positive for either antigliadin antibody, whereas none of the 103 patients tested positive for antiendomysial antibody." Rensch MJ, Szyjkowski R, Shaffer RT, Fink S, Kopecky C, Grissmer L, Enzenhauer R, Kadakia S. The prevalence of celiac disease autoantibodies in patients with systemic lupus erythematosus. *Am J Gastroenterol*. 2001 Apr;96(4):1113-5. For the authors to state that these patients did not have celiac disease simply because their intestinal biopsies were normal seems to indicate that the authors were ignorant of the modern paradigm of celiac disease which acknowledges that the disease can be present in the absence of gastrointestinal lesions.

[68] Vasquez A. Reducing Pain and Inflammation Naturally. Part 2: New Insights into Fatty Acid Supplementation and Its Effect on Eicosanoid Production and Genetic Expression. *Nutritional Perspectives* 2005; January: 5-16 www.optimalhealthresearch.com/part2

[69] Laidlaw M, Holub BJ. Effects of supplementation with fish oil-derived n-3 fatty acids and gamma-linolenic acid on circulating plasma lipids and fatty acid profiles in women. *Am J Clin Nutr*. 2003 Jan;77(1):37-42 http://www.ajcn.org/cgi/content/full/77/1/37

[70] Olthof MR, Brink EJ, Katan MB, Verhoef P. Choline supplemented as phosphatidylcholine decreases fasting and postmethionine-loading plasma homocysteine concentrations in healthy men. *Am J Clin Nutr*. 2005 Jul;82(1):111-7

[71] "These results show that policosanol-treated CHD patients improved clinical evolution, and exercise-ECG responses, owing to the amelioration of myocardial ischemia, even more when administered with aspirin." Stusser R, Batista J, Padron R, Sosa F, Pereztol O. Long-term therapy with policosanol improves treadmill exercise-ECG testing performance of coronary heart disease patients. *Int J Clin Pharmacol Ther*. 1998 Sep;36(9):469-73

[72] "Policosanol seems to be a very promising phytochemical alternative to classic lipid-lowering agents such as the statins and deserves further evaluation." Gouni-Berthold I, Berthold HK. Policosanol: clinical pharmacology and therapeutic significance of a new lipid-lowering agent. *Am Heart J*. 2002 Feb;143(2):356-65

standardized for content of octacosanol. In addition to its ability to favorably modulate lipid parameters, policosanol also exerts an anticoagulant effect and therefore exerts cardioprotective benefits independent from its lipid-lowering characteristics. Policosanol may be used with low-dose aspirin in this regard; in some cases, the cardioprotective/antithrombotic benefit of *low-dose* aspirin justifies its use despite its adverse effects, such as increased intestinal permeability.

- Alcohol/ethanol avoidance: Consumption of alcoholic beverages—even in low doses—increases intestinal permeability and can exacerbate inflammatory disorders, particularly those associated with food allergies, gastrointestinal dysbiosis, and/or overproduction of estrogen.

- Supplemented Paleo-Mediterranean diet: The health-promoting diet of choice for the majority of people is a diet based on abundant consumption of fruits, vegetables, seeds, nuts, omega-3 and monounsaturated fatty acids, and lean sources of protein such as lean meats, fatty cold-water fish, soy and whey proteins. This diet obviates overconsumption of chemical preservatives, artificial sweeteners, and carbohydrate-dominant foods such as candies, pastries, breads, potatoes, grains, and other foods with a high glycemic load and high glycemic index. This "Paleo-Mediterranean Diet" is a combination of the "Paleolithic" or "Paleo diet" and the well-known "Mediterranean diet", both of which are well described in peer-reviewed journals and the lay press. (See Chapter 2 and my other publications[73,74] for details). This diet is the most nutrient-dense diet available, and its benefits are further enhanced by supplementation with vitamins, minerals, probiotics, and the health-promoting fatty acids: ALA, GLA, EPA, DHA.

- Gluten-free vegetarian diet: Vegetarian/vegan diets have a place in the treatment plan of all patients with autoimmune/inflammatory disorders[75,76]; this is also true for patients for whom long-term exclusive reliance on a meat-free vegetarian diet is either not appropriate or not appealing. No legitimate scientist or literate clinician doubts the antirheumatic power and anti-inflammatory advantages of vegetarian diets, whether used short-term or long term.[77] The benefits of gluten-free vegetarian diets are well documented, and the mechanisms of action are well elucidated, including reduced intake of proinflammatory linoleic[78] and arachidonic acids[79], iron[80], common food antigens[81], gluten[82] and gliadin[83,84], proinflammatory sugars[85] and increased intake of omega-3 fatty acids and

[73] Vasquez A. A Five-Part Nutritional Protocol that Produces Consistently Positive Results. *Nutritional Wellness* 2005 September Available in the printed version and on-line at http://www.nutritionalwellness.com/archives/2005/sep/09_vasquez.php and http://optimalhealthresearch.com/protocol

[74] Vasquez A. Implementing the Five-Part Nutritional Wellness Protocol for the Treatment of Various Health Problems. *Nutritional Wellness* 2005 November. Available on-line at http://www.nutritionalwellness.com/archives/2005/nov/11_vasquez.php and http://optimalhealthresearch.com/protocol

[75] "After four weeks at the health farm the diet group showed a significant improvement in number of tender joints, Ritchie's articular index, number of swollen joints, pain score, duration of morning stiffness, grip strength, erythrocyte sedimentation rate, C-reactive protein, white blood cell count, and a health assessment questionnaire score." Kjeldsen-Kragh J, Haugen M, Borchgrevink CF, Laerum E, Eek M, Mowinkel P, Hovi K, Forre O. Controlled trial of fasting and one-year vegetarian diet in rheumatoid arthritis. *Lancet*. 1991 Oct 12;338(8772):899-902

[76] "During the vegan diet, both signs and symptoms returned in most patients, with the exception of some patients with psoriasis who experienced an improvement." Lithell H, Bruce A, Gustafsson IB, Hoglund NJ, Karlstrom B, Ljunghall K, Sjolin K, Venge P, Werner I, Vessby B. A fasting and vegetarian diet treatment trial on chronic inflammatory disorders. *Acta Derm Venereol*. 1983;63(5):397-403

[77] "For the patients who were randomised to the vegetarian diet there was a significant decrease in platelet count, leukocyte count, calprotectin, total IgG, IgM rheumatoid factor (RF), C3-activation products, and the complement components C3 and C4 after one month of treatment." Kjeldsen-Kragh J, Mellbye OJ, Haugen M, Mollnes TE, Hammer HB, Sioud M, Forre O. Changes in laboratory variables in rheumatoid arthritis patients during a trial of fasting and one-year vegetarian diet. *Scand J Rheumatol*. 1995;24(2):85-93

[78] Rusyn I, Bradham CA, Cohn L, Schoonhoven R, Swenberg JA, Brenner DA, Thurman RG. Corn oil rapidly activates nuclear factor-kappaB in hepatic Kupffer cells by oxidant-dependent mechanisms. *Carcinogenesis*. 1999 Nov;20(11):2095-100 http://carcin.oxfordjournals.org/cgi/content/full/20/11/2095

[79] Vasquez A. Reducing Pain and Inflammation Naturally. Part 2: New Insights into Fatty Acid Supplementation and Its Effect on Eicosanoid Production and Genetic Expression. *Nutritional Perspectives* 2005; January: 5-16 http://optimalhealthresearch.com/part2

[80] Dabbagh AJ, Trenam CW, Morris CJ, Blake DR. Iron in joint inflammation. *Ann Rheum Dis*. 1993 Jan;52(1):67-73

[81] Hafstrom I, Ringertz B, Spangberg A, von Zweigbergk L, Brannemark S, Nylander I, Ronnelid J, Laasonen L, Klareskog L. A vegan diet free of gluten improves the signs and symptoms of rheumatoid arthritis: the effects on arthritis correlate with a reduction in antibodies to food antigens. *Rheumatology* (Oxford). 2001 Oct;40(10):1175-9 http://rheumatology.oxfordjournals.org/cgi/reprint/40/10/1175

[82] "The data provide evidence that dietary modification may be of clinical benefit for certain RA patients, and that this benefit may be related to a reduction in immunoreactivity to food antigens eliminated by the change in diet." Hafstrom I, Ringertz B, Spangberg A, von Zweigbergk L, Brannemark S, Nylander I, Ronnelid J, Laasonen L, Klareskog L. A vegan diet free of gluten improves the signs and symptoms of rheumatoid arthritis: the effects on arthritis correlate with a reduction in antibodies to food antigens. *Rheumatology* (Oxford). 2001 Oct;40(10):1175-9

[83] "Despite the increased AGA [antigliadin antibodies] positivity found distinctively in patients with recent-onset RA, none of the RA patients showed clear evidence of coeliac disease." Paimela L, Kurki P, Leirisalo-Repo M, Piirainen H. Gliadin immune reactivity in patients with rheumatoid arthritis. Clin Exp Rheumatol. 1995 Sep-Oct;13(5):603-7

[84] "The median IgA antigliadin ELISA index was 7.1 (range 2.1-22.4) for the RA group and 3.1 (range 0.3-34.9) for the controls (p = 0.0001)." Koot VC, Van Straaten M, Hekkens WT, Collee G, Dijkmans BA. Elevated level of IgA gliadin antibodies in patients with rheumatoid arthritis. *Clin Exp Rheumatol*. 1989 Nov-Dec;7(6):623-6

[85] Seaman DR. The diet-induced proinflammatory state: a cause of chronic pain and other degenerative diseases? *J Manipulative Physiol Ther*. 2002 Mar-Apr;25(3):168-79

micronutrients[86], and anti-inflammatory and anti-oxidant phytonutrients[87]; vegetarian diets also effect profound changes—both *qualitative* and *quantitative*—in intestinal flora[88,89] that correlate with clinical improvement.[90] **Some patients diagnosed "systemic lupus erythematosus" have autoimmunity and systemic inflammation due to occult celiac disease, and they achieve complete remission of systemic inflammation and the ability to discontinue all anti-inflammatory drugs after avoiding gluten/gliadin-containing grains.**[91] Patients who rely on the Paleo-Mediterranean Diet can use vegetarian meals, on a daily basis or for days at a time, for example, by having a daily vegetarian meal, or one week per month of vegetarianism. Of course, some (not all) patients can use a purely vegetarian diet long-term provided that nutritional needs (especially protein and cobalamin) are consistently met.

- <u>Short-term fasting</u>: Whether the foundational diet is Paleo-Mediterranean, vegetarian, vegan, or a combination of all of these, autoimmune/inflammatory patients will still benefit from periodic fasting, whether on a weekly (e.g., every Saturday), monthly (every first week or weekend of the month, or every other month), or yearly (1-2 weeks of the year) basis. Since consumption of food—particularly unhealthy foods—induces an inflammatory effect[92], abstinence from food provides a relative anti-oxidative and anti-inflammatory benefit[93] with many of the antioxidant benefits beginning within 24 hours of the initiation of the fast.[94] Fasting indeed provides a distinct anti-inflammatory benefit and may help "re-calibrate" metabolic and homeostatic mechanisms by breaking self-perpetuating "vicious cycles"[95] that autonomously promote inflammation independent from proinflammatory stimuli. Of course, water-only fasting is completely hypoallergenic (assuming that the patient is not sensitive to chlorine, fluoride, or other contaminants), and subsequent re-introduction of foods provides the ideal opportunity to identify offending foods. Fasting deprives intestinal microbes of substrate[96], stimulates intestinal B-cell immunity[97], improves the bactericidal action of neutrophils[98], reduces lysozyme release and leukotriene formation[99], and ameliorates intestinal hyperpermeability.[100] In case reports and clinical trials, short-term fasting (or protein-sparing fasting)

[86] Hagfors L, Nilsson I, Skoldstam L, Johansson G. Fat intake and composition of fatty acids in serum phospholipids in a randomized, controlled, Mediterranean dietary intervention study on patients with rheumatoid arthritis. *Nutr Metab* (Lond). 2005 Oct 10;2:26 http://www.nutritionandmetabolism.com/content/2/1/26

[87] Liu RH. Health benefits of fruit and vegetables are from additive and synergistic combinations of phytochemicals. *Am J Clin Nutr* 2003;78(3 Suppl):517S-520S http://www.ajcn.org/cgi/content/full/78/3/517S

[88] "Significant alteration in the intestinal flora was observed when the patients changed from omnivorous to vegan diet. ... This finding of an association between intestinal flora and disease activity may have implications for our understanding of how diet can affect RA." Peltonen R, Kjeldsen-Kragh J, Haugen M, Tuominen J, Toivanen P, Forre O, Eerola E. Changes of faecal flora in rheumatoid arthritis during fasting and one-year vegetarian diet. *Br J Rheumatol*. 1994 Jul;33(7):638-43

[89] Toivanen P, Eerola E. A vegan diet changes the intestinal flora. *Rheumatology* (Oxford). 2002 Aug;41(8):950-1 http://rheumatology.oxfordjournals.org/cgi/reprint/41/8/950

[90] "We conclude that a vegan diet changes the faecal microbial flora in RA patients, and changes in the faecal flora are associated with improvement in RA activity." Peltonen R, Nenonen M, Helve T, Hanninen O, Toivanen P, Eerola E. Faecal microbial flora and disease activity in rheumatoid arthritis during a vegan diet. *Br J Rheumatol*. 1997 Jan;36(1):64-8 http://rheumatology.oxfordjournals.org/cgi/reprint/36/1/64

[91] "The immunological profile of IgA deficiency and/or raised double stranded DNA in the absence of antinuclear factor together with raised inflammatory markers and symptoms suggestive of an immune diathesis should alert the physician to the possibility of gluten sensitivity." Hadjivassiliou M, Sanders DS, Grunewald RA, Akil M. Gluten sensitivity masquerading as systemic lupus erythematosus. *Ann Rheum Dis*. 2004 Nov;63(11):1501-3 http://ard.bmjjournals.com/cgi/content/full/63/11/1501

[92] Aljada A, Mohanty P, Ghanim H, Abdo T, Tripathy D, Chaudhuri A, Dandona P. Increase in intranuclear nuclear factor kappaB and decrease in inhibitor kappaB in mononuclear cells after a mixed meal: evidence for a proinflammatory effect. *Am J Clin Nutr*. 2004 Apr;79(4):682-90 http://www.ajcn.org/cgi/content/full/79/4/682

[93] "This is the first demonstration of ...a decrease in reactive oxygen species generation by leukocytes and oxidative damage to lipids, proteins, and amino acids after dietary restriction and weight loss in the obese over a short period." Dandona P, Mohanty P, Ghanim H, Aljada A, Browne R, Hamouda W, Prabhala A, Afzal A, Garg R. The suppressive effect of dietary restriction and weight loss in the obese on the generation of reactive oxygen species by leukocytes, lipid peroxidation, and protein carbonylation. *J Clin Endocrinol Metab*. 2001 Jan;86(1):355-62 http://jcem.endojournals.org/cgi/content/full/86/1/355

[94] "Thus, a 48h fast may reduce ROS generation, total oxidative load and oxidative damage to amino acids." Dandona P, Mohanty P, Hamouda W, Ghanim H, Aljada A, Garg R, Kumar V. Inhibitory effect of a two day fast on reactive oxygen species (ROS) generation by leucocytes and plasma ortho-tyrosine and meta-tyrosine concentrations. *J Clin Endocrinol Metab*. 2001 Jun;86(6):2899-902 http://jcem.endojournals.org/cgi/content/abstract/86/6/2899

[95] "The ability of therapeutic fasts to break metabolic vicious cycles may also contribute to the efficacy of fasting in the treatment of type 2 diabetes and autoimmune disorders." McCarty MF. A preliminary fast may potentiate response to a subsequent low-salt, low-fat vegan diet in the management of hypertension - fasting as a strategy for breaking metabolic vicious cycles. *Med Hypotheses*. 2003 May;60(5):624-33

[96] Ramakrishnan T, Stokes P. Beneficial effects of fasting and low carbohydrate diet in D-lactic acidosis associated with short-bowel syndrome. *JPEN J Parenter Enteral Nutr*. 1985 May-Jun;9(3):361-3

[97] Trollmo C, Verdrengh M, Tarkowski A. Fasting enhances mucosal antigen specific B cell responses in rheumatoid arthritis. *Ann Rheum Dis*. 1997 Feb;56(2):130-4 http://ard.bmjjournals.com/cgi/content/full/56/2/130

[98] "An association was found between improvement in inflammatory activity of the joints and enhancement of neutrophil bactericidal capacity. Fasting appears to improve the clinical status of patients with RA." Uden AM, Trang L, Venizelos N, Palmblad J. Neutrophil functions and clinical performance after total fasting in patients with rheumatoid arthritis. *Ann Rheum Dis*. 1983 Feb;42(1):45-51

[99] "We thus conclude that a reduced ability to generate cytotaxins, reduced release of enzyme, and reduced leukotriene formation from RA neutrophils, together with an altered fatty acid composition of membrane phospholipids, may be mechanisms for the decrease of inflammatory symptoms that results from fasting." Hafstrom I, Ringertz B, Gyllenhammar H, Palmblad J, Harms-Ringdahl M. Effects of fasting on disease activity, neutrophil function, fatty acid composition, and leukotriene biosynthesis in patients with rheumatoid arthritis. *Arthritis Rheum*. 1988 May;31(5):585-92

[100] "The results indicate that, unlike lactovegetarian diet, fasting may ameliorate the disease activity and reduce both the intestinal and the non-intestinal permeability in rheumatoid arthritis." Sundqvist T, Lindstrom F, Magnusson KE, Skoldstam L, Stjernstrom I, Tagesson C. Influence of fasting on intestinal permeability and disease activity in patients with rheumatoid arthritis. *Scand J Rheumatol*. 1982;11(1):33-8

has been documented as safe and effective treatment for SLE[101], RA[102], and non-rheumatic diseases such as chronic severe hypertension[103], moderate hypertension[104], obesity[105,106], type-2 diabetes[107], and epilepsy.[108] **The combination of energy restriction and fish oil supplementation was shown highly beneficial in an animal model of SLE.**[109]

- Broad-spectrum fatty acid therapy with ALA, EPA, DHA, GLA and oleic acid: **Fish oil provides EPA and DHA which have well-proven anti-inflammatory benefits when used in the treatment of SLE.**[110,111,112] Fatty acid supplementation should be delivered in the form of combination therapy with ALA, GLA, DHA, and EPA. Given at doses of 3,000 – 9,000 mg per day, ALA from flax oil has impressive anti-inflammatory benefits demonstrated by its ability to halve prostaglandin production in humans.[113] Numerous studies have demonstrated the benefit of GLA in the treatment of rheumatoid arthritis when used at doses between 500 mg – 4,000 mg per day.[114,115] Fish oil provides EPA and DHA which have well-proven anti-inflammatory benefits in RA[116,117,118] and SLE.[119,120] ALA, EPA, DHA, and GLA need to be provided in the form of supplements; when using high doses of therapeutic oils, liquid supplements that can be mixed in juice or a smoothie are generally more convenient and palatable than capsules. Therapeutic amounts of oleic acid can be obtained from generous use of olive oil, preferably on fresh vegetables. Supplementation with polyunsaturated fatty acids warrants increased intake of antioxidants from diet, fruit and vegetable juices, and properly formulated supplements; since patients with systemic inflammation are generally in a pro-oxidative state, consideration must be given to the timing and starting dose of fatty acid supplementation and the need for anti-oxidant protection. See chapter on Therapeutics for more details and biochemical

[101] Fuhrman J, Sarter B, Calabro DJ. Brief case reports of medically supervised, water-only fasting associated with remission of autoimmune disease. *Altern Ther Health Med*. 2002 Jul-Aug;8(4):112, 110-1

[102] "An association was found between improvement in inflammatory activity of the joints and enhancement of neutrophil bactericidal capacity. Fasting appears to improve the clinical status of patients with RA." Uden AM, Trang L, Venizelos N, Palmblad J. Neutrophil functions and clinical performance after total fasting in patients with rheumatoid arthritis. *Ann Rheum Dis*. 1983 Feb;42(1):45-51

[103] "The average reduction in blood pressure was 37/13 mm Hg, with the greatest decrease being observed for subjects with the most severe hypertension. Patients with stage 3 hypertension (those with systolic blood pressure greater than 180 mg Hg, diastolic blood pressure greater than 110 mg Hg, or both) had an average reduction of 60/17 mm Hg at the conclusion of treatment." Goldhamer A, Lisle D, Parpia B, Anderson SV, Campbell TC. Medically supervised water-only fasting in the treatment of hypertension. *J Manipulative Physiol Ther*. 2001 Jun;24(5):335-9 http://www.healthpromoting.com/335-339Goldhamer115263.QXD.pdf

[104] "RESULTS: Approximately 82% of the subjects achieved BP at or below 120/80 mm Hg by the end of the treatment program. The mean BP reduction was 20/7 mm Hg, with the greatest decrease being observed for subjects with the highest baseline BP." Goldhamer AC, Lisle DJ, Sultana P, Anderson SV, Parpia B, Hughes B, Campbell TC. Medically supervised water-only fasting in the treatment of borderline hypertension. *J Altern Complement Med*. 2002 Oct;8(5):643-50

[105] Vertes V, Genuth SM, Hazelton IM. Supplemented fasting as a large-scale outpatient program. *JAMA*. 1977 Nov 14;238(20):2151-3

[106] Bauman WA, Schwartz E, Rose HG, Eisenstein HN, Johnson DW. Early and long-term effects of acute caloric deprivation in obese diabetic patients. *Am J Med*. 1988 Jul;85(1):38-46

[107] Goldhamer AC. Initial cost of care results in medically supervised water-only fasting for treating high blood pressure and diabetes. *J Altern Complement Med*. 2002 Dec;8(6):696-7

[108] "The ketogenic diet should be considered as alternative therapy for children with difficult-to-control seizures. It is more effective than many of the new anticonvulsant medications and is well tolerated by children and families when it is effective." Freeman JM, et al. The efficacy of the ketogenic diet-1998: a prospective evaluation of intervention in 150 children. *Pediatrics*. 1998 Dec;102(6):1358-63 http://pediatrics.aappublications.org/cgi/reprint/102/6/1358

[109] "In conclusion, our data strongly indicate that ER and FO maintain antioxidant status and GSH:GSSG ratio, thereby protecting against renal deterioration from oxidative insults during ageing." Kelley VE, Ferretti A, Izui S, Strom TB. A fish oil diet rich in eicosapentaenoic acid reduces cyclooxygenase metabolites, and suppresses lupus in MRL-lpr mice. *J Immunol*. 1985 Mar;134(3):1914-9

[110] "No major side effects were noted, and it is suggested that dietary modification with additional marine oil may be a useful way of modifying disease activity in systemic lupus erythematosus." Walton AJ, Snaith ML, Locniskar M, Cumberland AG, Morrow WJ, Isenberg DA. Dietary fish oil and the severity of symptoms in patients with systemic lupus erythematosus. *Ann Rheum Dis*. 1991 Jul;50(7):463-6

[111] "CONCLUSION: In the management of SLE, dietary supplementation with fish oil may be beneficial in modifying symptomatic disease activity." Duffy EM, Meenagh GK, McMillan SA, Strain JJ, Hannigan BM, Bell AL. The clinical effect of dietary supplementation with omega-3 fish oils and/or copper in systemic lupus erythematosus. *J Rheumatol*. 2004 Aug;31(8):1551-6 http://www.jrheum.com/subscribers/04/08/tables/PDF/1551.pdf

[112] "Oral supplementation of EPA and DHA induced prolonged remission of SLE in 10 consecutive patients without any side-effects. These results suggest that n-3 fatty acids, EPA and DHA, are useful in the management of SLE and possibly, other similar collagen vascular diseases." Das UN. Beneficial effect of eicosapentaenoic and docosahexaenoic acids in the management of systemic lupus erythematosus and its relationship to the cytokine network. *Prostaglandins Leukot Essent Fatty Acids*. 1994 Sep;51(3):207-13

[113] Adam O, Wolfram G, Zollner N. Effect of alpha-linolenic acid in the human diet on linoleic acid metabolism and prostaglandin biosynthesis. *J Lipid Res*. 1986 Apr;27(4):421-6 http://www.jlr.org/cgi/reprint/27/4/421

[114] "Other results showed a significant reduction in morning stiffness with gamma-linolenic acid at 3 months and reduction in pain and articular index at 6 months with olive oil." Brzeski M, Madhok R, Capell HA. Evening primrose oil in patients with rheumatoid arthritis and side-effects of non-steroidal anti-inflammatory drugs. *Br J Rheumatol*. 1991 Oct;30(5):370-2

[115] Rothman D, DeLuca P, Zurier RB. Botanical lipids: effects on inflammation, immune responses, and rheumatoid arthritis. *Semin Arthritis Rheum*. 1995 Oct;25(2):87-96

[116] Adam O, Beringer C, Kless T, Lemmen C, Adam A, Wiseman M, Adam P, Klimmek R, Forth W. Anti-inflammatory effects of a low arachidonic acid diet and fish oil in patients with rheumatoid arthritis. *Rheumatol Int*. 2003 Jan;23(1):27-36

[117] Lau CS, Morley KD, Belch JJ. Effects of fish oil supplementation on non-steroidal anti-inflammatory drug requirement in patients with mild rheumatoid arthritis--a double-blind placebo controlled study. *Br J Rheumatol*. 1993 Nov;32(11):982-9

[118] Kremer JM, Jubiz W, Michalek A, Rynes RI, Bartholomew LE, Bigaouette J, Timchalk M, Beeler D, Lininger L. Fish-oil fatty acid supplementation in active rheumatoid arthritis. A double-blinded, controlled, crossover study. *Ann Intern Med*. 1987 Apr;106(4):497-503

[119] Walton AJ, Snaith ML, Locniskar M, Cumberland AG, Morrow WJ, Isenberg DA. Dietary fish oil and the severity of symptoms in patients with systemic lupus erythematosus. *Ann Rheum Dis*. 1991 Jul;50(7):463-6

[120] Duffy EM, Meenagh GK, McMillan SA, Strain JJ, Hannigan BM, Bell AL. The clinical effect of dietary supplementation with omega-3 fish oils and/or copper in systemic lupus erythematosus. *J Rheumatol*. 2004 Aug;31(8):1551-6

pathways. Clinicians must realize that fatty acids are not clinically or biochemically interchangeable and that one fatty acid does not substitute for another; each of the fatty acids must be supplied in order for its benefits to be obtained.[121]

- Vitamin D3 supplementation with physiologic doses and/or tailored to serum 25(OH)D levels: Vitamin D deficiency is common in the general population and is even more common in patients with chronic illness and chronic musculoskeletal pain.[122] **At least 50% of patients with SLE are deficient in vitamin D.**[123] Correction of vitamin D deficiency supports normal immune function against infection and provides a clinically significant anti-inflammatory[124] and analgesic benefit in patients with back pain[125] and limb pain.[126] Reasonable daily doses for children and adults are 2,000 and 4,000 IU, respectively, as defined by Vasquez, et al.[127] Deficiency and response to treatment are monitored with serum 25(OH)vitamin D while safety is monitored with serum calcium; inflammatory granulomatous diseases and certain drugs such as hydrochlorothiazide greatly increase the propensity for hypercalcemia and warrant increment dosing and frequent monitoring of serum calcium.

- Assessment and treatment for dysbiosis: **Dysbiotic loci should be investigated as discussed previously in Chapter 4**. Recall that **patients with lupus have abnormal gastrointestinal bacteria** (decreased colonization resistance[128]), and some evidence suggests that **gastrointestinal bacteria in these patients may translocate into the systemic circulation to induce formation of antibodies that cross-react with double-stranded DNA to produce the clinical manifestations of the disease.**[129,130] Each cause—each contributor to disease—may in itself be "clinically insignificant" but when numerous "insignificant" additive and synergistic influences coalesce, we find ourselves confronted with an "idiopathic disease." We must then decide between the only two available options: 1) despair in the failure of our "one cause, one disease, one drug" paradigm, or 2) appreciate that numerous influences work together to disrupt physiologic function and produce the biologic dysfunction that we experience as disease. **Experimental evidence shows that exposure to single-stranded bacterial DNA can provoke formation of antibodies to single-stranded mammalian DNA. Human patients with SLE have a reduced ability to bind bacterial DNA with antibodies, thus allowing bacterial DNA to provoke an ongoing inflammatory response.**[131] Recall from Chapter 4 that stimulation of inflammation by bacterial DNA is one of the 17 pathomechanisms of autoimmune/inflammation induction by multifocal dysbiosis.

  ○ Sinorespiratory/nasopharyngeal and dermal dysbiosis: **Increased nasal colonization with *Staphylococcus aureus* has been noted in patients with SLE.**[132]

[121] Vasquez A. Reducing Pain and Inflammation Naturally. Part 2: New Insights into Fatty Acid Supplementation and Its Effect on Eicosanoid Production and Genetic Expression. *Nutritional Perspectives* 2005; January: 5-16 http://optimalhealthresearch.com/part2

[122] Plotnikoff GA, Quigley JM. Prevalence of severe hypovitaminosis D in patients with persistent, nonspecific musculoskeletal pain. *Mayo Clin Proc.* 2003 Dec;78(12):1463-70

[123] "CONCLUSION: Half the SLE and FM patients had 25(OH)-vitamin D levels < 50 nmol/l, a level at which PTH stimulation occurs. Our data suggest that in SLE patients HCQ might inhibit conversion of 25(OH)-vitamin D to 1,25(OH)2-vitamin D." Huisman AM, White KP, Algra A, Harth M, Vieth R, Jacobs JW, Bijlsma JW, Bell DA. Vitamin D levels in women with systemic lupus erythematosus and fibromyalgia. *J Rheumatol.* 2001 Nov;28(11):2535-9

[124] Timms PM, Mannan N, Hitman GA, Noonan K, Mills PG, Syndercombe-Court D, Aganna E, Price CP, Boucher BJ. Circulating MMP9, vitamin D and variation in the TIMP-1 response with VDR genotype: mechanisms for inflammatory damage in chronic disorders? *QJM.* 2002 Dec;95(12):787-96 http://qjmed.oxfordjournals.org/cgi/content/full/95/12/787

[125] Al Faraj S, Al Mutairi K. Vitamin D deficiency and chronic low back pain in Saudi Arabia. *Spine.* 2003 Jan 15;28(2):177-9

[126] Masood H, Narang AP, Bhat IA, Shah GN. Persistent limb pain and raised serum alkaline phosphatase the earliest markers of subclinical hypovitaminosis D in Kashmir. *Indian J Physiol Pharmacol.* 1989 Oct-Dec;33(4):259-61

[127] Vasquez A, Manso G, Cannell J. The clinical importance of vitamin D (cholecalciferol): a paradigm shift with implications for all healthcare providers. *Altern Ther Health Med.* 2004 Sep-Oct;10(5):28-36 http://optimalhealthresearch.com/monograph04

[128] "Colonization Resistance (CR)...tended to be lower in active SLE patients than in healthy individuals. This could indicate that in SLE more and different bacteria translocate across the gut wall due to a lower CR. Some of these may serve as polyclonal B cell activators or as antigens cross-reacting with DNA." Apperloo-Renkema HZ, Bootsma H, Mulder BI, Kallenberg CG, van der Waaij D. Host-microflora interaction in systemic lupus erythematosus (SLE): colonization resistance of the indigenous bacteria of the intestinal tract. *Epidemiol Infect.* 1994;112(2):367-73

[129] "The lower IgG antibacterial antibody titres in active SLE might possibly result from sequestration of these IgG antibodies in immune complexes, indicating a possible role for antibacterial antibodies in exacerbations of SLE." Apperloo-Renkema HZ, Bootsma H, Mulder BI, Kallenberg CG, van der Waaij D. Host-microflora interaction in systemic lupus erythematosus (SLE): circulating antibodies to the indigenous bacteria of the intestinal tract. *Epidemiol Infect.* 1995 Feb;114(1):133-41

[130] Pisetsky DS. Antibody responses to DNA in normal immunity and aberrant immunity. *Clin Diagn Lab Immunol.* 1998 Jan;5(1):1-6 http://cdli.asm.org/cgi/content/full/5/1/1

[131] Pisetsky DS. Antibody responses to DNA in normal immunity and aberrant immunity. *Clin Diagn Lab Immunol.* 1998 Jan;5(1):1-6 http://cdli.asm.org/cgi/content/full/5/1/1

[132] Medline abstract from Polish research: "In 9 from 14 patients with (64.3%) a.b. very massive growth of Staphylococcus aureus in culture from vestibulae of the nose swab was, in other cultures very massive growth of physiological flora was seen. ...clinical significance of asymptomatic bacteriuria and pathogenic bacteria colonisation of nostrils as a precedence to symptomatic infections needs further investigations." Koseda-Dragan M, Hebanowski M, Galinski J, Krzywinska E, Bakowska A. [Asymptomatic bacteriuria in women diagnosed with systemic lupus erythematosus (SLE)] *Pol Arch Med Wewn.* 1998 Oct;100(4):321-30.

- o <u>Gastrointestinal dysbiosis</u>: Yeast, bacteria, and parasites are treated as indicated based on identification and sensitivity results from comprehensive parasitology assessments.
- **<u>N-Acetyl-Cysteine (NAC) for antioxidant, antiviral, and mitochondrial-protective benefits</u>**: NAC provides cysteine for GSH production. NAC also inhibits NFkB. NAC inhibits viral replication (e.g., HIV) more effectively than and independently from its conversion to GSH. Recently, NAC at relatively high doses of 4,800mg/d in divided doses was shown to modulate mitochondrial hyperpolarization (by dissociating the generally resultant mTOR activation) and lead to very important clinical and immunological improvements in patients with SLE; NAC was shown to be safe and well-tolerated by all SLE patients up to 2.4g/d with reversible nausea in 33% of patients receiving 4.8g/d. This study by Lai, Hanczko, Bonilla, et al[133] is truly a landmark contribution and advance in the field of rheumatology and immunology because it proves 1) that mitochondrial dysfunction directly leads to an autoimmune phenotype, and 2) that inhibition of mTOR by NAC is safe and effective in patients with SLE; important insights from this remarkable work are as follows:
  - o NAC 4,800mg/d proved safe and clinically beneficial in patients with SLE, leading to reductions in disease activity and ANA levels.
  - o Mitochondrial hyperpolarization (MHP) causes mTOR activation which in turn suppresses the expression of the FoxP3 transcription factor necessary for induction of T-regulatory cells. Note that the mTOR activation is the cause of the FoxP3 suppression; ironically, NAC actually increases MHP but dissociates it from mTOR by having a greater effect on and via mTOR suppression. The nutritional supplement NAC works in a similar manner as does the immunosuppressive drug rapamycin, with a mechanism of suppression of mTOR and the effect of enhancing endogenous anti-inflammatory immunomodulation via CD4+ CD25+ FoxP3+ T-regulatory cells. Stated again and differently, NAC paradoxically worsens mitochondrial hyperpolarization in patients with SLE but does so at the same time that it has a more significant impact on mTOR; NAC's rapamycin-like targeting of mTOR dissociates mitochondrial hyperpolarization from mTOR activation. The reduction in mTOR activity (which is of greater consequence than the increase in MIM polarization) allows enhanced expression of FoxP3 for increased elaboration of T-regulatory cells, thereby providing endogenous immunoregulation.

> **Mechanistic and clinical proof that mitochondrial dysfunction directly contributes to autoimmunity**
>
> "Similar to the effect of rapamycin, **suppression of mTOR by NAC was accompanied by increased FoxP3 expression in CD4+/CD25+ T cells**. These results suggest that the effect of NAC on the immune system is 1) cell type-specific and 2) it occurs through disconnecting the activation of mTOR from the elevation of Δψm in lupus T cells, similar to the effect of rapamycin."
>
> Lai ZW, Hanczko R, Bonilla E, et al. N-acetylcysteine reduces disease activity by blocking mammalian target of rapamycin in T cells from systemic lupus erythematosus patients. *Arthritis Rheum*. 2012 Sep

  - o "MHP of lupus T cells, which most prominently affects DN [double-negative, autoimmunity-promoting] T cells, was associated with resistance to activation-induced apoptosis. In 27 SLE patients receiving daily NAC doses of 1.2 g, 2.4 g, and 4.8 g considered together, both **spontaneous and CD3/CD28-induced apoptosis of DN T cells were markedly increased** and the **expansion of these cells was effectively reversed**. The **elimination of DN T cells, which are known promote anti-DNA autoantibody production by B cells**, is likely to contribute to reduced anti-DNA titers and to the efficacy of NAC.
  - o "The therapeutic importance of NAC for SLE is reflected by: 1) achieving clinical improvement in two validated disease activity scores within 3 months; 2) diminishing fatigue (21), which is considered the most disabling symptom in a majority of SLE patients (22); 3) absence of significant side-effects; and 4) affordability of this medication. A monthly supply of 600-mg

---

[133] Lai ZW, Hanczko R, Bonilla E, et al. N-acetylcysteine reduces disease activity by blocking mammalian target of rapamycin in T cells from systemic lupus erythematosus patients: a randomized, double-blind, placebo-controlled trial. *Arthritis Rheum*. 2012 Sep;64(9):2937-46
http://www.ncbi.nlm.nih.gov/pmc/articles/PMC3411859/

NAC capsules (120–240 capsules) costs $15–$30 on the retail market. This sharply contrasts with average annual direct medical costs estimated to be ~$22,580 per patient in 2009. Thus, the cost of NAC at $180–$360/year would be negligible in comparison to the overall expenditures to society and the expected benefit in reducing the need for vastly more expensive medications burdened with potentially serious side-effects."

- **Orthoendocrinology**: Assess melatonin, prolactin, cortisol, DHEA, free and total testosterone, serum estradiol, and thyroid status (e.g., TSH, T4, *and* anti-thyroid peroxidase antibodies).
  - **Melatonin**: Melatonin is a pineal hormone with well-known sleep-inducing and immunomodulatory properties, and it is commonly administered in doses of 1-40 mg in the evening, before bedtime. Starting with a relatively low dose (e.g., 1-5 mg) and increasing as tolerated is recommended. Melatonin (20 mg hs) appears to have cured two patients with drug-resistant sarcoidosis[134] and 3 mg provided immediate short-term benefit to a patient with multiple sclerosis.[135]
  - **Prolactin (excess)**: **Prolactin has proinflammatory and immunodysregulatory actions and is commonly elevated—either overtly or latently—in patients with inflammatory/autoimmune disease.** Accordingly prolactin-lowering treatment shows safety and effectiveness in the treatment of numerous inflammatory/autoimmune diseases; often these results are noted even when the patient's prolactin level was not initially elevated, suggesting the alleviation of latent hyperprolactinemia and/or an inherent anti-inflammatory action of the prolactin-lowering treatment. According to clinical trials with small numbers of patients, whether prolactin levels are high or not, prolactin-lowering treatment (such as bromocriptine[136]) appears highly beneficial when used with other anti-rheumatic treatments ("...**drastic efficacy with spectacular improvement** in clinical, biological and occupational status..."[137]) in patients with psoriatic arthritis. Serum prolactin is the standard assessment of prolactin status. Since elevated prolactin may be a sign of pituitary tumor, assessment for headaches, visual deficits, other abnormalities of pituitary hormones (e.g., GH and TSH) should be performed and CT or MRI must be considered. Patients with prolactin levels less than 100 ng/mL and normal CT/MRI findings can be managed conservatively with effective prolactin-lowering treatment and annual radiologic assessment (less necessary with favorable serum response).[138, see review 139] **Patients with RA and SLE have higher basal and stress-induced levels of prolactin compared with normal controls.**[140,141] A normal serum prolactin level does not necessarily exclude the use of prolactin-lowering intervention, especially since many autoimmune patients have **latent hyperprolactinemia** which may not be detected with random serum measurement of prolactin. Specific treatment options include the following:
    - Thyroid hormone: Hypothyroidism frequently causes hyperprolactinemia which is reversible upon effective treatment of hypothyroidism. Obviously therefore, thyroid

---

[134] Cagnoni ML, Lombardi A, Cerinic MC, Dedola GL, Pignone A. Melatonin for treatment of chronic refractory sarcoidosis. *Lancet*. 1995 Nov 4;346(8984):1229-30

[135] "...administration of melatonin (3 mg, orally) at 2:00 p.m., when the patient experienced severe blurring of vision, resulted within 15 minutes in a dramatic improvement in visual acuity and in normalization of the visual evoked potential latency after stimulation of the left eye." Sandyk R. Diurnal variations in vision and relations to circadian melatonin secretion in multiple sclerosis. *Int J Neurosci*. 1995 Nov;83(1-2):1-6

[136] "In 2 cases of psoriatic arthritis, adding bromocriptine to gold salts and nonsteroidal anti-inflammatory drug was followed by a drastic efficacy with spectacular improvement in clinical, biological and occupational status. Because none of the cases had hyperprolactinaemia, bromocriptine acted probably had an intrinic anti-inflammatory effect independent of its antiprolactinic effect." Eulry F, Mayaudon H, Bauduceau B, Lechevalier D, Crozes P, Magnin J, Claude-Berthelot C. [Blood prolactin under the effect of protirelin in spondylarthropathies. Treatment trial of 4 cases of reactive arthritis and 2 cases of psoriatic arthritis with bromocriptine] *Ann Med Interne* (Paris). 1996;147(1):15-9. French.

[137] Abstract from article in French: "In 2 cases of psoriatic arthritis, adding bromocriptine to gold salts and nonsteroidal anti-inflammatory drug was followed by a drastic efficacy with spectacular improvement in clinical, biological and occupational status. Because none of the cases had hyperprolactinaemia, bromocriptine acted probably had an intrinic anti-inflammatory effect independent of its antiprolactinic effect." Eulry F, Mayaudon H, Bauduceau B, Lechevalier D, Crozes P, Magnin J, Claude-Berthelot C. [Blood prolactin under the effect of protirelin in spondylarthropathies. Treatment trial of 4 cases of reactive arthritis and 2 cases of psoriatic arthritis with bromocriptine] *Ann Med Interne* (Paris). 1996;147(1):15-9. French

[138] Beers MH, Berkow R (eds). The Merck Manual. Seventeenth Edition. Whitehouse Station; Merck Research Laboratories 1999 Page 77-78

[139] Serri O, Chik CL, Ur E, Ezzat S. Diagnosis and management of hyperprolactinemia. *CMAJ*. 2003 Sep 16;169(6):575-81 http://www.cmaj.ca/cgi/content/full/169/6/575

[140] Dostal C, Moszkorzova L, Musilova L, Lacinova Z, Marek J, Zvarova J. Serum prolactin stress values in patients with systemic lupus erythematosus. *Ann Rheum Dis*. 2003 May;62(5):487-8 http://ard.bmjjournals.com/cgi/content/full/62/5/487

[141] "RESULTS: A significantly higher rate of elevated PRL levels was found in SLE patients (40.0%) compared with the healthy controls (14.8%). No proof was found of association with the presence of anti-ds-DNA or with specific organ involvement. Similarly, elevated PRL levels were found in RA patients (39.3%)." Moszkorzova L, Lacinova Z, Marek J, Musilova L, Dohnalova A, Dostal C. Hyperprolactinaemia in patients with systemic lupus erythematosus. *Clin Exp Rheumatol*. 2002 Nov-Dec;20(6):807-12

status should be evaluated in all patients with hyperprolactinemia. Thyroid assessment and treatment is reviewed later in this section.

- *Vitex astus-cagnus* and other supporting botanicals and nutrients: **Vitex lowers serum prolactin in humans**[142,143] **via a dopaminergic effect.**[144] Vitex is considered safe for clinical use; mild and reversible adverse effects possibly associated with Vitex include nausea, headache, gastrointestinal disturbances, menstrual disorders, acne, pruritus and erythematous rash. No drug interactions are known, but given the herb's dopaminergic effect it should probably be used with some caution in patients treated with dopamine antagonists such as the so-called antipsychotic drugs (most of which do not work very well and/or carry intolerable adverse effects[145,146]). In a recent review, Bone[147] stated that daily doses of *Vitex* can range from 500 mg to 2,000 mg DHE (dry herb equivalent) and can be tailored to the suppression of prolactin. Due at least in part to its content of L-dopa, *Mucuna pruriens* **shows clinical dopaminergic activity** as evidenced by its effectiveness in Parkinson's disease[148]; up to 15-30 gm/d of mucuna has been used clinically but doses will be dependent on preparation and phytoconcentration.

- Bromocriptine: Bromocriptine has long been considered the pharmacologic treatment of choice for elevated prolactin.[149] Typical dose is 2.5 mg per day (effective against SLE[150]); gastrointestinal upset and sedation are common.[151] Clinical intervention with bromocriptine appears warranted in patients with RA, **SLE**, Reiter's syndrome, psoriatic arthritis, and probably multiple sclerosis and uveitis.[152] A normal serum prolactin level does not necessarily exclude the use of prolactin-lowering intervention, especially since many autoimmune patients have latent hyperprolactinemia which may not be detected with random serum measurement of prolactin.

- Cabergoline/Dostinex: Cabergoline/Dostinex is a newer dopamine agonist with few adverse effects; typical dose starts at 0.5 mg per week (0.25 mg twice per week).[153] Several studies have indicated that cabergoline is safer and more effective than bromocriptine for reducing prolactin levels[154] and the dose can often be reduced after

---

[142] "Since AC extracts were shown to have beneficial effects on premenstrual mastodynia serum prolactin levels in such patients were also studied in one double-blind, placebo-controlled clinical study. Serum prolactin levels were indeed reduced in the patients treated with the extract." Wuttke W, Jarry H, Christoffel V, Spengler B, Seidlova-Wuttke D. Chaste tree (Vitex agnus-castus)--pharmacology and clinical indications. *Phytomedicine*. 2003 May;10(4):348-57

[143] German abstract from Medline: "The prolactin release was reduced after 3 months, shortened luteal phases were normalised and deficits in the luteal progesterone synthesis were eliminated." Milewicz A, Gejdel E, Sworen H, Sienkiewicz K, Jedrzejak J, Teucher T, Schmitz H. [Vitex agnus castus extract in the treatment of luteal phase defects due to latent hyperprolactinemia. Results of a randomized placebo-controlled double-blind study] *Arzneimittelforschung*. 1993 Jul;43(7):752-6

[144] "Our results indicate a dopaminergic effect of Vitex agnus-castus extracts and suggest additional pharmacological actions via opioid receptors." Meier B, Berger D, Hoberg E, Sticher O, Schaffner W. Pharmacological activities of Vitex agnus-castus extracts in vitro. *Phytomedicine*. 2000 Oct;7(5):373-81

[145] "The majority of patients in each group discontinued their assigned treatment owing to inefficacy or intolerable side effects or for other reasons." Lieberman JA, Stroup TS, McEvoy JP, Swartz MS, Rosenheck RA, Perkins DO, Keefe RS, Davis SM, Davis CE, Lebowitz BD, Severe J, Hsiao JK; Clinical Antipsychotic Trials of Intervention Effectiveness (CATIE) Investigators. Effectiveness of antipsychotic drugs in patients with chronic schizophrenia. *N Engl J Med*. 2005 Sep 22;353(12):1209-23

[146] Whitaker R. The case against antipsychotic drugs: a 50-year record of doing more harm than good. *Med Hypotheses*. 2004;62(1):5-13

[147] "In conditions such as endometriosis and fibroids, for which a significant estrogen antagonist effect is needed, doses of at least 2 g/day DHE may be required and typically are used by professional herbalists." Bone K. New Insights Into Chaste Tree. *Nutritional Wellness* 2005 November http://www.nutritionalwellness.com/archives/2005/nov/11_bone.php

[148] "CONCLUSIONS: The rapid onset of action and longer on time without concomitant increase in dyskinesias on mucuna seed powder formulation suggest that this natural source of L-dopa might possess advantages over conventional L-dopa preparations in the long term management of PD." Katzenschlager R, Evans A, Manson A, Patsalos PN, Ratnaraj N, Watt H, Timmermann L, Van der Giessen R, Lees AJ. Mucuna pruriens in Parkinson's disease: a double blind clinical and pharmacological study. *J Neurol Neurosurg Psychiatry*. 2004 Dec;75(12):1672-7

[149] Beers MH, Berkow R (eds). The Merck Manual. Seventeenth Edition. Whitehouse Station; Merck Research Laboratories 1999 Page 77-78

[150] "A prospective, double-blind, randomized, placebo-controlled study compared BRC at a fixed daily dosage of 2.5 mg with placebo... Long term treatment with a low dose of BRC appears to be a safe and effective means of decreasing SLE flares in SLE patients." Alvarez-Nemegyei J, Cobarrubias-Cobos A, Escalante-Triay F, Sosa-Munoz J, Miranda JM, Jara LJ. Bromocriptine in systemic lupus erythematosus: a double-blind, randomized, placebo-controlled study. *Lupus*. 1998;7(6):414-9

[151] Serri O, Chik CL, Ur E, Ezzat S. Diagnosis and management of hyperprolactinemia. *CMAJ*. 2003 Sep 16;169(6):575-81 http://www.cmaj.ca/cgi/content/full/169/6/575

[152] "...clinical observations and trials support the use of bromocriptine as a nonstandard primary or adjunctive therapy in the treatment of recalcitrant RA, SLE, Reiter's syndrome, and psoriatic arthritis and associated conditions unresponsive to traditional approaches." McMurray RW. Bromocriptine in rheumatic and autoimmune diseases. *Semin Arthritis Rheum*. 2001 Aug;31(1):21-32

[153] Serri O, Chik CL, Ur E, Ezzat S. Diagnosis and management of hyperprolactinemia. *CMAJ*. 2003 Sep 16;169(6):575-81 http://www.cmaj.ca/cgi/content/full/169/6/575

[154] "CONCLUSION: These data indicate that cabergoline is a very effective agent for lowering the prolactin levels in hyperprolactinemic patients and that it appears to offer considerable advantage over bromocriptine in terms of efficacy and tolerability." Sabuncu T, Arikan E, Tasan E, Hatemi H. Comparison of the effects of cabergoline and bromocriptine on prolactin levels in hyperprolactinemic patients. *Intern Med*. 2001 Sep;40(9):857-61

successful prolactin reduction, allowing for reductions in cost and adverse effects.[155] Although fewer studies have been published supporting the antirheumatic benefits of cabergoline than those supporting bromocriptine; its antirheumatic benefits have indeed been documented.[156]

- o Estrogen (excess): A hormonal contribution to the immune dysfunction that underlies SLE is strongly suggested by the strong tendency of this disease to affect women, and by the timing of the onset of the disease during the years of highest estrogen levels and variability—generally *after menarche* and *before menopause*. **Men with rheumatoid arthritis show an excess of estradiol** and a decrease in DHEA, and the **excess estrogen is proportional to the degree of inflammation.**[157] Serum estradiol is commonly used to assess estrogen status; estrogens can also be measured in 24-hour urine samples. Beyond looking at estrogens from a *quantitative* standpoint, they can also be *qualitatively* analyzed with respect to the ratio of estrone:estradiol:estriol as well as the balance between the "good" 2-hydroxyestrone relative to the purportedly carcinogenic and proinflammatory 16-alpha-hydroxyestrone. Interventions to combat high estrogen levels may include any effective combination of the following:

  - Weight loss and weight optimization: In overweight patients, *weight loss* is the means to attaining the goal of *weight optimization*; the task is not complete until the body mass index is normalized/optimized. Excess adiposity and obesity raise estrogen levels due to high levels of aromatase (the hormone that makes estrogens from androgens) in adipose tissue; weight optimization and loss of excess fat helps normalize hormone levels and reduce inflammation.

  - Avoidance of ethanol: Estrogen production is stimulated by ethanol intake.

  - Consider surgical correction of varicocele in affected men: Men with varicocele have higher estrogen levels due to temperature-induced alterations in enzyme function in the testes; surgical correction of the varicocele lowers estrogen levels.

  - "Anti-estrogen diet": Foods and supplements such as green tea, diindolylmethane (DIM), indole-3-carbinol (I3C), licorice, and a high-fiber cruciter-based "anti-estrogenic diet" can also be used; monitoring clinical status and serum estradiol will prove or disprove efficacy. Whereas 16-alpha-hydroxyestrone is pro-inflammatory and immunodysregulatory, 2-hydroxyestrone has anti-inflammatory action[158] and been described as "the good estrogen"[159] due to its anticancer and comparatively health-preserving qualities. **In a recent short-term study using I3C in patients with SLE, I3C supplementation at 375 mg per day was well tolerated and resulted in modest treatment-dependent clinical improvement as well as favorable modification of estrogen metabolism away from 16-alpha-hydroxyestrone and toward 2-hydroxyestrone.**[160]

  - Anastrozole/Arimidex: In our office, we commonly measure serum estradiol in men and administer the aromatase inhibitor anastrozole/arimidex 1 mg (2-3 doses per

---

[155] "Cabergoline also normalized PRL in the majority of patients with known bromocriptine intolerance or -resistance. Once PRL secretion was adequately controlled, the dose of cabergoline could often be significantly decreased, which further reduced costs of therapy." Verhelst J, Abs R, Maiter D, van den Bruel A, Vandeweghe M, Velkeniers B, Mockel J, Lamberigts G, Petrossians P, Coremans P, Mahler C, Stevenaert A, Verlooy J, Raftopoulos C, Beckers A. Cabergoline in the treatment of hyperprolactinemia: a study in 455 patients. *J Clin Endocrinol Metab*. 1999 Jul;84(7):2518-22 http://jcem.endojournals.org/cgi/content/full/84/7/2518

[156] Erb N, Pace AV, Delamere JP, Kitas GD. Control of unremitting rheumatoid arthritis by the prolactin antagonist cabergoline. *Rheumatology* (Oxford). 2001 Feb;40(2):237-9 http://rheumatology.oxfordjournals.org/cgi/content/full/40/2/237

[157] "RESULTS: DHEAS and estrone concentrations were lower and estradiol was higher in patients compared with healthy controls. DHEAS differed between RF positive and RF negative patients. Estrone did not correlate with any disease variable, whereas estradiol correlated strongly and positively with all measured indices of inflammation." Tengstrand B, Carlstrom K, Fellander-Tsai L, Hafstrom I. Abnormal levels of serum dehydroepiandrosterone, estrone, and estradiol in men with rheumatoid arthritis: high correlation between serum estradiol and current degree of inflammation. *J Rheumatol*. 2003 Nov;30(11):2338-43

[158] "Micromolar concentrations of beta-estradiol, estrone, 16-alpha-hydroxyestrone and estriol enhance the oxidative metabolism of activated human PMNL's. The corresponding 2-hydroxylated estrogens 2-OH-estradiol, 2-OH-estrone and 2-OH-estriol act on the contrary as powerful inhibitors of cell activity." Jansson G. Oestrogen-induced enhancement of myeloperoxidase activity in human polymorphonuclear leukocytes--a possible cause of oxidative stress in inflammatory cells. *Free Radic Res Commun*. 1991;14(3):195-208

[159] "Even more dramatically, in the case of laryngeal papillomas induction of 2-hydroxylation with indole-3-carbinol (I3C) has resulted in inhibition of tumor growth during the time that the patients continue to take I3C or vegetables rich in this compound." Bradlow HL, Telang NT, Sepkovic DW, Osborne MP. 2-hydroxyestrone: the 'good' estrogen. *J Endocrinol*. 1996 Sep;150 Suppl:S259-65

[160] "Women with SLE can manifest a metabolic response to I3C and might benefit from its antiestrogenic effects." McAlindon TE, Gulin J, Chen T, Klug T, Lahita R, Nuite M. Indole-3-carbinol in women with SLE: effect on estrogen metabolism and disease activity. *Lupus*. 2001;10(11):779-83

week) to men whose estradiol level is greater than 32 picogram/mL. The Life Extension Foundation[161] advocates that the optimal serum estradiol level for a man is 10-30 picogram/mL. Clinical studies using anastrozole/arimidex in men have shown that aromatase blockade lowers estradiol and raises testosterone[162]; generally speaking, this is exactly the result that we want in patients with severe systemic autoimmunity. Frequency of dosing is based on serum and clinical response.

- o **Cortisol (insufficiency)**: Cortisol has immunoregulatory and "immunosuppressive" actions at physiological concentrations. Low adrenal function is common in patients with chronic inflammation.[163,164,165] Assessment of cortisol production and adrenal function was detailed in Chapter 4 under the section of Orthoendocrinology. Supplementation with 20 mg per day of cortisol/Cortef is physiologic; my preference is to dose 10 mg first thing in the morning, then 5 mg in late morning and 5 mg in midafternoon in an attempt to replicate the diurnal variation and normal morning peak of cortisol levels. In patients with hypoadrenalism, administration of pregnenolone in doses of 10-60 mg in the morning may also be beneficial.

- o **Testosterone (insufficiency)**: Androgen deficiencies predispose to, are exacerbated by, and contribute to autoimmune/inflammatory disorders. A large proportion of men with SLE or RA have low testosterone[166] and suffer the effects of hypogonadism: fatigue, weakness, depression, slow healing, low libido, and difficulties with sexual performance. Testosterone levels may rise following DHEA supplementation (especially in women) and can be elevated in men by the use of anastrozole/arimidex. Otherwise, transdermal testosterone such as Androgel or Testim can be applied as indicated. Wright[167] previously recommended 5-10 mg/day for females, 50-100 mg/day for males, if testosterone levels were low.

- o **DHEA**: DHEA is an anti-inflammatory and immunoregulatory hormone that is commonly deficient in patients with autoimmunity, including polymyalgia rheumatica, SLE, RA, and inflammatory arthritis.[168,169] DHEA levels are suppressed by prednisone[170], and DHEA has been shown to reverse the osteoporosis and loss of bone mass induced by corticosteroid treatment.[171] DHEA shows no acute or subacute toxicity even when used in supraphysiologic doses, even when used in sick patients. For example, in a study of 32 patients with HIV, DHEA doses of 750 mg – 2,250 mg per day were well-tolerated and produced no dose-limiting adverse effects.[172] This lack of toxicity compares favorably with any and all so-called

---

[161] Male Hormone Modulation Therapy, Page 4 Of 7: http://www.lef.org/protocols/prtcl-130c.shtml Accessed October 30, 2005

[162] "These data demonstrate that aromatase inhibition increases serum bioavailable and total testosterone levels to the youthful normal range in older men with mild hypogonadism." Leder BZ, Rohrer JL, Rubin SD, Gallo J, Longcope C. Effects of aromatase inhibition in elderly men with low or borderline-low serum testosterone levels. *J Clin Endocrinol Metab.* 2004 Mar;89(3):1174-80 http://jcem.endojournals.org/cgi/reprint/89/3/1174

[163] "Yet evidence that patients with rheumatoid arthritis improved with small, physiologic dosages of cortisol or cortisone acetate was reported over 25 years ago, and that patients with chronic allergic disorders or unexplained chronic fatigue also improved with administration of such small dosages was reported over 15 years ago..." Jefferies WM. Mild adrenocortical deficiency, chronic allergies, autoimmune disorders and the chronic fatigue syndrome: a continuation of the cortisone story. *Med Hypotheses.* 1994 Mar;42(3):183-9 http://www.thebuteykocentre.com/Irish_%20Buteykocenter_files/further_studies/med_hyp2.pdf http://members.westnet.com.au/pkolb/med_hyp2.pdf

[164] "The etiology of rheumatoid arthritis ...explained by a combination of three factors: (i) a relatively mild deficiency of cortisol, ..., (ii) a deficiency of DHEA, ...and (iii) infection by organisms such as mycoplasma,..." Jefferies WM. The etiology of rheumatoid arthritis. *Med Hypotheses.* 1998 Aug;51(2):111-4

[165] Jefferies W McK. Safe Uses of Cortisol. Second Edition. Springfield, CC Thomas, 1996

[166] Karagiannis A, Harsoulis F. Gonadal dysfunction in systemic diseases. *Eur J Endocrinol.* 2005 Apr;152(4):501-13 http://www.eje-online.org/cgi/content/full/152/4/501

[167] Gaby A, Wright JV. Nutritional Protocols. 1998 Nutrition Seminars

[168] "The low levels found in patients with PM:TA are in accordance with those previously reported in immune-mediated diseases such as systemic lupus erythematosus (SLE) and rheumatoid arthritis, suggesting that diminution of DHEAS is a constant endocrinologic feature in these categories of patients." Nilsson E, de la Torre B, Hedman M, Goobar J, Thorner A. Blood dehydroepiandrosterone sulphate (DHEAS) levels in polymyalgia rheumatica/giant cell arteritis and primary fibromyalgia. *Clin Exp Rheumatol.* 1994 Jul-Aug;12(4):415-7

[169] "DHEAS concentrations were significantly decreased in both women and men with inflammatory arthritis (IA) (P < 0.001)." Dessein PH, Joffe BI, Stanwix AE, Moomal Z. Hyposecretion of the adrenal androgen dehydroepiandrosterone sulfate and its relation to clinical variables in inflammatory arthritis. *Arthritis Res.* 2001;3(3):183-8. Epub 2001 Feb 21. http://arthritis-research.com/content/3/3/183

[170] "Basal serum DHEA and DHEAS concentrations were suppressed to a greater degree than was cortisol during both daily and alternate day prednisone treatments. ...Thus, adrenal androgen secretion was more easily suppressed than was cortisol secretion by this low dose of glucocorticoid, but there was no advantage to alternate day therapy." Rittmaster RS, Givner ML. Effect of daily and alternate day low dose prednisone on serum cortisol and adrenal androgens in hirsute women. *J Clin Endocrinol Metab.* 1988 Aug;67(2):400-3

[171] "CONCLUSION: Prasterone treatment prevented BMD loss and significantly increased BMD at both the lumbar spine and total hip in female patients with SLE receiving exogenous glucocorticoids." Mease PJ, Ginzler EM, Gluck OS, Schiff M, Goldman A, Greenwald M, Cohen S, Egan R, Quarles BJ, Schwartz KE. Effects of prasterone on bone mineral density in women with systemic lupus erythematosus receiving chronic glucocorticoid therapy. *J Rheumatol.* 2005 Apr;32(4):616-21

[172] "Thirty-one subjects were evaluated and monitored for safety and tolerance. The oral drug was administered three times daily in doses ranging from 750 mg/day to 2,250 mg/day for 16 weeks. ... The drug was well tolerated and no dose-limiting side effects were noted." Dyner TS, Lang W, Geaga J, Golub A, Stites D, Winger E, Galmarini M, Masterson J, Jacobson MA. An open-label dose-escalation trial of oral dehydroepiandrosterone tolerance and pharmacokinetics in patients with HIV disease. *J Acquir Immune Defic Syndr.* 1993 May;6(5):459-65

"antirheumatic" drugs, nearly all of which show impressive comparable toxicity. **High-dose supplemental DHEA has benefits in the treatment of SLE that are comparable to those obtained with antimalarial drugs.**[173] When used at doses of 200 mg per day, DHEA safely provides clinical benefit for patients with various autoimmune diseases, including ulcerative colitis, Crohn's disease[174], and SLE.[175] In patients with SLE, DHEA supplementation allows for reduced dosing of prednisone (thus avoiding its adverse effects) while providing symptomatic improvement.[176] Optimal clinical response appears to correlate with serum levels that are supraphysiologic[177], and therefore treatment may be implemented with little regard for initial/baseline DHEA levels provided that the patient is free of contraindications, particularly high risk for sex-hormone-dependent malignancy. Other than mild adverse effects predictable with any androgen (namely voice deepening, transient acne, and increased facial hair), DHEA supplementation does not cause serious adverse effects[178], and it is appropriate for routine clinical use particularly when 1) the dose of DHEA is kept as low as possible, 2) duration is kept as short as possible, 3) other interventions are used to address the underlying cause of the disease, 4) the patient is deriving benefit, and 5) the risk-to-benefit ratio is favorable.

- o Thyroid (insufficiency or autoimmunity): Overt or imminent hypothyroidism is suggested by TSH greater than 2 mU/L[179] or 3 mU/L[180], low T4 or T3, and/or the presence of anti-thyroid peroxidase antibodies.[181] Hypothyroidism can cause an inflammatory myopathy that can resemble polymyositis, and hypothyroidism is a frequent complication of any and all autoimmune diseases. Specific treatment considerations include the following:

  - Selenium: Supplementation with either selenomethonine[182] or sodium selenite[183,184] can reduce thyroid autoimmunity and improve peripheral conversion of T4 to T3. Selenium may be started at 500-800 mcg per day and tapered to 200-400 mcg per day for maintenance.[185]

  - L-thyroxine/levothyroxine/Synthroid—prescription synthetic T4: 25-50 mcg per day is a common starting dose which can be adjusted based on clinical and laboratory response. Thyroid hormone supplements must be consumed separately from soy products (by at least 1-2 hours) and preferably on an empty stomach to avoid absorption interference by food, fiber, and minerals, especially calcium. Doses are generally started at one-half of the daily dose for the first 10 days after which the full

[173] Tierney ML. McPhee SJ, Papadakis MA. Current Medical Diagnosis and Treatment 2006. 45th edition. New York; Lange Medical Books: 2006, pages 833-837

[174] "CONCLUSIONS: In a pilot study, dehydroepiandrosterone was effective and safe in patients with refractory Crohn's disease or ulcerative colitis." Andus T, Klebl F, Rogler G, Bregenzer N, Scholmerich J, Straub RH. Patients with refractory Crohn's disease or ulcerative colitis respond to dehydroepiandrosterone: a pilot study. *Aliment Pharmacol Ther.* 2003 Feb;17(3):409-14

[175] "CONCLUSION: The overall results confirm that DHEA treatment was well-tolerated, significantly reduced the number of SLE flares, and improved patient's global assessment of disease activity." Chang DM, Lan JL, Lin HY, Luo SF. Dehydroepiandrosterone treatment of women with mild-to-moderate systemic lupus erythematosus: a multicenter randomized, double-blind, placebo-controlled trial. *Arthritis Rheum.* 2002 Nov;46(11):2924-7

[176] "CONCLUSION: Among women with lupus disease activity, reducing the dosage of prednisone to < or = 7.5 mg/day for a sustained period of time while maintaining stabilization or a reduction of disease activity was possible in a significantly greater proportion of patients treated with oral prasterone, 200 mg once daily, compared with patients treated with placebo." Petri MA, Lahita RG, Van Vollenhoven RF, Merrill JT, Schiff M, Ginzler EM, Strand V, Kunz A, Gorelick KJ, Schwartz KE; GL601 Study Group. Effects of prasterone on corticosteroid requirements of women with systemic lupus erythematosus: a double-blind, randomized, placebo-controlled trial. *Arthritis Rheum.* 2002 Jul;46(7):1820-9

[177] "CONCLUSION: The clinical response to DHEA was not clearly dose dependent. Serum levels of DHEA and DHEAS correlated only weakly with lupus outcomes, but suggested an optimum serum DHEAS of 1000 microg/dl." Barry NN, McGuire JL, van Vollenhoven RF. Dehydroepiandrosterone in systemic lupus erythematosus: relationship between dosage, serum levels, and clinical response. *J Rheumatol.* 1998 Dec;25(12):2352-6

[178] Tierney ML. McPhee SJ, Papadakis MA. Current Medical Diagnosis and Treatment 2006. 45th edition. New York; Lange Medical Books: 2006, page 1721

[179] Weetman AP. Hypothyroidism: screening and subclinical disease. *BMJ.* 1997 Apr 19;314(7088):1175-8 http://bmj.bmjjournals.com/cgi/content/full/314/7088/1175

[180] "Now AACE encourages doctors to consider treatment for patients who test outside the boundaries of a narrower margin based on a target TSH level of 0.3 to 3.0. AACE believes the new range will result in proper diagnosis for millions of Americans who suffer from a mild thyroid disorder, but have gone untreated until now." American Association of Clinical Endocrinologists (AACE). 2003 Campaign Encourages Awareness of Mild Thyroid Failure, Importance of Routine Testing http://www.aace.com/pub/tam2003/press.php November 26, 2005

[181] Beers MH, Berkow R (eds). The Merck Manual. Seventeenth Edition. Whitehouse Station; Merck Research Laboratories 1999 Page 96

[182] Duntas LH, Mantzou E, Koutras DA. Effects of a six month treatment with selenomethionine in patients with autoimmune thyroiditis. *Eur J Endocrinol.* 2003 Apr;148(4):389-93 http://eje-online.org/cgi/reprint/148/4/389

[183] Gartner R, Gasnier BC, Dietrich JW, Krebs B, Angstwurm MW. Selenium supplementation in patients with autoimmune thyroiditis decreases thyroid peroxidase antibodies concentrations. *J Clin Endocrinol Metab.* 2002 Apr;87(4):1687-91 http://jcem.endojournals.org/cgi/content/full/87/4/1687

[184] "We recently conducted a prospective, placebo-controlled clinical study, where we could demonstrate, that a substitution of 200 wg sodium selenite for three months in patients with autoimmune thyroiditis reduced thyroid peroxidase antibody (TPO-Ab) concentrations significantly." Gartner R, Gasnier BC. Selenium in the treatment of autoimmune thyroiditis. *Biofactors.* 2003;19(3-4):165-70

[185] Bruns F, Micke O, Bremer M. Current status of selenium and other treatments for secondary lymphedema. *J Support Oncol.* 2003 Jul-Aug;1(2):121-30 http://www.supportiveoncology.net/journal/articles/0102121.pdf

dose is used. Caution must be applied in patients with adrenal insufficiency and/or those with cardiovascular disease.

- <u>Armour thyroid—prescription natural T4 and T3 from cow/pig thyroid gland</u>: 60 mg (one grain) is a common starting and maintenance dose. Due to the exacerbating effect on thyroid autoimmunity, Armour thyroid is never used in patients with thyroid autoimmunity.

- <u>Thyrolar/Liotrix—prescription synthetic T4 with T3</u>: Dosed as "1", "2", or "3." This product has been difficult to obtain for the past few years due to manufacturing problems (http://thyrolar.com/); previously it was my treatment of choice due to the combination of T4 and T3 and the lack of antigenicity compared to gland-derived products.

- <u>Liothyronine, Cytomel®</u>: Cytomel is prescription synthetic T3. Except in patients with myxedema for whom the appropriate starting dose is 5 mcg per day, treatment generally starts with 25 mcg per day and can be increased to 75 mcg per day; dose is adjusted based on clinical and laboratory response.[186] As stated previously, thyroid hormone supplements must be consumed separately from soy products (by at least 1-2 hours) and preferably on an empty stomach to avoid absorption interference by food, fiber, and minerals, especially calcium.

- <u>Thyroid glandular—nonprescription T3</u>: Producers of nutritional products are able to distribute T3 because it is not listed by the FDA as a prescription item. Nutritional supplement companies may start with Armour thyroid, remove the T4, and sell the thyroid glandular with active T3 thereby providing a nonprescription source of active thyroid hormone. For many patients, one tablet per day is at least as effective as a prescription source of thyroid hormone. Since it is derived from a glandular and therefore potentially antigenic source, thyroid glandular is not used in patients with thyroid autoimmunity due to its ability to induce increased production of anti-thyroid antibodies.

- <u>L-tyrosine and iodine</u>: Some patients with mild hypothyroidism respond to supplementation with L-tyrosine and iodine. Tyrosine is commonly used in doses of 4-9 grams per day in divided doses. According to Abraham and Wright[187], doses of iodine may be as high as 12.5 milligrams (12,500 micrograms), which is slightly less than the average daily intake in Japan at 13.8 mg per day.

- <u>Oral enzyme therapy with proteolytic/pancreatic enzymes</u>: Polyenzyme supplementation is used to ameliorate the pathophysiology induced by immune complexes, such as the related condition rheumatoid arthritis.[188]

- <u>CoQ10 (antihypertensive, renoprotective, and probably immunomodulatory)</u>: CoQ10 is a powerful antioxidant with a wide margin of safety and excellent clinical tolerability. **At least four studies have documented its powerful blood-pressure-lowering ability, which often surpasses the clinical effectiveness of antihypertensive drugs.[189,190,191,192] Furthermore, at least two published papers[193,194]**

[186] http://www.kingpharm.com/uploads/pdf_inserts/Cytomel_Web_PI.pdf
[187] Wright JV. Why you need 83 times more of this essential, cancer-fighting nutrient than the "experts" say you do. *Nutrition and Healing* 2005; volume 12, issue 4.
[188] Galebskaya LV, Ryumina EV, Niemerovsky VS, Matyukov AA. Human complement system state after wobenzyme intake. *VESTNIK MOSKOVSKOGO UNIVERSITETA. KHIMIYA.* 2000. Vol. 41, No. 6. Supplement. Pages 148-149
[189] Burke BE, Neuenschwander R, Olson RD. Randomized, double-blind, placebo-controlled trial of coenzyme Q10 in isolated systolic hypertension. *South Med J.* 2001 Nov;94(11):1112-7
[190] Singh RB, Niaz MA, Rastogi SS, Shukla PK, Thakur AS. Effect of hydrosoluble coenzyme Q10 on blood pressures and insulin resistance in hypertensive patients with coronary artery disease. *J Hum Hypertens.* 1999 Mar;13(3):203-8
[191] Digiesi V, Cantini F, Oradei A, Bisi G, Guarino GC, Brocchi A, Bellandi F, Mancini M, Littarru GP. Coenzyme Q10 in essential hypertension. *Mol Aspects Med.* 1994;15 Suppl:s257-63
[192] Langsjoen P, Langsjoen P, Willis R, Folkers K. Treatment of essential hypertension with coenzyme Q10. *Mol Aspects Med.* 1994;15 Suppl:S265-72
[193] Singh RB, Khanna HK, Niaz MA. Randomized, double-blind placebo-controlled trial of coenzyme Q10 in chronic renal failure: discovery of a new role. *J Nutr Environ Med* 2000;10:281-8
[194] Singh RB, Kumar A, Naiz MA, Singh RG, Gujrati S, Singh VP, Singh M, Singh UP, Taneja C, AND Rastogi SS. Randomized, Double-blind, Placebo-controlled Trial of Coenzyme Q10 in Patients with End-stage Renal Failure. *J Nutr Environ Med* 2003; Volume 13, Number 1: 13–22

and one case report[195] advocate that CoQ10 has powerful renoprotective benefits. CoQ10 levels are low in patients with allergies[196], and the symptomatic relief that many allergic patients experience following supplementation with CoQ10 suggests that CoQ10 has an immunomodulatory effect. Common doses start at > 100 mg per day with food; doses of 200 mg per day are not uncommon, and doses up to 1,000 mg per day are clinically well tolerated though the high financial toll resembles that of many pharmaceutical drugs.

- *Uncaria tomentosa, Uncaria guianensis*: Cat's claw has been safely and successfully used in the treatment of osteoarthritis[197] and rheumatoid arthritis.[198] High-quality extractions from reputable manufacturers used according to directions are recommended. Most products contain between 250-500 mg and are standardized to 3.0% alkaloids and 15% total polyphenols; QD-TID po dosing should be sufficient as *part* of a comprehensive plan.

- *Harpagophytum procumbens*: Harpagophytum is a moderately effective botanical analgesic for musculoskeletal pain.[199,200,201,202,203] Products are generally standardized for the content of harpagosides, with a target dose of 60 mg harpagoside per day.[204]

- Willow bark: Extracts from willow bark have proven safe and effective in the alleviation of moderate/severe low-back pain.[205,206] The mechanism of action appears to be inhibition of prostaglandin formation via inhibition of cyclooxygenase-2 gene transcription[207] by salicylates, phytonutrients which are widely present in fruits, vegetables, herbs and spices and which are partly responsible for the anti-cancer, anti-inflammatory, and health-promoting benefits of plant consumption.[208,209] According to a letter by Vasquez and Muanza[210], the only adverse effect that has been documented in association with willow bark was a single case of anaphylaxis in a patient previously sensitized to acetylsalicylic acid.

- *Boswellia serrata*: *Boswellia* shows clear anti-inflammatory and analgesic action via inhibition of 5-lipoxygenase[211] and clinical benefits have been demonstrated in patients with osteoarthritis of the knees[212] as well as asthma[213] and ulcerative colitis.[214] Products are generally standardized to contain 37.5–65% boswellic acids, with a target dose of approximately 150 mg of boswellic acids TID; dose and

[195] Singh RB, Singh MM. Effects of CoQ10 in new indications with antioxidant vitamin deficiency. *J Nutr Environ Med* 1999; 9:223-228

[196] Ye CQ, Folkers K, Tamagawa H, Pfeiffer C. A modified determination of coenzyme Q10 in human blood and CoQ10 blood levels in diverse patients with allergies. *Biofactors.* 1988 Dec;1(4):303-6

[197] Piscoya J, Rodriguez Z, Bustamante SA, Okuhama NN, Miller MJ, Sandoval M.Efficacy and safety of freeze-dried cat's claw in osteoarthritis of the knee: mechanisms of action of the species Uncaria guianensis. *Inflamm Res.* 2001 Sep;50(9):442-8

[198] "This small preliminary study demonstrates relative safety and modest benefit to the tender joint count of a highly purified extract from the pentacyclic chemotype of UT in patients with active RA taking sulfasalazine or hydroxychloroquine." Mur E, Hartig F, Eibl G, Schirmer M. Randomized double blind trial of an extract from the pentacyclic alkaloid-chemotype of uncaria tomentosa for the treatment of rheumatoid arthritis. *J Rheumatol.* 2002 Apr;29(4):678-81

[199] Chrubasik S, Thanner J, Kunzel O, Conradt C, Black A, Pollak S. Comparison of outcome measures during treatment with the proprietary Harpagophytum extract doloteffin in patients with pain in the lower back, knee or hip. *Phytomedicine* 2002 Apr;9(3):181-94

[200] Chantre P, Cappelaere A, Leblan D, Guedon D, Vandermander J, Fournie B. Efficacy and tolerance of Harpagophytum procumbens versus diacerhein in treatment of osteoarthritis. *Phytomedicine* 2000 Jun;7(3):177-83

[201] Leblan D, Chantre P, Fournie B. Harpagophytum procumbens in the treatment of knee and hip osteoarthritis. Four-month results of a prospective, multicenter, double-blind trial versus diacerhein. *Joint Bone Spine* 2000;67(5):462-7

[202] "…subgroup analyses suggested that the effect was confined to patients with more severe and radiating pain accompanied by neurological deficit. …a slightly different picture, with the benefits seeming, if anything, to be greatest in the H600 group and in patients without more severe pain, radiation or neurological deficit." Chrubasik S, Junck H, Breitschwerdt H, Conradt C, Zappe H. Effectiveness of Harpagophytum extract WS 1531 in the treatment of exacerbation of low back pain: a randomized, placebo-controlled, double-blind study. *Eur J Anaesthesiol* 1999 Feb;16(2):118-29

[203] Chrubasik S, Model A, Black A, Pollak S. A randomized double-blind pilot study comparing Doloteffin and Vioxx in the treatment of low back pain. *Rheumatology* (Oxford). 2003 Jan;42(1):141-8

[204] "They took an 8-week course of Doloteffin at a dose providing 60 mg harpagoside per day… Doloteffin is well worth considering for osteoarthritic knee and hip pain and nonspecific low back pain." Chrubasik S, Thanner J, Kunzel O, Conradt C, Black A, Pollak S. Comparison of outcome measures during treatment with the proprietary Harpagophytum extract doloteffin in patients with pain in the lower back, knee or hip. *Phytomedicine* 2002 Apr;9(3):181-94

[205] Chrubasik S, Eisenberg E, Balan E, Weinberger T, Luzzati R, Conradt C. Treatment of low-back pain exacerbations with willow bark extract: a randomized double-blind study. *Am J Med.* 2000;109:9-14

[206] Chrubasik S, Kunzel O, Model A, Conradt C, Black A. Treatment of low-back pain with a herbal or synthetic anti-rheumatic: a randomized controlled study. Willow bark extract for low-back pain. *Rheumatology* (Oxford). 2001;40:1388-93

[207] Hare LG, Woodside JV, Young IS. Dietary salicylates. *J Clin Pathol* 2003 Sep;56(9):649-50

[208] Lawrence JR, Peter R, Baxter GJ, Robson J, Graham AB, Paterson JR. Urinary excretion of salicyluric and salicylic acids by non-vegetarians, vegetarians, and patients taking low dose aspirin. *J Clin Pathol.* 2003 Sep;56(9):651-3

[209] Paterson JR, Lawrence JR. Salicylic acid: a link between aspirin, diet and the prevention of colorectal cancer. *QJM.* 2001 Aug;94(8):445-8

[210] Vasquez A, Muanza DN. Evaluation of Presence of Aspirin-Related Warnings with Willow Bark: Comment on the Article by Clauson et al. *Ann Pharmacotherapy* 2005 Oct;39(10):1763

[211] Wildfeuer A, Neu IS, Safayhi H, Metzger G, Wehrmann M, Vogel U, Ammon HP. Effects of boswellic acids extracted from a herbal medicine on the biosynthesis of leukotrienes and the course of experimental autoimmune encephalomyelitis. *Arzneimittelforschung* 1998 Jun;48(6):668-74

[212] Kimmatkar N, Thawani V, Hingorani L, Khiyani R. Efficacy and tolerability of Boswellia serrata extract in treatment of osteoarthritis of knee--a randomized double blind placebo controlled trial. *Phytomedicine.* 2003 Jan;10(1):3-7

[213] Gupta I, Gupta V, Parihar A, Gupta S, Ludtke R, Safayhi H, Ammon HP. Effects of Boswellia serrata gum resin in patients with bronchial asthma: results of a double-blind, placebo-controlled, 6-week clinical study. *Eur J Med Res.* 1998 Nov 17;3(11):511-4

[214] Gupta I, Parihar A, Malhotra P, Singh GB, Ludtke R, Safayhi H, Ammon HP. Effects of Boswellia serrata gum resin in patients with ulcerative colitis. *Eur J Med Res.* 1997 Jan;2(1):37-43

number of capsules/tablets will vary depending upon the concentration found in differing products. A German study showing that *Boswellia* was ineffective for rheumatoid arthritis[215] was poorly conducted, with inadequate follow-up, inadequate controls, and abnormal dosing of the herb.

- **Phytonutritional modulation of NF-kappaB**: As a stimulator of pro-inflammatory gene transcription, NF-kappaB is almost universally activated in conditions associated with inflammation.[216,217] Nutrients and botanicals which either directly or indirectly inhibit NF-kappaB for an anti-inflammatory benefit include vitamin D[218,219], curcumin[220] (requires piperine for absorption[221]), lipoic acid[222], green tea[223], ursolic acid[224] from rosemary[225], grape seed extract[226], propolis[227], zinc[228], high-dose selenium[229], indole-3-carbinol[230,231], N-acetyl-L-cysteine[232], resveratrol[233,234], isohumulones[235], GLA via PPAR-gamma[236]

[215] Sander O, Herborn G, Rau R. [Is H15 (resin extract of Boswellia serrata, "incense") a useful supplement to established drug therapy of chronic polyarthritis? Results of a double-blind pilot study] [Article in German] *Z Rheumatol*. 1998 Feb;57(1):11-6

[216] Tak PP, Firestein GS. NF-kappaB: a key role in inflammatory diseases. *J Clin Invest*. 2001 Jan;107(1):7-11 http://www.jci.org/cgi/content/full/107/1/7

[217] D'Acquisto F, May MJ, Ghosh S. Inhibition of Nuclear Factor KappaB (NF-B): An Emerging Theme in Anti-Inflammatory Therapies. *Mol Interv*. 2002 Feb;2(1):22-35 http://molinterv.aspetjournals.org/cgi/content/abstract/2/1/22

[218] "1Alpha,25-dihydroxyvitamin D3 (1,25-(OH)2-D3), the active metabolite of vitamin D, can inhibit NF-kappaB activity in human MRC-5 fibroblasts, targeting DNA binding of NF-kappaB but not translocation of its subunits p50 and p65." Harant H, Wolff B, Lindley IJ. 1Alpha,25-dihydroxyvitamin D3 decreases DNA binding of nuclear factor-kappaB in human fibroblasts. *FEBS Lett*. 1998 Oct 9;436(3):329-34

[219] "Thus, 1,25(OH)₂D₃ may negatively regulate IL-12 production by downregulation of NF-kB activation and binding to the p40-kB sequence." D'Ambrosio D, Cippitelli M, Cocciolo MG, Mazzeo D, Di Lucia P, Lang R, Sinigaglia F, Panina-Bordignon P. Inhibition of IL-12 production by 1,25-dihydroxyvitamin D3. Involvement of NF-kappaB downregulation in transcriptional repression of the p40 gene. *J Clin Invest*. 1998 Jan 1;101(1):252-62

[220] "Curcumin, EGCG and resveratrol have been shown to suppress activation of NF-kappa B." Surh YJ, Chun KS, Cha HH, Han SS, Keum YS, Park KK, Lee SS. Molecular mechanisms underlying chemopreventive activities of anti-inflammatory phytochemicals: down-regulation of COX-2 and iNOS through suppression of NF-kappa B activation. *Mutat Res*. 2001 Sep 1;480-481:243-68

[221] Shoba G, Joy D, Joseph T, Majeed M, Rajendran R, Srinivas PS. Influence of piperine on the pharmacokinetics of curcumin in animals and human volunteers. *Planta Med*. 1998 May;64(4):353-6

[222] "ALA reduced the TNF-alpha-stimulated ICAM-1 expression in a dose-dependent manner, to levels observed in unstimulated cells. Alpha-lipoic acid also reduced NF-kappaB activity in these cells in a dose-dependent manner." Lee HA, Hughes DA.Alpha-lipoic acid modulates NF-kappaB activity in human monocytic cells by direct interaction with DNA. *Exp Gerontol*. 2002 Jan-Mar;37(2-3):401-10

[223] "In conclusion, EGCG is an effective inhibitor of IKK activity. This may explain, at least in part, some of the reported anti-inflammatory and anticancer effects of green tea." Yang F, Oz HS, Barve S, de Villiers WJ, McClain CJ, Varilek GW. The green tea polyphenol (-)-epigallocatechin-3-gallate blocks nuclear factor-kappa B activation by inhibiting I kappa B kinase activity in the intestinal epithelial cell line IEC-6. *Mol Pharmacol*. 2001 Sep;60(3):528-33

[224] Shishodia S, Majumdar S, Banerjee S, Aggarwal BB. Ursolic acid inhibits nuclear factor-kappaB activation induced by carcinogenic agents through suppression of IkappaBalpha kinase and p65 phosphorylation: correlation with down-regulation of cyclooxygenase 2, matrix metalloproteinase 9, and cyclin D1. *Cancer Res*. 2003 Aug 1;63(15):4375-83 http://cancerres.aacrjournals.org/cgi/content/full/63/15/4375

[225] "These results suggest that carnosol suppresses the NO production and iNOS gene expression by inhibiting NF-kappaB activation, and provide possible mechanisms for its anti-inflammatory and chemopreventive action." Lo AH, Liang YC, Lin-Shiau SY, Ho CT, Lin JK. Carnosol, an antioxidant in rosemary, suppresses inducible nitric oxide synthase through down-regulating nuclear factor-kappaB in mouse macrophages. *Carcinogenesis*. 2002 Jun;23(6):983-91

[226] "Constitutive and TNFalpha-induced NF-kappaB DNA binding activity was inhibited by GSE at doses > or =50 microg/ml and treatments for > or =12 h." Dhanalakshmi S, Agarwal R, Agarwal C. Inhibition of NF-kappaB pathway in grape seed extract-induced apoptotic death of human prostate carcinoma DU145 cells. *Int J Oncol*. 2003 Sep;23(3):721-7

[227] "Caffeic acid phenethyl ester (CAPE) is an anti-inflammatory component of propolis (honeybee resin). CAPE is reportedly a specific inhibitor of nuclear factor-kappaB (NF-kappaB)." Fitzpatrick LR, Wang J, Le T. Caffeic acid phenethyl ester, an inhibitor of nuclear factor-kappaB, attenuates bacterial peptidoglycan polysaccharide-induced colitis in rats. *J Pharmacol Exp Ther*. 2001 Dec;299(3):915-20

[228] "Our results suggest that zinc supplementation may lead to downregulation of the inflammatory cytokines through upregulation of the negative feedback loop A20 to inhibit induced NF-kappaB activation." Prasad AS, Bao B, Beck FW, Kucuk O, Sarkar FH. Antioxidant effect of zinc in humans. *Free Radic Biol Med*. 2004 Oct 15;37(8):1182-90

[229] Note that the patients in this study received a very high dose of selenium: 960 micrograms per day. This is at the top—and some would say over the top—of the safe and reasonable dose for long-term supplementation. In this case, the study lasted for three months. "In patients receiving selenium supplementation, selenium NF-kappaB activity was significantly reduced, reaching the same level as the nondiabetic control group. CONCLUSION: In type 2 diabetic patients, activation of NF-kappaB measured in peripheral blood monocytes can be reduced by selenium supplementation, confirming its importance in the prevention of cardiovascular diseases." Faure P, Ramon O, Favier A, Halimi S. Selenium supplementation decreases nuclear factor-kappa B activity in peripheral blood mononuclear cells from type 2 diabetic patients. *Eur J Clin Invest*. 2004 Jul;34(7):475-81

[230] Takada Y, Andreeff M, Aggarwal BB. Indole-3-carbinol suppresses NF-{kappa}B and I{kappa}B{alpha} kinase activation causing inhibition of expression of NF-{kappa}B-regulated antiapoptotic and metastatic gene products and enhancement of apoptosis in myeloid and leukemia cells. *Blood*. 2005 Apr 5; [Epub ahead of print]

[231] "Overall, our results indicated that indole-3-carbinol inhibits NF-kappaB and NF-kappaB-regulated gene expression and that this mechanism may provide the molecular basis for its ability to suppress tumorigenesis." Takada Y, Andreeff M, Aggarwal BB. Indole-3-carbinol suppresses NF-kappaB and IkappaBalpha kinase activation, causing inhibition of expression of NF-kappaB-regulated antiapoptotic and metastatic gene products and enhancement of apoptosis in myeloid and leukemia cells. *Blood*. 2005 Jul 15;106(2):641-9. Epub 2005 Apr 5.

[232] "CONCLUSIONS: Administration of N-acetylcysteine results in decreased nuclear factor-kappa B activation in patients with sepsis, associated with decreases in interleukin-8 but not interleukin-6 or soluble intercellular adhesion molecule-1. These pilot data suggest that antioxidant therapy with N-acetylcysteine may be useful in blunting the inflammatory response to sepsis." Paterson RL, Galley HF, Webster NR. The effect of N-acetylcysteine on nuclear factor-kappa B activation, interleukin-6, interleukin-8, and intercellular adhesion molecule-1 expression in patients with sepsis. *Crit Care Med*. 2003 Nov;31(11):2574-8

[233] "Resveratrol's anticarcinogenic, anti-inflammatory, and growth-modulatory effects may thus be partially ascribed to the inhibition of activation of NF-kappaB and AP-1 and the associated kinases." Manna SK, Mukhopadhyay A, Aggarwal BB. Resveratrol suppresses TNF-induced activation of nuclear transcription factors NF-kappa B, activator protein-1, and apoptosis: potential role of reactive oxygen intermediates and lipid peroxidation. *J Immunol*. 2000 Jun 15;164(12):6509-19

[234] "Both resveratrol and quercetin inhibited NF-kappaB-, AP-1- and CREB-dependent transcription to a greater extent than the glucocorticosteroid, dexamethasone." Donnelly LE, Newton R, Kennedy GE, Fenwick PS, Leung RH, Ito K, Russell RE, Barnes PJ.Anti-inflammatory Effects of Resveratrol in Lung Epithelial Cells: Molecular Mechanisms. *Am J Physiol Lung Cell Mol Physiol*. 2004 Jun 4 [Epub ahead of print]

[235] Yajima H, Ikeshima E, Shiraki M, Kanaya T, Fujiwara D, Odai H, Tsuboyama-Kasaoka N, Ezaki O, Oikawa S, Kondo K. Isohumulones, bitter acids derived from hops, activate both peroxisome proliferator-activated receptor alpha and gamma and reduce insulin resistance. *J Biol Chem*. 2004 Aug 6;279(32):33456-62. Epub 2004 Jun 3. http://www.jbc.org/cgi/content/full/279/32/33456

[236] "Thus, PPAR gamma serves as the receptor for GLA in the regulation of gene expression in breast cancer cells. " Jiang WG, Redfern A, Bryce RP, Mansel RE. Peroxisome proliferator activated receptor-gamma (PPAR-gamma) mediates the action of gamma linolenic acid in breast cancer cells. *Prostaglandins Leukot Essent Fatty Acids*. 2000 Feb;62(2):119-27

and EPA via PPAR-alpha.[237] I have reviewed the phytonutritional modulation of NF-kappaB later in this text and elsewhere.[238] Several phytonutritional products targeting NF-kappaB are commercially available.

- Sunscreen: Sunscreen, long-sleeve shirts, and hats can be used to protect against photosensitivity; vitamin D needs can be met with supplementation at physiologic doses, generally 2,000-10,000 IU per day for adults.[239]

- Avoidance of *Echinacea*: *Echinacea* refers to a species of immunostimulating herbs with several valid clinical indications. However, its use has been anecdotally associated with flares of lupus nephritis in patients with previously quiescent lupus.[240]

- Anti-autoantibody interventions: **Patients with SLE have impaired ability to clear immune complexes via hepatic and splenic routes.**[241,242] Given that anti-DNA and related immune complexes and cryoglobulins are considered the most fundamental abnormalities in the pathogenesis of this disorder, we can explore at least three routes of clinical intervention based on this limited focus. First, therapeutic interventions might be used that inhibit the *de novo* formation of autoantibodies, particularly those that are directed against double-stranded DNA. This could be accomplished via bio-logical immunomodulation, pharmacologic/anti-biological immunosuppression, or by removing the underlying stimuli and predisposing factors ("etiologic approach"). Second, treatments might be implemented to nullify or diminish the adverse effects of these antibodies. Third, we might use interventions that remove the autoantibodies that are formed so that they are not significantly available to contribute to disease pathogenesis. As discussed previously in the section on treatments for multifocal dysbiosis, at least two primary mechanisms exist for the removal of autoantibody-containing immune complexes, namely 1) phagocytosis and proteolytic degradation by macrophages embedded in the liver and spleen, and 2) transport via hepatocytes directly into the bile for excretion. IgG double-stranded DNA antibodies are consumed and proteolytically/oxidatively/enzymatically degraded by monocytes/phagocytes[243] while IgA-containing immune complexes are preferentially consumed by hepatocytes and exported intact into the bile for excretion.

  o See table on following page; full-text article available online.

[237] "...EPA requires PPARalpha for its inhibitory effects on NF-kappaB." Mishra A, Chaudhary A, Sethi S. Oxidized omega-3 fatty acids inhibit NF-kappaB activation via a PPARalpha-dependent pathway. *Arterioscler Thromb Vasc Biol.* 2004 Sep;24(9):1621-7. Epub 2004 Jul 1. http://atvb.ahajournals.org/cgi/content/full/24/9/1621
[238] "Indeed, the previous view that nutrients only interact with human physiology at the metabolic/post-transcriptional level must be updated in light of current research showing that nutrients can, in fact, modify human physiology and phenotype at the genetic/pre-transcriptional level." Vasquez A. Reducing pain and inflammation naturally - part 4: nutritional and botanical inhibition of NF-kappaB, the major intracellular amplifier of the inflammatory cascade. A practical clinical strategy exemplifying anti-inflammatory nutrigenomics. *Nutritional Perspectives*, July 2005:5-12. www.OptimalHealthResearch.com/part4
[239] Vasquez A, Manso G, Cannell J. The clinical importance of vitamin D (cholecalciferol): a paradigm shift with implications for all healthcare providers. *Altern Ther Health Med.* 2004 Sep-Oct;10(5):28-36 http://optimalhealthresearch.com/monograph04
[240] Manzi S. Epidemiology of systemic lupus erythematosus. *Am J Manag Care.* 2001 Oct;7(16S):S474-9 ajmc.com/files/articlefiles/A01_131_2001octManziS474_9.pdf
[241] "These observations support the hypothesis that IC handling is abnormal in SLE." Davies KA, Peters AM, Beynon HL, Walport MJ. Immune complex processing in patients with systemic lupus erythematosus. In vivo imaging and clearance studies. *J Clin Invest.* 1992 Nov;90(5):2075-83
[242] "These results indicate that Fc-mediated clearance of ICs is defective in patients with SLE and suggest that ligation of ICs by Fc receptors is critical for their efficient binding and retention by the fixed MPS in the liver." Davies KA, Robson MG, Peters AM, Norsworthy P, Nash JT, Walport MJ. Defective Fc-dependent processing of immune complexes in patients with systemic lupus erythematosus. *Arthritis Rheum.* 2002 Apr;46(4):1028-38
[243] " In the presence of U937 [monocytic] cells, both the AHP-anti-dsDNA and C3b-opsonized ICs were rapidly removed from the erythrocytes; at 37 degrees C, more than half of the complexes were removed in 2 minutes." Craig ML, Bankovich AJ, McElhenny JL, Taylor RP. Clearance of anti-double-stranded DNA antibodies: the natural immune complex clearance mechanism. *Arthritis Rheum.* 2000 Oct;43(10):2265-75

Treatments to reduce the adverse effects of autoantibodies and immune complexes: a conceptual overview with interventional considerations		
Reduce *de novo* formation of autoantibodies	→ Biological immunomodulation	→ Orthoendocrinology, particularly supraphysiologic DHEA supplementation → Anti-inflammatory hypoallergenic diet → Anti-inflammatory nutrition: ALA, GLA, EPA, DHA, cholecalciferol, antioxidants, NF-kappaB inhibitors, and anti-inflammatory botanicals → Xenobiotic detoxification
	→ Pharmacologic immunosuppression	→ Prednisone and other corticosteroids → Antibiologics such as hydroxychloroquine which exert their clinical benefits via interfering with normal immunologic function, not by improving overall health or addressing underlying etiologic factors
	→ Removal/correction of primary stimuli for antibody formation *per patient*	→ Orthoendocrinology → Xenobiotic detoxification → Mitochondrial resuscitation → Antidysbiotic interventions: assessment and correction of multifocal dysbiosis
Reduce effects of autoantibodies	→ Anti-inflammatory treatments	→ Anti-inflammatory nutrition: ALA, GLA, EPA, DHA, cholecalciferol, antioxidants, NF-kappaB inhibitors, and anti-inflammatory botanicals
	→ Proteolytic enzymes	→ Proteolytic/pancreatic enzymes appear to reduce *de novo* formation of immune complexes
Enhance clearance of autoantibodies	→ Allopathic interventions	→ Immunoadsorption[244] → Plasmapheresis[245,246]
	→ Naturopathic interventions (theoretical[247])	→ Choleretic and cholagogic botanicals: beets, ginger[248], curcumin[249], *Picrorhiza*[250], milk thistle[251], *Andrographis paniculata*[252] and *Boerhaavia diffusa*.[253] → Low-volume enemas[254]

[244] Braun N, Erley C, Klein R, Kotter I, Saal J, Risler T. Immunoadsorption onto protein A induces remission in severe systemic lupus erythematosus. *Nephrol Dial Transplant*. 2000 Sep;15(9):1367-72 http://ndt.oxfordjournals.org/cgi/reprint/15/9/1367

[245] Santos-Ocampo AS, Mandell BF, Fessler BJ. Alveolar hemorrhage in systemic lupus erythematosus: presentation and management. *Chest*. 2000 Oct;118(4):1083-90

[246] Choi BG, Yoo WH. Successful treatment of pure red cell aplasia with plasmapheresis in a patient with systemic lupus erythematosus. *Yonsei Med J*. 2002 Apr;4):274-8

[247] Vasquez A. Do the Benefits of Botanical and Physiotherapeutic Hepatobiliary Stimulation Result From Enhanced Excretion of IgA Immune Complexes? *Naturopathy Digest* 2006; January: http://www.naturopathydigest.com/archives/2006/jan/vasquez_immune.php

[248] "Further analyses for the active constituents of the acetone extracts through column chromatography indicated that [6]-gingerol and [10]-gingerol, which are the pungent principles, are mainly responsible for the cholagogic effect of ginger." Yamahara J, Miki K, Chisaka T, Sawada T, Fujimura H, Tomimatsu T, Nakano K, Nohara T. Cholagogic effect of ginger and its active constituents. *J Ethnopharmacol*. 1985;13(2):217-25

[249] "On the basis of the present findings, it appears that curcumin induces contraction of the human gall-bladder." Rasyid A, Lelo A. The effect of curcumin and placebo on human gall-bladder function: an ultrasound study. *Aliment Pharmacol Ther*. 1999 Feb;13(2):245-9

[250] "Significant anticholestatic activity was also observed against carbon tetrachloride induced cholestasis in conscious rat, anaesthetized guinea pig and cat. Picroliv was more active than the known hepatoprotective drug silymarin." Saraswat B, Visen PK, Patnaik GK, Dhawan BN. Anticholestatic effect of picroliv, active hepatoprotective principle of Picrorhiza kurrooa, against carbon tetrachloride induced cholestasis. *Indian J Exp Biol*. 1993 Apr;31(4):316-8

[251] Crocenzi FA, Sanchez Pozzi EJ, Pellegrino JM, Rodriguez Garay EA, Mottino AD, Roma MG. Preventive effect of silymarin against taurolithocholate-induced cholestasis in the rat. *Biochem Pharmacol*. 2003 Jul 15;66(2):355-64

[252] Shukla B, Visen PK, Patnaik GK, Dhawan BN. Choleretic effect of andrographolide in rats and guinea pigs. *Planta Med*. 1992 Apr;58(2):146-9

[253] Chandan BK, Sharma AK, Anand KK. Boerhavia diffusa: a study of its hepatoprotective activity. *J Ethnopharmacol*. 1991 Mar;31(3):299-307

[254] Garbat AL, Jacobi HG. Secretion of Bile in Response to Rectal Installations. *Arch Intern Med* 1929; 44: 455-462

Do the Benefits of Botanical and Physiotherapeutic Hepatobiliary Stimulation Result From Enhanced Excretion of IgA Immune Complexes?

This article was originally published in *Naturopathy Digest*
http://www.naturopathydigest.com/archives/2006/jan/vasquez_immune.php

A cornerstone of science-based holistic health care, foremost among which is naturopathic medicine, is a profound and inviolable appreciation of the interconnected nature of various organs and body systems. By comparison, simplistic conceptualizations founded on the erroneous presumption that body systems function separately have become scientifically untenable and intellectually unsatisfying as biomedical research has continued to affirm holism and refute the isolationistic reductionism upon which the allopathic-pharmaceutical paradigm is founded. For example, these days, to think that the immune system functions separately from the body's ability to "detoxify" is clear indication of an incomplete education. The naturopathic profession is unique in its affirmation of holism in general and the importance of nutrition, gastrointestinal function and "detoxification" in particular. Within the profession, the importance of these tenets is accepted beyond the need for explication; however, a periodic review of these concepts and the ongoing molecular elucidation of the mechanisms involved is worthwhile, both for students and experienced clinicians.

The complete text is available online: naturopathydigest.com/archives/2006/jan/vasquez_immune.php

Scleroderma & Systemic Sclerosis

Introduction:
Scleroderma and systemic sclerosis are related conditions of either dermal or dermal+systemic fibrosis, respectively. A reasonable conceptualization is that of an inflammation-driven fibrotic response; the solution then—of course—is to address the disease-specific and patient-specific causes of excess inflammation and immune imbalance.

<u>Topics</u>:
- Introduction and Overview
- Clinical Presentation
- Prevalence, Symptoms, and Clinical Findings
- Pathophysiology
- Differential Diagnosis
- Diagnosis
- Standard Medical Treatment
- Therapeutic Interventions

Scleroderma
Systemic Sclerosis
Progressive Systemic Sclerosis

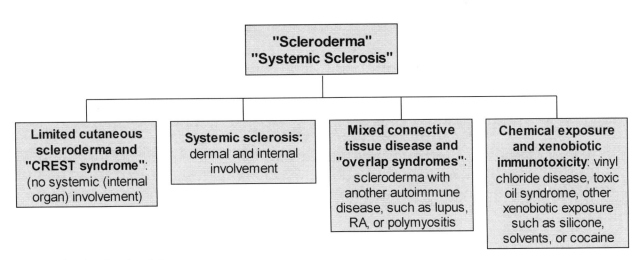

<u>Description/pathophysiology</u>:
- Generally considered "idiopathic." The terms *scleroderma* and *systemic sclerosis* are used somewhat interchangeably; yet, as these terms suggest, *scleroderma* is properly assigned to disease that is limited to the skin, while *systemic sclerosis* denotes visceral involvement in addition to skin changes. *Scleroderma* will be the default term in this section for linguistic expediency.
- **Characterized by fibrosis of the skin and internal organs, including the esophagus, intestines, lung, heart, and kidneys.** The condition can be mild and limited to the skin only, or it can be systemic and rapidly fatal due to internal organ involvement.

- Four subtypes:
  1. Limited cutaneous scleroderma: Only affecting the skin, especially of the fingers and face; relatively benign; **CREST syndrome:** calcinosis, Raynaud's phenomenon, esophageal dysmotility/dysfunction, sclerodactyly, telangiectasia
  2. Diffuse systemic sclerosis: Characterized by systemic fibrosis and degeneration of the skin (scleroderma) and internal organs; may rapidly progress to death.
  3. Mixed connective tissue disease and "overlap syndromes": Combination of scleroderma with another autoimmune disease, such as with dermatomyositis (sclerodermatomyositis) or with RA, SLE, or Sjogren's syndrome.
  4. Scleroderma secondary to xenobiotic immunotoxicity: Scleroderma can result from exposure to vinyl chloride, silicone, petroleum products, toxic oil syndrome, solvents, cocaine, and pesticides.
- Patients with scleroderma have evidence of **increased oxidative stress** demonstrated by a doubling of urinary isoprostane excretion.[1] Oxidative stress *results from* and *contributes to* systemic inflammation because 1) increased immune activity results in elaboration of oxidants, and 2) oxidative stress upregulates NF-kappaB (and other pathways) for additive immune activation; oxidative stress and inflammation both contribute to tissue fibrosis.

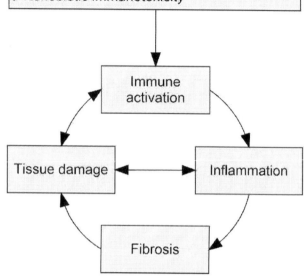

- Proinflammatory diet, nutritional imbalances
- Multifocal dysbiosis
- Immunophenotype imbalance due to malnutrition and dysbiosis
- Dysfunctional mitochondria
- Stress excess and sleep insufficiency
- Endocrine imbalances
- Xenobiotic immunotoxicity

Simple integrated model for scleroderma: Oxidative stress results from and contributes to systemic inflammation because 1) increased immune activity results in elaboration of oxidants, and 2) oxidative stress upregulates NF-kappaB (and other pathways) for additive immune activation; oxidative stress and inflammation both promote fibrosis.

Clinical presentations:
- 4x more common in women, general age of onset is 20-40 years.
- Skin changes: hyperpigmentation, tightness, tightness and thickening of the face results in "mask-like face", telangiectasia, may also have depigmentation; dermal ulceration of fingertips and extensor surfaces as skin loses elasticity. Swelling and thickening of the fingers: sclerodactyly.
- Soft tissue calcification: Especially in the hands; systemic calcification is also seen.
- Polyarthralgia: Affects 90% of patients; flexion contractures of the joints due to fibrosis is also common.
- Autonomic dysfunction: Raynaud's phenomenon: Seen in 90% of patients and often precedes sclerodermatous manifestations by a period of up to 5 years.
- Pulmonary: Dyspnea, pulmonary hypertension.
- Cardiac: Arrhythmias, CHF, hypertension, ECG abnormalities—may be fatal.
- Renal: Renal failure is a leading cause of death.

---

[1] "CONCLUSION: This study provides evidence of enhanced lipid peroxidation in both SSc and UCTD, and suggests a rationale for antioxidant treatment of SSc." Cracowski JL, Marpeau C, Carpentier PH, Imbert B, Hunt M, Stanke-Labesque F, Bessard G. Enhanced in vivo lipid peroxidation in scleroderma spectrum disorders. *Arthritis Rheum* 2001 May;44(5):1143-8

- GI disturbances:
  - Esophageal dysfunction and dysphagia eventually occur in most patients; histologic/biopsy examination reveals degeneration of intestinal nerves, vessels, and smooth muscle.[2]
  - Greatly increased risk for Barrett's esophagus (33% of all scleroderma patients) with a notably low risk of esophageal adenocarcinoma.
  - Slow intestinal transit—intestinal hypomotility in scleroderma promotes bacterial overgrowth of the small bowel, which probably contributes to the pathogenesis of the disease via the pro-inflammatory and immune activating effects discussed in Chapter 4. Treatment of bacterial overgrowth with antibiotics (ciprofloxacin 500 mg bid[3]) or promotility drugs (octreotide[4]) is effective treatment for scleroderma according to published case reports; **such research supports the hypothesis that intestinal dysbiosis—namely bacterial overgrowth—is an important contributor to the perpetuation of scleroderma**. Thus, *part of* the pathophysiology of scleroderma as related to bacterial overgrowth may be represented as follows:

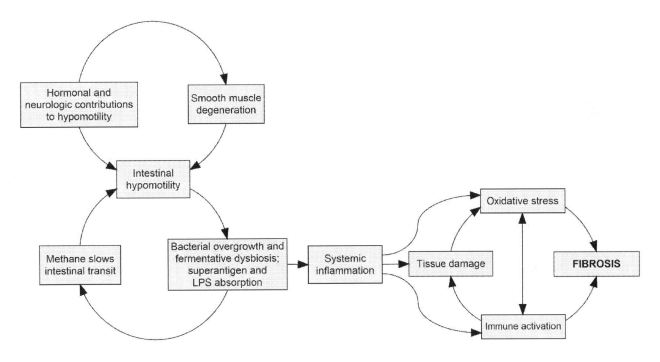

Aspects of scleroderma: diagram by Vasquez; quote from Radić et al[5]: "Systemic sclerosis is an autoimmune disease characterized by vascular obliteration, excessive extracellular matrix deposition and fibrosis of the connective tissues of the skin, lungs, gastrointestinal tract, heart, and kidneys. The pathogenesis of systemic sclerosis is extremely complex; at present, no single unifying hypothesis explains all aspects. **Over the last 20 years increasing evidence has accumulated to implicate infectious agents in the etiology of systemic sclerosis. Increased antibody titers, a preponderance of specific strains in patients with systemic sclerosis, and evidence of molecular mimicry inducing autoimmune responses suggest mechanisms by which infectious agents may contribute to the development and progression of systemic sclerosis.**"

---

[2] "We found ultrastructural signs of axonal degeneration and cytoskeletal abnormalities in the bundles of unmyelinated fibers. There was also focal degeneration of smooth muscle cells, often in association with the presence of partially degranulated mast cells." Malandrini A, Selvi E, Villanova M, Berti G, Sabadini L, Salvadori C, Gambelli S, De Stefano R, Vernillo R, Marcolongo R, Guazzi G. Autonomic nervous system and smooth muscle cell involvement in systemic sclerosis: ultrastructural study of 3 cases. *J Rheumatol*. 2000 May;27(5):1203-6

[3] Over KE, Bucknall RC. Regression of skin changes in a patient with systemic sclerosis following treatment for bacterial overgrowth with ciprofloxacin. *Br J Rheumatol*. 1998 Jun;37(6):696 http://rheumatology.oxfordjournals.org/cgi/reprint/37/6/696a

[4] "After 8 months of treatment, normal weight was obtained and skin induration was spectacularly reduced and pigmentation returned to a normal state." Descamps V, et al. Global improvement of systemic scleroderma under long-term administration of octreotide. *Eur J Dermatol* 1999 Sep;9(6):446-8

[5] Radić M, Martinović Kaliterna D, Radić J. Infectious disease as aetiological factor in the pathogenesis of systemic sclerosis. *Neth J Med*. 2010 Nov;68(11):348-53

Major differential diagnoses:
- Parkinson's disease: mask-like face
- Vinyl chloride disease: exposure to vinyl chloride (VC) monomer, a volatile substance mostly used for polyvinyl chloride (PVC) synthesis produces a scleroderma-like disorder that may be complicated by vasculitic and neurologic sequelae.[6,7,8]
- Toxic oil syndrome: A syndrome of incapacitating myalgias, marked peripheral eosinophilia, pulmonary infiltrates, and increased prevalence of scleroderma and neurologic disorders following consumption of contaminated oil.[9]
- Dermal infections and other diseases: Zygomycosis, sporotrichosis, cutaneous lymphoma
- Other autoimmune disorders: Overlap syndromes

Clinical assessments:
- **History/subjective**:
  - Symptoms and complications from dermal induration/hardening and fibrosis
  - Intestinal and digestive complaints
  - Areas affected, ROM, ADL, QOL
  - Xenobiotic exposure: Occupational exposure to silica is associated with scleroderma; some cases appear to be linked to silicone breast implants[10] (controversial[11]) and anti-silicate antibodies may be valuable for documenting humoral response to silicone.[12] Clinicians should ask about any history of iatrogenic, occupational, recreational or domestic xenobiotic exposure, such as to organic solvents[13], pesticides, epoxy resins[14], and other immunotoxins.[15] Use of cocaine can cause or exacerbate scleroderma.[16]
- **Physical examination/objective**: routine, including the following:
  - Dermal exam, including nailfold capillaroscopy: Symptoms and complications from dermal induration/hardening, swelling, and fibrosis: swollen fingers, tight skin on face and hands, dermal ulcerations and hypopigmentation. Nailfold capillaroscopy reveals microvascular changes consistent with autoimmunity and autoimmune-expedited cardiovascular disease. Per Cutolo et al[17], "Raynaud's phenomenon (RP) represents the most frequent clinical aspect of cardio/microvascular involvement and is a key feature of several autoimmune rheumatic diseases. Moreover, RP is associated in a statistically significant manner with many coronary diseases. In normal conditions or in primary RP (excluding during the cold-exposure test), the

[6] "Occupational exposure to vinyl chloride monomers is known to induce Raynaud's phenomenon, periportal fibrosis, liver angiosarcoma and scleroderma-like syndrome." Serratrice J, Granel B, Pache X, Disdier P, De Roux-Serratrice C, Pellissier JF, Weiller PJ. A case of polymyositis with anti-histidyl-t-RNA synthetase (Jo-1) antibody syndrome following extensive vinyl chloride exposure. *Clin Rheumatol.* 2001;20(5):379-82

[7] "An unusual case of systemic sclerosis occurring in a patient exposed to the vinyl chloride monomer (VCM) is presented." Ostlere LS, Harris D, Buckley C, Black C, Rustin MH. Atypical systemic sclerosis following exposure to vinyl chloride monomer. A case report and review of the cutaneous aspects of vinyl chloride disease. *Clin Exp Dermatol.* 1992 May;17(3):208-10

[8] "Angiosarcoma of the liver, Raynaud's phenomenon, scleroderma-like lesions, acroosteolysis and neuritis are known to be typical vinyl chloride-associated manifestations (VC disease)." Magnavita N, Bergamaschi A, Garcovich A, Giuliano G. Vasculitic purpura in vinyl chloride disease: a case report. *Angiology.* 1986 May;37(5):382-8

[9] "In 1981, in Spain, the ingestion of an oil fraudulently sold as olive oil caused an outbreak of a previously unrecorded condition, later known as toxic oil syndrome (TOS), clinically characterized by intense incapacitating myalgias, marked peripheral eosinophilia, and pulmonary infiltrates." Gelpi E, de la Paz MP, Terracini B, Abaitua I, de la Camara AG, Kilbourne EM, Lahoz C, Nemery B, Philen RM, Soldevilla L, Tarkowski S; WHO/CISAT Scientific Committee for the Toxic Oil Syndrome. Centro de Investigacion para el Sindrome del Aceite Toxico. The Spanish toxic oil syndrome 20 years after its onset: a multidisciplinary review of scientific knowledge. *Environ Health Perspect.* 2002 May;110(5):457-64 http://ehp.niehs.nih.gov/members/2002/110p457-464gelpi/gelpi-full.html

[10] "...idiopathic form of scleroderma and related conditions. CONCLUSION. These findings suggest that ANA positivity is relatively common in individuals with silicone breast implants, and may support the existence of autoimmune mechanisms in the pathogenesis of the clinical manifestations seen in this population." Cuellar ML, Scopelitis E, Tenenbaum SA, et al. Serum antinuclear antibodies in women with silicone breast implants. *J Rheumatol.* 1995 Feb;22(2):236-40

[11] "Neither the case-control studies nor the other epidemiologic data support the hypothesis that scleroderma is associated with or causally related to breast implants." Whorton D, Wong O. Scleroderma and silicone breast implants. West J Med 1997 Sep;167(3):159-65

[12] Shen GQ, Ojo-Amaize EA, Agopian MS, Peter JB.Silicate antibodies in women with silicone breast implants: development of an assay for detection of humoral immunity. *Clin Diagn Lab Immunol.* 1996 Mar;3(2):162-6 http://cdli.asm.org/cgi/reprint/3/2/162?view=reprint&pmid=8991630

[13] "We describe a sclerodermatous syndrome in a middle-aged man who had worked with a wide variety of organic solvents over a prolonged period." Bottomley WW, et al. A sclerodermatous syndrome with unusual features following prolonged occupational exposure to organic solvents. *Br J Dermatol* 1993 Feb;128(2):203-6

[14] "A new occupational disorder characterized by skin sclerosis is described. This disease developed acutely in workmen exposed to the vapor of epoxy resins." Yamakage A, et al. Occupational scleroderma-like disorder occurring in men engaged in the polymerization of epoxy resins. *Dermatologica.* 1980;161(1):33-44

[15] "There is growing concern about the association between systemic sclerosis and certain environmental and occupational risk factors, including exposures to vinyl chloride, adulterated cooking oils, L-tryptophan, silica, silicone breast implants, organic solvents, and other agents such as epoxy resins, pesticides, and hand/arm vibration." Nietert PJ, Silver RM. Systemic sclerosis: environmental and occupational risk factors. *Curr Opin Rheumatol* 2000 Nov;12(6):520-6

[16] "It has been reported that cocaine may initiate scleroderma in an already susceptible individual or unmask it at an earlier age in subclinical disease." Attoussi S, Faulkner ML, Oso A, Umoru B. Cocaine-induced scleroderma and scleroderma renal crisis. *South Med J* 1998 Oct;91(10):961-3

[17] Cutolo M, Sulli A, Secchi ME, Paolino S, Pizzorni C. Nailfold capillaroscopy is useful for the diagnosis and follow-up of autoimmune rheumatic diseases. A future tool for the analysis of microvascular heart involvement? *Rheumatology* (Oxford). 2006 Oct;45 Suppl 4:iv43-6 http://rheumatology.oxfordjournals.org/content/45/suppl_4/iv43.full.pdf

normal nailfold capillaroscopic pattern shows a regular disposition of the capillary loops along with the nailbed. On the contrary, in subjects suffering from secondary RP, one or more alterations of the capillaroscopic findings should alert the physician of the possibility of a connective tissue disease not yet detected. Nailfold capillaroscopy (NV) represents the best method to analyze microvascular abnormalities in autoimmune rheumatic diseases. Architectural disorganization, giant capillaries, hemorrhages, loss of capillaries, angiogenesis and avascular areas characterize >95% of patients with overt scleroderma (SSc)."

- o **Range of motion (ROM)**: Limited range of motion is characteristic secondary to a "straight jacket" effect secondary to tightened and fibrotic skin.
- o **Abdominal exam**: Abdominal exam, gastrointestinal motility
- o **Pulmonary exam**: Pulmonary examination and auscultation
- o **Cardiovascular exam**: Assessment for hypertension is mandatory
- **Laboratory assessments**: *lab assessments are only minimally supportive for the diagnosis, but are helpful to monitor for complications*
  - o **Urinalysis**: Screen for renal compromise as previously detailed
  - o **Chemistry panel**: Assess for renal and liver status, electrolytes, etc.
  - o **CBC**: May reveal anemia due to malabsorption-induced deficiencies of B12, folate, iron, hypoproliferation due to inflammation (i.e., the anemia of chronic disease).
  - o **Rheumatoid factor**: positive in 33%
  - o **Breath hydrogen/methane**: This test is used to assess for bacterial overgrowth
  - o **Lactulose and mannitol assay for "leaky gut" and malabsorption**: Abnormal results are likely due to bacterial overgrowth and/or celiac disease with resultant malabsorption and increased intestinal permeability.[18]
  - o **Leukocyte antigens**: Increased prevalence of HLA-DR5 and HLA-DR1
  - o *Helicobacter pylori* **detection**: Given the increased prevalence of *Helicobacter pylori* infection[19,20], the addition of antigen testing onto a comprehensive stool analysis and comprehensive parasitology examination is recommended.
  - o **Comprehensive stool analysis and comprehensive parasitology**: essential
  - o **ANA: positive in up to 96% of patients with scleroderma.**
  - o **Anticentromere antibody: positive in 50% with CREST; specific for scleroderma**; portends disease course limited to dermal involvement[21]
  - o **Anti-SCL-70 antibodies: positive in 20-30% of patients; specific for scleroderma**; portends disease course with internal organ involvement, particularly of the lungs
  - o **Antifibrillarin antibodies**: seen in a small portion (~4%) of patients with scleroderma and correlates with internal organ involvement[22]
- **Imaging**:
  - o ECG abnormalities are common and can include ventricular ectopy, which is correlated with sudden cardiac death
  - o Radiography, pulmonary function tests, and CT imaging may be used to detect fibrosing alveolitis and scleroderma-associated pulmonary decline

---

[18] "Coeliac disease may account for malabsorption in scleroderma patients even when test suggest bacterial overgrowth." Marguerie C, Kaye S, Vyse T, Mackworth-Young C, Walport MJ, Black C. Malabsorption caused by coeliac disease in patients who have scleroderma. *Br J Rheumatol*. 1995 Sep;34(9):858-61

[19] "Thus, the risk for gastric diseases caused by HP infection is enhanced in patients with systemic sclerosis compared with white healthy, asymptomatic persons examined in other studies." Reinauer S, Goerz G, Ruzicka T, Susanto F, Humfeld S, Reinauer H. Helicobacter pylori in patients with systemic sclerosis: detection with the 13C-urea breath test and eradication. *Acta Derm Venereol*. 1994 Sep;74(5):361-3

[20] "Patients with SSc have H. pylori infection at a higher prevalence than the general population." Yazawa N, Fujimoto M, Kikuchi K, Kubo M, Ihn H, Sato S, Tamaki T, Tamaki K. High seroprevalence of Helicobacter pylori infection in patients with systemic sclerosis: association with esophageal involvement. *J Rheumatol*. 1998 Apr;25(4):650-3

[21] Ho KT, Reveille JD. The clinical relevance of autoantibodies in scleroderma. Arthritis Res Ther. 2003;5(2):80-93. Epub 2003 Feb 12 http://arthritis-research.com/content/5/2/80

[22] "AFA identifies young SSc patients with frequent internal organ involvement, especially pulmonary hypertension, myositis and renal disease." Tormey VJ, Bunn CC, Denton CP, Black CM. Anti-fibrillarin antibodies in systemic sclerosis. *Rheumatology* (Oxford). 2001 Oct;40(10):1157-62 http://rheumatology.oxfordjournals.org/cgi/content/full/40/10/1157

- **Establishing the diagnosis**:
  - Clinical assessment is sufficient in patients with classic full-blown disease
  - Combination of serologic evidence of autoimmunity and dermal induration

Complications:
- 33% of patients will develop **Barrett's esophagus** and are at increased risk for cancer; periodic endoscopic surveillance is warranted; referral to gastroenterologist is recommended. To the extent possible, acid-blocking (proton pump-inhibiting) drugs should be avoided because the iatrogenic hypochlorhydria will exacerbate the small bowel bacterial overgrowth and thereby perpetuate the systemic inflammatory state.
- **Malabsorption** and resultant **malnutrition** due to intestinal hypomotility and dysbiosis
- **Sudden cardiac death**
- **Pulmonary hypertension and pulmonary failure**
- **Increased incidence of breast and lung cancer**
- **Hypertension**, secondary to scleroderma-induced renal damage

Clinical management:
- Address underlying causative contibutors; apply Functional Inflammology protocol.
- Monitor for complications such as systemic hypertension, pulmonary hypertension, renal failure.
- Referral if clinical outcome is unsatisfactory or if serious complications are possible/evident.
- Treat complications such as HTN and GERD.

Treatments:
- <u>Drug treatments</u>: "Treatment of progressive systemic sclerosis is symptomatic and supportive. ... Prednisone has little or no role in the treatment of scleroderma."[23] Other allopathic treatments have recently been reviewed in an article available for free on-line.[24]
  - <u>Prednisone</u> or other corticosteroid is used for myositis, MCTD, and arthritis
  - <u>Penicillamine</u> started at 250 mg/d and gradually increased to 0.5-1.0 g/d can reduce dermal and systemic involvement
  - <u>Tetracycline</u>: one gram per day for bacterial overgrowth[25]
  - <u>ACE inhibitors</u> are the drugs of choice for scleroderma renal disease and hypertension
- <u>Supplemented Paleo-Mediterranean diet</u>: The health-promoting diet of choice for the majority of people is a diet based on abundant consumption of fruits, vegetables, seeds, nuts, omega-3 and monounsaturated fatty acids, and lean sources of protein such as lean meats, fatty cold-water fish, soy and whey proteins. Although this diet is the most-nutrient dense diet available, rational supplementation with vitamins, minerals, and health promoting fatty acids (i.e., ALA, GLA, EPA, DHA) makes this the best practical diet that can possibly be conceived and implemented. **For scleroderma patients whose diets have habitually been low in fiber, dietary improvement which increases fiber consumption should be implemented slowly to avoid phytobezoar formation and intestinal obstruction**[26]**; consumption of water/fluids with meals is reasonable, as is periodic or regular use of osmotic laxative agents such as magnesium and ascorbate.**
- <u>Daily use of a broad-spectrum high-potency multivitamin and multimineral supplement</u>: **Vitamin and mineral supplementation is important for patients with scleroderma.** Vitamin supplementation (particularly with pyridoxine and riboflavin) appears warranted in patients with **systemic sclerosis** based on a small (n=5) study that documented the normalization of aberrant tryptophan metabolism in most patients following the administration of pyridoxine with riboflavin; the authors concluded

[23] Tierney ML. McPhee SJ, Papadakis MA (eds). Current Medical Diagnosis and Treatment. 35th edition. Stamford: Appleton and Lange, 1996 page 747

[24] Sapadin AN, Fleischmajer R. Treatment of scleroderma. *Arch Dermatol*. 2002 Jan;138(1):99-105. http://archderm.ama-assn.org/cgi/content/full/138/1/99 Accessed December 16, 2005

[25] Beers MH, Berkow R (eds). The Merck Manual. Seventeenth Edition. Whitehouse Station; Merck Research Laboratories 1999 Page 433

[26] Gough A, Sheeran T, Bacon P, Emery P. Dietary advice in systemic sclerosis: the dangers of a high fibre diet. *Ann Rheum Dis*. 1998;57(11):641-2 http://ard.bmjjournals.com/cgi/content/full/57/11/641

that this was evidence of combined vitamin deficiency in patients with scleroderma.[27] This combined deficiency is not surprising given the high incidence of bacterial overgrowth and malabsorption in scleroderma patients. Deficiencies of ascorbate and selenium have also been documented in patients with scleroderma.[28] Reduced folate and cobalamin and elevated homocysteine have also been noted in patients with scleroderma.[29]

- Avoidance of proinflammatory foods: Proinflammatory foods act *directly* or *indirectly*; direct mechanisms include activating Toll-like receptors or NF-kappaB or inducing oxidative stress, while indirect mechanisms include depleting the body of anti-inflammatory nutrients and displacing more nutritious anti-inflammatory foods. *See previous detailing in other chapters, especially Chapter 4.*

- Avoidance of allergenic foods: Any patient may be allergic to any food, even if the food is generally considered a health-promoting food. Generally speaking, the most notorious allergens are wheat, citrus (especially juice due to the industrial use of fungal hemicellulases), cow's milk, eggs, peanuts, chocolate, and yeast-containing foods; according to a study in patients with migraine, some patients will have to avoid as many as 10 specific foods in order to become symptom-free.[30] **Celiac disease is not uncommon in patients with scleroderma, and their scleroderma diagnosis may precede the recognition of celiac disease by many years.**[31,32] Clinicians must explain to their patients that celiac disease and wheat allergy are two different clinical entities and that exclusion of one does not exclude the other, and in neither case does mutual exclusion obviate the **promotion of intestinal bacterial overgrowth (i.e., proinflammatory dysbiosis) by indigestible wheat oligosaccharides.** Rapid implementation of high fiber diets may precipitate bowel obstruction.[33]

- Vitamin E: Morelli et al[34] describe a 60-year-old woman with **systemic sclerosis** complicated by hypertension, renal failure, and heart failure; although allopathic drug treatments were of no benefit, **the addition of "vitamin E (600 mg daily)" lead to rapid and significant clinical improvement.** Ayres and Mihan[35] wrote that vitamin E was effective in the clinical management of scleroderma, discoid lupus erythematosus[36], porphyria cutanea tarda, several types of vasculitis, and polymyositis.[37] Given that vitamin E is not a single compound but rather a family of closely related tocopherols, most clinicians prefer to use a source of "mixed tocopherols" inclusive of alpha, beta, delta, and—perhaps most importantly—gamma tocopherol.[38] Vitamin E has a wide margin of safety and although daily doses are kept in the range of 400-1200 IU, doses up to 3,200 IU are generally considered non-toxic.

- Vitamin D3 supplementation with physiologic doses and/or tailored to serum 25(OH)D and serum calcium levels: Vitamin D deficiency is common in the general population and is even more common

---

[27] "But the simultaneous administration of pyridoxine and nicotinamide to three of these patients normalized the excretory picture after tryptophan loading." De Antoni A, Muggeo M, Costa C, Allegri G, Crepaldi G. Tryptophan metabolism "via" nicotinic acid in patients with scleroderma. *Acta Vitaminol Enzymol.* 1976;30(4-6):134-9

[28] "Plasma ascorbic acid was reduced in all 3 groups of patients: median level 10.6 mg/l in controls, 4.8 mg/l in PRP (p < 0.01), 2.5 mg/l in lSSc (p < 0.01) and 6.8 mg/l in dSSc (p < 0.05). A reduction in serum selenium was especially found in dSSc (median 75 micrograms/l compared to 100 micrograms/l in controls, p < 0.05)." Herrick AL, Rieley F, Schofield D, Hollis S, Braganza JM, Jayson MI. Micronutrient antioxidant status in patients with primary Raynaud's phenomenon and systemic sclerosis. *J Rheumatol.* 1994 Aug;21(8):1477-83

[29] "Patients with SSc had higher Hcy and vWF concentrations than those with RP or controls. Folic acid and vitamin B12 were lower in SSc than in RP or controls." Marasini B, Casari S, Bestetti A, Maioli C, Cugno M, Zeni S, Turri O, Guagnellini E, Biondi ML. Homocysteine concentration in primary and systemic sclerosis associated Raynaud's phenomenon. *J Rheumatol.* 2000 Nov;27(11):2621-3

[30] Grant EC. Food allergies and migraine. *Lancet.* 1979 May 5;1(8123):966-9

[31] Gomez-Puerta JA, Gil V, Cervera R, Miquel R, Jimenez S, Ramos-Casals M, Font J. Coeliac disease associated with systemic sclerosis. *Ann Rheum Dis.* 2004 Jan;63(1):104-5 http://ard.bmjjournals.com/cgi/content/full/63/1/104

[32] "Coeliac disease may account for malabsorption in scleroderma patients even when test suggest bacterial overgrowth." Marguerie C, Kaye S, Vyse T, Mackworth-Young C, Walport MJ, Black C. Malabsorption caused by coeliac disease in patients who have scleroderma. *Br J Rheumatol.* 1995 Sep;34(9):858-61

[33] Gough A, Sheeran T, Bacon P, Emery P. Dietary advice in systemic sclerosis: the dangers of a high fibre diet. *Ann Rheum Dis.* 1998 Nov;57(11):641-2 http://ard.bmjjournals.com/cgi/content/full/57/11/641

[34] "Casually, vitamin E (600 mg daily) was added. After 6 months, clinical manifestations of heart failure were disappeared and the echocardiogram showed a normally-sized left ventricle with normal wall motion." Morelli S, Sgreccia A, Bernardo ML, Gurgo Di Castelmenardo A, Petrilli AC, De Leva R, Nuccio F, Calvieri S. Systemic sclerosis (scleroderma). A case of recovery of cardiomyopathy after vitamin E treatment. *Minerva Cardioangiol.* 2001 Apr;49(2):127-30

[35] "Among the diseases that were successfully controlled were a number in the autoimmune category, including scleroderma, discoid lupus erythematosus, porphyria cutanea tarda, several types of vasculitis, and polymyositis." Ayres S Jr, Mihan R. Is vitamin E involved in the autoimmune mechanism? *Cutis.* 1978 Mar;21(3):321-5

[36] "Despite conflicting opinions, our personal experience and a number of reviewed clinical reports indicate that vitamin E, properly administered in adequate doses, is a safe and effective treatment for chronic discoid lupus erythematosus, and may be of value in treating other types of the disease." Ayres S Jr, Mihan R. Lupus erythematosus and vitamin E: an effective and nontoxic therapy. *Cutis.* 1979;23(1):49-52, 54

[37] "She then made a dramatic improvement when large doses of vitamin E (d, alpha-tocopheryl acetate) were administered." Killeen RN, Ayres S Jr, Mihan R. Polymyositis: response to vitamin E. *South Med J.* 1976 Oct;69(10):1372-4

[38] Jiang Q, Christen S, Shigenaga MK, Ames BN. gamma-tocopherol, the major form of vitamin E in the US diet, deserves more attention. *Am J Clin Nutr.* 2001 Dec;74(6):714-22 http://www.ajcn.org/cgi/content/full/74/6/714

in patients with chronic illness and chronic musculoskeletal pain.[39] Correction of vitamin D deficiency provides a clinically significant anti-inflammatory and immunomodulatory benefit.[40] **Oral administration of active vitamin D3 (1,25-dihydroxyvitamin D) has lead to clinical improvement in patients with scleroderma.**[41] Reasonable daily doses for children and adults are 2,000 and 4,000 IU, respectively, as defined by Vasquez, et al.[42] Deficiency and response to treatment are monitored with serum 25(OH)vitamin D while safety is monitored with serum calcium; inflammatory granulomatous diseases and certain drugs such as hydrochlorothiazide greatly increase the propensity for hypercalcemia and warrant increment dosing and frequent monitoring of serum calcium.

- CoQ10: CoQ10 is a powerful antioxidant with a wide margin of safety and excellent clinical tolerability. **At least four studies have documented its powerful blood-pressure-lowering ability, which often surpasses the clinical effectiveness of antihypertensive drugs.**[43,44,45,46] **Furthermore, at least two published papers**[47,48] **and one case report**[49] **advocate that CoQ10 has powerful renoprotective benefits.** CoQ10 levels are low in patients with allergies[50], and the symptomatic relief that many allergic patients experience following supplementation with CoQ10 suggests that CoQ10 has an immunomodulatory effect. Common doses start at > 100 mg per day with food; doses of 200 mg per day are not uncommon, and doses up to 1,000 mg per day are clinically well tolerated though the high financial toll approximates that of many pharmaceutical drugs.

- N-acetyl-cysteine (NAC): **Oxidative stress promotes a fibrotic phenotype in scleroderma fibroblasts, which was normalized by administration of NAC** *in vitro*.[51] NAC is well-tolerated, inhibits NF-kappaB, functions as an antioxidant, and promotes detoxification via hepatoprotection and glutathione conjugation.

- Comprehensive antioxidation: **As previously mentioned, patients with scleroderma have evidence of increased oxidative stress demonstrated by a doubling of urinary isoprostane excretion**.[52] Oxidative stress results from and contributes to systemic inflammation because 1) increased immune activity results in elaboration of oxidants, and 2) oxidative stress upregulates NF-kappaB (and other pathways) for additive immune activation. *Antioxidant supplementation* alone is clinically and biochemically inferior to a *comprehensive program* that includes both antioxidant supplementation and dietary modification (i.e., the supplemented Paleo-Mediterranean diet, as described previously) that includes heavy reliance upon fruits, vegetables, low-glycemic juices, nuts, seeds, and berries for their additive and synergistic antioxidant benefits.[53]

---

[39] Plotnikoff GA, Quigley JM. Prevalence of severe hypovitaminosis D in patients with persistent, nonspecific musculoskeletal pain. *Mayo Clin Proc.* 2003 Dec;78(12):1463-70

[40] Timms PM, Mannan N, Hitman GA, Noonan K, Mills PG, Syndercombe-Court D, Aganna E, Price CP, Boucher BJ. Circulating MMP9, vitamin D and variation in the TIMP-1 response with VDR genotype: mechanisms for inflammatory damage in chronic disorders? *QJM.* 2002 Dec;95(12):787-96 http://qjmed.oxfordjournals.org/cgi/content/full/95/12/787

[41] "After the treatment period (6 months to 3 years), a significant improvement, as compared with baseline values, was observed. No serious side-effects were observed." Humbert P, Dupond JL, Agache P, Laurent R, Rochefort A, Drobacheff C, de Wazieres B, Aubin F. Treatment of scleroderma with oral 1,25-dihydroxyvitamin D3: evaluation of skin involvement using non-invasive techniques. Results of an open prospective trial. *Acta Derm Venereol.* 1993 Dec;73(6):449-51

[42] Vasquez A, Manso G, Cannell J. The clinical importance of vitamin D (cholecalciferol): a paradigm shift with implications for all healthcare providers. *Altern Ther Health Med.* 2004 Sep-Oct;10(5):28-36 http://InflammationMastery.com/monograph04

[43] Burke BE, Neuenschwander R, Olson RD. Randomized, double-blind, placebo-controlled trial of coenzyme Q10 in isolated systolic hypertension. *South Med J.* 2001 Nov;94(11):1112-7

[44] Singh RB, Niaz MA, Rastogi SS, Shukla PK, Thakur AS. Effect of hydrosoluble coenzyme Q10 on blood pressures and insulin resistance in hypertensive patients with coronary artery disease. *J Hum Hypertens.* 1999 Mar;13(3):203-8

[45] Digiesi V, Cantini F, Oradei A, Bisi G, Guarino GC, Brocchi A, Bellandi F, Mancini M, Littarru GP. Coenzyme Q10 in essential hypertension. *Mol Aspects Med.* 1994;15 Suppl:s257-63

[46] Langsjoen P, Langsjoen P, Willis R, Folkers K. Treatment of essential hypertension with coenzyme Q10. *Mol Aspects Med.* 1994;15 Suppl:S265-72

[47] Singh RB, Khanna HK, Niaz MA. Randomized, double-blind placebo-controlled trial of coenzyme Q10 in chronic renal failure: discovery of a new role. *J Nutr Environ Med* 2000;10:281-8

[48] Singh RB, Kumar A, Naiz MA, Singh RG, Gujrati S, Singh VP, Singh M, Singh UP, Taneja C, AND Rastogi SS. Randomized, Double-blind, Placebo-controlled Trial of Coenzyme Q10 in Patients with End-stage Renal Failure. *J Nutr Environ Med* 2003; Volume 13, Number 1: 13–22

[49] Singh RB, Singh MM. Effects of CoQ10 in new indications with antioxidant vitamin deficiency. *J Nutr Environ Med* 1999; 9:223-228

[50] Ye CQ, Folkers K, Tamagawa H, Pfeiffer C. A modified determination of coenzyme Q10 in human blood and CoQ10 blood levels in diverse patients with allergies. *Biofactors.* 1988 Dec;1(4):303-6

[51] "In contrast, treatment of SSc fibroblasts with the membrane-permeant antioxidant N-acetyl-L-cysteine inhibited ROS production, and this was accompanied by decreased proliferation of these cells and down-regulation of alpha1(I) and alpha2(I) collagen messenger RNA." Sambo P, Baroni SS, Luchetti M, Paroncini P, Dusi S, Orlandini G, Gabrielli A. Oxidative stress in scleroderma: maintenance of scleroderma fibroblast phenotype by the constitutive up-regulation of reactive oxygen species generation through the NADPH oxidase complex pathway. *Arthritis Rheum* 2001 Nov;44(11):2653-64

[52] "CONCLUSION: This study provides evidence of enhanced lipid peroxidation in both SSc and UCTD, and suggests a rationale for antioxidant treatment of SSc." Cracowski JL, Marpeau C, Carpentier PH, Imbert B, Hunt M, Stanke-Labesque F, Bessard G. Enhanced in vivo lipid peroxidation in scleroderma spectrum disorders. *Arthritis Rheum* 2001 May;44(5):1143-8

[53] Liu RH. Health benefits of fruit and vegetables are from additive and synergistic combinations of phytochemicals. *Am J Clin Nutr.* 2003 Sep;78(3 Suppl):517S-520S http://www.ajcn.org/cgi/content/full/78/3/517S

- Broad-spectrum fatty acid therapy with ALA, EPA, DHA, GLA and oleic acid: "Sophisticated manipulation of EFA metabolism" may prove clinically beneficial for **scleroderma** patients according to a review by the late David Horrobin[54]; however, a six-month clinical trial of fatty acid supplementation showed no benefit[55], thus proving the ineffectiveness of one-dimensional intervention and of fatty acid supplementation in a condition known to have a high prevalence of untreated malabsorption. Nonetheless, as part of a *comprehensive program*, fatty acid supplementation should be delivered in the form of combination therapy with ALA, GLA, DHA, and EPA. Fish oil provides EPA and DHA which have well-proven anti-inflammatory benefits in rheumatoid arthritis[56,57,58] and lupus.[59,60] ALA, EPA, DHA, and GLA need to be provided in the form of supplements; when using high doses of therapeutic oils, liquid supplements that can be mixed in juice or a smoothie are generally more convenient and palatable than capsules. Therapeutic amounts of oleic acid can be obtained from generous use of olive oil, preferably on fresh vegetables. Supplementation with polyunsaturated fatty acids warrants increased intake of antioxidants from diet, fruit and vegetable juices, and properly formulated supplements; since patients with systemic inflammation are generally in a pro-oxidative state, consideration must be given to the timing and starting dose of fatty acid supplementation and the need for antioxidant protection. See chapter on Therapeutics for more details and biochemical pathways. *See previous detailing in other chapters, especially Chapter 4.*

- Octreotide (prescription drug): Descamps et al[61] describe the case of a 53-year-old black woman with progressive and severe **systemic scleroderma**, with diffuse skin sclerosis, myositis with intestinal pseudo-obstruction and bacterial overgrowth who **experienced a "spectacular" normalization of clinical status and skin induration following several months of octreotide** (75 mug/d). This drug is a somatostatin analog used in the treatment of acromegaly[62] and it also promotes intestinal motility and thus reduces dysbiotic intestinal bacterial overgrowth in patients with scleroderma.[63] Efficacy of octreotide in improving clinical manifestations of scleroderma is probably mediated *at least in part* by reducing the pro-inflammatory effects of dysbiotic intestinal bacterial overgrowth, which can be addressed by other means as well.

- Assessment for dermal and gastrointestinal dysbiosis: A growing body of literature implicates infectious agents in the etiology of **scleroderma**.[64] Regarding dermal dysbiosis, several articles by Cantwell et al[65,66] suggest epidermal and/or intradermal dysbiosis with pleomorphic bacteria,

---

[54] "Controlled clinical trials of supplementation with gamma-linolenic acid (GLA) as evening primrose oil (Efamol) in both primary Sjogren's syndrome and systemic sclerosis have given positive results." Horrobin DF. Essential fatty acid and prostaglandin metabolism in Sjogren's syndrome, systemic sclerosis and rheumatoid arthritis. *Scand J Rheumatol* Suppl 1986;61:242-5

[55] "Dietary essential fatty acids have no role in the treatment of vascular symptoms in established systemic sclerosis." Stainforth JM, Layton AM, Goodfield MJ. Clinical aspects of the use of gamma linolenic acid in systemic sclerosis. *Acta Derm Venereol* 1996 Mar;76(2):144-6

[56] Adam O, Beringer C, Kless T, Lemmen C, Adam A, Wiseman M, Adam P, Klimmek R, Forth W. Anti-inflammatory effects of a low arachidonic acid diet and fish oil in patients with rheumatoid arthritis. *Rheumatol Int*. 2003 Jan;23(1):27-36

[57] Lau CS, Morley KD, Belch JJ. Effects of fish oil supplementation on non-steroidal anti-inflammatory drug requirement in patients with mild rheumatoid arthritis--a double-blind placebo controlled study. *Br J Rheumatol*. 1993 Nov;32(11):982-9

[58] Kremer JM, Jubiz W, Michalek A, Rynes RI, Bartholomew LE, Bigaouette J, Timchalk M, Beeler D, Lininger L. Fish-oil fatty acid supplementation in active rheumatoid arthritis. A double-blinded, controlled, crossover study. *Ann Intern Med*. 1987 Apr;106(4):497-503

[59] Walton AJ, Snaith ML, Locniskar M, Cumberland AG, Morrow WJ, Isenberg DA. Dietary fish oil and the severity of symptoms in patients with systemic lupus erythematosus. *Ann Rheum Dis*. 1991 Jul;50(7):463-6

[60] Duffy EM, Meenagh GK, McMillan SA, Strain JJ, Hannigan BM, Bell AL. The clinical effect of dietary supplementation with omega-3 fish oils and/or copper in systemic lupus erythematosus. *J Rheumatol*. 2004 Aug;31(8):1551-6

[61] "After 8 months of treatment, normal weight was obtained and skin induration was spectacularly reduced and pigmentation returned to a normal state." Descamps V, Duval X, Crickx B, Bouscarat F, Coffin B, Belaich S. Global improvement of systemic scleroderma under long-term administration of octreotide. *Eur J Dermatol* 1999 Sep;9(6):446-8

[62] http://www.us.sandostatin.com/info/about/home.jsp Accessed December 16, 2005

[63] "Octreotide stimulates intestinal motility in normal subjects and in patients with scleroderma. In such patients, the short-term administration of octreotide reduces bacterial overgrowth and improves abdominal symptoms." Soudah HC, Hasler WL, Owyang C. Effect of octreotide on intestinal motility and bacterial overgrowth in scleroderma. *N Engl J Med*. 1991 Nov 21;325(21):1461-7

[64] "...increasing evidence has accumulated to implicate infectious agents in the etiology of systemic sclerosis (SSc)... ...increased antibody titers, a preponderance of specific strains in patients with SSc, and evidence of molecular mimicry inducing autoimmune responses suggest mechanisms by which infectious agents may contribute to the development and progression of SSc." Hamamdzic D, Kasman LM, LeRoy EC. The role of infectious agents in the pathogenesis of systemic sclerosis. *Curr Opin Rheumatol*. 2002 Nov;14(6):694-8

[65] Disabling pansclerotic morphea (DPM): "The organism could be identified as Staphylococcus epidermidis, but it also had stages of growth with morphologic forms more characteristic of a Corynebacterium-like or actinomycetelike microbe." Cantwell AR Jr, Jones JE, Kelso DW. Pleomorphic, variably acid-fast bacteria in an adult patient with disabling pansclerotic morphea. *Arch Dermatol*. 1984 May;120(5):656-61

[66] "Variably acid-fast coccoid forms, suggestive of cell wall deficient forms of mycobacteria, were observed in the dermis in microscopic sections of skin from six patients with generalized scleroderma, 10 patients with localized scleroderma (morphea), and four patients with lichen sclerosus et atrophicus (LSA)." Cantwell AR Jr. Histologic observations of pleomorphic, variably acid-fast bacteria in scleroderma, morphea, and lichen sclerosus et atrophicus. *Int J Dermatol*. 1984 Jan-Feb;23(1):45-52

specifically acid-fast cell-wall-deficient mycobacteria. Regarding gastrointestinal dysbiosis, at the very least, we must acknowledge that 1) **bacterial overgrowth of the small bowel is common (33%) in patients with scleroderma**[67] due to impaired gastrointestinal motility, 2) **scleroderma patients show increased levels of deconjugating bacteria**[68], which inactivate bile acids and promote enterohepatic recirculation of endogenous and exogenous toxins, 3) **these patients have a high incidence of *Helicobacter pylori* infection (66% of patients with scleroderma, 78% of patients with scleroderma and Sicca syndrome**[69]), and 4) approximately **44% of scleroderma patients have esophageal overgrowth of *Candida albicans*.**[70] For these and other reasons (detailed in Chapter 4), **patients with scleroderma are presumed to have gastrointestinal dysbiosis until proven otherwise by the combination of 1) three-sample comprehensive parasitology examinations performed by a specialty laboratory and 2) clinical response to at least two 2-4 week courses of broad-spectrum antimicrobial treatment.** Yeast, bacteria, and parasites are treated as indicated based on identification and sensitivity results from comprehensive parasitology assessments. Breath hydrogen/methane testing is inferior to stool testing because it does not allow for identification and sensitivity testing of microbes. Other dysbiotic loci should be investigated as discussed in Chapter 4 in the section on multifocal dysbiosis. Attentive readers may have already surmised that treatment of gastrointestinal dysbiosis in patients with long-standing scleroderma is likely to be particularly difficult due to the neuropathic and myopathic **intestinal dysmotility**[71] **that will serve to perpetuate bacterial overgrowth and dysbiosis, thus necessitating vigilant and long-term treatment**; understanding and due persistence on the part of physician and patient are necessary to see this treatment through to completion—a combination of pharmaceutical/botanical antimicrobials and promotility agents, including the universally safe and effective osmotic laxative magnesium, is reasonable.

- o Gastrointestinal dysbiosis: Treatment for gastrointestinal dysbiosis should be guided by specific findings and sensitivity results from stool testing; the following are commonly employed treatments for dysbiosis:
  - **Ciprofloxacin: Over and Bucknall**[72] **published a case report of a progressive scleroderma patient who experienced marked clinical improvement and biopsy-proven regression of skin changes following administration of ciprofloxacin 500 mg bid which was eventually reduced to 250 mg/d. This case report strongly supports the theory that intestinal dysbiosis is a major contributor to scleroderma.** As with all antibacterial treatments, use empiric antifungal treatment with Nystatin 500,000 units bid and/or emulsified oregano 150 mg tid-qid.[73,74]
  - Oregano oil: Emulsified oil of oregano in a time-released tablet is proven effective in the eradication of harmful gastrointestinal microbes, including *Blastocystis hominis, Entamoeba*

[67] "Eight patients (33%) had significant bacterial counts: > 10(5) colony forming units per ml (cfu/ml) of jejunal fluid." Kaye SA, Lim SG, Taylor M, Patel S, Gillespie S, Black CM. Small bowel bacterial overgrowth in systemic sclerosis: detection using direct and indirect methods and treatment outcome. *Br J Rheumatol.* 1995 Mar;34(3):265-9

[68] "CONCLUSIONS: Our results demonstrated that some of the bacterial species that overgrow in the upper small intestine of patients with progressive systemic sclerosis can deconjugate bile acids, and that a shift to neutral pH in gastric juice, may promote the bacterial overgrowth related to their impaired peristaltic activity." Shindo K, Machida M, Koide K, Fukumura M, Yamazaki R. Deconjugation ability of bacteria isolated from the jejunal fluid of patients with progressive systemic sclerosis and its gastric pH. *Hepatogastroenterology.* 1998 Sep-Oct;45(23):1643-50

[69] "Urease test demonstrated the presence of HP in 23 patients out of 35 (66%); 12 of them were negative to colonization. A Sicca syndrome, with abnormal Schirmers test and dry mouth was detected in 66% of the patients. 78% of the patients with Sicca syndrome had a concomitant HP infection..." Farina G, Rosato E, Francia C, Proietti M, Donato G, Ammendolea C, Pisarri S, Salsano F. High incidence of Helicobacter pylori infection in patients with systemic sclerosis: association with Sicca Syndrome. *Int J Immunopathol Pharmacol.* 2001 May;14(2):81-85

[70] "Esophageal mucosal brushings from 51 consecutive patients with progressive systemic sclerosis (PSS) (group I), 18 PSS patients continuously treated with high-dose ranitidine or omeprazole (group II), 34 controls referred to the outpatient clinic for endoscopy (group III), and 10 patients receiving long-term potent antireflux therapy for idiopathic gastroesophageal reflux (group IV) were cultured for Candida albicans. There were 44%, 89%, 9%, and 0% Candida albicans culture-positive patients in groups I through IV, respectively." Hendel L, Svejgaard E, Walsoe I, Kieffer M, Stenderup A. Esophageal candidosis in progressive systemic sclerosis: occurrence, significance, and treatment with fluconazole. *Scand J Gastroenterol.* 1988 Dec;23(10):1182-6

[71] "We found ultrastructural signs of axonal degeneration and cytoskeletal abnormalities in the bundles of unmyelinated fibers. There was also focal degeneration of smooth muscle cells, often in association with the presence of partially degranulated mast cells." Malandrini A, Selvi E, Villanova M, Berti G, Sabadini L, Salvadori C, Gambelli S, De Stefano R, Vernillo R, Marcolongo R, Guazzi G. Autonomic nervous system and smooth muscle cell involvement in systemic sclerosis: ultrastructural study of 3 cases. *J Rheumatol.* 2000 May;27(5):1203-6

[72] Over KE, Bucknall RC. Regression of skin changes in a patient with systemic sclerosis following treatment for bacterial overgrowth with ciprofloxacin. *Br J Rheumatol.* 1998 Jun;37(6):696 http://rheumatology.oxfordjournals.org/cgi/reprint/37/6/696a

[73] Stiles JC, Sparks W, Ronzio RA. The inhibition of Candida albicans by oregano. *J Applied Nutr* 1995;47:96–102

[74] Force M, Sparks WS, Ronzio RA. Inhibition of enteric parasites by emulsified oil of oregano in vivo. *Phytother Res.* 2000 May;14(3):213-4

hartmanni, and *Endolimax nana.*[75] An *in vitro* study[76] and clinical experience support the use of emulsified oregano against *Candida albicans* and various bacteria. The common dose is 600 mg per day in divided doses for at least 6 weeks.[77]

- <u>Berberine</u>: Berberine is an alkaloid extracted from plants such as *Berberis vulgaris,* and *Hydrastis canadensis*, and it shows effectiveness against *Giardia, Candida,* and *Streptococcus* in addition to its direct anti-inflammatory and antidiarrheal actions. Oral dose of 400-1,5000 mg per day is common for adults.[78]

- *Artemisia annua*: Artemisinin has been safely used for centuries in Asia for the treatment of malaria, and it also has effectiveness against anaerobic bacteria due to the pro-oxidative sesquiterpene endoperoxide.[79,80] I commonly use artemisinin at 200 mg per day in divided doses for adults with dysbiosis. **Evidence of past/current H. pylori infection is common (~40-60%) in patients with scleroderma[81], and some doctors have reported anecdotally that *Artemisia annua* helps eradicate H. pylori**.

- <u>St. John's Wort (*Hypericum perforatum*)</u>: Hyperforin from *Hypericum perforatum* also shows impressive antibacterial action, particularly against gram-positive bacteria such as *Staphylococcus aureus, Streptococcus pyogenes, Streptococcus agalactiae*[82] and perhaps *Helicobacter pylori*.[83] Up to 600 mg three times per day of a 3% hyperforin standardized extract is customary in the treatment of depression.

- <u>Bismuth</u>: Bismuth is commonly used in the empiric treatment of diarrhea (e.g., "Pepto-Bismol") and is commonly combined with other antimicrobial agents to reduce drug resistance and increase antibiotic effectiveness.[84]

- <u>Undecylenic acid</u>: Derived from castor bean oil, undecylenic acid has antifungal properties and is commonly indicated by sensitivity results obtained by stool culture. Common dosages are 150-250 mg tid (up to 750 mg per day).[85]

- <u>Peppermint *(Mentha piperita)*</u>: Peppermint shows antimicrobial and antispasmodic actions and has demonstrated clinical effectiveness in patients with bacterial overgrowth of the small bowel.

- <u>Commonly used antibiotic/antifungal drugs</u>: The most commonly employed drugs for intestinal bacterial overgrowth are described here.[86] Treatment duration is generally at least 2 weeks and up to 8 weeks, depending on clinical response and the severity and diversity of the intestinal overgrowth. With all anti*bacterial* treatments, use empiric anti*fungal* treatment to prevent yeast overgrowth; some patients benefit from antifungal treatment that is continued for *months* and occasionally *years*. Drugs can generally be coadministered with natural antibiotics/antifungals for improved efficacy. Treatment can be guided by identification of the dysbiotic microbes and the results of culture and sensitivity tests.

[75] Force M, Sparks WS, Ronzio RA. Inhibition of enteric parasites by emulsified oil of oregano in vivo. *Phytother Res*. 2000 May;14(3):213-4

[76] Stiles JC, Sparks W, Ronzio RA. The inhibition of Candida albicans by oregano. *J Applied Nutr* 1995;47:96–102

[77] Force M, Sparks WS, Ronzio RA. Inhibition of enteric parasites by emulsified oil of oregano in vivo. *Phytother Res*. 2000 May;14(3):213-4

[78] Berberine. Altern Med Rev. 2000 Apr;5(2):175-7 http://www.thorne.com/altmedrev/.fulltext/5/2/175.pdf

[79] Dien TK, de Vries PJ, Khanh NX, Koopmans R, Binh LN, Duc DD, Kager PA, van Boxtel CJ. Effect of food intake on pharmacokinetics of oral artemisinin in healthy Vietnamese subjects. *Antimicrob Agents Chemother*. 1997 May;41(5):1069-72

[80] Giao PT, Binh TQ, Kager PA, Long HP, Van Thang N, Van Nam N, de Vries PJ. Artemisinin for treatment of uncomplicated falciparum malaria: is there a place for monotherapy? *Am J Trop Med Hyg*. 2001 Dec;65(6):690-5

[81] "Patients with SSc have H. pylori infection at a higher prevalence than the general population." Yazawa N, Fujimoto M, Kikuchi K, Kubo M, Ihn H, Sato S, Tamaki T, Tamaki K. High seroprevalence of Helicobacter pylori infection in patients with systemic sclerosis: association with esophageal involvement. *J Rheumatol*. 1998 Apr;25(4):650-3

[82] Schempp CM, Pelz K, Wittmer A, Schopf E, Simon JC. Antibacterial activity of hyperforin from St John's wort, against multiresistant Staphylococcus aureus and gram-positive bacteria. *Lancet*. 1999 Jun 19;353(9170):2129

[83] "A butanol fraction of St. John's Wort revealed anti-Helicobacter pylori activity with MIC values ranging between 15.6 and 31.2 microg/ml." Reichling J, Weseler A, Saller R. A current review of the antimicrobial activity of Hypericum perforatum L. *Pharmacopsychiatry*. 2001 Jul;34 Suppl 1:S116-8

[84] Veldhuyzen van Zanten SJ, Sherman PM, Hunt RH. Helicobacter pylori: new developments and treatments. *CMAJ*. 1997;156(11):1565-74 http://www.cmaj.ca/cgi/reprint/156/11/1565.pdf

[85] "Adult dosage is usually 450-750 mg undecylenic acid daily in three divided doses." Undecylenic acid. Monograph. *Altern Med Rev*. 2002 Feb;7(1):68-70 http://www.thorne.com/altmedrev/.fulltext/7/1/68.pdf

[86] Saltzman JR, Russell RM. Nutritional consequences of intestinal bacterial overgrowth. *Compr Ther*. 1994;20(9):523-30

⇒ Nonabsorbed antibiotics such as rifaxamin and vancomycin are particularly worthy of consideration.

⇒ Metronidazole: 250-500 mg BID-QID (generally limit to 1.5 g/d); metronidazole has systemic bioavailability and effectiveness against a wide range of dysbiotic microbes, including protozoans, amebas/Giardia, *H. pylori*, *Clostridium difficile* and most anaerobic gram-negative bacilli.[87] Adverse effects are generally limited to stomatitis, nausea, diarrhea, and—rarely and/or with long-term use—peripheral neuropathy, dizziness, and metallic taste; the drug must not be consumed with alcohol. Metronidazole resistance by *Blastocystis hominis* and other parasites has been noted.

⇒ **Erythromycin: 250-500 mg TID-QID; this drug is a widely used antibiotic that also has intestinal promotility benefits (thus making it an ideal treatment for intestinal bacterial overgrowth associated with or caused by intestinal dysmotility/hypomotility such as seen in scleroderma[88,89]).** Do not combine erythromycin with the promotility drug **cisapride** due to risk for serious cardiac arrhythmia.

⇒ Nystatin: Nystatin 500,000 units bid with food; duration of treatment begins with a minimum duration of 2-4 weeks and may continue as long as the patient is deriving benefit.

⇒ Ketoconazole: As a systemically bioavailable antifungal drug, ketoconazole has inherent anti-inflammatory benefits which may be helpful; however the drug inhibits androgen formation and may lead to exacerbation of the hypoandrogenism that is commonly seen in autoimmune patients and which contributes to the immune dysfunction.

▪ Probiotics: Live cultures in the form of tablets, capsules, yogurt, or kefir can be used per patient preference and tolerance. Obviously, dairy-based products should be avoided by patients with dairy allergy.

▪ Supplemented Paleo-Mediterranean diet / specific carbohydrate diet: The specifications of the specific carbohydrate diet detailed by Gottschall[90] are met with adherence to the Paleo diet by Cordain.[91] The combination of both approaches will give patients an excellent combination of informational understanding and culinary versatility. In accord with both of these dietary programs, the diet must remain free of gluten-containing grains such as wheat, since **some patients with scleroderma have celiac disease[92,93]**, and since **wheat, like most grains (except rice), promotes bacterial overgrowth of the intestine due to its high quantity of indigestible oligosaccharides.**[94]

• Orthoendocrinology: Assess **prolactin**, cortisol, **DHEA**, free and total testosterone, serum estradiol, and thyroid status (e.g., TSH, T4, free T3, *and* anti-thyroid peroxidase antibodies).

○ Melatonin: **In a recent *in vitro* study with fibroblasts from normal and scleroderma patients, melatonin was shown to inhibit fibroblast proliferation[95]**; future trials may demonstrate that

[87] Tierney ML. McPhee SJ, Papadakis MA. Current Medical Diagnosis and Treatment 2006. 45th edition. New York; Lange Medical Books: 2006, pages 1578-1577

[88] "Prokinetic agents effective in pseudoobstruction include metoclopramide, domperidone, cisapride, octreotide, and erythromycin. ... The combination of octreotide and erythromycin may be particularly effective in systemic sclerosis." Sjogren RW. Gastrointestinal features of scleroderma. *Curr Opin Rheumatol.* 1996 Nov;8(6):569-75

[89] "CONCLUSIONS: Erythromycin accelerates gastric and gallbladder emptying in scleroderma patients and might be helpful in the treatment of gastrointestinal motor abnormalities in these patients." Fiorucci S, Distrutti E, Bassotti G, Gerli R, Chiucchiu S, Betti L, Santucci L, Morelli A. Effect of erythromycin administration on upper gastrointestinal motility in scleroderma patients. *Scand J Gastroenterol.* 1994 Sep;29(9):807-13

[90] Gotschall E. Breaking the Vicious Cycle: Intestinal health though diet. Kirkton Press; Rev edition (August, 1994) http://www.scdiet.com/

[91] Cordain L: The Paleo Diet: Lose weight and get healthy by eating the food you were designed to eat. John Wiley & Sons Inc., New York 2002 http://thepaleodiet.com/

[92] "Coeliac disease may account for malabsorption in scleroderma patients even when test suggest bacterial overgrowth." Marguerie C, Kaye S, Vyse T, Mackworth-Young C, Walport MJ, Black C. Malabsorption caused by coeliac disease in patients who have scleroderma. *Br J Rheumatol.* 1995 Sep;34(9):858-61

[93] Gomez-Puerta JA, Gil V, Cervera R, Miquel R, Jimenez S, Ramos-Casals M, Font J. Coeliac disease associated with systemic sclerosis. *Ann Rheum Dis.* 2004 Jan;63(1):104-5 http://ard.bmjjournals.com/cgi/content/full/63/1/104

[94] "Short-chain fructooligosaccharides occur in a number of edible plants, such as chicory, onions, asparagus, wheat... Short-chain fructooligosaccharides, to a large extent, escape digestion in the human upper intestine and reach the colon where they are totally fermented mostly to lactate, short chain fatty acids (acetate, propionate and butyrate), and gas, like dietary fibres." Bornet FR, Brouns F, Tashiro Y, Duvillier V. Nutritional aspects of short-chain fructooligosaccharides: natural occurrence, chemistry, physiology and health implications. *Dig Liver Dis.* 2002 Sep;34 Suppl 2:S111-20

[95] "These results suggest that MLT, at higher dosages, is a potent inhibitor of the proliferation of fibroblasts derived from the skin of healthy and SSc patients." Carossino AM, et al. Effect of melatonin on normal and sclerodermic skin fibroblast proliferation. *Clin Exp Rheumatol.* 1996 Sep-Oct;14(5):493-8.

melatonin has an antifibrotic/antisclerodermatous benefit. Melatonin is a pineal hormone with well-known sleep-inducing and immunomodulatory properties, and it is commonly administered in doses of 1-40 mg in the evening, before bedtime. Its exceptional safety is well documented. In contrast to implementing treatment with high doses of 20-40 mg, starting with a relatively low dose (e.g., 1-5 mg) and increasing as tolerated is recommended.

> **Androgen and prolactin levels in systemic sclerosis**
>
> "The altered hormonal status could result in relative immunological hyperactivity contributing to enhance tissue damage and disease severity."
>
> Mirone, Barini, Barini. Androgen and prolactin levels in systemic sclerosis: relationship to disease severity. *Ann N Y Acad Sci* 2006

Melatonin (20 mg hs) appears to have cured two patients with drug-resistant sarcoidosis[96] and 3 mg provided immediate short-term benefit to a patient with multiple sclerosis.[97] Immunostimulatory anti-infective action of melatonin was demonstrated in a clinical trial wherein septic newborns administered 20 mg melatonin showed significantly increased survival over nontreated controls[98]; **given that scleroderma is associated with subclinical "infections", melatonin may provide therapeutic benefit by virtue of its anti-infective properties.**

- o Prolactin (excess): Serum prolactin is the standard assessment of prolactin status. Since elevated prolactin may be a sign of pituitary tumor, assessment for headaches, visual deficits, other abnormalities of pituitary hormones (e.g., GH and TSH) should be performed and CT or MRI must be considered. Patients with prolactin levels less than 100 ng/mL and normal CT/MRI findings can be managed conservatively with effective prolactin-lowering treatment and annual radiologic assessment (less necessary with favorable serum response).[99,100] Patients with RA and SLE have higher basal and stress-induced levels of prolactin compared with normal controls.[101,102] **Prolactin levels are high and DHEA levels are low in patients with scleroderma.**[103,104] Specific treatment options include the following:

  - ▪ Thyroid hormone: Hypothyroidism frequently causes hyperprolactinemia which is reversible upon effective treatment of hypothyroidism. Therefore, thyroid status should be evaluated in all patients with hyperprolactinemia.

  - ▪ Cabergoline/Dostinex: Cabergoline/Dostinex is a newer dopamine agonist with few adverse effects; typical dose starts at 0.5 mg per week (0.25 mg twice per week).[105] Several studies have indicated that cabergoline is safer and more effective than bromocriptine for reducing prolactin levels[106] and the dose can often be reduced after successful prolactin reduction, allowing for reductions in cost and adverse effects.[107] Although fewer studies

[96] Cagnoni ML, Lombardi A, Cerinic MC, Dedola GL, Pignone A. Melatonin for treatment of chronic refractory sarcoidosis. *Lancet.* 1995 Nov 4;346(8984):1229-30

[97] "...administration of melatonin (3 mg, orally) at 2:00 p.m., when the patient experienced severe blurring of vision, resulted within 15 minutes in a dramatic improvement in visual acuity and in normalization of the visual evoked potential latency after stimulation of the left eye." Sandyk R. Diurnal variations in vision and relations to circadian melatonin secretion in multiple sclerosis. *Int J Neurosci.* 1995 Nov;83(1-2):1-6

[98] Gitto E, Karbownik M, Reiter RJ, Tan DX, Cuzzocrea S, Chiurazzi P, Cordaro S, Corona G, Trimarchi G, Barberi I. Effects of melatonin treatment in septic newborns. *Pediatr Res.* 2001 Dec;50(6):756-60 http://www.pedresearch.org/cgi/content/full/50/6/756

[99] Beers MH, Berkow R (eds). The Merck Manual. Seventeenth Edition. Whitehouse Station; Merck Research Laboratories 1999 Page 77-78

[100] Serri O, Chik CL, Ur E, Ezzat S. Diagnosis and management of hyperprolactinemia. *CMAJ.* 2003 Sep 16;169(6):575-81 http://www.cmaj.ca/cgi/content/full/169/6/575

[101] Dostal C, Moszkorzova L, Musilova L, Lacinova Z, Marek J, Zvarova J. Serum prolactin stress values in patients with systemic lupus erythematosus. *Ann Rheum Dis.* 2003 May;62(5):487-8 http://ard.bmjjournals.com/cgi/content/full/62/5/487

[102] "RESULTS: A significantly higher rate of elevated PRL levels was found in SLE patients (40.0%) compared with the healthy controls (14.8%). No proof was found of association with the presence of anti-ds-DNA or with specific organ involvement. Similarly, elevated PRL levels were found in RA patients (39.3%)." Moszkorzova L, Lacinova Z, Marek J, et al. Hyperprolactinaemia in patients with systemic lupus erythematosus. *Clin Exp Rheumatol.* 2002 Nov-Dec;20(6):807-12

[103] "Compared to SSc with <9 disease manifestations, patients with > or =9 disease manifestations had higher PRL, higher soluble interleukin 2 receptor and vascular cell adhesion molecule, and lower DHEAS (P = 0.029)." Straub RH, Zeuner M, Lock G, Scholmerich J, Lang B. High prolactin and low dehydroepiandrosterone sulphate serum levels in patients with severe systemic sclerosis. *Br J Rheumatol.* 1997 Apr;36(4):426-32 http://rheumatology.oxfordjournals.org/cgi/reprint/36/4/426

[104] "The dysregulation of adrenal (DHEAS) and hypothalamic-pituitary function (Prl) is a characteristic feature of immune diseases." Mirone L, Barini A, Barini A. Androgen and prolactin (Prl) levels in systemic sclerosis (SSc): relationship to disease severity. *Ann N Y Acad Sci.* 2006 Jun;1069:257-62

[105] Serri O, Chik CL, Ur E, Ezzat S. Diagnosis and management of hyperprolactinemia. *CMAJ.* 2003 Sep 16;169(6):575-81 http://www.cmaj.ca/cgi/content/full/169/6/575

[106] "CONCLUSION: These data indicate that cabergoline is a very effective agent for lowering the prolactin levels in hyperprolactinemic patients and that it appears to offer considerable advantage over bromocriptine in terms of efficacy and tolerability." Sabuncu T, Arikan E, Tasan E, Hatemi H. Comparison of the effects of cabergoline and bromocriptine on prolactin levels in hyperprolactinemic patients. *Intern Med.* 2001 Sep;40(9):857-61

[107] "Cabergoline also normalized PRL in the majority of patients with known bromocriptine intolerance or -resistance. Once PRL secretion was adequately controlled, the dose of cabergoline could often be significantly decreased, which further reduced costs of therapy." Verhelst J, Abs R, Maiter D, van den Bruel A, Vandeweghe M, Velkeniers B, Mockel J, Lamberigts G, Petrossians P, Coremans P, Mahler C, Stevenaert A, Verlooy J, Raftopoulos C, Beckers A. Cabergoline in the treatment of hyperprolactinemia: a study in 455 patients. *J Clin Endocrinol Metab.* 1999 Jul;84(7):2518-22 http://jcem.endojournals.org/cgi/content/full/84/7/2518

have been published supporting the antirheumatic benefits of cabergoline than those supporting bromocriptine; its antirheumatic benefits have indeed been documented.[108]

- *Vitex astus-cagnus* and other supporting botanicals and nutrients: **Vitex lowers serum prolactin in humans[109,110] via a dopaminergic effect.[111]** Vitex is considered safe for clinical use; mild and reversible adverse effects possibly associated with Vitex include nausea, headache, gastrointestinal disturbances, menstrual disorders, acne, pruritus and erythematous rash.

- Bromocriptine: Bromocriptine has long been considered the pharmacologic treatment of choice for elevated prolactin.[112] Typical dose is 2.5 mg per day (effective against lupus[113]); gastrointestinal upset and sedation are common.[114] Clinical intervention with bromocriptine appears warranted in patients with RA, SLE, Reiter's syndrome, psoriatic arthritis, and probably multiple sclerosis and uveitis.[115]

o Estrogen (excess): **Research suggests that estrogen is immunodysregulatory and an important contributor to autoimmune disease**, perhaps explaining the greatly higher incidence of autoimmune diseases in women compared to men. So-called **"estrogen-replacement therapy" used in postmenopausal women increases the risk for lupus and scleroderma.[116]** Men with rheumatoid arthritis show an excess of estradiol and a decrease in DHEA, and the excess estrogen is proportional to the degree of inflammation.[117] Serum estradiol is commonly used to assess estrogen status; estrogens can also be measured in 24-hour urine samples. Interventions to combat high estrogen levels may include any effective combination of the following:

- Weight loss and weight optimization: In overweight patients, weight loss is the means to attaining the goal of weight optimization; the task is not complete until the body mass index is normalized/optimized. Excess adiposity and obesity raise estrogen levels due to high levels of aromatase (the hormone that makes estrogen) in adipose tissue; weight optimization and loss of excess fat helps normalize hormone levels and reduce inflammation.

- Avoidance of ethanol: Estrogen production is stimulated by ethanol intake.

- Consider surgical correction of varicocele in affected men: Men with varicocele have higher estrogen levels due to temperature-induced alterations in enzyme function in the testes; surgical correction of the varicocele lowers estrogen levels.

- "Anti-estrogen diet": Foods and supplements such as green tea, DIM, I3C, licorice, and a high-fiber "anti-estrogenic diet" can also be used; monitoring clinical status and serum estradiol will prove or disprove efficacy.

- Anastrozole/Arimidex: In our office, we commonly measure serum estradiol in men and administer the aromatase inhibitor anastrozole/arimidex 1 mg (2-3 doses per

[108] Erb N, Pace AV, Delamere JP, Kitas GD. Control of unremitting rheumatoid arthritis by the prolactin antagonist cabergoline. *Rheumatology* (Oxford). 2001 Feb;40(2):237-9 http://rheumatology.oxfordjournals.org/cgi/content/full/40/2/237

[109] "Since AC extracts were shown to have beneficial effects on premenstrual mastodynia serum prolactin levels in such patients were also studied in one double-blind, placebo-controlled clinical study. Serum prolactin levels were indeed reduced in the patients treated with the extract." Wuttke W, Jarry H, Christoffel V, Spengler B, Seidlova-Wuttke D. Chaste tree (Vitex agnus-castus)--pharmacology and clinical indications. *Phytomedicine*. 2003 May;10(4):348-57

[110] German abstract from Medline: "The prolactin release was reduced after 3 months, shortened luteal phases were normalised and deficits in the luteal progesterone synthesis were eliminated." Milewicz A, Gejdel E, Sworen H, Sienkiewicz K, Jedrzejak J, Teucher T, Schmitz H. [Vitex agnus castus extract in the treatment of luteal phase defects due to latent hyperprolactinemia. Results of a randomized placebo-controlled double-blind study] *Arzneimittelforschung*. 1993 Jul;43(7):752-6

[111] "Our results indicate a dopaminergic effect of Vitex agnus-castus extracts and suggest additional pharmacological actions via opioid receptors." Meier B, Berger D, Hoberg E, Sticher O, Schaffner W. Pharmacological activities of Vitex agnus-castus extracts in vitro. *Phytomedicine*. 2000 Oct;7(5):373-81

[112] Beers MH, Berkow R (eds). The Merck Manual. Seventeenth Edition. Whitehouse Station; Merck Research Laboratories 1999 Page 77-78

[113] "A prospective, double-blind, randomized, placebo-controlled study compared BRC at a fixed daily dosage of 2.5 mg with placebo... Long term treatment with a low dose of BRC appears to be a safe and effective means of decreasing SLE flares in SLE patients." Alvarez-Nemegyei J, Cobarrubias-Cobos A, Escalante-Triay F, Sosa-Munoz J, Miranda JM, Jara LJ. Bromocriptine in systemic lupus erythematosus: a double-blind, randomized, placebo-controlled study. *Lupus*. 1998;7(6):414-9

[114] Serri O, Chik CL, Ur E, Ezzat S. Diagnosis and management of hyperprolactinemia. *CMAJ*. 2003 Sep 16;169(6):575-81 http://www.cmaj.ca/cgi/content/full/169/6/575

[115] "...clinical observations and trials support the use of bromocriptine as a nonstandard primary or adjunctive therapy in the treatment of recalcitrant RA, SLE, Reiter's syndrome, and psoriatic arthritis and associated conditions unresponsive to traditional approaches." McMurray RW. Bromocriptine in rheumatic and autoimmune diseases. *Semin Arthritis Rheum*. 2001 Aug;31(1):21-32

[116] "These studies indicate that estrogen replacement therapy in postmenopausal women increases the risk of developing lupus, scleroderma, and Raynaud disease..." Mayes MD. Epidemiologic studies of environmental agents and systemic autoimmune diseases. *Environ Health Perspect*. 1999 Oct;107 Suppl 5:743-8

[117] "RESULTS: DHEAS and estrone concentrations were lower and estradiol was higher in patients compared with healthy controls. DHEAS differed between RF positive and RF negative patients. Estrone did not correlate with any disease variable, whereas estradiol correlated strongly and positively with all measured indices of inflammation." Tengstrand B, Carlstrom K, Fellander-Tsai L, Hafstrom I. Abnormal levels of serum dehydroepiandrosterone, estrone, and estradiol in men with rheumatoid arthritis: high correlation between serum estradiol and current degree of inflammation. *J Rheumatol*. 2003 Nov;30(11):2338-43

week) to men whose estradiol level is greater than 32 picogram/mL; we consider estradiol 10-24 picogram/mL to be optimal for a man.[118] Clinical studies using anastrozole/arimidex in men have shown that aromatase blockade lowers estradiol and raises testosterone[119]; generally speaking, this is exactly the result that we want in patients with severe systemic autoimmunity. Frequency of dosing is based on serum and clinical response.

- o Cortisol (insufficiency): Cortisol has immunoregulatory and "immunosuppressive" actions at physiological concentrations. Low adrenal function is common in patients with chronic inflammation[120,121,122] Assessment of cortisol production and adrenal function was detailed in Chapter 4 under the section of Orthoendocrinology. Supplementation with 20 mg per day of cortisol/Cortef is physiologic; my preference is to dose 10 mg first thing in the morning, then 5 mg in late morning and 5 mg in midafternoon in an attempt to replicate the diurnal variation and normal morning peak of cortisol levels. In patients with hypoadrenalism, administration of pregnenolone in doses of 10-60 mg in the morning may also be beneficial.

- o Testosterone (insufficiency): Androgen deficiencies predispose to, are exacerbated by, and contribute to autoimmune/inflammatory disorders. A large proportion of men with lupus or RA have low testosterone[123] and suffer the effects of hypogonadism: fatigue, weakness, depression, slow healing, low libido, and difficulties with sexual performance. Testosterone levels may rise following DHEA supplementation (especially in women) and can be elevated in men by the use of anastrozole/arimidex. Otherwise, transdermal testosterone such as Androgel or Testim can be applied as indicated.

- o DHEA (insufficiency / supraphysiologic supplementation): **Prolactin levels are high and DHEA levels are low in patients with scleroderma.**[124] DHEA is an anti-inflammatory and immunoregulatory hormone that is commonly deficient in patients with autoimmunity and inflammatory arthritis.[125] DHEA levels are suppressed by prednisone[126], and DHEA has been shown to reverse the osteoporosis and loss of bone mass induced by corticosteroid treatment.[127] DHEA shows no acute or subacute toxicity even when used in supraphysiologic doses, even when used in sick patients. For example, in a study of 32 patients with HIV, DHEA doses of 750 mg – 2,250 mg per day were well tolerated and produced no dose-limiting adverse effects.[128] This lack of toxicity compares favorably with any and all so-called "antirheumatic" drugs,

[118] Male Hormone Modulation Therapy, Page 4 Of 7: http://www.lef.org/protocols/prtcl-130c.shtml Accessed October 30, 2005

[119] "These data demonstrate that aromatase inhibition increases serum bioavailable and total testosterone levels to the youthful normal range in older men with mild hypogonadism." Leder BZ, Rohrer JL, Rubin SD, Gallo J, Longcope C. Effects of aromatase inhibition in elderly men with low or borderline-low serum testosterone levels. *J Clin Endocrinol Metab.* 2004 Mar;89(3):1174-80 http://jcem.endojournals.org/cgi/reprint/89/3/1174

[120] "Yet evidence that patients with rheumatoid arthritis improved with small, physiologic dosages of cortisol or cortisone acetate was reported over 25 years ago, and that patients with chronic allergic disorders or unexplained chronic fatigue also improved with administration of such small dosages was reported over 15 years ago..." Jefferies WM. Mild adrenocortical deficiency, chronic allergies, autoimmune disorders and the chronic fatigue syndrome: a continuation of the cortisone story. *Med Hypotheses.* 1994 Mar;42(3):183-9 http://www.thebuteykocentre.com/Irish_%20Buteykocenter_files/further_studies/med_hyp2.pdf http://members.westnet.com.au/pkolb/med_hyp2.pdf

[121] "The etiology of rheumatoid arthritis ...explained by a combination of three factors: (i) a relatively mild deficiency of cortisol, ..., (ii) a deficiency of DHEA, ...and (iii) infection by organisms such as mycoplasma,..." Jefferies WM. The etiology of rheumatoid arthritis. *Med Hypotheses.* 1998 Aug;51(2):111-4

[122] Jefferies W McK. Safe Uses of Cortisol. Second Edition. Springfield, CC Thomas, 1996

[123] Karagiannis A, Harsoulis F. Gonadal dysfunction in systemic diseases. *Eur J Endocrinol.* 2005 Apr;152(4):501-13 http://www.eje-online.org/cgi/content/full/152/4/501

[124] "Compared to SSc with <9 disease manifestations, patients with > or =9 disease manifestations had higher PRL, higher soluble interleukin 2 receptor and vascular cell adhesion molecule, and lower DHEAS (P = 0.029)." Straub RH, Zeuner M, Lock G, Scholmerich J, Lang B. High prolactin and low dehydroepiandrosterone sulphate serum levels in patients with severe systemic sclerosis. *Br J Rheumatol.* 1997 Apr;36(4):426-32 http://rheumatology.oxfordjournals.org/cgi/reprint/36/4/426 and http://rheumatology.oxfordjournals.org/cgi/content/abstract/36/4/426

[125] "DHEAS concentrations were significantly decreased in both women and men with inflammatory arthritis (IA) (P < 0.001)." Dessein PH, Joffe BI, Stanwix AE, Moomal Z. Hyposecretion of the adrenal androgen dehydroepiandrosterone sulfate and its relation to clinical variables in inflammatory arthritis. *Arthritis Res.* 2001;3(3):183-8. Epub 2001 Feb 21. http://arthritis-research.com/content/3/3/183

[126] "Basal serum DHEA and DHEAS concentrations were suppressed to a greater degree than was cortisol during both daily and alternate day prednisone treatments. ...Thus, adrenal androgen secretion was more easily suppressed than was cortisol secretion by this low dose of glucocorticoid, but there was no advantage to alternate day therapy." Rittmaster RS, Givner ML. Effect of daily and alternate day low dose prednisone on serum cortisol and adrenal androgens in hirsute women. *J Clin Endocrinol Metab.* 1988 Aug;67(2):400-3

[127] "CONCLUSION: Prasterone treatment prevented BMD loss and significantly increased BMD at both the lumbar spine and total hip in female patients with SLE receiving exogenous glucocorticoids." Mease PJ, Ginzler EM, Gluck OS, Schiff M, Goldman A, Greenwald M, Cohen S, Egan R, Quarles BJ, Schwartz KE. Effects of prasterone on bone mineral density in women with systemic lupus erythematosus receiving chronic glucocorticoid therapy. *J Rheumatol.* 2005 Apr;32(4):616-21

[128] "Thirty-one subjects were evaluated and monitored for safety and tolerance. The oral drug was administered three times daily in doses ranging from 750 mg/day to 2,250 mg/day for 16 weeks. ... The drug was well tolerated and no dose-limiting side effects were noted." Dyner TS, Lang W, Geaga J, Golub A, Stites D, Winger E, Galmarini M, Masterson J, Jacobson MA. An open-label dose-escalation trial of oral dehydroepiandrosterone tolerance and pharmacokinetics in patients with HIV disease. *J Acquir Immune Defic Syndr.* 1993 May;6(5):459-65

nearly all of which show impressive comparable toxicity. When used at doses of 200 mg per day, DHEA safely provides clinical benefit for patients with various autoimmune diseases, including ulcerative colitis, Crohn's disease[129], and SLE.[130] In patients with SLE, DHEA supplementation allows for reduced dosing of prednisone (thus avoiding its adverse effects) while providing symptomatic improvement.[131] Optimal clinical response appears to correlate with serum levels that are supraphysiologic[132], treatment may be implemented with little regard for initial DHEA levels, particularly when 1) the dose of DHEA is kept as low as possible, 2) duration is kept as short as possible, 3) other interventions are used to address the underlying cause of the disease, 4) the patient is deriving benefit and the risk-to-benefit ratio is favorable.

- o <u>Thyroid (insufficiency or autoimmunity)</u>: Overt or imminent hypothyroidism is suggested by TSH greater than 2 mU/L[133] or 3 mU/L[134], low T4 or T3, and/or the presence of anti-thyroid peroxidase antibodies.[135] Hypothyroidism can cause an inflammatory myopathy that can resemble polymyositis, and hypothyroidism is a frequent complication of any and all autoimmune diseases. Any hypothyroidism in patients with scleroderma should be treated (barring any contraindications) because hypothyroidism promotes SIBO via delayed intestinal transit; less important is the contribution of hypothyroidism to systemic edema.

- <u>Xenobiotic immunotoxicity</u>: Given that **antifibrillarin antibodies are specifically seen in patients with scleroderma**[136] and that **mercury exposure induces antifibrillarin autoimmunity in susceptible mice**[137], clinicians may be justified in searching for and treating evidence of mercury exposure in patients with autoimmunity in general and scleroderma in particular. Detailed history, dental examination for mercury-containing amalgams, and post-DMSA urine metal analysis are suggested.

- <u>Oral enzyme therapy with proteolytic/pancreatic enzymes</u>: Polyenzyme supplementation is used to ameliorate the pathophysiology induced by immune complexes.[138] Immune complexes are detected in the majority of patients with scleroderma[139] and correlate with disease severity and visceral involvement.[140] Orally administered polyenzyme preparations have an "immune stimulating" action[141] and promote degradation of microbial biofilms and increased immune and antimicrobial penetration into infectious foci.[142] Given that maldigestion, malabsorption, and pancreatic

---

[129] "CONCLUSIONS: In a pilot study, dehydroepiandrosterone was effective and safe in patients with refractory Crohn's disease or ulcerative colitis." Andus T, Klebl F, Rogler G, Bregenzer N, Scholmerich J, Straub RH. Patients with refractory Crohn's disease or ulcerative colitis respond to dehydroepiandrosterone: a pilot study. *Aliment Pharmacol Ther*. 2003 Feb;17(3):409-14

[130] "CONCLUSION: The overall results confirm that DHEA treatment was well-tolerated, significantly reduced the number of SLE flares, and improved patient's global assessment of disease activity." Chang DM, Lan JL, Lin HY, Luo SF. Dehydroepiandrosterone treatment of women with mild-to-moderate systemic lupus erythematosus: a multicenter randomized, double-blind, placebo-controlled trial. *Arthritis Rheum*. 2002 Nov;46(11):2924-7

[131] "CONCLUSION: Among women with lupus disease activity, reducing the dosage of prednisone to < or = 7.5 mg/day for a sustained period of time while maintaining stabilization or a reduction of disease activity was possible in a significantly greater proportion of patients treated with oral prasterone, 200 mg once daily, compared with patients treated with placebo." Petri MA, Lahita RG, Van Vollenhoven RF, Merrill JT, Schiff M, Ginzler EM, Strand V, Kunz A, Gorelick KJ, Schwartz KE; GL601 Study Group. Effects of prasterone on corticosteroid requirements of women with systemic lupus erythematosus: a double-blind, randomized, placebo-controlled trial. *Arthritis Rheum*. 2002 Jul;46(7):1820-9

[132] "CONCLUSION: The clinical response to DHEA was not clearly dose dependent. Serum levels of DHEA and DHEAS correlated only weakly with lupus outcomes, but suggested an optimum serum DHEAS of 1000 microg/dl." Barry NN, McGuire JL, van Vollenhoven RF. Dehydroepiandrosterone in systemic lupus erythematosus: relationship between dosage, serum levels, and clinical response. *J Rheumatol*. 1998 Dec;25(12):2352-6

[133] Weetman AP. Hypothyroidism: screening and subclinical disease. *BMJ*. 1997 Apr 19;314(7088):1175-8 http://bmj.bmjjournals.com/cgi/content/full/314/7088/1175

[134] "Now AACE encourages doctors to consider treatment for patients who test outside the boundaries of a narrower margin based on a target TSH level of 0.3 to 3.0. AACE believes the new range will result in proper diagnosis for millions of Americans who suffer from a mild thyroid disorder, but have gone untreated until now." American Association of Clinical Endocrinologists (AACE). 2003 Campaign Encourages Awareness of Mild Thyroid Failure, Importance of Routine Testing http://www.aace.com/pub/tam2003/press.php November 26, 2005

[135] Beers MH, Berkow R (eds). The Merck Manual. Seventeenth Edition. Whitehouse Station; Merck Research Laboratories 1999 Page 96

[136] "Since anti-fibrillarin antibodies are specific markers of scleroderma, the present animal model may be valuable for studies of the immunological aberrations which are likely to induce this autoimmune response." Hultman P, Enestrom S, Pollard KM, Tan EM. Anti-fibrillarin autoantibodies in mercury-treated mice. *Clin Exp Immunol*. 1989 Dec;78(3):470-7

[137] Nielsen JB, Hultman P. Mercury-induced autoimmunity in mice. Environ Health Perspect. 2002 Oct;110 Suppl 5:877-81 http://ehp.niehs.nih.gov/docs/2002/suppl-5/877-881nielsen/abstract.html

[138] Galebskaya LV, Ryumina EV, Niemerovsky VS, Matyukov AA. Human complement system state after wobenzyme intake. *VESTNIK MOSKOVSKOGO UNIVERSITETA. KHIMIYA*. 2000. Vol. 41, No. 6. Supplement. Pages 148-149

[139] "Serum immune complexes were measured in 92 patients with progressive systemic sclerosis, and elevated levels were found as follows: Raji cell assay 72% (59% after pronase treatment of Raji cell), agarose gel electrophoresis 52%, and C1q binding 24%." Seibold JR, Medsger TA Jr, Winkelstein A, Kelly RH, Rodnan GP. Immune complexes in progressive systemic sclerosis (scleroderma). *Arthritis Rheum*. 1982 Oct;25(10):1167-73

[140] "Patients with SS showed an incidence of circulating immune complexes comparable to that found in SLE, with 20 patients (58.5%),... ...associated with both elevation of serum IgG and IgA levels and extensive visceral involvement by the disease." Hughes P, Cunningham J, Day M, Fitzgerald JC, French MA, Wright JK, Rowell NR. Immune complexes in systemic sclerosis; detection by C1q binding, K-cell inhibition and Raji cell radioimmunoassays. *J Clin Lab Immunol*. 1983 Mar;10(3):133-8

[141] Zavadova E, Desser L, Mohr T. Stimulation of reactive oxygen species production and cytotoxicity in human neutrophils in vitro and after oral administration of a polyenzyme preparation. *Cancer Biother*. 1995 Summer;10(2):147-52

[142] "The enzymes were shown to inhibit the biofilm formation. When appllied to the formed associations, the enzymes potentiated the effect of antibiotics on the bacteria located in them." Tets VV, Knorring Glu, Artemenko NK, Zaslavskaia NV, Artemenko KL. [Impact of exogenic proteolytic enzymes on bacteria][Article in Russian] *Antibiot Khimioter*. 2004;49(12):9-13

insufficiency are not uncommon in patients with scleroderma[143], enzymes may be given with food for optimal benefit.

- PABA—para-amino benzoic acid: **Ninety percent of patients treated with PABA experience clinical benefit, namely skin softening.[144] PABA therapy prolongs survival in patients with scleroderma.[145]** "Potaba" is a well-tolerated prescription form of PABA.[146] Wright and Gaby[147] recommend "PABA, 2-3 g, 4 times a day." Adverse effects attributable to PABA are dose-dependent and include low blood sugar, rash, fever, and liver damage. Adverse effects may be seen with doses approximating or exceeding eight grams per day; thus serial serum chemistries (e.g., monthly at first, then bimonthly, then quarterly) are warranted, especially when using such high doses.

- *Centella asiatica* (Gotu cola): This botanical has been reported to favorably influence scleroderma.[148] Available forms include teas, tinctures, standardized capsules/tablets, topical ointments, and injectable preparations. The **proprietary product "Madecassol" containing madecassic acid, asiatic acid and asiaticoside has been used in several studies and has demonstrated clinical benefit in scleroderma**[149]; some preparations of this product apparently contain nitrofural, a topically and orally active antibiotic. Contact dermatitis has been reported.

- Raynaud's phenomenon—specific treatments: Treatment of Raynaud's phenomenon should not be trivialized as merely symptomatic; the pain experienced by some patients with Raynaud's phenomenon is truly excruciating. Additionally, a wonderfully insightful comment by Simonini et al[150] in 2000 stated that the tissue ischemia induced by Raynaud's phenomenon is *pathogenic* because it promotes oxidative stress and the vicious cycle of inflammation; the recurrent ischemia and reperfusion of hypoxic Raynaud's phenomenon could be thought of somewhat as a "recurrent, mild heart attack [or stroke] of the hands" causing tissue damage and cell apoptosis/necrosis leading to release of damage-associated molecular patterns (DAMP) and the resultant immune activation, systemic inflammation, mitochondrial dysfunction, proinflammatory immunophenotype switch toward Th1/Th2/Th17 and resultant fibrosis and autoimmunity. Remarkably, Mahoney et al[151] proposed a similar model in 2011 when they wrote, "We propose that a recent change in the conception of the role of type 1 interferon and the identification of adventitial stem cells suggests a unifying hypothesis for scleroderma. This hypothesis begins with vasospasm. Vasospasm is fully reversible unless, as proposed here, the resulting ischemia leads to apoptosis and activation of type 1 interferon. The interferon, we propose, initiates immune amplification, including characteristic scleroderma-specific antibodies." Thus, treatments to maintain vasodilation and quench the free radicals resultant from recurrent hypoxic events are necessary. Antioxidants have been discussed previously and should be common knowledge to readers of this text. Vasodilation in Raynaud's phenomenon can be supported with any/all of the following:

  o Eradication of *Helicobacter pylori*: Eradication of *Helicobacter pylori* is one of the most effective treatments of Raynaud's disease/syndrome/phenomenon and should therefore be pursued in all affected patients.

---

[143] Of 20 patients: "Three patients had very low levels of tryptic activity in their intestinal juice and only nine had results which were unequivocally normal." Cobden I, Axon AT, Rowell NR. Pancreatic exocrine function in systemic sclerosis. *Br J Dermatol* 1981 Aug;105(2):189-93

[144] "Ninety percent of 224 patients treated with KPAB experienced mild, moderate, or marked skin softening." Zarafonetis CJ, Dabich L, Skovronski JJ, DeVol EB, Negri D, Yuan W, Wolfe R. Retrospective studies in scleroderma: skin response to potassium para-aminobenzoate therapy. *Clin Exp Rheumatol*. 1988 Jul-Sep;6(3):261-8

[145] "For the entire group an estimated 81.4% survived 5 years from diagnosis and 69.4% survived 10 years. ...adequate treatment with potassium para-aminobenzoate (Potaba KPAB) was associated with improved survival (p less than 0.01); 88.5% 5 year survival rate and 76.6% 10 year survival rate for adequately treated patients." Zarafonetis CJ, Dabich L, Negri D, Skovronski JJ, DeVol EB, Wolfe R. Retrospective studies in scleroderma: effect of potassium para-aminobenzoate on survival. *J Clin Epidemiol*. 1988;41(2):193-205

[146] http://www.glenwood-llc.com/potaba.html

[147] Gaby A, Wright JV. Nutritional Protocols. © 1998 by Nutrition Seminars.

[148] "Titrated extract of Centella asiatica (TECA) contains three principal ingredients, asiaticoside (AS), asiatic acid (AA), and madecassic acid (MA). These components are known to be clinically effective on systemic scleroderma, abnormal scar formation, and keloids." Hong SS, Kim JH, Li H, Shim CK. Advanced formulation and pharmacological activity of hydrogel of the titrated extract of C. asiatica. *Arch Pharm Res*. 2005 Apr;28(4):502-8

[149] "Madecassol is effective and well tolerated and therefore recommended for oral and local use in combined treatment of SS adn FS." Guseva NG, Starovoitova MN, Mach ES. [Madecassol treatment of systemic and localized scleroderma]. *Ter Arkh*. 1998;70(5):58-61. Russian.

[150] "...daily episodes of hypoxia-reperfusion injury, produces several episodes of free radicals-mediated endothelial derangement. These events results in a positive feedback effect of luminal narrowing and ischemia and therefore to the birth of a vicious cycle of oxygen free radicals (OFR) generation, leading to endothelial damage, intimal thickening and fibrosis." Simonini G, Pignone A, Generini S, Falcini F, Cerinic MM. Emerging potentials for an antioxidant therapy as a new approach to the treatment of systemic sclerosis. *Toxicology*. 2000 Nov 30;155(1-3):1-15

[151] Mahoney WM Jr, Fleming JN, Schwartz SM. A unifying hypothesis for scleroderma: identifying a target cell for scleroderma. *Curr Rheumatol Rep*. 2011 Feb;13:28-36

- o Inositol hexaniacinate: 3,000-4,000 mg/d in divided doses[152,153,154]
- o *Ginkgo biloba*: Ginkgo reduces the number of daily Raynaud's attacks in patients with primary Raynaud's disease[155], and it is also an excellent antioxidant with potent anti-inflammatory benefits.
- o Magnesium: 300-500 mg/d or bowel tolerance; systemic alkalinization to achieve urine alkalinity of 7.5 promotes renal retention of magnesium and systemic cellular uptake.
- o Combination fatty acid therapy: must include GLA (minimum 500 mg) and EPA (minimum 2,000 mg)
- o L-arginine: L-arginine is the biochemical precursor to nitric oxide, which has vasodilating actions. L-arginine supplementation in patients with Raynaud's phenomenon showed benefit in one study[156] and no benefit in another.[157] However, arginine supplementation was tremendously beneficial in 4 case reports of scleroderma patients with Raynaud's-induced digital necrosis.[158] Excess arginine supplementation may lead to an overproduction of nitric oxide, which can be harmful in excess due to its free radical behavior and its contribution to peroxynitrite. Additionally, metabolism of arginine requires methyl groups, and therefore supplementation with methyl donors such as methylfolate/folinate, cobalamin, betaine, et al should be used anytime supplemental arginine is used for long periods of time; homocysteine levels should occasionally be measured.
- o NAC 500-1,500mg *po tid ic*: NAC is pleiotropically beneficial, via antiviral, antioxidant, GSH-supporting, and mTOR inhibiting actions.
  - ▪ Intravenous N-acetylcysteine for treatment of Raynaud's phenomenon secondary to systemic sclerosis (*J Rheumatol* 2001 Oct[159])—paraphrased/quoted as follows: "Twenty-two patients with RP secondary to SSc were enrolled in a multicenter, open clinical trial lasting 11 weeks and conducted in winter. Primary outcome measures were frequency and severity of RP attacks, and number of digital ulcers. Secondary outcome measure was improvement in digital cold challenge test assessed by photoelectric plethysmography. Patients received a continuous 5 day intravenous infusion of NAC starting with a 2 h loading dose of 150 mg/kg subsequently adjusted to 15 mg/kg/h. RESULTS: … Both frequency and severity of RP attacks decreased significantly compared to pretreatment values. Active ulcers were significantly less numerous at all follow-up visits (25% of baseline count on Day 33 from the beginning of infusion). In the cold challenge test, mean recovery time fell by 69%, 67%, 71%, and 71% on Days 12, 19, 33, and 61 from the beginning of treatment. Side effects were minor, easily controlled, and reversible. CONCLUSION: N-acetylcysteine appears to be safe for the treatment of RP secondary to SSc. These preliminary data warrant further controlled studies.
- o Acupuncture, biofeedback, counseling, stress reduction, cold avoidance, smoking cessation: Since stressful events, cold exposure, and cigarette smoking are all vasoconstrictive, these

[152] "It appears to be a safe and well tolerated drug, which, together with other symptomatic measures, merits to be used in the management of vasospastic disease of the extremities even in the presence of partial obliteration of the microcirculation." Holti G. An experimentally controlled evaluation of the effect of inositol nicotinate upon the digital blood flow in patients with Raynaud's phenomenon. *J Int Med Res*. 1979;7(6):473-83

[153] "Although the mechanism of action remains unclear Hexopal is safe and is effective in reducing the vasospasm of primary Raynaud's disease during the winter months." Sunderland GT, Belch JJ, Sturrock RD, Forbes CD, McKay AJ. A double blind randomised placebo controlled trial of hexopal in primary Raynaud's disease. *Clin Rheumatol*. 1988 Mar;7(1):46-9

[154] "It is suggested that long-term treatment with nicotinate acid derivatives may produce improvement in the peripheral circulation by a different mechanism than the transient effect detected by short-term studies." Ring EF, Bacon PA. Quantitative thermographic assessment of inositol nicotinate therapy in Raynaud's phenomena. J Int Med Res. 1977;5(4):217-22

[155] "Ginkgo biloba phytosome may be effective in reducing the number of Raynaud's attacks per week in patients suffering from Raynaud's disease." Muir AH, Robb R, McLaren M, Daly F, Belch JJ. The use of Ginkgo biloba in Raynaud's disease: a double-blind placebo-controlled trial. *Vasc Med*. 2002;7(4):265-7

[156] "After therapy, patients with Raynaud's phenomenon secondary to systemic sclerosis showed: (1) higher digital vasodilation after local warming, (2) cold-induced digital vasodilation, and (3) increase of plasma levels of tissue-type plasminogen activator." Agostoni A, Marasini B, Biondi ML, Bassani C, Cazzaniga A, Bottasso B, Cugno M. L-arginine therapy in Raynaud's phenomenon? *Int J Clin Lab Res*. 1991;21(2):202-3

[157] "L-arginine supplementation, however, had no significant effect on vascular responses to acetylcholine and sodium nitroprusside." Khan F, Belch JJ. Skin blood flow in patients with systemic sclerosis and Raynaud's phenomenon: effects of oral L-arginine supplementation. *J Rheumatol*. 1999 Nov;26(11):2389-94

[158] "We report two cases in which oral L-arginine reversed digital necrosis in Raynaud's phenomenon and two additional cases in which the symptoms of severe Raynaud's phenomenon were improved with oral L-arginine." Rembold CM, Ayers CR. Oral L-arginine can reverse digital necrosis in Raynaud's phenomenon. *Mol Cell Biochem*. 2003 Feb;244(1-2):139-41

[159] Sambo P, Amico D, Giacomelli R, Matucci-Cerinic M, Salsano F, Valentini G, Gabrielli A. Intravenous N-acetylcysteine for treatment of Raynaud's phenomenon secondary to systemic sclerosis: a pilot study. *J Rheumatol*. 2001 Oct;28(10):2257-62

should be avoided/modified to the highest extent possible. Stress reduction and modification of inter- and intra-personal socioemotional exchange would be beneficial for anyone.

- <u>Esophageal dysfunction and GERD—specific treatments:</u>
  - o <u>Low carbohydrate diet, specific carbohydrate diet:</u> The gastroesophageal dysfunction that contributes to the high incidence of Barrett's esophagus is likely the result of a confluence of different factors: neurogenic, myogenic, and dysbiotic. With regard to the latter, clinicians must be diligent in the eradication of small intestine bacterial overgrowth, since microbial products of fermentation lead to relaxation of the so-called lower esophageal sphincter.[160,161] This is why diets low in carbohydrate and fermentable fibers (such as those found in grains)—in other words: **"low fermentation diets"**—are effective in the treatment of esophageal reflux; low-carbohydrate diets deprive gut microbes of substrate for fermentation into metabolites that relax the lower esophageal sphincter and thereby contribute to symptomatic improvement in patients with gastroesophageal reflux.[162] This is part of the reason why the diet for these patients must be as low as possible in the difficult-to-digest and easy-to-ferment carbohydrates that are common in the Standard American Diet (SAD) from corn, potatoes, wheat, oats, and disaccharides such as lactose and sucrose; see *Breaking the Vicious Cycle*[163] by the late Elaine Gottschall for more details and recipes for the specific carbohydrate diet. Similarly, a low-carbohydrate Atkins-type low-carbohydrate diet[164] might also be considered, particularly for short-term use and particularly if modified away from proinflammatory saturated fats and arachidonic acid.
  - o <u>Alginate:</u> Alginate is a processed extract from seaweed that is the active ingredient in the FDA-approved OTC anti-heartburn drug Gaviscon.[165] When mixed with stomach acid, alginate forms a foam "raft" that creates a barrier of protection for the esophagus, and it significantly reduces the number of acidic reflux events. Clinical studies have proven the effectiveness of alginate for treating GERD; however pure supplements of sodium alginate may be preferred over Gaviscon due to the latter's inclusion of aluminum (hydroxide)[166], a metal correlated with adverse effects and increased risk for neurologic disease. Alginate is also said to bind toxic metals and may therefore reduce enterohepatic recirculation of these proinflammatory immunotoxins.
  - o <u>Betaine hydrochloric acid (betaine HCL):</u> Many patients with gastroesophageal reflux are cured with the administration of supplemental HCL. Although the addition of acid rather than the suppression of acid goes against the well-funded acid-blocking drug paradigm, the truth remains that—*physiologically*—gastric emptying is promoted by acidification and—*clinically*—the treatment works for a significant number of patients with GERD. Furthermore, correction of hypochlorhydria by supplementation with betaine HCL helps to reduce bacterial/yeast counts in the stomach and upper small intestine, thereby alleviating GERD by reducing the bacteria/yeast available for fermentation; recall that microbial fermentation is one of the primary driving influences for gastroesophageal reflux.[167]

---

[160] "Colonic fermentation of indigestible carbohydrates increases the rate of TLESRs [transient lower esophageal sphincter relaxations], the number of acid reflux episodes, and the symptoms of GERD." Piche T, des Varannes SB, Sacher-Huvelin S, Holst JJ, Cuber JC, Galmiche JP. Colonic fermentation influences lower esophageal sphincter function in gastroesophageal reflux disease. *Gastroenterology*. 2003 Apr;124(4):894-902

[161] Piche T, Zerbib F, Varannes SB, Cherbut C, Anini Y, Roze C, le Quellec A, Galmiche JP. Modulation by colonic fermentation of LES function in humans. *Am J Physiol Gastrointest Liver Physiol*. 2000 Apr;278(4):G578-84 http://ajpgi.physiology.org/cgi/content/full/278/4/G578

[162] "The 5 individuals described in these case reports experienced resolution of GERD symptoms after self-initiation of a low-carbohydrate diet." Yancy WS Jr, Provenzale D, Westman EC. Improvement of gastroesophageal reflux disease after initiation of a low-carbohydrate diet: five brief case reports. *Altern Ther Health Med*. 2001 Nov-Dec;7(6):120, 116-9

[163] Gotschall E. *Breaking the Vicious Cycle: Intestinal health though diet*. Kirkton Press; Rev edition (August, 1994) http://www.scdiet.com/

[164] Atkins, RC. Dr. Atkins' New Diet Revolution (revised and updated). New York: Avon Books, 1999

[165] "For this population, sodium alginate was assessed as significantly superior by both investigators and patients at week two (p < 0.001 and p = 0.004, respectively) and at week four (p = 0.001 and p < 0.001, respectively)." Chatfield S. A comparison of the efficacy of the alginate preparation, Gaviscon Advance, with placebo in the treatment of gastro-oesophageal reflux disease. *Curr Med Res Opin*. 1999;15(3):152-9

[166] http://www.gaviscon.com/info.htm

[167] "Colonic fermentation of indigestible carbohydrates increases the rate of TLESRs [transient lower esophageal sphincter relaxations], the number of acid reflux episodes, and the symptoms of GERD." Piche T, des Varannes SB, Sacher-Huvelin S, Holst JJ, Cuber JC, Galmiche JP. Colonic fermentation influences lower esophageal sphincter function in gastroesophageal reflux disease. *Gastroenterology*. 2003 Apr;124(4):894-902

- o <u>GLA</u>: Numerous studies have documented the anti-cancer effects of GLA, and these have specifically been documented in esophageal cancer cell lines.[168] Thus, GLA consumption may help protect against the development of esophageal cancer, in addition to its important anti-inflammatory and vasodilating actions.
- o <u>Vitamin B12</u>: Vitamin B-12 levels are low in patients with malabsorption, and vitamin B-12 administration (4,000 mcg/d orally, or 1,000-2,000 mcg intramuscularly/ 2-3 times weekly) promotes intestinal motility.

Twilight of the Idiopathic Era and the Dawn of New Possibilities in Health and Healthcare

Originally published in *Naturopathy Digest* in 2006, this essay was slightly edited in 2010.
http://www.naturopathydigest.com/archives/2006/mar/idiopathic.php

Among the perplexing paradoxes that exist in healthcare is coexistence of our adoration of allopathy for its "scientific method" along with the description of most chronic diseases as "idiopathic." If the allopathic use of the scientific method were so adroit, then why are so many conditions described as having "no known cause"? Is it that the scientific method is inadequate, or that the allopathic lens is incapable of bringing disease causation into focus? Perhaps a third option exists: that some groups—namely the allopaths and the pharmaceutical companies—benefit by convincing us that most diseases have "no known cause" and that therefore the best that doctors and patients can hope for is additive and endless pharmaceuticalization of all health problems. When the cause of our health problems is "unknown", we are disempowered, and we must depend on "experts" to help us. When the causes of our problems are known, we are empowered to take effective action. Certainly, some groups have financial and political interests in keeping us *as professionals* and *as patients* confused and disempowered.

<u>**The End of the Idiopathic Era**</u>: A stark contrast exists between primary research literature and the "facts" that are selectively reported in medical textbooks and which are used to buttress "conventional wisdom" and the resultant status quo. While I have been aware of this contrast for many years, the divergence was impressed upon me with renewed vigor during the preparation of a recent article[169] and the completion of my recent textbook <u>*Integrative Rheumatology*</u>.[170] Arthritis in general and autoimmune and rheumatic diseases in particular are frequently described as "idiopathic" and as having "no known cause" by most mainstream medical books like <u>*The Merck Manual*</u> and <u>*Current Medical Diagnosis and Treatment*</u>; these contentions are inconsistent with the abundant and diverse research showing that—rather than being *idiopathic*—most chronic musculoskeletal disorders are *multifactorial*. When a disease is codified as *idiopathic*, doctors lose their incentive to look for and treat the *causes* [plural] of the disease because the codified conventional wisdom has already stated that "The cause [singular] of the disease has not been identified." Similarly, patients are convinced to give up their hope of ever being *cured*; they chose what appears to be the second best option: lifelong medicalization. In these instances, acceptance of the codified conventional wisdom benefits doctors and patients by freeing them of the obligation to think, to mobilize their consciousness; the price paid for this exoneration from consciousness is perpetuated unconsciousness and drug dependence for doctors and patients. Being told by powerful institutions and ensconced authorities that "There's nothing else you can do, and nothing more to think about" lulls us all into apathy and conformity at the price of our individual and collective lives and consciousness.

<u>**Idiopathic, or Multifactorial?**</u>: Let's look at psoriasis and rheumatoid arthritis as two shining examples of *idiopathicity*. If one looks into a standard medical textbook, one sees that these conditions have no known cause and therefore the lifelong prescription of anti-inflammatory medications is presumptively justified. On the

---

[168] "A statistically highly significant growth-suppressive effect of the prostaglandin precursor gamma-linolenic acid (GLA) on MG63 human osteogenic sarcoma and oesophageal carcinoma cells in culture was found." Booyens J, Dippenaar N, Fabbri D, Engelbrecht P, Katzeff IE. The effect of gamma-linolenic acid on the growth of human osteogenic sarcoma and oesophageal carcinoma cells in culture. *S Afr Med J*. 1984 Feb 18;65(7):240-2

[169] Vasquez A. Nutritional and Botanical Treatments Against "Silent Infections" and Gastrointestinal Dysbiosis. *Nutritional Perspectives* 2006; January

[170] Vasquez A. *Integrative Rheumatology. The Art of Creating Wellness While Effectively Managing Acute and Chronic Musculoskeletal Disorders*. 2006

contrary, if one spends a few days in any medical library, one can find articles that point to the causes of these diseases and which then illuminate the path (and paths) by which doctors and patients can arrive at authentic improvement or permanent cure. Most patients can be cured of psoriasis, and a large percentage of rheumatoid arthritis patients can avoid the complications and medicalization associated with their disease, particularly if *the causes* of their condition are treated early. We now know that most autoimmune diseases are caused by and/or perpetuated by chronic infections, food allergies, a proinflammatory lifestyle, hormonal imbalances, and exposure to chemicals and metals that cause immune dysfunction. When the cause(s) of the disease is treated, the disease has the potential to be cured, provided that it is treated comprehensively and hopefully before the onset of irreversible damage. When the disease is cured, lifelong medicalization becomes unnecessary, the patient is free to fully resume his/her life, and doctors are liberated from their roles as drug representatives and can resume their proper positions as healers and creative free-thinking individuals.

Asserting an empowered stance toward disease prevention and treatment carries implications beyond those for the doctor and the patient. These implications also point to new ways of living and stewarding the world. When we look at a disease like Parkinson's disease and then determine that it is *idiopathic*, then nothing happens to change or shape our view of the world, our place in it, and the interconnected components of health and disease. Everyone agrees that that clinical manifestations of Parkinson's disease result from the death of dopaminergic neurons. From the allopathic perspective, the disease is *idiopathic*, while from an integrative naturopathic perspective, we see Parkinson's disease as a *multifaceted disorder* associated with defective mitochondrial function, impaired xenobiotic detoxification, and occupational and/or recreational exposure to toxicants, particularly pesticides. These associations align to create a new model for the illness based on exposure to neurotoxicants such as pesticides[171] which are ineffectively detoxified[172] and then accumulate in the brain[173] and induce mitochondrial dysfunction[174] and resultant oxidative stress[175] which leads to death of dopaminergic neurons. Therefore, from the perspective of both prevention and treatment, the clinical approach to Parkinson's disease would include pesticide avoidance and optimization of detoxification to prevent the neuronal accumulation of neurotoxic mitochondrial poisons. The plan must also include optimization of nutritional status, antioxidant capacity, and mitochondrial function.[176] Further, if our goal is to reduce the societal prevalence of Parkinson's disease, then we must begin living in better harmony with nature and thinking of ways to reduce our use of pesticides and herbicides, the chemicals that are consistently shown to cause premature neuronal death and which are increasingly pervasive in our home, work, and outdoor environments.

The Dawn of New Possibilities in Health and Healthcare: The time is now past when credible physicians can assert that most diseases are "of unknown origin." The truth is that we already have access to the information we need to help our patients. The truth is that we can often offer our patients the *probability of cure* rather than *lifelong and endless prescriptions for symptom-modifying drugs*. These truths imply that healthcare and our systems of healthcare delivery must change, because the pharmaceutical and medical icons that stand before us were built upon feet and legs of clay and interspersed lead. We stand at the dawn of a new era in healthcare—one in which patients with chronic diseases in general and autoimmune diseases in particular— have a tangible and authentic opportunity to regain their health.

[171] Ritz B, Yu F. Parkinson's disease mortality and pesticide exposure in California 1984-1994. *Int J Epidemiol.* 2000 Apr;29(2):323-9
[172] Menegon A, Board PG, Blackburn AC, et al. Parkinson's disease, pesticides, and glutathione transferase polymorphisms. *Lancet.* 1998;352(9137):1344-6
[173] Kamel F, Hoppin JA. Related Articles, Association of pesticide exposure with neurologic dysfunction and disease. *Environ Health Perspect.* 2004;112(9):950-8
[174] Parker WD Jr, Swerdlow RH. Mitochondrial dysfunction in idiopathic Parkinson disease. *Am J Hum Genet.* 1998;62(4):758-62
[175] Davey GP, Peuchen S, Clark JB. Energy thresholds in brain mitochondria. Potential involvement in neurodegeneration. *J Biol Chem.* 1998;273(21):12753-7
[176] Kidd PM. Parkinson's disease as multifactorial oxidative neurodegeneration: implications for integrative management. *Altern Med Rev.* 2000 Dec;5(6):502-29

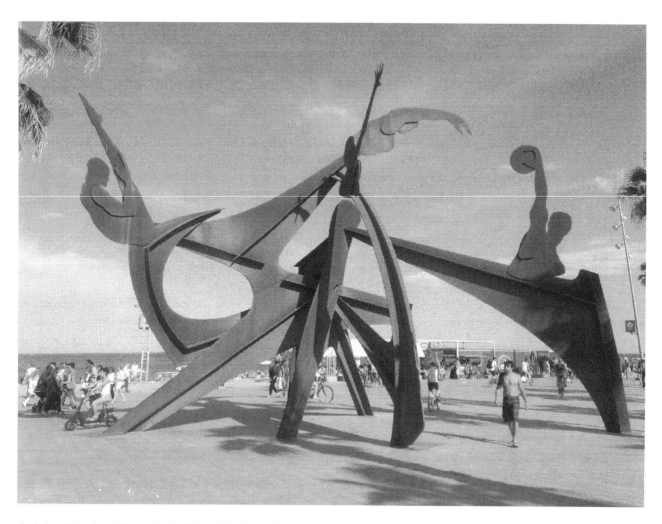

<u>Celebrating health and vitality</u>: Athletic metal sculpture by Alfredo Lanz on the promenade at Barceloneta, Barcelona, Cataluña. Photo by DrV.

Vasculitic Diseases & Wegener's Granulomatosis

Introduction:
Vasculitic diseases are largely considered to be mediated by deposition of circulating immune complexes (CIC) into/on the vascular endothelium, resulting in a localized activation of cell-mediated inflammation and activation of the complement cascade. From an allopathic perspective, these conditions are generally considered idiopathic and thus necessarily requiring long-term immunosuppression, in various forms. From the perspective of logic and with a desire to deconstruct complex clinical phenomena, one can approach diseases that are mediated by immune complex deposition by deciphering the components into their elemental parts. *Por ejemplo*/For example, given that vasculitic disease are mediated by endothelial deposition of immune complexes, and that immune complexes are chains of antigens and antibodies, one can then ask "*What are the major sources of antigens to which the immune system is exposed?*" and the correct answers are: "*Self, diet, microbes.*" One can then ponder the source of the antibodies, and ask if the presumed overproduction of antibodies is a *qualitative* problem or a *quantitative* problem, i.e., "Is the immune system 'wrong' in making antibodies to an antigen to which it is exposed [qualitative problem, error in action], *or* is the immune system 'correct' in its action but simply over-producing antibodies to perhaps otherwise benign antigens, whether these are self, diet, and/or microbes [quantitative problem, error in regulation]? From these questions, we arrive at answers other than crisis management and perpetual medicalization and pharmacologic immunosuppression; we arrive at the opportunity to reduce exposure to antigens from self (via antioxidant therapy to prevent molecular alteration of "self" structures), food (via food allergy avoidance and healing of intestinal hyperpermeability, and microbes (reducing dysbiosis and total microbial load [TML]) while also reducing the likely overzealous production of corresponding immunoglobulins via nutritional immunomodulation: induction of Treg for the reciprocal inhibition Th1, Th2, and Th17.

Topics:
- Introduction and Overview
- Clinical Presentation
- Prevalence, Symptoms, and Clinical Findings
- Pathophysiology
- Differential Diagnosis
- Diagnosis
- Standard Medical Treatment
- Therapeutic Interventions

Vasculitides and Vasculitis Syndromes

Description/pathophysiology, and clinical presentations:
- "Vasculitis" refers to a heterogeneous group of inflammatory disorders primarily affecting blood vessels, particularly the arteries and arterioles. Although the underlying pathomechanisms are similar among different disorders, these diseases differ in the location/size and number of affected vessels, and thus the clinical presentations and complications differ accordingly. Polymyalgia rheumatica / giant cell arteritis, Wegener's granulomatosis, and Behcet's disease are subtypes of vasculitis that are discussed in their respective chapters. As shown in the table at the

Overview of common inflammatory vasculopathic disorders
Primary vasculitides Large vessel diseases - Takayasu's arteritis - Behcet's disease Medium vessel diseases - Polyarteritis nodosa - Buerger's disease - Giant cell arteritis Small vessel diseases *Immune-complex mediated* - Cutaneous leukocystoclastic vasculitis - Henoch-Schonlein purpura - Cryoglobulinemia ANCA-associated disorders - Wegener's granulomatosis - Microscopic polyangiitis: microscopic polyarteritis, leukocytoclastic vasculitis ; variants include allergic granulomatosis and angiitis also known as Churg-Strauss syndrome **Secondary vasculitides** - Infections, dysbiosis - Other autoimmune disease - Crohn's disease or ulcerative colitis - Cancer - Drug reactions - Food allergies

right, several subtypes of vasculitis can be categorized based on the size/location of the vessel affected, and whether or not the cause of the vasculitis has been determined.

- Systemic manifestations are comparable to many other autoimmune disorders: insidious onset of fever, malaise, weight loss, generalized aches/pains;
- The autoimmune and immune-mediated pathogenesis of the vascultides includes the following:
  - ○ <u>Antibody-antigen binding</u>: *Example*: Goodpasture syndrome.
  - ○ <u>Delayed hypersensitivity reactions</u>: Especially in lesions characterized with granulomas formation. *Example*: temporal arteritis.
  - ○ <u>Deposition of circulating immune complexes</u>: The majority of the vascultides are characterized by intra-arterial deposition of circulating immune complexes, which provoke activation of the complement cascade and leukocyte migration and activation for the resultant vascular damage, which often includes necrosis, fibrinous occlusion, and thrombosis. *Example*: acute arteritis in SLE.

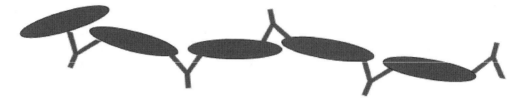

Schematized illustration of an immune complex: Immunoglobulins/antibodies—represented by the Y-shaped molecule—and antigens such as molecular fragments and peptides—represented by the ovoid molecule—form "chains" of alternating antigens-and-antibodies which in the circulation become lodged in the skin (dermatitis), vascular endothelium (vasculitis), kidney (nephritis), serosal surfaces (serositis), and synovial joints (arthritis). Readers must note that the location of the immune complex deposition is "innocent"; in immune complex disease, the location of the inflammation and complement activation (i.e., skin, vascular endothelium, kidney, synovial joints, serosa, and synovial joints) is simply a convenient molecular depot for the circulating immune complexes (CIC). Once deposited and following sufficient accumulation, immune complexes incite activation of the complement cascade and a local cell-mediated immune response, which causes local tissue inflammation and progressive destruction. Thus, for example, the joint or the skin or the kidney will be inflamed, but the actual problem of excess antigen exposure originated elsewhere, and the corresponding excess antibody production may have simply been a normal physiologic response to antigen exposure or may have been facilitated by a pro-inflammatory state and—synergistically yet distinctly—immunophenotypic imbalance.

<u>Major differential diagnoses</u>:
- <u>Infection</u>
- <u>Cancer</u>, especially leukemia, lymphoma, and multiple myeloma
- <u>Autoimmunity</u>: Concomitant or independent
- <u>Trauma or abuse</u>: Numerous unexplainable bruises/purpura may indicate abuse
- <u>Adverse drug reaction</u>
- <u>Atherosclerosis, peripheral vascular disease, aneuysm</u>

<u>Clinical assessments</u>:
- **History/subjective**:
  - ○ See clinical presentations
- **Physical examination/objective**:
  - ○ General physical examination with emphasis placed on symptomatic regions, circulatory examination, and dermal lesions

- **Laboratory assessments**:
  - Chemistry/metabolic panel: Assess for complications, especially renal insufficiency
  - Urinalysis: Assess for renal involvement
  - CRP/ESR: Generally elevated
  - Serum immune complexes: Most vasculopathies are due to immune complex deposition: Immune Complexes Reference Range (Raji cell technique, quantitative analysis):
    - Normal: ≤ 15.0 μg Eq/mL
    - Equivocal: 15.1-19.9 μg Eq/mL
    - Positive: ≥20.0 μg Eq/mL
  - Testing for multifocal dysbiosis: As discussed in Chapter 4
  - ANA
  - CH50: Complement levels may be low during exacerbations of immune complex mediated disease as the complement cascade is activated and complement proteins are consumed in the process, thus leading to a reduction in serum levels.
  - ANCA: Many of the vasculopathies, particularly those affecting the small vessels, are characterized by the presence of anti-neutrophilic cytoplasmic autoantibodies (ANCA), which can be segregated into two distinct subtypes: ❶ **cytoplasmic-ANCA** (C-ANCA, major antigen: proteinase 3) associated with Wegener granulomatosis, and ❷ **perinuclear-ANCA** (P-ANCA, major antigen: myeloperoxidase) associated with microscopic polyangiitis, or Churg-Strauss syndrome. Clinicians should note that neither P-ANCA nor C-ANCA is specific for a particular diagnosis, and that 10% of patients with biopsy-proved small vessel vasculitis do not show either ANCA subtype. In patients with small vessel vasculitis, levels of ANCA correlate with disease severity, especially C-ANCA in patients with Wegener granulomatosis.
- **Imaging and biopsy**:
  - Angiography is commonly used in the evaluation of vasculitic syndromes affecting larger vessels; Doppler ultrasound imaging can also be used.
  - Biopsy of dermal lesions, superficial arteries, and other tissues can support the diagnosis
- **Establishing the diagnosis**:
  - Based on clinical, laboratory, and biopsy/imaging findings

Major complications:

- Tissue necrosis: Complications depend on location of hypoxia and can include dermal necrosis, myocardial infarction, stroke, and intestinal infarction
- Infection secondary to immunosuppression
- Renal damage

Clinical management:

- Exacerbations are best managed pharmaceutically with appropriate immunosuppression. Patients may require hospital admission.
- An overview/survey of various inflammatory vascular disorders is presented on the following two pages.

> **Timely referral and comanagement**
> Generally speaking, patients with these conditions should be co-managed with a specialist (e.g., Internal Medicine, Rheumatology) because complications such as transverse myelitis and vascular occlusion leading to distal tissue ischemia—blindness, digital necrosis, mesenteric ischemia—can present quickly and require immediate immunosuppression in a hospital setting.

Overview of Vasculitic Diseases

Vasculitis subtype	Unique characteristics	Assessment and treatment considerations
Takayasu arteritis: "pulseless disease" • Leukocytic infiltration of the vasa vasorum followed by medial fibrosis and granulomatosis	• Granulomatous vasculitis of large and medium arteries • Fibrous thickening of the aortic arch and occlusion of large arteries • Presentation typically includes neuro-occular disturbances, reduced arm pulses; may include aortic valve insufficiency, and hypertension due to renal artery stenosis	• Clinical assessment with aortogram
Polyarteritis nodosa (PAN): • Immune-complex vasculitis • 10-30% of patients have Hepatitis B—testing for hepatitis B is mandatory[1] • Generally fatal if untreated; estimated 5-year survival 13% • Without treatment, only 20% of patients survive 5 years; with treatment, survival improves to 60-90% at 5 years	• Necrotizing vasculitic ischemia of numerous systems, thrombosis and ischemia at sites distal to lesion • <u>Gut</u>: abdominal pain, nausea, vomiting exacerbated by eating (due to ischemia) • <u>Nerves</u>: mononeuritis multiplex, vasculitic neuropathy; foot drop is most common manifestation • <u>Skin</u>: dermal lesions include sharply-demarcated nodules, erythema, and ulceration; lesions are **non-palpable** and are in **different stages** of development • <u>Kidneys</u>: hypertension due to renal involvement • *Pulmonary involvement is rare* • Can be categorized as *infectious and ANCA-negative* or *noninfectious and P-ANCA-positive*	• Clinical presentation is varied depending on location of arterial lesion(s) and severity of systemic inflammation; typical population is young adults • Anemia, elevated ESR, leukocytosis • Autoantibodies commonly normal or low-positive • Diagnosis is established with biopsy or angiogram • <u>Pharmacotherapy</u>: prednisone: 60 mg/d; pulsed methylprednisolone: 1 gram IV daily for 3 days; cyclophosphamide or other immunosuppressant drug • Plasmapheresis • Treatment of underlying hepatitis: must balance immunosuppression with anti-infective treatments
Mixed cryoglobulinemia: • Many patients have underlying hepatitis C • Many patient respond to avoidance of foods to which they are allergic	• Purpura • Peripheral neuropathy • Glomerulonephritis • Abdominal pain • Hepatitis • May have pulmonary involvement	• Diagnosis is based on clinical picture and serology for cryoglobulins • Testing for and treatment of underlying hepatitis is essential • Immunosuppression may exacerbate viral replication • **Avoidance of food allergens is highly beneficial[2,3]**
Henoch-Schonlein purpura: IgA vasculitis	• Dermal purpura • Abdominal pain • Arthritis • Hematuria associated with renal involvement; IgA nephropathy (Beuger's disease) is generally considered on a glomerular variant of with Henoch-Schonlein purpura	• The disease is generally self-limiting to 1-6 weeks, subsiding without complications if renal involvement is mild • Monitor renal function • No generally effective allopathic treatment is known

---

[1] Tierney ML. McPhee SJ, Papadakis MA (eds). *Current Medical Diagnosis and Treatment 2006. 45th edition*. New York; Lange Medical Books: 2006, pages 844-850
[2] "CONCLUSION: These data show that an LAC diet decreases the amount of circulating immune complexes in MC and can modify certain signs and symptoms of the disease." Ferri C, Pietrogrande M, Cecchetti R, et al. Low-antigen-content diet in the treatment of patients with mixed cryoglobulinemia. *Am J Med.* 1989 Nov;87:519-24
[3] Pietrogrande M, Cefalo A, Nicora F, Marchesini D. Dietetic treatment of essential mixed cryoglobulinemia. *Ric Clin Lab.* 1986 Apr-Jun;16(2):413-6

Overview of Vasculitic Diseases—*continued*

Vasculitis subtype	Unique characteristics	Assessment and treatment considerations
Giant Cell (Temporal) Arteritis: Three subtypes exist along a continuum: • Granulomatous vasculitis (2/3 of cases) • Leukocytic infiltration of vessel wall • Intimal fibrosis with lumenal narrowing	• GCA is the most common form of vasculitis; elevated ESR is classic • Granulomatous inflammation of medium and small arteries, particularly of the head; involvement of the aorta (giant cell aortitis) is a rare variant • Jaw claudication is highly suggestive • Classic presentation includes headache and facial pain; 50% of patients have PMR: polymyalgia rheumatica	• Biopsy is the gold standard for diagnosis, although it may be normal in one-third of patients due to lesion focality. • **Patients can transition from asymptomatic to blind—vision loss due to occlusion of ophthalmic artery—within days; therefore, this condition is generally considered a medical emergency/urgency mandating immediate implementation of prednisone, typically starting at 60 mg/d or 1 mg/kg/d.**
Microscopic polyangiitis, microscopic polyarteritis, leukocytoclastic vasculitis: • Affects small arterioles, capillaries, and venules; affected organs may include skin, lung, brain, heart, and kidneys (necrotizing glomerulonephritis) • Associated with relatively acute events, such as infection (including dysbiosis), drug administration, cancer, or administration of foreign protein	• Necrotizing vasculitis • Dermal lesions are differentiated from those of PAN because lesions of leukocytoclastic vasculitis are all at the **same stage of development** (due to acute event) and these lesions are **palpable due to acute inflammation** • P-ANCA is generally positive • Immune complexes are *not* characteristic of the vascular lesions	• P-ANCA is generally positive • "In general, the disease responds well to removal of the offending agent."[4]
Churg-Strauss syndrome, allergic granulomatous angiitis: affects small arteries all the way through to veins; variant of leukocytoclastic vasculitis	• Eosinophilia with bronchial asthma and sinusitis; mimics allergic sinusitis and allergic asthma • Pulmonary and splenic vessel involvement; granulomas • Associated with Henoch-Schonlein purpura, essential mixed cryoglobulinemia, and vasculitis of malignancy	• ANCA, particularly P-ANCA • Eosinophilia
Kawasaki disease; mucocutaneous lymph node syndrome: affects small-large arteries, classically the coronary arteries of children	• Arteritis of the coronary arteries in children • Mucocutaneous lymph node syndrome	• Coronary angiography • High-dose aspirin therapy
Wegener granulomatosis: affects small arteries all the way through to veins	• Granulomatous vasculitis affecting the upper respiratory tract	• Most patients have C-ANCA (cytoplasmic anti-proteinase 3 antibodies); small percentage of patients have P-ANCA (perinuclear anti-myeloperoxidase antibodies)

---

[4] Mitchell RN, et al. *Pocket Companion to Robbins and Cotran Pathologic Basis of Disease, Seventh Edition*. Philadelphia; Saunders Elsevier: 2006, page 279

Integrative and Nonpharmacologic Treatments:

- <u>Avoidance of allergenic foods</u>: **Hypoallergenic diets can benefit patients with immune-complex-mediated diseases such as mixed cryoglobulinemia[5,6], hypersensitivity vasculitis[7], and leukocystoclastic vasculitis with arthritis.[8]** Any patient may be allergic to any food, even if the food is generally considered a health-promoting food. Generally speaking, the most notorious allergens are wheat, citrus (especially juice due to the industrial use of fungal hemicellulases), cow's milk, eggs, peanuts, chocolate, and yeast-containing foods. According to a study in patients with migraine, some patients will have to avoid as many as 10 specific foods in order to become symptom-free.[9] **The severe wheat allergy** *celiac disease* **can present with inflammatory oligoarthritis[10,11], and celiac disease can also present as cryoglobulinemia and vasculitis[12], cutaneous leukocystoclastic vasculitis[13], including cerebral vasculitis[14] and pediatric stroke.[15]**

- <u>Avoidance of pro-inflammatory foods—detailed previously</u>: **High glycemic foods suppress immune function[16,17] and thus promote the perpetuation of infection/dysbiosis. Delivery of a high carbohydrate load to the gastrointestinal lumen promotes bacterial overgrowth[18,19], which is inherently pro-inflammatory[20,21] and which promotes immune complex formation.**

- <u>Alcohol/ethanol avoidance</u>: Consumption of alcoholic beverages—even in low doses—increases intestinal permeability and can exacerbate inflammatory disorders, particularly those associated with food allergies, gastrointestinal dysbiosis, and/or overproduction of estrogen.

- <u>Supplemented Paleo-Mediterranean diet</u>: The health-promoting diet of choice for the majority of people is a diet based on abundant consumption of fruits, vegetables, seeds, nuts, omega-3 and monounsaturated fatty acids, and lean sources of protein such as lean meats, fatty cold-water fish, soy and whey proteins. This diet obviates overconsumption of chemical preservatives, artificial sweeteners, and carbohydrate-dominant foods such as candies, pastries, breads, potatoes, grains, and other foods with a high glycemic load and high glycemic index. This "Paleo-Mediterranean Diet" is a combination of the "Paleolithic" or "Paleo diet" and the well-known "Mediterranean diet", both of which are well described in peer-reviewed journals and the lay press. (See Chapter 2 and my other publications[22,23] for details). This diet is the most nutrient-dense diet available, and its benefits are

---

[5] "CONCLUSION: These data show that an LAC diet decreases the amount of circulating immune complexes in MC and can modify certain signs and symptoms of the disease." Ferri C, Pietrogrande M, Cecchetti R, et al. Low-antigen-content diet in the treatment of patients with mixed cryoglobulinemia. *Am J Med.* 1989 Nov;87:519-24

[6] Pietrogrande M, Cefalo A, Nicora F, Marchesini D. Dietetic treatment of essential mixed cryoglobulinemia. *Ric Clin Lab.* 1986 Apr-Jun;16(2):413-6

[7] "In three cases the vasculitis relapsed following the introduction of food additives; in one case with the addition of potatoes and green vegetables (i.e., beans and green peas) and in the last case with the addition of eggs to the diet." Lunardi C, Bambara LM, Biasi D, Zagni P, Caramaschi P, Pacor ML. Elimination diet in the treatment of selected patients with hypersensitivity vasculitis. *Clin Exp Rheumatol.* 1992 Mar-Apr;10(2):131-5

[8] "Described in this report are two children with severe vasculitis caused by specific foods." Businco L, Falconieri P, Bellioni-Businco B, Bahna SL. Severe food-induced vasculitis in two children. *Pediatr Allergy Immunol.* 2002 Feb;13(1):68-71

[9] Grant EC. Food allergies and migraine. *Lancet.* 1979 May 5;1(8123):966-9

[10] "We report six patients with coeliac disease in whom arthritis was prominent at diagnosis and who improved with dietary therapy. Joint pain preceded diagnosis by up to three years in five patients and 15 years in one patient." Bourne JT, Kumar P, Huskisson EC, Mageed R, Unsworth DJ, Wojtulewski JA. Arthritis and coeliac disease. *Ann Rheum Dis.* 1985 Sep;44(9):592-8

[11] "A 15-year-old girl, with synovitis of the knees and ankles for 3 years before a diagnosis of gluten-sensitive enteropathy, is described." Pinals RS. Arthritis associated with gluten-sensitive enteropathy. *J Rheumatol.* 1986 Feb;13(1):201-4

[12] "Immunosuppressive treatment led to a normalization of transaminase levels and resolved the cryoglobulinaemic vasculitis. In addition, the patient exhibited low ferritin and iron levels, which led to the diagnosis of coeliac disease." Biecker E, Stieger M, Zimmermann A, Reichen J. Autoimmune hepatitis, cryoglobulinaemia and untreated coeliac disease: a case report. *Eur J Gastroenterol Hepatol.* 2003 Apr;15(4):423-7

[13] "A 38 year old female, with chronic uncontrolled coeliac disease, presented with the rare complication of cutaneous leucocytoclastic vasculitis." Meyers S, Dikman S, Spiera H, Schultz N, Janowitz HD. Cutaneous vasculitis complicating coeliac disease. *Gut.* 1981 Jan;22(1):61-4

[14] "A 51-year-old white man with celiac disease presented with seizures unresponsive to medical therapy." Rush PJ, Inman R, Bernstein M, Carlen P, Resch L. Isolated vasculitis of the central nervous system in a patient with celiac disease. *Am J Med.* 1986 Dec;81(6):1092-4

[15] "Because celiac disease is a potentially treatable cause of cerebral vasculopathy, serology-specifically antitissue transglutaminase antibodies-should be included in the evaluation for cryptogenic stroke in childhood, even in the absence of typical gut symptoms." Goodwin FC, Beattie RM, Millar J, Kirkham FJ.Celiac disease and childhood stroke. *Pediatr Neurol.* 2004 Aug;31(2):139-42

[16] Sanchez A, Reeser JL, Lau HS, et al. Role of sugars in human neutrophilic phagocytosis. *Am J Clin Nutr.* 1973 Nov;26(11):1180-4

[17] "Postoperative infusion of carbohydrate solution leads to moderate fall in the serum concentration of inorganic phosphate. ... The hypophosphatemia was associated with significant reduction of neutrophil phagocytosis, intracellular killing, consumption of oxygen and generation of superoxide during phagocytosis." Rasmussen A, Segel E, Hessov I, Borregaard N. Reduced function of neutrophils during routine postoperative glucose infusion. *Acta Chir Scand.* 1988 Jul-Aug;154(7-8):429-33

[18] Ramakrishnan T, Stokes P. Beneficial effects of fasting and low carbohydrate diet in D-lactic acidosis associated with short-bowel syndrome. *JPEN J Parenter Enteral Nutr.* 1985 May-Jun;9(3):361-3

[19] Gottschall E. *Breaking the Vicious Cycle: Intestinal Health Through Diet.* Kirkton Press; Rev edition (August 1, 1994)

[20] Lin HC. Small intestinal bacterial overgrowth: a framework for understanding irritable bowel syndrome. *JAMA.* 2004 Aug 18;292(7):852-8

[21] Lichtman SN, Wang J, Sartor RB, Zhang C, Bender D, Dalldorf FG, Schwab JH. Reactivation of arthritis induced by small bowel bacterial overgrowth in rats: role of cytokines, bacteria, and bacterial polymers. *Infect Immun.* 1995 Jun;63(6):2295-301

[22] Vasquez A. A Five-Part Nutritional Protocol that Produces Consistently Positive Results. *Nutritional Wellness* 2005 September

[23] Vasquez A. Implementing the Five-Part Nutritional Wellness Protocol for the Treatment of Various Health Problems. *Nutritional Wellness* 2005 Nov

further enhanced by supplementation with vitamins, minerals, probiotics, and the health-promoting fatty acids: ALA, GLA, EPA, DHA.

- Gluten-free vegetarian diet: **Wheat consumption induces formation for immune complexes in virtually everyone (i.e., people who are "apparently healthy")[24], including as expected (but certainly not limited to) patients with dermatitis herpetiformis.[25]** Vegetarian/vegan diets have a place in the treatment plan of all patients with autoimmune/inflammatory disorders[26,27]; this is also true for patients for whom long-term exclusive reliance on a meat-free vegetarian diet is either not appropriate or not appealing. No legitimate scientist or literate clinician doubts the antirheumatic power and anti-inflammatory advantages of vegetarian diets, whether used short-term or long term.[28] Patients who rely on the Paleo-Mediterranean Diet can use vegetarian meals, on a daily basis or for days at a time, for example, by having a daily vegetarian meal, or one week per month of vegetarianism. Of course, some (not all) patients can use a purely vegetarian diet long-term provided that nutritional needs (especially protein and cobalamin) are consistently met.

- Short-term fasting: Whether the foundational diet is Paleo-Mediterranean, vegetarian, vegan, or a combination of all of these, autoimmune/inflammatory patients will still benefit from periodic fasting, whether on a weekly

> **Wheat and circulating immune complexes in "healthy" disease-free persons**
>
> - Circulating immune complexes (CICs) in blood are associated with autoimmune-diseases such as systemic lupus erythematosus, immune complex glomerulonephritis, rheumatoid arthritis and vasculitis. However, slightly increased serum concentrations of such CICs are sometimes also found in healthy individuals. The objective of the current study was to assess whether food antigens could play a role in the formation of CICs.
> - MATERIAL AND METHODS: A total of **352 (265 F, 87 M), so far, healthy individuals** were tested for CICs containing C1q and immunoglobulin G (IgG) as well as for gliadin IgG antibodies using the ELISA technique. Additionally, fructose and lactose malabsorption was assessed using hydrogen breath tests.
> - RESULTS: In our study, 15.3% (54/352) of the patients presented with elevated CIC concentrations (above 50 microg/ml) and 6.5% (23/352) of the study population were positive for gliadin IgG antibodies (above 20 U/ml). **CIC concentration levels were significantly higher in the group with elevated gliadin IgG antibodies (CIC median: 49.0 microg/ml) compared with the group with normal levels of gliadin IgG antibodies** (CIC median: 30.0 microg/ml; Mann-Whitney U-test, U=1992; p <0.001). ...
> - CONCLUSIONS: **The results of this study indicate that certain food antigens (e.g. gluten) could play a role in the formation of CICs.** ...
>
> Eisenmann et al. *Scand J Gastroenterol*. 2009

(e.g., every Saturday), monthly (every first week or weekend of the month, or every other month), or yearly (1-2 weeks of the year) basis. Since consumption of food—particularly unhealthy foods—induces an inflammatory effect[29], abstinence from food provides a relative anti-oxidative and anti-inflammatory benefit[30] with many of the antioxidant benefits beginning within 24 hours of the initiation of the fast.[31] Fasting indeed provides a distinct anti-inflammatory benefit and may help "re-

---

[24] Eisenmann A, Murr C, Fuchs D, Ledochowski M. Gliadin IgG antibodies and circulating immune complexes. *Scand J Gastroenterol*. 2009;44(2):168-71

[25] Zone JJ, et al. Induction of IgA circulating immune complexes after wheat feeding in dermatitis herpetiformis patients. *J Invest Dermatol*. 1982 May;78(5):375-80

[26] "After four weeks at the health farm the diet group showed a significant improvement in number of tender joints, Ritchie's articular index, number of swollen joints, pain score, duration of morning stiffness, grip strength, erythrocyte sedimentation rate, C-reactive protein, white blood cell count, and a health assessment questionnaire score." Kjeldsen-Kragh J, et al. Controlled trial of fasting and one-year vegetarian diet in rheumatoid arthritis. *Lancet*. 1991 Oct 12;338(8772):899-902

[27] "During the vegan diet, both signs and symptoms returned in most patients, with the exception of some patients with psoriasis who experienced an improvement." Lithell H, Bruce A, Gustafsson IB, Hoglund NJ, Karlstrom B, Ljunghall K, Sjolin K, Venge P, Werner I, Vessby B. A fasting and vegetarian diet treatment trial on chronic inflammatory disorders. *Acta Derm Venereol*. 1983;63(5):397-403

[28] "For the patients who were randomised to the vegetarian diet there was a significant decrease in platelet count, leukocyte count, calprotectin, total IgG, IgM rheumatoid factor (RF), C3-activation products, and the complement components C3 and C4 after one month of treatment." Kjeldsen-Kragh J, Mellbye OJ, Haugen M, et al. Changes in laboratory variables in rheumatoid arthritis patients during a trial of fasting and one-year vegetarian diet. *Scand J Rheumatol*. 1995;24(2):85-93

[29] Aljada A, Mohanty P, Ghanim H, Abdo T, Tripathy D, Chaudhuri A, Dandona P. Increase in intranuclear nuclear factor kappaB and decrease in inhibitor kappaB in mononuclear cells after a mixed meal: evidence for a proinflammatory effect. *Am J Clin Nutr*. 2004 Apr;79(4):682-90 http://www.ajcn.org/cgi/content/full/79/4/682

[30] "This is the first demonstration of ...a decrease in reactive oxygen species generation by leukocytes and oxidative damage to lipids, proteins, and amino acids after dietary restriction and weight loss in the obese over a short period." Dandona P, Mohanty P, Ghanim H, Aljada A, Browne R, Hamouda W, Prabhala A, Afzal A, Garg R. The suppressive effect of dietary restriction and weight loss in the obese on the generation of reactive oxygen species by leukocytes, lipid peroxidation, and protein carbonylation. *J Clin Endocrinol Metab*. 2001 Jan;86(1):355-62 http://jcem.endojournals.org/cgi/content/full/86/1/355

[31] "Thus, a 48h fast may reduce ROS generation, total oxidative load and oxidative damage to amino acids." Dandona P, Mohanty P, Hamouda W, Ghanim H, Aljada A, Garg R, Kumar V. Inhibitory effect of a two day fast on reactive oxygen species (ROS) generation by leucocytes and plasma ortho-tyrosine and meta-tyrosine concentrations. *J Clin Endocrinol Metab*. 2001 Jun;86(6):2899-902 http://jcem.endojournals.org/cgi/content/abstract/86/6/2899

calibrate" metabolic and homeostatic mechanisms by breaking self-perpetuating "vicious cycles"[32] that autonomously promote inflammation independent from proinflammatory stimuli. Of course, water-only fasting is completely hypoallergenic (assuming that the patient is not sensitive to chlorine, fluoride, or other contaminants), and subsequent re-introduction of foods provides the ideal opportunity to identify offending foods. Fasting deprives intestinal microbes of substrate[33], stimulates intestinal B-cell immunity[34], improves the bactericidal action of neutrophils[35], reduces lysozyme release and leukotriene formation[36], and ameliorates intestinal hyperpermeability.[37] In case reports and clinical trials, short-term fasting (or protein-sparing fasting) has been documented as safe and effective treatment for SLE[38], RA[39], and non-rheumatic diseases such as chronic severe hypertension[40], moderate hypertension[41], obesity[42,43], type-2 diabetes[44], and epilepsy.[45]

- <u>Broad-spectrum fatty acid therapy with ALA, EPA, DHA, GLA and oleic acid—detailed previously</u>: **Fish oil provides EPA and DHA which have well-proven anti-inflammatory benefits when used in the treatment of various autoimmune and cardiovascular disorders.** Fatty acid supplementation should be delivered in the form of combination therapy with ALA, GLA, DHA, and EPA.

- <u>Vitamin D3 supplementation with physiologic doses and/or tailored to serum 25(OH)D levels</u>: Vitamin D deficiency is common in the general population and is even more common in patients with chronic illness and chronic musculoskeletal pain.[46] Correction of vitamin D deficiency supports normal immune function against infection and provides a clinically significant anti-inflammatory[47] and analgesic benefit in patients with back pain[48] and limb pain.[49] Reasonable daily doses for children and adults are 2,000 and 4,000 IU, respectively, as defined by Vasquez, et al.[50] Deficiency and response to treatment are monitored with serum 25(OH)vitamin D while safety is monitored with serum calcium; inflammatory granulomatous diseases and certain drugs such as hydrochlorothiazide greatly increase the propensity for hypercalcemia and warrant increment dosing and frequent monitoring of serum calcium.

---

[32] "The ability of therapeutic fasts to break metabolic vicious cycles may also contribute to the efficacy of fasting in the treatment of type 2 diabetes and autoimmune disorders." McCarty MF. A preliminary fast may potentiate response to a subsequent low-salt, low-fat vegan diet in the management of hypertension - fasting as a strategy for breaking metabolic vicious cycles. *Med Hypotheses*. 2003 May;60(5):624-33

[33] Ramakrishnan T, Stokes P. Beneficial effects of fasting and low carbohydrate diet in D-lactic acidosis associated with short-bowel syndrome. *JPEN J Parenter Enteral Nutr*. 1985 May-Jun;9(3):361-3

[34] Trollmo C, Verdrengh M, Tarkowski A. Fasting enhances mucosal antigen specific B cell responses in rheumatoid arthritis. *Ann Rheum Dis*. 1997 Feb;56(2):130-4

[35] "An association was found between improvement in inflammatory activity of the joints and enhancement of neutrophil bactericidal capacity. Fasting appears to improve the clinical status of patients with RA." Uden AM, Trang L, Venizelos N, Palmblad J. Neutrophil functions and clinical performance after total fasting in patients with rheumatoid arthritis. *Ann Rheum Dis*. 1983 Feb;42(1):45-51

[36] "We thus conclude that a reduced ability to generate cytotaxins, reduced release of enzyme, and reduced leukotriene formation from RA neutrophils, together with an altered fatty acid composition of membrane phospholipids, may be mechanisms for the decrease of inflammatory symptoms that results from fasting." Hafstrom I, Ringertz B, Gyllenhammar H, Palmblad J, Harms-Ringdahl M. Effects of fasting on disease activity, neutrophil function, fatty acid composition, and leukotriene biosynthesis in patients with rheumatoid arthritis. *Arthritis Rheum*. 1988 May;31(5):585-92

[37] "The results indicate that, unlike lactovegetarian diet, fasting may ameliorate the disease activity and reduce both the intestinal and the non-intestinal permeability in rheumatoid arthritis." Sundqvist T, Lindstrom F, Magnusson KE, Skoldstam L, Stjernstrom I, Tagesson C. Influence of fasting on intestinal permeability and disease activity in patients with rheumatoid arthritis. *Scand J Rheumatol*. 1982;11(1):33-8

[38] Fuhrman J, Sarter B, Calabro DJ. Brief case reports of medically supervised, water-only fasting associated with remission of autoimmune disease. *Altern Ther Health Med*. 2002 Jul-Aug;8(4):112, 110-1

[39] "An association was found between improvement in inflammatory activity of the joints and enhancement of neutrophil bactericidal capacity. Fasting appears to improve the clinical status of patients with RA." Uden AM, Trang L, Venizelos N, Palmblad J. Neutrophil functions and clinical performance after total fasting in patients with rheumatoid arthritis. *Ann Rheum Dis*. 1983 Feb;42(1):45-51

[40] "The average reduction in blood pressure was 37/13 mm Hg, with the greatest decrease being observed for subjects with the most severe hypertension. Patients with stage 3 hypertension (those with systolic blood pressure greater than 180 mg Hg, diastolic blood pressure greater than 110 mg Hg, or both) had an average reduction of 60/17 mm Hg at the conclusion of treatment." Goldhamer A, Lisle D, Parpia B, Anderson SV, Campbell TC. Medically supervised water-only fasting in the treatment of hypertension. *J Manipulative Physiol Ther*. 2001 Jun;24(5):335-9 http://www.healthpromoting.com/335-339Goldhamer115263.QXD.pdf

[41] "RESULTS: Approximately 82% of the subjects achieved BP at or below 120/80 mm Hg by the end of the treatment program. The mean BP reduction was 20/7 mm Hg, with the greatest decrease being observed for subjects with the highest baseline BP." Goldhamer AC, Lisle DJ, Sultana P, Anderson SV, Parpia B, Hughes B, Campbell TC. Medically supervised water-only fasting in the treatment of borderline hypertension. *J Altern Complement Med*. 2002 Oct;8(5):643-50

[42] Vertes V, Genuth SM, Hazelton IM. Supplemented fasting as a large-scale outpatient program. *JAMA*. 1977 Nov 14;238(20):2151-3

[43] Bauman WA, et al. Early and long-term effects of acute caloric deprivation in obese diabetic patients. *Am J Med*. 1988 Jul;85(1):38-46

[44] Goldhamer AC. Initial cost of care results in medically supervised water-only fasting for treating high blood pressure and diabetes. *J Altern Complement Med*. 2002 Dec;8(6):696-7 http://www.healthpromoting.com/Articles/pdf/Study%2032.pdf

[45] "The ketogenic diet should be considered as alternative therapy for children with difficult-to-control seizures. It is more effective than many of the new anticonvulsant medications and is well tolerated by children and families when it is effective." Freeman JM, Vining EP, Pillas DJ, Pyzik PL, Casey JC, Kelly LM. The efficacy of the ketogenic diet-1998: a prospective evaluation of intervention in 150 children. *Pediatrics*. 1998 Dec;102(6):1358-63

[46] Plotnikoff GA, Quigley JM. Prevalence of severe hypovitaminosis D in patients with persistent, nonspecific musculoskeletal pain. *Mayo Clin Proc*. 2003 Dec;78(12):1463-70

[47] Timms PM, et al. Circulating MMP9, vitamin D and variation in the TIMP-1 response with VDR genotype: mechanisms for inflammatory damage in chronic disorders? *QJM*. 2002 Dec;95(12):787-96 http://qjmed.oxfordjournals.org/cgi/content/full/95/12/787

[48] Al Faraj S, Al Mutairi K. Vitamin D deficiency and chronic low back pain in Saudi Arabia. *Spine*. 2003 Jan 15;28(2):177-9

[49] Masood H, Narang AP, Bhat IA, Shah GN. Persistent limb pain and raised serum alkaline phosphatase the earliest markers of subclinical hypovitaminosis D in Kashmir. *Indian J Physiol Pharmacol*. 1989 Oct-Dec;33(4):259-61

[50] Vasquez A, Manso G, Cannell J. The clinical importance of vitamin D (cholecalciferol): a paradigm shift with implications for all healthcare providers. *Altern Ther Health Med*. 2004 Sep-Oct;10(5):28-36

- Assessment and treatment for dysbiosis: **Dysbiotic loci should be investigated as discussed previously in Chapter 4**. Each cause—each contributor to disease—may in itself be "clinically insignificant" but when numerous "insignificant" additive and synergistic influences coalesce, we find ourselves confronted with an "idiopathic disease." We must then decide between the only two available options: 1) despair in the failure of our "one cause, one disease, one drug" paradigm, or 2) appreciate that numerous influences work together to disrupt physiologic function and produce the biologic dysfunction that we experience as disease.

- Orthoendocrinology: Assess melatonin, prolactin, cortisol, DHEA, free and total testosterone, serum estradiol, and thyroid status (e.g., TSH, T4, *and* anti-thyroid peroxidase antibodies). Treat accordingly as discussed in Chapter 4.

- Oral enzyme therapy with proteolytic/pancreatic enzymes: Polyenzyme supplementation is used to ameliorate the pathophysiology induced by immune complexes, such as rheumatoid arthritis.[51]

- CoQ10 (antihypertensive, renoprotective, and probably immunomodulatory): CoQ10 is a powerful antioxidant with a wide margin of safety and excellent clinical tolerability. **At least four studies have documented its powerful blood-pressure-lowering ability, which often surpasses the clinical effectiveness of antihypertensive drugs.[52,53,54,55] Furthermore, at least two published papers[56,57] and one case report[58] advocate that CoQ10 has powerful renoprotective benefits.** CoQ10 levels are low in patients with allergies[59], and the symptomatic relief that many allergic patients experience following supplementation with CoQ10 suggests that CoQ10 has an immunomodulatory effect. Common doses start at > 100 mg per day with food; doses of 200 mg per day are not uncommon, and doses up to 1,000 mg per day are clinically well tolerated though the high financial toll resembles that of many pharmaceutical drugs.

- Hepatobiliary stimulation—possible benefit, discussed previously: IgA immune complexes are removed from the serum by hepatocytes and transported intact into the bile.[60,61,62,63,64,65,66] Therefore, stimulating bile flow would be expected to expedite the removal of IgA immune complexes from the serum, thus lessening their clinical consequences. Dietary and botanical therapeutics that stimulate bile flow include beets, ginger, curcumin/turmeric, *Picrorhiza*, milk thistle, *Andrographis paniculata*, and *Boerhaavia diffusa*. Therapeutic enemas safely and effectively stimulate bile flow for 45-60 minutes following administration.[67]

[51] Galebskaya LV, Ryumina EV, Niemerovsky VS, Matyukov AA. Human complement system state after wobenzyme intake. *VESTNIK MOSKOVSKOGO UNIVERSITETA. KHIMIYA.* 2000. Vol. 41, No. 6. Supplement. 148-149

[52] Burke BE, et al. Randomized, double-blind, placebo-controlled trial of coenzyme Q10 in isolated systolic hypertension. *South Med J.* 2001 Nov;94(11):1112-7

[53] Singh RB, Niaz MA, Rastogi SS, Shukla PK, Thakur AS. Effect of hydrosoluble coenzyme Q10 on blood pressures and insulin resistance in hypertensive patients with coronary artery disease. *J Hum Hypertens.* 1999 Mar;13(3):203-8

[54] Digiesi V, Cantini F, Oradei A, et al. Coenzyme Q10 in essential hypertension. *Mol Aspects Med.* 1994;15 Suppl:s257-63

[55] Langsjoen P, Langsjoen P, Willis R, Folkers K. Treatment of essential hypertension with coenzyme Q10. *Mol Aspects Med.* 1994;15 Suppl:S265-72

[56] Singh RB, Khanna HK, Niaz MA. Randomized, double-blind placebo-controlled trial of coenzyme Q10 in chronic renal failure. *J Nutr Environ Med* 2000;10:281-8

[57] Singh RB, et al. Randomized, Double-blind, Placebo-controlled Trial of Coenzyme Q10 in Patients with End-stage Renal Failure. *J Nutr Environ Med* 2003;13: 13–22

[58] Singh RB, Singh MM. Effects of CoQ10 in new indications with antioxidant vitamin deficiency. *J Nutr Environ Med* 1999; 9:223-228

[59] Ye CQ, Folkers K, Tamagawa H, Pfeiffer C. A modified determination of coenzyme Q10 in human blood and CoQ10 blood levels in diverse patients with allergies. *Biofactors.* 1988 Dec;1(4):303-6

[60] Russell MW, Brown TA, Claflin JL, Schroer K, Mestecky J. Immunoglobulin A-mediated hepatobiliary transport constitutes a natural pathway for disposing of bacterial antigens. *Infect Immun.* 1983 Dec;42(3):1041-8 http://www.pubmedcentral.gov/articlerender.fcgi?tool=pubmed&pubmedid=6642659

[61] "The liver therefore appears to be singularly capable of transporting both free and complexed IgA into its secretion, the bile." Russell MW, Brown TA, Mestecky J. Preferential transport of IgA and IgA-immune complexes to bile compared with other external secretions. *Mol Immunol.* 1982 May;19(5):677-82

[62] "These results indicate that mouse hepatocytes are involved in the uptake and hepatobiliary transport of pIgA and pIgA-IC of low mol. wt." Phillips JO, Komiyama K, Epps JM, Russell MW, Mestecky J. Role of hepatocytes in the uptake of IgA and IgA-containing immune complexes in mice. *Mol Immunol.* 1988 Sep;25(9):873-9

[63] "Thus hepatobiliary transport appears to be the major pathway for the clearance of both IgA IC and free IgA from the circulation." Brown TA, Russell MW, Kulhavy R, Mestecky J. IgA-mediated elimination of antigens by the hepatobiliary route. *Fed Proc.* 1983 Dec;42(15):3218-21

[64] "Clearance of IgA immune complexes was delayed after bile duct ligation." Harmatz PR, Kleinman RE, Bunnell BW, McClenathan DT, Walker WA, Bloch KJ. The effect of bile duct obstruction on the clearance of circulating IgA immune complexes. *Hepatology.* 1984 Jan-Feb;4(1):96-100

[65] Lemaitre-Coelho I, Jackson GD, Vaerman JP. High levels of secretory IgA and free secretory component in the serum of rats with bile duct obstruction. *J Exp Med.* 1978 Mar 1;147(3):934-9 http://www.jem.org/cgi/reprint/147/3/934

[66] "CONCLUSIONS: Biliary obstruction secondary to both calculus or malignancy of the hepatobiliary system causes suppression of bile IgA secretion and elevated serum level of secretory IgA. Bile secretory IgA secretion recovers with endoscopic drainage of the obstructed system." Sung JJ, Leung JC, Tsui CP, Chung SS, Lai KN. Biliary IgA secretion in obstructive jaundice: the effects of endoscopic drainage. *Gastrointest Endosc.* 1995 Nov;42(5):439-44

[67] Garbat AL, Jacobi HG. Secretion of Bile in Response to Rectal Installations. *Arch Intern Med* 1929; 44: 455-462

Giant Cell Arteritis & Polymyalgia Rheumatica

Introduction:
Giant cell arteritis (previously called temporal arteritis) and polymyalgia rheumatica are related conditions characterized histopathologically by inflammatory occlusion of small arteries and arterioles in the upper body: head, neck, shoulders. The possibility of arterial occlusion leading to blindness due to occlusion of the ophthalmic artery mandates early implementation of immunosuppressive prednisone (generally at 60mg/d or 1mg/kg/d). These patients must be co-managed with an Internal Medicine or Rheumatology specialist, while components of the Functional Inflammology protocol are appropriately pursued (e.g., assessments detailed in Chapters 1 and 4) and implemented (e.g., treatments outlined in Chapter 4 as well as this chapter and throughout this book).

<u>Topics</u>:
- Introduction and Overview
- Clinical Presentation
- Prevalence, Symptoms, and Clinical Findings
- Pathophysiology
- Differential Diagnosis
- Diagnosis
- Standard Medical Treatment
- Therapeutic Interventions

Polymyalgia Rheumatica (PMR)
Giant Cell Arteritis (GCA)
Temporal Arteritis (previous term)

<u>Description/pathophysiology</u>:
- This group of tightly related and largely synonymous disorders is described as "idiopathic" by medical textbooks.
- **<u>Polymyalgia rheumatica (PMR)</u>**: This disorder typically presents with painful inflammation of the shoulder/neck and hip muscles along with systemic manifestations of fever, malaise, and weight loss. When present in isolation (i.e., not with giant cell arteritis), it does not lead to blindness, and the condition responds to low-dose (10-20 mg) prednisone.
- **<u>Giant Cell Arteritis (GCA):</u>** When treated allopathically, GCA requires higher daily doses (40-60 mg) of prednisone than PMR. GCA can result in rapid-onset blindness and therefore any evidence of ocular involvement in a patient with GCA must be treated as a medical emergency. **Indeed, the diagnosis of GCA itself is considered urgent due to ability of blindness to occur rapidly and without warning.** GCA was previously called temporal arteritis. Approximately 50% of patients with GCA have PMR.

<u>Clinical presentations</u>:
- Pain and stiffness in proximal muscle groups: shoulders, neck, and hips; weakness—if any—is secondary to pain, disuse atrophy, drug side-effect (e.g., "steroid myopathy"), or other concomitant disorder. Presentations are consistent with muscle/tissue ischemia due to the underlying panarteritis which results in vessel occlusion: head pain, jaw claudication, blindness.

- Generally presents after age 50 years. The later age of onset helps distinguish PMR from fibromyalgia, which generally affects young adult patients between the ages of 20-40 years.
- 2x more common in women than in men
- Typical autoimmune systemic manifestations: fatigue, malaise, fever, anorexia, and weight loss.
- Patients may have high fever and chills with disease initiation and/or exacerbation.

Major differential diagnoses:
- Fibromyalgia: ESR is normal, age of onset is nearly always before 50 years.
- Dermatomyositis, polymyositis: These conditions cause muscle weakness, which is characteristically absent in patients with PMR. Muscle enzymes are elevated in patients with dermatomyositis/polymyositis but are normal in patients with PMR.
- Cancer, particularly multiple myeloma
- Hypothyroidism: Hypothyroidism can easily mimic PMR by producing an inflammatory myopathy that affects the shoulder muscles and which remits following normalization of thyroid status.
- Rheumatoid arthritis, SLE, vasculitis, or other autoimmune disorder
- Infection: WBC count is normal in GCA/PMR and is generally elevated in patients with severe infection.
- Cervical spondylosis

Clinical assessments:
- **History/subjective**:
    o See clinical presentations
- **Physical examination/objective**:
    o Palpate pulses for strength and symmetry:
        - Carotid artery in the anterior neck
        - Axillary/brachial in the axilla and inner arm, respectively
        - Radial pulse at the distal radius
        - Aorta in the abdomen
        - Femoral pulses in the groin
        - Dorsalis pedis and posterior tibial arteries at the ankle/foot
- **Laboratory assessments**:
    o ESR: Most patients will have a very high ESR > 50 mm/h.
    o CBC: Anemia is common.
    o Chemistry/metabolic panel: Hepatic alkaline phosphatase is elevated in 20% of patients.
    o RF: generally negative
    o Muscle enzymes: are almost always normal.
    o Protein in urine, serum protein electrophoresis: No evidence of proteinuria or monoclonal gammopathy, as seen in MM.
- **Imaging**:
    o Not generally indicated except when looking for complications or concomitant disease
- **Establishing the diagnosis**:
    o PMR is a clinical diagnosis based on 1) painful inflammation of the shoulder/neck and hip muscles along with 2) systemic manifestations of fever, malaise, and weight loss and 3) the absence of evidence supporting an alternate diagnosis.[68]
    o GCA is classically diagnosed following biopsy of the temporal artery.
    o Clinical diagnosis: [69] Pattern recognition (proximal muscle pain with no other explanation) and evidence of inflammation in an elderly patient when other diseases have been ruled out.

---

[68] Tierney ML. McPhee SJ, Papadakis MA (eds). Current Medical Diagnosis and Treatment 2006. 45th edition. New York; Lange Medical Books: 2006, pages 486
[69] Tierney ML. McPhee SJ, Papadakis MA. Current Medical Diagnosis and Treatment. 35th edition. Stamford: Appleton and Lange, 1996 page 751

Complications:

- GCA can lead to blindness.
- Dry cough is seen in some patients and may be the presenting complaint.
- Mononeuritis multiplex may cause (shoulder) paralysis.
- Aneurysms of the thoracic aorta are 17x more common in patients with GCA than the general population

Clinical management:

- Referral if clinical outcome is unsatisfactory or if serious complications are possible/evident.
- Assess for temporal arteritis—educate patient about the significance of the onset of eye symptoms, headache, and jaw claudication.
- A few patients treated with prednisone will have permanent remission within 2 years.

Treatments: Use this section in association with previously mentioned assessments and interventions.

> *Drug treatments*: This condition requires early implementation of prednisone immunosuppression; comanagement with a specialist—Internal Medicine or Rheumatology—is mandatory.

- Prednisone (10-20 mg per day for PMR) should result in "dramatic improvement" within 72 hours.[70] Prednisone dose for GCA is typically 60 mg per day at the start of treatment in order to prevent one of the most feared complications—blindness. Dose is tapered after clinical remission. Low-dose aspirin appears to reduce the risk of blindness and stroke in GCA patients.
- **Presumptive treatment: In comparison with other, more common diseases such as SLE and RA, very little research has been done using non-pharmacologic treatments for PMR/GCA.**
- Orthoendocrinology: Assess prolactin, cortisol, DHEA, free and total testosterone, serum estradiol, and thyroid status (e.g., TSH, T4, *and* anti-thyroid peroxidase antibodies). Correct as indicated (see Chapter 4). **Prolactin levels are typically elevated in patients with PMR and correlate with clinical symptomatology.**[71] Adrenal hypofunction in patients with PR/GCA is suggested by the relative insufficiencies of cortisol and DHEA.[72] **DHEA (insufficiency and supraphysiologic supplementation):** Patients with autoimmunity should be tested for DHEA insufficiency by measurement of serum DHEA-sulfate; insufficiencies should generally be corrected except in cases of concomitant hormone-responsive cancer such as breast cancer or prostate cancer. The rationale for using high-dose DHEA in patients with autoimmune diseases is reviewed in Chapter 4.

Endocrine imbalance in PMR/GCA

"Patients with PMR/GCA with new-onset active disease before steroid treatment have inappropriately normal cortisol levels regarding the ongoing inflammation, and significantly lower levels of DHEAS compared to the age- and sex-matched healthy control subjects. These data support the existence of a relative adrenal hypofunction in PMR and GCA."

Narvaez et al. *J Rheumatol* 2006;33:1293-8

Is giant cell arteritis an infectious disease? Biological and epidemiological evidence

"Simultaneous occurrence of peaks of GCA/PMR and respiratory infections have been observed in Denmark. Several viruses have been suspected as triggers and assessed by serological testing, PCR or immunostaining on temporal artery biopsies, or both techniques: the hepatitis B virus can be ruled out, as well as Herpes simplex 1 and 2, Herpes varicellae, Epstein-Barr virus and cytomegalovirus. Recent studies focused on parainfluenza virus, Parvovirus B19 and Chlamydia pneumoniae. Immunological studies suggest, at the origin of the inflammatory reaction leading to the typical pathological features of giant cell arteritis, the existence of a triggering antigen of unknown nature activating T-cells in the artery wall."

Duhaut P, Bosshard S, Ducroix JP. Is giant cell arteritis an infectious disease? *Presse Med.* 2004 Nov 6;33(19 Pt 2):1403-8

---

[70] Tierney ML. McPhee SJ, Papadakis MA (eds). Current Medical Diagnosis and Treatment 2006. 45th edition. New York; Lange Medical Books: 2006, pages 487
[71] Straub RH, Georgi J, Helmke K, Vaith P, Lang B. In polymyalgia rheumatica serum prolactin is positively correlated with the number of typical symptoms but not with typical inflammatory markers. *Rheumatology* (Oxford). 2002 Apr;41(4):423-9 http://rheumatology.oxfordjournals.org/cgi/content/full/41/4/423
[72] "Patients with PMR/GCA with new-onset active disease before steroid treatment have inappropriately normal cortisol levels regarding the ongoing inflammation, and significantly lower levels of DHEAS compared to the age- and sex-matched healthy control subjects. These data support the existence of a relative adrenal hypofunction in PMR and GCA." Narvaez J, Bernad B, Diaz Torne C, Momplet JV, Montpel JZ, Nolla JM, Valverde-Garcia J. Low serum levels of DHEAS in untreated polymyalgia rheumatica/giant cell arteritis. *J Rheumatol.* 2006 Jul;33(7):1293-8. Epub 2006 Jun 15

Wegener's Granulomatosis

Introduction:

Wegener's is a granulomatous and vasculitic disease with a high mortality. Insight into the molecular basis of the condition—electrostatic haptenization of the *Staphylococcus aureus* enzyme acid phosphatase with endothelial cells—provides brilliant insight into the disease and its treatment. The possible role of other microbes, along with other factors such as immunophenotype imbalance should be intuitive by this time to readers who have read the other chapters.

<u>Topics</u>:
- Introduction and Overview
- Clinical Presentation
- Prevalence, Symptoms, and Clinical Findings
- Pathophysiology
- Differential Diagnosis
- Diagnosis
- Standard Medical Treatment
- Therapeutic Interventions

Wegener's Granulomatosis

<u>Description/pathophysiology</u>:
- This inflammatory condition generally begins with granulomatous involvement of the upper or lower respiratory tract and then progresses to systemic vasculitis and glomerulonephritis.
- Biopsy of nasopharyngeal/pulmonary/renal lesions reveals granulomatous/inflammatory tissue.
- Allopathic textbooks generally describe this condition as *idiopathic*, although the condition is increasingly associated with occult sinorespiratory dysbiosis with *Staphylococcus aureus*.[73,74] Additionally, *Klebsiella aerogenes, Haemophilus influenzae,* and *Bacillus subtilis* have been implicated.[75]
- Immune complexes contribute to pathophysiology

<u>Clinical presentations</u>:
- Twice as common in males as in females
- Sinorespiratory symptoms:
  - Mucosal ulcerations/friability, hemorrhagic rhinorrhea
  - Persistent sinusitis; increased incidence of otitis media
  - Cough, hemoptosis due to intraalveolar hemorrhage, pleuritis
- Renal complications are inevitable without effective/immunosuppressive treatment
- Typical autoimmune systemic manifestations: fatigue, malaise, low-grade fever, anorexia, and weight loss, polyarthritis.

<u>Major differential diagnoses</u>:
- Extramedullary plasmacytoma of multiple myeloma (typically occurs in the nasopharyngeal region)
- Sinus infection

---

[73] Brons RH, Bakker HI, Van Wijk RT, et al. Staphylococcal acid phosphatase binds to endothelial cells via charge interaction; a pathogenic role in Wegener's granulomatosis? *Clin Exp Immunol.* 2000 Mar;119(3):566-73 http://www.blackwell-synergy.com/doi/abs/10.1046/j.1365-2249.2000.01172.x
[74] Popa ER, et al. Staphylococcus aureus and Wegener's granulomatosis. *Arthritis Res.* 2002;4(2):77-9 arthritis-research.com/content/4/2/77
[75] George J, et al. Infections and Wegener's granulomatosis--a cause and effect relationship? *QJM.* 1997 May;90(5):367-73 qjmed.oxfordjournals.org/cgi/reprint/90/5/367

- Lung cancer
- Tuberculosis
- Septicemia or septic arthritis
- Lymphoma
- Other systemic/inflammatory disorder such as lupus (ANA and low complement)
- Bacterial endocarditis

Clinical assessments:
- **History/subjective**: See clinical presentations.
- **Physical examination/objective**:
  - Examination of oral and nasal mucosa
  - Pulmonary auscultation
  - Dermatologic screen for cutaneous vasculitis
- **Laboratory assessments**:
  - <u>Urinalysis</u> for assessment of renal status
  - <u>Chemistry/metabolic panel</u> for BUN and creatinine, etc.
  - <u>Microbial assessments</u>—reviewed in Chapters 1 and 4.
  - <u>Nasal culture</u> for *Staphylococcus aureus*[76] and other bacterial or fungal contaminants
  - <u>Complement</u> levels are normal or elevated
  - <u>ESR/CRP</u> is elevated
  - <u>CBC</u> may reveal leukocytosis and anemia
  - **<u>ANA (antinuclear antibodies) are generally absent</u>**
  - **<u>ANCA are almost always present and strongly support the diagnosis of this condition. The finding of the more specific C-ANCA is 97% specific for the diagnosis of Wegener's granulomatosis.</u>**[77] Interestingly, ANCA can also be induced by gastrointestinal parasitic infections.
- **Imaging**: Generally not required; only indicated as needed
- **Establishing the diagnosis**: Based on clinical, serologic, and biopsy findings.
  - Respiratory tract symptoms and mucosal lesions; biopsy of granulomas.
  - <u>C-ANCA</u>: positive C-ANCA result can replace biopsy in a patient with a clinical picture of Wegener's granulomatosis.[78]

Complications:
- Severe anemia requiring blood transfusion
- Secondary bacterial infections on ulcerated mucosa
- Respiratory and renal failure
- Hypoxic complications due to vasculitis

Clinical management:
- Referral to internist/rheumatologist for additional treatment and defensive management as indicated. Unless you are a specialist, you need to have a specialist as part of the care team who can help you manage acute exacerbations which can occur with any autoimmune/inflammatory disease.

Therapeutic considerations:
Medical treatment routinely includes the following:[79]
- <u>Cyclophosphamide</u>: 1-2 mg/kg/d PO or IV: associated with increased risk for cancer, particularly bladder cancer

---

[76] Brons RH, Bakker HI, Van Wijk RT, et al. Staphylococcal acid phosphatase binds to endothelial cells via charge interaction; a pathogenic role in Wegener's granulomatosis? *Clin Exp Immunol*. 2000 Mar;119(3):566-73 http://www.blackwell-synergy.com/doi/abs/10.1046/j.1365-2249.2000.01172.x P
[77] Beers MH, Berkow R (eds). The Merck Manual. Seventeenth Edition. Whitehouse Station; Merck Research Laboratories 1999 Page 443
[78] Shojania K. Rheumatology: 2. What laboratory tests are needed? *CMAJ*. 2000 Apr 18;162(8):1157-63 http://www.cmaj.ca/cgi/content/full/162/8/1157
[79] Beers MH, Berkow R (eds). The Merck Manual. Seventeenth Edition. Whitehouse Station; Merck Research Laboratories 1999 Page 443

- Prednisone: 1 mg/kg/d po; use the lowest dose possible
- Methotrexate: pulse treatment < 20-30 mg per week po
- **Antibiotic treatment: trimeth-sulfa 160/800 up to 480/2400 mg/d po**
- Blood transfusions for anemia
- **Assessment for multifocal dysbiosis: emphasis on gastrointestinal and sinorespiratory dysbiosis**
  - *Staphylococcus aureus*: **Produces an antigenic acid phosphatase which haptenizes with endothelial cells for the induction of autoimmune vasculitis in Wegener's granulomatosis.**[80] Antimicrobial treatment to eradicate *Staphylococcus aureus* results in clinical remission of the "autoimmune" disease, thus proving the microbe-rheumatic link.[81] Hyperforin from *Hypericum perforatum* is highly effective against *Staphylococcus aureus*[82] and can be used nasally and orally.
  - *Entamoeba histolytica*: **induces formation of antineutrophil cytoplasmic antibodies (ANCA)**.[83] Stool testing with a specialty laboratory is strongly recommended.
  - **Other microbes such as *Klebsiella aerogenes*, *Haemophilus influenzae* and *Bacillus subtilis*:** These have also been implicated.[84]
- Supplemented Paleo-Mediterranean diet: The health-promoting diet of choice for the majority of people is a diet based on abundant consumption of fruits, vegetables, seeds, nuts, omega-3 and monounsaturated fatty acids, and lean sources of protein such as lean meats, fatty cold-water fish, soy and whey proteins. (See Chapter 2 for details).
- Broad-spectrum fatty acid therapy with ALA, EPA, DHA, GLA and oleic acid: Fatty acid supplementation should be delivered in the form of combination therapy with ALA, GLA, DHA, EPA as described in this book and elsewhere.[85]
- Vitamin D3 supplementation with physiologic doses and/or tailored to serum 25(OH)D levels: **Since Wegener's *granulomatosis* is obviously a *granulomatous* disease, caution and frequent monitoring must be employed when optimizing vitamin D status to avoid hypercalcemia.** A reasonable clinical approach would be to start with a relatively low dose (1,000 – 2,000 IU cholecalciferol per day following the exclusion of hypercalcemia. Thereafter, serum calcium can be measured at 2 weeks, 4 weeks, 6 weeks, 8 weeks, and monthly thereafter. See Therapeutics section of this text and the review by Vasquez et al[86] for more details.
- Orthoendocrinology: Assess prolactin, cortisol, DHEA, free and total testosterone, serum estradiol, and thyroid status (e.g., TSH, T4, *and* anti-thyroid peroxidase antibodies). Correct effectively.
- Assess for heavy metals, especially mercury: **Exposure to mercury and lead is associated with increased risk of developing Wegener's granulomatosis.**[87] Consider urine toxic metal assessment following 10-30 mg/kg DMSA as described in Chapter 4 and as described elsewhere for the assessment of heavy metals in patients with autism.[88]
- Proteolytic enzymes: Wegener's granulomatosis is mediated in large part by IgG and IgA immune complexes, which directly contribute to vasculitis and nephritis.[89] Polyenzyme supplementation has been used to ameliorate the pathophysiology induced by immune complexes in other conditions.[90]

[80] Brons RH, Bakker HI, Van Wijk RT, et al. Staphylococcal acid phosphatase binds to endothelial cells via charge interaction; a pathogenic role in Wegener's granulomatosis? *Clin Exp Immunol.* 2000 Mar;119(3):566-73 http://www.blackwell-synergy.com/doi/abs/10.1046/j.1365-2249.2000.01172.x
[81] Popa ER, et al. Staphylococcus aureus and Wegener's granulomatosis. *Arthritis Res.* 2002;4(2):77-9 http://arthritis-research.com/content/4/2/077
[82] Schempp et al. Antibacterial activity of hyperforin from St John's wort, against multiresistant Staphylococcus aureus and gram-positive bacteria. *Lancet.* 1999 Jun 19;353(9170):2129
[83] George J, Levy Y, Kallenberg CG, Shoenfeld Y. Infections and Wegener's granulomatosis--a cause and effect relationship? QJM. 1997 May;90(5):367-73
[84] George J, Levy Y, Kallenberg CG, Shoenfeld Y. Infections and Wegener's granulomatosis--a cause and effect relationship? *QJM.* 1997 May;90(5):367-73
[85] Vasquez A. Reducing Pain and Inflammation Naturally. Part 2. *Nutritional Perspectives* 2005; January: 5-16
[86] Vasquez A, Manso G, Cannell J. The clinical importance of vitamin D (cholecalciferol). *Altern Ther Health Med.* 2004 Sep-Oct;10(5):28-36
[87] "Results suggest that mercury and perhaps lead exposure were positively associated with WG as compared with either control group, although the number of patients exposed was small... CONCLUSION: We conclude that heavy metal exposure and a prior history of allergy may play a role in the etiopathogenesis of Wegener's granulomatosis." Albert D, et al. Wegener's granulomatosis: Possible role of environmental agents in its pathogenesis. *Arthritis Rheum.* 2004 Aug 15;51(4):656-64
[88] Bradstreet J, Geier DA, Kartzinel JJ, Adams JB, Geier MR. A case-control study of mercury burden in children with autistic spectrum disorders. *Journal of American Physicians and Surgeons* 2003; 8: 76-79 http://www.jpands.org/vol8no3/geier.pdf
[89] "RESULTS: Four of 11 biopsies taken at initial presentation and four of 21 biopsies taken at the onset of a relapse of WG showed IgG and/or IgA containing immune deposits in the subepidermal blood vessels. ...CONCLUSION: A substantial number of skin biopsies showed immune deposits during active disease. These results could support the hypothesis that immune complexes may trigger vasculitic lesions in WG." Brons RH, et al. Detection of immune deposits in skin lesions of patients with Wegener's granulomatosis. *Ann Rheum Dis.* 2001 Dec;60(12):1097-102 http://ard.bmjjournals.com/cgi/content/full/60/12/1097
[90] Galebskaya et al. Human complement system state after wobenzyme intake. *Vestnik Moskovskogo Universiteta (Seriya 2: Khimiya).* 2000:41(6 Suppl): 148-149

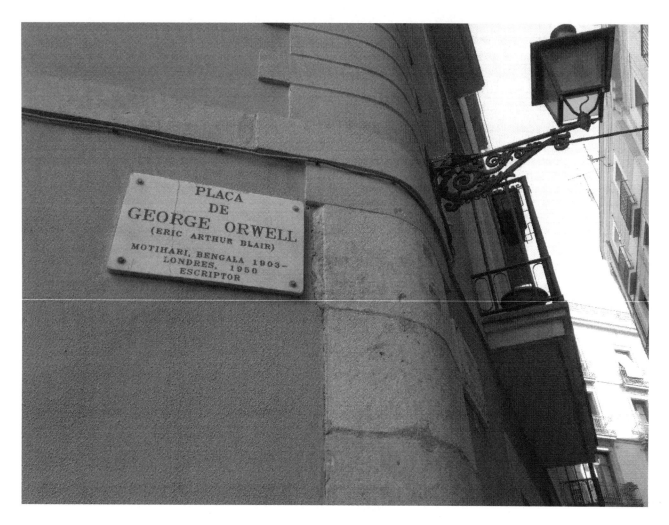

Homage to intellectuals: Intellectuals provide a great service to humanity by accumulating information and articulating that conjoined information in such a way as to extend beyond the information itself toward its current and future implications. Writers like George Orwell (Eric Blair) in *1984*, Aldous Huxley in *Brave New World*, and Friedrich Nietzsche in *Thus Spoke Zarathustra* articulated current and future social/political trends with prophetic insight. Barcelona Spain has a long-standing tradition of honoring intellectuals, as demonstrated in this photo by the naming of a modest neighborhood plaza for George Orwell, author of *Homage to Catalonia*, in which he describes his experience fighting fascism as a military volunteer from December 1936 until June 1937, during which time he received a (thankfully minor) gunshot wound to the neck by a sniper during the Spanish Civil War which lasted from July 1936 to 1 April 1939; he would later publish *1984* in 1949. Understanding the current state of the world is virtually impossible without a thorough reading of these books, appreciating that these authors used metaphors to brilliantly describe world-altering trends in society, politics, religion, and scientific thought. Reading of the paper versions of these works is indispensable for any intellectual today; additionally and conveniently, the audiobook versions of each of these masterworks brings new life to the books and enhances their accessibility and applicability. Recommended audio versions are as follows; of note, these are all annotated editions to compliment the original works in paper and also in audio:

- Thus Spoke Zarathustra: naxosaudiobooks.com/432512.htm
- 1984: audible.com/pd/Education/1984-Audiobook/B004RICKZ4/
- Brave New World: audible.com/pd/Sci-Fi-Fantasy/Brave-New-World-CliffsNotes-Audiobook/B004RR0T3K/

Spondyloarthropathies and Other Axial Inflammatory Conditions

---

Axial inflammation as yet another *pattern of inflammation*

Spinal/axial inflammatory conditions are patterns of inflammation with etiologic factors consistent with the pattern reviewed throughout this textbook and surveyed in Chapter 4; likewise therefore, similar therapeutic concepts are applicable. As always, pharmacologic immunosuppression may be urgently needed if a patient experiences exacerbation or inflammatory complication; however, routine "chronic" pharmacologic immunosuppression offers no hope of authentically curing the disease and correcting the underlying imbalances: it only suppresses manifestations of underlying physiologic imbalances.

Ankylosing spondylitis
Reactive arthritis (previously Reiter's syndrome)
Enteropathic spondyloarthropathy, enteropathic arthritis

<u>Topics:</u>
- Introduction and Overview
- Clinical Presentation
- Prevalence, Symptoms, and Clinical Findings
- Pathophysiology
- Differential Diagnosis
- Diagnosis
- Standard Medical Treatment
- Therapeutic Interventions

<u>Description/pathophysiology</u>:
- Inflammatory arthropathies affecting the spine and sacroiliac joints are termed "spondyloarthropathies" and like other arthritic conditions are termed *seronegative* if not related to rheumatoid arthritis in general and RF positivity in particular. **The spondyloarthropathies differ in some aspects of their etiologies, affected populations, clinical presentations, and treatment; however—regarding etiology and treatment—the similarities far outnumber the differences.** Regarding clinical management, from both allopathic and integrative/naturopathic perspectives, the treatment and management of these different conditions is virtually identical, save for a few important nuances.
- Spondyloarthropathies and reactive arthritis differ from the classic pattern of other autoimmune conditions in that 1) most patients affected are male, 2) they are highly correlated with HLA-B27, 3) serologic evidence of autoimmunity is generally absent, 4) they are strongly associated with dysbiosis, infections, and/or occult or overt enteropathy.[1,2]
- Some variation exists in the conditions that are included under the heading of *Spondyloarthropathies*. Most medical textbooks include four disorders under the heading of spondyloarthropathies: 1) ankylosing spondylitis, 2) psoriatic arthritis, 3) reactive arthritis, and 4) enteropathic spondyloarthropathy (ES), while a few others go on to include 5) juvenile spondyloarthropathy, and 6) rheumatoid arthritis. Psoriatic arthritis (PsA) and rheumatoid arthritis (RA) are detailed in their own chapters in this book and therefore will not be discussed in great detail here.

---

[1] Colmegna I, Cuchacovich R, Espinoza LR. HLA-B27-associated reactive arthritis: pathogenetic and clinical considerations. *Clin Microbiol Rev.* 2004 Apr;17(2):348-69 http://cmr.asm.org/cgi/content/full/17/2/348
[2] Ringrose JH. HLA-B27 associated spondyloarthropathy, an autoimmune disease based on crossreactivity between bacteria and HLA-B27? *Ann Rheum Dis.* 1999 Oct;58(10):598-610 http://ard.bmjjournals.com/cgi/content/full/58/10/598

- Although ankylosing spondylitis (AS) is the prototype of the spondyloarthropathies, reactive arthritis (ReA) is the best-known and most well accepted model for microbe-induced musculoskeletal autoimmunity. Despite nearly overwhelming research demonstrating that all of these conditions are triggered by exposure to microbes, major medical textbooks[3] still describe these conditions as *idiopathic*. Enteropathic arthritis and enteropathic spondyloarthropathy (EAES) demonstrate how gastrointestinal dysbiosis, hormonal imbalances, increased intestinal permeability ("leaky gut"), and non-musculoskeletal systemic inflammation can spill-over into peripheral and axial arthritis. As detailed in the separate chapter on psoriasis and psoriatic arthritis (PsA), PsA is clearly a microbe-triggered disease, and its similarity to AS suggests a common physiologic etiology. The common themes that weave these disorders together are 1) dysbiosis-induced musculoskeletal inflammation, 2) hormonal imbalances, and 3) increased intestinal/mucosal permeability—the latter is the most voluminous route of absorption of arthritogenic antigens, immunogens, and antimetabolites—see Chapter 4 for overview and details.

- All of these conditions are *systemic* inflammatory disorders that show clear evidence of immune-mediated tissue damage and are therefore worthy of being dubbed *autoimmune*. The systemic nature of these disorders carries important clinical implications because both doctor and patient need to be aware of *non-musculoskeletal* complications. Non-musculoskeletal complications of these disorders include renal failure secondary to amyloidosis[4,5], cardiovascular and pulmonary complications, and increased risk of trauma, violent death, poisonings, and alcohol misuse.[6,7,8] Not surprisingly, the risk of pulmonary, renal, neurologic, ocular and cardiac complications is increased in patients with long-standing and severe disease.

The use of a low starch diet in the treatment of patients suffering from ankylosing spondylitis: alleviation of dysbiosis and immune complex formation via nutritional intervention

"The majority of ankylosing spondylitis (AS) patients not only possess HLA-B27, but **during active phases of the disease have elevated levels of total serum IgA, suggesting that a microbe from the bowel flora is acting across the gut mucosa**. .... Furthermore **AS patients from 10 different countries have been found to have elevated levels of specific antibodies against Klebsiella bacteri**a. It has been suggested that these Klebsiella microbes, found in the bowel flora, might be the trigger factors in this disease and therefore **reduction in the size of the bowel flora could be of benefit in the treatment of AS patients**. Microbes from the bowel flora depend on dietary starch for their growth and therefore a reduction in starch intake might be beneficial in AS patients. **A "low starch diet" involving a reduced intake of "bread, potatoes, cakes and pasta"** has been devised and tested in healthy control subjects and AS patients. **The "low starch diet" leads to a reduction of total serum IgA in both healthy controls as well as patients, and furthermore to a decrease in inflammation and symptoms in the AS patients.** The role of a "low starch diet" in the management of AS requires further evaluation.

Ebringer A, Wilson C. The use of a low starch diet in the treatment of patients suffering from ankylosing spondylitis. *Clin Rheumatol*. 1996 Jan;15 Suppl 1:62-66

---

[3] Klippel JH (ed). *Primer on the rheumatic diseases. 11th edition*. Atlanta: Arthritis Foundation; 1997, page 181

[4] "The mechanism of death in these patients was secondary amyloidosis in 19, cardiovascular complications in six, fracture of the spine in one, and it was not known in one patient. Excess deaths due to circulatory, gastrointestinal and renal diseases, and violence were also observed." Lehtinen K. Mortality and causes of death in 398 patients admitted to hospital with ankylosing spondylitis. *Ann Rheum Dis*. 1993 Mar;52(3):174-6

[5] "During an outbreak of Yersinia pseudotuberculosis III, one of two HLA-B27 positive brothers developed reactive arthritis (ReA), mild at first, but later severely destructive and ultimately fatal. The reactivation of ReA was possibly triggered by an oral polio vaccine. The cause of death was severe secondary amyloidosis." Yli-Kerttula T, Mottonen T, Toivanen A. Different course of reactive arthritis in two HLA-B27 positive brothers with fatal outcome in one. *J Rheumatol*. 1997 Oct;24(10):2047-50

[6] "A marked sex-associated effect was noted among deaths caused by injuries/poisoning, since 6 of the deaths occurred in men and only 1 was in a woman. CONCLUSION: Patients with PsA are at an increased risk of death compared with the general population." Gladman DD, Farewell VT, Wong K, Husted J.Mortality studies in psoriatic arthritis: results from a single outpatient center. II. Prognostic indicators for death. *Arthritis Rheum*. 1998 Jun;41(6):1103-10

[7] "The 4 leading causes of death were diseases of the circulatory (36.2%) or respiratory (21.3%) system, malignant neoplasms (17.0%), and injuries/poisoning (14.9%). The SMR for the female cohort was 1.59, and for the men, it was 1.65, indicating a 59% and 65% increase in the death rate, respectively. Deaths due to respiratory causes were particularly increased in these patients." Wong K, Gladman DD, Husted J, Long JA, Farewell VT. Mortality studies in psoriatic arthritis: results from a single outpatient clinic. I. Causes and risk of death. *Arthritis Rheum*. 1997 Oct;40(10):1868-72

[8] "Subjects with ankylosing spondylitis (AS) have an increased incidence of deaths from accidents and violence, which is due in part, but perhaps not entirely, to the vulnerability of the affected spine to fractures... Uncontrolled use of alcohol is an important determinant in the surplus of deaths from accidents and violence in Finnish patients with AS." Myllykangas-Luosujarvi R, Aho K, Lehtinen K, Kautiainen H, Hakala M. Increased incidence of alcohol-related deaths from accidents and violence in subjects with ankylosing spondylitis. *Br J Rheumatol*. 1998 Jun;37(6):688-90 http://rheumatology.oxfordjournals.org/cgi/reprint/37/6/688

Differentiating Characteristics of the Spondyloarthropathies

Condition	Etiopathogenesis	Unique presentation	Specific emphasis
Ankylosing spondylitis	• *Allopathic*: idiopathic • *Integrative*: dysbiosis is paramount	• Insidious onset of low-back pain in young patient • Ankylosis begins in lumbopelvis and can progress to thorax, neck, hips and knees. • 90% positive HLA-B27	• *Allopathic*: anti-inflammatory drugs • *Integrative*: Antidysbiosis and orthoendocrinology are treatment cornerstones
Reactive arthritis (previously Reiter's syndrome[9])	• *Allopathic*: infection-triggered arthritis • *Integrative*: infection-triggered arthritis in a patient with dietary and endocrinologic predispositions.	• Classically associated with a recent infection, particularly a genitourinary infection or gastrointestinal infection. • Inflammation is characteristically located at the low-back, iris, and heels. • 75% positive HLA-B27	• Antimicrobial treatment for acute and chronic infections is the mainstay of treatment although in a large percentage of patients the arthropathy continues despite apparent clearance of the primary infection.
Enteropathic spondylo-arthropathy, enteropathic arthritis	• *Allopathic*: idiopathic • *Integrative*: dysbiosis-triggered arthritis in a patient with dietary and endocrinologic predispositions	• Arthropathy of the peripheral joints and/or spine in a patient with inflammatory bowel disease—Crohn's disease or ulcerative colitis • 50% positive HLA-B27	• *Allopathic*: anti-inflammatory drugs • *Integrative*: Antidysbiosis and orthoendocrinology are treatment cornerstones • Treatment is similar to other treatments except with a greater focus on addressing the intestinal lesions
Juvenile spondylo-arthropathy	• *Allopathic*: idiopathic • *Integrative*: dysbiosis[10]	• Generally occurs in boys aged 8-18 years • Peripheral arthritis (90%) is more common than spondylitis (50%)	• *Allopathic*: anti-inflammatory drugs • *Integrative*: Antidysbiosis
Psoriatic arthritis	• *Allopathic*: idiopathic • *Integrative*: Food allergies and dysbiosis are paramount	• Arthropathy of the peripheral joints and/or spine in a patient with psoriasis • 50% positive HLA-B27	• *Allopathic*: anti-inflammatory drugs • *Integrative*: Antidysbiosis and orthoendocrinology are treatment cornerstones
Rheumatoid arthritis	• *Allopathic*: idiopathic • *Integrative*: dysbiosis-triggered arthritis in a patient with dietary and endocrinologic predisposition	• Inflammatory peripheral arthropathy generally precedes axial joints • Sacroiliac joints are generally spared • RF is frequently positive	• *Allopathic*: anti-inflammatory drugs • *Integrative*: Antidysbiosis and orthoendocrinology are treatment cornerstones

[9] The term "Reiter's syndrome" has fallen out of favor due to the increasing acknowledgement that Dr Hans Reiter was affiliated with Nazi atrocities during World War II. See the following for additional information: "During World War II, Reiter, a physician leader of the Nazi party, authorized medical experiments on concentration camp prisoners." Lu DW, Katz KA. Declining use of the eponym "Reiter's syndrome" in the medical literature, 1998-2003. *J Am Acad Dermatol*. 2005 Oct;53(4):720-3 and "There is more than ample evidence that Hans Reiter, whose name has been eponymously linked to a rheumatologic syndrome, was a Nazi war criminal. He was responsible for heinous atrocities that violated the precepts of humanity, ethics, and professionalism." Panush RS, Paraschiv D, Dorff RE. The tainted legacy of Hans Reiter. *Semin Arthritis Rheum*. 2003 Feb;32(4):231-6

[10] "Our findings provide clear evidence of ReA diagnosis following an acute M. pneumoniae infection that in four patients progressed to chronic jSpA. Our results suggest that detecting M. pneumoniae-specific antibodies in serological screening of jSpA patients might be useful." Harjacek M, Ostojic J, Djakovic Rode O. Juvenile spondyloarthropathies associated with Mycoplasma pneumoniae infection. *Clin Rheumatol*. 2006 Jan 4;:1-6

<u>Clinical presentations</u>:

- <u>Musculoskeletal</u>:
    - o <u>Pain and limited motion in the low-back sacroiliac joints</u>: This is an aspect of all of the spondyloarthropathies, especially AS and ReA. Back pain is generally worse in the morning and alleviated by motion, including passive motion such as spinal manipulation.
    - o <u>Thoracic spine pain and decreased rib expansion/excursion</u>: Although it typically begins in the lumbar spine and sacroiliac joints, AS commonly progresses to involve the thoracic spine and rib cage. Decreased mobility of the ribs limit respiration, and thus respirometry is used in the clinical assessment of patients with AS.
    - o <u>Neck pain</u>: particularly common in RA and AS, two conditions associated with spontaneous atlantoaxial instability
    - o <u>Atlantoaxial instability</u>: May be the presenting manifestation of AS[11] and is a common long-term complication of RA. Particularly in patients with neck pain and/or long-standing inflammation, cervical radiographs including APOM and measurement of the atlantodental interval should be performed before the clinical use of forceful cervical spine manipulation as well as esophageal/tracheal endoscopy.
    - o <u>Enthesopathies</u>: Inflammation at the site of ligament insertion into bone—classically seen at the insertion of the Achilles' tendon at the calcaneus—is a characteristic finding and complaint in patients with ReA.
    - o <u>Non-erosive asymmetrical peripheral arthritis</u>: 50% of patients with AS experience a temporary peripheral arthritis, while in 25% of patients the peripheral arthritis is permanent.
- <u>Pulmonary</u>: Pleurisy (painful inflammation of the pleural lining of the internal thoracic cavity) may be a complication of nearly all rheumatic/inflammatory disorders. Patients with AS may develop pulmonary fibrosis.
- <u>Cardiac</u>: "Spondylitic heart disease" is seen in patients with AS and commonly includes atrioventricular conduction defects and aortic regurgitation.[12]
- <u>GI tract</u>: oral ulcers, intestinal inflammation, increased intestinal permeability
- <u>Skin/mucosal lesions</u>: Dermal lesions are particularly common in patients with ReA and PsA. Psoriatic lesions are typically well-demarcated erythematous patches with white/silvery scales. Dermal lesions of ReA can include pustular lesions on the feet and hands (palmoplantar pustulosis) in addition to genital lesions in patients with sexually transmitted diseases.
- <u>Renal complications</u>: These can be seen in nearly all rheumatic disorders, either as a result of the systemic inflammation (particularly immune complexes), amyloidosis, or as a result of NSAIDs or other pharmaceutical drugs.
- <u>Neurological complications</u>: Cerebral necrosis, corticosteroid psychosis, and transverse myelitis may occur. Atlantoaxial subluxation can present with myelopathic signs.
- <u>Ocular complications</u>: Anterior uveitis is seen in ~25% of patients with AS and is a characteristic finding in patients with ReA.

---

[11] Thompson GH, Khan MA, Bilenker RM. Spontaneous atlantoaxial subluxation as a presenting manifestation of juvenile ankylosing spondylitis. A case report. *Spine* 1982 Jan-Feb;7(1):78-9

[12] Tierney ML. McPhee SJ, Papadakis MA (eds). Current Medical Diagnosis and Treatment 2006. 45th edition. New York; Lange Medical Books: 2006, pages 851-855

Low Back Pain: Differential Diagnostic Considerations

	DDX Category	Examples:
V	Vascular	Aortic aneurysm
	Visceral referral	Pancreatic disease/cancer
I	Infectious	Ankylosing spondylitis, Reiter's syndrome
	Inflammatory	Rheumatoid arthritis
	Immunologic	Psoriatic arthritis
		Enteropathic spondyloarthropathy
		Lymphoma, leukemia
		Bone/ tissue infections
		Gastrointestinal disease
		Kidney infection
		Psoriatic arthritis
		Herpes zoster
N	Neurologic	Metastatic disease, primary bone tumors, multiple myeloma
	Nutritional	Herpes zoster
	New growth: neoplasia, pregnancy	Cauda equina syndrome
D	Deficiency	Degenerative joint/spine disease
	Degenerative	Congenital malformations of bones/ viscera
	Developmental	Scoliosis
		Postural syndromes
		Disc herniation
		Varicose veins in the leg mimicking sciatica
I	Iatrogenic (drug related)	Anticoagulants predispose to epidural or spinal cord bleeding[13]
	Intoxication	Prednisone use promotes osteoporosis and spinal fractures
	Idiosyncratic	Excess alcohol consumption[14]
C	Congenital	Congenital malformations of bones: hemivertebrae, leg length inequality, etc.
A	Allergy	Ankylosing spondylitis
	Autoimmune	Fractures, injuries
	Abuse	
T	Trauma	Fractures: injuries to vertebrae, ribs, muscles
E	Endocrine	Diabetes mellitus
	Exposure	
S	Subluxation	Segmental dysfunction of lumbar spine and pelvis
	Structural	Muscle tension
	Stress	
	Secondary gain	
M	Mental	Anxiety
	Malpractice	Depression
	Mental disorder	Endometriosis, hematocolpos[15]
	Malignancy	Ovarian tumor
	Metabolic disease	Nephrolithiasis
	Menstrual	Metastasis to spine
	Myofascial	Myofascial trigger points in quadratus lumborum, piriformis, iliacus, psoas

---

[13] Souza TA. Differential Diagnosis for the Chiropractor: Protocols and Algorithms. Gaithersburg: Aspen Publications. 1997 page 110
[14] "Alcohol abuse was significantly more frequent among the male low back patients." Sandstrom J, Andersson GB, Wallerstedt S. The role of alcohol abuse in working disability in patients with low back pain. *Scand J Rehabil Med*. 1984;16(4):147-9
[15] London NJ, Sefton GK. Hematocolpos. An unusual cause of sciatica in an adolescent girl. *Spine*. 1996 Jun 1;21(11):1381-2

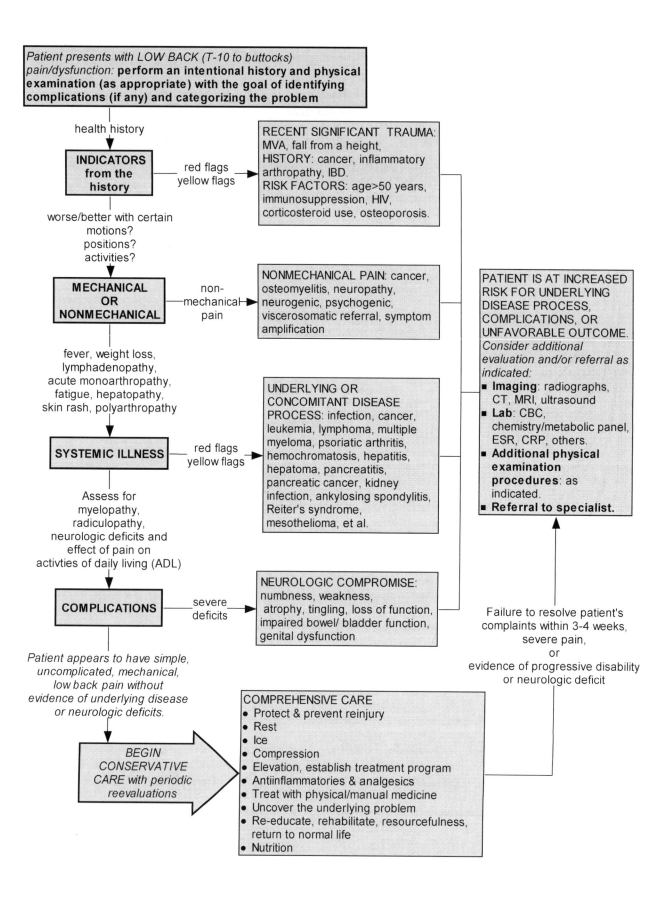

Algorithm for the Assessment and Management of Low Back Complaints

High-Risk Pain Patients

When a patient has musculoskeletal pain and any of the following characteristics, radiographs should be considered as an appropriate component of comprehensive evaluation. These considerations are particularly—though not exclusively—relevant for spine and low back pain.[16]

1. **More than 50 years of age**
2. **Physical trauma** (accident, fall, etc.)
3. **Pain at night**
4. **Back pain not relieved by lying supine**
5. **Neurologic deficits** (motor or sensory)
6. **Unexplained weight loss**
7. **Documentation or suspicion of inflammatory arthropathy**[17]
   - **Ankylosing spondylitis**
   - **Lupus**
   - **Rheumatoid arthritis**
   - **Juvenile rheumatoid arthritis**
   - **Psoriatic arthritis**

> Strongly consider the possibility of **osteoporotic fracture** in any patient—regardless of age or gender—who presents with spinal pain following multi-year use of **corticosteroids/prednisone** as treatment for a chronic inflammatory disorder.
>
> This applies both to *new patients with a previous history of long-term* pain as well as *long-term patients with new pain.*
>
> This continues to apply to patients for months and a few years after they have discontinued multi-year use of **corticosteroids/prednisone.**

8. **Drug or alcohol abuse** (increased risk of infection, nutritional deficiencies, anesthesia)
9. **History of cancer**
10. **Intravenous drug use**
11. **Immunosuppression, due to illness (e.g., HIV) or medications (e.g., steroids or cyclosporine)**
12. **History of corticosteroid use** (causes osteoporosis and increased risk for infection)
13. **Fever above 100° F or suspicion of septic arthritis or osteomyelitis**
14. **Diabetes** (increased risk of infection, nutritional deficiencies, anesthesia)
15. **Hypertension** (abdominal aneurysm: low back pain, nausea, pulsatile abdominal mass)
16. **Recent visit for same problem and not improved**
17. **Patient seeking compensation for pain/ injury** (increased need for documentation)
18. **Skin lesion** (psoriasis, melanoma, dermatomyositis, the butterfly rash of lupus, scars from previous surgery, accident, etc.…)
19. **Deformity or immobility**
20. **Lymphadenopathy** (suggests cancer or infection)
21. **Elevated ESR/CRP** (cancer, infection, inflammatory disorder)
22. **Elevated WBC count**
23. **Elevated alkaline phosphatase** (bone lesions, metabolic bone disease, hepatopathy)
24. **Elevated acid phosphatase** (occasionally used to monitor prostate cancer)
25. **Positive rheumatoid factor and/or CCP—cyclic citrullinated protein antibodies**
26. **Positive HLA-B27** (propensity for inflammatory arthropathies)
27. **Serum gammopathy** (multiple myeloma is the most common primary bone tumor)
28. **High-risk for disease:** *examples:*
    - Long-term heavy smoking of cigarettes
    - Long-term exposure to radiation
    - Obesity
29. **Strong family history of inflammatory, musculoskeletal, or malignant disease**

---

[16] Remember that metastasis often travel first from the primary site to bone, therefore bone pain may be an early manifestation of occult cancer. Most of the above are from "Table 1: The high-risk patient: clinical indications for radiography in low back pain patients." J Taylor, DC, DACBR, D Resnick, MD. Imaging decisions in the management of low back pain. Advances in Chiropractic. Mosby Year Book. 1994; 1-28

[17] Radiographs are often essential for diagnosis or to rule out complications of the disease. For example, in patients with inflammatory arthropathies such as these, spontaneous rupture of the transverse ligament (at the odontoid process) has been reported; although rare, this complication could be life-threatening if mismanaged or undiagnosed.

Major differential diagnoses:

- Initial evaluation of patients with spondyloarthropathy must include consideration of numerous differential diagnoses which may mimic or co-exist with inflammatory spondyloarthropathy. See table of *Differential Diagnoses* at the end of this chapter, as well as *algorithm for patient assessment and management*. Useful categories during the evaluation of low-back pain include the following:
    1. <u>Serious organic diseases requiring immediate attention</u>: Metastatic disease, viscerosomatic referral, osteomyelitis/discitis, aortic aneurysm.
    2. <u>Serious musculoskeletal disorders requiring immediate attention</u>: Recent fracture (pathologic fracture, osteoporosis, compression fracture, fall from a height, major motor vehicle accident), cauda equina syndrome, and severe radiculopathy (i.e., severe pain or progressive muscular deficits).
    3. <u>Rheumatologic disorders affecting the low back and pelvis</u>: Ankylosing spondylitis, reactive arthritis, enteropathic spondyloarthropathy, psoriatic arthritis, rheumatoid arthritis, and fibromyalgia.
    4. <u>Psychogenic</u>: Emotional overlay, symptom amplification, secondary gain, depression.
    5. <u>Benign musculoskeletal disorders requiring conservative treatment and monitoring</u>: Muscle spasm, facet irritation, disc injuries causing radiculitis or radiculopathy, self-limiting inflammation due to injury.
    6. <u>Functional, metabolic, allergic or nutritional causes of low-back pain</u>: Food allergies, obesity leading to a systemic inflammatory state as well as biomechanical stress on the lumbar spine, vitamin D deficiency[18], acidifying diet[19] (i.e., the Standard American Diet[20,21]).

<u>Specific differential diagnoses</u>

- <u>Mechanical low back pain</u>
- <u>Traumatic low back pain, spinal strain/sprain</u>
- <u>Cauda equina syndrome</u>
- <u>Vitamin D deficiency</u>: Vitamin D deficiency causes inflammation and low-back pain. Measure 25(OH)vitamin D in serum or supplement with 4,000-10,000 IU daily for at least three months[22] unless contraindicated by drugs (e.g., hydrochlorothiazide) or hypercalcemic condition (e.g., sarcoidosis, cancer, or hyperparathyroidism, etc.).[23]
- <u>Spinal degeneration, degenerative arthritis of the spine</u>
- <u>Spinal fracture</u>: Patients with AS may experience fracture following trivial "injury" such as rolling over in bed: **"Fracture should be suspected whenever a [AS] patient complains of new back pain."**[24]
- <u>Osteitis condensans ilii</u>
- <u>Cancer, malignant disease</u>
- <u>Vertebral osteomyelitis, infectious discitis</u>
- <u>Muscle spasm</u>
- <u>Developmental/congenital sacralization of the lumbar vertebrae</u>
- <u>Other autoimmune disease</u>
- <u>Lung disease</u>: asthma, COPD, bronchitis, tuberculosis
- <u>Iron overload</u>: Hemochromatosis may resemble ankylosing spondylitis clinically and radiographically.[25]
- <u>Fibromyalgia</u>: ESR, CRP, thyroid tests, ANA and most other 'basic' tests are normal; assess and treat for bacterial overgrowth of the small bowel.[26]

---

[18] Al Faraj S, Al Mutairi K. Vitamin D deficiency and chronic low back pain in Saudi Arabia. *Spine*. 2003 Jan 15;28(2):177-9

[19] "The results show that a disturbed acid-base balance may contribute to the symptoms of low back pain. The simple and safe addition of an alkaline multimineral preparate was able to reduce the pain symptoms in these patients with chronic low back pain." Vormann J,Worlitschek M,Goedecke T,Silver B. Supplementation with alkaline minerals reduces symptoms in patients with chronic low back pain. *J Trace Elem Med Biol*. 2001;15(2-3):179-83

[20] Seaman DR. The diet-induced proinflammatory state: a cause of chronic pain and other degenerative diseases? *J Manipulative Physiol Ther*. 2002 Mar-Apr;25(3):168-79

[21] Cordain L: *The Paleo Diet*. John Wiley & Sons Inc., New York 2002

[22] Al Faraj S, Al Mutairi K. Vitamin D deficiency and chronic low back pain in Saudi Arabia. *Spine*. 2003 Jan 15;28(2):177-9

[23] Vasquez A, Manso G, Cannell J. The clinical importance of vitamin D (cholecalciferol): a paradigm shift with implications for all healthcare providers. *Altern Ther Health Med*. 2004 Sep-Oct;10(5):28-36

[24] Harley JB, Scofield RH. The spectrum of ankylosing spondylitis. *Hosp Pract (Off Ed)* 1995 Jul 15;30(7):37-43, 46

[25] Bywaters EGL, Hamilton EBD, Williams R. The spine in idiopathic hemochromatosis. *Ann Rheum Dis* 1971; 30: 453-65

[26] Pimentel M, et al. A link between irritable bowel syndrome and fibromyalgia may be related to findings on lactulose breath testing. *Ann Rheum Dis*. 2004 Apr;63:450-2

- Diffuse idiopathic skeletal hyperostosis (DISH): DISH generally affects the longitudinal ligaments of the spine rather than the intervertebral discs. Cervical involvement generally precedes that of the lumbar spine, and the condition is strongly associated with diabetes mellitus.

Clinical assessments:
- **History/subjective**: See clinical presentations
  - **Typical presentation is that of dull achy pain in the low-back—worse in the morning and improving as the day progresses and/or with activity.**
  - **Systemic manifestations may or may not be present in the early stages of disease.**
- **Physical examination/objective**:
  - ROM, neurologic assessments; orthopedic assessments
  - Specialty examinations may be indicated:
    - Eye exam: for retinal and anterior chamber abnormalities; external exam for scleritis
    - Genital examination and/or assessment for UTI and STDs: Indicated in patients with ReA due to high association with sexually transmitted diseases. Urethral swab for culture and DNA probes are commonly indicated.
    - Cardiopulmonary assessment: common considerations include auscultation, measurement of thoracic excursion, and spirometry. Chest radiographs may be indicated.
    - Neurologic examination: A screening neurologic examination should be performed as part of the initial assessment of all patients and more detailed examinations are carried out when indicated.
    - Schober test: Draw a line over the spinous process of L5, then mark a line 10 cm above and 5 cm below; with lumbar flexion, the total distance should increase from 15 cm to 20 cm—less than 5 cm excursion indicates spinal rigidity, consistent with AS.
    - Occiput-to-wall distance: This assessment can be used to quantify progression/regression of cervical flexion in patients with AS.
    - Chest expansion: Use tape measure around lower thorax; measure chest circumference before and after inhalation; use along with spirometry to monitor thoracic stiffness in patients with AS.
- **Laboratory assessments**:
  - ESR or CRP: These are generally elevated, and neither test is superior to the other in the assessment of patients with AS. One study[27] used a unique approach to differentiate active disease from inactive disease in patients with AS; they added the ESR value (measured in mm/h) and CRP value (measured in mg/L) and classified patients as having active inflammatory disease if the total was greater than thirty (30).
  - Rheumatoid factor (RF): Characteristically **negative** *by definition* in patients with sero**negative** spondyloarthropathies. Positivity suggests rheumatoid spondylitis or concomitant RA with another spondyloarthropathy.
  - CBC: Look for evidence of true *infection* (in contrast to *dysbiosis*); also assess for anemia, which may be secondary to renal failure, NSAID gastropathy, chronic inflammation, or nutritional inadequacy.
  - Comprehensive metabolic panel: Assess as indicated for complications and concomitant disease.
  - Comprehensive stool analysis with comprehensive parasitology: **All patients with AS, RA, and PsA have gastrointestinal dysbiosis until proven otherwise.** Use of comprehensive stool tests should be the standard of care for all patients with AS, RA, PsA, and of course those with enteropathic spondyloarthropathy. Patients with ReA due to gastroenteritis or those

---

[27] Maki-Ikola O, Lehtinen K, Nissila M, Granfors K. IgM, IgA and IgG class serum antibodies against Klebsiella pneumoniae and Escherichia coli lipopolysaccharides in patients with ankylosing spondylitis. *Br J Rheumatol* 1994 Nov;33(11):1025-9

whose primary infection has not been identified/eliminated are also obvious candidates for stool testing; the most commonly implicated microbes are *Salmonella*, *Shigella*, and *Yersinia*. Regarding the etiopathogenesis of AS, the most commonly implicated microbes are *Klebsiella* and *E. coli*. However, it is more accurate to see that microbes incite autoimmunity/inflammation by numerous mechanisms and that exposure to numerous microbes—each one of which *in isolation* may be innocuous—in combination leads to additive and synergistic proinflammatory effects, as reviewed in Chapter 4 in the section on multifocal dysbiosis and elsewhere in a recent publication by the current author.[28]

Microorganisms clinically or molecularly associated with induction of seronegative spondyloarthropathy, ankylosing spondylitis, and reactive arthritis
• *Campylobacter* spp
• *Chlamydia trachomatis*
• *Citrobacter freundii*
• *E. coli*
• *Giardia lamblia*
• *Helicobacter pylori*
• *Klebsiella pneumoniae*
• *Mycoplasma* spp
• *Proteus mirabilis*
• *Salmonella typhimurium*
• *Shigella flexneri*
• *Shigella sonnei*
• *Staphylococcus aureus*
• *Streptococcus pyogenes*
• *Ureaplasma* spp
• *Yersinia enterocolitica*

o **Serologic and genital tests for sexually transmitted diseases**: These tests are particularly indicated in patients with ReA due to the frequent association of this disorder with genitourinary infections, particularly those caused by *Chlamydia*. Numerous articles have shown that patients with long-term idiopathic oligoarthritis harbor "silent infections"—otherwise known as dysbiosis—in the genitourinary and gastrointestinal tracts; the most commonly identified organisms are *Chlamydia trachomatis*, *Yersinia*, *Salmonella*, *Mycoplasma*, and *Ureaplasma*.[29,30]

o **Serum vitamin D**: Measure 25(OH)vitamin D in all patients and/or begin empiric treatment with physiologic doses of vitamin D3. Emulsified cholecalciferol is particularly efficacious in older patients and those with malabsorption due to enteropathy.[31] According to research by Falkenbach et al[32], **"Patients with ankylosing spondylitis may have extremely low levels of 25(OH)D."** Vitamin D deficiency appears common in patients with low-back pain[33], limb pain[34], chronic persistent musculoskeletal pain[35], and in general medical patients.[36] [37] In our review of the literature[38], we concluded that **optimal serum 25(OH)-vitamin D levels should be defined as 40 – 65 ng/mL (100 - 160 nmol/L)** and that, "Until proven otherwise, the balance of the research clearly indicates that oral supplementation in the range of 1,000 IU per day for infants, 2,000 IU per day for children and **4,000 IU per day for adults** is safe and reasonable to meet physiologic requirements, to promote optimal health, and to reduce the risk of several serious diseases. Safety and effectiveness of supplementation are assured by periodic monitoring of serum 25(OH)D and serum calcium." For additional research on the

[28] Vasquez A. Reducing Pain and Inflammation Naturally. Part 6: Nutritional and Botanical Treatments Against "Silent Infections" and Gastrointestinal Dysbiosis, Commonly Overlooked Causes of Neuromusculoskeletal Inflammation and Chronic Health Problems. *Nutritional Perspectives* 2006; January

[29] "Urogenital swab cultures showed a microbial infection in 44% of the patients with oligoarthritis (15% Chlamydia, 14% Mycoplasma, 28% Ureaplasma), whereas in the control group only 26% had a positive result (4% Chlamydia, 7% Mycoplasma, 21% Ureaplasma)." Erlacher L, Wintersberger W, Menschik M, Benke-Studnicka A, Machold K, Stanek G, Soltz-Szots J, Smolen J, Graninger W. Reactive arthritis: urogenital swab culture is the only useful diagnostic method for the detection of the arthritogenic infection in extra-articularly asymptomatic patients with undifferentiated oligoarthritis. *Br J Rheumatol.* 1995 Sep;34(9):838-42

[30] Fendler C, et al. Frequency of triggering bacteria in patients with reactive arthritis and undifferentiated oligoarthritis and the relative importance of the tests used for diagnosis. *Ann Rheum Dis.* 2001 Apr;60(4):337-43 http://ard.bmjjournals.com/cgi/content/full/60/4/337

[31] Vasquez A. Subphysiologic Doses of Vitamin D are Subtherapeutic: Comment on the Study by The Record Trial Group. *The Lancet* Published on-line May 6, 2005

[32] "Patients with ankylosing spondylitis may have extremely low levels of 25(OH)D." Falkenbach A, Tripathi R, Sedlmeyer A, Staudinger M, Herold M.Serum 25-hydroxyvitamin D and parathyroid hormone in patients with ankylosing spondylitis before and after a three-week rehabilitation treatment at high altitude during winter and spring. *Wien Klin Wochenschr.* 2001 Apr 30;113(9):328-32

[33] Al Faraj S, Al Mutairi K. Vitamin D deficiency and chronic low back pain in Saudi Arabia. *Spine.* 2003 Jan 15;28(2):177-9

[34] Masood H, Narang AP, Bhat IA, Shah GN. Persistent limb pain and raised serum alkaline phosphatase the earliest markers of subclinical hypovitaminosis D in Kashmir. *Indian J Physiol Pharmacol.* 1989 Oct-Dec;33(4):259-61

[35] Plotnikoff GA, Quigley JM. Prevalence of severe hypovitaminosis D in patients with persistent, nonspecific musculoskeletal pain. *Mayo Clin Proc.* 2003 Dec;78(12):1463-70

[36] Thomas MK, Lloyd-Jones DM, Thadhani RI, Shaw AC, Deraska DJ, Kitch BT, Vamvakas EC, Dick IM, Prince RL, Finkelstein JS. Hypovitaminosis D in medical inpatients. *N Engl J Med.* 1998 Mar 19;338(12):777-83

[37] Kauppinen-Makelin R, Tahtela R, Loyttyniemi E, Karkkainen J, Valimaki MJ. A high prevalence of hypovitaminosis D in Finnish medical in- and outpatients. *J Intern Med.* 2001 Jun;249(6):559-63

[38] Vasquez A, Manso G, Cannell J. The Clinical Importance of Vitamin D (Cholecalciferol): A Paradigm Shift with Implications for All Healthcare Providers. *Alternative Therapies in Health and Medicine* and *Integrative Medicine: A Clinician's Journal*

importance and safety of vitamin D, see the articles by Vieth[39], Heaney et al[40], Holick[41], and Vasquez, Manso, and Cannell.[42] Vitamin D supplementation 5,000 – 10,000 IU per day for adults was shown to alleviate low-back pain after 3 months in nearly all patients with low initial serum levels of vitamin D.[43]

- o Testing for multifocal dysbiosis: If the intestinal and genitourinary tracts appear clear of infection following direct testing, then empiric antimicrobial treatment should be considered. Following this, searching for other loci of infection—namely the mouth, throat, nose, sinuses, lungs, and skin—should be pursued as discussed in Chapter 4.
- o HLA-B27: This marker is seen with increased prevalence in patients with AS and ReA. The test can be used to support the diagnosis, particularly early in the course of the illness when radiographs are *negative*.
- o Hormone assessments: These should be performed as detailed in Chapter 4 and/or as indicated per patient.

- **Imaging**:
  - o Plain radiographs: In contrast to most of the other rheumatic disorders wherein radiographs are generally unnecessary in early stages of the disease, plain radiographs are of tremendous value in the assessment of spondylitis and sacroiliitis and are generally diagnostic once the diagnostic threshold has been crossed; i.e., they may be negative in early disease, but become positive after a given amount of time, which varies per patient and per disease. Characteristic initial findings in AS are lumbar syndesmophytes and sacroiliitis.
  - o MRI and CT imaging: Generally reserved for the evaluation of spinal stenosis and inflammatory myelopathy. **CT imaging is more sensitive than plain radiography for the initial evaluation of sacroiliitis.**[44] Also used for assessment of other complications as indicated.

- **Establishing the diagnosis**:
  - o Inflammatory spondyloarthropathy as a general term can be diagnosed with a combination of serologic, clinical, and radiographic findings. The subtype of spondyloarthropathy—AS, ReA, PsA, RA, ES, etc—is then distinguished based on the details of the clinical history (e.g., inflammatory bowel disease or recent infection), presentation, clinical findings, serologic tests, and radiographic characteristics.

Complications:

- Chronic pain, significant physical limitations and significant morbidity
- Renal failure, secondary to amyloidosis or medications such as sulfasalazine or NSAID's
- Spinal fracture (in patients with spinal ankylosis following minor trauma)
- Respiratory insufficiency
- Immobility
- Permanent disability due to rigid spinal flexion secondary to bony ankylosis resulting in loss of spinal motion
- Neurologic compromise: due to spinal stenosis, transverse myelopathy, atlantoaxial subluxation, cauda equina fibrosis[45], or cauda equina syndrome

[39] Vieth R. Vitamin D supplementation, 25-hydroxyvitamin D concentrations, and safety. *Am J Clin Nutr*. 1999 May;69(5):842-56
[40] Heaney RP, Davies KM, Chen TC, Holick MF, Barger-Lux MJ. Human serum 25-hydroxycholecalciferol response to extended oral dosing with cholecalciferol. *Am J Clin Nutr*. 2003 Jan;77(1):204-10
[41] Holick MF. Vitamin D: importance in the prevention of cancers, type 1 diabetes, heart disease, and osteoporosis. *Am J Clin Nutr*. 2004 Mar;79(3):362-71
[42] Vasquez A, Manso G, Cannell J. The Clinical Importance of Vitamin D (Cholecalciferol): A Paradigm Shift with Implications for All Healthcare Providers. *Alternative Therapies in Health and Medicine* and *Integrative Medicine: A Clinician's Journal* In press: See www.optimalhealthresearch.com/monograph04
[43] Al Faraj S, Al Mutairi K. Vitamin D deficiency and chronic low back pain in Saudi Arabia. *Spine*. 2003 Jan 15;28(2):177-9
[44] Tierney ML. McPhee SJ, Papadakis MA. Current Medical Diagnosis and Treatment 2006. 45th edition. New York; Lange Medical Books: 2006, pages 851-855
[45] Tierney ML. McPhee SJ, Papadakis MA. Current Medical Diagnosis and Treatment 2006. 45th edition. New York; Lange Medical Books: 2006, page 852

<u>Clinical management</u>:
- Referral if clinical outcome is unsatisfactory or as otherwise indicated.

<u>Treatments</u>[46]
- <u>NSAIDs</u>, especially <u>indomethacin</u> 25-50 mg thrice daily—"side effects" of indomethacin include headache, giddiness, psychosis, depression, nausea, vomiting, gastric ulcer, and renal impairment. <u>Sulfasalazine</u>: 1,000 mg twice daily.
- <u>Corticosteroids</u> are notably ineffective in the treatment of spondyloarthropathy, though they are commonly used against complications such as uveitis.
- <u>TNF inhibitors</u>: Etanercept 25 mg subcutaneously twice weekly, or <u>infliximab</u> 5 mg/kg every other month. These drugs are clinically effective from the perspective of anti-inflammation, but they are associated with increased risks for lymphoma, serious infections including pulmonary tuberculosis, congestive heart failure, demyelinating diseases, and systemic lupus erythematosus.
- <u>Methotrexate</u>: Used for recalcitrant psoriatic arthritis.[47]
- <u>Avoidance of pro-inflammatory foods</u>: Pro-inflammatory foods act *directly* and *indirectly* to promote and exacerbate systemic inflammation. *See previous detailing.*
- <u>Supplemented Paleo-Mediterranean diet</u>: The health-promoting diet of choice for the majority of people is a diet based on abundant consumption of fruits, vegetables, seeds, nuts, omega-3 and monounsaturated fatty acids, and lean sources of protein such as lean meats, fatty cold-water fish, soy and whey proteins. *See previous detailing.*
- <u>Avoidance of allergenic foods</u>: Any patient may be allergic to any food, even if the food is generally considered a health-promoting food. *See previous detailing.*
- <u>Gluten-free vegetarian/vegan diet</u>: Vegetarian/vegan diets have a place in the treatment plan of all patients with autoimmune/inflammatory disorders.[48,49,50,51] *See previous detailing.*
- <u>Short-term fasting</u>: Whether the foundational diet is Paleo-Mediterranean, vegetarian, vegan, or a combination of all of these, autoimmune/inflammatory patients will still benefit from periodic fasting, whether on a weekly (e.g., every Saturday), monthly (every first week or weekend of the month, or every other month), or yearly (1-2 weeks of the year) basis. *See previous detailing.*
- <u>Broad-spectrum fatty acid therapy with ALA, EPA, DHA, GLA and oleic acid</u>: Fatty acid supplementation should be delivered in the form of combination therapy with ALA, GLA, DHA, and EPA. *See previous detailing.*
- <u>Vitamin D3 supplementation with physiologic doses and/or tailored to serum 25(OH)D levels</u>: Vitamin D deficiency is common in the general population and is even more common in patients with chronic illness and chronic musculoskeletal pain.[52] Correction of vitamin D deficiency supports normal immune function against infection and provides a clinically significant anti-inflammatory[53]

[46] Tierney ML. McPhee SJ, Papadakis MA. Current Medical Diagnosis and Treatment 2006. 45th edition. New York; Lange Medical Books: 2006, pages 851-855
[47] Tierney ML. McPhee SJ, Papadakis MA. Current Medical Diagnosis and Treatment 2006. 45th edition. New York; Lange Medical Books: 2006, pages 851-855
[48] "The immunoglobulin G (IgG) antibody levels against gliadin and beta-lactoglobulin decreased in the responder subgroup in the vegan diet-treated patients, but not in the other analysed groups." Hafstrom I, Ringertz B, Spangberg A, von Zweigbergk L, Brannemark S, Nylander I, Ronnelid J, Laasonen L, Klareskog L. A vegan diet free of gluten improves the signs and symptoms of rheumatoid arthritis: the effects on arthritis correlate with a reduction in antibodies to food antigens. *Rheumatology* (Oxford). 2001 Oct;40(10):1175-9 http://rheumatology.oxfordjournals.org/cgi/content/abstract/40/10/1175
[49] "After four weeks at the health farm the diet group showed a significant improvement in number of tender joints, Ritchie's articular index, number of swollen joints, pain score, duration of morning stiffness, grip strength, erythrocyte sedimentation rate, C-reactive protein, white blood cell count, and a health assessment questionnaire score." Kjeldsen-Kragh J, Haugen M, Borchgrevink CF, Laerum E, Eek M, Mowinkel P, Hovi K, Forre O. Controlled trial of fasting and one-year vegetarian diet in rheumatoid arthritis. *Lancet*. 1991 Oct 12;338(8772):899-902
[50] "During fasting, arthralgia was less intense in many subjects. In some types of skin diseases (pustulosis palmaris et plantaris and atopic eczema) an improvement could be demonstrated during the fast. During the vegan diet, both signs and symptoms returned in most patients, with the exception of some patients with psoriasis who experienced an improvement." Lithell H, Bruce A, Gustafsson IB, Hoglund NJ, Karlstrom B, Ljunghall K, Sjolin K, Venge P, Werner I, Vessby B. A fasting and vegetarian diet treatment trial on chronic inflammatory disorders. *Acta Derm Venereol*. 1983;63(5):397-403
[51] Tanaka T, Kouda K, Kotani M, Takeuchi A, Tabei T, Masamoto Y, Nakamura H, Takigawa M, Suemura M, Takeuchi H, Kouda M. Vegetarian diet ameliorates symptoms of atopic dermatitis through reduction of the number of peripheral eosinophils and of PGE2 synthesis by monocytes. *J Physiol Anthropol Appl Human Sci*. 2001 Nov;20(6):353-61 http://www.jstage.jst.go.jp/article/jpa/20/6/20_353/_article/en
[52] Plotnikoff GA, Quigley JM. Prevalence of severe hypovitaminosis D in patients with persistent, nonspecific musculoskeletal pain. *Mayo Clin Proc*. 2003 Dec;78(12):1463-70
[53] Timms PM, Mannan N, Hitman GA, Noonan K, Mills PG, Syndercombe-Court D, Aganna E, Price CP, Boucher BJ. Circulating MMP9, vitamin D and variation in the TIMP-1 response with VDR genotype: mechanisms for inflammatory damage in chronic disorders? *QJM*. 2002 Dec;95(12):787-96 http://qjmed.oxfordjournals.org/cgi/content/full/95/12/787

and analgesic benefit in patients with back pain[54] and limb pain.[55] Reasonable daily doses for children and adults are 1,000-2,000 and 4,000 IU, respectively.[56] *See previous detailing.*

- **<u>Assessment for dysbiosis</u>: All patients with spondyloarthropathy and reactive arthritis have dysbiosis until proven otherwise by the combination of 1) three-sample comprehensive parasitology examinations performed by a specialty laboratory and 2) clinical response to at least two 2-4 week courses of broad-spectrum antimicrobial treatment.** Yeast, bacteria, and parasites are treated as indicated based on identification and sensitivity results from comprehensive parasitology assessments. Patients taking immunosuppressant drugs such as corticosteroids/prednisone have increased risk of intestinal bacterial overgrowth and translocation.[57,58] Other dysbiotic loci should be investigated as discussed in Chapter 4 in the section on multifocal dysbiosis. *See previous detailing.*

- <u>Orthoendocrinology</u>: Assess prolactin, cortisol, DHEA, free and total testosterone, serum estradiol, and thyroid status (e.g., TSH, T4, *and* anti-thyroid peroxidase antibodies). *See previous detailing.*

---

[54] Al Faraj S, Al Mutairi K. Vitamin D deficiency and chronic low back pain in Saudi Arabia. *Spine.* 2003 Jan 15;28(2):177-9

[55] Masood H, Narang AP, Bhat IA, Shah GN. Persistent limb pain and raised serum alkaline phosphatase the earliest markers of subclinical hypovitaminosis D in Kashmir. *Indian J Physiol Pharmacol.* 1989 Oct-Dec;33(4):259-61

[56] Vasquez A, Manso G, Cannell J. The clinical importance of vitamin D (cholecalciferol): a paradigm shift with implications for all healthcare providers. *Altern Ther Health Med.* 2004 Sep-Oct;10(5):28-36 http://optimalhealthresearch.com/monograph04

[57] "A 63-year-old man with systemic lupus erythematosus and selective IgA deficiency developed intractable diarrhoea the day after treatment with prednisone, 50 mg daily, was started. The diarrhoea was considered to be caused by bacterial overgrowth and was later successfully treated with doxycycline." Denison H, Wallerstedt S. Bacterial overgrowth after high-dose corticosteroid treatment. *Scand J Gastroenterol.* 1989 Jun;24(5):561-4

[58] "These bacteria also translocated to the mesenteric lymph nodes in mice injected with cyclophosphamide or prednisone." Berg RD, Wommack E, Deitch EA. Immunosuppression and intestinal bacterial overgrowth synergistically promote bacterial translocation. *Arch Surg.* 1988 Nov;123(11):1359-64

Vertebral Osteomyelitis
Infectious Discitis

Description/pathophysiology:
- Bacterial or fungal infection of the spine
- Back pain is common; spinal infection is relatively rare. Spinal infections are "a rare cause of common symptoms."[59]

Clinical presentations:
- Classic presentation: "...the diagnosis is suggested by the clinical findings: a sick patient with severe pain, a rigid back, fever, and a raised WBC and sedimentation rate."[60]
  - Patient generally appears sick with systemic manifestations: fatigue, sweats, anorexia, fever
  - Back/neck/spine pain (90%): Most common region for spinal osteomyelitis is the lumbar spine, followed by the thoracic spine, then the cervical spine. Cervical spine infections are more common in IV drug abusers
  - Pain may be acute, subacute, or chronic:
    - 30% of patients with vertebral osteomyelitis have had pain for 3 weeks to 3 months at time of diagnosis
    - 50% of patients with vertebral osteomyelitis have had pain for more than 3 months at time of diagnosis
  - Pain is continuous, intermittent, and/or "throbbing" and often worse at night
  - Pain is unrelated to motion or position (non-mechanical)
  - Localized stiffness
  - Elevated ESR/CRP
  - Vertebral osteomyelitis is more common in patients with a history of recurrent urinary tract infections and diabetes mellitus

> **Spinal infection is a medical urgency**
> "Up to 10-15% of patients with vertebral osteomyelitis will develop neurologic findings or frank spinal-cord compression."
>
> King RW, Johnson D. Osteomyelitis. Updated July 13, 2006. *eMedicine* emedicine.com/emerg/topic349.htm

- Atypical presentations: as many as 15% of affected patients
  - Little or no fever
  - Little or no back or neck pain
  - Little or no local tenderness
  - Cervical osteomyelitis may present with headache, dysphagia, sore throat rather than febrile neck pain
  - Vertebral osteomyelitis of the thoracic and lumbar spine may present with pain in the chest, shoulder, abdominal, hip or leg
  - Risk factors: IV drug use, DM, history of septicemia, spinal trauma, pulmonary tuberculosis, urinary tract infections, surgery, older men

Major differential diagnoses:
- Benign neck or back pain
- Degenerative disc disease
- Tumor
- Fracture
- Spondyloarthropathies: In particular, reactive arthritis is a difficult differential in this situation because of the concomitant infection (perhaps with fever and systemic symptoms) and back pain. Differentiation may be difficult, but is generally possible based on the severity of the systemic

---

[59] Strausbaugh LJ. Vertebral osteomyelitis. How to differentiate it from other causes of back and neck pain. *Postgrad Med* 1995 Jun;97(6):147-8, 151-4
[60] Macnab I, McCulloch J. Backache. Second Edition. Williams and Wilkins: Baltimore, 1990

manifestations and local examination findings. Patients with *focal pain*—particularly that which is exacerbated by vertebral percussion—should be further evaluated for osteomyelitis, fracture, or acute disc herniation

<u>Clinical assessment</u>:

- **<u>History/subjective</u>:**
  o Spinal pain
  o Malaise: may or may not have systemic symptoms
- **<u>Physical examination/objective</u>:**
  o Mild local tenderness
  o Paravertebral muscle spasm with limited ROM
  o Fever (50%)
  o Neurologic signs (20-40%)
  o Spinal percussion is positive for pain
  o May have painful and limited SLR due to hamstring spasm
- **<u>Imaging & laboratory assessments</u>:**
  o High ESR—elevated to 20-100 mm/hr in 90% of patients. ESR was considered "the most useful test for monitoring the disease activity and the efficacy of treatment."[61]
  o 50% have slight elevation of WBC.
  o The disc space is the first structure destroyed—the clinician and radiologist must not misinterpret early signs of infection with "degenerative disc disease."
  o **MRI has a sensitivity and specificity of >90% and also helps to assess epidural abscess.**
  o Radiographs are positive in 80% after the condition has been present for at least 10-14 days.
  o Bone scan is diagnostic in 90% of cases.
  o "Computed tomography is the imaging study of choice for preoperative evaluation and biopsy procedures. It is not a good screening test…"[62] and is generally used after routine radiographs and/or bone scan.

<u>Establishing the diagnosis</u>:
- Diagnosis is established based on a consistent spectrum of clinical signs and symptoms and is confirmed with imaging and/or biopsy, aspiration, and/or blood cultures

<u>Complications</u>:
- Abscesses
- Meningitis
- Vertebral collapse, fracture
- Neurologic injury: paralysis
- Septicemia and death

<u>Clinical management</u>:
- Immediate/urgent referral for diagnostic procedures, IV and oral antimicrobials, and surgery if needed

<u>Treatments</u>:
- **<u>Antimicrobial drugs</u>: Organism-specific IV/oral antimicrobials are often administered on an in-patient basis.**
- <u>Rest</u>: Bed rest, bracing, activity limitation

---

[61] Macnab I, McCulloch J. *Backache. Second Edition*. Williams and Wilkins: Baltimore, 1990
[62] Strausbaugh LJ. Vertebral osteomyelitis. How to differentiate it from other causes of back and neck pain. Postgrad Med 1995 Jun;97(6):147-8, 151-4

- <u>Surgery</u>: Surgery for debridement and complications such as cord compression, vertebral collapse or instability.
- **Immunonutrition:** Immunonutritional considerations are listed below; doses listed are for adults. General benefits derived from the use of immunonutrition are reductions in severity/frequency/duration of major infections, abbreviated hospitalization (i.e., early discharge due to expedited healing and recovery), reductions in the need for medications, significant improvements in survival, and hospital savings.[63,64,65,66,67,68,69]
  - <u>Paleo-Mediterranean diet</u>: As detailed later in this text and elsewhere[70,71]
  - <u>Vitamin and mineral supplementation</u>: anti-infective benefits shown in elderly diabetics[72]
  - <u>High-dose vitamin A</u>: Vitamin A shows potent immunosupportive benefits, and vitamin A stores are depleted by the stress of infection and injury. Consider 200,000-300,000 IU per day of retinol palmitate for 1-4 weeks, then taper; reduce dose or discontinue with onset of toxicity symptoms such as skin problems (dry skin, flaking skin, chapped or split lips, red skin rash, hair loss), joint pain, bone pain, headaches, anorexia (loss of appetite), edema (water retention, weight gain, swollen ankles, difficulty breathing), fatigue, and/or liver damage.
  - <u>Arginine</u>: Dose for adults is in the range of 5-10 grams daily
  - <u>Fatty acid supplementation</u>: In contrast to the higher doses used to provide an anti-inflammatory effect in patients with autoimmune/inflammatory disorders, doses used for immunosupportive treatments should be kept rather modest to avoid the *relative* immunosuppression that has been controversially reported in patients treated with EPA and DHA. Reasonable doses are in the following ranges for adults: EPA+DHA: 500-1,500, and GLA: 300-500 mg.
  - <u>Glutamine</u>: Glutamine enhances bacterial killing by neutrophils[73], and administration of 18 grams per day in divided doses to patients in intensive care units was shown to improve survival, expedite hospital discharge, and reduce total healthcare costs.[74] Another study using glutamine 12-18 grams per day showed no benefit in overall mortality but significant benefits in terms of reduced healthcare costs (-30%) and significantly reduced need for medical interventions.[75] After

---

[63] "To evaluate the metabolic and immune effects of dietary arginine, glutamine and omega-3 fatty acids (fish oil) supplementation, we performed a prospective study... CONCLUSIONS: The feeding of Neomune in critically injured patients was well tolerated as Traumacal and significant improvement was observed in serum protein. Shorten ICU stay and wean-off respirator day may benefit from using the immunonutrient formula." Chuntrasakul C, Siltham S, Sarasombath S, Sittapairochana C, Leowattana W, Chockvivatanavanit S, Bunnak A. Comparison of a immunonutrition formula enriched arginine, glutamine and omega-3 fatty acid, with a currently high-enriched enteral nutrition for trauma patients. *J Med Assoc Thai.* 2003 Jun;86(6):552-6

[64] "CONCLUSIONS: In conclusion, arginine-enhanced formula improves fistula rates in postoperative head and neck cancer patients and decreases length of stay." de Luis DA, Izaola O, Cuellar L, Terroba MC, Aller R. Randomized clinical trial with an enteral arginine-enhanced formula in early postsurgical head and neck cancer patients. *Eur J Clin Nutr.* 2004;58(11):1505-8

[65] "In this prospective, randomised, double-blind, placebo-controlled study, we randomly assigned 50 patients who were scheduled to undergo coronary artery bypass to receive either an oral immune-enhancing nutritional supplement containing L-arginine, omega3 polyunsaturated fatty acids, and yeast RNA (n=25), or a control (n=25) for a minimum of 5 days... Intake of an oral immune-enhancing nutritional supplement for a minimum of 5 days before surgery can improve outlook in high-risk patients who are undergoing elective cardiac surgery." Tepaske R, Velthuis H, Oudemans-van Straaten HM, Heisterkamp SH, van Deventer SJ, Ince C, Eysman L, Kesecioglu J. Effect of preoperative oral immune-enhancing nutritional supplement on patients at high risk of infection after cardiac surgery: a randomised placebo-controlled trial. *Lancet.* 2001 Sep 1;358(9283):696-701

[66] "The feeding of IMMUNE FORMULA was well tolerated and significant improvement was observed in nutritional and immunologic parameters as in other immunoenhancing diets. Further clinical trials of prospective double-blind randomized design are necessary to address the so that the necessity of using immunonutrition in critically ill patients will be clarified." Chuntrasakul C, Siltharm S, Sarasombath S, Sittapairochana C, Leowattana W, Chockvivatanavanit S, Bunnak A. Metabolic and immune effects of dietary arginine, glutamine and omega-3 fatty acids supplementation in immunocompromised patients. *J Med Assoc Thai.* 1998 May;81(5):334-43

[67] "enteral diet supplemented with arginine, dietary nucleotides, and omega-3 fatty acids (IMPACT, Sandoz Nutrition, Bern, Switzerland) " Senkal M, Mumme A, Eickhoff U, Geier B, Spath G, Wulfert D, Joosten U, Frei A, Kemen M. Early postoperative enteral immunonutrition: clinical outcome and cost-comparison analysis in surgical patients. *Crit Care Med* 1997;25(9):1489-96

[68] "supplemented diet with glutamine, arginine and omega-3-fatty acids... It was clearly established in this trial that early postoperative enteral feeding is safe in patients who have undergone major operations for gastrointestinal cancer. Supplementation of enteral nutrition with glutamine, arginine, and omega-3-fatty acids positively modulated postsurgical immunosuppressive and inflammatory responses." Wu GH, Zhang YW, Wu ZH. Modulation of postoperative immune and inflammatory response by immune-enhancing enteral diet in gastrointestinal cancer patients. *World J Gastroenterol.* 2001 Jun;7(3):357-62 http://www.wjgnet.com/1007-9327/7/357.pdf

[69] "using a formula supplemented with arginine, mRNA, and omega-3 fatty acids from fish oil (Impact)... CONCLUSIONS: Immune-enhancing enteral nutrition resulted in a significant reduction in the mortality rate and infection rate in septic patients admitted to the ICU. These reductions were greater for patients with less severe illness." Galban C, Montejo JC, Mesejo A, Marco P, Celaya S, Sanchez-Segura JM, Farre M, Bryg DJ. An immune-enhancing enteral diet reduces mortality rate and episodes of bacteremia in septic intensive care unit patients. *Crit Care Med.* 2000 Mar;28(3):643-8

[70] Vasquez A. A Five-Part Nutritional Protocol that Produces Consistently Positive Results. *Nutritional Wellness* 2005 September

[71] Vasquez A. Implementing the Five-Part Nutritional Wellness Protocol for the Treatment of Various Health Problems. *Nutritional Wellness* 2005 November.

[72] "CONCLUSIONS: A multivitamin and mineral supplement reduced the incidence of participant-reported infection and related absenteeism in a sample of participants with type 2 diabetes mellitus and a high prevalence of subclinical micronutrient deficiency." Barringer TA et al. Effect of a multivitamin and mineral supplement on infection and quality of life. A randomized, double-blind, placebo-controlled trial. *Ann Intern Med.* 2003 Mar 4;138(5):365-71 http://www.annals.org/cgi/reprint/138/5/365

[73] Furukawa S, Saito H, Fukatsu K, Hashiguchi Y, Inaba T, Lin MT, Inoue T, Han I, Matsuda T, Muto T. Glutamine-enhanced bacterial killing by neutrophils from postoperative patients. *Nutrition* 1997;13(10):863-9. *In vitro* study.

[74] Griffiths RD, Jones C, Palmer TE. Six-month outcome of critically ill patients given glutamine-supplemented parenteral nutrition. *Nutrition* 1997 Apr;13(4):295-302

[75] "There was no mortality difference between those patients receiving glutamine-containing enteral feed and the controls. However, there was a significant reduction in the median postintervention ICU and hospital patient costs in the glutamine recipients $23 000 versus $30 900 in the control patients." Jones C, Palmer TE, Griffiths RD. Randomized clinical outcome study of critically ill patients given glutamine-supplemented enteral nutrition. *Nutrition.* 1999 Feb;15(2):108-15

administering glutamine 26 grams/d to severely burned patients, Garrel et al[76] concluded that glutamine reduced the risk of infection by 3-fold and that oral glutamine "may be a life-saving intervention" in patients with severe burns. A dose of 30 grams/d was used in a recent clinical trial showing hemodynamic benefit in patients with sickle cell anemia.[77] The highest glutamine dose that the current author is aware of is the study by Scheltinga et al[78] who used 0.57 gm/kg/day in cancer patients following chemotherapy administration; for a 220-lb-pt, this would be approximately 57 grams of glutamine per day.

- o <u>Melatonin</u>: 20-40 mg hs (*hora somni*—Latin: sleep time). Immunostimulatory anti-infective action of melatonin was demonstrated in a small clinical trial wherein septic newborns administered 20 mg melatonin showed significantly increased survival over nontreated controls.[79]

---

[76] The glutamine dose in this study was "a total of 26 g/day" administered in four divided doses. CONCLUSION: "The results of this prospective randomized clinical trial show that enteral G reduces blood culture positivity, particularly with P. aeruginosa, in adults with severe burns and may be a life-saving intervention." Garrel D, Patenaude J, Nedelec B, Samson L, Dorais J, Champoux J, D'Elia M, Bernier J. Decreased mortality and infectious morbidity in adult burn patients given enteral glutamine supplements: a prospective, controlled, randomized clinical trial. *Crit Care Med.* 2003 Oct;31(10):2444-9

[77] Niihara Y, Matsui NM, Shen YM, et al. L-glutamine therapy reduces endothelial adhesion of sickle red blood cells to human umbilical vein endothelial cells. *BMC Blood Disord.* 2005 Jul 25;5:4 http://www.biomedcentral.com.proxy.hsc.unt.edu/1471-2326/5/4

[78] "Subjects with hematologic malignancies in remission underwent a standard treatment of high-dose chemotherapy and total body irradiation before bone marrow transplantation. After completion of this regimen, they were randomized to receive either standard parenteral nutrition (STD, n = 10) or an isocaloric, isonitrogenous nutrient solution enriched with crystalline L-glutamine (0.57 g/kg/day, GLN, n = 10)." Scheltinga MR, Young LS, Benfell K, Bye RL, Ziegler TR, Santos AA, Antin JH, Schloerb PR, Wilmore DW. Glutamine-enriched intravenous feedings attenuate extracellular fluid expansion after a standard stress. *Ann Surg.* 1991 Oct;214(4):385-93; discussion 393-5 http://www.pubmedcentral.nih.gov/articlerender.fcgi?tool=pubmed&pubmedid=1953094 For additional review, see Ziegler TR. Glutamine supplementation in cancer patients receiving bone marrow transplantation and high dose chemotherapy. *J Nutr.* 2001 Sep;131(9 Suppl):2578S-84S http://jn.nutrition.org/cgi/content/full/131/9/2578S

[79] Gitto E, Karbownik M, Reiter RJ, Tan DX, Cuzzocrea S, Chiurazzi P, Cordaro S, Corona G, Trimarchi G, Barberi I. Effects of melatonin treatment in septic newborns. *Pediatr Res.* 2001 Dec;50(6):756-60 http://www.pedresearch.org/cgi/content/full/50/6/756

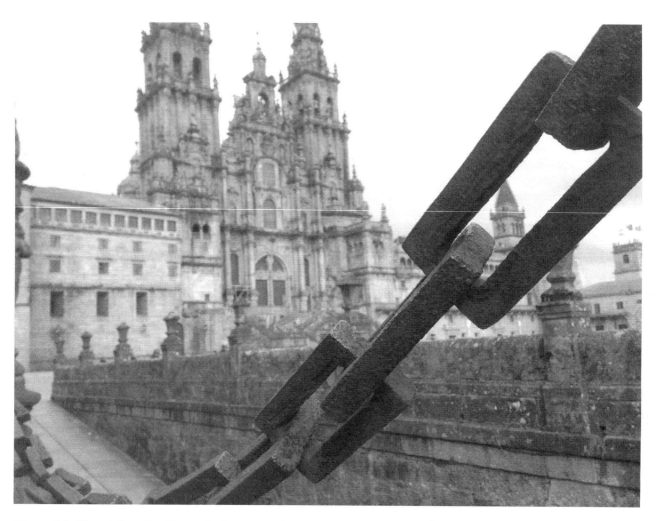

Plaza del Obradoiro, Santiago de Compostela, northern Spain (photo by Dr Vasquez, June 2013):
- "Many chains have been laid upon man so that he should no longer behave like an animal: and he has in truth become gentler, more spiritual, more joyful, more reflective than any animal is. Now, however, he suffers from having worn his chains for so long, from being deprived for so long of clean air and free movement... Only when this sickness from one's chains has also been overcome will the first great goal have truly been attained: the separation of man from the animals." Nietzsche FW. _The Wanderer and His Shadow_. #350
- "Emancipate yourself from mental slavery; none but ourselves can free our minds." Marley B ☺

Sjögren Syndrome/Disease

Introduction:
Sjögren Syndrome/Disease is a sustained inflammatory disorder characterized by inflammatory and destructive lymphocytic infiltrates in exocrine organs, leading to failure of these glands and the resultant complications reviewed in the section that follows. Common to other inflammatory and autoimmune disorders, the condition is multifactorial in accord with most of the categories addressed by the Functional Inflammology protocol and recalled by the FINDSEX acronym detailed in Chapter 4 and the accompanying videos. Readers are expected to have read Chapters 1 and 4 so that this chapter can focus on the more salient points specific for Sjögren Syndrome/Disease.
The condition is inaccurately named a "syndrome"—implying that it is a "group of symptoms that collectively indicate or characterize a disease or disorder"; however, this condition—like fibromyalgia—has distinct clinical and histopathological findings and is therefore more accurately described and legitimized as a "disease", which it properly is.

<u>Topics</u>:
- Introduction and Overview
- Clinical Presentation
- Prevalence, Symptoms, and Clinical Findings
- Pathophysiology
- Differential Diagnosis
- Diagnosis
- Standard Medical Treatment
- Therapeutic Interventions

Sjögren Syndrome/Disease

<u>Description/pathophysiology</u>:
- **Autoimmune condition affecting the exocrine glands; mucosal surfaces become dry, irritated and prone to microbial colonization.** Clinically manifested as "*sicca* syndrome" which implies a group of symptoms caused by *dryness* of mucosal surfaces.
- Like most conditions, it is generally described as "idiopathic" by medical textbooks and journal articles.[1] More common than SLE, less common than RA; Sjogren's syndrome is considered by some references to be as common as RA.
- <u>Occurs in two general forms</u>:
    1. <u>Primary</u>—only Sjogren's/Sicca syndrome *without evidence of systemic autoimmunity*
    2. <u>Secondary</u>—the occurrence of Sjogren's syndrome *along with another autoimmune disease*, especially rheumatoid arthritis, but also SLE, systemic sclerosis, primary biliary cirrhosis, polymyositis, Hashimoto's thyroiditis, polyarteritis, interstitial pulmonary fibrosis

<u>Clinical presentations</u>:
- Much more common in women—90% of patients with Sjogren's disease are female[2]
- Average age of onset is 50 years (typical range 40-60 years)
- **"Sicca syndrome"** denotes dryness of mucus membranes:

---

[1] "In spite of [the fact that we have no evidence-based solutions to the etiology and pathogenesis of autoimmune diseases], consensus is often taken as a truth, which may hamper the production, funding and/or publication of new and original ideas and views." Konttinen YT, Kasna-Ronkainen L. Sjogren's syndrome: viewpoint on pathogenesis. One of the reasons I was never asked to write a textbook chapter on it. *Scand J Rheumatol Suppl* 2002;(116):15-22

[2] Tierney ML. McPhee SJ, Papadakis MA. *Current Medical Diagnosis and Treatment 2006. 45ᵗʰ edition*. New York; Lange Medical Books: 2006, pages 842-843

- o <u>Dry eyes, keratoconjunctivitis sicca</u>: Lymphocyte and plasma cells cause destruction of lacrimal glands; subjective complaints are more prominent than objective evidence: dry eyes, burning, itching, inability to wear contact lenses, thick mucus, photophobia, corneal ulceration—the latter can lead to infection, vision loss.
    - o <u>Dry mouth, xerostomia</u>: this is generally more problematic than keratoconjunctivitis sicca; dental carries ("cavities") are greatly increased; 33% of patients will have parotid gland tenderness (can be treated with analgesics) and fluctuations in gland size.
    - o Nose, throat, bronchi, and vagina may also be affected.
- <u>Joint pain</u>: Similar distribution to RA but less severe and nondestructive; minimal swelling: PIP and knees most common
- <u>Classic presentation</u>: Woman (90%) aged 40-60 years with dry mouth, dry eyes, and arthritis that mimics RA; other common presentations include:
    - o Photosensitivity, skin rash
    - o Hair loss
    - o Mouth lesions
    - o Chest pain
    - o Raynaud's phenomenon

<u>Major differential diagnoses</u>:
- Dehydration
- Exposure to excessively dry air (furnaces, dehumidifiers, etc.)
- Another autoimmune disease may mimic or occur concomitantly: RA, SLE, scleroderma, polymyositis, autoimmune thyroid disease, arteritis—none of these conditions by itself will cause sicca/dryness.
- Medication side effects (dry eyes and dry mouth are common side effects of many drugs)
- HIV
- Lymphoma
- Sarcoidosis
- Hepatitis C—may possibly induce Sjogren's syndrome[3]
- Mumps
- Menopause
- Normal aging
- Salivary gland atrophy/fibrosis due to previous radiation to head and neck

<u>Clinical assessments</u>:
- **<u>History/subjective</u>**:
    - o See clinical presentations
- **<u>Physical examination/objective</u>**:
    - o <u>Schirmer test</u>: Use filter paper to assess adequacy of lacrimation for 5 minutes; less than 5 mm of wetness is abnormal
    - o <u>Rose Bengal staining</u>: Used to assess the health of the cornea and to thus search for objective evidence of keratoconjunctivitis sicca
- **<u>Laboratory assessments</u>**:
    - o <u>ANA</u>: positive in >95%
        - ▪ If ANA is negative, consider HIV, lymphoma, sarcoidosis, hepatitis C.
        - ▪ Supportive evidence with **anti-SS-A (anti-Ro)** and **anti-SS-B (anti-La)**, neither of which are specific
        - ▪ Autoimmunity directed toward glands/tissues such as stomach, adrenal, and neurons may also be noted[4]

[3] Siegel LB, Gall EP. Viral infection as a cause of arthritis. *Am Fam Physician* 1996 Nov 1;54(6):2009-15
[4] Rehman HU. Sjogren's syndrome. *Yonsei Med J*. 2003 Dec 30;44(6):947-54 http://www.eymj.org/2003/pdf/12947.pdf

- o <u>RF</u>: Positive in 70%
- o <u>ESR</u>: Elevated in 70%
- o <u>CBC</u>: Shows anemia (33%), leukopenia and eosinophilia (25%)
- o <u>Thyroid disorders</u>: Thyroid autoimmunity is common in patients with Sjogren's syndrome; test anti-thyroid peroxidase antibodies and anti-thyroglobulin antibodies along with TSH, T4, and perhaps T3—see Chapter 1 for discussions on thyroid assessments and interventions.
- o <u>HLA markers</u>: DR2 and DR3 are more common in patients who have Sjogren's syndrome *without rheumatoid arthritis*.
- o <u>Schirmer test</u>: Measures quantity of tears and thus objectively quantifies keratoconjunctivitis sicca.
- o <u>Salivary gland biopsy</u>: Not commonly performed except for atypical presentations such as unilateral involvement and to exclude malignancy.
- o <u>Anti-parietal cell antibodies</u>: Noted in various autoimmune conditions (e.g., approximately 33% of patients with Hashimoto thyroiditis); leads to gastric atrophy and associated hypochlorhydria, cobalamin malabsorption, and microbial overgrowth.
- o Assess patient as indicated for other conditions and complications.
- • **Imaging**: Used as indicated per patient; generally not part of assessment
- • **Establishing the diagnosis**: Both of the following must be present:
  1. <u>Autoantibodies—ANA or variant</u>: Preferably in combination with the gold standard in allopathic medicine: salivary gland biopsy—this is necessary for "definite diagnosis" but is not necessary for clinical purposes based on "probable diagnosis."
  2. <u>Evidence of exocrine damage</u>: keratoconjunctivitis sicca and/or xerostomia.

Complications:

- • Vision impairment, vision loss due to corneal lesion, ulceration and secondary infection
- • Dental carries
- • Malnutrition, especially vitamin B-12 deficiency
- • Inflammatory polyarthropathy
- • Salivary stones
- • Pneumonia: can be fatal
- • Pancreatitis
- • Raynaud's phenomenon is seen in ~20%
- • Sensory neuropathy, peripheral neuropathy: immune complex neuropathy, nutrient/B12 deficiencies
- • Renal tubular acidosis
- • Renal insufficiency and failure: can be fatal
- • Nephritis (immune complex disorder)
- • Vasculitis (immune complex disorder)
- • Cryoglobulinemia (immune complex disorder)
- • **Lymphoma: Up to 3-10% of patients with Sjogren's syndrome develop lymphoma**; risk is increased in patients with severe dryness and systemic complications such as vasculitis, splenomegaly, and cryoglobulinemia.
- • Waldenstrom's macroglobulinemia

<u>Clinical management</u>:
- <u>Medical treatment</u>:
    - o "Treatment is symptomatic and supportive."[5]
    - o "There is no specific [allopathic] treatment for the basic process. Local manifestations can be treated symptomatically."[6]
- Referral if clinical outcome is unsatisfactory or if serious complications are possible.

<u>Treatments</u>:
- Drug treatments include pilocarpine (5 mg 4 times daily) and/or cevimeline (30 mg three times daily) to promote salivation. Associated rheumatic diseases are treated as indicated; prednisone is commonly used.
- <u>Eye drops</u>: Consider vitamin-A-containing eye drops, available OTC or by a compounding pharmacist
- <u>For dry mouth</u>:
    - o Sip fluids throughout the day.
    - o Chew sugarless gum to promote saliva flow; xylitol chewing gum can stimulate saliva flow and inhibit the growth of cariogenic bacteria.
    - o Saliva substitute with carboxymethylcellulose.
    - o Fastidious oral hygiene (brushing, flossing, oral antiseptics) and regular dental care are important.
    - o Liquid folic acid supplementation swished in the mouth may help alleviate mouth sores; likewise, topical vitamin E and glutamine may help (as they do with chemotherapy-induced mucositis); chewable deglycyrrhizinated licorice benefits some patients.
    - o Acupuncture improves salivary flow rates in patients with Sjogren's syndrome.[7,8]
- <u>Avoidance of allergenic foods</u>: Any patient may be allergic to any food, even if the food is generally considered a health-promoting food. Generally speaking, the most notorious allergens are wheat, citrus (especially juice due to the industrial use of fungal hemicellulases), cow's milk, eggs, peanuts, chocolate, and yeast-containing foods. **Patients with celiac disease have an increased prevalence of Sjogren's syndrome[9], and patients with Sjogren's syndrome have an increased prevalence of celiac disease.[10] In one study, the estimated prevalence of celiac disease in Sjogren's patients was nearly 1 in 20.[11]** Celiac disease can present with inflammatory oligoarthritis that resembles rheumatoid arthritis and which remits with avoidance of wheat/gluten; the inflammatory arthropathy of celiac disease has preceded bowel symptoms and/or an accurate diagnosis by as many as 3-15 years.[12,13] Clinicians must explain to their patients that celiac disease and wheat allergy are two different clinical entities and that exclusion of one does not exclude the other, and in neither case does mutual exclusion obviate the promotion of intestinal bacterial overgrowth (i.e., proinflammatory dysbiosis) by indigestible wheat oligosaccharides.
- <u>Avoidance of proinflammatory foods</u>: Proinflammatory foods act *directly* or *indirectly*; direct mechanisms include activating Toll-like receptors or NF-kappaB or inducing oxidative stress, while

---

[5] Tierney ML. McPhee SJ, Papadakis MA. *Current Medical Diagnosis and Treatment. 35th edition*. Stamford: Appleton and Lange, 1996 page 749 and Tierney ML. McPhee SJ, Papadakis MA. *Current Medical Diagnosis and Treatment 2006. 45th edition*. New York; Lange Medical Books: 2006, pages 842-843

[6] Beers MH, Berkow R (eds). *The Merck Manual. Seventeenth Edition*. Whitehouse Station; Merck Research Laboratories 1999 Page 424

[7] "CONCLUSIONS: This study shows that acupuncture treatment results in statistically significant improvements in SFR in patients with xerostomia up to 6 months. It suggests that additional acupuncture therapy can maintain this improvement in SFR for up to 3 years. "Blom M, Lundeberg T. Long-term follow-up of patients treated with acupuncture for xerostomia and the influence of additional treatment. *Oral Dis* 2000 Jan;6(1):15-24

[8] "A majority of the patients subjectively reported some improvement after treatment, and a significant increase in paraffin-stimulated saliva secretion was found after treatment." List T, Lundeberg T, Lundstrom I, Lindstrom F, Ravald N. The effect of acupuncture in the treatment of patients with primary Sjogren's syndrome. A controlled study. *Acta Odontol Scand* 1998 Apr;56(2):95-9

[9] "Sjogren's syndrome occurred in 3.3% of coeliac patients and in 0.3% of controls (p = 0.0059)." Collin P, Reunala T, Pukkala E, Laippala P, Keyrilainen O, Pasternack A. Coeliac disease--associated disorders and survival. *Gut*. 1994 Sep;35(9):1215-8.

[10] "Further, our study shows that anti-tTG is more prevalent in SS than in other systemic rheumatic diseases." Luft LM, Barr SG, Martin LO, Chan EK, Fritzler MJ. Autoantibodies to tissue transglutaminase in Sjogren's syndrome and related rheumatic diseases. *J Rheumatol*. 2003 Dec;30(12):2613-9

[11] "The frequency of CD in the SS population was significantly higher than in the non-SS European population (4.5:100 vs 4.5-5.5:1,000)." Szodoray P, Barta Z, Lakos G, Szakall S, Zeher M. Coeliac disease in Sjogren's syndrome--a study of 111 Hungarian patients. Rheumatol Int. 2004 Sep;24(5):278-82. Epub 2003 Sep 17.

[12] "We report six patients with coeliac disease in whom arthritis was prominent at diagnosis and who improved with dietary therapy. Joint pain preceded diagnosis by up to three years in five patients and 15 years in one patient." Bourne JT, Kumar P, Huskisson EC, et al. Arthritis and coeliac disease. *Ann Rheum Dis*. 1985 Sep;44(9):592-8

[13] "A 15-year-old girl, with synovitis of the knees and ankles for 3 years before a diagnosis of gluten-sensitive enteropathy, is described." Pinals RS. Arthritis associated with gluten-sensitive enteropathy. *J Rheumatol*. 1986 Feb;13(1):201-4

indirect mechanisms include depleting the body of anti-inflammatory nutrients and displacing more nutritious anti-inflammatory foods.

- <u>Broad-spectrum fatty acid therapy with ALA, EPA, DHA, GLA and oleic acid</u>: Fatty acid supplementation should be delivered in the form of combination therapy with ALA, GLA, DHA, and EPA. Given at doses of 3,000 – 9,000 mg per day, ALA from flax oil has impressive anti-inflammatory benefits demonstrated by its ability to halve prostaglandin production in humans.[14] **Patients with Sjogren's syndrome have lower levels of GLA/DGLA[15] and fatty acid supplementation—particularly with GLA (along with vitamin C)—is safe and may be beneficial (positive reports[16,17], neutral report[18], negative report[19]).**

- <u>Assess for and treat dysbiosis</u>: Insufficient flow of saliva and other fluids promotes microbial colonization of mucosal surfaces, particularly the digestive and respiratory tracts. **Gastrointestinal infection/dysbiosis can cause nutrient malabsorption, and the resultant nutritional insufficiencies can exacerbate the sicca symptoms.[20] Patients with Sjogren's syndrome may have an increased prevalence of infection/colonization with *H. pylori*[21],** an organism known to incite systemic inflammation and to produce pro-inflammatory endotoxin and antigens; eradication of this microbe—or others per patient—may alleviate clinical manifestations by addressing one of the inciting causes. Of particular note is that *H. pylori* promotes gastric autoimmunity, sicca syndrome, as well as intestinal lymphoma—all of which are noted in Sjogren's syndrome.

  - <u>*H pylori* and gastrointestinal cancer</u>: "*H. pylori* infection is a major cause of gastric (stomach) cancer, specifically non-cardia gastric cancer (cancer in all areas of the stomach, except for the top portion near where it joins the esophagus). *H. pylori* infection also causes gastric mucosa-associated lymphoid tissue (MALT) lymphoma. *H. pylori* infection is associated with a decreased risk of some other cancers, including gastric cardia cancer (cancer in the top portion of the stomach) and esophageal adenocarcinoma."[22]

- <u>Vitamin D3 supplementation with physiologic doses and/or tailored to serum 25(OH)D levels</u>: **Vitamin D insufficiency has been reported in patients with Sjogren's syndrome, presumably due to reduced intake and/or malabsorption.** Vitamin D deficiency is common in the general population and is even more common in patients with chronic illness and chronic musculoskeletal pain.[23] Correction of vitamin D deficiency supports normal immune function against infection and provides a clinically significant anti-inflammatory[24] and analgesic benefit in patients with back pain[25] and limb pain.[26] **Vitamin D status is inversely associated with inflammation in patients with Sjogren's**

[14] Adam O, Wolfram G, Zollner N. Effect of alpha-linolenic acid in the human diet on linoleic acid metabolism and prostaglandin biosynthesis. *J Lipid Res.* 1986 Apr;27(4):421-6 http://www.jlr.org/cgi/reprint/27/4/421
[15] "We found MD levels of 20:3n6 (dihommo-gamma-linolenic acid), and basal and indomethacin-enhanced NK cell activity significantly reduced, in 10 primary Sjogren's syndrome patients as compared with 10 healthy controls." Oxholm P, Pedersen BK, Horrobin DF.Natural killer cell functions are related to the cell membrane composition of essential fatty acids: differences in healthy persons and patients with primary Sjogren's syndrome. *Clin Exp Rheumatol.* 1992 May-Jun;10(3):229-34
[16] "An attempt to treat humans with Sjogren's syndrome by raising endogenous PGE1 production by administration of essential fatty acid PGE1 precursors, of pyridoxine and of vitamin C was successful in raising the rates of tear and saliva production." Horrobin DF, Campbell A. Sjogren's syndrome and the sicca syndrome: the role of prostaglandin E1 deficiency. Treatment with essential fatty acids and vitamin C. *Med Hypotheses.* 1980 Mar;6(3):225-32
[17] "Efamol treatment improved the Schirmer-I-test..." Manthorpe R, Hagen Petersen S, Prause JU. Primary Sjogren's syndrome treated with Efamol/Efavit. A double-blind cross-over investigation. *Rheumatol Int.* 1984;4(4):165-7. The duration of this study was ridiculously short—only 3 weeks.
[18] "The objective ocular status, evaluated by a combined ocular score, including the results from Schirmer-I test, break-up time and van Bijsterveld score, improved significantly during Efamol treatment when compared with Efamol start-values (p less than 0.05), but not when compared with placebo values (p less than 0.2)." Oxholm P, Manthorpe R, Prause JU, Horrobin D. Patients with primary Sjogren's syndrome treated for two months with evening primrose oil. *Scand J Rheumatol.* 1986;15:103-8
[19] "There was no significant improvement in any of the patients during the treatment period compared to assessments done pre and post treatment." McKendry RJ. Treatment of Sjogren's syndrome with essential fatty acids, pyridoxine and vitamin C. *Prostaglandins Leukot Med.* 1982 Apr;8(4):403-8
[20] Bosman C, Boldrini R, Borsetti G, Morelli S, Paglia MG, Visca P. Sicca syndrome associated with Tropheryma whipplei intestinal infection. *J Clin Microbiol.* 2002 Aug;40(8):3104-6 http://jcm.asm.org/cgi/content/full/40/8/3104?view=long&pmid=12149393
[21] "Patients with SS are more prone to have H. pylori infection in comparison to other connective tissue diseases. Serum antibody titer to H. pylori correlated with index for clinical disease manifestations, age, disease duration and CRP." El Miedany YM, Baddour M, Ahmed I, Fahmy H. Sjogren's syndrome: concomitant H. pylori infection and possible correlation with clinical parameters. *Joint Bone Spine.* 2005 Mar;72(2):135-41
[22] http://www.cancer.gov/cancertopics/factsheet/Risk/h-pylori-cancer
[23] Plotnikoff GA, Quigley JM. Prevalence of severe hypovitaminosis D in patients with persistent, nonspecific musculoskeletal pain. *Mayo Clin Proc.* 2003 Dec;78(12):1463-70
[24] Timms PM, et al. Circulating MMP9, vitamin D and variation in the TIMP-1 response with VDR genotype: mechanisms for inflammatory damage in chronic disorders? *QJM.* 2002 Dec;95(12):787-96 http://qjmed.oxfordjournals.org/cgi/content/full/95/12/787
[25] Al Faraj S, Al Mutairi K. Vitamin D deficiency and chronic low back pain in Saudi Arabia. *Spine.* 2003 Jan 15;28(2):177-9
[26] Masood H, Narang AP, Bhat IA, Shah GN. Persistent limb pain and raised serum alkaline phosphatase the earliest markers of subclinical hypovitaminosis D in Kashmir. *Indian J Physiol Pharmacol.* 1989 Oct-Dec;33(4):259-61

syndrome.[27,28] Reasonable daily doses for children and adults are 2,000 and 4,000 IU, respectively, as defined by Vasquez, et al.[29] Deficiency and response to treatment are monitored with serum 25(OH)vitamin D while safety is monitored with serum calcium; inflammatory granulomatous diseases and certain drugs such as hydrochlorothiazide greatly increase the propensity for hypercalcemia and warrant increment dosing and frequent monitoring of serum calcium.

- Supplemented Paleo-Mediterranean diet: The health-promoting diet of choice for the majority of people is a diet based on abundant consumption of fruits, vegetables, seeds, nuts, omega-3 and monounsaturated fatty acids, and lean sources of protein such as lean meats, fatty cold-water fish, soy and whey proteins. Rational supplementation with vitamins, minerals, and health promoting fatty acids (i.e., ALA, GLA, EPA, DHA) makes this the best practical diet that can possibly be conceived and implemented.

- Orthoendocrinology: Assess and treat per patient. As noted with most other autoimmune/inflammatory diseases, patients with Sjogren's syndrome have elevated levels of pro-inflammatory prolactin that correlate with disease activity.[30]

- Raynaud's phenomenon—specific treatments: *See Chapter on Raynaud's phenomenon.*

- Green tea, green tea extract (EGCG), and other phytonutritional antioxidants and anti-inflammatories: **Very interestingly, an *in vitro* study[31] showed that epigallocatechin gallate inhibited the expression of major autoantigens, including those which are characteristic of Sjogren's syndrome: SS-B/La, SS-A/Ro. Given its antioxidant properties and anti-inflammatory actions (specifically via inhibition of NF-kappaB[32]), green tea and related supplements may prove beneficial for patients with Sjogren's syndrome.**

- High-dose short-term oral vitamin A: **Szocsik et al[33] administered vitamin A 100,000 IU per day for two weeks and obtained improved immune function, such as improved natural killer cell function, in patients with Sjogren's syndrome.**

- Individualized homeopathy: A small randomized placebo-controlled trial found homeopathy beneficial for xerostomia.[34]

- Replacement of gastric HCL: Tablets/capsules of betaine HCL may improve digestion, nutrient assimilation, and also alleviate intestinal microbial overgrowth; antiparietal cell antibodies may be noted.

---

[27] "In conclusion the inverse correlations found between levels of 25 OH D and measures of clinical and immunoinflammatory status support the notion that vitamin D metabolism may be involved in the pathogenesis of primary SS." Bang B, Asmussen K, Sorensen OH, Oxholm P. Reduced 25-hydroxyvitamin D levels in primary Sjogren's syndrome. Correlations to disease manifestations. *Scand J Rheumatol.* 1999;28(3):180-3

[28] "Among patients with increased concentrations of IgM rheumatoid factor there was a significant negative correlation between the serum titres of IgM rheumatoid factor and 25-OHD3 concentrations." Muller K, et al. Abnormal vitamin D3 metabolism in patients with primary Sjogren's syndrome. *Ann Rheum Dis.* 1990 Sep;49(9):682-4

[29] Vasquez A, Manso G, Cannell J. The clinical importance of vitamin D (cholecalciferol): a paradigm shift with implications for all healthcare providers. *Altern Ther Health Med.* 2004 Sep-Oct;10(5):28-36

[30] "Patients with primary SS have moderately increased levels of serum PRL, especially evident in patients diagnosed at a young age with active immunological disease." Haga HJ, Rygh T. The prevalence of hyperprolactinemia in patients with primary Sjogren's syndrome. *J Rheumatol.* 1999 Jun;26(6):1291-5

[31] "EGCG inhibited the transcription and translation of major autoantigens, including SS-B/La, SS-A/Ro, coilin, DNA topoisomerase I, and alpha-fodrin. These findings, taken together with green tea's anti-inflammatory and antiapoptotic effects, suggest that green tea polyphenols could serve as an important component in novel approaches to combat autoimmune disorders in humans." Hsu S, Dickinson DP, Qin H, Lapp C, Lapp D, Borke J, Walsh DS, Bollag WB, Stoppler H, Yamamoto T, Osaki T, Schuster G. Inhibition of autoantigen expression by (-)-epigallocatechin-3-gallate (the major constituent of green tea) in normal human cells. *J Pharmacol Exp Ther.* 2005 Nov;315(2):805-11. Epub 2005 Jul 26

[32] "In conclusion, EGCG is an effective inhibitor of IKK activity. This may explain, at least in part, some of the reported anti-inflammatory and anti-cancer effects of green tea." Yang F, Oz HS, Barve S, de Villiers WJ, McClain CJ, Varilek GW. The green tea polyphenol (-)-epigallocatechin-3-gallate blocks nuclear factor-kappa B activation by inhibiting I kappa B kinase activity in the intestinal epithelial cell line IEC-6. *Mol Pharmacol.* 2001 Sep;60(3):528-33

[33] "Patients with Sjogren's syndrome were treated with vitamin A (100,000 U) daily during a two-week period. The vitamin treatment significantly elevated their ADCC and NK activity." Szocsik K, Gonzalez-Cabello R, Vien CV, Mezes M, Szongoth M, Gergely P. Effect of vitamin A treatment on immune reactivity and lipid peroxidation in patients with Sjogren's syndrome. *Clin Rheumatol.* 1988 Dec;7(4):514-9

[34] "Our results suggest that individually prescribed homeopathic medicine could be a valuable adjunct to the treatment of oral discomfort and xerostomic symptoms." Haila S, Koskinen A, Tenovuo J. Effects of homeopathic treatment on salivary flow rate and subjective symptoms in patients with oral dryness: a randomized trial. *Homeopathy.* 2005 Jul;94(3):175-81

Raynaud's Syndrome/Phenomenon/Disorder

> ### Introduction:
> Raynaud's Syndrome/Phenomenon/Disorder is a disorder of periodic vasoconstriction mainly affecting the hands/fingers; it is a manifestation of autonomic dysfunction associated with and often preceding autoimmune diseases, especially scleroderma. Per the 2010 criteria for fibromyalgia (FM), Raynaud's is now associated with that condition as well; this is utterly absurd except that both Raynaud's and FM are causatively associated with microbial dysbiosis, especially in the intestines, i.e., *Helicobacter pylori* with Raynaud's and SIBO with FM. The condition responds poorly to medical/pharmacologic treatment that focuses on vasodilation; the condition responds very well to integrative treatment, especially that which focuses on dysbiosis eradication, antioxidant supplementation, and other components of the Functional Inflammology protocol.

Introduction and Diagnosis

- Introduction and terminology: Raynaud's phenomenon is periodic recurrent severe vasoconstriction-induced hypoperfusion accompanied by discomfort most commonly affecting the fingers.
  - Primary Raynaud's phenomenon: Not associated with a concomitant disease.
  - Secondary Raynaud's phenomenon, Raynaud's syndrome: Associated with a concomitant disease, especially autoimmunity, especially scleroderma.
- Diagnosis and Evaluation: Assessment for the presence/absence of systemic disease is important; Raynaud's can precede systemic autoimmunity by several years, for example in scleroderma.
  - Digital artery blood pressure: A decrease of > 15 mmHg is consistent with vasoconstriction.
  - Doppler ultrasound: Can be used to measure blood flow.
  - Routine labs: CBC, chemistry/metabolic panel, ANA, CRP, and the full thyroid evaluation previously discussed.
  - Nailfold capillaroscopy: Reveals microvascular changes consistent with autoimmunity and autoimmune-expedited cardiovascular disease. Per Cutolo et al[1], "Raynaud's phenomenon (RP) represents the most frequent clinical aspect of cardio/microvascular involvement and is a key feature of several autoimmune rheumatic diseases. Moreover, RP is associated in a statistically significant manner with many coronary diseases. In normal conditions or in primary RP (excluding during the cold-exposure test), the normal nailfold capillaroscopic pattern shows a regular disposition of the capillary loops along with the nailbed. On the contrary, in subjects suffering from secondary RP, one or more alterations of the capillaroscopic findings should alert the physician of the possibility of a connective tissue disease not yet detected. Nailfold capillaroscopy (NV) represents the best method to analyze microvascular abnormalities in autoimmune rheumatic diseases. Architectural disorganization, giant capillaries, hemorrhages, loss of capillaries, angiogenesis and avascular areas characterize >95% of patients with overt scleroderma (SSc)."
- Complications: Long-term recurrent vasoconstriction can result in atrophy of the skin and subcutaneous tissues including muscle; digital ulceration and ischemic gangrene can result. Recurrent vasospasm-induced tissue hypoxia appears to increase inflammation via oxidative stress and possibly via elaboration of damage-associated molecular patterns.

---

[1] Cutolo M, Sulli A, Secchi ME, Paolino S, Pizzorni C. Nailfold capillaroscopy is useful for the diagnosis and follow-up of autoimmune rheumatic diseases. A future tool for the analysis of microvascular heart involvement? *Rheumatology* (Oxford). 2006 Oct;45 Suppl 4:iv43-6 http://rheumatology.oxfordjournals.org/content/45/suppl_4/iv43.full.pdf

Clinical Applications and Interventions

- <u>Raynaud's phenomenon—specific treatments</u>: Treatment of Raynaud's phenomenon should not be trivialized as merely symptomatic; the pain experienced by some patients with Raynaud's phenomenon is truly excruciating. Additionally, a wonderfully insightful comment by Simonini et al[2] in 2000 stated that the tissue ischemia induced by Raynaud's phenomenon is *pathogenic* because it promotes oxidative stress and the vicious cycle of inflammation; the recurrent ischemia and reperfusion of hypoxic Raynaud's phenomenon could be thought of somewhat as a "recurrent, mild heart attack [or stroke] of the hands" causing tissue damage and cell apoptosis/necrosis leading to release of damage-associated molecular patterns (DAMP) and the resultant immune activation, systemic inflammation, mitochondrial dysfunction, proinflammatory immunophenotype switch toward Th1/Th2/Th17 and resultant fibrosis and autoimmunity. Remarkably, Mahoney et al[3] proposed a similar model in 2011 when they wrote, "We propose that a recent change in the conception of the role of type 1 interferon and the identification of adventitial stem cells suggests a unifying hypothesis for scleroderma. This hypothesis begins with vasospasm. Vasospasm is fully reversible unless, as proposed here, the resulting ischemia leads to apoptosis and activation of type 1 interferon. The interferon, we propose, initiates immune amplification, including characteristic scleroderma-specific antibodies." Thus, treatments to maintain vasodilation and quench the free radicals resultant from recurrent hypoxic events are necessary. Antioxidants have been discussed previously and should be common knowledge to readers of this text. Vasodilation in Raynaud's phenomenon can be supported with any/all of the following:
  - <u>Eradication of *Helicobacter pylori*</u>: Eradication of *Helicobacter pylori* is one of the most effective treatments of Raynaud's disease/syndrome/phenomenon and should therefore be pursued in all affected patients.
    - Helicobacter pylori eradication ameliorates primary Raynaud's phenomenon (*Dig Dis Sci* 1998 Aug[4]): "Forty-six patients affected by primary Raynaud's phenomenon were evaluated. *H. pylori* infection was assessed by [13C]urea breath test. Eradication therapy was given to infected patients for seven days. ... **Attacks of Raynaud's phenomenon completely disappeared in 17% of the patients with *H. pylori* eradication. Discomfort and the duration and frequency of attacks of Raynaud's phenomenon were significantly reduced in 72% of the remaining patients.** ... The study shows that *H. pylori* eradication causes a significant decrease in clinical attacks of Raynaud's disease. The reduction of vasoactive substances determined by the eradication of the bacterium may be the pathogenetic mechanism underlying the phenomenon."
  - <u>Inositol hexaniacinate</u>: 3,000-4,000 mg/d *po* in divided doses[5,6,7]
  - <u>*Ginkgo biloba*</u>: Ginkgo reduces the number of daily Raynaud's attacks in patients with primary Raynaud's disease[8], and it is also an excellent antioxidant with potent anti-inflammatory benefits.
  - <u>Magnesium</u>: 300-500 mg/d or bowel tolerance; systemic alkalinization to achieve urine alkalinity of 7.5 promotes renal retention of magnesium and systemic cellular uptake.

---

[2] "...daily episodes of hypoxia-reperfusion injury, produces several episodes of free radicals-mediated endothelial derangement. These events results in a positive feedback effect of luminal narrowing and ischemia and therefore to the birth of a vicious cycle of oxygen free radicals (OFR) generation, leading to endothelial damage, intimal thickening and fibrosis." Simonini G, Pignone A, Generini S, Falcini F, Cerinic MM. Emerging potentials for an antioxidant therapy as a new approach to the treatment of systemic sclerosis. *Toxicology*. 2000 Nov 30;155(1-3):1-15

[3] Mahoney WM Jr, Fleming JN, Schwartz SM. A unifying hypothesis for scleroderma: identifying a target cell for scleroderma. *Curr Rheumatol Rep*. 2011 Feb;13:28-36

[4] Gasbarrini A et al. Helicobacter pylori eradication ameliorates primary Raynaud's phenomenon. *Dig Dis Sci*. 1998 Aug;43(8):1641-5

[5] "It appears to be a safe and well tolerated drug, which, together with other symptomatic measures, merits to be used in the management of vasospastic disease of the extremities even in the presence of partial obliteration of the microcirculation." Holti G. An experimentally controlled evaluation of the effect of inositol nicotinate upon the digital blood flow in patients with Raynaud's phenomenon. *J Int Med Res*. 1979;7(6):473-83

[6] "Although the mechanism of action remains unclear Hexopal is safe and is effective in reducing the vasospasm of primary Raynaud's disease during the winter months." Sunderland GT, Belch JJ, Sturrock RD, Forbes CD, McKay AJ. A double blind randomised placebo controlled trial of hexopal in primary Raynaud's disease. *Clin Rheumatol*. 1988 Mar;7(1):46-9

[7] "It is suggested that long-term treatment with nicotinate acid derivatives may produce improvement in the peripheral circulation by a different mechanism than the transient effect detected by short-term studies." Ring EF, Bacon PA. Quantitative thermographic assessment of inositol nicotinate therapy in Raynaud's phenomena. J Int Med Res. 1977;5(4):217-22

[8] "Ginkgo biloba phytosome may be effective in reducing the number of Raynaud's attacks per week in patients suffering from Raynaud's disease." Muir AH, Robb R, McLaren M, Daly F, Belch JJ. The use of Ginkgo biloba in Raynaud's disease: a double-blind placebo-controlled trial. *Vasc Med*. 2002;7(4):265-7

- o **Combination fatty acid therapy**: must include GLA (minimum 500 mg) and EPA (minimum 2,000 mg)
- o **L-arginine**: L-arginine is the biochemical precursor to nitric oxide, which has vasodilating actions. L-arginine supplementation in patients with Raynaud's phenomenon showed benefit in one study[9] and no benefit in another.[10] However, arginine supplementation was tremendously beneficial in 4 case reports of scleroderma patients with Raynaud's-induced digital necrosis.[11] Excess arginine supplementation may lead to an overproduction of nitric oxide, which can be harmful in excess due to its free radical behavior and its contribution to peroxynitrite. Additionally, metabolism of arginine requires methyl groups, and therefore supplementation with methyl donors such as methylfolate/folinate, cobalamin, betaine, et al should be used anytime supplemental arginine is used for long periods of time; homocysteine levels should occasionally be measured.
- o **NAC 500-1,500mg *po tid ic***: NAC is pleiotropically beneficial, via antiviral, antioxidant, GSH-supporting, and mTOR inhibiting actions.
  - ▪ **Intravenous N-acetylcysteine for treatment of Raynaud's phenomenon secondary to systemic sclerosis (*J Rheumatol* 2001 Oct[12])**—paraphrased/quoted as follows: "Twenty-two patients with RP secondary to SSc were enrolled in a multicenter, open clinical trial lasting 11 weeks and conducted in winter. Primary outcome measures were frequency and severity of RP attacks, and number of digital ulcers. Secondary outcome measure was improvement in digital cold challenge test assessed by photoelectric plethysmography. Patients received a continuous 5 day intravenous infusion of NAC starting with a 2 h loading dose of 150 mg/kg subsequently adjusted to 15 mg/kg/h. RESULTS: ... Both frequency and severity of RP attacks decreased significantly compared to pretreatment values. Active ulcers were significantly less numerous at all follow-up visits (25% of baseline count on Day 33 from the beginning of infusion). In the cold challenge test, mean recovery time fell by 69%, 67%, 71%, and 71% on Days 12, 19, 33, and 61 from the beginning of treatment. Side effects were minor, easily controlled, and reversible. CONCLUSION: N-acetylcysteine appears to be safe for the treatment of RP secondary to SSc. These preliminary data warrant further controlled studies.
- o **Acupuncture, biofeedback, counseling, stress reduction, cold avoidance, smoking cessation**: Since stressful events, cold exposure, and cigarette smoking are all vasoconstrictive, these should be avoided/modified to the highest extent possible. Stress reduction and modification of inter- and intra-personal socioemotional exchange would be beneficial for anyone.

[9] "After therapy, patients with Raynaud's phenomenon secondary to systemic sclerosis showed: (1) higher digital vasodilation after local warming, (2) cold-induced digital vasodilation, and (3) increase of plasma levels of tissue-type plasminogen activator." Agostoni A, Marasini B, Biondi ML, Bassani C, Cazzaniga A, Bottasso B, Cugno M. L-arginine therapy in Raynaud's phenomenon? *Int J Clin Lab Res*. 1991;21(2):202-3
[10] "L-arginine supplementation, however, had no significant effect on vascular responses to acetylcholine and sodium nitroprusside." Khan F, Belch JJ. Skin blood flow in patients with systemic sclerosis and Raynaud's phenomenon: effects of oral L-arginine supplementation. *J Rheumatol*. 1999 Nov;26(11):2389-94
[11] "We report two cases in which oral L-arginine reversed digital necrosis in Raynaud's phenomenon and two additional cases in which the symptoms of severe Raynaud's phenomenon were improved with oral L-arginine." Rembold CM, Ayers CR. Oral L-arginine can reverse digital necrosis in Raynaud's phenomenon. *Mol Cell Biochem*. 2003 Feb;244(1-2):139-41
[12] Sambo P, Amico D, Giacomelli R, Matucci-Cerinic M, Salsano F, Valentini G, Gabrielli A. Intravenous N-acetylcysteine for treatment of Raynaud's phenomenon secondary to systemic sclerosis: a pilot study. *J Rheumatol*. 2001 Oct;28(10):2257-62

The End
<ul><li>"It was during the years of my lowest vitality that I ceased to be a pessimist. The instinct of self restoration forbade me a philosophy of poverty and discouragement. As it were, that is how those years appear to me now. I soon discovered life anew…including myself. I turned my will to health, to life, into a philosophy….into the will to power."</li><li>"The time is now past when accidents could befall me; and what *could* now fall to my lot which has not already be my own!? It returns only, it comes home to me at last—mine own Self. And such of it as has been long abroad, and scattered among things and accidents. And one thing more do I know: I stand now before my last summit, and before that which has been longest reserved for me."</li><li>"You have within you the power to merge everything you have lived through – attempts, false starts, errors, delusions, passions, your loves and your hopes – into your highest goal, with nothing left over."</li><li>"At every step one has to wrestle for truth; one has to surrender for it almost everything to which the heart, to which our love, our trust in life, cling otherwise. That requires greatness of soul: the service of truth is the hardest service…"</li><li>"With your love go into your isolation and with your creativity, my brother; and only later will justice limp after you.</li><li>"What makes a person heroic?" Answer: "To simultaneously face one's greatest fear and one's highest hope."</li><li>"My principle article of faith is that one can only flourish among people who share the identical ideas and the identical will."</li><li>"Not around the inventors of new noise but around the inventors of new values does the world revolve."</li></ul> Friedrich Nietzsche (German classical Scholar, Philosopher and Critic of culture, 1844-1900)

Index: